Discovering
Nutrition

Sixth Edition

Paul Insel
Stanford University

Don Ross
California Institute of Human Nutrition

Kimberley McMahon
Logan University

Melissa Bernstein
Chicago Medical School

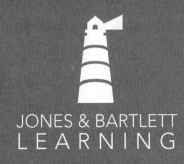

JONES & BARTLETT
LEARNING

World Headquarters
Jones & Bartlett Learning
5 Wall Street
Burlington, MA 01803
978-443-5000
info@jblearning.com
www.jblearning.com

Jones & Bartlett Learning books and products are available through most bookstores and online booksellers. To contact Jones & Bartlett Learning directly, call 800-832-0034, fax 978-443-8000, or visit our website, www.jblearning.com.

Substantial discounts on bulk quantities of Jones & Bartlett Learning publications are available to corporations, professional associations, and other qualified organizations. For details and specific discount information, contact the special sales department at Jones & Bartlett Learning via the above contact information or send an email to specialsales@jblearning.com.

13956-3

Production Credits

VP, Product Management: David D. Cella
Director of Product Management: Cathy L. Esperti
Product Manager: Sean Fabery
Senior Developmental Editor: Jennifer Angel
Associate Production Editor: Rachel DiMaggio
Associate Production Editor: Jamie Reynolds
Director of Marketing: Andrea DeFronzo
VP, Manufacturing and Inventory Control: Therese Connell

Composition: SourceHOV LLC
Cover and Text Design: Kristin E. Parker
Director of Rights & Media: Joanna Gallant
Rights & Media Specialist: Merideth Tumasz
Media Development Editor: Shannon Sheehan
Cover Image: © Greentellect Studio/Shutterstock
Printing and Binding: LSC Communications
Cover Printing: LSC Communications

Library of Congress Cataloging-in-Publication Data

Names: Insel, Paul M., author. | Ross, Don, 1952- , author. | McMahon, Kimberley, author. | Bernstein, Melissa, author.
Title: Discovering nutrition / Paul Insel, Don Ross, Kimberley McMahon, Melissa Bernstein.
Description: Sixth edition. | Burlington, MA : Jones & Bartlett Learning, [2019] | Includes bibliographical references and index.
Identifiers: LCCN 2017039397 | ISBN 9781284139464 (paperback)
Subjects: | MESH: Nutritional Physiological Phenomena | Diet
Classification: LCC QP141 | NLM QU 145 | DDC 613.2--dc23
LC record available at https://lccn.loc.gov/2017039397

6048

Printed in the United States of America
22 21 20 19 18   10 9 8 7 6 5 4 3 2

Brief Contents

© Greentellect Studio/Shutterstock.

Contents

©Greentellect Studio/Shutterstock.

Preface

Welcome to the sixth edition of *Discovering Nutrition*.

With changes in nutrition-related information having never been more exciting or important than they are today, learning about nutrition should be stimulating and engaging. With that in mind, *Discovering Nutrition* takes students on a fascinating journey beginning with curiosity and ending with solid knowledge and a healthy dose of skepticism. Knowledge is power, and our mission is to offer students the tools to logically interpret nutrition information provided by the news media, popular entertainment, food labels, and government agencies. Our goal is to create sophisticated consumers of nutritional science as well as nutrition information.

Discovering Nutrition is unique in its behavioral approach, challenging students not just to memorize material, but to act on it. Familiar experiences and choices beckon students into each chapter. Analogies illuminate difficult concepts. We address important topics that students are curious about, ranging from functional foods and supplements to vegetarianism, athlete diets, and linkages between diet and chronic disease. In special spotlights, we focus attention on topics like alcohol, eating disorders, obesity, and complementary nutrition. For those instructors wishing to cover metabolism, we also include a "Spotlight on Metabolism and Energy Balance" that provides a friendly tour of the metabolic pathways. For this edition, we have significantly revised two areas that are of especially high interest, Chapter 9 "Nutrition for Physical Performance" and the "Spotlight on Eating Disorders," to reflect the current state of knowledge.

Accessible Science

Discovering Nutrition makes use of the latest in learning theory and balances the behavioral aspects of nutrition with an accessible approach to scientific concepts. This text is intended to be a comprehensive resource that communicates nutrition both graphically and personally. We present technical concepts in an engaging and friendly way with an appealing, stepwise, and parallel development of text and annotated illustrations. Illustrations in all chapters use consistent representations. Each type of nutrient, for example, has a distinct color and shape. Icons of an amino acid, a protein, a triglyceride, and a glucose molecule represent "characters" in the nutrition story and are instantly recognizable as they appear throughout the text.

This text leads the way in depicting important biological and physiological phenomena, such as emulsification, glucose regulation, digestion and absorption, and fetal development. Extensive graphic presentations make nutrition and physiological principles come alive.

2015–2020 Dietary Guidelines for Americans

The eighth edition of the *Dietary Guidelines for Americans* emphasizes following a healthy and varied eating pattern that limits calories from added sugars and saturated fats, reduces sodium intake, and incorporates more vegetables and whole grains. On the whole, this edition reflects advances in the scientific understanding of the importance of improving diets and increasing physical activity, two of the most important factors in reducing obesity and preventing chronic diseases in Americans. Focused on science-based recommendations on food and nutrition, the *Dietary Guidelines* empowers the American public to make shifts in what they eat and drink in favor of good health. As you read this text, look for key recommendations of the *Dietary Guidelines* highlighted in the margins.

Food Labeling

The Food and Drug Administration announced a new and redesigned Nutrition Facts label that will be required on most packaged food by January 2020. In an effort to encourage consumers to make more informed decisions, changes on the new label include such things as highlighting calories per serving and serving sizes more prominently, featuring a separate line showing how much sugar has been added to the food, and including updated Dietary Value information. The new label is discussed in Chapter 2 and has been incorporated into all Label to Table features found throughout the text.

New to This Edition

For this edition, the latest scientific evidence, recommendations, and national standards have been incorporated throughout the text.

Key Highlights

- Updated content reflects the *2015–2020 Dietary Guidelines for Americans*, as well as the redesigned Nutrition Facts label.
- The new "Why Is This Important?" feature, tied to the majority of major headings in the text, breaks down the practical importance and value of the key concepts students are learning.
- The new "Getting Personal" feature, found in most of the end-of-chapter Learning Portfolios, encourages students to apply their nutritional knowledge to understanding their own diets.
- Revised statistics and data incorporated throughout the text reflect the current state of nutrition in the United States and the world.
- Revised food source charts in Chapters 7 and 8 more clearly convey common sources for vitamins and minerals.
- Updated Position Statements from the Academy of Nutrition and Dietetics, the American Heart Association, and other organizations appear throughout the text.
- Updated references utilize the latest science in the field.
- New and updated FYI and Quick Bite features provide in-depth discussions of controversial issues and topics for classroom discussion.
- The redesigned Nutrition Facts label has been incorporated into the Label to Table features found throughout the text.

Chapter 1—Food Choices: Nutrients and Nourishment

- Updated discussion of the effects TV advertisements have on childhood nutrition
- Updated coverage of the impact of eating away from home
- Updated section comparing the "healthfulness" of the American diet versus the recommendations of the *2015–2020 Dietary Guidelines for Americans*
- New comparison of phytochemicals and zoochemicals
- New comparison of the terms *kilocalorie* and *calorie*

- New features presenting excerpts from the Academy of Nutrition and Dietetics' practice papers on social media and communicating accurate food and nutrition information
- New Quick Bite feature "Correlation or Causation?"

Chapter 2—Nutrition Guidelines: Tools for a Healthful Diet

- Inclusion of the key recommendations and overarching guidelines of the *2015–2020 Dietary Guidelines for Americans*
- Revised description and discussion of the Nutrition Facts label, reflecting changes announced in 2016
- New Quick Bites features "Early 'Laws' of Health," "SuperTracker: My Foods, My Fitness, My Health" and "Underconsumption of Nutrients"
- Revised FYI feature "Portion Distortion"

Chapter 3—The Human Body: From Food to Fuel

- New section on gut microbiota
- Heavily revised FYI feature "Microbiota Out of Whack? Pre- and Probiotics May Help"
- Expanded description of passive diffusion

Chapter 4—Carbohydrates: Simple Sugars and Complex Chains

- New coverage of agave sweeteners
- New figure summarizing types of carbohydrates
- New table recapping common nonnutritive sweeteners
- New table summarizing the health benefits of fiber, as well as its effects in the gastrointestinal tract
- Heavily revised FYI feature "Is the Glycemic Index a Useful Tool for Constructing a Healthy Diet with Carbohydrates?"
- Expanded discussion of glycemic load
- New Quick Bite feature "Low-Carb Diets"

Spotlight on Alcohol

- Updated description and statistics about college drinking behaviors
- Expanded Quick Bite feature "Energy Drinks + Alcohol = A Recipe for Disaster"

Chapter 5—Lipids: Not Just Fat

- Updated sections providing recommendations for omega fatty acid intake and summarizing the health effects of omega-3 fatty acids
- New table listing good food sources of omega-3 fatty acids
- Updated consideration of seafood consumption guidelines, along with a new figure illustrating healthy and safe fish options for pregnant and breastfeeding women
- Revised FYI feature "Fats on the Health Food Store Shelf" that includes a new section on coconut and grapeseed oil
- New description of fat's structural role in the brain
- New discussion of the lack of a UL for fat, trans fat, or cholesterol

Chapter 6—Proteins and Amino Acids: Function Follows Form

- New FYI feature "Celiac Disease and Gluten Sensitivity"
- New discussion about the lack of evidence for gluten-free diets impacting weight loss
- Updated consideration of protein recommendations for athletes
- Updated discussion of the health benefits and risks of vegetarian diets, including a new table providing healthy tips for vegetarians
- New Position Statement from the Academy of Nutrition and Dietetics on vegetarian diets

Chapter 7—Vitamins: Vital Keys to Health

- Expanded presentation of the impact of vitamin A deficiency on skin and other epithelial cells
- Expanded discussion of vitamin B_{12} deficiency, including atrophic gastritis
- New Quick Bite features "Help the Vitamins Go Down" and "A Yellowish-Orange Hue"

Spotlight on Dietary Supplements and Functional Foods

- Significantly revised FYI feature "Defining Complementary and Integrative Health: How Does Nutrition Fit In?"
- Expanded discussion of fad diets and critical appraisal of diets, foods, and supplements

Chapter 8—Water and Minerals: The Ocean Within

- Revised FYI feature "Tap, Filtered, or Bottled: Which Water Is Best?" that considers current statistics surrounding bottled water use and things to keep in mind when selecting vitamin waters, supplements, or bottled waters
- New table summarizing macronutrients and micronutrients
- New discussion about the controversy surrounding the American Heart Association's suggestion and the *Dietary Guidelines*' recommendation to reduce sodium
- New Quick Bite feature "Processed Foods and Salt"

Spotlight on Metabolism and Energy Balance

- Updated section on portion size based on recent studies
- Revised FYI feature "What's Neat About NEAT?" that expands on sedentary behavior in the workplace
- New Quick Bite feature "Is Tom Brady Too Fat?"

Chapter 9—Nutrition for Physical Performance

- Incorporates new suggestions for eating and drinking before, during, and after exercise
- Expanded discussion of dehydration, including ways to check your hydration status
- New consideration of energy availability
- New section describing how vitamin D may support athletic performance
- New section on the vegetarian athlete
- New table presenting the Physical Activity Guidelines for Americans
- New table summarizing the American College of Sports Medicine's position on the amount and type of fluid to consume before, during, and after activity
- New table presenting a summary of generalized carbohydrate intake by athletes
- Added clarification regarding the distinction between lactic acid and lactate
- New FYI feature "When Are Sports Drinks Recommended?"

- New Position Statement from the Academy of Nutrition and Dietetics on nutrition and athletic performance
- New Quick Bite feature "Alligator Water?"

Spotlight on Eating Disorders

- Reflects the diagnostic criteria presented in the *Diagnostic and Statistical Manual of Mental Disorders, Fifth Edition (DSM-V)*
- Incorporates current theories of causes of eating disorders
- Added background on binge-eating disorder
- New section on the prevalence of eating disorders
- New section elaborating on the consequences of eating disorders
- New FYI features "Exploring the Connection Between Negative Affect and Eating Disorders" and "Night-Eating Syndrome: Not an Eating Disorder, But Sometimes a Concern"
- New Quick Bite features "Body Dysmorphic Disorder," "A Matter of Degree," "Estimates for Prevalence of Binge-Eating Disorder May Soon Rise," and "Changing the Perception of Exercise to Help Combat an Eating Disorder"

Chapter 10—Diet and Health

- New section on the link between diet and cardiometabolic disease, including a table outlining the top five dietary factors associated with cardiometabolic deaths
- Enhanced description of personalized nutrition
- Updated section on the possible link between diet and cancer, including a new table summarizing dietary components and cancer risk

Spotlight on Obesity and Weight Management

- Updated statistics about obesity and overweight rates in the United States
- Expanded discussion of the role of social networks in obesity
- New section on smartphone-based interventions
- New section on weight-loss devices
- Revised FYI feature "Childhood and Teenage Obesity" that includes a discussion of taxes on sugary beverages

- New Position Statement from the Academy of Nutrition and Dietetics on interventions for the treatment of overweight and obesity in adults
- New Quick Bite feature "Dangerous Caloric Restriction"

Chapter 11—Life Cycle: Maternal and Infant Nutrition

- New FYI feature "New Guidelines for Introducing Peanut Products"
- New Quick Bite feature "Would It Be Healthier to Menstruate Less Often?"

Chapter 12—Life Cycle: From Childhood Through Adulthood

- New FYI features "Farmers' Markets" and "School Vending Machines and the Teen Diet"
- Updated American Heart Association recommendations for fiber consumption
- Updated figures showing MyPlate meal and snack patterns for preschoolers and the modified MyPlate for older adults

Spotlight on World Nutrition: The Faces of Global Malnutrition

- Updated statistics regarding world hunger, homelessness in the United States, and malnutrition in the United States
- Updated U.S. poverty guidelines
- Expanded description of food deserts
- New Quick Bite features "Is There a Food Desert Near You?" and "To Breastfeed or Not?"

Chapter 13—Food Safety and Technology: Microbial Threats and Genetic Engineering

- Expanded coverage of natural toxins and food allergies
- Expanded coverage of the benefits and risks of genetic engineering
- New Quick Bite features "Flesh-Eating Bacteria?" and "Is It Stomach Flu or Food Poisoning?"

The Pedagogy

Discovering Nutrition focuses on teaching behavioral change, personal decision making, and up-to-date scientific concepts in a number of novel ways. This interactive approach addresses different learning styles, making it the ideal text to ensure mastery of key concepts. Beginning with Chapter 1, the material engages students in considering their own behavior in light of the knowledge they are gaining. The pedagogical aids that appear in most chapters include the following:

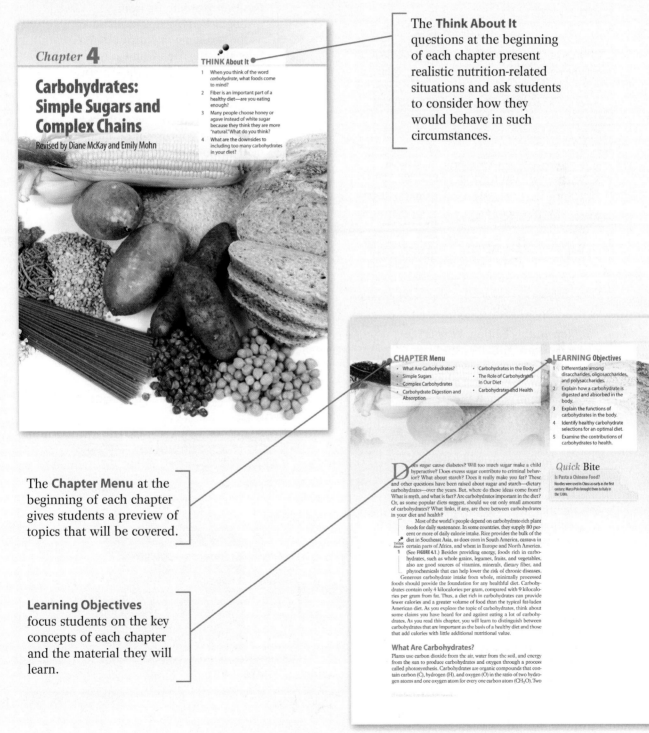

The **Think About It** questions at the beginning of each chapter present realistic nutrition-related situations and ask students to consider how they would behave in such circumstances.

The **Chapter Menu** at the beginning of each chapter gives students a preview of topics that will be covered.

Learning Objectives focus students on the key concepts of each chapter and the material they will learn.

obese older adults.[92] The presence of nutritional deficiencies in overweight and obese older adults can be a consequence of the long-term consumption of a high-calorie, poor-nutrient diet and a physically inactive lifestyle.[93]

Key Concepts Oral health, vision, and bone health all decline with aging. Tooth loss and oral pain can reduce food intake and nutrient quality. Loss of vision can make food shopping and preparation difficult. Osteoporosis, most common in postmenopausal women, can cause debilitating fractures. Alzheimer's disease eventually destroys the ability to obtain, prepare, and consume an optimal diet. Overweight and obesity are increasingly common and significantly affect the quality of life and health of older adults. Management of these conditions depends first on their identification by healthcare professionals.

Meal Management for Mature Adults

Many older adults are at nutritional risk because of economics, social isolation, physical restrictions, inability to shop for or prepare food, and medical conditions. Fortunately, there are a number of ways that older adults can remain independent and have access to an adequate diet.

Managing Independently

Independent and assisted-living programs allow people to live relatively carefree yet independent lives. Senior citizen apartment buildings and retirement villages offer a variety of services, including balanced meals. Programs such as **Meals on Wheels** and the **Older Americans Act Nutrition Program** (formerly known as the Elderly Nutrition Program) provide meals to home-bound people as well as those in congregate (group) settings. Most programs provide meals at least five times per week. The Older Americans Act Nutrition Program is supported primarily with federal funds: volunteer time, in-kind donations, and participant contributions make up the remainder. The **Supplemental Nutrition Assistance Program (SNAP)**, formerly the Food Stamp Program, is another option that provides low-income older adults with the means to purchase food. Unfortunately, because SNAP carries a "welfare" stigma, some older adults are reluctant to participate. In addition, many people who need some help buying food do not meet the eligibility requirements.

An evaluation of the Older Americans Act Nutrition Program showed that program participants had higher nutrient intake levels than nonparticipants and had a higher number of regular social contacts—another important factor in eating well.[94] Participation in food assistance programs can reduce the incidence of depression and overweight associated with food insecurity.[95]

Wise Eating for One or Two

Preparing meals that are healthful and tasty is a challenge for those living alone or in small households. As discussed earlier in this chapter, our nutrition needs—with the exception of calories—do not decrease as we age, but our ability to meet them does. Reliance on convenience foods, fast foods, and eating out can adversely affect the nutritional status of older adults. Men who live alone are especially likely to eat out or skip meals rather than prepare food for themselves. For both men and women, physical disability or illness can diminish the desire to prepare and eat meals.

▶ **Meals on Wheels** A voluntary, not-for-profit organization established to provide nutritious meals to homebound people (regardless of age) so they can maintain their independence and quality of life.

▶ **Older Americans Act Nutrition Program** A federally funded program (formerly known as the Elderly Nutrition Program) that provide older persons with nutritionally sound meals through home-delivered nutrition services, congregate nutrition services, and the nutrition services' incentive.

▶ **Supplemental Nutrition Assistance Program (SNAP)** A USDA program that helps single people and families with little or no income to buy food. Formerly known as the Food Stamp Program.

Position Statement: Academy of Nutrition and Dietetics

Food and Nutrition for Older Adults: Promoting Health and Wellness

It is the position of the Academy of Nutrition and Dietetics that all Americans aged 60 years and older receive appropriate nutrition care; have access to coordinated, comprehensive food and nutrition services; and receive the benefits of ongoing research to identify the most effective food and nutrition programs, interventions, and therapies.

Source: Reprinted from *Journal of the Academy of Nutrition and Dietetics*, 112(8), Melissa Bernstein, Nancy Munoz, Position of the Academy of Nutrition and Dietetics: Food and Nutrition for Older Adults: Promoting Health and Wellness, Page no. 1255-1277, 2014, with permission from Elsevier.

Key Concepts summarize previous text and highlight important information.

Position Statements from distinguished organizations such as the Academy of Nutrition and Dietetics, the American College of Sports Medicine, and the American Heart Association relate to the chapter topics and bolster the assertions made by the authors by showcasing concurrent opinions held by some of the leading organizations in nutrition and health.

Genetics and Disease

Why Is This Important? Nutritionists are combining genetic data with behavioral data, such as personal dietary practices, to find new connections to health and disease. Understanding the basics of genetics will help you appreciate the latest research findings.

In the last several years, knowledge has exploded regarding the relationship between our genetic makeup and disease. We now recognize that nearly all diseases have some genetic component. Most human illnesses occur because of the interaction of many genetic, environmental, nutritional, and lifestyle factors. (See FIGURE 10.2.) As the number one killer in the United States, cardiovascular disease is a good example of how genetic influences affect the development of disease.[12] A family history of heart disease indicates genetic vulnerability and is an important risk factor for developing the disease. Although some cancers, for example, breast cancer, have a genetic basis and affect many members of a given family, most cancers seem to be caused by a variety of factors.

Understanding how our genes influence our risk for disease has been a major goal of the **Human Genome Project**, an international effort spearheaded by the U.S. National Institutes of Health (NIH). The Human Genome Project is providing scientists with clues to the genetic variations that are responsible for common illnesses. Understanding the genetics of diseases will allow researchers to develop more effective medications and may lead to routine gene-based treatments.[13]

THINK About It 1

▶ **genes** Sections of DNA that contain hereditary information. Most genes contain information for making proteins.

▶ **Human Genome Project** An effort coordinated by the Department of Energy and the National Institutes of Health to map the genes in human DNA.

Quick Bite

Biological Blueprint
Nearly all 100 trillion cells in the human body contain a copy of the entire human genome, the complete set of genetic instructions necessary to build a human being.

FIGURE 10.2 **Risk factors for chronic diseases.** Diet, lifestyle choices, and genetics interact to shape a person's risk profile.

New to this edition, **Why Is This Important?** provides students with a brief overview of the practical importance and value of the information they're learning.

Key Terms are in boldface type the first time they are mentioned. Their definitions also appear in the margins near the relevant textual discussion, making it easy for students to review material.

Quick Bites sprinkled throughout the text offer fun facts about nutrition-related topics such as unique foods, social customs, origins of phrases, folk remedies, medical history, and so on.

Is the Glycemic Index a Useful Tool for Constructing a Healthy Diet with Carbohydrates?

The glycemic index is a valuable tool and easy-to-use concept that may be important for individuals with diabetes to help fine tune their blood glucose control.[a] Several popular weight-loss diets use the glycemic index to guide food choices.

How Is the Glycemic Index Measured?
The glycemic index compares the change in blood glucose after eating a sample food to the change expected from eating an equal amount of available carbohydrate from a standard food, such as white bread or from pure glucose. Therefore, the glycemic index is expressed as a percentage, ranging from 1–100, with 100 being the standard food.[b]

Foods with a high glycemic index trigger a sharp rise in blood glucose, followed by a dramatic fall, often to levels that are below normal. This explains why these foods could be undesirable for a person with diabetes. In contrast, low-glycemic-index foods trigger slower and more modest changes in blood glucose levels, thereby making blood glucose easier to manage. However, the effects of high or low glycemic index foods on people without diabetes are questionable, especially when eating a mixed diet.

What Factors Affect the Glycemic Index of a Food or Meal?
The glycemic index of a food is not always easy to predict. Would you expect a sweet food such as ice cream to have a high glycemic index? Ice cream actually has a low glycemic value because its fat slows sugar absorption. On the other hand, wouldn't you expect complex carbohydrates such as bread or potatoes to have a low glycemic index? In fact, the starch in white bread and cooked potatoes is readily absorbed, so each has a high value. The glycemic indices of some common foods are listed in **TABLE A**, and lower-glycemic-index substitutions are provided in **TABLE B**.

The type of carbohydrate, the cooking process, and the presence of fat, dietary fiber, and other food components in a meal or snack all affect the glycemic response.[d,e] In a person's diet, it is the glycemic index of mixed meals, referred to as the glycemic load, that is more important than the effect of individual foods on blood glucose.[f] Specifically, the glycemic load takes into account the amount of carbohydrate consumed. Glycemic load is calculated by multiplying the glycemic index of a food by the amount of carbohydrate in a serving. Because the glycemic index is a percentage, the resulting value is divided by 100. High-glycemic-index foods do not necessarily have high glycemic loads if there is a relatively small amount of carbohydrate in one serving. For example, watermelon has a high glycemic index (72), but it mostly consists of water, and there is only a small amount of carbohydrate per serving.

Why Do Some Researchers Believe the Glycemic Index Is Useful?
Health benefits of following a low-glycemic-index diet can be significant. Diets that emphasize low-glycemic-index foods decrease the risk of developing type 2 diabetes and improve blood glucose control in people who are already afflicted.[g,h] Epidemiological studies suggest that such diets also reduce the risk of colon and other cancers and may help reduce the risk of heart disease.[i] Diets with a low glycemic load are associated with favorable blood lipid profiles.[k] Also, studies indicate that the effectiveness of low-fat, high-carbohydrate diets for weight loss can be improved by reducing the glycemic load.[l]

Why Do Some Researchers Believe the Glycemic Index Is Useless?
Whether a person is diabetic trying to control blood glucose levels, attempting weight loss, or reducing risk for heart disease, there is no "best way" to improve your diet. Some researchers question the usefulness of conclusions drawn primarily from epidemiological studies, given that these studies can show an association but cannot prove the cause. Additionally, results on the effectiveness of low glycemic index/load diets on health outcomes have been mixed.[m,n]

TABLE A
Glycemic Index of Some Foods Compared to Pure Glucose*

Food	Glycemic Index	Food	Glycemic Index
Bakery Products		*Fruits*	
Vanilla cake	42 ± 4	Apples	39 ± 3
Doughnut	75 ± 7	Watermelon	72 ± 13
Bread/Breakfast Foods		Dates	42 ± 4
Bagel	69	*Legumes*	
Wheat and rye bread	40	Baked beans	40 ± 3
Pita bread	68 ± 5	Black-eyed peas	38
All-Bran®	44 ± 6	Pinto beans	33
Froot Loops®	69 ± 9	*Pasta*	
Porridge	55 ± 2	Lasagna	53
Cereal Grains		Spaghetti	49 ± 3
Couscous	65 ± 7	*Vegetables*	
Sweet corn	52 ± 5	Pumpkin	64
Japonica short-grain brown rice	62 ± 5	Carrots	39 ± 4
Instant white rice	87 ± 2	Baked potato	86 ± 6
Dairy Foods		*Candy*	
Ice cream	57	Marshmallow	62 ± 6
Full-fat milk	41 ± 2	M&M's®, peanut	33 ± 3

* Glycemic response to pure glucose is 100.
Data from Atkinson FS, Foster-Powell K, Brand-Miller. International Tables of Glycemic Index Values: 2008. 2008 Diab Care; 31(12).

FYI (For Your Information) offers more in-depth discussions of controversial and timely topics, such as claims about the effects of sugar, the protein needs of athletes, and the usefulness of the glycemic index.

Label to Table helps students apply their new decision-making skills at the supermarket. It walks students through the various types of information that appear on food labels, including government-mandated terminology, misleading advertising phrases, and amounts of ingredients. This feature has been updated for this edition to reflect the new labeling guidelines released by the FDA in May 2016.

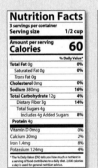

Label to Table

Sodium is found naturally in many foods, but processed foods account for most of the salt and sodium Americans consume. Processed foods with high amounts of salt include regular canned vegetables and soups, frozen dinners, lunch meats, instant and ready-to-eat cereals, and salty chips and other snacks. You can use food labels to choose products lower in sodium.

Compare Labels
Which of these two items is lower in sodium? To tell, check the Percent Daily Value.

The frozen peas are lower in sodium, with just 5 percent of the DV per 1/2 cup serving. The canned peas have three times more sodium than the frozen peas: 16 percent of the DV in one serving. Sodium is found in many foods that might surprise you, such as baking soda, soy sauce, and monosodium glutamate (MSG). Sodium is even found in some antacids—the range is wide. Before trying salt substitutes, check with your doctor, especially if you have high blood pressure. Many salt substitutes contain potassium chloride and can be harmful for individuals who have certain medical conditions or who take diuretic medications.

Nutrition Facts
3 servings per container
Serving size 1/2 cup

Amount per serving
Calories 60

% Daily Value*

Total Fat 0g	0%
Saturated Fat 0g	0%
Trans Fat 0g	
Cholesterol 0mg	0%
Sodium 380mg	16%
Total Carbohydrate 12g	4%
Dietary Fiber 3g	14%
Total Sugars 4g	
Includes 4g Added Sugars	8%
Protein 4g	
Vitamin D 0mcg	0%
Calcium 20mg	2%
Iron 1.4mg	8%
Potassium 124mg	4%

* The % Daily Value (DV) tells you how much a nutrient in a serving of food contributes to a daily diet. 2,000 calories a day is used for general nutrition advice.

Nutrition Facts
3 servings per container
Serving size 1/2 cup

Amount per serving
Calories 60

% Daily Value*

Total Fat 0g	0%
Saturated Fat 0g	0%
Trans Fat 0g	
Cholesterol 0mg	0%
Sodium 125mg	5%
Total Carbohydrate 11g	4%
Dietary Fiber 6g	22%
Total Sugars 5g	
Includes 5g Added Sugars	10%
Protein 5g	
Vitamin D 0mcg	0%
Calcium 300mg	30%
Iron 1.1mg	6%
Potassium 87mg	2%

* The % Daily Value (DV) tells you how much a nutrient in a serving of food contributes to a daily diet. 2,000 calories a day is used for general nutrition advice.

The **Learning Portfolio** at the end of each chapter condenses all aspects of nutrition information that students need to solidify their understanding of the material. The various formats will appeal to students according to their individual learning and studying styles.

Key Terms list all new vocabulary alphabetically with the page number of the first appearance. This arrangement allows students to review any term they do not recall and turn immediately to the definition and discussion of it in the chapter. This approach also promotes the acquisition of knowledge, not simply memorization.

Study Points summarize the content of each chapter with a synopsis of each major topic. The points are in the order in which they appear in the chapter, so related concepts flow together.

Study Questions encourage students to probe deeper into the chapter content, making connections and gaining new insights. Although these questions can be used for pop quizzes, they will also help students to review, especially students who study by writing out material.

---

662   CHAPTER 12   LIFE CYCLE: FROM CHILDHOOD TO ADULTHOOD

Learning Portfolio

Key Terms

	page
acne	641
adolescence	629
Alzheimer's disease (AD)	658
anorexia of aging	656
childhood	629
epiphyses	638
hyperactivity	634
hypervitaminosis	653
macular degeneration	657
Meals on Wheels	659
menarche	638
Older Americans Act Nutrition Program	659
puberty	637
Supplemental Nutrition Assistance Program (SNAP)	659
taste threshold	647
urinary tract infection (UTI)	646

Study Points

- For children and adolescents, growth is the key determinant of nutrient needs. If diets are planned carefully, children do not need vitamin/mineral supplementation.
- Federally funded nutrition and feeding programs reduce malnutrition and hunger among U.S. children.
- Adoption of adult food plans to reduce risk of chronic disease should begin gradually after the age of 2.
- The prevalence of obesity and eating disorders is rising among U.S. children and teens; treatment programs should address food choices and activity levels rather than impose strict calorie limits. Vegetarian diets for children need to be planned carefully to avoid nutrient deficiencies.
- The total energy and nutrient needs of adolescents are high to support growth and maturation. Girls need more iron than boys do to compensate for losses after the onset of menstruation. Active teens need more calories and nutrients than sedentary teens; fluid intake is also a priority.
- Nutrition and physical activity are two important controllable components of a healthy life and healthful aging. Moreover, numerous physiological and psychological aspects of the aging process affect food intake and nutritional status.
- Energy needs decline with age, reflecting loss of lean body mass and reduced physical activity.

The protein RDA and the recommended balance of carbohydrate and fat calories in the diet are similar for young and older adults. Fluid intake needs special attention because of the reduced thirst response that occurs with age.

- Because of reduced intake, synthesis, and activation, vitamin D status declines with age; recommended intake levels are therefore raised. Vitamin B_{12} status might be compromised by inadequate absorption. Antioxidants can help in the protection against degenerative diseases.
- Calcium and zinc intakes are likely to be marginal in the diets of older adults. Iron also remains important.
- Dietary supplements, both vitamin/mineral and herbal/botanical, should be used with caution, preferably with professional advice.
- Because many older adults take multiple medications, they are at risk for drug–nutrient, food–drug, and drug–drug interactions. Anorexia of aging is also a major public health problem.
- Arthritis is a prevalent chronic health problem in this age group. Weight management is a key element of arthritis treatment.
- Chronic constipation is a common complaint among older adults. Fluids, fiber, and regular exercise can reduce the likelihood of constipation.
- Poor oral and visual health both can compromise the ability of older adults to consume a nutritionally adequate diet.
- Osteoporosis is a major health problem that can be addressed through adequate calcium and vitamin D, regular weight-bearing exercise, and medication if needed.
- Adults can maintain independence while aging but may require special assistance to obtain and prepare food. Community resources can help respond to the needs of older adults and those of their caretakers and family.

Study Questions

1. Which vitamins and minerals are most likely to be deficient in a child's diet?
2. Identify several chronic nutrition problems that can affect children. How can these problems be avoided?

LEARNING PORTFOLIO **663**

3. What are typical nutritional concerns for adolescents?

4. What are some consequences of decreased immunity among older adults?

5. Compared with a younger adult, does a person older than 65 years need more, less, or about the same amount of protein?

6. Why are older adults at risk of vitamin D deficiency?

7. Discuss minerals that may need special attention in assessment of an older adult's nutrition status.

8. What problems might older adults encounter with dietary supplements?

9. What is the role of physical activity in osteoporosis prevention? What nutritional factors are important?

Try This ●

Eat Like a Kid

Children, especially toddlers, tend to be exploratory and take in the sensory nature of food—the textures, smells, and tastes. In fact, you were probably once this way. The purpose of this exercise is to eat a meal like a kid and gain an appreciation of food's textures and taste. Make some mashed potatoes, macaroni and cheese, buttered peas, or spaghetti (favorite "kid food") and eat it with your fingers. Explore your food and play with it. Try mixing foods. How does this experience make you feel?

Aging Simulation

The purpose of this exercise is to simulate what it can be like to age and experience age-related declines in health. Have you ever thought of how difficult it is to be an older person with health problems and do routine tasks? Invite a few friends over and do the following:

■ Put gloves on to simulate the difficulty of losing sensitivity in your hands.

■ Use cotton balls in your ears to decrease your hearing ability.

■ Apply some petroleum jelly to a pair of glasses or sunglasses to give yourself poor vision.

Now try a simple activity. Make a salad, send a text message, or play a video. After completing the activity, switch disabilities with your friends so that everyone has experienced each of the limitations. What is it like to do these activities with your impairment?

Getting Personal ●

You have just graduated. Revisit your eating habits as a child, teenager, and college student, and assign the most appropriate descriptor to each item. Consider how your past nutritional behavior has helped determine your current health status.

0 = seldom or never true

1 = sometimes true

2 = frequently true

As a child,

1. I was a picky eater, rejecting the food usually offered.

2. I was not permitted to decide how much to eat.

3. I rarely drank milk.

4. I ate candy every day.

As an adolescent,

5. I let peer pressure influence my nutrition choices.

6. I ate in front of the TV.

7. I worried about my weight.

As a college student,

8. I didn't think about healthy food choices.

9. I resisted changing my eating habits.

10. I was influenced by food fads.

Add up your score. Scores over 12 should signal that your healthy nutrition behavior can be improved. Highlight the items you feel can be affected by behavior change.

References

1. Institute of Medicine. Food and Nutrition Board. *Dietary Reference Intakes for Energy, Carbohydrate, Fiber, Fat, Fatty Acids, Cholesterol, Protein, and Amino Acids*. Washington, DC: National Academies Press; 2005.

2. Kleinman RE, Greer FR, eds. *Pediatric Nutrition Handbook*. 7th ed. Elk Grove Village, IL: American Academy of Pediatrics; 2014.

3. Ogata B, Hayes D. Position of the Academy of Nutrition and Dietetics: nutrition guidance for healthy children ages 2 to 11 years. *J Acad Nutr Diet*. 2014;114:1257-1276.

4. Kumar J, Muntner P, Kaskel FJ, et al. Prevalence and associations of 25-hydroxyvitamin D deficiency in U.S. children: NHANES 2001–2004. *Pediatrics*. 2009;124(3):e362-e370.

5. Ogata B. Hayes D. Op. cit.

6. Kleinman RE, Greer FR. Op. cit.

7. Ogata B. Hayes D. Op. cit.

8. Neelon SE, Briley ME. Position of the American Dietetic Association: benchmarks for nutrition in child care. *J Am Diet Assoc*. 2011;111:607-615.

9. Pearson N, Biddle SJ. Sedentary behavior and dietary intake in children, adolescents, and adults: a systematic review. *Am J Prev Med*. 2011;41(2):178-188.

Getting Personal encourages students to consider their newly gained knowledge in the context of their own diets.

Try This activities provide suggestions for hands-on activities that encourage students to put theory into practice. It will especially help students whose major learning style is experimental.

The Integrated Learning and Teaching Package

Jones & Bartlett Learning provides a full suite of instructor resources for *Discovering Nutrition, Sixth Edition*, which qualified instructors can receive by contacting their Account Manager. Available resources include:

- Test Bank, including more than 850 questions
- Slides in PowerPoint format, featuring more than 500 slides
- Instructor's Manual, containing lecture outlines, discussion questions, and answers to the in-text Study Questions
- Image Bank, supplying key figures from the text
- Sample Syllabus, showing how a course can be structured around this text
- Transition Guide, providing guidance in switching from the previous edition

In addition, *Discovering Nutrition* is available in a variety of eBook formats, including as a Navigate 2 Advantage eBook containing 36 scientifically based animations that give students an accurate, accessible explanation of the major scientific concepts and physiological principles presented in this text.

About the Authors

The *Discovering Nutrition* author team represents a culmination of years of teaching and research in nutrition science and psychology. The combined experience of the authors yields a balanced presentation of both the science of nutrition and the components of behavioral change.

Dr. Paul Insel is Adjunct Professor of Psychiatry and the Behavioral Sciences at Stanford University (Stanford, California). In addition to being the principal investigator on several nutrition projects for the National Institutes of Health (NIH), he is the senior author of the seminal text in health education and has co-authored several best-selling nutrition books.

Don Ross is Director of the California Institute of Human Nutrition (Redwood City, California). For more than 30 years he has co-authored multiple textbooks and created educational materials about health and nutrition for consumers, professionals, and college students. He has special expertise in communicating complicated physiological processes with easily understood graphical presentations. The National Institutes of Health selected his *Travels with Cholesterol* for distribution to consumers. His multidisciplinary focus brings together the fields of psychology, nutrition, biochemistry, biology, and medicine.

Kimberley McMahon, MDA, RD, received her registration with the Academy of Nutrition and Dietetics upon completion of a nutrition program at Montana State University and a dietetic internship at Miami Valley Hospital in Dayton, Ohio. Her graduate studies at Utah State University investigated a person's success with behavior and weight management as it relates to personality psychology and the extent to which individuals believe they can control events affecting their lives. Kimberley has taught nutrition courses for more than 18 years in both traditional and online settings, including basic nutrition, advanced nutrition, medical terminology, nutrition for exercise and sport, dietetics administration, and clinical nutrition. She has been an instructor at Utah State University and Northern Kentucky University, and currently teaches in the Master of Science Degree in Nutrition and Human Performance program at Logan University (Chesterfield, Missouri). In addition to *Discovering Nutrition*, she is a co-author of *Nutrition*, *Nutrition Across Life Stages*, and *Eat Right! Healthy Eating in College and Beyond*. Her interests and experience are in the areas of wellness, weight management, sports nutrition, and eating disorders. Kimberley is currently licensed as a Dietitian in the state of Indiana.

Dr. Melissa Bernstein is a Registered Dietitian Nutritionist, Licensed Dietitian, and Fellow of the Academy of Nutrition and Dietetics. She received her doctoral degree from the Gerald J. and Dorothy R. Friedman School of Nutrition Science and Policy at Tufts University (Boston, Massachusetts). As an Assistant Professor in the Department of Nutrition at Chicago Medical School, Dr. Bernstein is innovative in creating engaging and challenging nutrition courses. Her interests include introductory nutrition, health and wellness, geriatric nutrition, physical activity, and nutritional biochemistry. In addition to co-authoring leading nutrition textbooks—including *Nutrition*, *Discovering Nutrition*, *Nutrition Across Life Stages*, *Nutrition for the Older Adult*, and *Nutrition Assessment: Clinical and Research Applications*—Dr. Bernstein has reviewed and authored textbook chapters, position statements, and peer-reviewed journal publications on the topics of nutrition and nutrition for older adults. She is the co-author of the *Position of the Academy of Nutrition and Dietetics: Food and Nutrition for Older Adults: Promoting Health and Wellness*. She serves on review and advisory committees for the Academy's Evidence Analysis Library and as a reviewer for upcoming position statements.

Contributors

© Greentellect Studio/Shutterstock.

The authors would like to acknowledge the valuable contributions of the following:

Feon Cheng, PhD, MPH, RDN, CHTS-CP

Academy of Nutrition and Dietetics
Chapter 7, "Vitamins"

Brian Cook, PhD

California State University, Monterey Bay
"Spotlight on Eating Disorders"

Carolyn Dunn, PhD, RD

North Carolina State University
"Spotlight on Alcohol"
Chapter 8, "Water and Minerals"

Fabio Giallongo, PhD

Chapter 7, "Vitamins"

Diane L. McKay, PhD, FACN

Tufts University
Chapter 4, "Carbohydrates"

Emily Mohn, PhD

Tufts University
Chapter 4, "Carbohydrates"

Tara LaRowe, PhD, RDN, CD

University of Wisconsin–Madison
"Spotlight on World Nutrition"

Contributors from past editions include the following:

Nancy K. Amy, PhD, University of California, Berkeley

Janine T. Baer, PhD, RD, University of Dayton

Katherine Beals, PhD, RD, FACSM, University of Utah

Hope McClusky Bilyk, MS, RD, LDN, Rosalind Franklin University of Medicine and Science

Toni Bloom, MS, RD, CDE, San Jose State University

Pat Brown, MS, RD, Cuesta College

Boyce W. Burge, PhD, California Institute of Human Nutrition

Robert DiSilvestro, PhD, The Ohio State University

Eileen G. Ford, MS, RD, Drexel University

Ellen B. Fung, PhD, RD, University of Pennsylvania

Michael I. Goran, PhD, University of Southern California

Nancy J. Gustafson, MS, RD, FADA, Sawyer County (WI) Aging Unit

Rita H. Herskovitz, MS, University of Pennsylvania

Nancy I. Kemp, MD, University of California, San Francisco

Sarah Harding Laidlaw, MS, RD, MPA, Dietitians in Integrative and Functional Medicine DPG #18

Sally A. Lederman, PhD, Columbia University

Rick D. Mattes, MPH, PhD, RD, Purdue University

Alexandria Miller, PhD, RD/LD, Northeastern State University

Carla Miller, PhD, The Ohio State University

Nancy Munoz, DCN, MHA, RD

Maye Musk, MS, RD, Past President of the Consulting Dietitians of Canada

Joyce D. Nash, PhD

Marcia Nelms, PhD, RD, Missouri State University

C.J. Nieves, MS, University of Florida

Elizabeth Quintana, MS, RD, LD, CDE, West Virginia University School of Medicine

Barbara Reynolds, MS, RD, College of the Sequoias

Mackinnon Ross, MPH, California Institute of Human Nutrition

Sylvia Santosa, PhD, Concordia University

Helen Spremulli, RN, CP, Dr. Dario Del Rizzo Professional Medicine Corporation

Rachel Stern, MS, RD, CNS, North Jersey Community Research Initiative

Lisa Stollman, MA, RD, CDE, CDN, State University of New York at Stony Brook

Barbara Sutherland, PhD, University of California, Davis

R. Elaine Turner, PhD, University of Florida

Debra M. Vinci, PhD, RD, CD, Appalachian State University

Stella L. Volpe, PhD, RD, FACSM, University of Massachusetts

Paula Kurtzweil Walter, MS, RD, Federal Trade Commission

Reviewers

The authors would like to thank the following for their assistance in providing feedback that informed the revisions for this edition:

Reviewers of the *Sixth Edition*

Patricia Abraham, MPH, RD, CNS, LD, Arkansas State University

Diane Anderson, DNP, MSN, RN, CNE, Chamberlain University

Dorothy Chen-Maynard, PhD, RDN, FAND, California State University, San Bernardino

Brian Cook, PhD, California State University, Monterey Bay

Linda DeTurk, MS, Mid-Plains Community College

Elizabeth T. Dixon, DrPH, BSN, RN, MHA, Armstrong Atlantic University

Johanna Donnenfield, MS, RD, Scottsdale Community College

Michelle Eggers, RD, CDE, MEd, CCC-SLP, Appalachian State University

Marianne Heffrin, MS, RD, LD, Endicott College

Cynthia Heiss, PhD, RD, LD, University of the Incarnate Word

Sharon Himmelstein, PhD, MNS, RDN, Central New Mexico Community College

Arlene J. Hoogewerf, PhD, Calvin College

Kathleen M. Laquale, PhD, ATC, LAT, LDN, Bridgewater State University

Maryln Lehmkuhl, RDN, MS, Alexandria Technical and Community College

Lindsay Malone, MS, RD, CSO, LD, Case Western Reserve University

Mary Martinez, MS, RDN, LD, Central New Mexico Community College

Sara S. Plaspohl, DrPH, CHES, Armstrong State University

Robin Polokoff, PhD, Las Positas College

Vidya Sharma, MA, RD, LD, CDE, University of the Incarnate Word

Ellen Thompson, RDN, LD, Cedarville University

Belinda Zeidler, MST, Portland State University

Reviewers of Previous Editions

Donna L. Acox, MA, MS, RD, CD/N, Syracuse University

Helen C. Alexanderson-Lee, PhD, RD, California State University, Long Beach

Betty B. Alford, PhD, RD, LD, Texas Women's University

Nancy K. Amy, PhD, University of California at Berkeley

Susan I. Barr, PhD, RDN, University of British Columbia

Renee Barrile, PhD, RD, University of Massachusetts–Lowell

Richard C. Baybutt, PhD, Kansas State University

Kristen Beavers, PhD, MPH, RD, Wake Forest University

Beverly A. Benes, PhD, RD, University of Nebraska at Lincoln

Orville Bigelow, MS, RD, Mohave Community College

Teresa Blair, MS, RD, LD, CDE, Eastern Kentucky University

Cynthia Blanton, PhD, RD, Idaho State University

Virginia C. Bragg, MS, RD, CD, Utah State University

Dr. Michele Brandenburger, BS, DC, MS, Presentation College

Katie Brown, BS, MS, Central Missouri State University

Lisa Burgoon, MS, RD, CSSD, LDN, University of Illinois at Urbana-Champaign

Melanie Tracy Burns, PhD, RD, Eastern Illinois University

N. Joanne Caid, PhD, California State University, Fresno

Deborah Cheater, MS, RN, Carl Albert State College

Sai Chidambaram, Canisius College

Alana D. Cline, PhD, RD, University of Northern Colorado

Janet Colson, PhD, RD, Middle Tennessee State University

Marisela Contreras, PhD, Richland College

Holly A. Dieken, PhD, MS, BS, RD, University of Tennessee at Chattanooga

Judy A. Driskell, PhD, RD, University of Nebraska

Liz Emery, MS, RD, CNSD, Drexel University

Dorelle Engel, MS, Montgomery College

Joan Fischer, PhD, RD, LD, University of Georgia

Jeanne Freeman, PhD, CHES, Butte-Glenn Community College

Bernard L. Frye, PhD, University of Texas at Arlington

Amy Gannon, MS, RD, LD, Marshall University

Esperanza Garza, MS, RD, LD, South Texas College

Shelby Goldberg, RD, CDE, Pima Community College

Christine Goodner, MS, RD, Winthrop University

Michael I. Goran, PhD, University of Southern California

Margaret Gunther, PhD, Palomar Community College

Nancy J. Guthrie, MA, Pierce College

Lisa P. Hall, MHA, MS, RD LD, CDE, Fayette County Memorial Hospital

Julia Halterman, PhD, Eastern Mennonite University

Shelley R. Hancock, MS, RD, LD, University of Alabama

Thomas P. Harnden, PhD, Georgia Highlands College

Nancy Gordon Harris, MS, RD, LDN, East Carolina University

Mary K. Head, PhD, RD, LD, University of West Virginia

Deloy G. Hendricks, PhD, CNS, Utah State University

Sharon Himmelstein, PhD, MNS, RD, LD, Albuquerque Technical Vocational Institute

Cathy Hix-Cunningham, PhD, RD, LDN, Tennessee Technological University

Carolyn Holcroft-Burns, BSN, PhD, Foothill College

Claire B. Hollenbeck, PhD, San Jose State University

Kevin Huggins, PhD, Auburn University

Donna Huisenga, MS, RD, LDN, Illinois Central College

Craig T. Hunt, RDN, Eastern Washington University

Michael Jenkins, Kent State University

Amy Kelly, MS, RD, LDN, Illinois Central College

Zaheer Ali Kirmani, PhD, RD, LD, Sam Houston State University

Mark E. Knauss, PhD, Georgia Highlands College

Laura Freeland Kull, MS, RD, Madonna University

Colleen Kvaska, MA, RD, CDE, Fullerton College

Sarah Harding Laidlaw, MS, RD, MPA, CDE

Janet Levins, PhD, RD, LD, Pensacola Junior College

David Lightsey, MS, Bakersfield College

Samantha R. Logan, DrPH, RD, University of Massachusetts

Lynne Marie LoPresto, MS, RD, Dominican University of California

Lourdes Lore, MS, Henry Ford Community College

Michael P. Maina, PhD, Valdosta State University

Patricia Z. Marincic, PhD, RD, LD, CLE, College of Saint Benedict/Saint John's University

Melissa J. Martilotta, MS, RD, Pennsylvania State University

Laura H. May, RD, Mesa Community College

Jennifer McLean, MSPH, Corning Community College

Brett R. Merklet, MSN, RN, LDS Business College

Mark S. Meskin, PhD, RD, California State Polytechnic University at Pomona

Stella Miller, BA, MA, Mount San Antonio College

Kristin Moline, MSEd, Lourdes University

Marilyn Mook, BS, MS, Michigan State University

Mary W. Murimi, PhD, Louisiana Technical University

Lisa M. Murray, MS, Pierce College

Katherine O. Musgrave, MS, RD, CAS, University of Maine at Orono

Joyce D. Nash, PhD

J. Dirk Nelson, PhD, Missouri Southern State College

Karen Nguyen-Garcia, Community College of Denver

Nora Norback, MPH, RD, CDE, City College of San Francisco

Veronica J. Oates, PhD, RDN, LDN, Tennessee State University

Anne O'Donnell, MS, MPH, RD, Santa Rosa Junior College

Esther Okeiyi, PhD, RD, LDN, North Carolina Central University

Nancy Peterson, PhD, North Central College

Scott Peterson, MS, Hill College

Rebecca S. Pobocik, PhD, RD, Bowling Green State University

Roseanne L. Poole, MS, RD, LD/N, Tallahassee Community College

Elizabeth Quintana, MS, RD, LD, CDE, West Virginia University School of Medicine

Amy F. Reeder, MS, RD, University of Utah

Robert D. Reynolds, PhD, University of Illinois at Chicago

Lois A. Ritter, EdD, MS, California State University at East Bay

Becky Sander, MS, RD, LD, Miami University

Stephen W. Sansone, BS, EdM, Chemekata Community College

Lisa Sasson, MS, RD, New York University

Susan T. Saylor, RD, EdD, Shelton State University

Donal Scheidel, DDS, University of South Dakota

Stephanie Schroeder, PhD, Webster University

Shannon Seal, MS, RD, Front Range Community College

Brian Luke Seaward, PhD, University of Colorado at Boulder

Mohammad R. Shayesteh, PhD, RD, LD, Youngstown State University

Melissa Shock, PhD, RD, University of Central Arkansas

LuAnn Soliah, PhD, RD, Baylor University

Bernice Gales Spurlock, PhD, Hinds Community College

Christine Stapell, MS, RD, LDN, Tallahassee Community College

Barbara A. Stettler, MEd, Bluffton College

Beth Stewart, PhD, RD, University of Arizona

Rhoada Tanenbaum, EdD, Long Island University at CW Post

Kathy Timperman, MS, West Virginia University

Annette R. Tommerdahl, PhD, University of Louisiana at Monroe

Norman R. Trezek, MS, Pima Community College

Duane Trogdon, EdD, LeTourneau University

Anna Sumabat Turner, MEd, Bob Jones University

Karen M. Ulrich, BS, Paul Smith's College of Arts and Sciences

Amy A. Vaughn, MS, Radford University

Andrea M. Villarreal, MS, RD, Phoenix College

Debra M. Vinci, DrPh, RD, LDN, University of West Florida

Janelle Walter, PhD, Baylor University

Claire E. Watson, PhD, St. Bonaventure University

Beverly G. Webber, MS, RD, CD, University of Utah

Jennifer Weddig, MS, RD, Metropolitan State College of Denver

Acknowledgments

We would like to thank the following people for their hard work and dedication. They have helped make this new edition a reality. A special thank you to Sean Fabery and our entire editorial staff from Jones & Bartlett Learning, including Taylor Maurice and Jennifer Angel. We would also like to acknowledge and express our thanks to Rachel DiMaggio for her production help, Andrea DeFronzo for marketing our texts, Shannon Sheehan for her assistance with the artwork, Merideth Tumasz for her photo research and permissions work, as well as Toni Ackley, copyeditor, and Susan Beckett, proofreader, for their exceptional assistance with content and grammar. We thank you all for your efforts, dedication, and guidance.

Thanks to Diane L. McKay, Emily Mohn, Carolyn Dunn, Brian Cook, Feon Cheng, Fabio Giallongo, and Tara LaRowe for their contributions to this edition. The authors would like to acknowledge Feon Cheng and Fabio Giallongo for their work updating the Test Bank, Instructor's Manual, and Slides in PowerPoint format, as well as Mackinnon Ross for her research assistance.

Finally, we would like to thank all of the instructors and students who were involved in the process of developing our introductory text for majors, *Nutrition*, without whose involvement the creation of *Discovering Nutrition* would not have been possible.

Chapter 1

Food Choices: Nutrients and Nourishment

Revised by Kimberley McMahon

THINK About It

1   What, if anything, might persuade or influence you to change your food preferences?

2   Are there some foods you definitely avoid? If so, do you know why?

3   How do you define nutrients?

4   How do you determine if the nutrition information you read is accurate?

LEARNING Objectives

1 Define nutrition.
2 List factors that influence food choices.
3 Describe the standard American diet.
4 List the six classes of nutrients essential for health.
5 Outline the basic steps in the nutrition research process.
6 Recognize credible scientific research and reliable sources of nutrition information.

Consider these scenarios. A group of friends goes out for pizza every Thursday night. A young man greets his girlfriend with a box of chocolates. A 5-year-old shakes salt on her meal after watching her parents do this. A man says hot dogs are his favorite food because they remind him of going to baseball games with his father. A parent punishes a misbehaving child by withholding dessert. What do all of these people have in common? They are all using food for something other than its nutrient value. Can you think of a holiday that is not celebrated with food? For most of us, food is more than a collection of nutrients. Many factors affect what we choose to eat. Many of the foods people choose are nourishing and contribute to good health. The same, of course, may be true of the foods we reject.

The science of **nutrition** helps us improve our food choices by identifying the amounts of nutrients we need, the best food sources of those nutrients, and the other components in foods that may be helpful or harmful. The U.S. National Library of Medicine defines nutrition as the science of food; the nutrients and other substances therein; their action, interaction, and balance in relation to health and disease; and the processes by which we ingest, absorb, transport, utilize, and excrete food substances.[1] Learning about nutrition will help us to be informed and more likely to make good nutrition choices, which in turn may not only improve our health, but also reduce our risk of some diseases and may even help us to live longer. Keep in mind, though, that no matter how much you know about nutrition, you are still likely to choose some foods regardless of the nutrients they provide, simply for their taste or just because it makes you feel good to eat them.

▶ **nutrition** The science of foods and their components (nutrients and other substances), including the relationships to health and disease (actions, interactions, and balances); processes within the body (ingestion, digestion, absorption, transport, functions, and disposal of end products); and the social, economic, cultural, and psychological implications of eating.

Why Do We Eat the Way We Do?

🍎 **Why Is This Important?** Many different factors play a role in determining why we choose to eat certain foods and avoid others. Understanding the influence of these factors can shape the way we eat and help us make more healthful food choices.

Do you "eat to live" or "live to eat"? For all of us, the first is certainly true—you must eat to live. But there may be times when our enjoyment of food is more important to us than the nourishment we get from it. We use food to project a desired image, forge relationships, express friendship, show creativity, and disclose our feelings. We cope with anxiety or stress by eating or not eating; we reward ourselves with food for a good grade or a job well done; or, in extreme cases, we punish failures by denying ourselves the benefit and comfort of eating. Factors such as age, gender, genetic makeup, occupation, lifestyle, family, and cultural background can all affect our daily and habitual food choices. In this book we refer to these daily and habitual food choices as a person's "diet." Unless otherwise indicated, the term *diet* is not used to describe a regimen of eating and drinking for the purpose of weight loss, such as "dieting to lose weight," but rather the term *diet* will refer to daily and habitual food choices that a person makes.

Personal Preferences

What we eat reveals much about who we are. Food preferences begin early in life and then change as we interact with parents, friends, and peers. Further experiences with different people, places, and situations often cause us to expand or change our preferences. Taste and other sensory factors such as texture are some of the most important things that influence our food choices; cost and convenience are important, too.[2]

THINK
About It

1

Age is another factor in food choices. Consider taste preferences and how they might be influenced even before birth. Science shows that, when compared to adults, children naturally prefer higher levels of sweet and salty tastes and reject bitter tastes.[3] This might help explain why children are drawn to more unhealthy food choices. In support of this idea, studies have found that sensory experiences, beginning early in life, can shape preferences in both a positive and a negative way. For example, an expecting mother who consumes a diet rich in healthy foods can help develop her child's taste preferences in a positive way because flavors from foods that the mother eats are transmitted to amniotic fluid and to mother's milk, creating an environment in which breastfed infants are more accepting of these flavors.[4] In contrast, infants fed formula learn to prefer its unique flavor profile and may have more difficulty initially accepting flavors not found in formula, such as those of fruit and vegetables.[5] Having healthy food experiences early in life may go a long way toward promoting healthy eating throughout a person's life span.

Although young children prefer sweet or familiar foods, babies and toddlers are generally willing to try new things. (See **FIGURE 1.1**.) Experimental evidence suggests that when children are repeatedly exposed to a variety of foods, they are more likely to accept those foods, thus adding more variety to their diet and eating more healthfully. This result is even stronger for children whose willingness to try new foods is encouraged by their caregivers.[6]

Preschoolers typically go through a period of food **neophobia**, a dislike for anything new or unfamiliar. School-age children tend to accept a wider array of foods, and teenagers are strongly influenced by the preferences and habits of their peers. If you track the kinds of foods you have eaten in the past year, you might be surprised to discover how few basic foods your diet includes. By the time we reach adulthood,

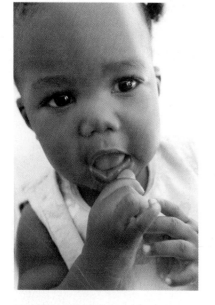

FIGURE 1.1 Adventures in eating. Babies and toddlers are willing to try new things, generally after repeat exposure.
© Monkey Business Images/Shutterstock.

▶ **neophobia** A dislike for anything new or unfamiliar.

we have formed a core group of foods we prefer. Of this group, only about 100 basic items account for 75 percent of our food intake.

Like many aspects of human behavior, food choices are influenced by many interrelated factors. Generally, hunger and satiety (the feeling of being full) dictate when we eat, but what we choose to eat is not always determined by physiological or nutritional needs. When we consider that our food preferences are also dictated by factors such as sensory properties of foods (taste, smell, and texture), emotional and cognitive factors (habits, comfort/discomfort foods, food advertising and promotion, eating away from home, etc.), and environmental factors (economics, lifestyle, food availability, culture, religion, and socioeconomics), we can better understand why we choose to eat the foods that we do. (See **FIGURE 1.2**.)

THiNK
About It
2

Sensory Influence
Taste
Smell
Texture

Environmental Factors
Economic
Lifestyle
Food availability
Culture
Religion
Geographic location
Environment

Social, Emotional, and Cognitive Factors
Habits
Food likes and dislikes
Knowledge and attitudes related to diet and health
Personal values
Comfort/discomfort foods
Food marketing, advertising, and promotion
Food and diet trends

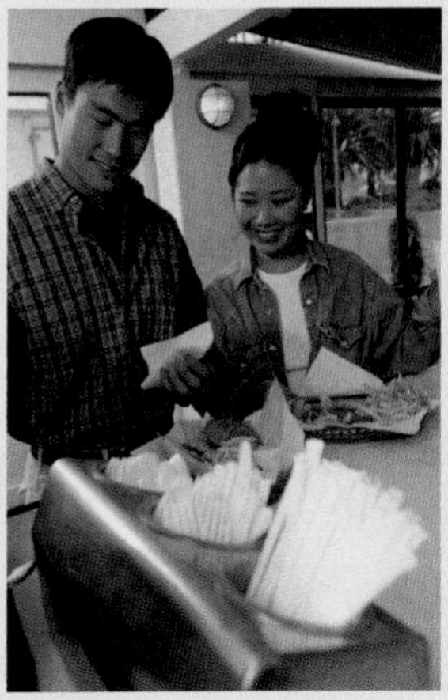

FIGURE 1.2 Factors that affect food choices. We often select a food to eat automatically without thought. But in fact, our choices are complex events involving the interactions of a multitude of factors.
© Photodisc.

Sensory Influences: Taste, Smell, and Texture

In making food choices, what appeals to our senses also contributes to our personal preferences. People often refer to **flavor** as a collective experience that describes both taste and smell. Texture also plays a part. You may prefer foods that have a crisp, chewy, or smooth texture. You may reject foods that feel grainy, slimy, or rubbery. Other sensory characteristics that affect food choice are color, moisture, and temperature.

We are familiar with the classic four tastes—sweet, sour, bitter, and salty—but do you know that there are more? One of these additional taste sensations is **umami**. Umami is a Japanese term used to describe the taste produced by glutamate.[7] It is the brothy, meaty, savory flavor in foods such as meat, seafood, and vegetables. A seasoning commonly added to Chinese food, canned vegetables, soups, and processed meats, called monosodium glutamate (MSG), enhances this umami flavor. Despite many people identifying themselves as being sensitive to MSG, the Food and Drug Administration (FDA) considers that adding MSG to foods is "generally recognized as safe." People who claim sensitivity report symptoms such as headache, flushing, sweating, and nausea; however, studies have not been able to consistently trigger these reactions.[8]

Emotional and Cognitive Influences

Habits

Your eating and cooking habits likely reflect what you learned from your parents. We typically learn to eat three meals a day, at about the same times each day. Quite often we eat the same foods, particularly for breakfast (e.g., cereal and milk) and lunch (e.g., sandwiches). This routine makes life convenient, and we don't have to think much about when or what to eat. But we don't have to follow this routine. How would you feel about eating mashed potatoes for breakfast and cereal for dinner? Some people might get a stomach-ache just thinking about

Quick **Bite**

Try it Again, You Just Might Like It
Studies have found that children between the ages of 2 and 6 years commonly dislike things that are new or unfamiliar. This is also the age when kids are most likely to reject vegetables. Kids have a better chance to overcome this tendency if they are repeatedly exposed to the food they initially reject—somewhere between 5 and 15 exposures should do it.

▶ **flavor** The collective experience that describes both taste and smell.

▶ **umami [ooh-MA-mee]** A Japanese term that describes a delicious meaty or savory sensation. Chemically, this taste detects the presence of glutamate.

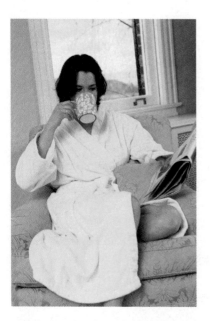

FIGURE 1.3 Comfort foods. Depending on your childhood food experiences, a bowl of traditional soup, a remembered sweet, or a mug of hot chocolate can provide comfort in times of stress.

© Jules Frazier/Photodisc/Getty Images.

it, whereas others may enjoy the prospect of doing things differently. Look at your eating habits and see how often you make the same choices every single day.

Comfort/Discomfort Foods

Our desire for particular foods often is based on behavioral motives, even though we may not be aware of them. For some people, food becomes an emotional security blanket. Consuming our favorite foods can make us feel better, relieve stress, and allay anxiety. (See **FIGURE 1.3**.) Starting with the first days of life, food and affection are intertwined. Breastfed infants, for example, experience physical, emotional, and psychological satisfaction when nursing. As we grow older, this experience is continually reinforced. For example, chicken soup and hot tea with honey may be favorites when we feel ill because someone had prepared those foods for us when we were not feeling well. If we were rewarded for good behavior with a particular food (e.g., ice cream, candy, cookies), our positive feelings about that food may persist for a lifetime.

In contrast, at some point you may have gotten sick soon after eating a certain food, and you still avoid that food.

Food Advertising and Promotion

Aggressive and sometimes deceptive advertising can influence a person's food-buying decisions; therefore, it may not surprise you that some of the most popular food purchases are high-fat and high-sugar baked goods and alcoholic beverages. According to the Federal Trade Commission (FTC), businesses spend $9.6 billion annually marketing food and beverages, both on television and online. More than $1.79 billion specifically targets children and adolescents, promoting items such as sugared breakfast cereals, fast food, and soft drinks.[9] Exposure to food advertising increases the preference and purchase of the advertised foods, particularly by overweight or obese adults and children.[10]

Food and beverage advertising greatly influences children's eating behavior. Children and teens see about 12–16 TV advertisements per day for products generally high in saturated fat, sugar, and/or sodium.[11] One study suggests that advertising changes the way children consider the importance of taste when making food choices: after watching food commercials, children rely less on health values for their food choices, and instead place significantly more importance on taste.[12] In another study, children consumed 14% more high-sugar breakfast cereal for every 10 advertisements seen for that kind of cereal.[13]

Although the majority of food advertisements are for less healthy foods, positive food advertising also exists. We are seeing more innovative advertising that promotes locally grown, hormone- and pesticide-free foods, plus whole grains, nuts, berries, vegetarian foods, and other nutrient-dense products.

Eating Meals Prepared Outside the Home

In recent years there has been a general shift away from domestic cooking and toward the use of pre-prepared and ultra-processed foods. There has also been an upsurge in time and money devoted to dining out. In all, Americans spend almost half of their food budget on foods prepared away from home, however, they also underestimate the amount of calories and fat in these foods, which is likely contributing to increasing weight and obesity.[14] This trend has promoted an increased interest in information on calories, fat, sodium, and other nutrients on menus. When calories are present on menus, people order foods with fewer calories compared to those ordering from menus without calories identified, and parents order foods with fewer calories for their children.[15] The Food and Drug Administration (FDA) has implemented guidelines in which nutrition labeling in chain restaurants and similar food establishments will provide consumers with clear and consistent nutrition information in a direct and accessible manner.

Food and Diet Trends

The popularity of different diets can influence changes in food product consumption. Beginning in the late 1980s, low-fat diets became popular and were accompanied by an explosion of reduced-fat, low-fat, and fat-free products. When the low-carbohydrate diet became popular, there was a rise in low-carb and no-carb products. Diet and health-related products also compete for consumer dollars. For example, sales of gluten-free products in the United States continue to rise due to the increased diagnosis of celiac disease and the unproven belief that eliminating gluten, a protein found in wheat and related grains such as barley and rye, from the diet will treat other conditions as well. Some notable food trends of the last decade include organic foods, locally grown and prepared foods, fermented foods that contain live cultures, and "craft foods" that hail from a particular locale and claim to have unique tastes. Other trends relate more to our behaviors than particular foods, but they ultimately affect our food purchases; they include snacking throughout the day, using online grocery shopping and delivery services, using apps to calculate the exact nutritional content of meals, and shopping at supermarkets converted into socializing spaces. (See **FIGURE 1.4.**)

Social Factors

Social factors exert a powerful influence on food choice. Food is often at the center of family gatherings, social events, and office parties. Perhaps even more influential, though, are the messages from peers about what to eat or how to eat.

As **FIGURE 1.5** illustrates, eating is a social event that brings together people for a variety of purposes (e.g., religious or cultural celebrations, business meetings, family dinners). Social pressures, however, also can restrict our food intake and selection. We might, for example, order nonmeat dishes when dining with a group of vegetarian friends.

Knowledge of Health and Nutrition

Many people select and emphasize certain foods they think are "good for them." (See **FIGURE 1.6.**) Consumer health beliefs, perceptions of disease susceptibility, and desires to take action to prevent or delay disease onset can have powerful influences

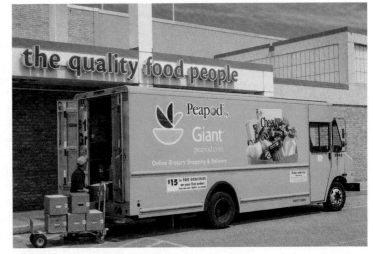

FIGURE 1.4 Food and Diet Trends. Online grocery shopping and delivery are becoming popular across the United States.
© J.D. Maman/Shutterstock.

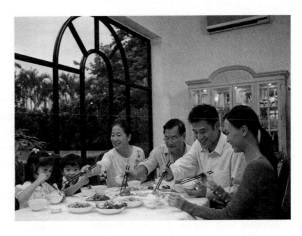

FIGURE 1.5 Social facilitation. Interactions with others can affect your eating behaviors.
© Fuse/Thinkstock.

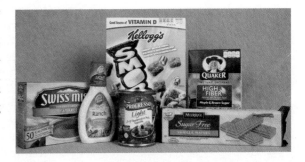

FIGURE 1.6 Where do you get your nutrition information? We are constantly bombarded by food messages. Which sources do you find most influential? Are they also the most reliable?
© Jones & Bartlett Learning. Photographed by Sarah Cebulski.

on diet and food choices. For example, people who feel vulnerable to disease and believe that dietary change might lead to positive results are more likely to pay attention to information about links among dietary choices, dietary fat, and health risks. A desire to lose weight or alter one's physical appearance also can be a powerful force shaping decisions to accept or reject particular foods. Furthermore, consumers are placing a higher priority on foods for health and seeking foods with more protein, less sugar, and minimal processing.[16]

How nutrition information is delivered to consumers may also play a role in food choices. One study that compared the type of nutrition information provided, education levels, and obesity predominance in three different countries (France, Canada, and the United States) supported the idea that a "scientific" or nutrient-based approach to food might not result in the most beneficial food choices, indicating that in these instances consumers lose sight of the big picture. It has been suggested that nutrition education that focuses on overall results, or how current nutrition decisions will effect overall health, may lead to better overall food choices.[17]

> **Key Concepts** Many factors influence our decisions about what to eat and when to eat. Some of the main factors include personal preferences such as taste, texture, and smell; our habits with eating; the emotional connections of comfort or discomfort that are linked to certain foods; advertisements and promotions; whether we choose to eat our meals at home or away from home; and knowledge of health and nutrition. The cultural environment in which people live also has a major influence on what foods they choose to eat.

Environment

Your environment—where you live, how you live, whom you live with—has a lot to do with what you choose to eat. People around us influence our food choices, and we generally prefer the foods we grew up eating. Environmental factors that influence our food choices include economics, food availability, culture, and religion. In the United States, our environment and the choices we make play a significant role in the current obesity epidemic. We live in what has been termed an **obesogenic environment**; in other words, an environment that promotes gaining weight and one that is not conducive to weight loss within the home or workplace.[18]

▶ **obesogenic environment** Circumstances in which a person lives, works, and plays in a way that promotes the overconsumption of calories and discourages physical activity and calorie expenditure.

Economics

Where you live not only influences which foods are most accessible to you, but also affects food costs, which are a major determinant of food choice. You may have "lobster taste" but a "hot dog budget." The types of foods purchased and the percentage of income used for food are affected by total income. Households spend more money on food when incomes rise. In 2014, middle income families spent an average of $5,992 on food, representing about 13 percent of income, whereas the lowest income households spent an average of $3,667 on food, representing 34 percent of income.[19] Rising food prices and falling incomes put pressure on food budgets. How much does it cost to follow dietary recommendations? For adults on a 2,000-calorie diet, the cost of meeting the *2015–2020 Dietary Guidelines for Americans* recommendations for fruit and vegetable consumption is $2.00 to $2.50 per day, according to an analysis by the U.S. Department of Agriculture (USDA).[20]

Food Availability

Poor access to healthy, nutritious foods can negatively affect food choices, and therefore health and well-being. Approximately 23.5 million Americans, including 6.5 million children, live in nutritional wastelands commonly referred to as **food deserts**.[21] Food deserts are low-income areas where residents lack access to a supermarket or large grocery store to buy affordable fruits, vegetables, whole grains, low-fat milk, and other foods that make up the full range of a healthy diet.[22]

Not only do many people who live in food deserts lack the ability to get fresh, healthy, and affordable foods easily, but they often rely on "quick markets" that offer a lot of highly processed, high-sugar, and high-fat foods. Their communities often lack healthy food providers, such as grocery stores and farmers' markets. In these neighborhoods, food needs typically are served by inexpensive restaurants and convenience stores, which offer few fresh foods.

Cultural Influences

One of the strongest influences on food preferences is tradition or cultural background. In all societies, no matter how simple or complex, eating is the primary way of initiating and maintaining human relationships.

To a large extent, culture defines our attitudes. "One man's food is another man's poison." Look at **FIGURE 1.7**. How does the photo make you feel? Insects, maggots, and entrails are delicacies to some, whereas just the thought of ingesting them is enough to make others cringe. Cultural forces are so powerful that if you were permitted only a single question to establish someone's food preferences, a good choice would be "What is your ethnic background?" (See the FYI feature "Food and Culture.")

Knowledge, beliefs, customs, and habits all are defining elements of human culture. Although genetic characteristics tie people of ethnic groups together, culture is a learned behavior and, consequently, can be modified through education, experience, and social and political trends.[24]

In many cultures, food has symbolic meanings related to family traditions, social status, and even health. In fact, many folk remedies rely on food. Some of these have gained wide acceptance, such as the use of spices and herbal teas for purposes ranging from allaying anxiety to preventing cancer and heart disease. Just as cultural distinctions eventually blur when ethnic groups take part in the larger American culture, so do many of the unique expectations about the ability of certain foods to prevent disease, restore health among those with various afflictions, or enhance longevity. However, food habits may be among the last practices to change when an immigrant adapts to a new culture.

Religion

Food is an important part of religious rites, symbols, and customs. Some religious rules apply to everyday eating, whereas others are concerned with special celebrations. Christianity, Judaism, Hinduism, Buddhism, and Islam, for example, all have distinct dietary laws, but within each religion different interpretations of these laws give rise to variations in dietary practices.

Social-Ecological Model

The social-ecological model included in the *2015–2020 Dietary Guidelines for Americans* is designed to illustrate how individual factors, environmental settings, various sectors of influence, and social and

▶ **food deserts** Low income areas where it is difficult to purchase food that is fresh, of good-quality, and affordable.

Quick **Bite**

Bad Food Habits Are Hard to Break

Bad habits like eating while watching TV, eating in the car, skipping breakfast, or eating too quickly are easy to develop and hard to break. But being aware of your behavior can help you take some steps toward positive change. For example, if you are guilty of eating too quickly, slow down, relax, chew your food, and enjoy the taste of what you are eating. It takes about 20 minutes for your stomach to tell your brain that it is full. If you wait to stop eating until you actually feel full, you have already overeaten!

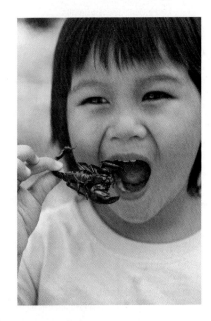

FIGURE 1.7 Cultural influences. If you were visiting China, would you sample the local delicacy—deep-fried scorpion?
© DK. Khattiya/Alamy Images.

Quick **Bite**

Nerve Poison for Dinner?

The puffer fish is a delicacy in Japan. Danger is part of its appeal; eating a puffer fish can be life threatening! The puffer fish contains a poison called tetrodotoxin (TTX), which blocks the transmission of nerve signals and can lead to death. Chefs who prepare the puffer fish must have special training and licenses to prepare the fish properly, so diners feel nothing more than a slight numbing feeling.

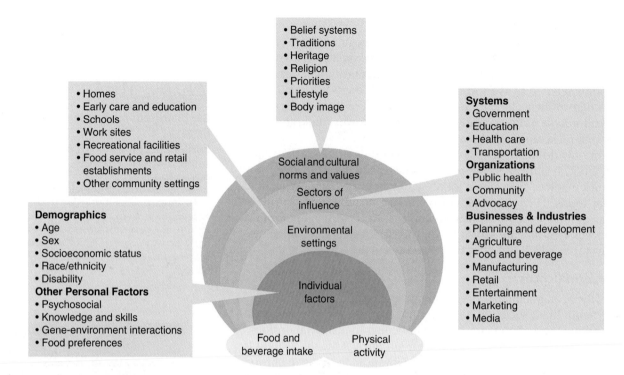

FIGURE 1.8 A social-ecological model. A framework for nutrition and physical activity decisions.

Modified from: (1) Centers for Disease Control and Prevention. Division of Nutrition, Physical Activity, and Obesity. *State Nutrition, Physical Activity and Obesity (NPAO) Program: Technical Assistance Manual.* January 2008, page 36. Accessed April 21, 2010. http://www.cdc.gov/obesity/ downloads/TA_Manual_1_31_08.pdf. (2) Institute of Medicine. *Preventing Childhood Obesity: Health in the Balance.* Washington (DC): The National Academies Press; 2005, page 85. (3) Story M, Kaphingst KM, Robinson-O'Brien R, Glanz K. Creating healthy food and eating environments: Policy and environmental approaches. *Annu Rev Public Health* 2008;29:253-272.

Quick Bite

Does Being Overweight Spread from Person to Person?

The spread of obesity in social networks appears to be a factor in the obesity epidemic. Likewise, this also suggests that it may be possible that peers can have the same effect in the opposite direction, slowing the spread of obesity.

cultural elements of society overlap to form the food and physical activity choices for an individual.[25] The social-ecological model illustrates that implementing multiple changes at various levels is an effective way to improve eating and physical activity behavior. (See **FIGURE 1.8**.)

Key Concepts The cultural environments in which people grow up have a major influence on what foods they prefer, what foods they consider edible, and what foods they eat in combination and at what time of day. Many factors work to define a group's culture: environment, economics, access to food, lifestyle, traditions, and religious beliefs. As people from other cultures immigrate to new lands, they will adopt new behaviors consistent with their new homes. However, food habits are among the last to change. The social-ecological model can be used to help us understand how layers of influence converge to influence a person's food and physical activity choices.

The Standard American Diet

What is a typical *American diet*? As a country influenced by the practices of so many cultures, religions, backgrounds, and lifestyles, there is no easy or single answer to this question. The U.S. diet is as diverse as Americans themselves, even though many people around the world imagine that the American diet consists mainly of hamburgers, french fries, and cola drinks. Our fondness for fast food and the marketability of such restaurants overseas make them seem like icons of American culture—and many of the stereotypes are true.

So, how healthful is the "American" diet? The average American falls short of the USDA's MyPlate recommendations for vegetables, dairy, and fruit. **TABLE 1.1** shows average U.S. consumption compared to the MyPlate recommendations.

For individuals age 2 years and older, the estimated average total intakes of the following foods are all well below the *Dietary Guidelines for Americans*: fruit intake is 1.03 cups, with 33 percent consumed as fruit juice; vegetable intake is 1.47 cups, of which 22 percent is potatoes and 20 percent is tomatoes; whole grains consumption is less than 1 ounce; average dairy intake is 1.8 cups, of which 44 percent is cheese and 51 percent is fluid milk; average solid fat intake is 37 grams, oil is 25 grams, and sugar intake is estimated to be 18.4 teaspoon equivalents. (See **TABLE 1.2**.) Americans are not eating enough nutrient-dense foods and eating too much of the foods known to be harmful. Together, solid fats and added sugars contribute nearly 800 calories per day while providing minimal important nutrients.[26] Soda, sugar-sweetened beverages, and grain-based desserts are the major sources of added sugars for many Americans. Regular cheese, grain-based desserts, and pizza are the top contributors of solid and saturated fat in the American diet. In addition, Americans of all age groups are eating more than the recommended amounts of sodium, mainly in the form of processed foods.[27]

Although good health and nutrition information can be found in multiple publications and at a variety of venues, this doesn't necessarily translate into better food choices. People are not natural nutritionists, and they generally don't know instinctively which foods to choose for good health. So, it is not surprising when national surveys indicate that although Americans know that nutrition and food choices are important factors in health, few have made the recommended changes, such as eating less fat, sugar, and salt, and eating more fruits and vegetables.

You are in a position to gather more information than the average consumer. By taking this course in nutrition, you will be getting the full story: the nutrients we need for good health, the science behind the health messages, and the food choices it will take to implement them. Whether you use this information is up to you, but at least you will be a well-informed consumer.

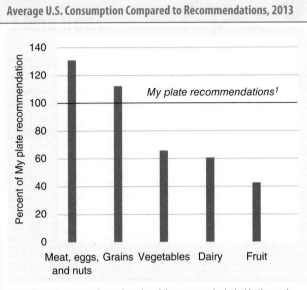

TABLE 1.1
Average U.S. Consumption Compared to Recommendations, 2013

Note: Rice data were discontinued and thus are not included in the grains group.
[1]Based on a 2,000-calorie diet.
Reproduced from USDA, Economic Research Service, Loss-adjusted Food Availability Data.

Reproduced from USDA, Economic Research Service, Loss-Adjusted Food Availability Data.

TABLE 1.2
Estimated Average Intake Compared to the *Dietary Guidelines for Americans*, 2015–2020

	Estimated Average Intake	**Recommended Intake**
Fruit	1.03 cups	2 cups per day
Vegetables	1.47 cups	2 ½ cups per day
Whole grains	< 1 ounce per day	> 3 ounces per day
Dairy	1.8 cups	3 cups per day
Solid fat intake	37 grams	Limit solid fat intake
Sugar	18.4 teaspoon equivalents	< 10% of calories per day

Data from Bowman S, Clemens J, Friday J, Moshfegh A. Food Patterns Equivalents Intakes from Food: Mean Amounts Consumer per Individual, What We Eat in America, NHANES 2011-12; Tables 1-4. http://www.ars.usda.gov/research/publications/publications.htm?seq_no_115=312662.

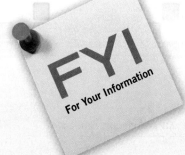

Food and Culture

Do you ever wonder why people choose prickly pears over apples or pomegranates over blueberries? For the most part, food choices are a result of what people are accustomed to or what they have learned. Dietary habits are as diverse as individuals, and culture plays a key role in the food choices people make. Cultural influences often determine what roles various foods play in dietary habits, health beliefs, and everyday behaviors. Beliefs and traditions may be modified by geography, economics, or experiences, but core values and customs typically remain similar within a specific group.[a-b] However, as cultural diversity becomes more common among populations, regional food favorites become less foreign.

Food plays a major role in most religions and religious customs. Religious beliefs usually are learned early and can define certain dietary habits. For example, Jewish dietary laws specify that foods must be *kosher*. To be kosher, meat must come from animals that chew their cud, have split hooves, and are free from blemishes to their internal organs. Fish must have fins and scales. Pork, crustaceans and shellfish, and birds of prey are not kosher. Kosher laws prohibit eating meat and milk at the same meal or even preparing or serving them with the same dishes and utensils. Islam identifies acceptable foods as *halal* and has rules similar to those of Judaism for the slaughtering of animals. Islam prohibits the consumption of pork, the flesh of clawed animals, alcohol, and other intoxicating drugs. The Church of Jesus Christ of Latter Day Saints disapproves of coffee, tea, and alcoholic beverages. Most Hindus are vegetarians and do not eat eggs, and some avoid onions and garlic. The Orthodox Jain religion in India forbids eating meat or animal products (e.g., milk, eggs) and any root vegetables (e.g., potatoes, carrots, garlic). In Buddhism, mind-altering substances or intoxicating beverages are prohibited, but dietary habits vary considerably based on the sect and geographic location.[c] Some Buddhists follow strict forms of vegetarianism whereas others do not. In Christianity and many other religions, food plays a key role in religious ceremonies and various religious holidays, from what foods may or may not be eaten (e.g., no meat on Fridays during Lent) to when foods can be consumed (e.g., only from sundown to sunrise during Islam's Ramadan). Food plays an important role not only in physical survival, but also in many people's spiritualism.

Many cultures have traditional medical practices based on the belief that nature is composed of two opposing forces. In traditional Chinese medicine, for example, these forces, called *yin* and *yang*, must be in proper balance for good health.[d] It is believed that excesses in either direction cause illness. The illness must then be treated by eating foods of the opposite force. This idea of balance or harmony, accompanied by terms describing illness and foods as either cold (e.g., banana, fish, juices) or hot (e.g., beef, nuts, ginger) or yin or yang, also is found in other Asian countries, including India and the Philippines, and in Latin American cultures and ethnicities.

Numerous cultures view a variety of foods as having medicinal properties. Treatments commonly include assorted herbs, herbal teas, and special foods. From generation to generation, knowledge of such remedies is passed on. Remarkably, various cultures all over the world use remedies based on similar common substances, such as chamomile, garlic, and honey. These familiar substances often are more trusted and are considered safer than modern medicines. In addition to traditions and culture, the complete array of herbs and foods used daily and also as medicines is based on the geographic region, growing conditions, and climate.

The interplay of diet and culture helps to define a person's values, preferences, and practices. As a result, even in the face of changing world events and populations, neither is abandoned easily or quickly. Just as there is diversity in individuals and families, there is also diversity within cultures. One must be alert to avoid the assumption that all people of a specific culture eat, believe, or follow traditions in the exact same manner. Even so, the question arises: What impact will our increasing mobility and globalization have on food choice? Undoubtedly, cultural interactions and exposure to various cuisines will increase. Will this expand our appreciation and preservation of cultural culinary practices and result in the formation of new hybrid cuisines?

a   Food Culture and Tradition. Food, people and culture resources. http://www.food-links.com. Accessed August 12, 2017.
b   Ethnomed. Cultures. http://ethnomed.org/culture. Accessed August 12, 2017.
c   HerbMed. Top 20 herbs. http://www.herbmed.org/#param.wapp?sw_page=top20. Accessed August 12, 2017.
d   China Highlights. Chinese medicinal cuisine/food therapy—healthy seasonal recipes. http://www.chinahighlights.com/travelguide/chinese-food/medicinal-cuisine.htm. Accessed August 12, 2017.

Key Concepts "American" cuisine is truly a melting pot of cultural contributions to foods and tastes. Although Americans receive and believe many messages about the role of diet in good health, these beliefs do not always translate into better food choices. The typical American diet contains too much sodium, solid fat, saturated fat, and sugar and not enough fruits, vegetables, low-fat dairy, and whole-grain foods.

Introducing the Nutrients

Why Is This Important? The body is made up of millions of cells that grow and change every day. Nutrients from foods that we eat provide the building blocks to replace cells when they die. Nutrients also provide the energy necessary to all body functions. Therefore, knowing about nutrients helps us understand their role in keeping us alive and healthy.

Although we give food meaning through our culture and experience and make dietary decisions based on many factors, ultimately the reason for eating is to obtain nourishment—nutrition.

Food is a mixture of chemicals called **nutrients**. You need nutrients for normal growth and development, for maintaining cells and tissues, for fuel to perform physical and metabolic work, and for regulating the hundreds of thousands of body processes that go on inside of you every second of every day. Some nutrients either exist in the body or the body can synthesize them. Examples of these nutrient are the amino acids alanine, arginine, asparagine, and others. These nutrients are referred to as **nonessential nutrients** because it is not necessary to obtain these nutrients from foods that we eat. On the other hand, there are nutrients that the body cannot synthesize, or cannot make enough of, and that must be provided through foods that we eat. These nutrients are termed **essential nutrients**. There are six classes of essential nutrients: carbohydrates, lipids (fats and oils), proteins, vitamins, minerals, and water. (See **FIGURE 1.9**.) The minimum diet for human growth, development, and maintenance must supply about 45 essential nutrients. Although termed nonessential and essential, all nutrients are required by the body for supporting daily processes and to maintain health. Adequate amounts of both nonessential and essential nutrients are necessary for optimal health.

Definition of Nutrients

In studying nutrition, we focus on the functions of nutrients in the body so that we can see why they are important in the diet. However, to define a nutrient in technical terms, we focus on what happens in its absence. A nutrient is a chemical whose absence from the diet for a long enough time results in a specific change in health; we say that a person has a deficiency of that nutrient. A lack of vitamin C, for example, can eventually lead to scurvy. A diet with too little iron will result in iron-deficiency anemia. To complete the definition of a nutrient, it also must be true that putting the essential chemical back in the diet will reverse the change in health, if done before permanent damage occurs. If taken early enough, supplements of vitamin A can reverse the effects of deficiency on the eyes. If not, prolonged vitamin A deficiency can cause permanent blindness.

THINK About It 3

Nutrients are not the only chemicals in food. Other substances add flavor and color, some contribute to texture, and others like caffeine have physiological effects on the body. **Phytochemicals** are compounds in plants that are believed to provide health benefits beyond those provided by traditional nutrients. **Zoochemicals** are the animal equivalent of phytochemicals in plants; that is, they are found in animal tissues that we consume. Although not nutrients, nor considered essential in the diet, phyto- and zoochemicals have important health benefits. For instance, research suggests that phytochemicals in fruit and vegetables provide **antioxidant** activity, which may reduce risk for heart disease or cancer.[29]

The six classes of nutrients serve three general functions: They provide energy, regulate body processes, and contribute to body structures (see **FIGURE 1.10**). Although virtually all nutrients can be said to regulate

▶ **nutrients** Any substances in food that the body can use to obtain energy, synthesize tissues, or regulate functions.

▶ **nonessential nutrients** Those nutrients that can be made by the body.

▶ **essential nutrients** Substances that must be obtained in the diet because the body either cannot make them or cannot make adequate amounts of them.

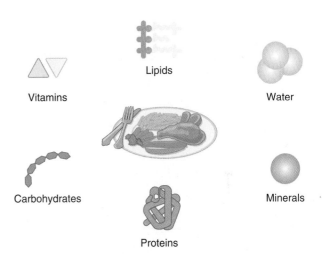

FIGURE 1.9 The six classes of nutrients. Water is the most important nutrient, and we cannot survive long without it. Because our bodies need large quantities of carbohydrate, protein, and fat, they are called macronutrients. Our bodies need comparatively small amounts of vitamins and minerals, so they are called micronutrients.

▶ **phytochemicals** Substances in plants that may possess health-protective effects, even though they are not essential for life.

▶ **zoochemicals** The animal equivalent of phytochemicals in plants that are believed to provide health benefits beyond the traditional nutrients that foods contain.

▶ **antioxidant** A substance that combines with or otherwise neutralizes a free radical, thus preventing oxidative damage to cells and tissues.

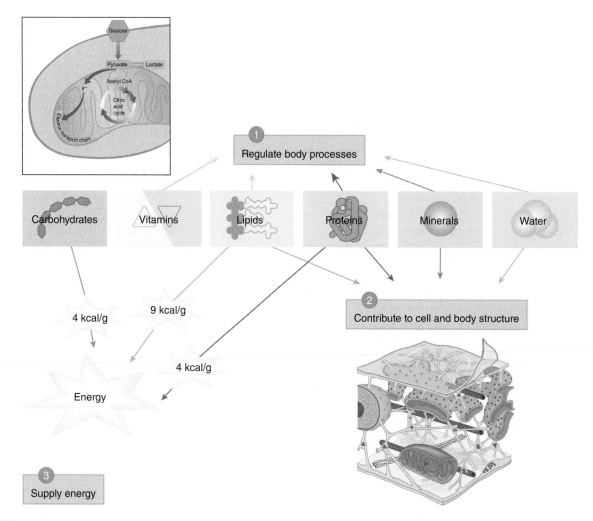

FIGURE 1.10 Nutrients have three general functions in your body. (1) Micronutrients, some lipids and proteins, and water help regulate body processes such as blood pressure, energy production, and temperature. (2) Lipids, proteins, minerals, and water help provide structure to bone, muscle, and other cells. (3) Macronutrients supply energy to power muscle contractions and cellular functions.

▶ **macronutrients** Nutrients, such as carbohydrate, fat, or protein, that are needed in relatively large amounts in the diet.

▶ **micronutrients** Nutrients, such as vitamins and minerals, that are needed in relatively small amounts in the diet.

▶ **organic** In chemistry, any compound that contains carbon, except carbon oxides (e.g., carbon dioxide) and sulfides and metal carbonates (e.g., potassium carbonate). The term *organic* also is used to denote crops that are grown without synthetic fertilizers or chemicals.

▶ **inorganic** Any substance that does not contain carbon, excepting certain simple carbon compounds such as carbon dioxide and carbon monoxide. Common examples include table salt (sodium chloride) and baking soda (sodium bicarbonate).

body processes, and many contribute to body structures, only proteins, carbohydrates, and fats are sources of energy.

Because the body needs large quantities of carbohydrates, proteins, and fats, they are called **macronutrients**; vitamins and minerals are called **micronutrients** because the body needs comparatively small amounts of these nutrients. Even though micronutrients are needed in far smaller amounts than macronutrients, a healthy diet must supply both in adequate amounts.

In addition to their functions, there are several other key differences among the classes of nutrients. First, the chemical composition of nutrients varies widely. One way to divide the nutrient groups is based on whether the compounds contain the element carbon. Substances that contain carbon are **organic** substances; those that do not are **inorganic**. Carbohydrates, lipids, proteins, and vitamins are all organic; minerals and water are not. Structurally, nutrients can be very simple—minerals such as sodium are single elements, although we often consume them as larger compounds (e.g., sodium chloride, which is table salt). Water also is very simple in structure. The organic nutrients have more complex structures—the carbohydrates, lipids, and proteins we eat are made of smaller building blocks whereas the vitamins are elaborately structured compounds.

It is rare for a food to contain just one nutrient. Meat is not just protein and bread is not solely carbohydrate. Foods contain mixtures of nutrients, although in most cases protein, fat, or carbohydrate dominates. So although bread is certainly rich in carbohydrates, it also contains some protein, a little fat, and many vitamins and minerals. If it's whole-grain bread you're eating, you also get fiber, which is not technically a nutrient, but is an important compound for good health nonetheless.

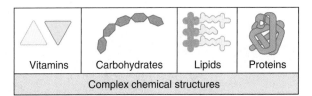

Vitamins	Carbohydrates	Lipids	Proteins
Complex chemical structures			

Organic – contains carbon

Minerals	Water
Simple chemical structures	

Inorganic – no carbon

Key Concepts Nutrients are the essential chemicals in food that the body needs for normal functioning and good health and that must come from the diet because they either cannot be made in the body or cannot be made in sufficient quantities. Six classes of nutrients—carbohydrates, proteins, lipids, vitamins, minerals, and water—can be described by their composition or by their function in the body.

Carbohydrates

If you think of water when you hear the word *hydrate*, then the word *carbohydrate*—or literally "hydrate of carbon"—tells you exactly what this nutrient is made of. **Carbohydrates** are made of carbon, hydrogen, and oxygen and are a major source of fuel for the body. Dietary carbohydrates are the starches and sugars found in grains, vegetables, **legumes** (dry beans and peas), and fruits. We also get carbohydrates from dairy products and from fiber, a type of carbohydrate made up of long chains of sugars that cannot be broken down by human digestive enzymes. Although fiber doesn't fit the classical definition of a nutrient, it plays important roles in the body, especially in improving digestive function. Your body converts most nonfiber dietary carbohydrates to glucose, a simple sugar compound that provides a source of energy for cells and tissues. **Circulation** moves glucose and other substances through the vessels of the cardiovascular or lymphatic system. Carbohydrates provide approximately 4 calories per gram.

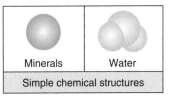

Whenever you see this icon, we'll be talking about **carbohydrates.**

Provide:
Energy (4 kcal/g)

© Photodisc

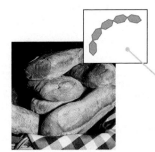

Whenever you see one of these three icons, we'll be talking about **lipids.**

Provide:
Energy (9 kcal/g)
Structure
Regulation
(hormones)

© Photodisc

Lipids

The term **lipids** refers to substances we know as fats and oils but also to fatlike substances in foods, such as cholesterol and phospholipids. Lipids are organic compounds and, like carbohydrates, contain carbon, hydrogen, and oxygen. Fats and oils—or, more correctly, **triglycerides**—are another major fuel source for the body. In addition, triglycerides, cholesterol, and phospholipids have other important functions: providing structure for body cells, carrying the fat-soluble vitamins (A, D, E, and K), and providing the starting material (cholesterol) for making many **hormones**. Dietary sources of lipids include the fats and oils we cook with or add to foods, the naturally occurring fats in meats and dairy products, and less obvious plant sources, such as coconut, olives, and avocado. Lipids provide approximately 9 calories per gram.

▶ **carbohydrates** Compounds, including sugars, starches, and dietary fibers, that usually have the general chemical formula $(CH_2O)_n$, where n represents the number of CH_2O units in the molecule. Carbohydrates are a major source of energy for body functions.

▶ **legumes** A family of plants with edible seed pods, such as peas, beans, lentils, and soybeans. Also called *pulses*.

▶ **circulation** Movement of substances through the vessels of the cardiovascular or lymphatic system.

▶ **lipids** A group of fat-soluble compounds that includes triglycerides, sterols, and phospholipids.

▶ **triglycerides** Fats composed of three fatty acid chains linked to a glycerol molecule.

▶ **hormones** Chemical messengers that are secreted into the blood by one tissue and act on cells in another part of the body.

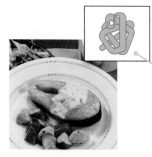

Whenever you see this icon, we'll be talking about **proteins**.

Provide:
Energy (4 kcal/g)
Structure
Regulation

© Photodisc.

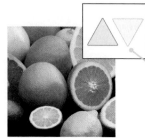

Whenever you see these icons, we'll be talking about **vitamins**.

Provide:
Regulation

© Photodisc.

▶ **proteins**   Large, complex compounds consisting of many amino acids connected in varying sequences and forming unique shapes.

▶ **amino acids**   Compounds that function as the building blocks of protein.

▶ **vitamins**   Organic compounds necessary for reproduction, growth, and maintenance of the body. Vitamins are required in miniscule amounts.

▶ **minerals**   Inorganic compounds needed for growth and for regulation of body processes.

▶ **macrominerals**   Major minerals required in the diet and present in the body in large amounts compared with trace minerals.

▶ **microminerals**   See *trace minerals*.

▶ **trace minerals**   Those minerals present in the body and required in the diet in relatively small amounts compared with major minerals. Also known as *microminerals*.

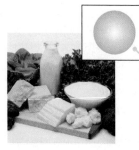

Whenever you see this icon, we'll be talking about **minerals**.

Provide:
Regulation
Structure

© Photodisc.

Proteins

Proteins are organic compounds made of smaller building blocks called **amino acids**. Unlike carbohydrates and lipids, amino acids contain nitrogen as well as carbon, hydrogen, and oxygen. Proteins are found in a variety of foods. Meats and dairy products are concentrated sources of protein. Grains, legumes, and vegetables are also sources of protein, whereas fruits contribute negligible amounts. The amino acids that we get from dairy protein combine with the amino acids made in the body to make hundreds of different body proteins. Proteins are the main structural material in the body. They are also important components in blood, cell membranes, enzymes, and immune factors. Proteins regulate body processes and can also be used for energy. They provide approximately 4 calories per gram.

Vitamins

Vitamins are organic compounds that contain carbon and hydrogen and perhaps nitrogen, oxygen, phosphorus, sulfur, or other elements. The main function of vitamins is to help regulate many body processes such as energy production, blood clotting, and calcium balance. Vitamins help to keep organs and tissues functioning and healthy. Because vitamins have such diverse functions, a lack of a particular vitamin can have widespread effects. Although the body does not break down vitamins to yield energy, vitamins have vital roles in the extraction of energy from carbohydrate, fat, and protein.

Each of the 13 vitamins belong to one of two groups: fat-soluble or water-soluble. The four fat-soluble vitamins—A, D, E, and K—have very diverse roles. What they have in common is the way they are absorbed and transported in the body and the fact that they are more likely to be stored in larger quantities than the water-soluble vitamins. The water-soluble vitamins include vitamin C and eight B vitamins: thiamin, riboflavin, niacin, pyridoxine (B_6), cobalamin (B_{12}), folate, pantothenic acid, and biotin. Most of the B vitamins are involved in some way with the pathways for energy metabolism.

Vitamins are found in a wide variety of foods, not just fruits and vegetables—although these are important sources—but also meats, grains, legumes, dairy products, and even fats. Choosing a well-balanced diet usually makes vitamin supplements unnecessary. In fact, when taken in large doses, vitamin supplements (especially those containing vitamins A, D, B_6, or niacin) can be harmful.

Minerals

Structurally, **minerals** are simple, inorganic substances. Minerals are important for keeping your body healthy, and your body uses minerals for many different functions. There are two kinds of minerals: macrominerals and trace minerals. **Macrominerals** are minerals your body needs in relatively large amounts compared to other minerals; these include calcium, phosphorus, magnesium, sodium, potassium, chloride, and sulfur. The body needs the remaining minerals only in very small amounts. These **microminerals**, or **trace minerals**, include iron, zinc, copper, manganese, molybdenum, selenium, iodine, and fluoride. As with vitamins, the functions of minerals are diverse. Minerals can be found in structural roles (e.g., calcium, phosphorus, and fluoride in bones and teeth) as well as regulatory roles (e.g., control of fluid balance, regulation of muscle contraction).

Food sources of minerals are just as diverse as mineral functions. Although we often associate minerals with animal foods, such as meats and milk, plant foods are important sources as well. Deficiencies of minerals—with the exception of iron, calcium, iodine (in patients with cystic fibrosis or pregnancy), and selenium—are generally uncommon. A balanced diet provides enough minerals for most people. However, individuals with iron-deficiency anemia may need iron supplements, and others may need calcium supplements if they cannot or will not drink milk or eat dairy products. As is true for vitamins, excessive intake of some minerals as supplements can be toxic.

Water

Water is the most essential nutrient. We can survive far longer without any of the other nutrients in the diet, indeed without food at all, than we can without water. Like minerals, water is inorganic. Water has many roles in the body, including temperature control, lubrication of joints, and transportation of nutrients and wastes.

Because your body is nearly 60 percent water, regular fluid intake to maintain adequate hydration is important. Water is found not only in beverages, but also in most food products. Fruits and vegetables in particular are high in water content. Through many chemical reactions, the body makes some of its own water, but this is only a fraction of the amount needed for normal function.

Whenever you see this icon, we'll be talking about **water**.

Provides:
Regulation
Structure

© Nancy R. Choen/Photodisc/Getty Images.

> **Key Concepts**   The body needs larger amounts of carbohydrates, lipids, and proteins (macronutrients) than vitamins and minerals (micronutrients). Carbohydrates, lipids, and proteins provide energy; proteins, vitamins, minerals, water, and some fatty acids regulate body processes; and proteins, lipids, minerals, and water contribute to body structure.

Nutrients and Energy

One major reason we eat food, and the nutrients it contains, is for **energy**. Every cellular reaction, every muscle movement, and every nerve impulse requires energy. Three of the nutrient classes—carbohydrates, lipids (triglycerides only), and proteins—are energy sources. Although not considered a nutrient, another energy source is alcohol. When we speak of the energy in foods, we are really talking about the *potential* energy that foods contain.

Different scientific disciplines use different measures of energy. In nutrition, we discuss the potential energy in food, or the body's use of energy, in units of heat called **kilocalories** (1,000 calories). One kilocalorie (or kcal) is the amount of energy (heat) it would take to raise the temperature of 1 kilogram (kg) of water by 1 degree Celsius. For now, this may be an abstract concept, but, as you learn more about nutrition, you will discover how much energy you likely need to fuel your daily activities. You also will learn about the amounts of potential energy in various foods. You'll find that food labels, diet books, and other sources of nutrition information generally use the term **calorie** rather than *kilocalorie*. Technically, the potential energy in foods is best measured in kilocalories; however, the term *calorie* has become familiar and commonplace. Throughout the text we will use the terms *calorie* and *kilocalorie (kcal)* to mean generally the same thing.

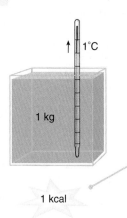

1°C

1 kg

1 kcal is the amount of energy that will raise the temperature of 1 kg of water by 1° Celsius

1 kcal

▶ **energy**   The capacity to do work. The energy in food is chemical energy, which the body converts to mechanical, electrical, or heat energy.

▶ **kilocalories (kcal) [KILL-oh-kal-oh-rees]**   Units used to measure food energy (1,000 calories = 1 kilocalorie).

▶ **calorie**   The general term for energy in food and used synonymously with the term *energy*. Often used instead of kilocalorie on food labels, in diet books, and in other sources of nutrition information.

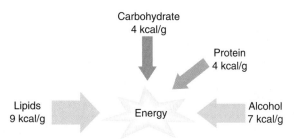

FIGURE 1.11 Energy sources. Carbohydrate, fat, protein, and alcohol provide different amounts of energy per gram.

Energy in Foods

Energy is available from foods because foods contain carbohydrate, fat, and protein. These nutrients can be broken down completely (metabolized) to yield energy in a form that cells can use. When completely metabolized in the body, carbohydrate and protein yield 4 kilocalories of energy for every gram (g) consumed; fat yields 9 kilocalories per gram; and alcohol contributes 7 kilocalories per gram. (See **FIGURE 1.11**.) Therefore, the energy available from a given food or from a total diet is determined by the amount of each of these substances consumed. Because fat is a concentrated source of energy, adding or removing fat from the diet can have a big effect on available energy.

How Can We Calculate the Energy Available from Foods?

To calculate the energy available from food, multiply the number of grams of fat, carbohydrate, and protein by 9, 4, and 4, respectively; then add the results.

Here is an example:

One bagel with cream cheese contains 39 grams of carbohydrate, 10 grams of protein, and 16 grams of fat; thus, we can determine the available energy from each component.

39 g carbohydrate × 4 kcal/g	=	156 kcal
10 g protein × 4 kcal/g	=	40 kcal
16 g fat × 9 kcal/g	=	144 kcal
Total	=	340 kcal

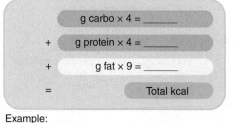

CALCULATING THE ENERGY
AVAILABLE FROM FOODS

g carbo × 4 = _____

+   g protein × 4 = _____

+   g fat × 9 = _____

=   Total kcal

Example:
275 g carbohydrate × 4 kcal/g = 1,100 kcal
75 g protein × 4 kcal/g = 300 kcal
67 g fat × 9 kcal/g = 600 kcal (rounded
from 603 kcal)

Printing Office, December 2010.   Total = 2,000 kcal

Be Food Smart: Calculate the Percentages of Calories in Food

To calculate the *percentage* of calories that carbohydrate, protein, and fat each contributes to the total, divide the amount of kcal from each nutrient by the total amount of kcal and then multiply by 100.

For example, to determine the percentage of calories from fat in the bagel with cream cheese example:

% of energy as carbohydrates	=	156 kcal/340 kcal	=	0.459 × 100	=	46% kcal from carbohydrate
% of energy from protein	=	40 kcal/340 kcal	=	0.118 × 100	=	12% kcal from protein
% of energy from fat	=	144 kcal/340 kcal	=	0.423 × 100	=	42% kcal from fat

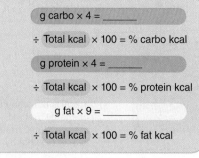

CALCULATING THE PERCENTAGE OF
KILOCALORIES FROM NUTRIENTS

g carbo × 4 = _____

÷ Total kcal × 100 = % carbo kcal

g protein × 4 = _____

÷ Total kcal × 100 = % protein kcal

g fat × 9 = _____

÷ Total kcal × 100 = % fat kcal

Example:
275 g carbohydrate × 4 = 1,100 kcal
1,100 kcal ÷ 2,000 kcal × 100 = 55% carbo kcal

75 g protein × 4 = 300 kcal
300 kcal ÷ 2,000 kcal × 100 = 15% protein kcal

67 g fat × 9 = 600 kcal (rounded
from 603 kcal)
600 kcal ÷ 2,000 kcal × 100 = 30% fat kcal

Current health recommendations suggest limiting fat intake to about 20 to 35 percent of *total* energy intake. You can monitor this for yourself in two ways. If you like counting fat grams, you can first determine your suggested maximum fat intake. For example, if you need to eat 2,000 kilocalories each day to maintain your current weight, at most 35 percent of those calories can come from fat:

2,000 kcal × 0.35	=	700 kcal from fat
700 kcal from fat ÷ 9 kcal/g	=	77.8 g of fat

Therefore, your maximum fat intake should be about 78 grams. You can check food labels to see how many fat grams you typically eat.

Another way to monitor your fat intake is to know the percentage of calories that come from fat in various foods. If the proportion of fat in each food choice throughout the day exceeds 35 percent of calories, then the day's total of fat will be too high as well. Some foods contain virtually no fat calories (e.g., fruits, vegetables) whereas others are nearly 100 percent fat calories (e.g., margarine, salad dressing). Being aware that a snack like the bagel with cream cheese provides 42 percent of its calories from fat can help you select lower-fat foods at other times of the day.

Diet and Health

What does it mean to be healthy? The World Health Organization (WHO) defines health as "a state of complete physical, mental, and social well-being and not merely the absence of disease or infirmity."[28] Although we often focus on the last part of that definition, "the absence of disease or infirmity," the first part is equally important. As you have learned, nutrition is an important part of physical, mental, and social well-being. It also is important for preventing disease.

Disease can be defined as "an impairment of the normal state of the living animal or plant body or one of its parts that interrupts or modifies the performance of the vital functions"[29] and can arise from environmental factors or specific infectious agents, such as bacteria or viruses. Diseases can be *acute* (short-lived illnesses that arise and resolve quickly) or *chronic* (diseases with a slow onset and long duration). Although nutrition can affect our susceptibility to acute diseases—and contaminated food is certainly a source of acute disease—our food choices are more likely to affect our risk for developing chronic diseases such as heart disease or cancer. Other lifestyle factors, such as smoking and exercise, in addition to genetic factors, also may determine who gets sick and who remains healthy. The 10 leading causes of death are listed in **TABLE 1.3**. Nutrition plays a role in the prevention or treatment of more than half of the conditions listed. Heart disease and cancer, together, account for almost half of all deaths.[30]

The foods we choose do more than provide us with an adequate diet. The balance of energy sources can affect our risk of chronic disease. For example, high-fat diets have been linked to heart disease and cancer. Excess calories contribute to obesity, which also increases disease risk. Other nutrients, such as the minerals sodium, chloride, calcium, and magnesium, affect blood pressure whereas a lack of the vitamin folate prior to conception and in early pregnancy can cause serious birth defects. Nonnutrient components in the diet (e.g., phytochemicals) may have antioxidant or immune-enhancing properties that also can keep us healthy. The choices we make can reduce our disease risk, as well as provide energy and essential nutrients.

Physical Activity

A sedentary lifestyle is a significant risk factor for chronic disease. Physically active people generally outlive those who are inactive, and, as a risk factor for heart disease, inactivity can be almost as significant as high blood pressure, smoking, or high blood cholesterol. Physical activity also plays a significant role in long-term weight management. Current physical activity guidelines recommend that children and adolescents do 60 minutes or more of physical activity each day. Children should be encouraged to participate in activities that are age-appropriate, are enjoyable, and offer variety. Aerobic activity should make up most of a child's activity time, but muscle strengthening, such as gymnastics or doing push-ups, and bone strengthening, such as jumping rope or

▶ **disease** A particular quality, habit, or disposition regarded as adversely affecting a person or group of people.

TABLE 1.3
Leading Causes of Death: United States

Rank	Cause of Death
1	Heart disease[a]
2	Cancer[a]
3	Chronic lower respiratory diseases
4	Accidents (unintentional injuries)
5	Stroke
6	Alzheimer's disease
7	Diabetes mellitus[a]
8	Influenza and pneumonia
9	Kidney disease[a]
10	Intentional self-harm (suicide)

[a] Causes for which nutrition is thought to be important in the prevention or treatment of the condition.

Reproduced from Centers for Disease Control and Prevention. National Center for Health Statistics. Leading Causes of Death. Data from 2015. https://www.cdc.gov/nchs/fastats/leading-causes-of-death.htm. Accessed August 18, 2017.

running, count as well. For adults, the Centers for Disease Control and Prevention set the recommendations to be measured as a weekly total, with the understanding that one can reach the suggested weekly time goals by breaking up exercise time into shorter increments of time. Recommendations for adults include 150 minutes of moderate-intensity aerobic activity every week and muscle-strengthening activity on 2 or more days a week, or 75 minutes of vigorous-intensity aerobic activity every week and muscle-strengthening activities on 2 or more days a week.[31]

> **Key Concepts** All cells and tissues need energy to keep the body functioning. Energy in foods and in the body is measured in kilocalories. The carbohydrates, lipids, and proteins in food are potential sources of energy, meaning that the body can extract energy from them. Excess energy intake is a contributing factor to obesity, a major public health issue. All individuals should aim to be physically active.

Applying the Scientific Process to Nutrition

🍎 **Why Should I Know This?** Good nutrition research follows a specific process, which is important to understand in order to determine the validity of studies conducted.

Whether it's identifying essential nutrients, establishing recommended intake levels, or exploring the effects of vitamins on cancer risk, scientific studies are the cornerstone of nutrition. Although we may use creative, artistic talents to choose and serve a pleasing array of healthful foods, the fundamentals of nutrition are developed through the scientific process of observation and inquiry.

The scientific process enables researchers to test the validity of a **hypothesis** that arises from observations of natural phenomena. A hypothesis is a supposition or proposed explanation made on the basis of limited evidence as a starting point for further investigation. For example, it was common knowledge in the eighteenth century that sailors on long voyages would likely develop scurvy (which we now know results from a deficiency of vitamin C). Scurvy had been recognized since ancient times, and its common symptoms—pinpoint skin hemorrhages, swollen and bleeding gums, joint pain, fatigue and lethargy, and psychological changes such as depression and hysteria—were well known. Native populations discovered plant foods that would cure this illness; among Native Americans these included cranberries in the Northeast and many tree extracts in other parts of the country. From observations such as these, that certain plant foods would cure scurvy, come questions that lead to hypotheses, or "educated guesses," about factors that might be responsible for the observed phenomenon. Scientists then test hypotheses using appropriate research designs. Poorly designed research can produce useless results or false conclusions.

By following the steps of the scientific process (**FIGURE 1.12**), researchers can minimize influences that may arise during a research study (such as bias, prejudice, or coincidence). The scientific process (also referred to as the scientific method) follows these general steps: (1) make observations, ask questions, or describe phenomena; (2) formulate a hypothesis to explain the observation, question, or phenomena; (3) test the hypothesis by conducting an experiment; (4) analyze data and draw conclusions; and (5) communicate results indicating whether the hypothesis is accepted or not.

▶ **hypothesis** A supposition or proposed explanation made on the basis of limited evidence as a starting point for further investigation.

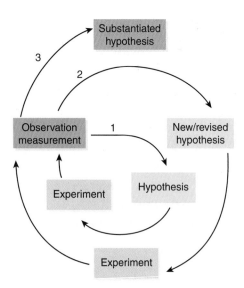

FIGURE 1.12 The scientific process. The scientific process follows these general steps: (1) make observations; (2) formulate a hypothesis; (3) test the hypothesis; (4) analyze data; and (5) communicate results.

TABLE 1.4
Common Study Designs Used in Nutrition Research

Human Studies
Epidemiological studies compare disease rates among population groups and attempt to identify related conditions or behaviors such as diet and smoking habits. Epidemiological studies can provide useful information about relationships but often do not clarify cause and effect. The results of these studies show **correlations**—relationships between two or more factors; however, they do not establish nor address cause and effect. Epidemiological studies can provide important clues that lead to animal and human studies that can further clarify diet and disease relationships.

Case Control Studies
Case control studies are small-scale epidemiological studies in which individuals who have a condition (e.g., breast cancer) are compared with similar individuals who do not have the condition. Researchers then identify factors other than the disease in question that differ between the two groups. These factors provide researchers with clues about the cause, progression, and prevention of the disease.

Clinical Trials
Clinical trials, also called **intervention studies**, are controlled studies where some type of intervention (e.g., a nutrient supplement, a controlled diet, or an exercise program) is used to determine its impact on certain health parameters. These studies include an **experimental group** (people who experience the intervention) and a **control group** (similar people who are not treated). Scientists measure aspects of health or disease in each group and compare the results.

Animal Studies
Animal studies can provide preliminary data that lead to human studies or can be used to study hypotheses that cannot be tested on humans. Although animal studies give scientists important information that furthers nutrition knowledge, the results of animal studies cannot be extrapolated directly to humans. Animal studies need to be followed with cell culture studies and ultimately human clinical studies to determine specific effects in humans.

Cell Culture Studies
Another way to study nutrition is to isolate specific types of cells and grow them in the laboratory. Scientists then can use these cells to study the effects of nutrients or other components on metabolic processes in the cell. An important area of nutrition research, called **nutrigenomics**, explores the effect of specific nutrients and other chemical compounds on gene expression. This area of molecular biology will help us explain individual differences in chronic disease risk factors and may lead to designing diets based on an individual's genetic profile.

▶ **correlations** Connections co-occurring more frequently than can be explained by chance or coincidence but without a proven cause.

▶ **case control studies** Investigations that use a group of people with a particular condition rather than a randomly selected population. These cases are compared with a control group of people who do not have the condition.

▶ **clinical trials** Studies that collect large amounts of data to evaluate the effectiveness of a treatment.

▶ **intervention studies** See *clinical trials*.

▶ **experimental group** A set of people being studied to evaluate the effect of an event, substance, or technique.

▶ **control group** A set of people used as a standard of comparison to the experimental group. The people in the control group have characteristics similar to those in the experimental group and are selected at random.

▶ **nutrigenomics** The study of how nutrition interacts with specific genes to influence a person's health.

Nutrition research is exciting. Scientists ask questions to be answered and define problems to be solved. Investigators choose a study design that will best answer their research question or hypothesis. Throughout the research process, researchers must follow ethical procedures in all areas of the study design. Common study designs used in nutrition research are defined in **TABLE 1.4**.

James Lind's experiments with sailors aboard the *Salisbury* in 1747 are considered to be the first dietary clinical trial. (See **FIGURE 1.13**.) His observation that oranges and lemons were the only dietary elements that seemed to cure scurvy was an important finding. However, it took more than 40 years before the British Navy began routinely giving all sailors citrus juice or fruit, such as lemons or limes—a practice that led to the nickname "limeys" when referring to British sailors. It took nearly 200 years (until the 1930s) for scientists to isolate the compound we call vitamin C and show that it had antiscurvy activity. The chemical name for vitamin C, ascorbic acid, comes from its role as an antiscorbutic (antiscurvy) compound.

Modern clinical trials include several important elements: random assignment to groups, use of placebos, and the double-blind method. Subjects are assigned randomly—as by the flip of a coin—to the experimental group or the control group. Randomization potentially reduces,

1. **Observation**
   Sailors on long voyages all became ill with scurvy.
2. **Hypothesis**
   Lack of certain foods causes scurvy.
3. **Experimentation**
   Experiment to test hypothesis.
   Predicts that some dietary element will cure scurvy.

Key

Controlled variables
Experimental variables
Results
Conclusions

James Lind: A Treatise of the Scurvy in Three Parts. Containing an inquiry into the Nature, Causes and Cure of that Disease, together with a Critical and Chronological View of what has been published on the subject. A. Millar, London, 1753.

On the 20th May, 1747, I took twelve patients in the scurvy on board the Salisbury at sea. Their cases were as similar as I could have them. They all in general had putrid gums, the spots and lassitude, with weakness of their knees. They lay together in one place, being a proper apartment for the sick in the fore-hold; and had one diet in common to all, viz., water gruel sweetened with sugar in the morning; fresh mutton broth often times for dinner; at other times puddings, boiled biscuit with sugar ect.; and for supper barley, raisins, rice and currants, sago and wine, or the like. Two of these were ordered each, a quart of cyder a day. Two others took twenty five gutts of elixir vitriol three times a day upon an empty stomach, using a gargle strongly acidulated with it for their mouths. Two others took two spoonfuls of vinegar three times a day upon an empty stomach, having their gruels and their other food well acidulated with it, as also the gargle for the mouth.

The consequence was that the most sudden and visible good effects were perceived from the use of the oranges and lemons; one of those who had taken them being at the end of six days fit four duty. The spots were not indeed at that time quite off his body, nor his gums sound; but without any other medicine than a gargarism or, elixir of vitriol he became quite healthy before we came into Plymouth, which was on the 16th June. The other was the best recovered of any in his condition, and being now deemed pretty well was appointed nurse to the rest of the sick...

As I shall have occasion elsewhere to take notice of the effects of other medicines in this disease, I shall here only observe that the result of all my experiments was that oranges and lemons were the most effectual remedies for this distemper at sea. I am apt to think oranges preferable to lemons...

4. **Publication**
   Publication subjects the findings to peer review by fellow scientists.
5. **More experiments**
   Further experiments replicate the findings and extend knowledge.
6. **Theory**
   Scientists consolidate acquired knowledge into a theory that explains the observed phenomenon.

FIGURE 1.13 The first clinical trial. In 1758, physician James Lind reported the careful process of his clinical trial among British sailors afflicted with scurvy.

▶ **placebo** An inactive substance that is outwardly indistinguishable from the active substance whose effects are being studied.

minimizes, or eliminates selection and volunteer bias. People in the experimental group receive the treatment or specific protocol (e.g., consuming a certain nutrient at a specific level). People in the control group do not receive the treatment but usually receive a placebo. A **placebo** is an imitation treatment (such as a sugar pill) that looks the same as the experimental treatment but has no effect. The placebo also is important for reducing bias because subjects do not know if they are receiving the intervention and are less inclined to alter their responses or reported symptoms based on what they think should happen. The *expectation* that a medication will be effective can be nearly as effective as the medication itself—a phenomenon called the **placebo effect**. Because the placebo effect can exert a powerful influence, research studies must take it into account.

When the members of neither the experimental nor the control group know what treatment they are receiving, we say the subjects are "blinded" to the treatment. If a clinical trial is designed so neither the subjects nor the researchers collecting data are aware of the subjects' group assignments (experimental or control), the study is called a **double-blind study**. This reduces the possibility that researchers will see the results they want to see even if these results do not occur. In this case, another member of the research team holds the code for subject assignments and does not participate in the data collection. Double-blind, placebo-controlled clinical trials are considered the "gold standard" of nutrition studies. These studies can show clear cause-and-effect relationships but often require large numbers of subjects and are expensive and time consuming to conduct.

> **placebo effect** A physical or emotional change that is not due to properties of an administered substance. The change reflects participants' expectations.

> **double-blind study** A research study set up so that neither the subjects nor the investigators know which study group is receiving the placebo and which is receiving the active substance.

Quick Bite

Controlling the Pesky Placebo

When researchers tested the effectiveness of a medication in reducing binge eating among people with bulimia, they used a double-blind, placebo-controlled study to eliminate the placebo effect. After a baseline number of binge-eating episodes was determined, 22 women with bulimia were given the medication or a placebo. After a period of time, the number of binge-eating episodes was reassessed. The group taking the medication had a 78 percent reduction in binge-eating episodes. Sounds good, right? But, the placebo group had a similar reduction of 70 percent. The placebo effect was nearly as powerful as the medication.

Key Concepts The scientific method is used to expand our nutrition knowledge. Hypotheses are formed from observations and are then tested by experiments. Epidemiological studies observe patterns in populations. Animal and cell culture studies can test the effects of various treatments. For human studies, randomized, double-blind, placebo-controlled clinical trials are the best research tools for determining cause-and-effect relationships.

From Research Study to Headline

🍎 **Why Should I Know This?** Media headlines are written to grab your interest, but they can often be misleading. Having the tools to identify which headlines and stories are generated from sound nutrition research can go a long way in helping you assess nutrition information in the media.

How can you evaluate the nutrition and health headlines you see online or on television, or hear about from friends or family? Consumers often are confused by what they see as the "wishy-washiness" of scientists—for example, coffee is good, then coffee is bad. Margarine is better than butter. . . . No wait, maybe butter is better after all. These contradictions, despite the confusion they cause, show us that nutrition is truly a science: dynamic, changing, and growing with each new finding. Let's take a look at what happens (or what *should* happen) before nutrition information becomes news.

Publishing Experimental Results

Once an experiment is complete, scientists publish the results in a scientific journal to communicate new information to other people who work in that field of study. Generally, before articles are published in scientific journals, other scientists who have expert knowledge of the subject critically review them. This **peer review** greatly reduces the chance that low-quality research is published. Examples of peer-reviewed journals are the *American Journal of Clinical Nutrition* and the *Journal of the Academy of Nutrition and Dietetics*.

> **peer review** An appraisal of research against accepted standards by professionals in the field.

SCIENTISTS DISPUTE CLAIMS OF GINKGO BILOBA EFFECTIVENESS

Researchers Link Caffeine and Cancer

Some Say Ginkgo Biloba Improves Memory

Cancer and Vitamin E Link Disputed

Vitamin E Reduces Risk of Cancer

Practice Paper: Academy of Nutrition and Dietetics

Communicating Accurate Food and Nutrition Information

Consumers are increasingly interested in food and nutrition information, and the channels for receiving information are expanding at a fast pace. In this paper, the Academy of Nutrition and Dietetics shows registered dietitian nutritionists (RDNs) how to reach diverse audiences with credible nutrition messages by providing guidelines. RDNs must actively take steps to position themselves as reliable sources of science-based food and nutrition information and communicate through a variety of new media and traditional channels. RDNs are uniquely qualified to evaluate and interpret nutrition research and appropriately translate the findings into positive and practical food and diet advice for the public.

Reprinted from *Journal of the Academy of Nutrition and Dietetics*, 112(5), Diane Quagliani and Mindy Hermann, Practice Paper of the Academy of Nutrition and Dietetics Abstract: Communicating Accurate Food and Nutrition Information, Page no. 759, 2012, with permission from Elsevier.

From Journals to the Public

Let's examine the process by which the results of primary nutrition research reach most of us. There are usual several steps involved. Typically, secondary sources of information (e.g., scientific magazines such as *Discover* or *Scientific American*) will gather information from the primary-source journal article. This information is further translated into articles in general magazines (e.g., *Time*) and newspapers. Finally, mass-media outlets—such as various websites, nightly news broadcasts, and tabloids—will present the information. By this last step in the chain of information, the original research may have become a 30-second sound bite or a "click bait" headline that fails to reflect the caveats or limitations of the original study. In some cases, the study may be distorted, with its results misstated or overstated. (See **FIGURE 1.14**.)

Sorting Facts and Fallacies in the Media

Even when it has no basis in fact, a claim can seem credible if heard often enough. For example, do you believe that sugar makes kids hyperactive? There is no scientific evidence to support this claim. Although news stories may be based on reports in the scientific literature, the media may distort the facts through omission of details. The results of studies on certain hot topics, such as weight loss and which foods contribute to hyperactivity in children, are frequently taken out of context and presented as nutrition advice that may be ineffective or even harmful.

Evaluating Information on the Internet

Using the Internet has made life easier in many ways. You can buy a car, check stock prices, search out sources for a paper you're writing, chat with like-minded people, and stay up-to-date on news or sports scores. Hundreds of websites are devoted to nutrition and health topics. How do you evaluate the quality of information obtained online? Can you trust what you read?

First, it's important to remember that there are no rules for posting information online. Although the Health on the Net Foundation has set up a Code of Conduct for medical and health websites, following its eight principles is completely voluntary.[32]

Second, consider the source—if you can tell what it is. Many websites do not specify where the content came from, who is responsible for it, or how often it is updated. If the site lists the authors, what are their credentials? Who sponsors the site? Educational institutions (.edu), government agencies (.gov), and organizations (.org) generally have more credibility than commercial (.com) sites, where selling rather than educating may be the primary motive. Identifying the purpose for a site can give you more clues about the validity of its content.

Third, when you see claims for nutrients, dietary supplements, or other products and the results of studies or other information, keep in mind the scientific method and the basics of sound science. Who did the study? What type of study was it? How many subjects were included? Was it a double-blind study? Were the results published in a peer-reviewed journal? Think critically about the content, look at other sources, and ask questions of experts before you accept information as truth. What is true of books, magazines, and newspapers also applies to the Internet: Just because it is in print or online doesn't mean it's true.

As scientific information is made accessible to more and more people, less detail is provided and more opinion and sensationalism are introduced.

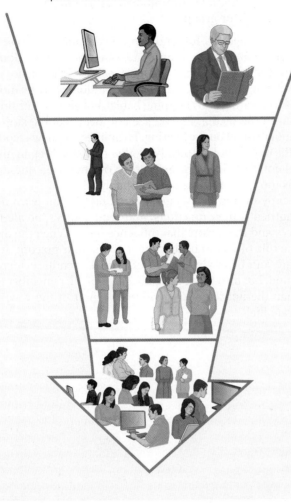

Primary sources: Professional journals in print and on the Internet

Secondary sources: Scientific magazines with articles based on primary source material written by specialists

Science writing: Generalist magazines and newspapers' science pages; articles written by science writers

Mass media: Nightly news bites; "instant books;" unattributed Internet sites

FIGURE 1.14 Sifting facts and fallacies. From original research to the evening news, each step along the way introduces biases as information is summarized and restated. Whether on television, radio, or the Internet, or in print, the best consumer information cites sources for reported facts.

THINK About It 4 Finally, be on the lookout for "junk science"—sloppy methods, interpretations, and claims that lead to public misinformation. The Food and Nutrition Science Alliance (FANSA) is a coalition of several health organizations, including the Academy of Nutrition and Dietetics. FANSA has developed the "10 Red Flags of Junk Science" to help consumers identify potential misinformation. Use these red flags to evaluate websites.

The 10 Red Flags of Junk Science[33]

1. Recommendations that promise a quick fix
2. Dire warnings of danger from a single product or regimen
3. Claims that sound too good to be true
4. Simplistic conclusions drawn from a complex study
5. Recommendations based on a single study
6. Statements refuted by reputable scientific organizations
7. Lists of "good" and "bad" foods

Practice Paper: Academy of Nutrition and Dietetics

Social Media and the Dietetics Practitioner: Opportunities, Challenges, and Best Practices

The potential role of social media in the profession of dietetics is far reaching, yet there are important guidelines to follow related to ethics and professionalism. When using social media, nutrition and dietetics practitioners must remember that they are governed by the same Code of Ethics that guides all other aspects of practice. The use of digital technologies can help practitioners connect with colleagues, promote public health, advocate for a cause, and advance their own careers. Social media policies, education, and peer-to-peer mentoring can help maximize the potential of social media, while maintaining ethical standards and professionalism.

Data from Academy of Nutrition and Dietetics. *Practice Paper: Social Media and the Dietetics Practitioner: Opportunities, Challenges and Best Practices.* 2016;116(11):1825-1835.

8. Recommendations made to help sell a product
9. Recommendations based on studies that are not peer reviewed
10. Recommendations from studies that ignore differences among individuals or groups

Use the Internet; it's fun and can be educational. However, treat claims as "guilty until proven innocent"—in other words, don't accept what you read at face value until you have evaluated the science behind it.

As you learn about nutrition, you will undoubtedly be more aware not only of your eating and shopping habits, but also of nutrition-related information in the media. As you see and hear reports, stop to think carefully about what you are hearing. Headlines and news reports often overstate the findings of a study. Two other things to keep in mind: One study does not provide all the answers to our nutrition questions; and if it sounds too good to be true, it probably is!

Your study of nutrition is just beginning. As you learn about the essential nutrients, their functions, and food sources, be alert to your food choices and the factors that influence them. When the discussion turns to the role of diet in health, think about your preconceived ideas and evaluate your beliefs in the light of current scientific evidence. Keep an open mind, but also think critically. Most of all, remember that food is more than the nutrients it provides; it is part of the way we enjoy and celebrate life!

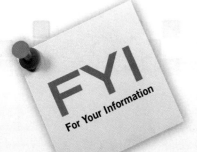

The Affordable Care Act and Nutrition

The Affordable Care Act (ACA), also known as Obamacare, was signed into law on March 23, 2010. By 2014, much of the new policy had been implemented. Here is a brief summary of healthcare coverage, costs, and care provided by the law.[a]

Coverage

- *Ends preexisting condition exclusions:* Health plans can no longer deny or limit benefits due to a preexisting condition.
- *Keeps young adults covered:* If you are under 26, you may be eligible to be covered under your parents' health plan.
- *Ends arbitrary withdrawals of insurance coverage:* Insurers can no longer cancel your coverage just because you made an honest mistake.
- *Guarantees the right to appeal:* You now have the right to ask that your plan reconsider its denial of payment.

Costs

- *Ends lifetime limits on coverage:* There are no longer limits on the amount paid out for most benefits over a lifetime.
- *Reviews premium increases:* Insurance companies must now publicly justify any unreasonable rate hikes.
- *Helps you get the most from your premium dollars:* The majority of your premium dollars (amount charged for your plan) must be spent primarily on health care—not administrative costs.

Care

- *Covers preventive care at no cost to you:* You may be eligible for recommended preventive health services with no copayment.
- *Protects your choice of doctors:* From your plan's network, you can choose the primary care doctor you want.
- *Removes insurance company barriers to emergency services:* You can seek emergency care at a hospital outside of your health plan's network.[b]

Benefits to College Students

Before the ACA, what was health insurance like for college students? Most colleges required students to either purchase health insurance or continue enrollment in their parents' plans. As previously mentioned, under the ACA students are now able to stay on their parents' health insurance plans until age 26—even if they are married or have coverage through employers.

Since 2014, college students, like other sectors of the population, have had to abide by the "individual mandate" in the ACA, which requires most people to obtain insurance or pay tax penalties. That's where the "exchanges" come in for students who aren't on their parents' plans and don't want to purchase insurance through their schools: Each state provides health insurance exchanges for qualified Americans to purchase affordable coverage. Each state also has its own exchange that offers a variety of coverage options from private, state-regulated insurance companies—often cheaper than other options. However, the National Center for Public Policy calculated that a college student's penalty for nonenrollment ($325 or 2% of income in 2015) could be cheaper in the short term (if they didn't get sick) than paying for health insurance. Alternatively, students who can't afford insurance may qualify for Medicaid if their income is below a certain threshold. To see whether you're eligible, check with your state department of health insurance.

Another option for those under 30 is to purchase a "catastrophic" health plan. These plans usually feature low monthly premiums, but the insured are required to pay all their medical costs up to a certain amount, usually several thousand dollars. The insurance company pays for essential health benefits over that amount, essentially providing participants with protection in the event of serious accidents or illnesses.

Finally, individuals with nonimmigrant status, including people on worker visas and student visas, can qualify for insurance coverage through the exchanges.[c]

Healthcare Reform, Preventive Care, and Nutrition

The ACA emphasizes prevention through wellness plans, outreach campaigns, and more opportunities to see registered dietitian nutritionists. The law supports counseling and behavioral interventions in the areas of obesity, breastfeeding, chronic diseases, blood pressure, and cholesterol. It requires most plans to cover calcium and vitamin D testing for women over 60 at risk for osteoporosis, anemia screening for most pregnant women, folic acid pills, and type 2 diabetes screening for adults with high blood pressure.

The ACA also requires proper nutrition labeling in chain restaurants and vending machines, which informs consumers about calories so that they will be aware of the recommended daily caloric intake and its effect on obesity. Should the consumer request it, the following information must be available on menus or display items: total calories, calories from fat, total fat, saturated fat, cholesterol, trans fat, sodium, total carbohydrates, sugars, dietary fiber, and protein.[d,e]

References

a U.S. Department of Health and Human Services, Health Resources and Services Administration, Maternal and Child Health. The Affordable Care Act (ACA) and the nutrition workforce: a summary report. http://www.mchb.hrsa.gov/training/pgm-hi-nutri.asp. Accessed August 13, 2017.

b Healthcare.gov. Accessed August 13, 2017.

c *Christian Science Monitor.* Obamacare 101: what to know if you opt out of buying health insurance. http://www.csmonitor.com/USA/DC-Decoder/2013/1001/Obamacare-101-What-to-know-if-you-opt-out-of-buying-health-insurance. Accessed August 13, 2015.

d Obamacare Facts. Summary of provisions in the Patient Protection and Affordable Care Act. http://obamacarefacts.com/summary-of-provisions-patient-protection-and-affordable-care-act. Accessed August 13, 2017.

e U.S. Department of Health & Human Services. About the Affordable Care Act. https://www.hhs.gov/healthcare/about-the-aca/index.html. Accessed September 11, 2017.

Learning Portfolio

Key Terms

	page
amino acids	16
antioxidant	13
calorie	17
carbohydrates	15
case control studies	21
circulation	15
clinical trials	21
control group	21
correlations	21
disease	19
double-blind study	23
energy	17
essential nutrients	13
experimental group	21
flavor	5
food deserts	9
hormones	15
hypothesis	20
inorganic	14
intervention studies	21
kilocalories (kcal) [KILL-oh-kal-oh-rees]	17
legumes	15
lipids	15
macrominerals	16
macronutrients	14
microminerals	16
micronutrients	14
minerals	16
neophobia	4
nonessential nutrients	13
nutrients	13
nutrigenomics	21
nutrition	3
obesogenic environment	8
organic	14
peer review	23
phytochemicals	13
placebo	22
placebo effect	23
proteins	16
trace minerals	16
triglycerides	15
umami [ooh-MA-mee]	5
vitamins	16
zoochemicals	13

Study Points

- Most people make food choices for reasons other than nutrient value.

- Taste and texture are the two most important factors that influence food choices.

- In all cultures, eating is the primary way of maintaining social relationships.

- Although most North Americans know about healthful food choices, their eating habits do not always reflect this knowledge.

- Food is a mixture of chemicals. Essential chemicals in food are called nutrients.

- Carbohydrates, lipids, proteins, vitamins, minerals, and water are the six classes of nutrients found in food.

- Nutrients have three general functions in the body: They serve as energy sources, structural components, and regulators of metabolic processes.

- Vitamins regulate body processes such as energy metabolism, blood clotting, and calcium balance.

- Minerals contribute to body structures and to regulating processes such as fluid balance.

- Water is the most important nutrient in the body. We can survive much longer without the other nutrients than we can without water.

- Energy in foods and the body is measured in kilocalories. Carbohydrates, fats, and proteins are sources of energy.

- Carbohydrate and protein have a potential energy value of 4 kilocalories per gram, and fat provides 9 kilocalories per gram.

- Scientific studies are the cornerstone of nutrition. The scientific method uses observation and inquiry to test hypotheses.

- Double-blind, placebo-controlled clinical trials are considered the "gold standard" of nutrition studies.

- Research designs used to test hypotheses include epidemiological, animal, cell culture, and human studies.

- Information in the public media is not always an accurate or complete representation of the current state of the science on a particular topic.

Study Questions

1. Name three sensory aspects of food that influence our food choices.

2. How do our health beliefs affect our food choices?

3. List and describe the main role of each class of nutrients in a healthy diet.

4. List the 13 vitamins.

5. What determines whether a mineral is a macromineral or a micro- (trace) mineral?

6. How many kilocalories are in 1 gram of carbohydrate, of protein, and of fat?

7. What is an epidemiological study?

8. What is the difference between an experimental and control group?

9. Describe how a placebo is used in research studies.

Try This

Try a New Cuisine Challenge

Expand your culinary taste buds and try a new cuisine. Go to the grocery store or a nearby restaurant and select a cuisine you are not very familiar with. If you go out to eat, take some friends along so you can order and share more than one dish. While you're there, don't be afraid to ask questions about the menu, so you can gain a better understanding of the foods, preparation techniques, spices, and even the cultural meaning attached to some of the dishes. If you select food from the grocery store, choose food or dishes that require you to do minimal preparation—maybe something from the frozen section. As you try the new food(s), think about your eating experience in terms of sensory properties. Are the smells, flavors, and textures different from what you are used to eating? Do you like the new foods you are trying, or do you think that after multiple exposures to the food you would learn to like it?

Food Label Puzzle

The purpose of this exercise is to put the individual pieces of the food label together to determine how many kilocalories are in a serving. Pick six foods that have complete food labels. On a separate sheet of paper, write down the value for grams of total carbohydrate, protein, and fat in one serving. Now, using information from this chapter, calculate the amount of calories per serving, using the macronutrient amounts. Check your answer against the package information. Remember that the term *calories* on a food label is really referring to kilocalories. If you need help, review this chapter and pay close attention to the section on the energy-yielding nutrients. How many kilocalories does each have per gram? You may find that the results of your calculations don't exactly match the numbers on the label. Within labeling guidelines, food manufacturers can round values.

Getting Personal

Why Are You Eating?

Choose one day this week to evaluate why you are eating. Using the table below, list all of the foods and drinks that you consume in a 24-hour period. Select a day where your schedule is fairly predictable and you are eating what is considered normal for you. Using factors that influence food choices as discussed in the

Time	Food or Drink	Amount	Why I Ate	Hunger and Fullness Rating: Before	Hunger and Fullness Rating: After

Learning Portfolio (continued)

section "Why Do We Eat the Way We Do?," identify why you consumed each food that you ate. Example reasons could be: you felt hungry; you wanted the flavor of a particular food that was available; it is a habit to eat at that particular time; or everyone else was eating right then. Keep in mind that there may be more than one reason for eating. Also, using the Hunger/Fullness scale below, rate how hungry you were before you started eating and rate how full you were after you finished eating.

Rating System to Determine How Hungry and How Full You Are Feeling

0 or 1: Empty feeling in your stomach; you feel grumpy and irritable.

2 or 3: Feeling very hungry; you want to eat just about any type of food.

4: Feeling some hunger pangs; particular foods are starting to sound good to you.

5: Neutral; you have no strong feelings of hunger or fullness.

6 or 7: Satisfied; you are content with your recent food choices and the amount of food that you have eaten.

8: Full; you feel like you may have overeaten just a bit.

9: Stuffed; you feel like you have overeaten.

10: Sick feeling in your stomach; you feel like you ate much more than you should have.

Upon completion of the exercise, ask yourself the following questions:

■ Was there one reason that you ate that appeared more often than any other? If so, what was that reason?

■ Are health and nutrition concerns ever a reason for your eating? If not, how can you make eating for health and nutrition concerns a priority?

■ Looking at your hunger and fullness ratings, are you eating when you are hungry and stopping when you are satisfied? What changes can you make to become a more mindful and healthy eater?

Adapted from Tribole E, Resch E. *Intuitive Eating: A Revolutionary Program That Works.* New York: St. Martin's Griffin; 2003.

References

1. National Institutes of Health, U.S. National Library of Medicine. Definitions of health terms: nutrition. https://medlineplus.gov/definitions/nutritiondefinitions.html. Accessed August 13, 2017.
2. Kittler PG, Sucher KP, Nelms M. *Food and Culture.* 6th ed. Belmont, CA: Wadsworth; 2011.
3. Mennella JA. Ontogeny of taste preferences: basic biology and implications for health. *Am J Clin Nutr.* 2014;99(3):704S-711S. Epub 2014 Jan 22.
4. Ibid.
5. Ibid.
6. Ibid.
7. Bachmanov AA, Bosak NP, Lin C, et al. Genetics of taste receptors. *Curr Pharm Des.* 2014;20(16):2669-2683.
8. U.S. Department of Health and Human Services. Questions and answers on monosodium glutamate (MSG). November 19, 2012. http://www.fda.gov/Food/IngredientsPackagingLabeling/FoodAdditivesIngredients/ucm328728.htm. Accessed August 13, 2017.
9. Federal Trade Commission. FTC releases follow-up study detailing promotional activities, expenditures, and nutritional profiles of food marketed to children and adolescents. December 2012. http://www.ftc.gov/news-events/press-releases/2012/12/ftc-releases-follow-study-detailing-promotional-activities. Accessed August 13, 2017.
10. Bacardi-Gascon M, Jimenez-Cruz A. TV food advertising geared to children in Latin-American countries and Hispanics in the USA: a review. *Nutr Hosp.* 2015;31(5):1928-1935.
11. Powell LM, Harris JL, Fox T. Food marketing expenditures aimed at youth: putting the numbers in context. *Am J Prev Med.* 2013;45(4):453-461.
12. Bruce AS, Pruitt SW, Ha OR, et al. The influence of televised food commercials on children's food choices: evidence from ventromedial prefrontal cortex activations. *J Pediatr.* 2016;177:27-32.
13. U.S. Department of Agriculture. Food prices and spending. http://www.ers.usda.gov/data-products/ag-and-food-statistics-charting-the-essentials/food-prices-and-spending.aspx#.UznDOyjPCLE. Accessed August 13, 2017.
14. U.S. Department of Agriculture. Food away from home. https://www.ers.usda.gov/topics/food-choices-health/food-consumption-demand/food-away-from-home.aspx. Accessed September 27, 2017.
15. Larson N, Story M. *Menu Labeling: Does Providing Nutrition Information at the Point of Purchase Affect Customer Behavior? A Research Synthesis.* Princeton, NJ: Robert Wood Johnson Foundation; 2009.
16. Layman DK. Eating patterns, diet quality and energy balance: a perspective about applications and future directions for the food industry. *Physiol Behav.* 2014;134:126-130.
17. Laulais L, Doyon M, Ruffeux B, Kaiser H. Consumer knowledge about dietary fats: another French paradox? *Br Food J.* 2012;114(1):108-120.
18. Lake A, Townshend T. Obesogenic environments: exploring the built and food environments. *J R Soc Promot Health.* 2006;126(6):262-267.
19. U.S. Department of Agriculture. Food prices and spending. https://www.ers.usda.gov/data-products/ag-and-food-statistics-charting-the-essentials/food-prices-and-spending.aspx. Accessed August 13, 2017.
20. Hayden S, Hyman J, Buzby JC, Frazão E, Carlson A. *How Much Do Fruits and Vegetables Cost?* Economic Information Bulletin No. (EIB-71). Washington, DC: USDA, Economic Research Service; 2011. https://www.ers.usda.gov/webdocs/publications/44518/7967_eib71.pdf?v=42192. Accessed April 1, 2014.
21. Economic Research Service. Food access research atlas. http://www.ers.usda.gov/data-products/food-access-research-atlas.aspx. Accessed August 13, 2017.

22. U.S. Department of Agriculture. Providing affordable, healthy food options in food deserts. March 7, 2016. https://nifa.usda.gov/announcement /providing-affordable-healthy-food-options-food-deserts. Accessed August 13, 2017.

23. Bryant CA, DeWalt KM, Courtney A, Schwartz J. *The Cultural Feast: An Introduction to Food and Society.* 2nd ed. Belmont, CA: Wadsworth; 2004.

24. U.S. Department of Agriculture, U.S. Department of Health and Human Services. *Dietary Guidelines for Americans, 2015–2020.* 8th ed. Washington, DC: U.S. Government Printing Office; December 2014.

25. Ibid.

26. Ibid.

27. U.S. Food and Drug Administration. Survey shows gains in food-label use, health/diet awareness. https://www.fda.gov/ForConsumers/ConsumerUp dates/ucm202611.htm. Accessed August 13, 2017.

28. World Health Organization. Health education. http://www.who.int /topics/health_education/en/. Accessed August 13, 2017.

29. Ross A, Caballero B, Cousins R, Tucker K, Ziegler T. *Modern Nutrition in Health and Disease.* 11th ed. Philadelphia: Lippincott Williams & Wilkins; 2014.

30. Centers for Disease Control and Prevention, National Centers for Health Statistics. Leading causes of death. https://www.cdc.gov/nchs/fastats /leading-causes-of-death.htm. Accessed August 13, 2017.

31. U.S. Department of Health and Human Services. *Physical Activity Guidelines for Americans*: chapter 4: active adults. http://www.health.gov /paguidelines/guidelines/chapter4.aspx. Accessed August 13, 2017.

32. Health on the Net Foundation. The HON Code of Conduct for medical and health websites (HONcode). http://www.hon.ch/HONcode/Conduct .html. Accessed August 13, 2017.

33. Position of the American Dietetic Association: food and nutrition misinformation. *J Am Diet Assoc.* 2006;106:601-607.

Chapter 2

Nutrition Guidelines: Tools for a Healthful Diet

Revised by Kimberley McMahon

THINK About It

1   Do you think that the food choices you make today will affect your future health?

2   How much variety do you have in your diet? Do you consider your diet healthy because you eat the same foods on most days?

3   Do you understand how nutrition and physical activity can help promote health and reduce the risk for major chronic diseases throughout life?

4   Think about your eating habits. What suggestions from *The 2015–2020 Dietary Guidelines for Americans* can you incorporate into your diet to make it more healthy?

CHAPTER Menu

- Linking Nutrients, Foods, and Health
- Dietary Guidelines
- Recommendations for Nutrient Intake: The DRIs
- Food Labels

LEARNING Objectives

1 Describe and discuss the nutrition concepts of adequacy, balance, calorie control, nutrient density, moderation, and variety.

2 List the key recommendations of the *2015–2020 Dietary Guidelines for Americans*.

3 Define the Dietary Reference Intake values: DRI, EAR, RDA, AI, and DV.

4 Identify five mandatory components of a food label.

5 List and describe four major factors in nutrition assessment of an individual.

So, you want to be healthier—maybe that's why you are taking this course! Although we know that the foods we choose to eat have a major impact on our health, we aren't always certain about what choices to make. Choosing the right foods isn't made any easier when we are bombarded by headlines and advertisements: Eat less fat! Get more fiber in your diet! Moderation is the key! Build strong bones with calcium!

For many Americans, nutrition is simply a lot of hearsay, or maybe the latest slogan coined from last week's news headlines. Conversations about nutrition start with "*They* say you should . . ." or "Now *they* think that . . ." Have you ever wondered who "they" are and why "they" are telling you what to eat or what not to eat?

It's no secret that a healthy population is a more productive population, so many of our nutrition guidelines come from the federal government's efforts to improve our overall health. Thus, the government is one "they." Undernutrition and overnutrition are examples of two nutrition problems that government policy has addressed.

Many important elements of nutrition policy focus on relieving **undernutrition** in some population groups. Let's look at some examples. To prevent widespread deficiencies, the government requires food manufacturers to add nutrients to certain foods: iodine to salt, vitamin D to milk, and thiamin, riboflavin, niacin, iron, and folic acid to enriched grains. Another example is the creation of dietary standards, such as the Dietary Reference Intakes, which make it easier to define adequate diets for large groups of people.

Overnutrition, or the excessive intake of food, especially in unbalanced proportions, has led to changes in public policy as well. Health researchers have discovered links between diet and obesity, high blood pressure, cancer, and heart disease. As a result, nutritionists suggest that individuals make informed food choices by reducing intake of excess calories, sodium, saturated fats, added sugar, refined grains, and trans fats, and at the same time, be physically active. Another aspect of nutrition policy is shaped by the public's desire to know what is in the food we eat. This need has led to increased nutrition information on food labels. Public education efforts have resulted in the development of teaching tools such as **MyPlate**.

▶ **undernutrition** Poor health resulting from depletion of nutrients caused by inadequate nutrient intake over time. It is now most often associated with poverty, alcoholism, and some types of eating disorders.

▶ **overnutrition** The long-term consumption of an excess of nutrients. The most common type of overnutrition in the United States results from the regular consumption of excess calories, fats, saturated fats, and cholesterol.

▶ **MyPlate** The current nutrition guide published by the United States Department of Agriculture, presented in the format of an easy-to-understand visual image intended to empower people with the information they need to make healthy food choices and create eating habits consistent with the *Dietary Guidelines for Americans, 2015–2020*.

New information about diet and health will continue to drive public policy. This chapter explores diet-planning tools, dietary guidelines, and current dietary standards, in addition to discussing how to evaluate nutritional health. As you study this chapter, think about how your diet compares to the current guidelines and standards.

Linking Nutrients, Foods, and Health

🍎 **Why Is This Important?** Your future health depends on today's lifestyle choices, including your food choices. Nutrition science identifies essential nutrients and the foods in which they are found. Understanding the link between nutrients and food, together with diet planning principles, will allow you to make the best food choices.

We know that what we eat affects our health. For example, eating foods with all of the essential nutrients prevents nutritional deficiencies such as scurvy (vitamin C deficiency) or pellagra (deficiency of the B vitamin niacin). In the United States, few people suffer nutritional deficiencies as a result of dietary inadequacies. More often, Americans suffer from chronic diseases such as heart disease, cancer, hypertension, and diabetes—all linked to overconsumption of particular nutrients and lifestyle choices.

THINK
About It
1

Living in a high-tech world, we expect immediate solutions to long-term problems. Wouldn't it be interesting if we could avoid the consequences of overeating by taking a pill or drinking a beverage? As you know, no magic food, nutrient, or drug exists. Instead, we have to rely on healthful foods, exercise, and lifestyle choices to reduce our risk of chronic disease—a task that challenges many Americans. Tools are available to help us select healthful foods to eat, such as the U.S. Department of Agriculture's MyPlate food guidance system. MyPlate relies on the core nutrition concepts of adequacy, balance, calorie (energy) control, nutrient density, moderation, and variety. These underlying concepts help to keep the focus of healthy eating on a total diet approach.[1] Let's look at how each concept can shape our eating patterns.

Adequacy

Having an adequate diet means that the foods you choose to eat provide all the essential nutrients, fiber, and energy in amounts sufficient to support growth and maintain health.[2] Many Americans consume more calories than they need without getting 100 percent of the recommended intakes for a number of nutrients. Take, for example, a meal of soda pop, two hard-shell beef tacos, and cinnamon breadsticks. Although this meal provides foods from different food groups, it is high in sugar and fat and low in many of the vitamins and minerals found in fruits and vegetables. Occasionally skipping fruits and vegetables at a meal does not create a vitamin or mineral deficiency; however, dietary habits that skimp on fruits and vegetables most of the time provide an overall inadequate diet. Most people could improve the adequacy of their diet by choosing meals and snacks that are high in vitamins and minerals but low to moderate in energy (calorie) content. Doing so offers important benefits: normal growth and development of children, health promotion for people of all ages, and reduction of risk for a number of chronic diseases that are major public health problems.[3]

Quick **Bite**

Early "Laws" of Health

Galen, a Greek physician, surgeon, and philosopher of the second century, and arguably the most accomplished of all medical researchers, expounded his "laws of health"—eat proper foods, drink the right beverages, exercise, breathe fresh air, get enough sleep, have a daily bowel movement, and control your emotions. Isn't it interesting that these core concepts are still recommended today?

Balance

A healthful diet requires a balance of a variety of foods (grains, vegetables, fruits, oil, milk, and meat and beans), energy sources (carbohydrate, protein, and fat), and other nutrients (vitamins and minerals). Your diet can also be balanced in a complementary way when the foods you choose to eat provide you with adequate nutrients. The trick is to consume enough, but not too much, from all the different food groups.

Calorie Control

For many years, research supported the idea that weight loss and subsequent weight maintenance rely on energy balance, which is the net difference between energy intake and energy expenditure.[4] Current research is challenging this simplistic mathematic equation of calories in vs. calories out and focusing more on diet composition, rather than just total calories. In this chapter, we focus on how to choose foods by learning how to get the most nutrients without wasting calories. This is a lesson on budgeting: You should demand value for your expenditures. Just as each of us has a monetary budget—a limited amount of money to spend on things such as food, rent, books, and transportation—in a sense we all have a calorie budget as well. Every time you eat, you are choosing to spend some of your calorie budget for that day. Those who spend their budget wisely tend to be healthier than those who do not. Let's put the concept of calorie control together with nutrient density to see how it works.

Nutrient Density

The concern that Americans' diets are becoming increasingly energy-rich but nutrient-poor has focused attention on the nutrient content of individual foods relative to the energy they provide.[5] Understanding nutrient density can help explain how overeating can nevertheless result in undernutrition, and it also can help people make informed food choices.

The **nutrient density** of food is the ratio of nutrient content to energy content; this measurement helps determine how "healthy" a food is. Nutrient-dense foods provide substantial amounts of vitamins and minerals and relatively few calories.[6] Foods that are energy-dense (low in nutrient density) supply calories but relatively small amounts of vitamins and minerals, or sometimes none at all.[7]

Consider a potato as an example. We can prepare a potato in many different ways. We can eat baked potatoes, mashed potatoes with toppings, or french fries. Depending on how it is cooked and what is added to it before we eat it, the nutrient density of a potato changes. The most nutrient-dense form of this potato would be a plain baked potato, which provides the most vitamins and minerals with relatively few calories. The least nutrient-dense version of this potato is french fries, because frying a food adds a lot more calories without adding more vitamins and minerals. In this case, the proportion of vitamins and minerals is low compared to the overall higher calorie content. French fries are not nutrient dense (See **FIGURE 2.1**).

Some foods with little or no added sugar or fat are high-nutrient-density food choices. For example, you might decide to eat an apple instead of a handful of caramel corn. Both provide about the same amount of calories. By choosing to eat the apple instead of the caramel

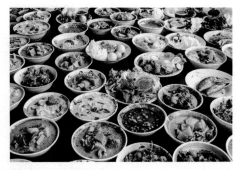

Aryut Tantisoontornchai/Shutterstock.

▶ **nutrient density** A description of the healthfulness of foods. Foods high in nutrient density are those that provide substantial amounts of vitamins and minerals and relatively few calories; foods low in nutrient density are those that supply calories but relatively small amounts of vitamins and minerals (or none at all).

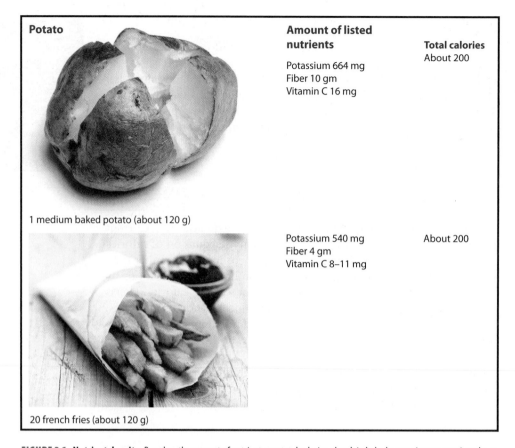

Potato	Amount of listed nutrients	Total calories
1 medium baked potato (about 120 g)	Potassium 664 mg Fiber 10 gm Vitamin C 16 mg	About 200
20 french fries (about 120 g)	Potassium 540 mg Fiber 4 gm Vitamin C 8–11 mg	About 200

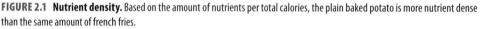

FIGURE 2.1 **Nutrient density.** Based on the amount of nutrients per total calories, the plain baked potato is more nutrient dense than the same amount of french fries.
Baked potato: © Joe Gough/Shutterstock; Fries and ketchup: © Elena Shashkina/Shutterstock.

corn, however, you are working toward meeting your daily nutrient needs while gaining more nutrients within the calories consumed, thereby selecting a more nutrient-dense and overall more healthy food choice.

Moderation

Not too much or too little—that's what moderation means. Moderation does not mean that you have to eliminate low-nutrient-density foods from your diet, such as soft drinks and candy, but rather that you can include them occasionally. Moderation entails not taking anything to extremes. You probably have heard that vitamin C has positive effects on your health, but that doesn't mean huge doses of this essential nutrient are appropriate for you. It's also important to remember that substances that are healthful in small amounts can sometimes be dangerous in large quantities. For example, the body needs zinc for hundreds of chemical reactions, including those that support normal growth, development, and immune function. Too much zinc, however, can cause deficiency of copper, another essential mineral, which can lead to impaired immune function. Being moderate in your diet means that you do not restrict or completely eliminate any one type of food, but rather that all types of food can fit into a healthful diet.

Food guides and their graphics convey the message of moderation by showing suggested amounts of different food groups. Appearing in

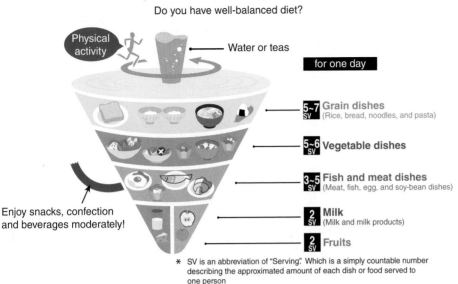

Japanese Food Guide Spinning Top

Do you have well-balanced diet?

Physical activity

Water or teas

for one day

5~7 SV **Grain dishes** (Rice, bread, noodles, and pasta)

5~6 SV **Vegetable dishes**

3~5 SV **Fish and meat dishes** (Meat, fish, egg, and soy-bean dishes)

2 SV **Milk** (Milk and milk products)

2 SV **Fruits**

Enjoy snacks, confection and beverages moderately!

* SV is an abbreviation of "Serving". Which is a simply countable number describing the approximated amount of each dish or food served to one person

FIGURE 2.2 Dietary guidelines around the world. Global differences in environment, culture, socioeconomics, and behavior create significant differences in the foods that make up our diets. Despite this, dietary guidelines from one country to the next show surprising similarities. Whether a country has only 3 guidelines or as many as 23, all share similar basic recommendations. For example, the Japanese dietary guidelines use a spinning top. The United States uses a plate, and Canada uses a rainbow. Mexico and most European countries use a circular form.

Courtesy of the Japanese Ministry of Health, Labor and Welfare/USDA.

diverse shapes, food guides from other countries reflect their cultural contexts. Japan, for example, uses the shape of a spinning top (see **FIGURE 2.2**).

Variety

THINK About It **2**

How many different foods do you eat on a daily basis? Ten? Fifteen? Variety means including a lot of different foods in the diet: not just different food groups such as fruits, vegetables, and grains, but also different foods from each group. Eating two bananas and three carrots each and every day might give you the minimum number of recommended daily servings of fruits and vegetables, but it doesn't add much variety.

Variety is important for a number of reasons. Eating a variety of fruits, for example, provides a broader mix of vitamins, minerals, and phytochemicals than if you eat the same one or two fruits most of the time. Choosing a variety of protein sources gives you a different balance of fats and other nutrients. Variety can add interest and excitement to your meals while preventing boredom with your diet. Perhaps most important, variety in your diet helps ensure that you get all the nutrients you need. Studies have shown that people who have varied diets are more likely to meet their overall nutrient needs.[8]

There are no magic diets, foods, or supplements. Instead, your overall, long-term food choices can bring you the benefits of a nutritious diet. A healthful diet is something you create over time, not the way you eat on any given day. Using the principles of adequacy, balance, calorie (energy) control, nutrient density, moderation, and variety can help you attain and achieve healthy eating habits, which in turn will contribute to your overall healthy lifestyle. Let's take a look at some general guidance for making those food choices.

Quick Bite

Variety Is Key

Mothers often say, "Eat your vegetables." Studies show that adding variety in the vegetables you eat is a good indicator of overall increased vegetable consumption. It may cost a little more today, but eating different types of vegetables is related to better overall diet quality and a larger quantity of vegetables consumed. The small increase in cost at the grocery store now likely will save you more than money in the future. So, experiment a little, and try something other than your usual carrots and green beans at dinner.

▶ **U.S. Department of Agriculture (USDA)** The government agency that monitors the production of eggs, poultry, and meat for adherence to standards of quality and wholesomeness. The USDA also provides public nutrition education, performs nutrition research, and administers the WIC program.

▶ **U.S. Department of Health and Human Services (DHHS)** The principal federal agency responsible for protecting the health of all Americans and providing essential human services. The agency is especially concerned with those Americans who are least able to help themselves.

▶ **2015–2020 Dietary Guidelines for Americans** The foundation of federal nutrition policy; they are developed by the U.S. Department of Agriculture (USDA) and the U.S. Department of Health and Human Services (DHHS). These science-based guidelines are intended to reduce the number of Americans who develop chronic diseases such as hypertension, diabetes, cardiovascular disease, obesity, and alcoholism.

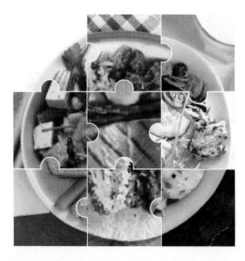

FIGURE 2.3 *Dietary Guidelines for Americans.* A revised *Dietary Guidelines for Americans* was released in 2015. The *2015–2020 Dietary Guidelines for Americans* recommends reducing intake of sodium (salt), added sugars (e.g., cookies), and refined grains (e.g., white bread). Reducing alcohol intake (e.g., beer) is a strategy that adults can use to reduce calorie consumption.

Reproduced from U.S. Department of Health and Human Services and U.S. Department of Agriculture. *Dietary Guidelines for Americans, 2015–2020.* 8th ed. Washington, DC: U.S. Government Printing Office; 2015.

Key Concepts Food and nutrient intake play a major role in health and risk of disease. For most Americans, overnutrition is more of a problem than undernutrition. The diet-planning principles of adequacy, balance, calorie (energy) control, nutrient density, moderation, and variety are important concepts in choosing a healthful diet.

Dietary Guidelines

🍎 **Why Is This Important?** At times it may be difficult to know what advice about eating and physical activity to follow. The *Dietary Guidelines for Americans* and Canada's *Guidelines for Healthy Eating*, which are written by teams of experts, provide nutrition and physical activity advice intended to promote individual health and prevent chronic disease.

To help individuals evaluate and improve their overall health, the United States and many other countries have developed dietary guidelines—simple, easy-to-understand statements about food choices, food safety, and physical activity. This section examines dietary guidelines for the United States and Canada.

Dietary Guidelines for Americans

In 1980, the **U.S. Department of Agriculture (USDA)** and the **U.S. Department of Health and Human Services (DHHS)** jointly released the first edition of the *Dietary Guidelines for Americans.* The *Dietary Guidelines for Americans* provides science-based advice that suggests how nutrition and physical activity can help promote health across the lifespan and reduce the risk for major chronic diseases in the U.S. population ages 2 years and older.[9]

THINK About It 3

By law, the *Dietary Guidelines for Americans* is reviewed, updated if necessary, and published every five years. The ***2015–2020 Dietary Guidelines for Americans*** (see **FIGURE 2.3**) is designed as a tool for professionals to help individuals and their families consume a healthy, nutritionally adequate diet. The *Dietary Guidelines for Americans* is based on research that looks at the relationship among overall eating patterns, health, and risk of chronic disease. Advances in research have provided a greater understanding of, and focus on, the importance of healthy eating patterns as a whole, and how foods and beverages act in combination to affect health. Recommendations within the *Guidelines* are what experts have determined to be the best advice for Americans to reduce the risk for chronic diseases such as heart disease, cancer, diabetes, stroke, osteoporosis, and obesity. These guidelines are the cornerstone of federal nutrition policy and education. They are used to develop educational materials and to aid in the design and implementation of nutrition-related programs, such as the National School Lunch Program and Meals on Wheels. The *Dietary Guidelines for Americans* serves as the basis for nutrition messages and consumer materials developed by nutrition educators and health professionals for the general public.[10]

Lifestyle choices, including a poor diet and lack of physical activity, are significant factors contributing to the overweight and obesity epidemic that is currently affecting men, women, and children throughout the United States. Even for individuals who are not overweight, a poor diet and physical inactivity are well known to be associated with the major causes of morbidity and mortality. The number of Americans who are overweight or obese is high; as a consequence, the risk for various chronic diseases is also on the rise. Furthermore, among the population of overweight and obese individuals, many are undernourished in several key nutrients.

In an effort to address this growing problem, the *2015–2020 Dietary Guidelines for Americans* focuses on the integration of government, agriculture, health care, business, educators, and communities working together to encourage individuals to make healthy lifestyle changes.[11] The main objective of these guidelines is to encourage healthy eating patterns and regular physical activity for the American people. These guidelines emphasize a total diet approach by encouraging us to think holistically about what we eat and drink. They also emphasize meeting nutritional needs by including nutrient-dense foods that contain essential vitamins and minerals, dietary fiber, and other naturally occurring substances that have positive health effects. The guidelines offer practical tips for how people can make changes within their own diet as a way to integrate healthier choices. Examples of these practical tips include: consuming more vegetables, fruits, whole grains, fat-free and low-fat dairy products, and seafood; consuming foods with less sodium, saturated and trans fats, added sugars, and refined grains; and increasing daily physical activity.

The *2015–2020 Dietary Guidelines for Americans* provides five overarching guidelines that encourage healthy eating patterns, recognizing that individuals will need to make shifts in their food and beverage choices to achieve a healthy pattern, and acknowledge that all segments of our society—food producers, grocery stores, restaurants, families, and policymakers—have a role to play in supporting healthy choices. These guidelines also emphasize that a healthy eating pattern is not a rigid prescription, but rather an adaptable framework in which individuals can enjoy foods that meet their personal, cultural, and traditional preferences and fit within their budget and lifestyle.

Overarching Guidelines

The *2015–2020 Dietary Guidelines for Americans* include a section called the overarching Guidelines. These Guidelines urge individuals to develop healthy eating patterns by making necessary changes to food and beverage consumption, and remind readers that all segments of our society have a role to play in supporting healthy choices. Below lists the 5 Overarching Guidelines of *The 2015–2020 Dietary Guidelines for Americans*.

1. *Follow a healthy eating pattern across the lifespan.* All food and beverage choices matter. Choose a healthy eating pattern at an appropriate calorie level to help achieve and maintain a healthy body weight, support nutrient adequacy, and reduce the risk of chronic disease.
2. *Focus on variety, nutrient density, and amount.* To meet nutrient needs within calorie limits, choose a variety of nutrient-dense foods across and within all food groups in recommended amounts.
3. *Limit calories from added sugars and saturated fats and reduce sodium intake.* Consume foods low in added sugars, saturated fats, and sodium. Cut back on foods and beverages higher in these components to amounts that fit within healthy eating patterns.

4. *Shift to healthier food and beverage choices.* Choose nutrient-dense foods and beverages across and within all food groups in place of less healthy choices. Consider cultural and personal preferences to make these shifts easier to accomplish and maintain.

5. *Support healthy eating patterns for all.* Everyone has a role in helping to create and support healthy eating patterns in multiple settings nationwide, from home to school to work to communities.

Key Recommendations from the 2015–2020 Dietary Guidelines for Americans

Key recommendations provide further guidance on how individuals can follow the five guidelines. These should be applied in their entirety, given the interconnected relationship that each dietary component can have with others.

- Follow a healthy eating pattern that accounts for all foods and beverages within an appropriate calorie level.
- Consume less than 10 percent of calorie per day from added sugars.
- Consume less than 10 percent of calories per day from saturated fats.
- Consume less than 2,300 mg per day of sodium.
- If alcohol is consumed, it should be consumed in moderation—up to one drink per day for women and up to two drinks per day for men—and only by adults of legal drinking age.
- Meet the *Physical Activity Guidelines for Americans.*

Looking further into the *Dietary Guidelines,* you can determine what foods to increase in your diet as well as what foods to limit. For most Americans, foods to eat more of include the following:

- A variety of vegetables from all of the subgroups—dark green, red and orange, legumes (beans and peas), starchy, and other types
- Fruits, especially whole fruits
- Grains, at least half of which are whole grains
- Fat-free or low-fat dairy, including milk, yogurt, cheese, and/or fortified soy beverages
- A variety of protein foods, including seafood, lean meats and poultry, eggs, legumes, and nuts, seeds, and soy products
- Oils

In order to follow healthy eating patterns, individuals should limit the following foods:

- Saturated fats and trans fats
- Added sugars
- Sodium

The relationship between diet and physical activity contributes to calorie balance and managing body weight. The *Physical Activity Guidelines for Americans* suggests that adults should do the equivalent of 150 minutes of moderate-intensity aerobic activity each week—that's an average of only 30 minutes a day, five days a week. For children and adolescents age 6 years or older, the recommendation is 60 minutes or more of physical activity per day.[11]

The environment in which many Americans live, work, learn, and play can be a roadblock for many people trying to achieve or maintain

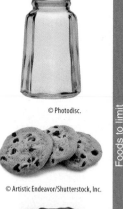

© Photodisc.

© Artistic Endeavor/Shutterstock, Inc.

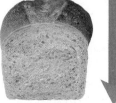

© Photodisc.

Foods to limit

a healthy body weight. Having been described as an obesogenic environment, this way of life is a significant contributor to America's obesity epidemic because it affects both sides of the calorie balance equation.[12] In our modern lifestyle, the availability of high-calorie, palatable, inexpensive food is coupled with many mechanized labor-saving devices. The result is that we live in an environment that often promotes overeating while at the same time discourages physical activity.

Ways to Incorporate the Dietary Guidelines into Your Daily Life

THINK About It 4

Think about your diet and consider your overall food intake to determine whether it is consistent with the *2015–2020 Dietary Guidelines for Americans*. Choose more fruits, vegetables, and whole grains to make sure you are getting all the nutrients you need while lowering your intake of saturated fat, trans fat, added sugar, and sodium. Eat fewer high-fat and fried foods to help you balance energy intake and expenditure. Exercise regularly. Drink water more often than soft drinks, and if you choose to drink alcohol at all, use caution.

Using the *Dietary Guidelines* as your road map for finding a healthier way of eating, you might find it easier to meet your nutrition needs while also protecting your health and achieving or maintaining a healthy weight along the way. **TABLE 2.1** suggests things you might be able to change in your own diet or lifestyle. Pick one or two suggestions or come up with some simple changes of your own to try to incorporate the *2015–2020 Dietary Guidelines for Americans* into your daily life. **TABLE 2.2** summarizes daily limits or targets for a number of nutrients addressed in the *Dietary Guidelines*.

TABLE 2.1
2015–2020 Dietary Guidelines for Americans: Benefits, Behaviors, and Tips

Action	Reasoning for Implementing the Action	Goals or Behaviors That Could Make You Healthier	How to Implement the Action
Follow a healthy eating pattern across the lifespan.	• Individuals throughout all stages of the lifespan should have eating patterns that promote overall health and help prevent chronic disease. • Choose a healthy eating pattern at an appropriate calorie level to help achieve and maintain a healthy body weight, support nutrient adequacy, and reduce the risk of chronic disease.	• Consume foods and drinks to meet, not exceed, calorie needs. • Plan ahead to make healthy food choices. • Track food and calorie intake. • Reduce portion sizes, especially of high-calorie foods. • Choose healthy food options when eating away from home.	• Know your calorie needs. • Prepare and pack healthy snacks at home to eat at school or work.
Focus on variety, nutrient density, and amount.	• Choose a variety of nutrient-dense foods across and within all food groups in recommended amounts.	• Eat five or more servings of vegetables and fruit daily, made up of a variety of choices. • Choose foods that contain nutrients and other beneficial substances that have not been "diluted" by the addition of calories from added solid fats, sugars, or refined starches, or by the solid fats naturally present in food.	• Add dark-green, red, and orange vegetables to soups, stews, casseroles, and stir-fries and other main and side dishes. • Add beans or peas to salads, soups, and side dishes, or serve as a main dish. • Have raw, cut-up vegetables and fruit handy for a quick side dish, snack, salad, or dessert. • When eating out, choose a vegetable as a side dish.

(continued)

TABLE 2.1 (continued)
2015–2020 Dietary Guidelines for Americans: Benefits, Behaviors, and Tips

Action	Reasoning for Implementing the Action	Goals or Behaviors That Could Make You Healthier	How to Implement the Action
Limit calories from added sugars and saturated fats and reduce sodium intake.	• Cut back on foods and beverages high in added sugars, saturated fats, and sodium to amounts that fit within healthy eating patterns. • Limit added sugars to less than 10% of calories per day. • Limit saturated fat intake to less than 10% of calories per day. • Limit sodium to less than 2,300 mg per day (adults). • Eating a diet that includes saturated fat, trans fat, and dietary cholesterol raises low-density lipoprotein (LDL), or "bad" cholesterol levels, which increases the risk of coronary heart disease (CHD).	• Replace saturated fats with polyunsaturated fats. • Be aware of the most likely sources of trans fat in your diet, such as many pastry items and donuts, deep-fried foods, many types of snack chips, cookies, and crackers.	• Eat less cake, cookies, ice cream, other desserts, and candy. • Include foods that provide monounsaturated and polyunsaturated fats, such as olive oil and nuts, in your diet. • Limit intake of foods high in saturated and trans fats such as ground beef and full-fat dairy products.
Shift to healthier food and beverage choices.	• Choose nutrient-dense foods and beverages across and within all food groups. • Excessive alcohol consumption has no benefits, and the health and social hazards of heavy alcohol intake are numerous and well known.	• Drink an adequate amount of water each day. • Choose foods and drinks with added sugars or caloric sweeteners (sugar-sweetened beverages) less frequently. • If you are of legal drinking age and you consume alcohol, do so in moderation. • Mixing alcohol and caffeine is not recognized as safe by the FDA.	• Drink few or no regular sodas, sports drinks, energy drinks, and fruit drinks. • Choose water, fat-free milk, 100 percent fruit juice, or unsweetened tea or coffee as drinks. • If you consume alcohol, limit it to no more than one drink per day for women and two drinks per day for men. • Avoid excessive (heavy or binge) drinking. • Avoid alcohol if you are pregnant or may become pregnant.
Support healthy eating patterns for all.	• Everyone has a role in helping to create and support healthy eating patterns in multiple settings.	• Systems, organizations, and businesses and industries all have an important role to play in helping individuals make healthy choices. • Professionals can work with individuals in a variety of settings to adapt their choices to develop a healthy eating pattern tailored to accommodate physical health; cultural, ethnic, traditional, and personal preferences; and personal food budgets and other issues of accessibility.	• Make healthy food choices at home and away from home.

Modified from U.S. Department of Health and Human Services and U.S. Department of Agriculture. *2015–2020 Dietary Guidelines for Americans.* 8th Edition. December 2015. Available at http://health.gov/dietaryguidelines/2015/guidelines/. Accessed August 15, 2017.

Key Concepts Dietary guidelines are recommendations based on current science that guide people toward more healthful choices. The *2015–2020 Dietary Guidelines for Americans* provides five overarching guidelines that encourage healthy eating patterns, recognize that individuals will need to make shifts in their food and beverage choices to achieve a healthy pattern, and acknowledge that all segments of our society have a role to play in supporting healthy choices.

From Dietary Guidelines to Planning: What You Will Eat

🍎 **Why Is This Important?** By understanding the *Dietary Guidelines for Americans*, you will be able to identify characteristics of a diet that make it healthy. The next step is to translate your knowledge into healthful food choices.

TABLE 2.2

Daily Targets for Nutrients as Addressed in the *2015–2020 Dietary Guidelines for Americans*

Nutrient or Food Group	Target Amount per Day for Adult Females Ages 19–30
Protein	46 g (10–35% kcal)
Carbohydrate	130 g (45–65% kcal)
Dietary fiber	28 g
Added sugars	< 10% kcal
Total fat	20–35% kcal
Saturated fat	< 10% kcal
Linoleic acid	12 g
Linolenic acid	1.1 g
Calcium	1,000 mg
Iron	18 mg
Magnesium	310 mg
Phosphorus	700 mg
Potassium	4,700 mg
Sodium	2,300 mg
Vitamin A	700 mg RAE
Vitamin E	15 mg AT
Vitamin D	600 IU
Vitamin C	75 mg

Data from U.S. Department of Agriculture and U.S. Department of Health and Human Services. *Dietary Guidelines for Americans, 2015–2020.* 8th ed. Washington, DC: U.S. Government Printing Office; 2015.

For many years, nutritionists and teachers have used **food groups** to illustrate the proper combination of foods in a healthful diet. Even young children can sort food into groups and fill a plate with foods from each group. The foods within each group are similar because of their origins—fruits, for example, all come from the same part of different plants. But from a nutritional perspective, what fruits have in common is the balance of macronutrients and the similarities in micronutrient composition. Even so, the foods in one group can differ significantly in their vitamin and mineral profiles; for example, some fruits (e.g., citrus, strawberries, and kiwi) are rich in vitamin C, whereas others (e.g., apples, bananas) have very little. Here again, we can see the importance of variety, of not simply including different food groups but also choosing a variety of foods *within* each group.

Canada's Food Guide

Promoting healthy eating habits among Canadians has been a priority of Health Canada for many years. Health Canada is the federal department responsible for helping the people of Canada maintain and improve their health. In the 1980s, a high priority was given to developing a single set of dietary guidelines. The results of this effort

Quick Bite

How Well Do School Cafeterias Follow Nutrition Guidelines?

About one in three kids and teenagers is obese, and high-fat school lunches may be contributing to the problem. With the majority of school-age kids and teens getting 30 to 50 percent of their total calories from cafeteria meals each day, it's important that these meals be as healthy as possible. The Healthy, Hunger-Free Kids Act, which was passed in 2010, (1) boosts the nutrition quality of school lunches by requiring fewer calories, less sodium, and more fresh fruits, vegetables, and whole grains; (2) expands the number of students enrolled in free- and reduced-cost meals; and (3) puts into place a plan to eliminate things like vending machines from school cafeterias.

Position Statement: Academy of Nutrition and Dietetics

Total Diet Approach to Communicating Food and Nutrition Information

It is the position of the Academy of Nutrition and Dietetics that the total diet or overall pattern of food eaten is the most important focus of a healthful eating style. All foods can fit within this pattern, if consumed in moderation with appropriate portion size and combined with regular physical activity. The Academy of Nutrition and Dietetics strives to communicate healthful eating messages to the public that emphasize a balance of food and beverages, rather than any one food or meal.

Reprinted from *Journal of the Academy of Nutrition and Dietetics*, 113(2), Jeanne H. Freeland-Graves and Susan Nitzke, Position of the Academy of Nutrition and Dietetics: Total Diet Approach to Healthy Eating, Page no. 307-317, 2013, with permission from Elsevier.

▶ **food groups** Categories of similar foods, such as fruits or vegetables.

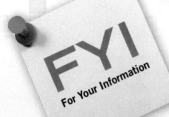

MyPlate: Foods, Serving Sizes, and Tips

Grains	Amount Equal to 1 Ounce	Common Portions and Ounce Equivalents
Bagels	1 "mini" bagel	1 large bagel = 4 ounce equivalents
Biscuits	1 small (2" diameter)	1 large (3") = 2 ounce equivalents
Breads	1 regular slice	2 regular slices = 2 ounce equivalents
Bulgur	½ cup cooked	
Cornbread	1 small piece (2½" × 1¼" × 1¼")	1 medium piece = 2 ounce equivalents
English muffins	½ muffin	1 muffin = 2 ounce equivalents
Muffins	1 small (2½" diameter)	1 large (3½" diameter) = 3 ounce equivalents
Oatmeal	½ cup cooked	
Pancakes	1 pancake (4½" diameter)	3 pancakes (4½" diameter) = 3 ounce equivalents
Popcorn	3 cups, popped	1 microwave bag, popped = 4 ounce equivalents
Ready-to-eat cereals	1 cup flakes; 1¼ cups puffed	
Rice	½ cup cooked (1 ounce dry)	1 cup cooked = 2 ounce equivalents
Pasta	½ cup cooked (1 ounce dry)	1 cup cooked = 2 ounce equivalents
Tortillas	1 small (6" diameter)	1 large (12" diameter) = 4 ounce equivalents

Tips: Make at least half your grains whole grains. Choose foods that name one of the following first on the label's ingredient list: brown rice, bulgur, graham flour, oatmeal, whole oats, whole rye, whole wheat, wild rice. Go easy on high-fat or sugary toppings.

Vegetables	Amount Equal to 1 Cup of Vegetables	Vegetables	Amount Equal to 1 Cup of Vegetables
Dark-Green Vegetables		**Starchy Vegetables**	
Spinach, romaine, collards, mustard greens, kale, other leafy greens	2 cups raw or 1 cup cooked	Corn	1 cup or 1 large ear (8" to 9" long)
		Green peas	1 cup
Broccoli	1 cup chopped or florets	White potatoes	1 cup diced or mashed 1 medium potato, boiled or baked
Orange Vegetables		**Other Vegetables**	
Carrots	1 cup raw or cooked 2 medium whole 1 cup baby chopped, sliced, or cooked	Bean sprouts	1 cup cooked
		Green beans	1 cup cooked
		Tomatoes	1 large raw whole (3")
Pumpkin, sweet potato, winter squash	1 cup chopped, sliced, or cooked		

Tips: Vary your veggies. Make half your plate fruits and vegetables. Eat more dark-green vegetables, more orange vegetables, and more dry beans. Buy fresh vegetables in season for best taste and lowest cost. Buy vegetables that are easy to prepare.

Fruit	Amount Equal to 1 Cup of Fruit	Milk	Amount Equal to 1 Cup of Milk
Apple	1 small	Milk	1 cup
Applesauce	1 cup	Yogurt	1 regular container (8 ounces) or 1 cup yogurt
Banana	1 large (8" to 9" long)	Cheese	1½ ounces hard cheese
Melon	1 cup diced or melon balls		⅓ cup shredded cheese
Grapes	1 cup whole; 32 seedless grapes		2 ounces processed cheese
Canned fruit or diced raw fruit	1 cup		2 cups cottage cheese
Orange or peach	1 large	Milk-based desserts	1 cup pudding made with milk
Strawberries	About 8 large berries		1 cup frozen yogurt
100% fruit juice	1 cup	Soymilk	1 cup calcium-fortified soymilk

Tips: Focus on fruit. Make half your plate fruits and vegetables. Eat a variety of fruit. Choose fresh, frozen, canned, or dried fruit. Go easy on juices. When choosing a juice, look for "100% juice" on the label.

Tips: Get your calcium-rich foods. Switch to fat-free or low-fat milk. If you don't or can't consume milk, get your calcium-rich foods by choosing lactose-free or other calcium sources such as calcium-fortified juices, cereals, breads, soy beverages, or rice beverages.

Meat and Beans	Amount Equal to 1 Ounce	Common Portions and Ounce Equivalents
Cooked lean beef, pork, or ham	1 ounce	1 small steak = 3½ to 4 ounce equivalents 1 small lean hamburger = 2 to 3 ounce equivalents
Cooked chicken or turkey without skin	1 ounce	1 small chicken breast half = 3 ounce equivalents
Cooked fish or shellfish	1 ounce	1 can tuna, drained = 3 to 4 ounce equivalents 1 salmon steak = 4 to 6 ounce equivalents 1 small trout = 3 ounce equivalents
Eggs	1 egg	
Nuts and seeds	½ ounce of nuts (12 almonds, 24 pistachios, 7 walnut halves) ½ ounce of seeds, roasted 1 tablespoon of peanut butter	
Dry beans and peas	¼ cup cooked beans or peas ¼ cup baked beans, refried beans ¼ cup tofu 1 ounce tempeh 2 tablespoons hummus	

Tips: Go lean with protein. Choose low-fat or lean meats and poultry. Bake it, broil it, or grill it. Vary your choices, with more fish, beans, peas, nuts, and seeds.

Oils
Common oils: Vegetable oils (canola, corn, cottonseed, olive, safflower, soybean, sunflower)
Foods naturally high in oils: Nuts, olives, some fish, avocados

Tips: Know your oils. Oils are not a food group, but they provide essential nutrients. Make most of your fat sources from fish, nuts, and vegetable oils. Limit solid fats such as butter, stick margarine, shortening, and lard.

Modified from U.S. Department of Agriculture Center for Nutrition Policy and Promotion. Food Groups, MyPlate. Available at http://www.choosemyplate.gov/food-groups. Accessed August 15, 2017.

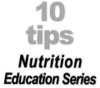

10 tips

Nutrition Education Series

liven up your meals with vegetables and fruits

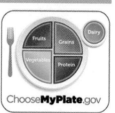

ChooseMyPlate.gov

10 tips to improve your meals with vegetables and fruits

Discover the many benefits of adding vegetables and fruits to your meals. They are low in fat and calories, while providing fiber and other key nutrients. Most Americans should eat more than 3 cups—and for some, up to 6 cups—of vegetables and fruits each day. Vegetables and fruits don't just add nutrition to meals. They can also add color, flavor, and texture. Explore these creative ways to bring healthy foods to your table.

1 fire up the grill
Use the grill to cook vegetables and fruits. Try grilling mushrooms, carrots, peppers, or potatoes on a kabob skewer. Brush with oil to keep them from drying out. Grilled fruits like peaches, pineapple, or mangos add great flavor to a cookout.

2 expand the flavor of your casseroles
Mix vegetables such as sauteed onions, peas, pinto beans, or tomatoes into your favorite dish for that extra flavor.

3 planning something Italian?
Add extra vegetables to your pasta dish. Slip some peppers, spinach, red beans, onions, or cherry tomatoes into your traditional tomato sauce. Vegetables provide texture and low-calorie bulk that satisfies.

4 get creative with your salad
Toss in shredded carrots, strawberries, spinach, watercress, orange segments, or sweet peas for a flavorful, fun salad.

5 salad bars aren't just for salads
Try eating sliced fruit from the salad bar as your dessert when dining out. This will help you avoid any baked desserts that are high in calories.

6 get in on the stir-frying fun
Try something new! Stir-fry your veggies—like broccoli, carrots, sugar snap peas, mushrooms, or green beans—for a quick-and-easy addition to any meal.

7 add them to your sandwiches
Whether it is a sandwich or wrap, vegetables make great additions to both. Try sliced tomatoes, romaine lettuce, or avocado on your everday sandwich or wrap for extra flavor.

8 be creative with your baked goods
Add apples, bananas, blueberries, or pears to your favorite muffin recipe for a treat.

9 make a tasty fruit smoothie
For dessert, blend strawberries, blueberries, or raspberries with frozen bananas and 100% fruit juice for a delicious frozen fruit smoothie.

10 liven up an omelet
Boost the color and flavor of your morning omelet with vegetables. Simply chop, saute, and add them to the egg as it cooks. Try combining different vegetables, such as mushrooms, spinach, onions, or bell peppers.

Go to www.ChooseMyPlate.gov for more information.

Reproduced from U.S. Department of Agriculture and U.S. Department of Health and Human Services. Dietary Guidelines Tip Sheet No. 10. Washington, DC: U.S. Government Printing Office; 2011.

were the *Nutrition Recommendations for Canadians* and *Canada's Guidelines for Healthy Eating*. These reports updated the existing dietary standards and provided a scientific description of the characteristics of a healthy dietary pattern.

Canada's official food rules have evolved into *Eating Well with Canada's Food Guide*. (See **FIGURE 2.4**.) The amounts and types of foods recommended in the *Food Guide* are based on the nutrient reference values of the Dietary Reference Intakes (DRIs). The foods pictured in the *Food Guide* reflect the diversity of foods available in Canada. The "rainbow" used by the *Food Guide* places foods into four groups: Vegetables and Fruit, Grain Products, Milk and Alternatives, and Meat and Alternatives. The *Food Guide* describes the kinds of foods to choose from each group. For example, under the Milk and Alternatives group, the *Food Guide* suggests, "Drink fortified soy beverages if you do not drink milk." *Eating Well with Canada's Food Guide* illustrates that vegetables, fruits, and grains should be the major part of the diet, with milk products and meats consumed in smaller amounts.

The *Food Guide* also provides a "bar" that shows how many daily servings are recommended for each age group and gives examples of serving sizes. The *Food Guide* provides specific advice for different ages and stages. Limiting foods and beverages high in calories, fat, sugar, or salt is recommended, as is label-reading.

The current edition of *Eating Well with Canada's Food Guide* recommends that Canadians do the following[13]:

- Eat at least one dark-green and one orange vegetable each day.
- Enjoy vegetables and fruit prepared with little or no added fat, sugar, or salt.
- Eat vegetables and fruits more often than juice.
- Select whole grains for at least half of one's grain products.
- Choose grain products that are low in fat, sugar, or salt.
- Drink skim, 1 percent, or 2 percent milk each day.
- Consume meat alternatives, such as beans, lentils, and tofu, often.
- Eat at least two *Food Guide* servings of fish each week.
- Select lean meat and alternatives prepared with little or no added fat or salt.
- Include a small amount of unsaturated fat each day.
- Satisfy thirst with water.
- Limit foods and beverages high in calories, fat, sugar, or salt.
- Be active every day.

Following the eating pattern of *Canada's Food Guide* will help people to get enough vitamins, minerals, and other nutrients; reduce the risk of obesity, type 2 diabetes, heart disease, certain types of cancer, and osteoporosis; and achieve overall health and vitality. The Health Canada website (www.canada.ca/en/health-canada/services/canada-food-guides.html) includes a link to My Food Guide, which is an interactive tool for personalizing the information in *Canada's Food Guide*.

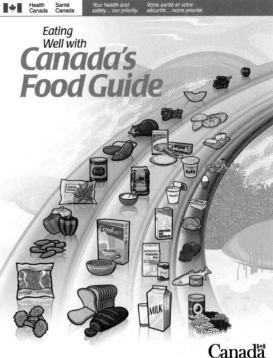

FIGURE 2.4 *Eating Well with Canada's Food Guide.* The rainbow portion of *Canada's Food Guide* sorts food into groups from which people can make wise food choices.

Quick Bite

SuperTracker: My Foods, My Fitness, My Health

The MyPlate website includes an interactive diet and physical activity tool called SuperTracker. You can use it to get your own personalized nutrition and physical activity plan. Track your foods and physical activities to see how they stack up to recommendations. Get tips and support to help you make healthier choices and plan ahead. Visit www.supertracker.usda.gov.

▶ **Nutrition Recommendations for Canadians** A set of scientific statements that provide guidance to Canadians for a dietary pattern that will supply recommended amounts of all essential nutrients while reducing the risk of chronic disease.

▶ **Canada's Guidelines for Healthy Eating** Key messages that are based on the 1990 *Nutrition Recommendations for Canadians* and that provide positive, action-oriented, scientifically accurate eating advice to Canadians.

▶ **Eating Well with Canada's Food Guide** Recommendations to help Canadians select foods to meet energy and nutrient needs while reducing the risk of chronic disease. The *Food Guide* is based on the *Nutrition Recommendations for Canadians* and *Canada's Guidelines for Healthy Eating* and is a key nutrition education tool for Canadians age 4 years or older.

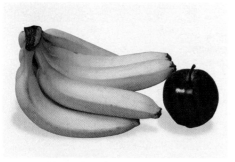

© Digital Stock

Canada's Physical Activity Guide, released by the Canadian Society for Exercise Physiology, outlines recommendations for infants to adults 65 years old or older. Infants and toddlers should get physical activity several times per day, progressing toward at least 60 minutes of energetic play by 5 years of age. Children ages 5 to 11 and youth ages 12 to 17 should get at least 60 minutes of moderate- to vigorous-intensity physical activity daily. Adults ages 18 to 64 and older adults age 65 or older should get at least 150 minutes of moderate- to vigorous-intensity aerobic physical activity per week, in bouts of 10 minutes or more.

Using MyPlate or *Canada's Food Guide* in Diet Planning

The first step in using MyPlate or *Canada's Food Guide* for diet planning is to determine the amount of calories you should eat each day. **TABLE 2.3** shows the recommended amounts of food for three calorie-intake levels. It also gives you an idea of how MyPlate varies with different energy needs. Next, become familiar with the types of food in each group, the number of recommended servings, and the appropriate serving sizes. For an intuitive guide to serving sizes, see **TABLE 2.4**, and plan your meals and snacks using the suggested serving sizes for your appropriate calorie level.

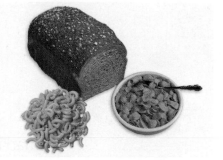

© Digital Stock

Using a 2,000-calorie diet as a sample, refer to **TABLE 2.5** to see how this can work. Beginning with breakfast, you could plan to have the following: 1 cup (1 oz) of ready-to-eat cereal, ½ cup of skim milk, 1 slice of whole wheat toast with 1 teaspoon of butter, and 1 cup of orange juice. Continue to plan your meals and snacks for the rest of the day with the amount of servings you have remaining for each food

TABLE 2.3
MyPlate Suggested Daily Amounts for Three Levels of Energy Intake

Food Group	Energy Intake Level		
	Low (1,400 kcal)[a]	Moderate (2,000 kcal)[b]	High (2,800 kcal)[c]
Grains	5 oz eq	6 oz eq	10 oz eq
Vegetables	1½ cups	2½ cups	3½ cups
Fruits	1½ cups	2 cups	2½ cups
Milk	2 cups	3 cups	3 cups
Meat and beans	4 oz eq	5½ oz eq	7 oz eq
Oils	4 teaspoons	6 teaspoons	8 teaspoons
Empty calories allowed[d]	117 kilocalories	270 kilocalories	426 kilocalories

[a] 1,400 kilocalories is about right for many young children.

[b] 2,000 kilocalories is about right for teenage girls, active women, and many sedentary men.

[c] 2,800 kilocalories is about right for teenage boys and many active men.

[d] Empty calorie allowance is the remaining amount of calories needed for all food groups, assuming that those choices are fat-free or low-fat and with no added sugars.

Note: Your calorie needs may be higher or lower than those shown. Women may need more calories when they are pregnant or breastfeeding.

Modified from *Dietary Guidelines for Americans 2010*, 7th ed., U.S. Government Printing Office, 2010. Courtesy of U.S. Department of Agriculture and U.S. Department of Health and Human Services.

TABLE 2.4
Playing with MyPlate Portions: Your Favorite Sports and Games Can Help You Visualize MyPlate Portion Sizes

Grains	1 cup dry cereal	2-ounce bagel	½ cup cooked cereal, rice, or pasta
	4 golf balls	1 hockey puck	1 tennis ball
Vegetables	1 cup of vegetables		
	1 baseball		
Fruits	1 medium fruit (equivalent of 1 cup of fruit)		
	1 baseball		
Oils	1 teaspoon vegetable oil	1 tablespoon salad dressing	
	1 die (11/16" size)	1 jacks ball	
Milk	1 ½ ounces of hard cheese	1/3 cup of shredded cheese	
	6 dice (11/16" size)	1 billiard ball or racquetball	
Meat and beans	3 ounces cooked meat	2 tablespoons hummus	
	1 deck of playing cards	1 ping-pong ball	

group. Keep in mind that what you consider a serving might differ from the sizes defined in MyPlate. Research shows that Americans' serving sizes for common foods such as pasta, cookies, cereal, soft drinks, and french fries have increased significantly.[14] Do large portions promote overeating and obesity? See the FYI feature "Portion Distortion" for a scientific exploration related to this question.

TABLE 2.5
Sample 2,000-Calorie Diet

Food Group	Total Recommended for 2,000-Calorie Diet	Amount Used at Breakfast	Amount Left for Remainder of the Day
Grains	6 oz eq	2 oz eq	4 oz eq
Vegetables	2½ cups	0	2½ cups
Fruits	2 cups	1 cup	1 cup
Meat, poultry, eggs	3½ cups	½ cup	2 cups
Nuts, seeds, and soy products	5 oz eq/wk	0	5 oz/wk
Oils	6 tsp	1 tsp	5 tsp
Limit on calories for other uses	270 calories	0	270 calories

Data from U.S. Department of Agriculture, U.S. Department of Health and Human Services. *2015–2020 Dietary Guidelines for Americans.* 8th ed. Washington, DC: U.S. Government Printing Office; 2015. https://health.gov/dietaryguidelines/2015/guidelines/chapter-1/a-closer-look-inside-healthy-eating-patterns/#table-1-1. Accessed September 14, 2017.

Sometimes it's difficult to figure out how to account for foods that are mixtures of different groups—lasagna, casseroles, or pizza, for example. Try separating such foods into their ingredients (e.g., pizza contains crust, tomato sauce, cheese, and toppings, which might be meats or vegetables) to estimate the amounts. You should be able to come up with a reasonable approximation. All in all, MyPlate and *Canada's Food Guide* are easy-to-use guidelines that can help you select a variety of foods.

Be aware of foods that contain many calories but have little or no nutrients, such as cookies, pastries, and donuts. Note in Table 2.5 that for a 2,000-calorie food plan, 270 calories are remaining and allowed to be used even when all the other food groups are accounted for. However, this accounting with leftover calories assumes that all food choices are fat-free or low-fat and do not have added sugars. What does this mean? If you are already in the habit of choosing low-fat and low-sugar options, you have a few calories to play with each day. These calories can be used for a higher-fat choice or for some sugar in your iced tea. But watch out! Those calories can get used up quickly. One regular 12-ounce soft drink would take up 150 discretionary calories; an extra tablespoon of dressing on your salad can add 100 more calories.

Using the ChooseMyPlate.gov website is easy and informative. Getting a personalized plan, learning healthy eating tips, getting weight loss information, planning a healthy menu, and analyzing your diet are examples of what ChooseMyPlate.gov offers. The website is an excellent way to help guide you through the necessary steps of putting the *Dietary Guidelines* into practice, while at the same time teaching good nutrition and providing appropriate physical activity information.

Key Concepts MyPlate is a complete food guidance system based on the *Dietary Guidelines for Americans* and Dietary Reference Intakes to help Americans make healthy food choices and remind them to be active every day. The interactive tools on the ChooseMyPlate.gov website can help you monitor your food choices. *Eating Well with Canada's Food Guide* illustrates the dietary guidelines for Canadians and the Dietary Reference Intakes. These graphic tools show the appropriate balance of food groups in a healthful diet: more whole grains, low-fat dairy, vegetables, and fruits; less meat and added fats and sugars.

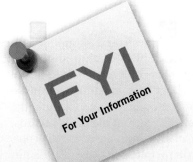

Portion Distortion

How do portions and serving sizes differ? According to the National Institutes of Health, a *portion* of food is defined as the amount of food that you choose to eat at one time, whereas a *serving* is a specific amount of food or drink.[a] Many foods that are packaged as a single portion actually contain multiple servings. Sometimes the portion size and serving size are the same, but not always. Check the food label to see how many servings are in the portion of food that you like to eat.

Over the past few years, portions have grown significantly in supermarkets, restaurants, and even in our own homes.[b]

Many factors contribute to Americans' growing waistlines, but one observation in particular cannot be overlooked: The incidence of obesity has increased in parallel with increasing portion sizes.[c] Consider this: Adults today consume an average of 300 more calories per day than they did in the year 1985.[d] Is this just a coincidence, or do larger portion sizes have something to do with it? In almost every eating situation, we are now confronted by huge portions, which are perceived as "normal" or "a great value." Americans have created the perception that large portion sizes are appropriate, creating an environment of *portion distortion*.[e] We find portion distortions in restaurants, where the jumbo-sized portions are consistently 250 percent larger than the regular portions.[f] We even find portion distortions in our homes, where the sizes of our bowls and glasses have steadily increased and where the surface area of the average dinner plate has increased 36 percent since 1960.[g] Research shows that people unintentionally consume more calories when offered larger portions.[h] Consuming larger portion sizes can contribute to positive energy balance, which, over time, leads to weight gain and ultimately can result in obesity.

The phenomenon of portion distortion has the potential to hinder weight loss, weight maintenance, and health improvement efforts. Consider right-sizing the portions of food that you choose to eat. This just might bring super-size benefits to your health.

To see whether you know how today's portions compare to the portions available 20 years ago, take the interactive portion distortion quizzes on the National Heart, Lung, and Blood Institute's Portion Distortion webpage (www.nhlbi.nih.gov/health/educational/wecan/eat-right/portion-distortion.htm). You can also learn about the amount of physical activity required to burn off the extra calories provided by today's portions.

a American Heart Association, Robert Wood Johnson Foundation. A nation at risk: obesity in the United States. http://www.ca-ilg.org/sites/main/files/file-attachments/resources__26310.NationAtRisk.ObesityEpidemic.pdf. Accessed August 15, 2017.

b Ibid.

c Schwartz J, Byrd-Bredbenner C. Portion distortion: typical portion sizes selected by young adults. *J Am Diet Assoc.* 2006;106(9):1412-1418.

d American Heart Association, Robert Wood Johnson Foundation. Op cit.

e Wansink B, van Ittersum K. Portion size me: downsizing our consumption norms. *J Am Diet Assoc.* 2007;7(7):1103-1106.

f Ibid.

g Ibid.

h Herman P, Polivy J, Pliner P, Vartanian L. Mechanisms underlying the portion-size effect. *Physiol Behav.* 2015;144:129-136. Epub 2015 March 20.

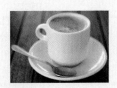

8-oz coffee with milk and sugar
© holbox/Shutterstock, Inc.

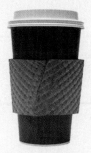

16-oz mocha coffee
© iStockphoto/Thinkstock.

Recommendations for Nutrient Intake: The DRIs

🍎 **Why Is This Important?** Before you can choose foods that meet your needs for specific nutrients, you need to know how much of each nutrient is required daily. Understanding dietary standards will allow you to make these assessments.

Understanding Dietary Standards

So far, the tools described (*Dietary Guidelines for Americans*, MyPlate, and *Eating Well with Canada's Food Guide*) deal with whole foods and food groups rather than individual nutrient values; after all, foods are

▶ **dietary standards** A set of values for the recommended intake of nutrients.

▶ **Dietary Reference Intakes (DRIs)** A framework of dietary standards that includes Estimated Average Requirement (EAR), Recommended Dietary Allowance (RDA), Adequate Intake (AI), and Tolerable Upper Intake Level (UL).

▶ **Recommended Nutrient Intakes (RNIs)** Canadian dietary standards that have been replaced by Dietary Reference Intakes.

▶ **Recommended Dietary Allowances (RDAs)** The nutrient intake levels that meet the nutrient needs of almost all (97 to 98 percent) individuals in a life-stage and gender group.

▶ **Food and Nutrition Board** A board within the Institute of Medicine of the National Academy of Sciences. It is responsible for assembling the group of nutrition scientists who review available scientific data to determine appropriate intake levels of the known essential nutrients.

▶ **requirement** The lowest continuing intake level of a nutrient that prevents deficiency in an individual.

Quick **Bite**

Underconsumption of Nutrients

Although diseases caused by nutrient deficiencies are generally uncommon in the United States, underconsumption of many nutrients does exist and can lead to chronic health conditions. Current dietary guidelines identify these nutrients and make suggestions for intake of each.

what we think about in planning our daily meals and shopping lists. Sometimes, though, we need more specific information about our nutritional needs. **Dietary standards** are sets of recommended intake values for nutrients. These standards tell us how much of each nutrient we should have in our diets. In the United States and Canada, the **Dietary Reference Intakes (DRIs)** are the current dietary standards.

Consider the following scenario. You are running a research center located in Antarctica that is staffed by 60 people. Because staff will not be able to leave the site to get meals, you must provide all their food. You must keep the group adequately nourished; you certainly don't want anyone to become ill as a result of a nutrient deficiency. How would you (or the nutritionist you hire) start planning? How can you be sure to provide adequate amounts of the essential nutrients? The most important tool would be a set of dietary standards! Essentially the same scenario faces those who plan and provide food for groups of people in more routine circumstances—the military, prisons, and even schools. To assess nutritional adequacy, diet planners can compare the nutrient composition of their food plans to recommended intake values.

A Brief History of Dietary Standards

Beginning in 1938, Health Canada published dietary standards called **Recommended Nutrient Intakes (RNIs)**. In the United States, the **Recommended Dietary Allowances (RDAs)** were first published in 1941. By the 1940s, nutrition scientists had been able to isolate and identify many of the nutrients in food. They were able to measure the amounts of these nutrients in foods and to recommend daily intake levels. These levels became the first RNI and RDA values. Committees of scientists regularly reviewed the standards and published revised editions; for example, the tenth (and final) edition of RDAs was published in 1989.

In the mid-1990s, the **Food and Nutrition Board** of the National Academy of Sciences began a partnership with Health Canada to make fundamental changes in the approach to setting dietary standards and to replace the RDAs and RNIs. In 1997, the first set of DRIs was published. The DRIs suggest intake levels not just for dietary adequacy, but also for optimal nutrition.

Dietary Reference Intakes

Since the inception of the RDAs and RNIs, we have learned more about the relationships between diet and chronic disease; hence, changes in food production have been implemented (such as folic acid fortification), and nutrient-deficiency diseases have become rare in the United States.

The DRIs are reference values for nutrient intakes to be used in assessing and planning diets for healthy people (see **FIGURE 2.5**). The DRIs include four basic elements: Estimated Average Requirement (EAR), Recommended Dietary Allowance (RDA), Adequate Intake (AI), and Tolerable Upper Intake Level (UL). Underlying each of these values is the definition of a **requirement** as the "lowest continuing intake level of a nutrient that, for a specific indicator of adequacy, will maintain a defined level of nutrition in an individual."[15-18] In other words, a requirement is the smallest amount of a nutrient you should take in on a regular basis to remain healthy. In the DRI report on macronutrients, two other concepts were introduced: the Estimated Energy Requirement (EER) and the Acceptable Macronutrient Distribution Ranges (AMDRs).[19]

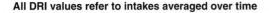

All DRI values refer to intakes averaged over time

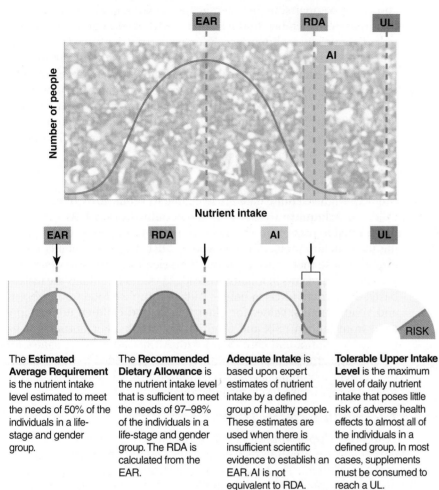

The **Estimated Average Requirement** is the nutrient intake level estimated to meet the needs of 50% of the individuals in a life-stage and gender group.

The **Recommended Dietary Allowance** is the nutrient intake level that is sufficient to meet the needs of 97–98% of the individuals in a life-stage and gender group. The RDA is calculated from the EAR.

Adequate Intake is based upon expert estimates of nutrient intake by a defined group of healthy people. These estimates are used when there is insufficient scientific evidence to establish an EAR. AI is not equivalent to RDA.

Tolerable Upper Intake Level is the maximum level of daily nutrient intake that poses little risk of adverse health effects to almost all of the individuals in a defined group. In most cases, supplements must be consumed to reach a UL.

FIGURE 2.5 Dietary Reference Intakes. The Dietary Reference Intakes are a set of dietary standards that include Estimated Average Requirement (EAR), Recommended Dietary Allowance (RDA), Adequate Intake (AI), and Tolerable Upper Intake Level (UL).

© Photodisc.

Estimated Average Requirement

The **Estimated Average Requirement (EAR)** reflects the amount of a nutrient that would meet the needs of 50 percent of the people in a particular life-stage (age) and gender group. For each nutrient, this requirement is defined using a specific indicator of dietary adequacy. This indicator could be the level of the nutrient or one of its breakdown products in the blood, or the amount of an enzyme associated with that nutrient.[20] The EAR is used to set the RDA; EAR values also can be used to assess dietary adequacy or to plan diets for groups of people.

Recommended Dietary Allowance

The Recommended Dietary Allowance (RDA) is the daily intake level that meets the needs of most people (97 to 98 percent) in a life-stage and gender group. The RDA is set at two standard deviations above the EAR. A nutrient will not have an RDA value if there are not enough scientific data available to set an EAR value.

▶ **Estimated Average Requirement (EAR)** The intake value that meets the estimated nutrient needs of 50 percent of individuals in a specific life-stage and gender group.

People can use the RDA value as a target or goal for dietary intake and make comparisons between actual intake and RDA values. It is important to remember, however, that the RDAs do not define an *individual's* nutrient requirements. Your actual nutrient needs might be much lower than average, and therefore the RDA would be more than you need. An analysis of your diet might show, for example, that you consume 45 percent of the RDA for a certain vitamin, but that might be adequate for your needs. Only specific laboratory or other tests can determine a person's true nutrient requirements and actual nutritional status; however, an intake that is consistently at or near the RDA level is likely to be meeting your needs.

Adequate Intake

If not enough scientific data are available to set an EAR level, a value called an **Adequate Intake (AI)** is determined instead. AI values are determined in part by observing healthy groups of people and estimating their dietary intake. All the current DRI values for infants are AI levels because there have been too few scientific studies to determine specific requirements in infants. Instead, AI values for infants are usually based on nutrient levels in human milk, a complete food for newborns and young infants. Values for older infants and children are extrapolated from human milk and from data on adults. For nutrients (e.g., vitamin K, biotin, and chromium) with AI instead of RDA values for all life-stage groups, more scientific research is needed to better define the nutrient requirements of population groups. AI values can be considered target intake levels for individuals.

Tolerable Upper Intake Level

Tolerable Upper Intake Levels (ULs) have been defined for many nutrients. Consumption of a nutrient in amounts higher than the UL could be harmful. The ULs have been developed partly in response to the growing interest in dietary supplements that contain large amounts of essential nutrients. The UL is *not* to be used as a target for intake but rather should be a cautionary level for people who regularly take nutrient supplements.

Estimated Energy Requirement

The **Estimated Energy Requirement (EER)** is defined as the energy intake that is estimated to maintain energy balance in healthy, normal-weight individuals. It is determined using an equation that considers weight, height, age, and physical activity. Different equations are used for males and females and for different age groups.

Acceptable Macronutrient Distribution Ranges

Acceptable Macronutrient Distribution Ranges (AMDRs) indicate the recommended balance of energy sources in a healthful diet. These values consider the amounts of macronutrients needed to provide adequate intake of essential nutrients while reducing the risk for chronic disease. The AMDRs are shown in **TABLE 2.6**.

Use of Dietary Standards

The most appropriate use of DRIs is to plan and evaluate diets for large groups of people. Remember the Antarctica scenario at the beginning of this section? If you had planned menus and evaluated the nutrient composition of the foods that would be included, and if the average

▶ **Adequate Intake (AI)** The nutrient intake that appears to sustain a defined nutritional state or some other indicator of health (e.g., growth rate or normal circulating nutrient values) in a specific population or subgroup. AI is used when there is insufficient scientific evidence to establish an EAR.

▶ **Tolerable Upper Intake Levels (ULs)** The maximum levels of daily nutrient intakes that are unlikely to pose health risks to almost all of the individuals in the group for whom they are designed.

▶ **Estimated Energy Requirement (EER)** Dietary energy intake that is predicted to maintain energy balance in a healthy adult of a defined age, gender, weight, height, and level of physical activity consistent with good health.

▶ **Acceptable Macronutrient Distribution Ranges (AMDRs)** Range of intakes for a particular energy source that are associated with reduced risk of chronic disease while providing adequate intakes of essential nutrients.

TABLE 2.6
Acceptable Macronutrient Distribution Ranges (AMDRs) for Adults

Macronutrient	Recommended Percentage of Diet	Equivalent Number of Calories or Grams in a 2,000-Calorie Diet
Fat	20–35%	400–700 calories or 44–78 grams
Carbohydrate	45–65%	900–1,300 calories or 225–325 grams
Protein	10–35%	200–700 calories or 50–175 grams
Omega-6 polyunsaturated fatty acids	5–10%	100–200 calories or 11–22 grams
Alpha-linolenic acid	0.6–1.2%	12–24 grams or 1–3 grams

Note: % values are percentage of energy intake. To convert % macronutrients to calories, use the total daily calorie amount divided by percent of macronutrient, multiplied by calories per gram for each macronutrient.

Reproduced from Institute of Medicine, Food and Nutrition Board. *Dietary Reference Intakes for Energy, Carbohydrate, Fiber, Fat, Fatty Acids, Cholesterol, Protein, and Amino Acids.* Copyright © 2005 by the National Academy of Sciences, courtesy of the National Academies Press, Washington, DC.

nutrient levels of those daily menus met or exceeded the RDA/AI levels, you could be confident that your group would be adequately nourished. If you had a very large group—thousands of soldiers, for instance—the EAR would be a more appropriate guide.

Dietary standards are also used to make decisions about nutrition policy. The Special Supplemental Food Program for Women, Infants, and Children (WIC), for example, takes into account the DRIs as it provides food or vouchers for food. The goal of this federally funded supplemental feeding program is to improve the nutrient intake of low-income pregnant and breastfeeding women, their infants, and young children. The guidelines for school lunch and breakfast programs are also based on DRI values.

Often, we use dietary standards as comparison values for individual diets. It can be interesting to see how your daily intake of a nutrient compares with the RDA or AI. However, an intake that is less than the RDA/AI doesn't necessarily mean deficiency; your individual requirement for a nutrient can be less than the RDA/AI value. You can use the RDA/AI values as targets for dietary intake, while avoiding nutrient intake that exceeds the UL.

Key Concepts Dietary standards are levels of nutrient intake recommended for healthy people. These standards help the government set nutrition policy and also can be used to guide the planning and evaluation of diets for groups and individuals. The Dietary Reference Intakes are the dietary standards for the United States and Canada. These standards focus on maintaining optimal health and lowering the risks of chronic disease, rather than simply on dietary adequacy.

Food Labels

Why Is This Important? Food labels are very useful tools in making food decisions. They provide standard information regarding important nutrients in a serving of packaged food. This information can be helpful when looking for a particular type of food or nutrient (such as carbohydrates), when categorizing foods (such as "high fiber"), and in comparing similar food products.

Now that you understand diet-planning tools and dietary standards, let's focus on your use of these tools—for example, when making decisions

▶ **food label** Label required by law on virtually all packaged foods and having five requirements: (1) a statement of identity; (2) the net contents (by weight, volume, or measure) of the package; (3) the name and address of the manufacturer, packer, or distributor; (4) a list of ingredients; and (5) nutrition information.

▶ **Food and Drug Administration (FDA)** The federal agency responsible for ensuring that foods sold in the United States (except for eggs, poultry, and meat, which are monitored by the U.S. Department of Agriculture [USDA]) are safe, wholesome, and labeled properly. The FDA sets standards for the composition of some foods, inspects food plants, and monitors imported foods. The FDA is an agency of the U.S. Department of Health and Human Services (DHHS).

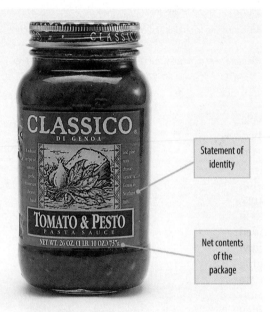

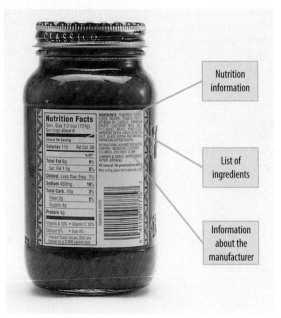

FIGURE 2.6 The five mandatory requirements for food labels.
Federal regulations determine what may and may not appear on food labels.

at the grocery store. One of the most useful tools in planning a healthful diet is the **food label**.

Specific federal regulations control what may and may not appear on a food label and what must appear on it. The **Food and Drug Administration (FDA)** is responsible for ensuring that foods sold in the United States are safe, wholesome, and properly labeled. The Health Products and Food Branch of Health Canada has similar responsibilities.

Only a small category of foods, such as spices and flavorings, is not required by the FDA to have a particular food label. Such foods are exempted because they do not provide a significant amount of nutrients. Deli items and ready-to-eat foods that are prepared and sold in retail establishments also do not require a food label.[21] Raw fruits and vegetables and fresh fish generally do not carry food labels either; however, these foods fall under the FDA's voluntary, point-of-purchase nutrition information program, which establishes that the nutrition information for grocery stores' most commonly purchased items must be posted somewhere near where that food is sold.[22] The FDA's jurisdiction applies to packaged foods except for certain meat, poultry and processed egg products, because these foods are regulated by the U.S. Department of Agriculture Food Safety and Inspection Service.

In May 2016 the FDA introduced updates to the Nutrition Facts panel. Until then, and aside from adding trans fat to the list of required nutrients in 2006, the Nutrition Facts Label had not changed since 1994. Food manufacturers have time to implement the required label changes; therefore, although less common, it is possible for consumers to still see the old version of the Nutrition Facts panel. Let's take a closer look at food labels.

Ingredients and Other Basic Information

The label on a food you buy today has been shaped by many sets of regulations. As **FIGURE 2.6** shows, food labels have five mandatory components:

1. A statement of identity/name of the food
2. The net weight of the food contained inside of the package, not including the weight of the package
3. The name and address of the manufacturer, packer, or distributor
4. A list of ingredients in descending order by weight
5. Nutrition information

The **statement of identity** requirement means that the product must prominently display the common or usual name of the product or identify the food with an "appropriately descriptive term." For example, it would be misleading to label a fruit beverage containing only 10 percent fruit juice as a "juice." The statement of net package contents must accurately reflect the quantity in terms of weight, volume, measure, or numerical count. Information about the manufacturer, packer, or distributor gives consumers a way to contact someone in case they have questions about the product.

Ingredients must be listed by common or usual name, in descending order by weight; thus, the first ingredient listed is the primary ingredient in that food product. Let's compare the ingredient list of two cereals:

Cereal A ingredients: Milled corn, sugar, salt, malt flavoring, high-fructose corn syrup

Cereal B ingredients: Sugar, yellow corn flour, rice flour, wheat flour, whole oat flour, partially hydrogenated vegetable oil (contains one or more of the following oils: canola, soybean, cottonseed), salt, cocoa, artificial favor, corn syrup

In Cereal B, the first ingredient listed is sugar, which means this cereal contains more sugar by weight than any other ingredient. Cereal A's primary ingredient is milled corn. That can make quite a difference in the amount (grams) of sugar a cereal contains.

Also, preservatives and other additives in foods must be listed, along with an explanation of their function. Accurate and complete ingredient information is vital for people with food allergies who must avoid certain food components. The labels of foods that contain any of the eight major food allergens (egg, wheat, peanuts, milk, tree nuts, soy, fish, and crustaceans) are required to include common names when listing these ingredients.

Nutrition Facts Panel

The **Nutrition Facts panel** informs the consumer about the nutritional value of a food product, enabling an informed shopper to compare similar products.

Take a closer look at the elements making up the new and the older version of the Nutrition Facts panel. (See **FIGURE 2.7**.) The heading "Nutrition Facts" stands out clearly. Just under the heading is information about the number of servings and serving size per container. It is important to note the serving size because all the nutrient information that follows is based on that amount of food, and the listed serving size might be different from what you usually eat. One change to the new label is that the serving sizes described on the package are required to more closely reflect the amount of that food that people typically eat, something that has certainly changed since the last serving size requirements were published in 1993. People should recognize that the serving size does not necessarily reflect the recommended portion size, but rather the amount of that food that is generally eaten in one sitting. In addition, calories and nutrition information must be declared for the entire package.

The next part of the label shows a list of nutrients with % Daily Values. "Calories from Fat" has been removed from the new label because research shows that the type of fat is more important than the total amount. Total Fat, Saturated Fat, Trans Fat, and Cholesterol will continue to be required on the label. In addition, Sodium, Total Carbohydrates, Dietary Fiber, Total Sugars, Added Sugars, and Protein are included on this part of the label. This information is given both in quantity (grams or milligrams per serving) and as a percentage of the Daily Value—a comparison standard specifically for food labels. (This standard is described in the following section.) Listed next are percentages of Daily Values for vitamin D, calcium, iron, and potassium. which are the only micronutrients that must appear on all standard labels. People tend not to get enough vitamin D and

▶ **statement of identity** A mandate that commercial food products prominently display the common or usual name of the product or identify the food with an "appropriately descriptive term."

▶ **Nutrition Facts panel** A portion of the food label that states the content of selected nutrients in a food in a standard way prescribed by the Food and Drug Administration. By law, Nutrition Facts must appear on nearly all processed food products in the United States. The new Nutrition Facts panel is intended to make it easier for consumers to make informed decisions about the foods they are eating. For example, the new panel includes nutrients that better reflect people's adequate consumption, overconsumption, or underconsumption of nutrients and vitamins such as added sugar, Vitamin D, and potassium.

Quick **Bite**

PKU Warning

As you may have noticed, when an ingredient list includes the artificial sweetener aspartame, it also displays a warning statement. This is because aspartame contains phenylalanine, which individuals with the rare hereditary disease known as phenylketonuria (PKU) have a difficult time metabolizing. These individuals must control their intake of phenylalanine from all sources, including aspartame.

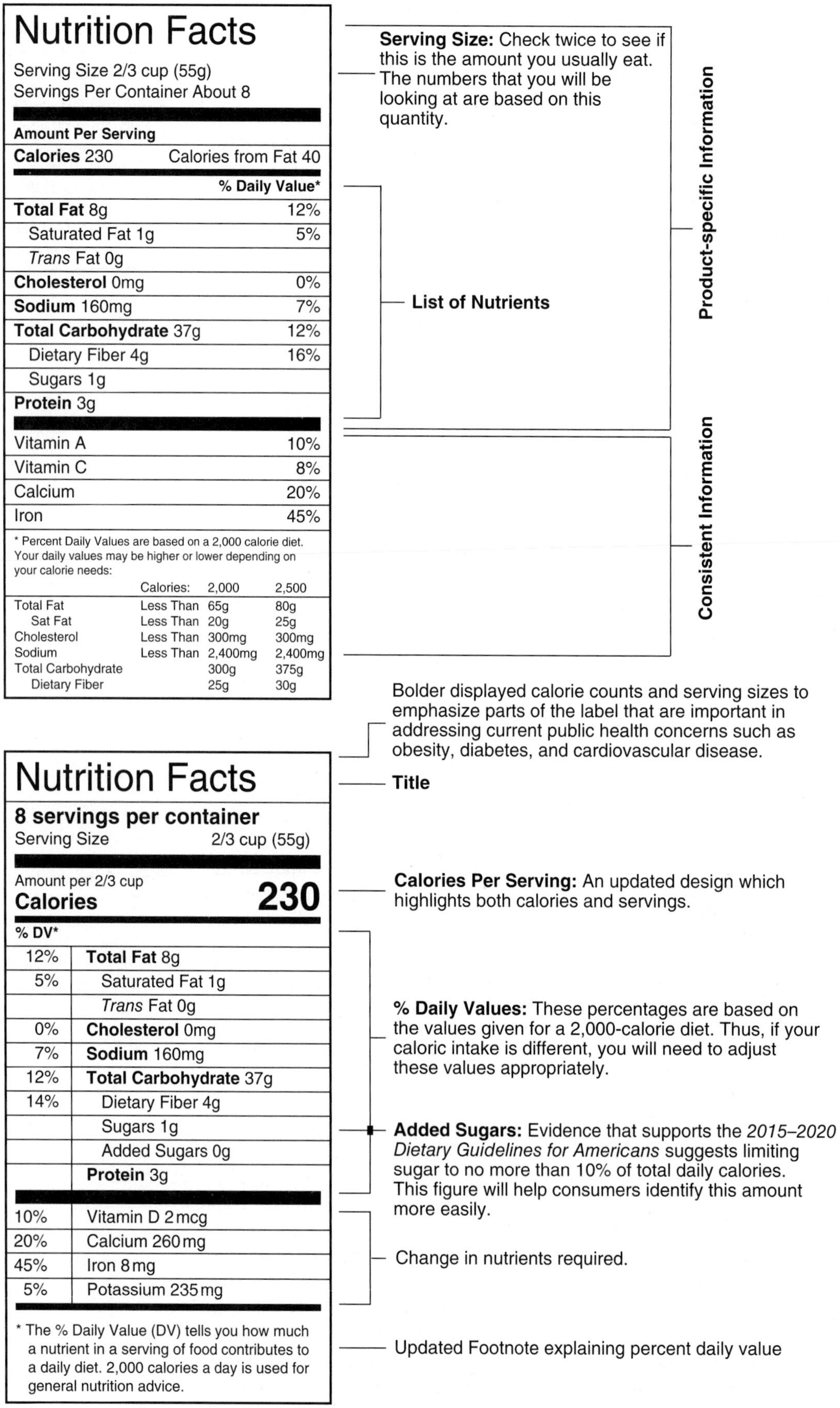

Nutrition Facts

Serving Size 2/3 cup (55g)
Servings Per Container About 8

Amount Per Serving

Calories 230	Calories from Fat 40

	% Daily Value*
Total Fat 8g	12%
Saturated Fat 1g	5%
Trans Fat 0g	
Cholesterol 0mg	0%
Sodium 160mg	7%
Total Carbohydrate 37g	12%
Dietary Fiber 4g	16%
Sugars 1g	
Protein 3g	

Vitamin A	10%
Vitamin C	8%
Calcium	20%
Iron	45%

* Percent Daily Values are based on a 2,000 calorie diet.
Your daily values may be higher or lower depending on
your calorie needs:

	Calories:	2,000	2,500
Total Fat	Less Than	65g	80g
Sat Fat	Less Than	20g	25g
Cholesterol	Less Than	300mg	300mg
Sodium	Less Than	2,400mg	2,400mg
Total Carbohydrate		300g	375g
Dietary Fiber		25g	30g

Serving Size: Check twice to see if this is the amount you usually eat. The numbers that you will be looking at are based on this quantity.

List of Nutrients

Product-specific Information

Consistent Information

Bolder displayed calorie counts and serving sizes to emphasize parts of the label that are important in addressing current public health concerns such as obesity, diabetes, and cardiovascular disease.

Nutrition Facts

8 servings per container

Serving Size	2/3 cup (55g)

Amount per 2/3 cup
Calories	**230**

% DV*		
12%	**Total Fat** 8g	
5%	Saturated Fat 1g	
	Trans Fat 0g	
0%	**Cholesterol** 0mg	
7%	**Sodium** 160mg	
12%	**Total Carbohydrate** 37g	
14%	Dietary Fiber 4g	
	Sugars 1g	
	Added Sugars 0g	
	Protein 3g	

10%	Vitamin D 2mcg
20%	Calcium 260mg
45%	Iron 8mg
5%	Potassium 235mg

* The % Daily Value (DV) tells you how much
a nutrient in a serving of food contributes to
a daily diet. 2,000 calories a day is used for
general nutrition advice.

Title

Calories Per Serving: An updated design which highlights both calories and servings.

% Daily Values: These percentages are based on the values given for a 2,000-calorie diet. Thus, if your caloric intake is different, you will need to adjust these values appropriately.

Added Sugars: Evidence that supports the *2015–2020 Dietary Guidelines for Americans* suggests limiting sugar to no more than 10% of total daily calories. This figure will help consumers identify this amount more easily.

Change in nutrients required.

Updated Footnote explaining percent daily value

FIGURE 2.7 The Nutrition Facts panel. Comparison of the previous and new Nutrition Facts panel.

potassium; therefore, these nutrients have been added to the label. Vitamins A and C will no longer be required because deficiencies of these vitamins are rare. These nutrients can be included on a voluntary basis. The % Daily Values for calcium and iron will continue to be required, along with the actual gram amounts. Manufacturers can choose to include information about other nutrients, such as polyunsaturated fat, additional vitamins, or other minerals, in the Nutrition Facts panel. However, if they make a claim about an optional component (e.g., "good source of vitamin E") or **enrich** or **fortify** the food, the manufacturers must include specific nutrition information for these added nutrients. This information must be included even when government regulations require enrichment or fortification, such as the fortification of milk with vitamin D to prevent rickets (a bone disease in children that results from vitamin D deficiency) and the fortification of grain products with folic acid to reduce the risk of birth defects. Updated daily values for the nutrients sodium, dietary fiber, vitamin D, and potassium on the new label will now be consistent with the Institute of Medicine recommendations and the *2015–2020 Dietary Guidelines for Americans*.

Food products that come in small packages (e.g., gum, candy, tuna) or that have little nutritional value (e.g., diet soft drinks) can have abbreviated versions of the Nutrition Facts on the label, as **FIGURE 2.8** shows.

▶ **enrich** To add vitamins and minerals lost or diminished during food processing, particularly the addition of thiamin, riboflavin, niacin, folic acid, and iron to grain products.

▶ **fortify** Refers to the addition of vitamins or minerals that were not originally present in a food.

▶ **Daily Values (DVs)** A single set of nutrient intake standards developed by the Food and Drug Administration to represent the needs of the "typical" consumer; used as standards for expressing nutrient content on food labels.

▶ **nutrient content claims** These claims describe the level of a nutrient or dietary substance in the product, using terms such as *good source*, *high*, or *free*.

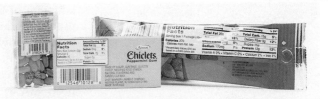

FIGURE 2.8 Nutrition Facts on small packages. When a product package has insufficient space to display a full Nutrition Facts panel, manufacturers may use an abbreviated version.

Daily Values

Let's come back to the Daily Values part of the label. The **Daily Values (DVs)** are a set of dietary standards used to compare the amount of a nutrient (or other component) in a serving of food to the amount recommended for daily consumption. Nutrients are listed as a percentage of the food's Daily Value on the Nutrition Facts panel; the Percent Daily Values (%DV) are based on a 2,000-calorie diet. Your estimated needs may be more or less than 2,000 calories per day, but you can still use the %DV as a guide. The %DV helps you determine if a serving of a food is high or low in a nutrient. In other words, you can see if this food contributes a lot or a little to your daily recommended allowance. Let's say you rely on your breakfast cereal as a major source of dietary fiber intake. Comparing two packages, you find that a serving of cornflakes cereal has 4 percent of the DV for dietary fiber, but choosing bran-flakes cereal gives you 20 percent. By eating one serving of the cornflakes, you will get 4 percent of an estimated 100 percent of your fiber needs for the day. If you choose to eat the bran flakes, you will get 20 percent of the 100 percent estimated needs of fiber for the day. You don't have to know anything about grams to see which food is higher in fiber.

Nutrient Content Claims

The Nutrition Labeling and Education Act (NLEA) and the associated FDA regulations allow food manufacturers to make **nutrient content claims** using a variety of descriptive terms on labels, such as *low fat* and *high fiber*. The FYI feature "Definitions for Nutrient Content Claims on Food Labels" contains a list of terms that may be used. The FDA has made an effort to make the terms meaningful, and the regulations have reduced the number of potentially misleading label

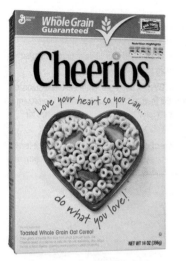

© smartstock/iStockphoto.com.

▶ **health claim** Any statement that associates a food or a substance in a food with a disease or health-related condition. The FDA authorizes health claims.

statements. It would be misleading, for example, to print "cholesterol free" on a can of vegetable shortening—a food that is 100 percent fat and high in saturated and trans-fatty acids (types of fat that raise blood cholesterol levels). Although true, this type of statement misleads consumers who associate "cholesterol free" with "heart healthy." Under the NLEA regulations, statements about low cholesterol content can be used only when the product is also low in saturated fat (less than 2 grams per serving).

The FDA recently made a ruling on food labels for the term *gluten-free*. The rule will be helpful for people who have celiac disease, a digestive and autoimmune disorder that results in damage to the lining of the small intestine when foods with gluten are eaten. Gluten is a protein that occurs naturally in wheat, rye, barley, and cross-bred hybrids of these grains. The rule requires that to be labeled "gluten-free," each kilogram of the product must contain less than 20 milligrams of the protein, and the food cannot contain any of the following: an ingredient that is any type of wheat, rye, barley, or cross-breeds of these grains; an ingredient derived from these grains that has not been processed to remove gluten; or an ingredient derived from these grains that has been processed to remove gluten, if it results in the food containing 20 or more parts per million of gluten.[23] Most people with a gluten allergy can tolerate gluten in small amounts, and this amount is consistent with the threshold established by other countries and international bodies that set food safety standards.[24]

In addition to the content claims defined in the regulations, companies may submit to the FDA a notification of a new nutrient content claim based on "an authoritative statement from an appropriate scientific body of the United States Government or the National Academy of Sciences."[25]

Health Claims

With the passage of the NLEA, manufacturers also were allowed to add health claims to food labels. A **health claim** is a statement that links one or more dietary components to reduced risk of disease—such as a claim that calcium helps reduce the risk of osteoporosis. Before the NLEA was passed, products making such claims were considered drugs, not foods.

A health claim must be supported by scientifically valid evidence for it to be approved for use on a food label. Regulations require a finding of "significant scientific agreement" before the FDA may authorize a new health claim. In addition, there are specific criteria for the use of claims. For example, a high-fiber food that is also high in fat is not eligible for a health claim. So far, the FDA has approved the following health claims:

- *Calcium, vitamin D, and osteoporosis:* Adequate calcium and vitamin D along with regular exercise may reduce the risk of osteoporosis.
- *Dietary fat and cancer:* Low-fat diets may reduce the risk for some types of cancer.
- *Dietary fiber, such as that found in whole oats, barley, and psyllium seed husk, and coronary heart disease (CHD):* Diets low in fat and rich in these types of fiber can help reduce the risk of heart disease.
- *Dietary noncarcinogenic carbohydrate sweeteners and dental caries (tooth decay):* Foods sweetened with sugar alcohols do not promote tooth decay.

- *Dietary saturated fat and cholesterol and coronary heart disease (CHD):* Diets high in saturated fat and cholesterol increase risk for heart disease.
- *Dietary saturated fat, cholesterol, and trans fat and heart disease:* Diets low in saturated fat and cholesterol and as low as possible in trans fat may reduce the risk of heart disease.
- *Fiber-containing grain products, fruits, and vegetables and cancer:* Diets low in fat and rich in high-fiber foods may reduce the risk of certain cancers.
- *Fluoridated water and dental caries:* Drinking fluoridated water may reduce the risk of dental caries.
- *Folate and neural tube defects:* Adequate folate intake prior to and early in pregnancy may reduce the risk of neural tube defects (a birth defect).
- *Fruits and vegetables and cancer:* Diets low in fat and rich in fruits and vegetables may reduce the risk of certain cancers.
- *Fruits, vegetables, and grain products that contain fiber, particularly pectins, gums, and mucilages, and CHD:* Diets low in fat and rich in these types of fiber may reduce the risk of heart disease.
- *Plant sterol/stanol esters and CHD:* Diets low in saturated fat and cholesterol that contain significant amounts of these additives may reduce the risk of heart disease.
- *Potassium and high blood pressure/stroke:* Diets that contain good sources of potassium may reduce the risk of high blood pressure and stroke.
- *Sodium and hypertension (high blood pressure):* Low-sodium diets may help lower blood pressure.
- *Soy protein and CHD:* Foods rich in soy protein as part of a low-fat diet may help reduce the risk of heart disease.
- *Substitution of saturated fat with unsaturated fat and heart disease:* Replacing saturated fat with similar amounts of unsaturated fats may reduce the risk of heart disease.
- *Whole-grain foods and CHD or cancer:* Diets high in whole-grain foods and other plant foods and low in total fat, saturated fat, and cholesterol may help reduce the risk of heart disease and certain cancers.

A new health claim may be proposed at any time, so this list might expand in the future. The most current information on label statements and claims can be found on the Food tab of the FDA website at www.fda.gov.

Structure/Function Claims

Food labels also may contain **structure/function claims** that describe potential effects of a food, food component, or dietary supplement component on body structures or functions, such as bone health, muscle strength, and digestion. As long as the label does not claim to diagnose, cure, mitigate, treat, or prevent a disease, a manufacturer can claim that a product "helps promote immune health" or is an "energizer" if *some* evidence can be provided to support the claim. Currently, structure/function claims on foods must be related to the food's nutritive value. Many scientists are concerned about the lack of a consistent scientific standard for both health claims and structure/function claims.

PER 1 CUP SERVING

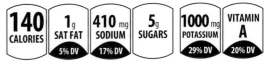

| 140 CALORIES | 1 g SAT FAT 5% DV | 410 mg SODIUM 17% DV | 5 g SUGARS | 1000 mg POTASSIUM 29% DV | VITAMIN A 20% DV |

Facts Up Front is a voluntary food and beverage industry nutrient-based labeling initiative that summarizes important nutrition information on the front of food packages with the intention of helping busy consumers make healthier food choices.

Courtesy of Grocery Manufacturers Association, available at http://www.factsupfront.org.

▶ **structure/function claims** These statements may claim a benefit related to a nutrient-deficiency disease (e.g., *Vitamin C prevents scurvy*) or describe the role of a nutrient or dietary ingredient intended to affect a structure or function in humans (e.g., *Calcium helps build strong bones*).

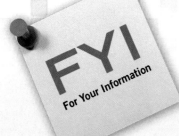

Definitions for Nutrient Content Claims on Food Labels

Free: Food contains no amount (or trivial or "physiologically inconsequential" amounts). May be used with one or more of the following: fat, saturated fat, cholesterol, sodium, sugar, and calories. Synonyms include *without, no, and zero*.

Fat-free: Less than 0.5 gram of fat per serving.

Saturated fat-free: Less than 0.5 gram of saturated fat per serving, and less than 0.5 gram of trans fatty acids per serving.

Cholesterol-free: Less than 2 milligrams of cholesterol and 2 grams or less of saturated fat per serving.

Sodium-free: Less than 5 milligrams of sodium per serving.

Sugar-free: Less than 0.5 gram of sugar per serving.

Calorie-free: Fewer than 5 calories per serving.

Low: Food can be eaten frequently without exceeding dietary guidelines for one or more of these components: fat, saturated fat, cholesterol, sodium, and calories. Synonyms include *little, few,* and *low source of.*

Low-fat: 3 grams or less per serving.

Low-saturated-fat: 1 gram or less of saturated fat per serving; no more than 15 percent of calories from saturated fat.

Low-cholesterol: 20 milligrams or less of cholesterol and 2 grams or less of saturated fat per serving.

Low-sodium: 140 milligrams or less per serving.

Very-low-sodium: 35 milligrams or less per serving.

Low-calorie: 40 calories or less per serving.

Lean and extra lean: Describe the fat content of meal and main dish products, seafood, and game meat products.

Lean: Less than 10 grams of fat, 4.5 grams or less of saturated fat, and less than 95 milligrams of cholesterol per serving and per 100 grams.

Extra lean: Less than 5 grams of fat, less than 2 grams of saturated fat, and less than 95 milligrams of cholesterol per serving and per 100 grams.

High: Food contains 20 percent or more of the Daily Value for a particular nutrient in a serving.

Good source: Food contains 10 to 19 percent of the Daily Value for a particular nutrient in one serving.

Reduced: Nutritionally altered product containing at least 25 percent less of a nutrient or of calories than the regular or reference product. *Note:* A "reduced" claim cannot be used if the reference product already meets the requirement for "low."

Less: Food, whether altered or not, contains 25 percent less of a nutrient or of calories than the reference food. *Fewer* is an acceptable synonym.

Light: This descriptor can have two meanings:

1. A nutritionally altered product contains one-third fewer calories or half the fat of the reference food. If the reference food derives 50 percent or more of its calories from fat, the "light" version must contain 25 percent or less calories (which is 50 percent of the reference food fat content) from fat.

2. The sodium content of a low-calorie, low-fat food has been reduced by 50 percent. Also, *light in sodium* may be used on a food in which the sodium content has been reduced by at least 50 percent.

Note: The term *light* can still be used to describe such properties as texture and color as long as the label clearly explains its meaning (e.g., *light brown sugar, light and fluffy*).

More: A serving of food, whether altered or not, contains more of a nutrient that is at least 10 percent of the Daily Value more than the reference food. This also applies to *fortified, enriched,* and *added* claims, but in those cases, the food must be altered.

Healthy: A *healthy* food must be low in fat and saturated fat and contain limited amounts of cholesterol (less than 60 milligrams) and sodium (less than 360 milligrams for individual foods and less than 480 milligrams for meal-type products). In addition, a single-item food must provide at least 10 percent or more of one of the following: vitamin A or C, iron, calcium, protein, or fiber. A meal-type product, such as a frozen entrée or dinner, must provide 10 percent of two or more of these vitamins or minerals, or protein or fiber, in addition to meeting the other criteria. Additional regulations allow the term *healthy* to be applied to raw, canned, or frozen fruits and vegetables and enriched grains even if the 10 percent nutrient content rule is not met. However, frozen or canned fruits or vegetables cannot contain ingredients that would change the nutrient profile.

Fresh: Food is raw, has never been frozen or heated, and contains no preservatives. *Fresh frozen, frozen fresh,* and *freshly frozen* can be used for foods that are quickly frozen while still fresh. Blanched foods also can be called fresh.

Percent fat-free: Food must be a low-fat or a fat-free product. In addition, the claim must reflect accurately the amount of nonfat ingredients in 100 grams of food.

Implied claims: These are prohibited when they wrongfully imply that a food contains or does not contain a meaningful level of a nutrient. For example, a product cannot claim to be made with an ingredient known to be a source of fiber (such as "made with oat bran") unless the product contains enough of that ingredient (e.g., oat bran) to meet the definition for "good source" of fiber. As another example, a claim that a product contains "no tropical oils" is allowed, but only on foods that are "low" in saturated fat, because consumers have come to equate tropical oils with high levels of saturated fat.

Data from Food and Drug Administration. Guidance for industry: a food labeling guide (9. Appendix A: definitions of nutrient content claims). October 2009. http://www.fda.gov/food/guidanceregulation/guidancedocumentsregulatoryinformation/labelingnutrition/ucm064911.htm. Accessed February 12, 2017.

Using Labels to Make Healthful Food Choices

What's the best way to start using information on food labels to make food choices? Let's look at a couple examples. Perhaps one of your goals is to add more iron to your diet. Compare the cereal labels in **FIGURE 2.9**. Which cereal contains a higher percentage of the Daily Value for iron? How do they compare in terms of sugar content? What about vitamins and other minerals?

Maybe it's a frozen entrée you're after. Look at the two examples in Figure 2.9. Which is the best choice nutritionally? Are you sure? Sometimes the answer is not clear-cut. Product A is higher in sodium, whereas Product B has more saturated and trans fat. It would be important to know about the rest of your dietary intake before deciding. Do you already have quite a bit of sodium in your diet, or are you likely to add salt at the table? Maybe you never salt your food, so a bit extra in your entrée is okay. If you know that your saturated fat intake is already a bit high, however, Product A might be a better choice. To make the best choice, you should know which substances are most important in terms of your own health risks. The label is there to help you make these types of food decisions.

Key Concepts Making food choices at the grocery store is your opportunity to implement the *Dietary Guidelines for Americans* and your MyPlate-planned diet. The Nutrition Facts panel on most packaged foods contains not only specific amounts of nutrients shown in grams or milligrams, but also comparisons between amounts of nutrients in a food and recommended intake values. These comparisons are reported as %DV (Daily Values). The %DV information can be used to compare two products or to see how individual foods contribute to the total diet.

Nutrition Facts
8 servings per container
Serving size   2/3 cup (55g)

Amount per serving
Calories **230**

	% Daily Value*
Total Fat 8g	10%
Saturated Fat 1g	5%
Trans Fat 0g	
Cholesterol 0mg	0%
Sodium 160mg	7%
Total Carbohydrate 37g	13%
Dietary Fiber 4g	14%
Total Sugars 12g	
Includes 10g Added Sugars	20%
Protein 3g	
Vitamin D 2mcg	10%
Calcium 260mg	20%
Iron 8mg	45%
Potassium 235mg	6%

* The % Daily Value (DV) tells you how much a nutrient in a serving of food contributes to a daily diet. 2,000 calories a day is used for general nutrition advice.

Nutrition Facts
8 servings per container
Serving size   2/3 cup (55g)

Amount per serving
Calories **250**

	% Daily Value*
Total Fat 10g	13%
Saturated Fat 3g	15%
Trans Fat 0g	
Cholesterol 0mg	0%
Sodium 220mg	9%
Total Carbohydrate 37g	13%
Dietary Fiber 4g	14%
Total Sugars 12g	
Includes 10g Added Sugars	20%
Protein 4g	
Vitamin D 2mcg	10%
Calcium 260mg	20%
Iron 8mg	45%
Potassium 235mg	6%

* The % Daily Value (DV) tells you how much a nutrient in a serving of food contributes to a daily diet. 2,000 calories a day is used for general nutrition advice.

FIGURE 2.9 Comparing product labels. Labels might looks similar, but appearances can be deceptive. Compare the amounts of saturated fat and sodium in these two products.

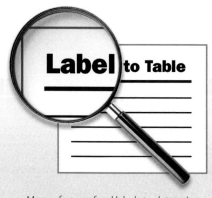

Label to Table

Many of us use food labels to determine such things as how many calories are in a food, how many grams of carbohydrate it provides, or how much saturated fat it contains. Sometimes we overlook the serving size that these numbers are based on and just assume that the amount we eat is considered one serving. Although the amount equal to one serving on food labels is intended to be realistic to what one person generally consumes in one sitting, it may be a good idea to check what actually constitutes a serving, especially with foods that you eat most often.

Consider snack crackers. About how much would you eat at one time? Not sure? Pour your typical serving into a bowl. Now, use a measuring cup to measure how much you have. Look at the serving size listed on the food's label. Is the amount you will eat smaller, larger, or the same as the serving size listed? Remember that the amounts of each nutrient listed on the food's Nutrition Facts panel, as well as the %DVs, are based on the listed serving size, so you may have to recalculate those numbers based on the actual size of your serving to get more accurate nutrient values.

Learning Portfolio

Key Terms

	page
Acceptable Macronutrient Distribution Ranges (AMDRs)	54
Adequate Intake (AI)	54
Canada's Guidelines for Healthy Eating	47
Daily Values (DVs)	59
Dietary Guidelines for Americans, 2015–2020	38
Dietary Reference Intakes (DRIs)	52
dietary standards	52
Eating Well with Canada's Food Guide	47
enrich	59
Estimated Average Requirement (EAR)	53
Estimated Energy Requirement (EER)	54
Food and Drug Administration (FDA)	56
Food and Nutrition Board	52
food groups	43
food label	56
fortify	59
health claim	60
MyPlate	33
nutrient content claims	59
nutrient density	35
Nutrition Facts panel	57
Nutrition Recommendations for Canadians	47
overnutrition	33
Recommended Dietary Allowances (RDAs)	52
Recommended Nutrient Intakes (RNIs)	52
requirement	52
statement of identity	57
structure/function claims	61
Tolerable Upper Intake Levels (ULs)	54
undernutrition	33
U.S. Department of Agriculture (USDA)	38
U.S. Department of Health and Human Services (DHHS)	38

Study Points

- The diet-planning principles of adequacy, balance, calorie (energy) control, nutrient density, moderation, and variety are important concepts in choosing a healthful diet.

- The *Dietary Guidelines for Americans* gives consumers advice regarding general components of the diet.

- *Nutrition Recommendations for Canadians*, and *Canada's Guidelines for Healthy Eating* are provided by the Canadian government in an effort to help people maintain and improve their health.

- MyPlate is a graphic representation of a food guidance system that supports the principles of the *Dietary Guidelines for Americans*.

- Each food group in MyPlate has a recommended daily amount based on calorie needs. A variety of foods from each group can supply all the nutrients.

- Dietary standards are values for individual nutrients that reflect recommended intake levels. These values are used for planning and evaluating diets for groups and individuals.

- The Dietary Reference Intakes are the current dietary standards in the United States and Canada. The DRIs consist of several types of values: EAR, RDA, AI, UL, EER, and AMDR.

- Nutrition information on food labels can be used to determine a more healthful diet.

- Label information not only provides the gram or milligram amounts of the nutrients present, but also gives a percentage of Daily Values so that the consumer can compare the amount in the food to the amount recommended for consumption each day.

Study Questions

1. Define undernutrition and overnutrition.
2. What is the purpose of the *Dietary Guidelines for Americans*?
3. What are the recommended amounts for each food group of MyPlate for a 2,000-calorie diet?
4. List and define four main Dietary Reference Intake categories.
5. List five mandatory components found on all food labels.
6. The newer version of the Nutrition Facts panel shows information on which nutrients?
7. What is the purpose of the % Daily Value listed next to most nutrients on food labels?
8. Define three types of claims that might be found on food labels.

Learning Portfolio (continued)

Try This

Are You a MyPlate Pleaser?

Keep a detailed food diary for three days. Make sure to include things you drink, along with the amounts (e.g., cups, ounces, tablespoons) of each food or beverage. How well do you think your intake matches the *Dietary Guidelines* and MyPlate recommendations? To find out, go to ChooseMyPlate.gov and click on SuperTracker, and then on Food Tracker. This feature allows you to do an online assessment of your food intake. Follow the instructions to Create Your Profile. Then, click on Proceed to Food Intake and enter each food you ate for all three days. When you are done, you can click on Analyze Your Food Intake and see the comparisons to the *Dietary Guidelines* and MyPlate.

How did you do? From which groups did you tend to eat more than is recommended? Were there any groups for which you did not meet the recommendations? Was there a day-to-day variation in the number of servings you ate of each group? Use the results of this activity to plan ways you can improve your diet. You might want to visit this site frequently to monitor changes you are making in your food intake.

Food Label Scavenger Hunt

On your next trip to the grocery store, or in your own food pantry, find a food item that has any number other than a "0" listed for all four of the vitamins and minerals that are required to be listed on the food label. This information is near the bottom of the Nutrition Facts panel and include: Vitamin D, Calcium, Iron, and Potassium. It doesn't matter whether you choose a cereal, soup, cracker, or snack item, as long as it has numbers other than "0" for all four items. Assume that you eat one serving of the product selected. Using the mg per serving and the %DV amount, calculate how much of each of these nutrients (Vitamin D, Calcium, Iron, and Potassium) you should eat today in order to fulfill 100% of the suggested DV for each.

Getting Personal

How Well Are You Following the *Dietary Guidelines*?

Advice provided by the *Dietary Guidelines for Americans* can help you determine the healthfulness of your diet. Using these guidelines as an evaluation tool can also help identify shifts you can make on the road to a healthier lifestyle.

Food Group	Suggested Amount/Day Based on 2,000-Calorie Level	Other Calorie Level Suggestions	My Intake Each Day	Did I Meet the Recommendations?	
				Yes	No
Dark-green vegetables	2½ cups				
Red and orange vegetables	5½ cups				
Legumes (beans and peas)	1½ cups				
Starchy vegetables	5 cups				
Other vegetables	4 cups				
Fruits	2 cups				
Grains	6 oz				
Dairy	3 cups				
Protein foods	5½ oz				
• Seafood	8 oz/wk				
• Meats, poultry, eggs	26 oz/wk				
• Nuts, seeds, soy products	5 oz/wk				
Oil	27 g				
Limit on calories for other uses	270 kcal or 14% of calorie intake				
Physical activity guidelines	Equivalent of 150 minutes of moderate-intensity aerobic activity each week				

Using the checklist below, consider your own eating habits and evaluate them against the recommendations. An example 2,000-calorie level is provided. Table A3-1 of the *2015–2020 Dietary Guidelines for Americans* provides recommendations for a variety of calorie levels.

For each of the food groups for which you did not meet the recommended intake amounts each day, consider shifts you can make in your eating habits that will improve your intake. List three measurable goals to help achieve these changes:

To make my diet and lifestyle healthier, I can:

1. _____
2. _____
3. _____

Serving Sizes and Equivalents

Food Group	Serving Sizes and Equivalents
Grains	1 ounce-equivalent = 1 slice of bread; 1 small muffin; 1 cup ready-to-eat cereal flakes; or ½ cup cooked cereal, rice, grains, or pasta
Vegetables	1 cup or equivalent (1 serving) = 1 cup raw or cooked vegetables; 2 cups raw leafy salad greens; or 1 cup vegetable juice
Fruits	1 cup or equivalent (1 serving) = 1 cup fresh, canned, or frozen fruit; 1 cup fruit juice; 1 small whole fruit; or ½ cup dried fruit
Dairy	1 cup or equivalent = 1 cup milk or yogurt; 1½ oz natural cheese; or 2 oz processed cheese
Protein foods	1 ounce-equivalent = 1 oz lean meat, poultry, or fish; ¼ cup cooked dry beans or tofu; 1 egg; 1 tablespoon peanut butter; or ½ oz nuts or seeds
Oils	1 teaspoon or equivalent = 1 teaspoon vegetable oil or 1 tablespoon mayonnaise-type salad dressing

References

1. Freeland-Graves JH, Nitzke S; Academy of Nutrition and Dietetics. Position of the Academy of Nutrition and Dietetics: total diet approach to healthy eating. *J Acad Nutr Diet*. 2013;113(2):307-317.

2. Schwartz C, Scholtens PA, Lalanne A, et al. Development of healthy eating habits early in life. Review of recent evidence and selected guidelines. *Appetite*. 2011;57(3):796-807.

3. U.S. Department of Agriculture, U.S. Department of Health and Human Services. *2015–2020 Dietary Guidelines for Americans*. 8th ed. Washington, DC: U.S. Government Printing Office; 2015.

4. Drenowatz C. Reciprocal compensation to changes in dietary intake and energy expenditure within the concept of energy balance. *Adv Nutr*. 2015;6(5):592-599.

5. U.S. Department of Agriculture, U.S. Department of Health and Human Services. *2015–2020 Dietary Guidelines for Americans*. Op. cit.

6. Hingle M, Kandiah J, Maggi A. Practice paper of the American Dietetic Association: nutrient density—selecting nutrient-dense foods for good health. *J Am Diet Assoc*. 2016;116(9):1473-1480.

7. Ibid.

8. Vadiveloo M, Dixon LB, Mijanovich T, et al. Dietary variety is inversely associated with body adiposity among US adults using a novel food diversity index. *J Nutr*. 2015;145(3):555-563.

9. Office of Disease Prevention and Health Promotion. Scientific report of the 2015 Dietary Guidelines Advisory Committee. http://www.health.gov/dietaryguidelines/2015-scientific-report/04-integration.asp. Accessed August 16, 2017.

10. Ibid.

11. U.S. Department of Health and Human Services. *Physical Activity Guidelines for Americans*. Washington, DC: Author; 2008. http://www.health.gov/paguidelines/guidelines. Accessed August 16, 2017.

12. U.S. Department of Agriculture, U.S. Department of Health and Human Services. *2015–2020 Dietary Guidelines for Americans*. Op. cit.

13. Health Canada. Eating well with Canada's food guide. https://www.canada.ca/content/dam/hc-sc/migration/hc-sc/fn-an/alt_formats/hpfb-dgpsa/pdf/food-guide-aliment/view_eatwell_vue_bienmang-eng.pdf. Accessed September 14, 2017.

14. Burger KS, Kern M, Coleman KJ. Characteristics of self-selected portion size in young adults. *J Am Diet Assoc*. 2007;3:611-618.

15. Institute of Medicine, Food and Nutrition Board. *Dietary Reference Intakes for Calcium, Phosphorus, Magnesium, Vitamin D, and Fluoride*. Washington, DC: National Academies Press; 1997.

16. Institute of Medicine, Food and Nutrition Board. *Dietary Reference Intakes for Thiamin, Riboflavin, Niacin, Vitamin B-6, Folate, Vitamin B-12, Pantothenic Acid, Biotin, and Choline*. Washington, DC: National Academies Press; 1998.

17. Institute of Medicine, Food and Nutrition Board. *Dietary Reference Intakes for Vitamin C, Vitamin E, Selenium, and Carotenoids*. Washington, DC: National Academies Press; 2000.

18. Institute of Medicine, Food and Nutrition Board. *Dietary Reference Intakes for Vitamin A, Vitamin K, Arsenic, Boron, Chromium, Copper, Iodine, Iron, Molybdenum, Nickel, Silicon, Vanadium, and Zinc*. Washington, DC: National Academies Press; 2001.

19. Institute of Medicine, Food and Nutrition Board. *Dietary Reference Intakes for Energy, Carbohydrate, Fiber, Fat, Fatty Acids, Cholesterol, Protein, and Amino Acids*. Washington, DC: National Academies Press; 2005.

20. Institute of Medicine Subcommittee on Interpretation and Uses of Dietary Reference Intakes. *Institute of Medicine Standing Committee on the Scientific Evaluation of Dietary Reference Intakes*. Washington, DC: National Academies Press; 2000. Using the Estimated Average Requirements for Nutrient Assessment of Groups. https://www.ncbi.nlm.nih.gov/books/NBK222898/. Accessed September 27, 2017.

21. Ibid.

22. Ibid.

23. U.S. Food and Drug Administration. 'Gluten-free' now means what it says. http://www.fda.gov/ForConsumers/ConsumerUpdates/ucm363069.htm. Accessed August 16, 2017.

24. Taylor MR. A new era of "gluten-free" labeling. FDA Voice. August 5, 2014. http://blogs.fda.gov/fdavoice/index.php/2014/08/a-new-era-of-gluten-free-labeling. Accessed August 16, 2017.

25. U.S. Food and Drug Administration. FDA proposed updates to Nutrition Facts label on food packages. Op. cit.

Chapter 3

The Human Body: From Food to Fuel

Revised by Melissa Bernstein

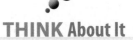

THINK About It

1   Your friend warns you that eating some foods at the same time is not healthful. Is this likely to change your eating behavior?

2   How good are you at identifying tastes?

3   Have you ever noticed that food sometimes tastes sweet after you've chewed it for a while?

4   You feel particularly happy, and you find that a meal prepared by your friend tastes especially good. Any connection?

LEARNING Objectives

1   Discuss the basic components and functions of digestive system organs.
2   Sequence the steps for digestion of food and absorption of nutrients through the digestive system.
3   Explain the role of enzymes and hormones required for digestion and absorption of nutrients.
4   Explain how nutrients are absorbed, circulated through, and eliminated from the body.
5   Identify factors that influence digestion, absorption, and nutrient transport in the body.
6   Describe common nutritional and digestive system disorders and approaches to prevention and treatment.

The aroma of food you like to eat fills the air—maybe it's sautéed onion and garlic, fresh baked bread, or chocolate chip cookies. You start to anticipate a delicious food experience (after all, you haven't eaten for six or seven hours), and all of a sudden your mouth waters as your digestive juices are turned on. Is this virtual reality? Not at all! Before you eat a morsel, your brain signals your body to prepare for food. The process of digestion begins even before you eat, with your sense of taste and smell attracting you to certain foods, and it continues until all of the food you have eaten has moved from your mouth through the gastrointestinal tract.

Your body's mechanisms for processing food and turning it into nutrients are both efficient and elegant. The action unfolds in the digestive tract in two stages: **digestion**—the breaking apart of foods into smaller and smaller units—and **absorption**—the movement of those small units from the gut into the bloodstream or lymphatic system for circulation. Your digestive system is designed to digest carbohydrates, proteins, and fats simultaneously, while preparing other substances—vitamins, minerals, and cholesterol, for example—for absorption. Remarkably, your digestive system doesn't need any help. Despite promotions for enzyme supplements and diet books that recommend consuming food or nutrient groups separately, scientific research does not support these claims. Unless you have a specific medical condition, your digestive system is able to digest and absorb the foods you eat, in whatever combination you eat them.

THINK About It
1

▶ **digestion** The process of transforming the foods we eat into units for absorption.

▶ **absorption** The movement of substances into or across tissues; in particular, the passage of nutrients and other substances into the walls of the gastrointestinal tract and then into the bloodstream.

The Gastrointestinal Tract

🍎 **Why Is This Important?** The GI starts at the mouth and ends at the anus. How food is broken down, moved along the GI tract, and moved into the body's tissues along the way is the process of digestion and absorption.

Even before you take the first bite of food, digestion has started! The sight, smell, thought, taste, and, in some cases, even the sound of food being prepared can trigger a set of responses that prepare the digestive tract to receive food.[1] Your mouth begins to water, and stomach

RESPONSE   STIMULUS

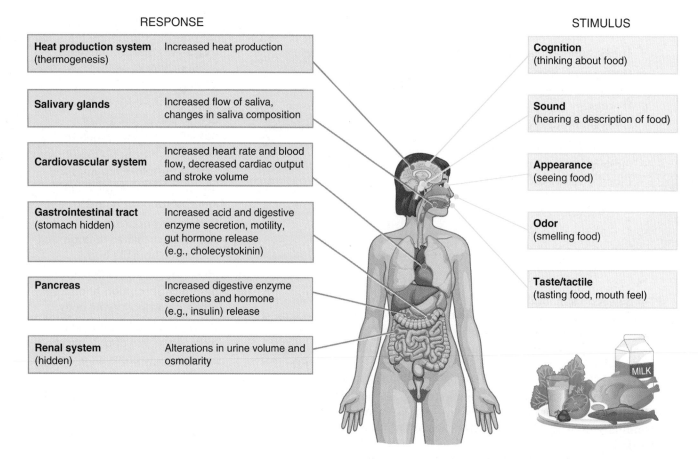

FIGURE 3.1 **Are you ready to eat?** In response to the sight and smell of food, as well as other sensory experiences, your body primes its resources to better digest, absorb, and use anticipated nutrients.

secretions flow. (See **FIGURE 3.1**.) If no food is consumed, the response diminishes. If, instead of teasing the body with mere sights and smells, we actually sit down to a meal and experience the full flavor and texture of foods, the real work of the digestive tract begins. For the food we eat to nourish our bodies, we need to digest it (break it down into smaller units), absorb it (move it from the gut into circulation), and finally transport it to the tissues and cells of the body.

The digestive process starts in the mouth and continues as food journeys down the gastrointestinal (GI) tract. In the mouth, tastes, as well as texture and temperature, combine with odors to produce a perception of flavor. It is flavor that lets us know whether we are eating a pear or an apple. You recognize flavors mainly through the sense of smell. If you hold your nose while eating chocolate, for example, you will have trouble identifying it—even though you can distinguish the food's sweetness or bitterness. That's because the familiar flavor of chocolate is sensed largely by odor, as is the well-known flavor of coffee.

THINK About It 2

At various points along the GI tract, nutrients are absorbed, meaning they move from the GI tract into circulatory systems so they can be transported throughout the body. If there are problems along the way, with either incomplete digestion or inadequate absorption, the cells will not receive the nutrients they need to grow, perform daily activities, fight infection, and maintain health. A closer look at the gastrointestinal tract will help you see just how amazing this organ system is.

▶ **gastrointestinal (GI) tract** [GAS-troh-in-TES-tin-al] The connected series of organs and structures used for digestion of food and absorption of nutrients. Also called the *alimentary canal* or the *digestive tract*.

▶ **accessory organs** Organs that assist in the digestion and absorption of foods and nutrients.

▶ **elimination** The removal of undigested food from the body.

Organization of the GI Tract

The **gastrointestinal (GI) tract**, also known as the alimentary canal, is a long, hollow tube that begins at the mouth and ends at the anus. The specific parts include the mouth, esophagus, stomach, small intestine, large intestine, and rectum. (See **FIGURE 3.2.**) With the help of the **accessory organs**—the salivary glands, liver, gallbladder, and pancreas—the GI tract turns food into small molecules that the body can absorb and use. The GI tract has an amazing variety of functions, including:

- Ingestion (the receipt and softening of food)
- Transport of ingested food
- Secretion of digestive enzymes, acid, mucus, and bile
- Absorption of end products of digestion
- Movement of undigested material
- **Elimination** of waste products

Because of its basic shape, the GI tract is often described as a hollow tube; however, its structure is really much more complex. As you can see in **FIGURE 3.3**, there are several layers to this tube. The innermost layer, called the **mucosa**, is lined with glands and absorptive cells (epithelial cells). Layers of **circular muscle** and **longitudinal muscle** help mix and move the food we eat.

At points along the tract, where one organ connects with another (e.g., where the esophagus meets the stomach), the muscles are thicker and form **sphincters**. (See **FIGURE 3.4.**) A sphincter acts as a valve that controls the movement of food material so it travels through the GI tract in only one direction. By alternately contracting and relaxing, these muscular rings act like one-way doors, allowing the mixture of food and digestive juices to flow progressively along the GI tract into an organ but not back out.

Functional Organization	Anatomical Organization	Organ's Role in Digestion
Ingestion	Mouth	Breakdown of food. With the enzyme amylase, starch digestion begins here.
	Esophagus	Moves food from the mouth to the stomach.
Digestion and Absorption	Stomach	Secretes gastric juices and acid, which aid in digestion. Mixes food and converts it into liquid chyme. Kills pathogenic (disease-causing) bacteria that might have been ingested. Starts the digestion of protein. Starts the digestion of fat Secretes intrinsic factor which is necessary for vitamin B$_{12}$ absorption. Slowly releases chyme into the small intestine.
	Small intestine	Where the digestion of protein, fat, and carbohydrates is completed. Where the majority of nutrients are absorbed.
	Large intestine	Absorbs water and electrolytes. Forms and stores feces. Where most gut microbiota exist.
Assisting Organs	Salivary glands	Secrete saliva which moistens food, allowing for easier swallowing.
	Liver	Produces bile, which aids in the digestion and absorption of fat.
	Gallbladder	Stores and concentrates bile from the liver.
	Pancreas	Secretes enzymes that affect digestion and absorption. Releases hormones which help to regulate metabolism and how nutrients are used in the body.
Elimination	Rectum	Holds and releases feces via the anus.

FIGURE 3.2 Anatomical and functional organization of the GI tract. Although digestion begins in the mouth, most digestion occurs in the stomach and small intestine. Absorption takes place primarily in the small and large intestines.

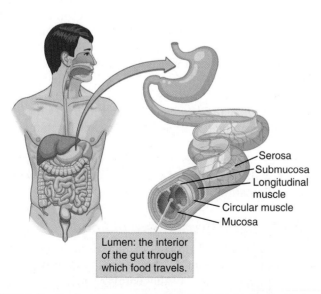

Serosa
Submucosa
Longitudinal muscle
Circular muscle
Mucosa

Lumen: the interior of the gut through which food travels.

FIGURE 3.3 Structural organization of the GI tract wall. Your intestinal tract is a long hollow tube lined with mucosal cells and surrounded by layers of muscle cells.

▶ **mucosa [myu-KO-sa]** The innermost layer of a cavity. The inner layer of the gastrointestinal tract (the intestinal wall). It is composed of epithelial cells and glands.

▶ **circular muscle** Layers of smooth muscle that surround organs, including the stomach and the small intestine.

▶ **longitudinal muscle** Muscle fibers aligned lengthwise.

▶ **sphincters [SFINGK-ters]** Circular bands of muscle fibers that surround the entrance or exit of a hollow body structure (e.g., the stomach) and act as valves to control the flow of material.

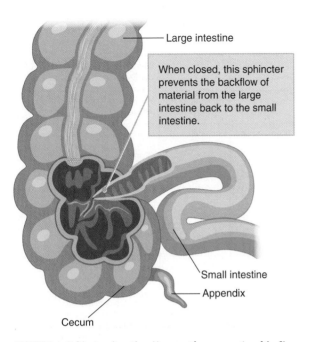

Large intestine

When closed, this sphincter prevents the backflow of material from the large intestine back to the small intestine.

Small intestine

Appendix

Cecum

FIGURE 3.4 Sphincters in action. Movement from one section of the GI tract to the next is controlled by muscular valves called sphincters.

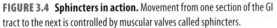

PERISTALSIS

Longitudinal (lengthwise) muscles relax while circular muscles contract, pushing the bolus ahead.

Relaxed longitudinal muscles

Contracted circular muscles

Bolus

Sphincter closed

Sphincter open

SEGMENTATION

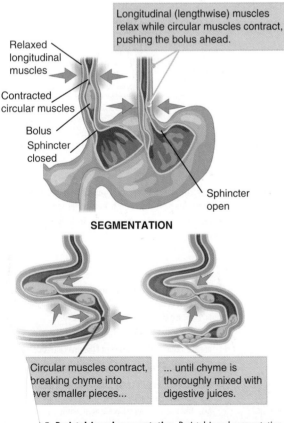

Circular muscles contract, breaking chyme into ever smaller pieces...

... until chyme is thoroughly mixed with digestive juices.

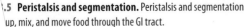

.5 Peristalsis and segmentation. Peristalsis and segmentation up, mix, and move food through the GI tract.

Key Concepts The gastrointestinal tract consists of the mouth, esophagus, stomach, small intestine, large intestine, and rectum. In the mouth, sensory responses to food stimulate other body systems and the organs along the GI tract. The functions of the GI tract are to ingest, digest, and absorb nutrients and to eliminate waste. The general structure of the GI tract consists of many layers, including the mucosa, the inner lining of glands, and absorptive cells. Sphincters are muscular valves along the GI tract that control movement from one part to the next.

Overview of Digestion: Physical and Chemical Processes

🍎 **Why Is This Important?** Both physical and chemical processes break down nutrients from food. It is important to know how the muscular contractions and digestive juices of the GI tract work together to turn food into smaller units for absorption.

The breakdown of food into smaller, absorbable nutrients involves both chemical and physical processes. The physical process comes first, as food is broken up into smaller pieces. Chewing starts the breakup, and muscular contractions of the GI tract continue it. As the GI tract breaks up food, it mixes the food with various secretions and moves the mixture (called **chyme**) along the tract. Enzymes, along with other chemicals, help complete the breakdown process and promote absorption of nutrients.

The Physical Movement and Breakdown of Food

Distinct muscular actions of the GI tract take the food on its long journey. From mouth to anus, waves of muscular contractions, called **peristalsis**, transport food and nutrients along the length of the GI tract. Peristaltic waves from the stomach muscles occur about three times per minute. In the small intestine, circular and longitudinal bands of muscle contract approximately every four to five seconds. Peristaltic contractions of the small intestine often are continuations of contractions that began in the stomach. The large intestine uses slow peristalsis to move the waste products of digestion (feces).

Segmentation, a series of muscular contractions that occur in the small intestine, divides and mixes the chyme. Every few centimeters along the gut wall, alternating constrictions "chop" the contents into smaller portions. Segmentation also increases absorption by bringing chyme into contact with the intestinal wall. **FIGURE 3.5** shows peristalsis and segmentation.

The Chemical Breakdown of Food

During the chemical process of digestion, enzymes divide nutrients into compounds small enough for absorption.

Enzymes are proteins that **catalyze**, or speed up, chemical reactions but are not themselves altered in the process. Enzymes act in part by bringing the reacting molecules close together. In digestion, these chemical reactions divide

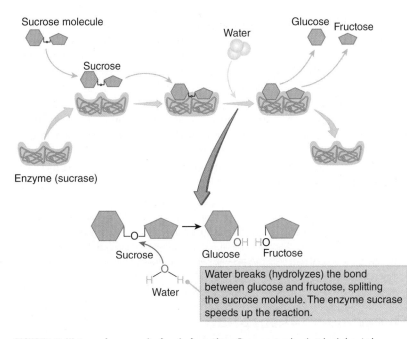

Sucrose molecule

Glucose Fructose

Water

Sucrose

Enzyme (sucrase)

Sucrose

Glucose   Fructose

Water

Water breaks (hydrolyzes) the bond between glucose and fructose, splitting the sucrose molecule. The enzyme sucrase speeds up the reaction.

FIGURE 3.6 Water and enzymes in chemical reactions. Enzymes speed up (catalyze) chemical reactions. When water breaks a chemical bond, the action is called hydrolysis.

substances into smaller compounds by a process called **hydrolysis** (breaking apart by water), as **FIGURE 3.6** shows. The function of most digestive enzymes can be identified by their names, which commonly end in –*ase* (amylase, lipase, and so on). For example, the enzyme needed to digest sucr*ose* is sucr*ase*.

▶ **chyme [KIME]** A mass of partially digested food and digestive juices moving from the stomach into the small intestine.

▶ **peristalsis [per-ih-STAHL-sis]** The wavelike, rhythmic muscular contractions of the GI tract that propel its contents down the tract.

▶ **segmentation** Periodic muscle contractions at intervals along the GI tract that alternate forward and backward movement of the contents, thereby breaking apart chunks of the food mass and mixing in digestive juices.

▶ **enzymes [EN-zimes]** Proteins in the body that speed up the rate of chemical reactions but are not altered in the process.

▶ **catalyze** To speed up a chemical reaction.

▶ **hydrolysis** A reaction that breaks apart a compound through the addition of water.

SALIVARY GLANDS

Secretion of lubricating fluid containing enzymes that break down carbohydrates

ORAL CAVITY, TEETH, TONGUE

Mechanical processing, moistening, mixing with salivary secretions

PHARYNX

Pharyngeal muscles propel materials into the esophagus

LIVER

Secretion of bile (important for lipid digestion), storage of nutrients, many other vital functions

ESOPHAGUS

Transport of materials to the stomach

GALLBLADDER

Storage and concentration of bile

STOMACH

Chemical breakdown of materials via acid and enzymes, mechanical processing through muscular contractions

LARGE INTESTINE

Dehydration and compaction of indigestible materials in preparation for elimination

PANCREAS

Exocrine cells secrete buffers and digestive enzymes, endocrine cells secrete hormones

SMALL INTESTINE

Enzymatic digestion and absorption of water, organic substrates vitamins, and ions

▶ **mucus** A slippery substance secreted in the GI tract (and other body linings) that protects cells from irritants.

In addition to enzymes, other chemicals are part of the digestive process. These include acid in the stomach, a neutralizing base in the small intestine, bile that prepares fat for digestion, and **mucus** secreted along the GI tract. This mucus does not break down food but lubricates it and protects the cells that line the GI tract from the strong digestive chemicals. Along the GI tract, fluids containing various enzymes and other substances are added to the consumed food. In fact, the digestive secretions (about 8 L/day) account for a much greater portion of the water that passes through and is absorbed by the GI tract than the water consumed in foods (about 1 L/day) and beverages (about 2–3 L/day).[2]

> **Key Concepts** Digestion involves both physical and chemical activity. Physical activity includes chewing and the movement of muscles along the GI tract that break food into smaller pieces and mix it with digestive secretions. Chemical digestion includes the breaking of bonds in nutrients, such as carbohydrates or proteins, to produce smaller units. Enzymes—proteins that encourage chemical processes—catalyze these reactions.

Overview of Absorption

🍎 **Why Is This Important?** Once food is broken down, it is ready to be absorbed. Describing the different absorptive processes is important for understanding how nutrients move from the GI tract into the body's circulation.

Food is broken apart during digestion and moved from the GI tract into circulation and on to the cells. Many of the nutrients—vitamins, minerals, and water—do not need to be digested before they are absorbed. But the energy-yielding nutrients—carbohydrate, fat, and protein—are too large to be absorbed intact and must be digested first. When ready for absorption, how are nutrients moved from the interior, or **lumen**, of the gut through the lining cells (mucosa) and into circulation?

The Roads to Nutrient Absorption

▶ **lumen** Cavity or hollow channel in any organ or structure of the body.

▶ **passive diffusion** The movement of substances into or out of cells without the expenditure of energy or the involvement of transport proteins in the cell membrane. Also called *simple diffusion*.

▶ **concentration gradients** Differences between the solute concentrations of two solutions.

▶ **facilitated diffusion** A process by which carrier (transport) proteins in the cell membrane transport substances into or out of cells down a concentration gradient.

Three main processes allow nutrients to be absorbed from the GI tract into circulation: passive diffusion, facilitated diffusion, and active transport. (See **FIGURE 3.7**.) Let's take a look at each one.

Passive diffusion is the movement of molecules through the cell membrane without the expenditure of energy. **Concentration gradients** (e.g., a high outside concentration and a low inside concentration of molecules) drive passive diffusion. Molecules cross permeable cell membranes as a result of random movements that tend to equalize the concentration of substances on both sides of a membrane. The larger the concentration of molecules on one side of the cell membrane, the faster those molecules move across the membrane to the area of lower concentration.

Because the cell membrane consists mainly of fat-soluble substances, it welcomes fats and other fat-soluble molecules. Oxygen, nitrogen, carbon dioxide, and alcohols are highly soluble in fat and readily dissolve in the cell membrane and diffuse across it. Although water crosses cell membranes easily, most water-soluble nutrients need additional help.

In **facilitated diffusion**, special protein carriers and channels help substances cross the cell membrane. The facilitating carriers are proteins that reside in the cell membrane. The diffusing molecule becomes lightly

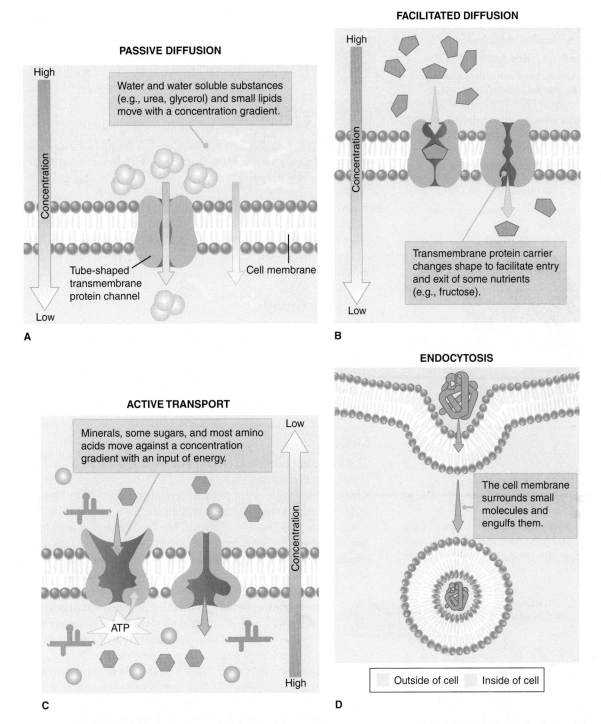

FIGURE 3.7 **a. Passive diffusion.** Using passive diffusion, some substances easily move into and out of cells, either through protein channels or directly through the cell membrane. **b. Facilitated diffusion.** Some substances need a little assistance to enter and exit cells. A transmembrane protein helps out by changing shape. **c. Active transport.** Some substances need a lot of assistance to enter cells. Just as in swimming upstream, energy is needed for the substance to get through an unfavorable concentration gradient. **d. Endocytosis.** Cells can use their cell membranes to engulf a particle and bring it inside the cell. The engulfing portion of the membrane separates from the cell wall and encases the particle in a vesicle.

bound to a protein channel that changes shape to open a pathway and allow diffusing molecules to enter or exit the cell.

Some substances need energy to move across a cell membrane, a process called **active transport.** Substances that usually require active transport across some cell membranes include many minerals, several sugars, and most amino acids (simple components of protein).

▶ **active transport** The movement of substances into or out of cells against a concentration gradient. Active transport requires energy (ATP) and involves carrier (transport) proteins in the cell membrane.

▶ **emulsifiers** Agents that blend fatty and watery liquids by promoting the breakup of fat into small particles and stabilizing their suspension in a watery solution.

▶ **salivary glands** Glands in the mouth that release saliva.

▶ **liver** The largest glandular organ in the body, it produces and secretes bile, detoxifies harmful substances, and helps metabolize carbohydrates, lipids, proteins, and micronutrients.

▶ **bile** An alkaline, yellow-green fluid that is produced in the liver and stored in the gallbladder. Bile emulsifies dietary fats, aiding fat digestion and absorption.

▶ **enterohepatic circulation [EN-ter-oh-heh-PAT-ik]** Recycling of certain compounds between the small intestine and the liver.

▶ **excretion** The process of separating and removing waste products of metabolism.

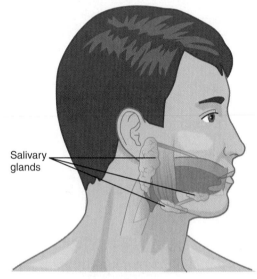

FIGURE 3.8 The salivary glands. The three pairs of salivary glands supply saliva, which moistens and lubricates food. Saliva also contains salivary enzymes that begin the digestion of starch.

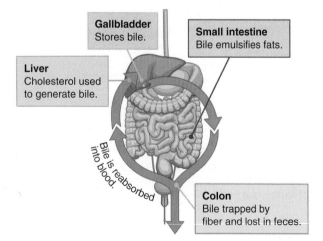

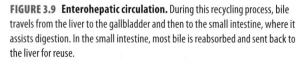

FIGURE 3.9 Enterohepatic circulation. During this recycling process, bile travels from the liver to the gallbladder and then to the small intestine, where it assists digestion. In the small intestine, most bile is reabsorbed and sent back to the liver for reuse.

Key Concepts Absorption through the GI cell membranes occurs by one of three basic processes. In passive diffusion, nutrients such as water permeate the intestinal wall without a carrier or energy expenditure. In facilitated diffusion, a protein carrier helps bring substances into the absorptive intestinal cell without expending energy. Active transport requires energy to transport a substance across a cell membrane.

Accessory Organs

🍎 **Why Is This Important?** There are many organs that assist the GI tract in digestion and absorption. Explaining how the accessory organs work together to break down food is important to understanding the digestive system.

Although food does not pass through them, the accessory organs—the salivary glands, liver, gallbladder, and pancreas—all have critical roles in the digestive process. The GI tract works together with these organs, which assist digestion by providing fluid, acid neutralizers, enzymes, and **emulsifiers**.

Salivary Glands

We have three pairs of **salivary glands**, located in or near the mouth, that secrete saliva into the oral cavity. (See **FIGURE 3.8**.) Saliva moistens food, lubricating it for easy swallowing. Saliva also contains enzymes that begin the process of chemical digestion. We secrete approximately 1,500 milliliters (about 1 1/2 quarts) of saliva each day. The mere sight, smell, or thought of food can start the flow of saliva.

Liver

The **liver** produces and secretes 600 to 1,000 milliliters of bile daily. **Bile** is a yellow-green, pasty material that helps digest fat. It contains water, bile salts and acids, pigments, cholesterol, phospholipids (a type of fat molecule), and electrolytes (electrically charged minerals). Bile tastes bitter, which is why the word *bile* has come to denote bitterness. Bile acts as an emulsifier by reducing large globs of fat to smaller globs, similar to how dish soap separates a layer of fat into smaller particles.

This process of emulsification breaks no bonds in fat molecules, but rather increases the surface area of fat, allowing more contact between fat molecules and enzymes in the small intestine. Emulsification makes fat digestion more efficient.

Bile is stored and concentrated in your gallbladder, which releases it to the small intestine on demand. After bile has done its work, most is reabsorbed and returned to the liver for recycling. This recirculation is known as the **enterohepatic circulation** (*entero* meaning "intestines," *hepatic* referring to the liver) of bile. (See **FIGURE 3.9**.)

The liver also is a detoxification center that filters toxic substances from the blood and alters their chemical form. These altered substances may be sent to the kidneys for **excretion** or carried by bile to the small intestine and removed from the body in feces. The liver is analogous to a chemical factory; it performs over 500 chemical functions, including the production of blood proteins, cholesterol, and sugars. The liver also is like an active warehouse, because it stores vitamins, hormones, minerals, and sugars, and it releases them into the bloodstream as needed.

Gallbladder

The primary function of the **gallbladder** is to store and concentrate bile from the liver. The gallbladder is a small, muscular, pear-shaped sac nestled in a depression on the right underside of the liver. This organ holds about a quarter of a cup of bile and is the storage stop for bile between the liver and the small intestine. The gallbladder fills with bile and thickens it until a hormone released after eating signals the gallbladder to squirt out its contents.

The gallbladder is normally relaxed and full between meals. When dietary fats enter the small intestine, they trigger the contraction of the gallbladder. Like a squeeze bulb, the gallbladder squirts bile through the common bile duct into the upper part of the small intestine. The common bile duct also carries digestive enzymes from the pancreas.

▶ **gallbladder** A pear-shaped sac that stores and concentrates bile from the liver.

Pancreas

The **pancreas** secretes enzymes that affect the digestion and absorption of nutrients in the small intestine. During the course of a day, the pancreas secretes about 1,500 milliliters of fluid, which contains mostly water, bicarbonate, and digestive enzymes. The pancreas also releases hormones that are involved in other aspects of nutrient use by the body. For example, the pancreatic hormones insulin and glucagon regulate blood glucose levels. The combination of these two functions makes the pancreas one of the most important organs in the digestion and use of food.

▶ **pancreas** An organ that secretes enzymes that affect the digestion and absorption of nutrients and that releases hormones, such as insulin, that regulate metabolism as well as the way nutrients are used in the body.

> **Key Concepts** The salivary glands, liver, gallbladder, and pancreas all make important contributions to the digestive process. The salivary glands release saliva, which contains mucus and enzymes, into the mouth. The liver produces bile, which is stored in the gallbladder and released into the small intestine, where the bile then helps to prepare fats for digestion. The pancreas secretes liquid that contains bicarbonate and several types of enzymes into the small intestine.

Putting It All Together: Digestion and Absorption

🍎 **Why Is This Important?** Understanding how the digestive system turns the foods we eat into the nutrients used by our body for growth, development, and maintenance is the foundation for learning about human nutrition.

Up to this point, we have focused on structures, mechanisms, and processes to give you a general idea of the workings of the GI tract. Now you're ready for a complete tour—a journey along the GI tract—to see what happens and how digestion and absorption are accomplished.

Mouth

As soon as you put food in your mouth the digestive process begins. As you chew, you break down the food into smaller pieces, increasing the surface area available to enzymes. Saliva contains the enzyme **salivary amylase**, which breaks down starch into small sugar molecules. Food remains in the mouth for just a short time, so only about 5 percent of the starch is completely broken down. The next time you eat a cracker or a piece of bread, chew slowly and notice the change in the way it tastes. It gets sweeter. That's the salivary amylase breaking down the starch into sugar. Salivary amylase continues to work until the strong acid content of the stomach deactivates it. To start the process of fat digestion, the cells at the base of the tongue secrete another

THINK About It 3

▶ **salivary amylase [AM-ih-lace]** An enzyme that catalyzes the hydrolysis of amylose, a starch. Also called *ptyalin*.

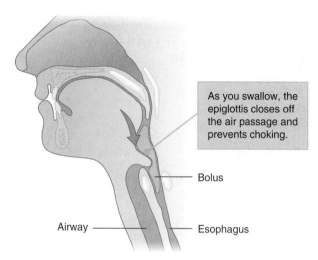

FIGURE 3.10 Swallowing. Your epiglottis didn't completely do its job if you have ever choked on a drink that went "down the wrong pipe."

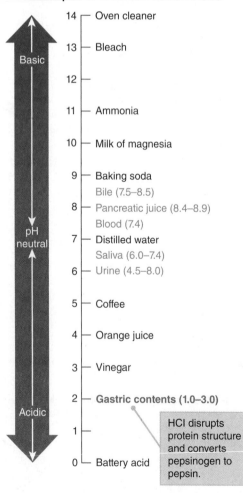

FIGURE 3.11 The pH scale. Because pancreatic juice has a pH around 8, it can neutralize the acidic chyme, which leaves the stomach with a pH around 2.

enzyme, **lingual lipase**. The overall impact of lingual lipase on fat digestion, though, is small.

Saliva and other fluids, including mucus, blend with the food to form a **bolus**, a chewed, moistened lump of food that is soft and easy to swallow. When you swallow, the bolus slides past the epiglottis—a valve-like flap of tissue that closes off your air passages so you don't choke. The bolus then moves rapidly through the **esophagus** to the stomach, where it will be digested further. **FIGURE 3.10** shows the process of swallowing.

Stomach

The bolus enters the **stomach** through the **esophageal sphincter**, also called the cardiac sphincter, which immediately closes to keep the bolus from sliding back into the esophagus. This sphincter needs to close quickly and completely to prevent the acidic stomach contents from backing up into the esophagus, causing the pain and tissue damage called **heartburn**.

Nutrient Digestion in the Stomach

The stomach cells produce secretions that are collectively called gastric juice. Included in this mixture are water, hydrochloric acid, mucus, pepsinogen (the inactive form of the enzyme pepsin), the enzyme gastric lipase, the hormone gastrin, and intrinsic factor.

- **Hydrochloric acid (gastric acid)** makes the stomach contents extremely acidic—dropping the **pH** to 2, compared to a neutral pH of 7. (See the pH scale in **FIGURE 3.11**.) This acidic environment kills many pathogenic (disease-causing) bacteria that may have been ingested and also aids in the digestion of protein. Mucus secreted by the stomach cells coats the stomach lining, protecting these cells from damage by the strong gastric juice.
- Hydrochloric acid works in protein digestion in two ways. First, it demolishes the functional, three-dimensional shape of proteins, unfolding them into linear chains; this increases their vulnerability to attacking enzymes. Second, it promotes the breakdown of proteins by converting **pepsinogen**, an enzyme **precursor**, to **pepsin**, its active form.
- Pepsin then begins breaking the links in protein chains, cutting dietary proteins into smaller and smaller pieces.
- Stomach cells also produce an enzyme called **gastric lipase**. It has a minor role in the digestion of lipids, specifically butterfat.
- **Gastrin**, another component of gastric juice, is a hormone that stimulates gastric secretion and movement.
- **Intrinsic factor** is a substance necessary for the absorption of vitamin B_{12} that occurs farther down the GI tract, near the end of the small intestine. In the absence of intrinsic factor, only about one-fiftieth of ingested vitamin B_{12} is absorbed.

Recall that salivary amylase begins to break down carbohydrates in the mouth. After you swallow, salivary amylase continues its work to digest carbohydrates. About an hour later, acidic stomach secretions become well mixed with the food. This increases the acidity of the food and effectively blocks further salivary amylase activity.

Do you sometimes feel your stomach churning? The stomach works to continue mixing food with GI secretions and produces the semiliquid chyme. To accomplish this, the stomach has an extra layer of muscles. These diagonal muscles, along with the circular and longitudinal muscles, contract and relax to mix food completely. The bolus of food is ground to a size of less than 2 mm in diameter to easily pass into the small intestine.[3] The stomach slowly releases the chyme through the **pyloric sphincter** and into the small intestine, normally at a rate of 2 mL/min.[4] When closed, the pyloric sphincter prevents the chyme from returning to the stomach. (See **FIGURE 3.12**.)

The stomach normally empties in one to four hours, depending on the types and amounts of food eaten. Carbohydrates speed through the stomach in the shortest time, followed by protein and fat. Thus, the higher the fat content of a meal, the longer it will take to leave the stomach.

Nutrient Absorption in the Stomach

Although much digestion has been accomplished by the time chyme leaves the stomach, very little absorption has occurred. The stomach absorbs weak acids, such as alcohol and aspirin, and only a few fat-soluble compounds. Chyme moves on to the small intestine, the digestive and absorptive workhorse of the gut.

▶ **lingual lipase** A fat-splitting enzyme secreted by cells at the base of the tongue.

▶ **bolus [BOH-lus]** A chewed, moistened lump of food that is ready to be swallowed.

▶ **esophagus [ee-SOFF-uh-gus]** The food pipe that extends from the pharynx to the stomach.

▶ **stomach** The enlarged, muscular, saclike portion of the digestive tract between the esophagus and the small intestine, with a capacity of about 1 quart.

▶ **esophageal sphincter** The opening between the esophagus and the stomach that relaxes and opens to allow the bolus to travel into the stomach, and then closes behind it. Acts as a barrier to prevent the reflux of gastric contents. Also called the *cardiac sphincter*.

▶ **heartburn** Burning pain behind the breastbone area caused by acidic stomach contents backing up into the esophagus.

▶ **hydrochloric acid (gastric acid)** A very strong acid of chloride and hydrogen atoms made by stomach glands and secreted into the stomach. Also called *gastric acid*.

▶ **pH** A measurement of the hydrogen ion concentration, or acidity, of a solution.

▶ **pepsinogen** The inactive form of the enzyme pepsin.

▶ **precursor** A substance that is converted into another active substance. Enzyme precursors also are called *proenzymes*.

▶ **pepsin** A protein-digesting enzyme produced by the stomach.

▶ **gastric lipase** An enzyme in the stomach that primarily breaks down butterfat.

▶ **gastrin [GAS-trin]** A hormone released from the walls of the stomach and duodenum that stimulates gastric secretions and motility.

▶ **intrinsic factor** A glycoprotein released from parietal cells in the stomach wall that binds to and aids in absorption of vitamin B_{12}.

▶ **pyloric sphincter** A circular muscle that forms the opening between the duodenum and the stomach. It regulates the passage of food into the small intestine.

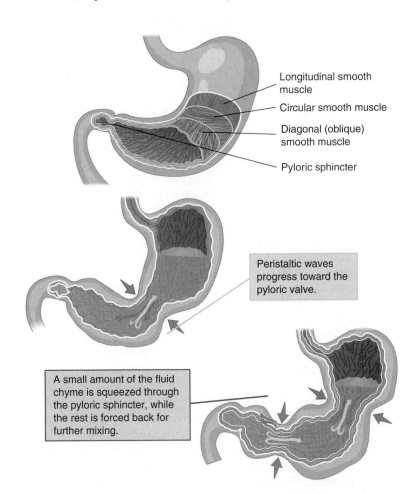

Longitudinal smooth muscle

Circular smooth muscle

Diagonal (oblique) smooth muscle

Pyloric sphincter

Peristaltic waves progress toward the pyloric valve.

A small amount of the fluid chyme is squeezed through the pyloric sphincter, while the rest is forced back for further mixing.

FIGURE 3.12 The stomach. The stomach churns and mixes food with stomach secretions. Hydrochloric acid unfolds proteins and stops salivary amylase action while pepsin begins protein digestion. The pyloric sphincter controls movement of chyme from the stomach to the small intestine.

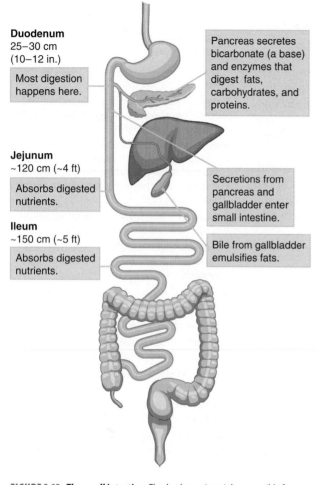

Duodenum
25–30 cm
(10–12 in.)

Most digestion happens here.

Pancreas secretes bicarbonate (a base) and enzymes that digest fats, carbohydrates, and proteins.

Jejunum
~120 cm (~4 ft)

Absorbs digested nutrients.

Secretions from pancreas and gallbladder enter small intestine.

Ileum
~150 cm (~5 ft)

Absorbs digested nutrients.

Bile from gallbladder emulsifies fats.

FIGURE 3.13 The small intestine. The duodenum is mainly responsible for digesting food; the jejunum and ileum primarily deal with the absorption of nutrients. In addition to receiving the digestive juices from accessory organs, the duodenum secretes mucus, enzymes, and hormones to aid digestion. All along the intestinal walls, nutrients are absorbed into blood and lymph. Undigested materials are passed on to the large intestine.

▶ **small intestine** Where the digestion of protein, fat, and carbohydrate is completed and where the majority of nutrients are absorbed. The small intestine is approximately 3 meters [10 ft] long and is divided into three parts: the duodenum, the jejunum, and the ileum.

▶ **duodenum [doo-oh-DEE-num]** The portion of the small intestine closest to the stomach. The duodenum is 25 to 30 cm (10 to 12 in.) long and wider than the remainder of the small intestine.

▶ **jejunum [je-JOON-um]** The middle section (about 4 feet or 122 cm) of the small intestine, lying between the duodenum and ileum.

▶ **ileum [ILL-ee-um]** The terminal segment (about 5 feet or 152 cm) of the small intestine, which opens into the large intestine.

▶ **digestive secretions** Substances released at different places in the GI tract to speed the breakdown of ingested carbohydrates, fats, and proteins.

▶ **villi** Small fingerlike projections that blanket the folds in the lining of the small intestine. Singular is *villus*.

Small Intestine

The **small intestine** completes the digestion of protein, fat, and nearly all carbohydrates, and it absorbs most nutrients. As you can see in **FIGURE 3.13**, the small intestine is a tube approximately 3 meters long (about 10 feet), divided into three parts:

- **Duodenum** (the first 25 to 30 centimeters—10 to 12 inches)
- **Jejunum** (about 120 centimeters—about 4 feet)
- **Ileum** (about 150 centimeters—about 5 feet)

Most digestion occurs in the duodenum, where the small intestine receives **digestive secretions** from the pancreas, gallbladder, and its own glands. The remainder of the small intestine primarily absorbs previously digested nutrients.

Nutrient Digestion in the Small Intestine

In the duodenum, bicarbonate from the pancreas neutralizes the acidic chyme from the stomach. This is important because the enzymes of the small intestine need a more neutral environment to work effectively. Pancreatic juice contains a variety of digestive enzymes that help to digest fats, carbohydrates, and proteins. Secretions from the intestinal wall cells add enzymes to complete carbohydrate digestion.

The presence of fat in the duodenum stimulates the release of stored bile by the gallbladder. Lipids ordinarily do not mix with water, but bile acts as an emulsifier, keeping lipid molecules mixed with the watery chyme and digestive secretions. Without the action of bile, lipids might not come into contact with pancreatic lipase, and digestion would be incomplete.

With the pancreatic and intestinal enzymes working together, digestion progresses nicely, leaving smaller protein, carbohydrate, and lipid compounds ready for absorption. Other nutrients, such as vitamins, minerals, and cholesterol, are not digested and generally are absorbed unchanged. Most of the dietary fat, carbohydrates, and protein are completely digested and absorbed in the small intestine.

Just as the small intestine accomplishes much of the nutrient digestion, it is also responsible for most nutrient absorption. Its structure makes the process of absorption efficient and complete. In most cases, more than 90 percent of ingested carbohydrate, fat, and protein gets absorbed. To see how this is possible, we need to examine the structure of the small intestine.

Absorptive Structures of the Small Intestine

The small intestine packs a gigantic surface area into a small space. As you can see in **FIGURE 3.14**, the interior surface of the small intestine is wrinkled into folds, tripling the absorptive surface area. These folds are carpeted with fingerlike projections called **villi** that expand the absorptive area another 10-fold. Each cell lining the surface of each villus is covered with a "brush border" containing as many as 1,000 hair-like projections called **microvilli**. The microvilli increase the surface area another 20 times. Taken together, the folds plus the villi and microvilli yield a

600-fold increase in surface area. In fact, your 10-foot-long (3-meter-long) small intestine has an absorptive surface area of more than 300 square yards (more than 250 square meters)—equivalent to the surface of a tennis court!

Nutrient Absorption in the Small Intestine

As nutrients journey through the small intestine, they are trapped in the folds and projections of the intestinal wall and absorbed through the microvilli into the lining cells. Depending on your diet, each day your small intestine absorbs several hundred grams of carbohydrates, 60 or more grams of fat, 50 to 100 grams of amino acids, and 7 to 8 liters of water. But the total absorptive capacity of the healthy small intestine is far greater. Approximately 85 percent of the water absorption by the gut takes place in the jejunum and ileum.[5]

Nutrients absorbed through the intestinal lining pass into the interior of the villi. Each villus contains blood vessels (veins, arteries, and capillaries) and a **lymph** vessel (known as a **lacteal**) that transport nutrients to other parts of your body. Water-soluble nutrients are absorbed directly into the bloodstream. Fat-soluble lipid compounds are absorbed into the lymph rather than directly into the blood. Most vitamin absorption takes place in the small intestine, but although water-soluble vitamins are absorbed easily, often less than half of dietary fat-soluble vitamins get absorbed.[6] Unlike other nutrients, the absorption of some minerals is regulated by the level of reserves in the body to prevent toxicity. Additionally, minerals can compete for absorption, and the absorption of one mineral can decrease the absorption of another.

The small intestine suffers constant wear and tear as it propels and digests the chyme. The intestinal lining is renewed continually as the mucosal cells are replaced every two to five days. When the chyme has completed its 3- to 10-hour journey through the small intestine, it passes through the ileocecal valve, the connection to the large intestine.

Large Intestine

The chyme's next stop is the **large intestine**. As **FIGURE 3.15** shows, this 5-foot-long tube includes the **cecum**, **colon**, **rectum**, and anal canal. As chyme fills the cecum, a local reflex signals the ileocecal valve to close, preventing material from reentering the ileum of the small intestine.

Digestion in the Large Intestine

The peristaltic movements of the large intestine are sluggish compared with those of the small intestine. Normally 18 to 24 hours are required for material to travel its length. During that time, the colon's large population of bacteria digests small amounts of fiber,[7] providing a negligible number of calories daily. Other substances formed by this bacterial activity—including several vitamins, short-chain fatty acids, and various gases—can contribute to **flatulence**. Other than bacterial action, no further digestion occurs in the large intestine.

Nutrient Absorption in the Large Intestine

Nutrient absorption in the large intestine is minimal, limited to water, sodium, chloride, potassium, and some of the vitamin K

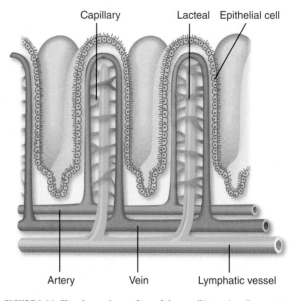

Capillary   Lacteal   Epithelial cell

Artery   Vein   Lymphatic vessel

FIGURE 3.14 The absorptive surface of the small intestine. To maximize the absorptive surface area, the small intestine is folded and lined with villi. You have a surface area the size of a tennis court packed into your gut.

▶ **microvilli** Minute, hairlike projections that extend from the surface of absorptive cells facing the intestinal lumen.

▶ **lymph** Fluid that travels through the lymphatic system, made up of fluid drained from between cells and large fat particles.

▶ **lacteal** A small lymphatic vessel in the interior of each intestinal villus that picks up chylomicrons and fat-soluble vitamins from intestinal cells.

▶ **large intestine** The tube (about 5 feet or 152 cm long) extending from the ileum of the small intestine to the anus. The large intestine includes the appendix, cecum, colon, rectum, and anal canal.

▶ **cecum** The blind pouch at the beginning of the large intestine into which the ileum opens from one side and that is continuous with the colon.

▶ **colon** The portion of the large intestine extending from the cecum to the rectum. It is made up of four parts: the ascending, transverse, descending, and sigmoid colons.

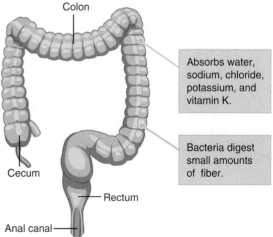

Colon

Absorbs water, sodium, chloride, potassium, and vitamin K.

Bacteria digest small amounts of fiber.

Cecum

Rectum

Anal canal

FIGURE 3.15 The large intestine. As the large intestine absorbs water, it forms undigested materials into feces for elimination.

▶ **rectum** The muscular final segment of the intestine, extending from the sigmoid colon to the anus.

▶ **flatulence** The presence of excessive amounts of air or other gases in the stomach or intestines.

produced by intestinal bacteria. Although the colon's bacteria also produce vitamin B_{12}, it is not absorbed. The colon dehydrates the watery chyme, removing and absorbing most of the fluid. Of the approximately 1,000 milliliters of material that enters the large intestine, only about 150 milliliters remain for elimination as feces. The semisolid feces, consisting of roughly 60 percent solid matter (e.g., dietary fiber, bacteria, digestive secretions) and 40 percent water, then pass into the rectum. In the rectum, strong muscles hold back the waste until it is time to defecate. The rectal muscles then relax, and the anal sphincter opens to allow passage of the stool out the anal canal. **FIGURE 3.16** summarizes nutrient absorption along the gastrointestinal tract.

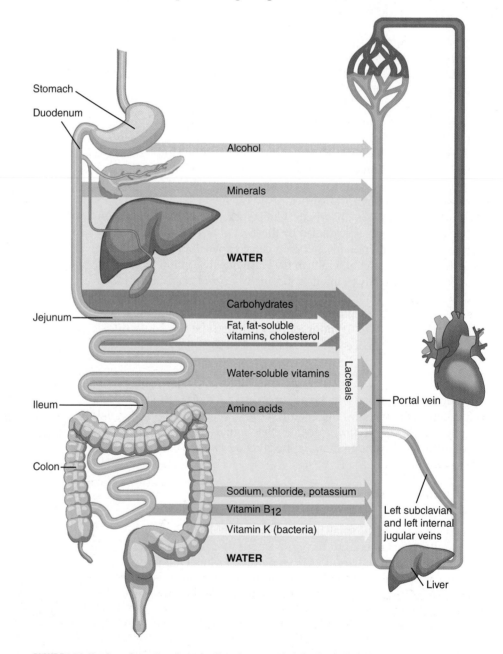

FIGURE 3.16 Nutrient absorption along the digestive tract. Alcohol is absorbed quickly in the stomach. The small intestine is the absorptive site for carbohydrate, amino acids, fats, and most vitamins. Absorption of some vitamins and minerals takes place in the large intestine. Both the small and large intestines absorb water.

Gut Microbiota

The human gastrointestinal tract contains microorganisms—including bacteria, fungi and viruses—collectively called the **gut microbiota**. In fact, there are 100 trillion bacterial cells (representing more than 1,000 species) in the human intestines.[8] The majority of these microorganisms live in the colon, where the ileocecal valve prevents the movement of colon-dwelling microbes into the small intestine. The intestinal mucosal layer also provides a layer of protection between the contents of the gut and the body's circulation.

A healthy gut flora is largely responsible for the overall health of the host.[9] Gut microbiota are able to interact with each other and the human host in mutually beneficial processes of energy metabolism and in facilitating chemical reactions. For example, gut microbiota extract energy from dietary compounds that are not digestible by the human gut, synthesize essential vitamins, and provide immune benefits to their human hosts.[10] Gut microbiota are currently being investigated for their role in the development and prevention of metabolic diseases, including obesity and glucose regulation.[11,12] Some types of gut bacteria may even produce compounds that reduce risk of colon cancer; for example, acids produced by colon bacteria change the pH of the colon, which may interfere with the development of cancer.

The relationship between humans and their gut microbiota is not always beneficial, however. Some species of bacteria can cause infections or even produce cancer-causing substances, emphasizing the need for a healthy balance of intestinal microorganisms. The types of microbiota in the gut are influenced by age, what we eat, and the medicines we take. Antibiotics used to treat bacterial infections can disrupt a healthy balance of gut microbiota for two to four years.[13]

Probiotics and **prebiotics** affect the microbiota of the gut in specific ways to provide health benefits. The key difference between probiotics and prebiotics are that probiotics are living microbes in the diet, whereas prebiotics can be thought of as the "food" for the probiotics. Prebiotics are nondigestible substances in foods, such as certain types of plant fiber, that are fermented by gut bacteria. They have been shown to increase the number of beneficial bacteria in the human gut.[14] Together, prebiotics and probiotics promote a balance of intestinal bacteria for a healthy gut microbiota, boost immunity, and improve general health, especially that of the digestive system. (See the FYI feature "Microbiota Out of Whack? Pre- and Probiotics May Help.")

▶ **gut microbiota** The population of microorganisms living in the digestive tract.

▶ **probiotics** Living microorganisms that provide health benefits when ingested, either directly through interactions with host cells or indirectly through effects on other bacterial species. Also known as *live cultures*.

▶ **prebiotics** Natural, nondigestible components of food that promote the growth of healthy bacteria in the gut and overall health.

Quick **Bite**

The Clever Colon
Although it has been presumed that the colon has no digestive function, research shows that the human colon can be an important digestive site. Fiber and other undigested carbohydrates are metabolized by bacteria living in the colon. The products of this fermentation process can be absorbed to nourish the cells of the colon and may even affect the whole body's nutrition and metabolic processes.

Key Concepts Digestion begins in the mouth with the action of salivary amylase. Food material next moves down the esophagus to the stomach, where it mixes with gastric secretions. Protein digestion begins with the action of pepsin, while salivary amylase action ceases due to the low pH level of the stomach. The liquid material (chyme) next moves to the small intestine. Here, secretions from the gallbladder, pancreas, and intestinal lining cells complete the digestion of carbohydrates, proteins, and fats. The end products of digestion, along with vitamins, minerals, water, and other compounds, are absorbed through the intestinal wall and into circulation. Undigested material and some liquid move on to the large intestine, where water and electrolytes are absorbed, leaving waste material to be excreted as feces. Gut microbiota function as part of the intestinal ecosystem, interacting with the rest of the body in numerous metabolic and nutritional roles.

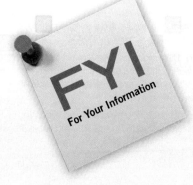

Gut Microbiota Out of Whack? Pre- and Probiotics May Help

Have you ever wondered why your doctor recommended eating yogurt with "live active cultures" while you took a course of antibiotics? Perhaps she said it would help prevent an upset stomach or constipation. What's the connection? Antibiotics may kill the nasty bacteria causing your strep throat or other infection, but are likely to kill many of your helpful gut microbiota as well. The reason your doctor recommended the yogurt was to boost the number of "good guys" in your gut after their knockdown by the antibiotic drug. Many types of bacteria found in yogurt are categorized as probiotics, and most fall into one of two groups: *Lactobacillus* and *Bifidobacterium*. Probiotics can be helpful in other situations besides when you are taking antibiotics. For example, studies in young children show that supplementation with *Lactobacillus* reduced the severity and duration of diarrhea caused by rotavirus, a common infectious agent in daycare centers.

Feeding the bacteria in your gut with *prebiotics* can also improve your health. Encouraging the growth of helpful bacteria allows them to outnumber (and out-eat) disease-causing bacteria, thus reducing the likelihood of foodborne illness and other infections. In addition, some prebiotics have been shown to enhance absorption of calcium and magnesium. Other prebiotics inhibit growth of lesions in the gut, which in turn reduces colorectal cancer risk. Lipid-lowering effects have also been attributed to prebiotics; however, the limited data available show inconsistent effects on cholesterol and triglycerides.

So, how can you incorporate more pre- and probiotics in your diet? Fermented milk products such as yogurt, kefir, or aged cheeses are good sources; nondairy products such as miso, pickles, sauerkraut, and kimchi are good sources, too. In yogurts, look for a seal adopted by the National Yogurt Association to identify products that contain a minimum of 100 million live lactic acid bacteria per gram of yogurt. Not all brands of yogurt contain live, active cultures. Probiotics also can be taken as a dietary supplement. However, probiotics in supplement form must have sufficient numbers of live bacteria to be useful; currently, identification and standardization procedures are lacking. Probiotics occur naturally in onions, garlic, tomatoes, asparagus, soybeans, bananas, and whole-wheat foods.

Prebiotics are the subject of intense and promising research. Although results are preliminary, food and supplement sources of prebiotics may be another useful way to improve gut microbiota and overall health. Common prebiotics include inulin fiber from chicory root, leeks, onions, garlic, banana, plantains, wheat, and resistant starches (fibers that resist digestion) from oats, legumes, potatoes, and rice.

Circulation of Nutrients

🍎 **Why Is This Important?** Once nutrients are absorbed into the bloodstream, they have to reach their intended destination in the body. This occurs by the process of circulation in the blood or the lymph system, depending on the nutrient being transported.

After foods are digested and nutrients are absorbed, they are transported via the vascular and lymphatic systems to specific destinations throughout the body. Let's take a closer look at how each of these circulatory systems delivers nutrients to the places they are needed.

Vascular System

▶ **vascular system** A network of veins and arteries through which the blood carries nutrients. Also called the *blood circulatory system*.

The **vascular system**, or blood circulatory system, is a network of veins and arteries through which the blood carries nutrients. (See **FIGURE 3.17**.) The heart is the pump that keeps the blood circulating through the body. Water-soluble nutrients are absorbed directly from intestinal cells into tiny capillary tributaries of the bloodstream, which carries them to the liver before they are dispersed throughout the body. Blood carries oxygen from the lungs and nutrients from the GI system to all body

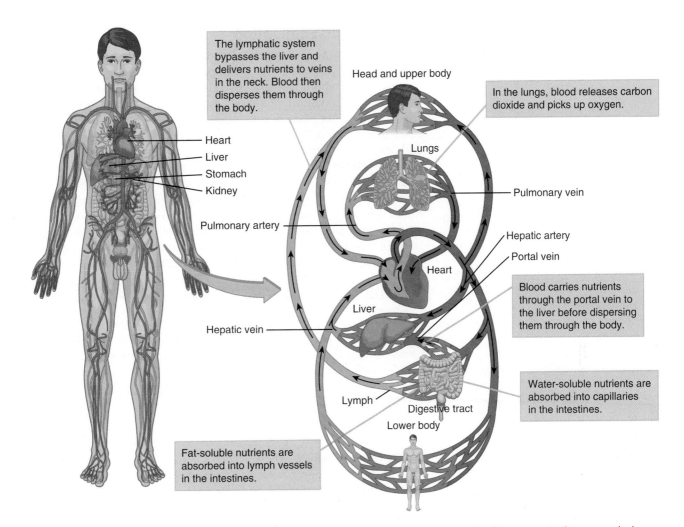

FIGURE 3.17 Circulation. Blood carries oxygen from the lungs and nutrients from the GI system to all body tissues. The lymphatic system, a circulatory system that bypasses the liver before connecting to the bloodstream, carries fat-soluble nutrients.

tissues. Once the destination cells have used the oxygen and nutrients, carbon dioxide and waste products are picked up by the blood and transported to the lungs and kidneys, respectively, for excretion.

Lymphatic System

The **lymphatic system** is a network of vessels that drain lymph, the clear fluid formed in the spaces between cells. Lymph moves through this system and eventually empties into the bloodstream near the neck. Lymph vessels in the small intestine carry fat-soluble nutrients and most end products of fat digestion. After a fatty meal, lymph can become as much as 1 to 2 percent fat. Nutrients absorbed into the lymphatic system, unlike those absorbed directly into the vascular system, bypass the liver before entering the bloodstream.

Unlike the vascular system, the lymphatic system has no pumping organ. The major lymph vessels contain one-way valves; when the vessels are filled with lymph, smooth muscles in the vessel walls contract and pump the lymph forward. The succession of valves allows each segment of the vessel to act as an independent pump. Lymph also is moved along by skeletal muscle contractions that squeeze the vessels.

▶ **lymphatic system** A system of small vessels, ducts, valves, and organized tissue (e.g., lymph nodes) through which lymph moves from its origin in the tissues toward the heart.

Excretion and Elimination

Excretion regulates the concentrations of minerals and other substances in the body and removes the waste products of metabolism. Do not confuse the metabolic waste removed by excretion with digestive waste removed by elimination. Metabolic waste arises from all the chemical reactions that take place in cells throughout the body. Digestive waste never passes into cells—it is the unabsorbed "leftovers" that pass along and out of the GI tract.

The primary organs of excretion are the lungs and kidneys. The lungs excrete water and carbon dioxide. The kidneys filter the blood and excrete substances to remove waste and maintain the body's water and ion balance. The kidneys excrete salts, nitrogen-containing wastes such as urea, small amounts of other substances, and water. This watery mix is called urine. The kidneys vary the amount and concentration of urine to help maintain constant physiological conditions within the body.

> **Key Concepts** Absorbed nutrients are carried by either the vascular or lymphatic system. Water-soluble nutrients are absorbed directly into the bloodstream, carried to the liver, and then distributed around the body. Fat-soluble vitamins and large lipid molecules are absorbed into the lymphatic vessels and carried by this system before entering the vascular system. The main excretory organs are the lungs and kidneys. The lungs excrete carbon dioxide and water. The kidneys excrete salts, metabolic wastes, and water.

Signaling Systems: Command, Control, and Defense

> 🍎 **Why Is This Important?** The process of digestion, absorption, and transport of nutrients is controlled by the nervous system through signals and messengers. The GI tract also plays an important role in defending the body from potential sources of infection.

How does your body keep the complex processes of digestion, absorption, and nutrient transport running smoothly? The nervous system, your body's communication network, carries commands and feedback to and from tissues throughout the body. Signals delivered by the nervous system can trigger the release of hormones—chemical messengers that control and coordinate biological activities. The gastrointestinal tract also is a major player in your immune system, a coordinated system of cells and tissues that defends against invading microorganisms.

Nervous System

Nerves carry information back and forth between tissues and the brain. Chemicals called neurotransmitters send signals to either excite or suppress nerves, thereby stimulating or inhibiting activity in various parts of the body.

The **central nervous system (CNS)** regulates GI activity in two ways. The **enteric nervous system** is a local system of nerves in the gut wall that is stimulated both by the chemical composition of chyme and by the stretching of the GI lumen that results from food in the GI tract. This stimulation leads to nerve impulses that enhance secretions and muscle movement along the tract. The enteric nervous system plays an essential role in controlling movement, blood flow, water and electrolyte transport, and acid secretion in the GI tract. A branch of the **autonomic nervous system** (the portion of the CNS that controls organ function) responds to the sight, smell, and thought of food. This branch of the

▶ **central nervous system (CNS)** The brain and the spinal cord. The central nervous system transmits signals that control muscular actions and glandular secretions along the entire GI tract.

▶ **enteric nervous system** A network of nerves located in the gastrointestinal wall.

▶ **autonomic nervous system (ANS)** The part of the central nervous system that regulates the automatic responses of the body; consists of the sympathetic and parasympathetic systems.

CNS carries signals to and from the GI tract through the vagus nerve and enhances GI motility and secretion. In the past, treatments for some ulcers and other GI ailments included severing the vagus nerve, a measure that brought temporary, but not long-term, relief from pain.

Hormonal System

Hormones also are involved in GI regulation. Hormones are chemical messengers that generally are produced at one location and travel in the bloodstream to affect another location in the body. Gastrointestinal hormonal signals increase or decrease GI motility and secretions and influence your appetite by sending signals to the central nervous system. Some GI hormones function as growth factors for the gastrointestinal mucosa and pancreas.

Taken together, nerve cells and hormones coordinate the movement and secretions of the GI tract so that enzymes are released when and where they are needed. A healthy GI system functions at a rate that will make digestion and absorption most efficient.

Immune System

The immune system protects us from foreign invaders. A healthy immune system can detect and fight off potential sources of infection, recognize the difference between foreign cells and the body's own cells, recognize and react when it encounters a microbe it has seen before, and then scale back its response when the foreign agent has been dealt with.[15]

Our first line of defense is preventing infectious agents from entering the body. That's the job of the skin and the mucous membranes that line the gastrointestinal, respiratory, and reproductive systems. Of these, the gastrointestinal system is the largest barrier. The normal structure and activities of the gastrointestinal system are a major part of the body's defense—tight junctions between the cells that line the intestines, normal peristalsis, and intestinal secretions all work to keep foreign bodies out. Other tissues involved in the immune system are the lymph nodes, located along the lymphatic system, and the spleen.

Different types of white blood cells carry out the immune response. Some travel the bloodstream to areas of invasion, attacking and ingesting pathogens. **Natural killer cells** attack virus-infected cells and cells that have turned cancerous. **Macrophages**, or "big eaters," take up stations in tissues and act as scavengers, devouring pathogens and worn-out cells. Macrophages congregate in the lymph nodes, where they filter bacteria and other substances from lymph. **Lymphocytes**—white blood cells of the immune system—travel in both the bloodstream and lymphatic system. Some types of lymphocytes produce **antibodies**. Others remember a prior invader, enabling the body to mount a rapid response should the same invader appear again. Upon recognizing an invasion, helper cells trigger the mass production of killer cells. When the danger is over, suppressor cells halt the immune response.

Quick **Bite**

Halt! Who Goes There?
Be they friend or foe, antibiotics kill microorganisms in your GI tract, frequently causing diarrhea. About half of pharmaceutical drugs have gastrointestinal side effects.

▶ **natural killer cells** Nonspecific lymphocytes that spontaneously attack and kill cancer cells and cells infected by microorganisms. They are "natural" killers because they do not need to recognize a specific antigen in order to attack and kill.

▶ **macrophages** Large immune system cells that function as patrol cells and engulf and kill foreign invaders.

▶ **lymphocytes** White blood cells that are primarily responsible for immune responses. Present in the blood and lymph.

▶ **antibodies [AN-tih-bod-eez]** Infection-fighting protein molecules in blood or secretory fluids that tag, neutralize, and help destroy pathogenic microorganisms (e.g., bacteria, viruses) or toxins.

Key Concepts Both hormonal and nervous system signals regulate gastrointestinal activity. Nerve cells in both the enteric and autonomic nervous systems control muscle movement and secretions. Key hormones coordinate GI movement and secretion for optimal digestion and absorption of nutrients. The GI tract also is a major player in the immune system.

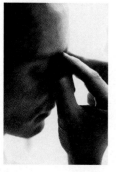
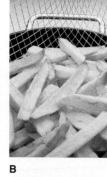
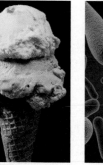
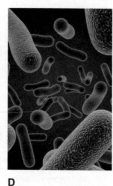

A B C D

FIGURE 3.18 Negative factors for digestion. Several factors can reduce digestive secretions that interfere with digestion and absorption. Such factors include a. stress, b. high-temperature fat frying, c. cold foods, and d. some species of bacteria.

(a) © Corbis; (b) © Photodisc; (c) © Photodisc; (d) © Tischenko Irina/Shutterstock, Inc.

▶ **acrolein** A pungent decomposition product of fats, generated from dehydrating the glycerol component of fats; responsible for the coughing attacks caused by the fumes released by burning fat. This toxic water-soluble liquid vaporizes easily and is highly flammable.

Influences on Digestion and Absorption

🍎 **Why Is This Important?** Learning about the psychological, chemical, and bacterial influences on digestion and absorption is important for understanding the full range of factors that impact the digestion and absorption of foods and nutrients.

Psychological Influences

The taste, smell, and presentation of foods can have a positive effect on digestion. Just the thought of food can trigger saliva production and peristalsis. Stressful emotions such as depression and fear can have the reverse effect (see **FIGURE 3.18**); they stimulate the brain to activate the autonomic nervous system. This results in decreased gastric acid secretion, reduced blood flow to the stomach, inhibition of peristalsis, and reduced propulsion of food.[16] The next time you sit down to a holiday meal, notice how you feel at the sight and smells of your family's traditional foods as well as smells from your childhood. Happiness and positive memories add to the enjoyment of food, whereas unhappiness can bring on a poor appetite or stomach upset.

THINK About It 4

Chemical Influences

The type of protein you eat and the way it is prepared affect digestion. Plant proteins tend to be less digestible than animal proteins. Cooking food usually denatures protein (uncoils its three-dimensional structure), which increases digestibility. Cooking meat softens its connective tissue, making chewing easier and increasing the ability of digestive enzymes to break the meat down into absorbable nutrients. Food processing produces chemicals that may influence digestive secretions. For example, whereas meat extracts may stimulate digestion, frying foods in fat at very high temperatures produces small amounts of **acrolein**,[17] a chemical that decreases the flow of digestive secretions.

The physical condition of a food also sometimes causes problems with digestion. Cold foods, for example, may cause intestinal spasms in people who suffer from irritable bowel syndrome or Crohn's disease. Stomach contents can affect absorption. When food is consumed on an empty stomach, it has more contact with gastric secretions and will be absorbed faster than if it was consumed on a full stomach. Certain medicines can also affect food absorption. For example, the medication Reglan (a drug used to treat heartburn) increases GI motility, which decreases food absorption. In turn, certain foods can enhance, delay, or decrease drug absorption.

Bacterial Influences

In the healthy stomach, hydrochloric acid kills most bacteria. In conditions where there is a lower concentration of hydrochloric acid, more bacteria can survive and multiply. Harmful bacteria can cause gastritis (an inflammation of the stomach lining) and peptic ulcer (a wound in the mucous membranes lining the stomach or duodenum). Bacteria that cause foodborne illness can resist the germicidal effects of hydrochloric acid, so they survive to wreak havoc on the digestive process.

The large intestine maintains a large population of bacteria—they are part of the gut microbiota. In addition to various functions described earlier, these bacteria digest small amounts of fiber, producing a small amount of energy. These bacteria also synthesize gases, such as hydrogen, ammonia, and methane, as well as acids and various substances that contribute to the odor of feces. If the digestion and absorption of food in the small intestine are incomplete, the undigested material enters the large intestine, where bacterial action produces excessive gas and possibly bloating and pain.

Key Concepts Psychological, chemical, and bacterial factors can influence the processes of digestion and absorption. Emotions can influence GI motility and secretion. The temperature and form of food also can affect digestive secretions. Although stomach acid kills many types of bacteria, some are resistant to acid and cause foodborne illness. Helpful bacteria in the large intestine can cause bloating and gas if they receive and begin to digest food components that are normally digested in the small intestine.

Nutrition and GI Disorders

Why Is This Important? A healthy, functioning GI tract is important for overall well-being. Knowing about common problems in the digestive system can help you to reduce your risk.

"I have butterflies in my stomach." "It was a gut-wrenching experience." Our language contains many references to the connection between emotional distress and the GI tract. Most of us have experienced a queasy stomach or intestinal pain right before an important event such as a special date, big exam, or job interview. Through its many neurochemical connections with the gut, the brain exerts a profound influence on GI function. Nearly all GI disorders are influenced to some degree by emotional state. However, a number of illnesses that were once attributed largely to emotional stress, such as peptic ulcer disease, have been shown to be caused primarily by infection and other physical causes. **FIGURE 3.19** shows some common ailments that affect the GI tract.

Although stress management might help and medical intervention might be required, we can prevent and manage most GI disorders with diet. For instance, adding fiber-rich foods (see **TABLE 3.1**) and water to the diet reduces intestinal pressure, decreases the time food by-products remain in the colon, and promotes bowel regularity. Eating a healthful diet, exercising, and maintaining a healthy weight are all good ways to help prevent and/or manage most GI disorders.

Constipation

Constipation is defined as having a bowel movement fewer than three times per week.[18] With constipation, stools are usually hard, dry, small in size, and difficult to eliminate. People who are constipated may find it painful to have a bowel movement and often experience straining, bloating, and the sensation of a full bowel.

Constipation is a symptom, not a disease. Almost everyone experiences constipation at some point. Although stress, inactivity, cessation of smoking, or various illnesses can lead to constipation, a diet that is low in fiber and water and high in fats is a common cause. Some fibers, such as the pectins in fruits and gums in beans, dissolve easily in water and take on a soft, gel-like texture in the intestines. Other fibers, such as cellulose in wheat bran, pass almost unchanged through the intestines. The bulk and soft texture of fiber help prevent hard, dry stools that are difficult to pass. People who eat plenty of high-fiber foods are not likely to become constipated. When eating a

▶ **constipation** Infrequent and difficult bowel movements, followed by a sensation of incomplete evacuation.

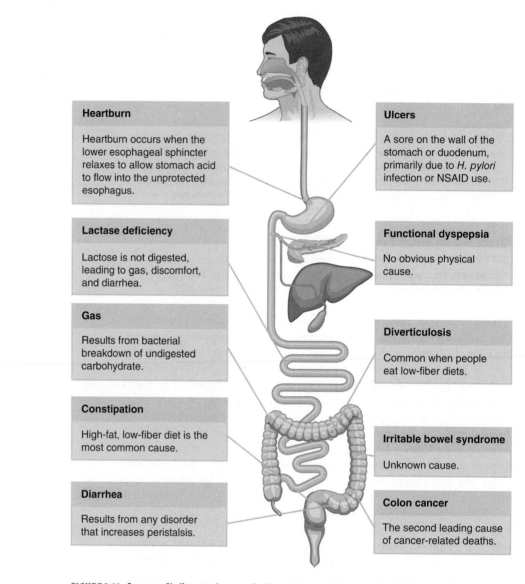

Heartburn

Heartburn occurs when the lower esophageal sphincter relaxes to allow stomach acid to flow into the unprotected esophagus.

Lactase deficiency

Lactose is not digested, leading to gas, discomfort, and diarrhea.

Gas

Results from bacterial breakdown of undigested carbohydrate.

Constipation

High-fat, low-fiber diet is the most common cause.

Diarrhea

Results from any disorder that increases peristalsis.

Ulcers

A sore on the wall of the stomach or duodenum, primarily due to *H. pylori* infection or NSAID use.

Functional dyspepsia

No obvious physical cause.

Diverticulosis

Common when people eat low-fiber diets.

Irritable bowel syndrome

Unknown cause.

Colon cancer

The second leading cause of cancer-related deaths.

FIGURE 3.19 Common GI ailments. Beans are familiar culprits in what is perhaps the most common GI ailment—gas. Rice is the only starch that does not cause gas.

high-fiber diet, one should also include plenty of liquids. Liquids such as water and juice add fluid to the colon and bulk to stools, making bowel movements softer and easier to pass. The caffeine in many liquids (e.g., coffee, tea, many soft drinks) is a mild diuretic (a substance that increases urine production).

Although treatment of constipation is determined by the cause, severity, and duration, in most cases dietary changes help relieve symptoms and prevent constipation. Also, regular exercise helps keep all the body's muscles healthy, including the GI tract muscles, and will help promote regularity.

Diarrhea

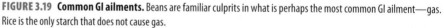

▶ **diarrhea** Watery stools due to reduced absorption of water.

Diarrhea—loose, watery stools that occur more than three times in one day—is caused by digestive products moving through the large intestine too rapidly for sufficient water to be reabsorbed.

TABLE 3.1
Examples of Foods That Contain Fiber

Food	Standard Size Portion	Dietary Fiber in Standard Portion (g)[a]
High-fiber bran ready-to-eat cereal	⅓–¾ cup	9.1–14.3
Shredded wheat ready-to-eat cereal (various)	1–1¼ cup	5.0–9.0
Chickpeas, canned	½ cup	8.1
Lentils, cooked	½ cup	7.8
Black beans, cooked	½ cup	7.5
White beans, canned	½ cup	6.3
Wheat bran flakes ready-to-eat cereal (various)	¾ cup	4.9–5.5
Pear, raw	1 medium	5.5
Baked beans, canned, plain	½ cup	5.2
Soybeans, cooked	½ cup	5.2
Avocado	½ cup	5.0
Apple, with skin	1 medium	4.4
Green peas, cooked (fresh, frozen, canned)	½ cup	3.5–4.4
Chia seeds, dried	1 Tbsp	4.1
Bulgur, cooked	½ cup	4.1
Raspberries	½ cup	4.0
Sweet potato, baked in skin	1 medium	3.8
Pumpkin, canned	½ cup	3.6
Popcorn, air-popped	3 cups	3.5
Almonds	1 ounce	3.5
Orange	1 medium	3.1
Banana	1 medium	3.1
Pearled barley, cooked	½ cup	3.0
Winter squash, cooked	½ cup	2.9
Dates	¼ cup	2.9
Peanuts, oil roasted	1 ounce	2.7
Quinoa, cooked	½ cup	2.6

[a] Data from U.S. Department of Agriculture, Agricultural Research Service, Nutrient Data Laboratory. 2014. USDA National Nutrient Database for Standard Reference, Release 27. Available at: http://www.ars.usda.gov/nutrientdata

Diarrhea is a symptom of many disorders that cause increased peristalsis. Culprits include stress, intestinal irritation or damage, side effects of medications, and intolerance to gluten (a protein in wheat), fat, or lactose (the natural sugar in milk). Eating food contaminated with bacteria or viruses often causes diarrhea when the digestive tract speeds the offending food along the alimentary canal and out of the body. Diarrhea can cause dehydration, which means the body lacks enough fluid to function properly. Dehydration is particularly dangerous in children and the elderly, and it must be treated promptly to avoid serious health problems.

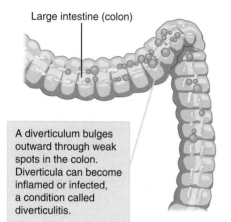

Large intestine (colon)

A diverticulum bulges outward through weak spots in the colon. Diverticula can become inflamed or infected, a condition called diverticulitis.

FIGURE 3.20 Diverticulosis. In industrialized nations, diverticulosis is common in older people. It is unusual in developing countries where people eat high-fiber diets.

▶ **diverticulosis [dy-vur-tik-yoo-LOH-sis]** A condition that occurs when small pouches (diverticula) push outward through weak spots in the colon.

▶ **diverticulitis [dy-vur-tik-yoo-LY-tis]** A condition that occurs when small pouches in the colon (diverticula) become infected or irritated. Also called *left-sided appendicitis*.

Quick **Bite**

Short Bowel Syndrome

Patients who suffer from short bowel syndrome, a condition where a large portion of the intestine has been surgically removed because of illness or injury, commonly have difficulty absorbing fat-soluble vitamins. To enhance absorption, treatment includes taking a fat-soluble vitamin supplement that easily mingles with water. These patients also may need to take intramuscular shots of B_{12} because they are unable to absorb this water-soluble vitamin.

A diet of broth, tea, toast, and other low-fiber foods, along with avoidance of lactose, fructose, caffeine, and sugar alcohols such as sorbitol, can help reduce diarrhea until it subsides. As stools form, you can gradually introduce more foods. Pectin, a form of dietary fiber found in apples and citrus peel, may be helpful, along with foods high in potassium—if they are tolerated—to replace lost electrolytes. Fluid replacement also is important to avoid dehydration.

Diverticulosis

As people age, the colon develops small pouches that bulge outward through weak spots on the digestive tract. (See **FIGURE 3.20**.) Known as **diverticulosis**, this condition afflicts about half of all Americans ages 60 to 80 and almost everyone over age 80. One contributor to this condition is a low-fiber diet, which you read previously can make stools hard and difficult to pass. If the stool is too hard, muscles must strain to move it, increasing pressure in the colon and causing weak spots to bulge outward. Although the bulging pouches usually cause few problems, in 10 to 25 percent of these people, the pouches become infected or inflamed—a painful condition called **diverticulitis**. Symptoms of diverticulitis include abdominal pain, usually along the upper left side of the lower abdomen. If the area is infected, fever, nausea, vomiting, chills, cramping, constipation, or bleeding may develop. Treatment of diverticulitis depends on its severity. Generally, this condition can be managed with diet, but serious cases of diverticulitis may require surgery to remove the affected part of the colon.

Diverticulosis and diverticulitis are common in developed or industrialized countries—particularly the United States, England, and Australia—where low-fiber diets are common. Diverticular disease is rare in countries of Asia and Africa, where people eat high-fiber, vegetable-based diets.

Increasing the amount of fiber in the diet, along with adequate fluid intake, may reduce symptoms of diverticulosis and prevent complications such as diverticulitis. During acute attacks of diverticulitis, following a low-fiber diet and avoiding foods that may contribute to nausea or pain, such as caffeine, spicy foods, chocolate, and milk products, is recommended. Once symptoms of diverticulitis have subsided, gradual transition to a high-fiber diet (25–35 grams per day) is recommended. Some benefits of fiber are listed in **TABLE 3.2**.

TABLE 3.2 **Benefits of Fiber**
• Helps control weight by delaying gastric emptying and providing a feeling of fullness
• Improves glucose tolerance by delaying the movement of carbohydrate into the small intestine
• Reduces risk of heart disease by binding with bile (which contains cholesterol) in the intestine and causing it to be excreted, which in turn helps to lower blood cholesterol levels
• Promotes regularity and reduces constipation by increasing stool weight and decreasing transit time
• Reduces the risk of diverticulosis by decreasing pressure within the colon, decreasing transit time, and increasing stool weight

Data from Institute of Medicine, Food and Nutrition Board. *Dietary Reference Intakes for Energy, Carbohydrate, Fiber, Fat, Fatty Acids, Cholesterol, Protein, and Amino Acids (Macronutrients)*. Washington, DC: National Academies Press; 2002.

Heartburn and Gastroesophageal Reflux Disease

Heartburn occurs when the sphincter between the esophagus and stomach relaxes inappropriately, allowing the stomach's contents to flow back into the esophagus. Unlike the stomach, the esophagus has no protective mucous lining, so acid can damage it quickly and cause pain. Many people experience occasional heartburn, referred to as gastroesophageal reflux (GER), but for some, heartburn is a chronic, often daily, event and a symptom of a more serious disorder called **gastroesophageal reflux disease (GERD)**. GERD, along with obesity, is a key risk factor for esophageal cancer.[19] GERD has a variety of causes, and many treatment strategies involve lifestyle and nutrition.

▶ **gastroesophageal reflux disease (GERD)** A backflow of stomach contents into the esophagus, accompanied by a burning pain because of the acidity of the gastric juices.

Dietary recommendations include avoiding foods and beverages that can weaken the esophageal sphincter, including chocolate, peppermint, fatty foods, coffee, and alcoholic beverages. Foods and beverages that can irritate a damaged esophageal lining, such as citrus fruits and juices, tomato products, and pepper, also should be avoided.

Decreasing both the portion size and the fat content of meals may help. High-fat meals remain in the stomach longer than low-fat meals. This creates back pressure on the esophageal sphincter. Eating meals at least two to three hours before bedtime may reduce reflux problems by allowing partial emptying and a decrease in stomach acidity. Elevating the head of the bed 4 to 8 inches or sleeping on a specially designed wedge reduces heartburn by allowing gravity to minimize reflux of stomach contents into the esophagus.

In addition, cigarette smoking weakens the esophageal sphincter, and being overweight or obese often worsens symptoms. Smokers have various reasons to stop, including GERD, and many overweight people find relief when they lose weight.

Irritable Bowel Syndrome

About 10–15 percent of adults in the U.S. suffer from **irritable bowel syndrome (IBS)**, a poorly understood condition that causes abdominal pain, altered bowel habits (such as diarrhea or constipation), and cramps.[20] Often IBS is just a mild annoyance, but for some people it can be disabling.

▶ **irritable bowel syndrome (IBS)** A disruptive state of intestinal motility with no known cause. Symptoms include constipation, abdominal pain, and episodic diarrhea.

The cause of IBS remains a mystery, but emotional stress and specific foods clearly aggravate the symptoms in most sufferers.[21] Beans, chocolate, milk products, and large amounts of alcohol are frequent offenders. Fat in any form (animal or vegetable) is a strong stimulus of colonic contractions after a meal. Caffeine causes loose stools in many people, but it is more likely to affect those with IBS. Women with IBS may have more symptoms during their menstrual periods, suggesting that reproductive hormones can increase IBS symptoms.

The good news about IBS is that although its symptoms can be uncomfortable, it does not shorten life span or progress to more serious illness. IBS can usually be controlled with diet and lifestyle modifications, as well as judicious use of medication. A diet strategy referred to as FODMAP (low fermentable oligosaccharides, disaccharides, monosaccharides, and polyol diet) has been shown to decrease symptoms caused by IBS. The short-chain carbohydrates (oligo-, di-, and monosaccharides) are incompletely absorbed in the GI tract and can easily be fermented by gut bacteria. This fermentation and osmosis caused by these undigested sugars are a cause of IBS symptoms such as gas, pain, and diarrhea,[22] and eliminating these foods from the diet can help prevent such undesirable symptoms. Stress management is an important part of treatment for IBS as well. This includes stress reduction training and relaxation therapies, such as meditation, counseling and support, regular exercise, changes to stressful situations in your life, and adequate sleep.[23]

Colorectal Cancer

After lung cancer, colorectal cancer—cancer of the colon or rectum—is the second leading cause of cancer-related deaths in the United States.[24] Many studies suggest that consumption of large amounts of red and processed meats, along with low intake of fiber and the protective phytochemicals found in fruits, vegetables, and whole grains, might be responsible for the high incidence of colorectal cancer.[25] It is important to recognize, however, that other dietary factors (i.e., Western lifestyle; high intake of refined sugars and alcohol; and low intake of fruits, vegetables, and fiber) and behavioral factors (i.e., low physical activity, high smoking prevalence, high body mass index) limit the ability to isolate the effects of red meat consumption from other factors.[26] The link between colorectal cancer and the consumption of cooked and processed red meat is attributed to chemical carcinogens that arise during the cooking process.[27]

Observational and case control studies support the idea that fiber-rich diets reduce colorectal cancer risk, and scientists have hypothesized a number of possible ways that fiber might be protective.[28] These include dilution of carcinogens in a bulkier stool, more rapid transit of carcinogens through the GI tract, and lower colon pH due to bacterial fermentation of fiber.

Gas

Everyone has gas and eliminates it by burping or passing it through the rectum. Gas is made primarily of odorless vapors. Flatulence has an unpleasant odor because bacteria in the large intestine release small amounts of gases that contain sulfur. Although having gas is common, it can be uncomfortable and embarrassing.

Gas in the stomach is commonly caused by swallowing air. We all swallow small amounts of air when we eat and drink. However, eating or drinking rapidly, chewing gum, smoking, or wearing loose dentures can cause us to take in more air. Burping is the way most swallowed air leaves the stomach. The remaining gas moves into the small intestine, where it is partially absorbed. A small amount travels into the large intestine for release through the rectum. (The stomach also releases carbon dioxide when stomach acid and bicarbonate mix, but most of this gas is absorbed into the bloodstream and does not enter the large intestine.)

Frequent passage of rectal gas may be annoying, but it is seldom a symptom of serious disease. **Flatus** (lower intestinal gas) composition depends to a great extent on your carbohydrate intake and the activity of the colon's bacterial population.

Most foods that contain carbohydrates can cause gas. By contrast, fats and proteins cause little gas. In the large intestine, bacteria partially break down undigested carbohydrate, producing hydrogen, carbon dioxide, and, in about one-third of people, methane. Eventually these gases exit through the rectum.

Foods that produce gas in one person may not cause gas in another. Some common bacteria in the large intestine can destroy the hydrogen

▶ **flatus** Lower intestinal gas that is expelled through the rectum.

that other bacteria produce. The balance of the two types of bacteria may explain why some people have more gas than others.

Carbohydrates that commonly cause gas are (1) raffinose and stachyose, found in large quantities in beans; (2) fructose, a common sweetener in soft drinks and fruit drinks; (3) lactose; and (4) sorbitol. Most starches, including potatoes, corn, noodles, and wheat, produce gas as they are broken down in the large intestine. Rice is the only starch that does not cause gas.

The fiber in oat bran, beans, peas, and most fruits is broken down in the large intestine, where digestion causes gas. In contrast, the fiber in wheat bran and some vegetables, such as green beans, cauliflower, zucchini, and celery, passes essentially unchanged through the intestines and produces little gas.

Ulcers

A gnawing, burning pain in the upper abdomen is the classic sign of a peptic **ulcer**, which also can cause nausea, vomiting, loss of appetite, and weight loss. A peptic ulcer is a sore that forms in the duodenum (duodenal ulcer) or the lining of the stomach (gastric ulcer).

It was once assumed that stress was a major factor in the development of ulcers, particularly in people with "intense" personalities. Diet was also thought to be important, with spicy foods often cast as a major villain. But much to the amazement of most of the medical community, research in the 1980s and 1990s confirmed that infection with the bacterium *Helicobacter pylori* actually causes most ulcers. *H. pylori* are spiral-shaped bacteria found in the stomach that can cause ulcers by damaging the mucous coating that protects the lining of the stomach and duodenum. Once *H. pylori* have damaged the mucous coating, powerful stomach acid can penetrate and irritate the lining of the stomach and duodenum, causing an ulcer.[29]

Excessive use of nonsteroidal anti-inflammatory drugs (NSAIDs), such as aspirin, ibuprofen, and naproxen sodium, is also a common cause of ulcers. NSAIDs cause ulcers by interfering with the GI tract's ability to protect itself from acidic stomach juices. Normally the stomach and duodenum employ three defenses against digestive juices: mucus that coats the lining and shields it from stomach acid, the chemical bicarbonate that neutralizes acid, and blood circulation that aids in cell renewal and repair. NSAIDs hinder all these protective mechanisms. With the defenses down, digestive juices can cause ulcers by damaging the sensitive lining of the stomach and duodenum. Fortunately, NSAID-induced ulcers usually heal once the person stops taking the medication.

If you had ulcers in the 1950s, you would have been told to quit your high-stress job and switch to a bland diet. Today, patients with ulcers are usually treated with proton pump inhibitors or histamine receptor blockers and also possibly a protectant such as sucralfate. Antibiotics are used for those cases that test positive for *H. pylori*.[30] Although personality and life stress are no longer considered significant factors in the development of most ulcers, relapse after treatment is more common in people who are emotionally stressed or suffering from depression.

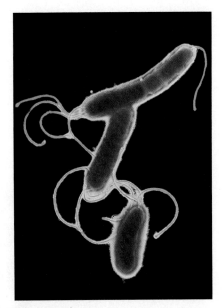

Helicobacter pylori.
© A.B. Dowsett/SPL/Photo Researchers, Inc.

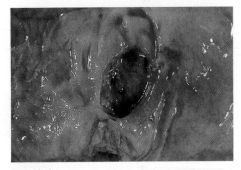

Stomach ulcer.
© Dr. E. Walker/Science Photo Library/Photo Researchers, Inc.

▶ **ulcer** A craterlike lesion that occurs in the lining of the stomach or duodenum; also called a *peptic ulcer* to distinguish it from a skin ulcer.

Key Concepts GI disorders generally produce uncomfortable symptoms such as abdominal pain, gas, bloating, and change in elimination patterns. Some GI disorders, such as diarrhea, are generally symptoms of some other illness. Although medications are useful in reducing symptoms, many GI disorders are treatable with changes in diet, especially the addition of adequate fiber and fluids.

Quick Bite

Flatulence Facts

Researchers studying pilots and astronauts during the 1960s made some interesting discoveries. The average person inadvertently swallows air with food and drink, and subsequently expels approximately 1 pint of gas per day, composed of 50 percent nitrogen. Another 40 percent is composed of carbon dioxide and the products of aerobic bacteria in the intestine.

As you have seen, the gastrointestinal tract is the key to turning food and its nutrients into nourishment for our bodies. **FIGURE 3.21** shows the sites for digestion and absorption of the macronutrients, using a piece of pizza as an example of a food that would contain substantial amounts of carbohydrate, fat, and protein. A healthy GI tract is an important factor in our overall health and well-being.

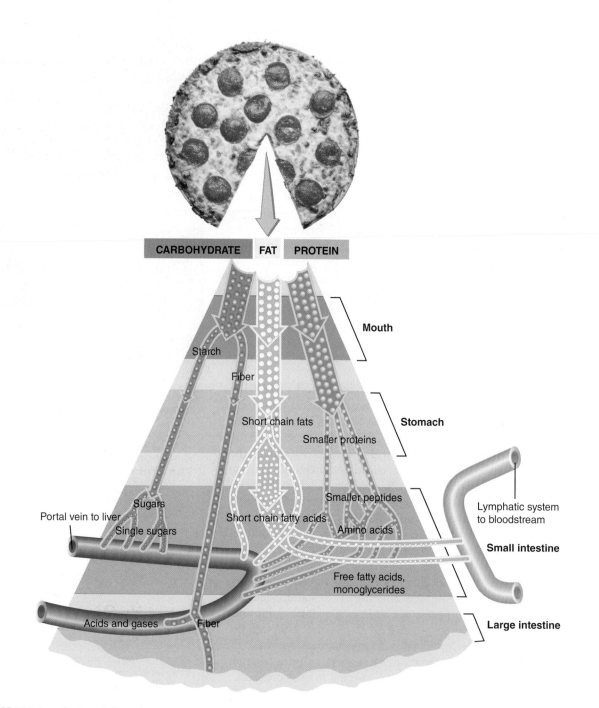

FIGURE 3.21 Fate of a piece of pizza. When you eat a piece of pizza, what happens to the carbohydrate, fat, and protein?

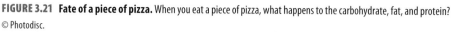

© Photodisc.

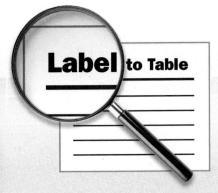

Label to Table

As you've learned in this chapter, fiber is one of the few things you do not digest fully. Instead, fiber moves through the GI tract, and most of it leaves the body in feces. If it's not digested, then why all the fuss about eating more fiber? A healthy intake of fiber can lower your risk of cancer and heart disease and help with bowel regularity. So, how do you know which foods have fiber? You have to check out the food label!

This Nutrition Facts panel is from the label on a loaf of whole-wheat bread. The highlighted sections show you that every slice of bread contains 3 grams of fiber. The 12% listed to the right of that refers to the Daily Values below. The Daily Value (25 g) is for a person who consumes about 2,000 kilocalories per day. It should be no surprise that if you are consuming more calories,

you should also be consuming more fiber. The 12% Daily Value is calculated using the 2,000-kilocalorie fiber guideline as follows:

$$\frac{3\text{ grams fiber per slice}}{25\text{ grams Daily Value}} = 0.12,\text{ or }12\%$$

This means if you make a sandwich with two slices of whole-wheat bread, you're getting 6 grams of fiber and almost one-quarter (24% Daily Value) of your fiber needs per day. Not bad! Be careful, though; many people inadvertently buy wheat bread thinking that it's as high in fiber as *whole-wheat* bread, but it's not. Whole-wheat bread contains the whole (complete) grain, but wheat bread often is stripped of its fiber. Check the label before you buy your next loaf.

Nutrition Facts

16 servings per container
Serving size   1 slice (43g)

Amount per serving
Calories   **100**

	% Daily Value*
Total Fat 2g	3%
Saturated Fat 0g	0%
Trans Fat 0g	
Cholesterol 0mg	0%
Sodium 230mg	
Total Carbohydrate 18g	9%
Dietary Fiber 3g	6%
Total Sugars 2g	12%
Includes 1g Added Sugars	0%
Protein 5g	
Vitamin D 0mcg	0%
Calcium 60mg	6%
Iron 1mg	6%
Potassium 144mg	4%
Niacin 2mg	10%

* The % Daily Value (DV) tells you how much a nutrient in a serving of food contributes to a daily diet. 2,000 calories a day is used for general nutrition advice.

INGREDIENTS: STONE GROUND WHOLE WHEAT FLOUR, WATER, HIGH FRUCTOSE CORN SYRUP, WHEAT GLUTEN, WHEAT BRAN, CONTAINS 2% OR LESS OF EACH OF THE FOLLOWING: YEAST, SALT, PARTIALLY HYDROGENATED SOYBEAN OIL, HONEY, MOLASSES, RAISIN JUICE CONCENTRATE, DOUGH CONDITIONERS (MAY CONTAIN ONE OR MORE OF EACH OF THE FOLLOWING: MONO- AND DIGLYCERIDES, CALCIUM AND SODIUM STEAROYL LACTYLATES, CALCIUM PEROXIDE), WHEAT GERM, WHEY, CORNSTARCH, YEAST NUTRIENTS (MONOCALCIUM PHOSPHATE, CALCIUM SULFATE, AMMONIUM SULFATE).

Learning Portfolio

Key Terms

	page		page
absorption	69	gut microbiota	83
accessory organs	70	heartburn	79
acrolein	88	hydrochloric acid (gastric acid)	79
active transport	75	hydrolysis	73
antibodies [AN-tih-bod-eez]	87	ileum [ILL-ee-um]	80
autonomic nervous system (ANS)	86	intrinsic factor	79
bile	76	irritable bowel syndrome (IBS)	93
bolus [BOH-lus]	79	jejunum [je-JOON-um]	80
catalyze	73	lacteal	81
cecum	81	large intestine	81
central nervous system (CNS)	86	lingual lipase	79
chyme [KIME]	73	liver	76
circular muscle	71	longitudinal muscle	71
colon	81	lumen	74
concentration gradients	74	lymph	81
constipation	89	lymphatic system	85
diarrhea	90	lymphocytes	87
digestion	69	macrophages	87
digestive secretions	80	microvilli	81
diverticulitis [dy-vur-tik-yoo-LY-tis]	92	mucosa [myu-KO-sa]	71
diverticulosis [dy-vur-tik-yoo-LOH-sis]	92	mucus	74
duodenum [doo-oh-DEE-num]	80	natural killer cells	87
elimination	70	pancreas	77
emulsifiers	76	passive diffusion	74
enteric nervous system	86	pepsin	79
enterohepatic circulation [EN-ter-oh-heh-PAT-ik]	76	pepsinogen	79
enzymes [EN-zimes]	73	peristalsis [per-ih-STAHL-sis]	73
esophageal sphincter	79	pH	79
esophagus [ee-SOFF-uh-gus]	79	prebiotics	83
excretion	76	precursor	79
facilitated diffusion	74	probiotics	83
flatulence	82	pyloric sphincter	79
flatus	94	rectum	82
gallbladder	77	salivary amylase [AM-ih-lace]	77
gastric lipase	79	salivary glands	76
gastrin [GAS-trin]	79	segmentation	73
gastroesophageal reflux disease (GERD)	93	small intestine	80
gastrointestinal (GI) tract	70	sphincters [SFINGK-ters]	71
		stomach	79
		ulcer	96
		vascular system	84
		villi	80

Study Points

- The GI tract is a tube that can be divided into regions: the mouth, esophagus, stomach, small intestine, large intestine, and rectum.

- Digestion and absorption of the nutrients in foods occur at various sites along the GI tract.

- Digestion involves both physical processes (e.g., chewing, peristalsis, and segmentation) and chemical processes (e.g., the hydrolytic action of enzymes).

- Absorption is the movement of molecules across the lining of the GI tract and into circulation.

- The major mechanisms involved in nutrient absorption are passive diffusion, facilitated diffusion, and active transport.

- In the mouth, food is mixed with saliva for lubrication. Salivary amylase begins the digestion of starch.

- Acid and enzyme secretions from the stomach lower the pH of stomach contents and begin the digestion of proteins.

- The pancreas and gallbladder secrete material into the small intestine to help with digestion.

- Most chemical digestion and nutrient absorption occur in the small intestine.

- Electrolytes and water are absorbed from the large intestine. Remaining material—waste—is excreted as feces.

- Gut microbiota are microorganisms living in the digestive tract that interact with each other and the human host in mutually beneficial processes. Gut microbiota are currently being investigated for their role in the development and prevention of metabolic diseases, including obesity and glucose regulation.

- Both the nervous system and the hormonal system regulate GI tract processes.

- Numerous factors affect GI tract functioning, including psychological, chemical, and bacterial factors.

- Problems that occur along the GI tract can affect digestion and absorption of nutrients. Dietary changes are important in the treatment of GI disorders.

Study Questions

1. List the organs (in order) that make up the GI tract.

2. Name the four "assisting" organs that are not part of the GI tract but are needed for proper digestion. What are their roles in digestion?

3. What substance makes the stomach contents acidic? What substance protects stomach cells from the low pH of stomach contents?

4. Where in the GI tract does the majority of nutrient digestion and absorption take place?

5. What two circulatory systems transport absorbed nutrients around the body?

6. Increasing fiber in the diet may decrease symptoms of the GI disorder diverticulosis. List other benefits of eating a high-fiber diet.

Try This

The Saltine Cracker Experiment

This experiment will help you understand the effect of salivary amylase. Remember, salivary amylase is the starch-digesting enzyme produced by the salivary glands. Chew two saltine crackers until a watery texture forms in your mouth. You have to fight the urge to swallow so you can pay attention to the taste of the crackers. Do you notice a change in the taste?

The crackers first taste salty and "starchy," but as amylase is secreted it begins to break the chains of starch into sugar. As it does this, the saltines begin to taste sweet like animal crackers.

Getting Personal

Are you following a diet that helps to keep your gut healthy? What we usually eat can either help maintain a healthy GI tract or cause GI trouble.

For each of the following questions, determine if this is a dietary habit you "usually do," you "sometimes do," or you "never do." To ensure that you are eating a diet that keeps your GI tract healthy, consider improving those things that you sometimes or never do by turning them into eating habits that you usually do.

Learning Portfolio (continued)

Eating Habits	Usually Do	Sometimes Do	Never Do
I eat at least seven servings of fruits and vegetables every day.			
For breakfast I choose whole grains, nuts, and berries instead of foods like low-fiber, refined cereal.			
For lunch I select sandwiches or wraps on a whole-grain tortilla or whole-grain bread and add veggies.			
For a snack I choose fresh veggies, fruit, whole-grain crackers, almonds, avocado, or air-popped popcorn.			
I drink 8–10 cups of water each day.			
I limit foods that are high in fat, and if I eat meat, I choose lean cuts.			
I include probiotics (such as low-fat yogurt) in my diet.			
I exercise regularly, getting at least 30 minutes of exercise each day.			

References

1. Smeets PA, Erkner A, deGraaf C. Cephalic phase responses and appetite. *Nutr Rev.* 2010;68(1):643-655.
2. Popkin BM, D'Anci KE, Rosenberg IH. Water, hydration and health. *Nutr Rev.* 2010;68(8):439-458. doi: 10.1111/j.1753-4887.2010.00304.x
3. Sullivan S, Alpers DH, Klein S. Nutritional physiology of the alimentary tract. In: Ross AC, Cabellero B, Cousins RJ, et al., eds. *Modern Nutrition in Health and Disease.* 11th ed. Philadelphia: Lippincott Williams & Wilkins; 2014: 540-574.
4. Ibid.
5. Ibid.
6. Ibid.
7. El Kaoutari A, Armougom F, Raoult D, Henrissat B. Gut microbiota and digestion of polysaccharides. *Med Sci (Paris).* 2014;30(3):259-265.
8. Kich DM, Vincenzi A, Majolo F, Volken de Souza CF, Goettert MI. Probiotic: effectiveness nutrition in cancer treatment and prevention. *Nutr Hosp.* 2016;33(6):1430-1437. doi: 10.20960/nh.806.
9. Jandhyala SM, Talukdar R, Subramanyam C, Vuyyuru H, Sasikala M, Reddy DN. Role of the normal gut microbiota. *World J Gastroenterol.* 2015;21(29):8787-8803. doi:10.3748/wjg.v21.i29.8787.
10. Lozupone CA, Stombaugh JI, Gordon JI, Jansson JK, Knight R. Diversity, stability and resilience of the human gut microbiota. *Nature.* 2012;489:220-230.
11. Martinez KB, Leone V, Chang EB. Western diets, gut dysbiosis, and metabolic diseases: are they linked? *Gut Microbes.* 2017;8(2):1-13. doi: 10.1080/19490976.2016.1270811.and
12. Brahe LK, Astrup A, Larsen LH. Can we prevent obesity-related metabolic diseases by dietary modulation of the gut microbiota? *Adv Nutr.* 2016;7:90-101.
13. Jandhyala SM, Talukdar R, Subramanyam C, Vuyyuru H, Sasikala M, Reddy DN. Role of the normal gut microbiota. Op. cit.
14. Tejero S, Rowland IR, Rastall R, Gibson GR. Probiotics and prebiotics as modulators of the gut microbiota. In: Ross AC, Cabellero B, Cousins RJ, et al., eds. *Modern Nutrition in Health and Disease.* 11th ed. Philadelphia: Lippincott Williams & Wilkins; 2014: 506-512.
15. Marraffini LA, Sontheimer EJ. Self versus non-self discrimination during CRISPR RNA-directed immunity. *Nature.* 2010;463(7280):568-571.

16. Konturek PC, Brzozowski T, Konturek SJ. Stress and the gut: pathophysiology, clinical consequences, diagnostic approach and treatment options. *J Physiol Pharmacol*. 2011;62(6):591-599.

17. U.S. Public Health Service, U.S. Department of Health and Human Services, Agency for Toxic Substances and Disease Registry. Toxicological profile for acrolein. 2007. http://www.atsdr.cdc.gov/toxprofiles/tp.asp?id=557&tid=102. Accessed August 17, 2017.

18. National Institute of Diabetes and Digestive and Kidney Diseases, National Institutes of Health. Constipation. https://www.niddk.nih.gov/health-information/digestive-diseases/constipation. Accessed August 17, 2017.

19. Nam SY. Obesity-related digestive diseases and their pathophysiology. *Gut Liver*. 2017;11(3):323-334. http://www.gutnliver.org/journal/view.html?doi=10.5009/gnl15557. Accessed August 17, 2017.

20. National Institute of Diabetes and Digestive and Kidney Diseases, National Institutes of Health. Definitions & facts for irritable bowel syndrome. https://www.niddk.nih.gov/health-information/digestive-diseases/irritable-bowel-syndrome/definition-facts. Accessed August 17, 2017.

21. Ibid.

22. Shephard SJ, Halmos E, Glance S. The role of FODMAPS in irritable bowel syndrome. *Curr Opin Clin Nutr Metab Care*. 2014;17(6):605-609.

23. National Institute of Diabetes and Digestive and Kidney Diseases, National Institutes of Health. Irritable bowel syndrome. Op. cit.

24. Centers for Disease Control and Prevention. Colorectal (colon) cancer. http://www.cdc.gov/cancer/colorectal. Accessed August 17, 2017.

25. Durko L, Malecka-Panas E. Lifestyle modifications and colorectal cancer. *Curr Colorect Cancer Rep*. 2014;10:45-54.

26. Alexander DD, Cushing CA. Red meat and colorectal cancer: a critical summary of prospective epidemiologic studies. *Obesity Rev*. 2011;12(Suppl):e472-e493.

27. National Cancer Institute. Chemicals in meat cooked at high temperatures and cancer risk. https://www.cancer.gov/about-cancer/causes-prevention/risk/diet/cooked-meats-fact-sheet. Accessed August 17, 2017.

28. Kunzmann AT, Coleman HG, Huang WY, Kitahara CM, Cantwell MM, Berndt SI. Dietary fiber intake and risk of colorectal cancer and incident and recurrent adenoma in the Prostate, Lung, Colorectal, and Ovarian Cancer Screening Trial. *Am J Clin Nutr*. 2015;102(4):881-890.

29. National Institute of Diabetes and Digestive and Kidney Diseases, National Institutes of Health. Peptic ulcers (stomach ulcers). https://www.niddk.nih.gov/health-information/digestive-diseases/peptic-ulcers-stomach-ulcers. Accessed August 17, 2017.

30. Ibid.

Chapter 4

Carbohydrates: Simple Sugars and Complex Chains

Revised by Diane McKay and Emily Mohn

THINK About It

1. When you think of the word *carbohydrate*, what foods come to mind?

2. Fiber is an important part of a healthy diet—are you eating enough?

3. Many people choose honey or agave instead of white sugar because they think they are more "natural." What do you think?

4. What are the downsides to including too many carbohydrates in your diet?

LEARNING Objectives

1 Differentiate among disaccharides, oligosaccharides, and polysaccharides.
2 Explain how a carbohydrate is digested and absorbed in the body.
3 Explain the functions of carbohydrates in the body.
4 Identify healthy carbohydrate selections for an optimal diet.
5 Examine the contributions of carbohydrates to health.

Does sugar cause diabetes? Will too much sugar make a child hyperactive? Does excess sugar contribute to criminal behavior? What about starch? Does it really make you fat? These and other questions have been raised about sugar and starch—dietary carbohydrates—over the years. But, where do these ideas come from? What is myth, and what is fact? Are carbohydrates important in the diet? Or, as some popular diets suggest, should we eat only small amounts of carbohydrates? What links, if any, are there between carbohydrates in your diet and health?

THINK About It

1

Most of the world's people depend on carbohydrate-rich plant foods for daily sustenance. In some countries, they supply 80 percent or more of daily calorie intake. Rice provides the bulk of the diet in Southeast Asia, as does corn in South America, cassava in certain parts of Africa, and wheat in Europe and North America. (See **FIGURE 4.1**.) Besides providing energy, foods rich in carbohydrates, such as whole grains, legumes, fruits, and vegetables, also are good sources of vitamins, minerals, dietary fiber, and phytochemicals that can help lower the risk of chronic diseases.

Generous carbohydrate intake from whole, minimally processed foods should provide the foundation for any healthful diet. Carbohydrates contain only 4 kilocalories per gram, compared with 9 kilocalories per gram from fat. Thus, a diet rich in carbohydrates can provide fewer calories and a greater volume of food than the typical fat-laden American diet. As you explore the topic of carbohydrates, think about some claims you have heard for and against eating a lot of carbohydrates. As you read this chapter, you will learn to distinguish between carbohydrates that are important as the basis of a healthy diet and those that add calories with little additional nutritional value.

What Are Carbohydrates?

Plants use carbon dioxide from the air, water from the soil, and energy from the sun to produce carbohydrates and oxygen through a process called photosynthesis. Carbohydrates are organic compounds that contain carbon (C), hydrogen (H), and oxygen (O) in the ratio of two hydrogen atoms and one oxygen atom for every one carbon atom (CH_2O). Two

Quick Bite

Is Pasta a Chinese Food?
Noodles were used in China as early as the first century; Marco Polo brought them to Italy in the 1300s.

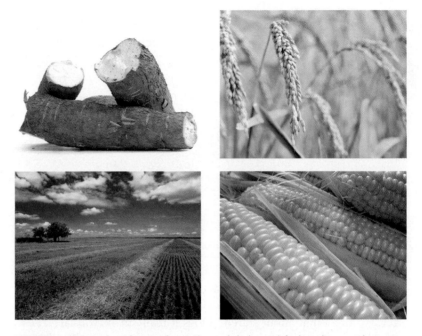

FIGURE 4.1 Cassava, rice, wheat, and corn. These carbohydrate-rich foods are dietary staples in many parts of the world.

Cassava: © Vinicius Tupinamba/Shutterstock; rice: © Mircea BEZERGHEANU/Shutterstock; wheat: © Ayd/Shutterstock; corn: © Krunoslav Cestar/Shutterstock.

or more sugar molecules can be assembled to form increasingly complex carbohydrates. The two main types of carbohydrates in food are simple carbohydrates (sugars) and complex carbohydrates (starches and fiber).

Simple Sugars

🍎 **Why Is This Important?** The media often discuss "carbs" and "sugars" as a single entity, but sugars are just one family of carbs. Learning how to identify members of the sugar family (and distinguish them from other carbohydrates) will help you understand that not all sugars are created equal and that the consumption of each type has different effects on our bodies.

▶ **simple carbohydrates** Sugars composed of a single sugar molecule (a monosaccharide) or two joined sugar molecules (a disaccharide).

▶ **monosaccharides [mon-uh-SACK-uh-rides]** Any sugars that are not broken down further during digestion and have the general formula $C_nH_{2n}O_n$, where $n = 3$ to 7. The common monosaccharides glucose, fructose, and galactose all have six carbon atoms ($n = 6$).

▶ **disaccharides [dye-SACK-uh-rides]** Carbohydrates composed of two monosaccharide units linked by a glycosidic bond. They include sucrose (common table sugar), lactose (milk sugar), and maltose.

Simple carbohydrates are naturally present as simple sugars in fruits, milk, and other foods. Plant carbohydrates also can be refined to produce sugar products such as table sugar or corn syrup. The two main types of sugars are monosaccharides and disaccharides. **Monosaccharides** consist of a single sugar molecule (*mono* meaning "one" and *saccharide* meaning "sugar"). **Disaccharides** consist of two sugar molecules chemically joined together (*di* meaning "two"). Monosaccharides and disaccharides give various degrees of sweetness to foods.

Monosaccharides: The Single Sugars

The most common monosaccharides in the human diet are the following:

- Glucose
- Fructose
- Galactose

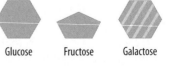

Glucose   Fructose   Galactose

All three monosaccharides have six carbons, and all have the chemical formula $C_6H_{12}O_6$, but each has a different arrangement of these atoms. The carbon and oxygen atoms of glucose and galactose form a six-sided ring.

Glucose

The monosaccharide **glucose** is the most abundant simple carbohydrate unit in nature. Also referred to as dextrose, glucose plays a key role in both foods and the body. Glucose gives food a mildly sweet flavor. It doesn't usually exist as a monosaccharide in food but is instead joined to other sugars to form disaccharides, starch, or dietary fiber. Glucose makes up at least one of the two sugar molecules in every disaccharide.

In the body, glucose supplies energy to cells. The body closely regulates blood glucose (blood sugar) levels to ensure a constant fuel source for vital body functions. Glucose is virtually the only fuel used by the brain, except during prolonged starvation, when the glucose supply is low.

Fructose

Fruit sugar, **fructose**, tastes the sweetest of all the sugars and occurs naturally in fruits and vegetables. Although the sugar in honey is about half fructose and half glucose, fructose is the primary source of its sweet taste. Food manufacturers use high-fructose corn syrup as an additive to sweeten many foods, including soft drinks, fruit beverages, desserts, candies, jellies, and jams. The term *high fructose* is a little misleading—the fructose content of this sweetener is around 50 percent.

Galactose

Galactose rarely occurs as a monosaccharide in food. It usually is chemically bonded to glucose to form lactose, the primary sugar in milk and dairy products.

Disaccharides: The Double Sugars

Disaccharides consist of two monosaccharides linked together. The following disaccharides (see **FIGURE 4.2**) are important in human nutrition:

- Sucrose (common table sugar)
- Lactose (major sugar in milk)
- Maltose (product of starch digestion)

Sucrose

Sucrose, most familiar to us as table sugar, is made up of one molecule of glucose and one molecule of fructose. Sucrose provides some of the natural sweetness of honey, maple syrup, fruits, and vegetables. Manufacturers use a refining process to extract sucrose from the juices of sugar cane or sugar beets. Full refining removes impurities; white sugar and powdered sugar are so highly refined that they are virtually 100 percent sucrose. When a food label lists sugar as an ingredient, the term refers to sucrose.

Lactose

Lactose, or milk sugar, is composed of one molecule of glucose and one molecule of galactose. Lactose gives milk and other dairy products a slightly sweet taste. Human milk has a higher concentration (approximately 7 grams per 100 milliliters) of lactose than cow's

▶ **glucose [GLOO-kose]** A common monosaccharide containing six carbons that is present in the blood. It is a component of the disaccharides sucrose, lactose, and maltose and various complex carbohydrates. Also known as *dextrose* or *blood sugar*.

▶ **fructose [FROOK-tose]** A common monosaccharide containing six carbons that is naturally present in honey and many fruits; often added to foods in the form of high-fructose corn syrup. Also called *levulose* or *fruit sugar*.

▶ **galactose [gah-LAK-tose]** A monosaccharide containing six carbons that can be converted into glucose in the body. In foods and living systems, galactose usually is joined with other monosaccharides.

▶ **sucrose [SOO-crose]** A disaccharide composed of one molecule of glucose and one molecule of fructose joined together. Also known as *table sugar*.

▶ **lactose [LAK-tose]** A disaccharide composed of glucose and galactose. Also called *milk sugar* because it is the major sugar in milk and dairy products.

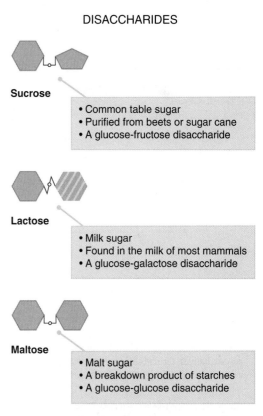

DISACCHARIDES

Sucrose
- Common table sugar
- Purified from beets or sugar cane
- A glucose-fructose disaccharide

Lactose
- Milk sugar
- Found in the milk of most mammals
- A glucose-galactose disaccharide

Maltose
- Malt sugar
- A breakdown product of starches
- A glucose-glucose disaccharide

FIGURE 4.2 The disaccharides: sucrose, lactose, and maltose. The three monosaccharides pair up in different combinations to form the three disaccharides.

milk (approximately 4.5 grams per 100 milliliters), so human milk tastes sweeter than cow's milk.

Maltose

Maltose is composed of two glucose molecules. Maltose seldom occurs naturally in foods, but is formed whenever long molecules of starch break down. Human digestive enzymes in the mouth and small intestine break starch down into maltose. When you chew a slice of fresh bread, you may detect a slightly sweet taste as starch breaks down into maltose. Starch also breaks down into maltose in germinating seeds. Maltose is fermented in the production of beer.

> **Key Concepts** Carbohydrates can be categorized as simple or complex. Simple carbohydrates include monosaccharides and disaccharides. The monosaccharides glucose, fructose, and galactose are single sugar molecules. The disaccharides sucrose, lactose, and maltose are double sugar molecules.

Complex Carbohydrates

Why Is This Important The complex carbohydrates are a large family of molecules that range from as few as three linked monosaccharides to hundreds or even thousands of linked monosaccharides. Some we can digest, others we cannot. Learning where to find complex carbohydrates in your diet and how they differ in structure will help you understand how they influence health in different ways.

Complex carbohydrates are chains of more than two sugar molecules. Short carbohydrate chains are called oligosaccharides and contain 3 to 10 sugar molecules. Long carbohydrate chains can contain hundreds or even thousands of monosaccharide units.

Oligosaccharides

Oligosaccharides (*oligo* meaning "scant") are short carbohydrate chains of 3 to 10 sugar molecules. Dried beans, peas, and lentils contain the two most common oligosaccharides—raffinose and stachyose.[1] Raffinose is formed from three monosaccharide molecules—one galactose, one glucose, and one fructose. Stachyose is formed from four monosaccharide molecules—two galactose, one glucose, and one fructose. The body cannot break down raffinose or stachyose, but they are readily broken down by intestinal bacteria and are responsible for the familiar gaseous effects of foods such as beans.

Human milk contains more than 200 different oligosaccharides, which vary according to the length of a woman's pregnancy, how long she has been nursing, and her genetic makeup.[2] For breastfed infants, oligosaccharides serve a function similar to dietary fiber in adults—making stools easier to pass. Certain human milk oligosaccharides act as prebiotics—they resist digestion in the small intestine, and after reaching the large intestine they become a food source for the "good bacteria" that are part of the gut microbiota.[3] Milk oligosaccharides also play important roles in children's diets; they can protect infants from disease-causing agents by binding to these agents in the intestines, and they provide sialic acid, a compound essential for normal brain development.[4]

Polysaccharides

Polysaccharides (*poly* meaning "many") are long carbohydrate chains of monosaccharides. Some polysaccharides form straight chains whereas

▶ **maltose [MALL-tose]** A disaccharide composed of two glucose molecules. Maltose seldom occurs naturally in foods but is formed whenever long molecules of starch break down. Sometimes called *malt sugar*.

▶ **complex carbohydrates** Chains of more than two monosaccharides. May be oligosaccharides or polysaccharides.

▶ **oligosaccharides** Short carbohydrate chains composed of 3 to 10 sugar molecules.

▶ **polysaccharides** Long carbohydrate chains composed of more than 10 sugar molecules. Polysaccharides can be straight or branched.

▶ **starch** The major storage form of carbohydrate in plants; starch is composed of long chains of glucose molecules in a straight (amylose) or branching (amylopectin) arrangement.

▶ **amylose [AM-ih-los]** A straight-chain polysaccharide composed of glucose units.

others branch off in all directions. Such structural differences affect how the polysaccharide behaves in water and with heating. The way the monosaccharides within them are linked makes the polysaccharides either digestible (e.g., starch) or indigestible (e.g., fiber).

Starch

Plants store energy as **starch** for use during growth and reproduction. Rich sources of starch include (1) grains, such as wheat, rice, corn, oats, millet, and barley; (2) legumes, such as peas, beans, and lentils; and (3) tubers, such as potatoes, yams, and cassava. Starch imparts a moist, gelatinous texture to food; for example, it makes the inside of a baked potato moist, thick, and almost sticky. The starch in flour absorbs moisture and thickens gravy.

Starch takes two main forms in plants: amylose and amylopectin. **Amylose** is made up of long, unbranched chains of glucose molecules, whereas **amylopectin** is made up of branched chains of glucose molecules. (See **FIGURE 4.3**.) Wheat flour contains a higher proportion of amylose, whereas cornstarch contains a higher proportion of amylopectin.

In the body, amylopectin is digested more rapidly than amylose.[5] Although the body easily digests most starches, a small portion of the starch in plants may remain enclosed in cell structures and escape digestion in the small intestine. Starch that is not digested is called **resistant starch**. Green bananas and cooked legumes such as peas are high in resistant starch.[6] Foods such as potatoes, rice, pasta, breakfast cereals, and bread are low in resistant starch; however, resistant starch forms when these types of foods are cooked and subsequently cooled.

Glycogen

Living animals, including humans, store carbohydrate in the form of **glycogen**, also called animal starch. Although some organ meats, such as kidney, heart, and liver, contain small amounts of carbohydrate, meat from muscle contains none.[7] This is because after an animal is slaughtered, enzymes in the muscle tissue break down most glycogen within 24 hours. Plant foods also do not contain glycogen, so it is a negligible carbohydrate source in our diets. Glycogen does, however, play an important role in our bodies as a readily mobilized store of glucose.

Glycogen is composed of long, highly branched chains of glucose molecules. Its structure is similar to amylopectin, but glycogen is much more highly branched. When we need extra glucose, for example during exercise, the glycogen in our cells can be broken down rapidly into single glucose molecules. Because enzymes can attack only the ends of glycogen chains, the highly branched structure of glycogen multiplies the number of sites available for enzyme activity.

Most glycogen is stored in skeletal muscle and the liver. In muscle cells, glycogen provides a supply of glucose for its own cells involved in strenuous muscular activity. Liver cells also use glycogen to regulate blood glucose levels throughout the body. Normally, the body can store only about 200 to 500 grams of glycogen at a time.[8] Some athletes practice a carbohydrate-loading regimen, which increases the amount of stored glycogen by 20 to 40 percent above normal, providing a competitive edge for marathon running and other endurance events.[9,10]

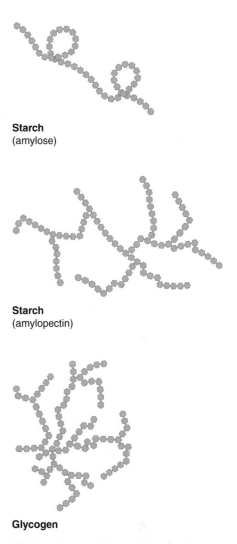

Starch
(amylose)

Starch
(amylopectin)

Glycogen

FIGURE 4.3 Starch and glycogen. Plants have two main types of starch—amylose, which has long unbranched chains of glucose, and amylopectin, which has branched chains. Animals store glucose in highly branched chains called glycogen.

Quick **Bite**

Banana Facts
You may know that bananas are high in potassium, but did you also know that they have an unusually high carbohydrate content? Before ripening, a banana is almost entirely starch. After ripening, certain bananas are almost entirely sugar—as much as 20 percent by weight.

▶ **amylopectin [am-ih-low-PEK-tin]** A branched-chain polysaccharide composed of glucose units.

▶ **resistant starch** A starch that is not digested.

▶ **glycogen [GLY-ko-jen]** A very large, highly branched polysaccharide composed of multiple glucose units. Sometimes called *animal starch*, glycogen is the primary storage form of glucose in animals.

▶ **dietary fiber** Carbohydrates and lignins that are naturally in plants and are nondigestible; that is, they are not digested and absorbed in the human small intestine.

▶ **functional fiber** Isolated nondigestible carbohydrates, including some manufactured carbohydrates, that have beneficial effects in humans.

▶ **soluble fiber** Nondigestible carbohydrates that dissolve in water.

▶ **insoluble fiber** Nondigestible carbohydrates that do not dissolve in water.

▶ **cellulose [SELL-you-los]** A straight-chain polysaccharide composed of hundreds of glucose units linked by beta bonds. It is nondigestible by humans and is a component of dietary fiber.

Fiber

All types of plant foods—including fruits, vegetables, legumes, and whole grains—contain dietary fiber. Animal sources of food, such as beef, pork, chicken, and eggs, do not contain fiber. **Dietary fiber** consists of indigestible carbohydrates and lignins that are intact and intrinsic in plants. Although not digested by the human gastrointestinal system and used as an energy source, these indigestible carbohydrates can enhance the process of digestion and provide other health benefits. **Functional fiber** refers to isolated, indigestible carbohydrates that have beneficial physiological effects in humans. Examples of functional fiber include extracted plant pectins, gums and resistant starches, chitin and chitosan, and commercially produced nondigestible polysaccharides.

Many types of dietary fiber resemble starches—they are polysaccharides, but they are not digested in the human GI tract. Fiber is often classified as being either soluble or insoluble. **Soluble fiber** dissolves easily in water. When it attracts water in the GI tract, it becomes gel-like, slowing digestion and absorption. Examples of soluble fiber include oligosaccharides, some hemicelluloses and beta-glucans (ß-glucans), pectins, gums, and mucilages. Conversely, **insoluble fiber** does not dissolve in water. This type of fiber adds bulk to stools and speeds up their passage through the digestive tract. Examples of insoluble fiber include cellulose, some hemicelluloses and β-glucans, and lignins. Whole-grain foods such as brown rice, rolled oats, and whole-wheat breads and cereals; legumes such as kidney beans, garbanzo beans (chickpeas), peas, and lentils; fruits; and vegetables are all rich sources of dietary fiber (see **TABLE 4.1**).

Cellulose

In plants, **cellulose** makes the walls of cells strong and rigid. It forms the woody fibers that support tall trees. It also forms the brittle shafts of hay and straw and the stringy threads in celery. Cellulose is made up of long, straight chains of glucose molecules. (See **FIGURE 4.4**.) Grains, fruits, vegetables, and nuts all contain cellulose.

TABLE 4.1
Foods Rich in Dietary Fiber

Fruits		Nuts and Seeds	
Apples	Grapefruit	Almonds	Sesame seeds
Bananas	Mangos	Peanuts	Sunflower seeds
Berries	Oranges	Pecans	Walnuts
Cherries	Pears	**Legumes**	
Cranberries		Most legumes	
Vegetables		**Grains**	
Asparagus	Green peppers	Brown rice	Wheat-bran cereals
Broccoli	Red cabbage	Oat bran	Wheat-bran breads
Carrots	Sprouts		

Modified from Shils ME, Shike M, Ross AC, Cabellero B, Cousins RJ, eds. *Modern Nutrition in Health and Disease.* 11th ed. Philadephia: Lippincott Williams & Wilkins; 2013.

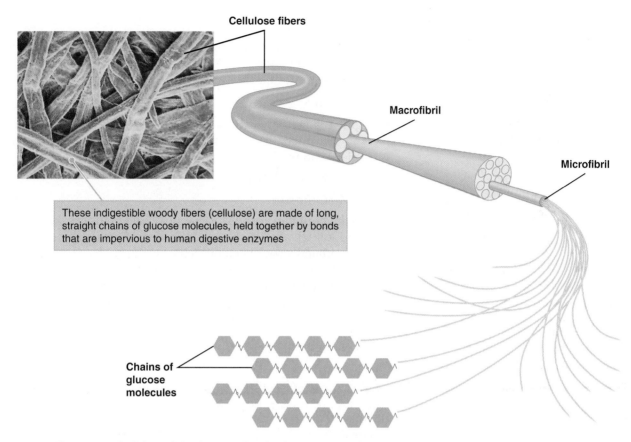

Cellulose fibers

Macrofibril

Microfibril

These indigestible woody fibers (cellulose) are made of long, straight chains of glucose molecules, held together by bonds that are impervious to human digestive enzymes

Chains of glucose molecules

FIGURE 4.4 The structure of cellulose. Cellulose forms the indigestible, fibrous component of plants and is part of grasses, trees, fruits, and vegetables.
© J.D. Litvay/Visuals Unlimited.

Hemicelluloses

The **hemicelluloses** are a diverse group of polysaccharides that vary from plant to plant. They are mixed with cellulose in plant cell walls.[11] Hemicelluloses are composed of a variety of monosaccharides with many branching side chains. The outer bran layer on many cereal grains is rich in hemicelluloses, as are legumes, vegetables, and nuts.

Pectins

Found in all plants, but especially fruits, **pectins** are gel-forming polysaccharides. The pectin in fruits acts like a cement that gives body to fruits and helps them keep their shape. When fruit becomes overripe, pectin breaks down into monosaccharides and the fruit becomes mushy. When mixed with sugar and acid, pectin forms a gel used to add firmness to jellies, jams, sauces, and salad dressings.

Gums and Mucilages

Like pectin, **gums** and **mucilages** are thick, gel-forming fibers that help hold plant cells together. The food industry uses plant gums (gum arabic, guar gum, locust bean gum, and xanthan gum, for example) and mucilages (such as carrageenan) to thicken, stabilize, or add texture to foods such as salad dressings, puddings, pie fillings, candies, sauces, and even drinks. **Psyllium** (the husk of psyllium seeds) is a mucilage that becomes very viscous (thick and sticky) when mixed with water. It is the main component in the laxative Metamucil and is added to some breakfast cereals.

▶ **hemicellulose [hem-ih-SELL-you-los-es]** A group of large polysaccharides in dietary fiber that are fermented more easily than cellulose.

▶ **pectin** A type of dietary fiber found in fruits.

▶ **gums** Dietary fibers, which contain galactose and other monosaccharides, found between plant cell walls.

▶ **mucilage** Gelatinous soluble fiber containing galactose, mannose, and other monosaccharides; found in seaweed.

▶ **psyllium** The dried husk of the psyllium seed.

▶ **lignin [LIG-nin]** Insoluble fiber composed of multi-ring alcohol units that constitute the only noncarbohydrate component of dietary fiber.

▶ **beta-glucan** Functional fiber, consisting of branched polysaccharide chains of glucose, that helps lower blood cholesterol levels; found in barley and oats.

▶ **chitin** A long-chain structural polysaccharide of slightly modified glucose. Found in the hard exterior skeletons of insects, crustaceans, and other invertebrates; also occurs in the cell walls of fungi.

▶ **chitosan** Polysaccharide derived from chitin.

Lignins

Not actually carbohydrates, **lignins** are indigestible substances that make up the woody parts of vegetables such as carrots and broccoli and the seeds of fruits such as strawberries.

Beta-glucans

Beta-glucans are polysaccharides of branched glucose units. These fibers are found in large amounts in barley and oats. Beta-glucan fiber is especially effective in lowering blood cholesterol levels (see the "Carbohydrates and Health" section later in this chapter).

Chitin and Chitosan

Chitin and **chitosan** are polysaccharides found in the exoskeletons of crabs and lobsters, and in the cell walls of most fungi. Chitin and chitosan are primarily consumed in supplement form. Marketed as being useful for weight control, chitosan supplements may impair the absorption of fat-soluble vitamins and some minerals[12]; however, published research has identified concerns with using chitosan supplements, such as their interacting with vitamins and causing malabsorption issues.[13] (See **FIGURE 4.5** for a summary classification of the most important dietary carbohydrates.)

Quick Bite

"An Apple a Day Keeps the Doctor Away"
Most likely this adage persisted over time because of the actual health benefits from apples. Apples have a lot of pectin, which is a soluble fiber known to be effective as a GI tract regulator.

Key Concepts Complex carbohydrates include starch, glycogen, and dietary fiber. Starch is composed of straight or branched chains of glucose molecules and is the storage form of energy in plants. Glycogen is composed of highly branched chains of glucose molecules and is the storage form of energy in humans and animals. Fibers include many different substances (both polysaccharides and oligosaccharides) that cannot be digested by enzymes in the human intestinal tract and are found in plant foods, such as whole grains, legumes, vegetables, and fruits.

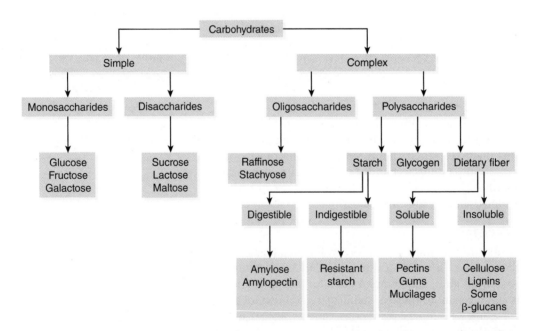

FIGURE 4.5 Summary of types of carbohydrates. Carbohydrates are classified as simple or complex. Simple carbohydrates include monosaccharides, such as glucose, fructose, and galactose, and disaccharides, such as sucrose, lactose, and maltose. Complex carbohydrates include oligosaccharides, such as raffinose and stachyose, as well as polysaccharides, such as glycogen, digestible starch (amylose and amylopectin), indigestible (resistant) starch, soluble dietary fiber (e.g. pectins), and insoluble dietary fiber (e.g. cellulose).

Carbohydrate Digestion and Absorption

🍎 **Why Is This Important?** Before carbohydrates are used as an energy source, you must first digest, absorb, and convert them into glucose molecules. Learning the steps of carbohydrate digestion and absorption can help you better understand why some foods are digested more quickly than others, why certain foods may make you feel full longer after eating, and why some people can enjoy foods like milk and cheese while others must avoid them.

Although glucose is a key building block of carbohydrates, you can't exactly find it on the menu at your favorite restaurant. You must first drink that chocolate milkshake or eat that hamburger bun so that your body can convert the food carbohydrate into glucose in the body. Let's see what happens to the carbohydrate foods you eat.

Digestion of Carbohydrates

Carbohydrate digestion begins in the mouth, where the starch-digesting enzyme salivary amylase breaks down starch into shorter polysaccharides and maltose. Chewing stimulates saliva production and mixes salivary amylase with food. Disaccharides, unlike starch, are not digested in the mouth. In fact, only about 5 percent of the starches in food are broken down by the time the food is swallowed. **FIGURE 4.6** provides an overview of the digestive process.

When carbohydrate enters the stomach, the acidity of stomach juices eventually halts the action of salivary amylase by causing the enzyme (a

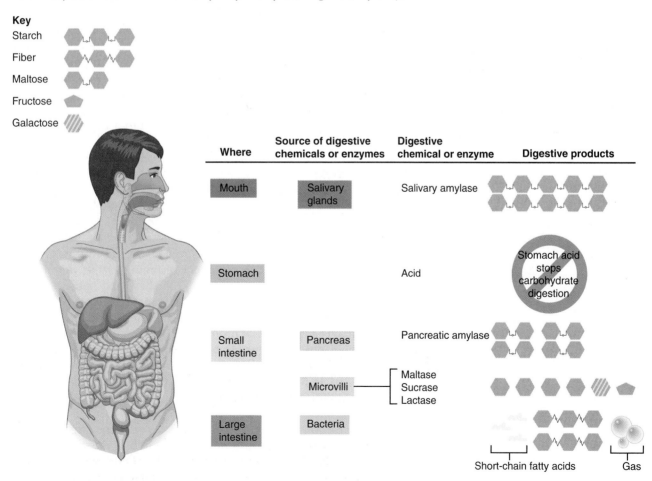

FIGURE 4.6 Carbohydrate digestion. Most carbohydrate digestion takes place in the small intestine.

▶ **pancreatic amylase** Starch-digesting enzyme secreted by the pancreas.

▶ **alpha (α) bonds** Chemical bonds linking monosaccharides, which can be broken by human intestinal enzymes, releasing the individual monosaccharides. Starch, maltose, and sucrose contain alpha bonds.

▶ **beta (β) bonds** Chemical bonds linking monosaccharides, which sometimes can be broken by human intestinal enzymes. Lactose contains digestible beta bonds, and cellulose contains nondigestible beta bonds.

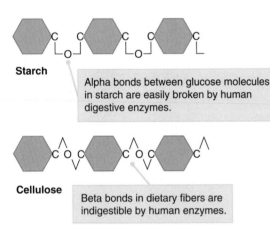

Starch

Alpha bonds between glucose molecules in starch are easily broken by human digestive enzymes.

Cellulose

Beta bonds in dietary fibers are indigestible by human enzymes.

FIGURE 4.7 Alpha bonds and beta bonds. Human digestive enzymes can easily break the alpha bonds in starch, but they cannot break the beta bonds in cellulose.

▶ **lactose intolerance** The inability to digest lactose, leading to diarrhea, bloating, and gas whenever lactose-containing foods are consumed.

protein) to lose its shape and function. Carbohydrate digestion starts again in the small intestine. This is how soluble fibers, such as pectins and gums, provide a feeling of fullness—they attract water and tend to delay digestive activity by slowing stomach emptying.

Most carbohydrate digestion takes place in the small intestine. As the stomach contents enter the small intestine, the pancreas secretes pancreatic amylase into the small intestine. **Pancreatic amylase** continues the digestion of starch, breaking it into many units of the disaccharide maltose. Meanwhile, enzymes attached to the brush border (microvilli) of the mucosal cells lining the intestinal tract go to work. These digestive enzymes break disaccharides into monosaccharides for absorption. The enzyme maltase splits maltose into two glucose molecules. The enzyme sucrase splits sucrose into glucose and fructose. The enzyme lactase splits lactose into glucose and galactose.

The bonds that link glucose molecules in complex carbohydrates are called glycosidic bonds. This type of covalent bond joins two simple sugars within a disaccharide or polysaccharide. Depending on the position of the OH group on the first carbon atom of the monosaccharide, the bond itself is identified as either an **alpha (α) bond** or a **beta (β) bond**. (See **FIGURE 4.7**.)

Human enzymes easily break alpha bonds, making glucose available from the polysaccharides starch and glycogen. Beta links are stronger than alpha links because they are more stable. Our bodies don't have enzymes to break most beta bonds, such as those that link the glucose molecules in cellulose, an insoluble fiber. Fiber remaining intact in the small intestine acts as a bulky barrier between certain nutrients (for example, glucose) and digestive enzymes, delaying their digestion and absorption. Additionally, soluble fiber can bind cholesterol and bile in the small intestine, inhibiting its absorption. This can lead to lower blood cholesterol levels, which is linked to a decreased risk for cardiovascular disease.

Beta bonds also link the galactose and glucose molecules in the disaccharide lactose, but the enzyme lactase is specifically tailored to attack this small molecule. People with a sufficient supply of the enzyme lactase can break these bonds; however, people with **lactose intolerance** do not have adequate lactase enzymes, so the beta bonds remain unbroken and lactose remains undigested until it interacts with bacteria in the colon. Symptoms associated with lactose intolerance can occur 30 minutes to 2 hours after consuming lactose, and include abdominal pain, bloating, flatulence, diarrhea, and nausea. People who are not able to make enough lactase can take lactase pills to aid in the digestion of lactose, thereby reducing the symptoms of lactose intolerance. The commercial product Beano is another example of an enzyme preparation designed to break down larger sugars (in this case, oligosaccharides in beans) into monosaccharides so that the body can absorb them. In this way, Beano also helps to minimize the flatulence caused by nondigestible carbohydrates reaching gas-producing bacteria in the large intestine.

Some carbohydrate remains intact as it enters the large intestine. This carbohydrate may be fiber or resistant starch, or the small intestine may have lacked the necessary enzymes to break it down. In the large intestine, bacteria partially ferment (break down) undigested carbohydrate and produce gas plus a few short-chain fatty acids. These fatty

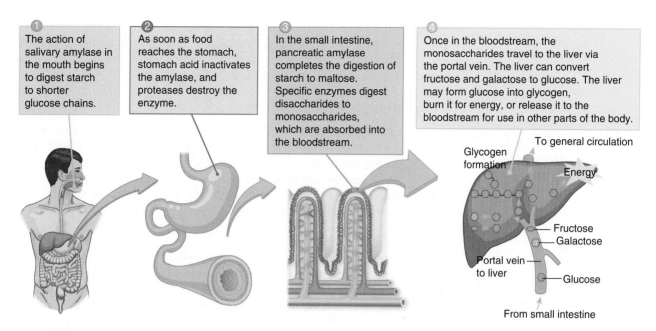

① The action of salivary amylase in the mouth begins to digest starch to shorter glucose chains.

② As soon as food reaches the stomach, stomach acid inactivates the amylase, and proteases destroy the enzyme.

③ In the small intestine, pancreatic amylase completes the digestion of starch to maltose. Specific enzymes digest disaccharides to monosaccharides, which are absorbed into the bloodstream.

④ Once in the bloodstream, the monosaccharides travel to the liver via the portal vein. The liver can convert fructose and galactose to glucose. The liver may form glucose into glycogen, burn it for energy, or release it to the bloodstream for use in other parts of the body.

To general circulation

Glycogen formation

Energy

Fructose
Galactose

Portal vein to liver

Glucose

From small intestine

FIGURE 4.8 **Travels with carbohydrate.** 1. Carbohydrate digestion begins in the mouth. 2. Stomach acid halts carbohydrate digestion. 3. Carbohydrate digestion resumes in the small intestine, where monosaccharides are absorbed. 4. The liver converts fructose and galactose to glucose, which it can assemble into chains of glycogen, release to the blood, or use for energy.

acids are absorbed into the colon and are used for energy by the colon cells. In addition, these fatty acids change the composition of the GI tract flora, which contributes to reduced risk of developing gastrointestinal disorders, cancers, and cardiovascular disease.[14]

Some fibers, particularly cellulose and psyllium, pass through the large intestine unchanged and therefore produce little gas. Instead, these fibers add to the stool weight and water content, making it easier to pass.

Absorption

Monosaccharides are absorbed into the mucosal cells lining the small intestine by two different mechanisms that you learned about in Chapter 3. Glucose and galactose are absorbed via active transport, which requires energy in the form of adenosine triphosphate (ATP). Fructose, on the other hand, is absorbed via facilitated diffusion. After absorption, glucose, galactose, and fructose molecules travel to the liver through the portal vein, where galactose and fructose are converted to glucose. The liver stores and releases glucose as needed to maintain constant blood glucose levels. **FIGURE 4.8** summarizes the digestion and absorption of carbohydrates.

Key Concepts Carbohydrate digestion takes place primarily in the small intestine, where digestible carbohydrates are broken down and absorbed as monosaccharides. Bacteria in the large intestine partially ferment resistant starch and certain types of fiber, producing gas and a few short-chain fatty acids that can be absorbed by the large intestine and used for energy. The liver converts absorbed monosaccharides into glucose.

Carbohydrates in the Body

🍎 **Why Is This Important?** In order to fully appreciate glucose's role as the primary energy source for cells (as opposed to fat and protein), it's important to understand the mechanisms by which your body regulates glucose levels in response to food intake and what happens when these processes go awry.

Through the processes of digestion and absorption, most of the carbohydrates in our diet from vegetables, fruits, grains, and milk becomes glucose. (The exceptions are fiber and resistant starch.) Glucose has one major role—to supply energy for the body.

Roles of Glucose

Cells throughout the body depend on glucose for energy to drive chemical processes. Although most—but not all—cells also can burn fat for energy, the body needs some glucose to burn fat efficiently.

When we eat food, our bodies immediately use some glucose to maintain normal blood glucose levels. We store excess glucose as glycogen in liver and muscle tissue.

Using Glucose for Energy

Glucose is the primary fuel for most cells in the body and the preferred fuel for the brain, red blood cells, and nervous system, as well as for the fetus and placenta in a pregnant woman. Even when fat is burned for energy, a small amount of glucose is needed to break down fat completely. To obtain energy from glucose, cells must first take up glucose from the blood. Once glucose enters cells, a series of reactions breaks it down into carbon dioxide and water, releasing energy in a form that is usable by the body.[15]

Storing Glucose as Glycogen

To store excess glucose, the body assembles it into the long, branched chains of glycogen. Glycogen can be broken down quickly, releasing glucose for energy when needed. Liver glycogen stores are used to maintain normal blood glucose levels throughout the body. Liver glycogen accounts for about one-third of the body's total glycogen stores. Muscle glycogen stores are used to fuel muscle activity, and account for about two-thirds of the body's total glycogen stores.[16] The body can store only limited amounts of glycogen—usually enough to last from a few hours to one day, depending on activity level.[17]

Sparing Body Protein

If carbohydrate is not available, both protein and fat can be used for energy. Although most cells can break down fat for energy, brain cells and developing red blood cells require a constant supply of glucose.[18] The availability of glucose for the brain is critical for survival because it takes an extended period of starvation for the brain to be able to use some by-products of fat breakdown for part of its energy needs. What happens if glucose stores (glycogen in liver and muscles) are depleted and the diet supplies no carbohydrate? To maintain blood glucose levels and supply glucose to the brain, the body can make glucose from body proteins. Adequate consumption of dietary carbohydrate spares body proteins from being broken down and used to make glucose.

Preventing Ketosis

Even when fat provides fuel for the body, the cells will still require a small amount of carbohydrate, in the form of glucose, to completely break down fat to release energy. When no carbohydrate is available, the liver cannot break down fat completely. Instead, it produces small compounds called **ketone bodies**.[19] Most cells can use ketone bodies for energy. The ability of the body to successfully produce and use ketone bodies from fat is essential for the body to adapt to times of inadequate energy and essential to survival during starvation.

Glucose

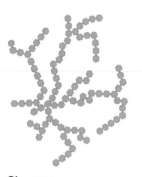

Glycogen

Glucose and Glycogen

▶ **ketone bodies** Molecules formed when insufficient carbohydrate is available to completely metabolize fat. Formation of ketone bodies is promoted by a low glucose level and high acetyl CoA level within cells. Acetone, acetoacetate, and beta-hydroxybutyrate are ketone bodies. Beta-hydroxybutyrate is sometimes improperly called a ketone.

Ketone bodies are produced normally in very small amounts. Increased production of ketones is most commonly caused by very low carbohydrate diets, starvation, and chronic alcoholism. To prevent **ketosis**, the buildup of ketone bodies, the body needs a minimum of 50 to 100 grams of carbohydrate daily.[20]

> **Key Concepts**   Glucose circulates in the blood to provide immediate energy to cells. The body stores excess glucose in the liver and muscle as glycogen. The body needs adequate carbohydrate intake so that body proteins are not broken down to fulfill energy needs. The body requires some carbohydrate to completely break down fat and prevent the buildup of ketone bodies in the blood.

Regulating Blood Glucose Levels

The body closely regulates blood glucose levels (also known as blood sugar levels) to maintain an adequate supply of glucose for cells. If blood glucose levels drop too low, a person becomes shaky and weak. If blood glucose levels rise too high, a person becomes sluggish and confused and may have difficulty breathing.

Two hormones produced by the pancreas, insulin and glucagon, tightly control blood glucose levels.[21] When blood glucose levels rise after a meal, special pancreatic cells called beta cells release the hormone insulin into the blood. **Insulin's** action can be thought of like a key, "unlocking" the cells of the body and allowing glucose to enter and fuel them. It also stimulates liver and muscle cells to store glucose as glycogen. As glucose enters cells to deliver energy or be stored as glycogen, blood glucose levels return to normal. (See **FIGURE 4.9**.)

When an individual has not eaten for a number of hours and blood glucose levels begin to fall, the pancreas releases another hormone, **glucagon**. Glucagon stimulates the body to break down stored liver glycogen, releasing glucose into the bloodstream. (See Figure 4.9b.) It also stimulates the synthesis of glucose from protein by a process called gluconeogenesis. Another hormone, **epinephrine** (also called

▶ **ketosis [kee-TOE-sis]**   Abnormally high concentration of ketone bodies in body tissues and fluids.

▶ **insulin [IN-suh-lin]**   Produced by beta cells in the pancreas, this polypeptide hormone stimulates the uptake of blood glucose into muscle and adipose cells, the synthesis of glycogen in the liver, and various other processes.

▶ **glucagon [GLOO-kuh-gon]**   Produced by alpha cells in the pancreas, this polypeptide hormone promotes the breakdown of liver glycogen to glucose, thereby increasing blood glucose. Glucagon secretion is stimulated by low blood glucose levels and by growth hormone.

▶ **epinephrine**   A hormone released in response to stress or sudden danger, epinephrine raises blood glucose levels to ready the body for "fight or flight." Also called *adrenaline*.

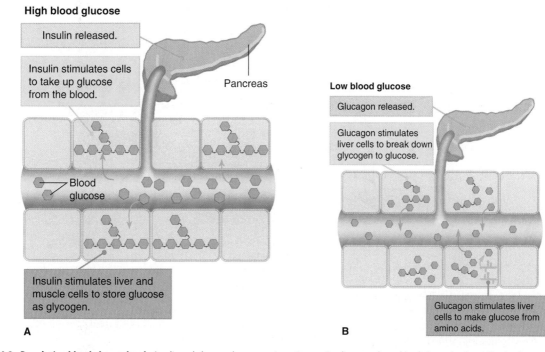

FIGURE 4.9   Regulating blood glucose levels. Insulin and glucagon have opposing actions. **a.** Insulin acts to lower blood glucose levels, and **b.** glucagon acts to raise them.

▶ **diabetes mellitus** A chronic disease in which uptake of glucose into body cells is impaired, resulting in higher glucose levels in blood and urine. Type 1 is caused by impaired insulin release from the pancreas. Type 2 occurs when body cells, such as fat and muscle cells, have an impaired response to insulin.

▶ **glycemic index** Measures the effect of food on blood glucose levels. It is the ratio of blood glucose response after eating a test food to blood glucose response after eating the same amount of white bread or glucose.

adrenaline), exerts effects similar to glucagon to ensure that all body cells have adequate energy for emergencies. Released by the adrenal glands in response to sudden stress or danger, epinephrine is called the fight-or-flight hormone.

Diabetes mellitus is a chronic disease in which blood glucose levels are not properly regulated. People suffering from this condition have impaired uptake of blood glucose by body cells, resulting in high glucose levels in their blood and urine. There are two types of diabetes mellitus. Type 1 diabetes is caused by decreased release of insulin from the pancreas. In type 2 diabetes, body cells, such as liver and muscle cells, do not respond normally to insulin action.

Glycemic Index of Foods

Different foods vary in their effect on blood glucose levels. The **glycemic index** measures the effect of a food on blood glucose levels (see **FIGURE 4.10**).

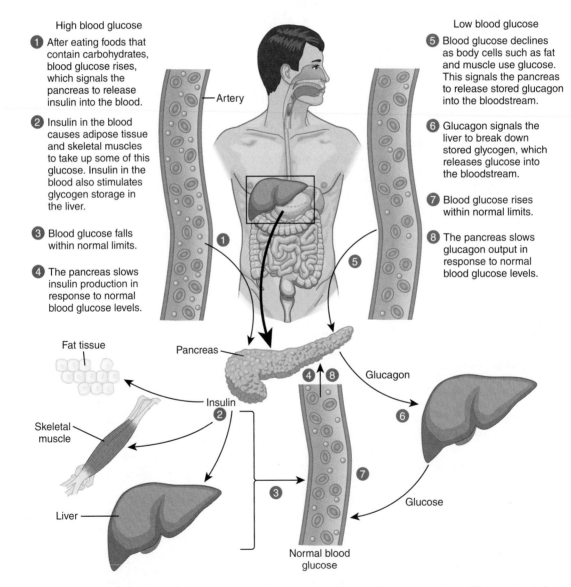

High blood glucose

1 After eating foods that contain carbohydrates, blood glucose rises, which signals the pancreas to release insulin into the blood.

2 Insulin in the blood causes adipose tissue and skeletal muscles to take up some of this glucose. Insulin in the blood also stimulates glycogen storage in the liver.

3 Blood glucose falls within normal limits.

4 The pancreas slows insulin production in response to normal blood glucose levels.

Low blood glucose

5 Blood glucose declines as body cells such as fat and muscle use glucose. This signals the pancreas to release stored glucagon into the bloodstream.

6 Glucagon signals the liver to break down stored glycogen, which releases glucose into the bloodstream.

7 Blood glucose rises within normal limits.

8 The pancreas slows glucagon output in response to normal blood glucose levels.

Artery

Fat tissue

Skeletal muscle

Liver

Pancreas

Insulin

Glucagon

Glucose

Normal blood glucose

FIGURE 4.10 Blood glucose regulation. The regulatory system for normal blood glucose comes by way of the pancreas monitoring blood glucose and adjusting its concentration as necessary, using the action of two opposing hormones: insulin and glucagon. When blood glucose is too high, the pancreas releases insulin and glucose is shifted to other cells, which helps to decrease blood glucose levels. When insulin is too low, the pancreas releases glucagon, which signals the liver to break down stored glycogen, which releases glucose into the bloodstream. Both actions work to bring blood glucose levels back to normal.

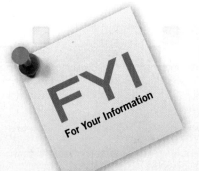

Is the Glycemic Index a Useful Tool for Constructing a Healthy Diet with Carbohydrates?

The glycemic index is a valuable tool and easy-to-use concept that may be important for individuals with diabetes to help fine tune their blood glucose control.[a] Several popular weight-loss diets use the glycemic index to guide food choices.

How Is the Glycemic Index Measured?

The glycemic index compares the change in blood glucose after eating a sample food to the change expected from eating an equal amount of available carbohydrate from a standard food, such as white bread, or from pure glucose. Therefore, the glycemic index is expressed as a percentage, ranging from 1–100, with 100 being the standard food.[b]

Foods with a high glycemic index trigger a sharp rise in blood glucose, followed by a dramatic fall, often to levels that are below normal. This explains why these foods could be undesirable for a person with diabetes. In contrast, low-glycemic-index foods trigger slower and more modest changes in blood glucose levels, thereby making blood glucose easier to manage. However, the effects of high or low glycemic index foods on people without diabetes are questionable, especially when eating a mixed diet.

What Factors Affect the Glycemic Index of a Food or Meal?

The glycemic index of a food is not always easy to predict. Would you expect a sweet food such as ice cream to have a high glycemic index? Ice cream actually has a low glycemic value because its fat slows sugar absorption. On the other hand, wouldn't you expect complex carbohydrates such as bread or potatoes to have a low glycemic index? In fact, the starch in white bread and cooked potatoes is readily absorbed, so each has a high value.[c] The glycemic indices of some common foods are listed in **TABLE A**, and lower-glycemic-index substitutions are provided in **TABLE B**.

The type of carbohydrate, the cooking process, and the presence of fat, dietary fiber, and other food components in a meal or snack all affect the glycemic response.[d,e] In a person's diet, it is the glycemic index of mixed meals, referred to as the glycemic load, that is more important than the effect of individual foods on blood glucose.[f] Specifically, the glycemic load takes into account the amount of carbohydrate consumed. Glycemic load is calculated by multiplying the glycemic index of a food by the amount of carbohydrate in a serving. Because the glycemic index is a percentage, the resulting value is divided by 100. High-glycemic-index foods do not necessarily have high glycemic loads if there is a relatively small amount of carbohydrate in one serving. For example, watermelon has a high glycemic index (72), but it mostly consists of water, and there is only a small amount of carbohydrate per serving.

Why Do Some Researchers Believe the Glycemic Index Is Useful?

Health benefits of following a low-glycemic-index diet can be significant. Diets that emphasize low-glycemic-index foods decrease the risk of developing type 2 diabetes and improve blood glucose control in people who are already afflicted.[g,h] Epidemiological studies suggest that such diets also reduce the risk of colon and other cancers and may help reduce the risk of heart disease.[i,j] Diets with a low glycemic load are associated with favorable blood lipid profiles.[k] Also, studies indicate that the effectiveness of low-fat, high-carbohydrate diets for weight loss can be improved by reducing the glycemic load.[l]

TABLE A
Glycemic Index of Some Foods Compared to Pure Glucose*

Food	Glycemic Index	Food	Glycemic Index
Bakery Products		***Fruits***	
Vanilla cake	42 ± 4	Apples	39 ± 3
Doughnut	75 ± 7	Watermelon	72 ± 13
Bread/Breakfast Foods		Dates	42 ± 4
Bagel	69	***Legumes***	
Wheat and rye bread	40	Baked beans	40 ± 3
Pita bread	68 ± 5	Black-eyed peas	38
All-Bran®	44 ± 6	Pinto beans	33
Froot Loops®	69 ± 9	***Pasta***	
Porridge	55 ± 2	Lasagna	53
Cereal Grains		Spaghetti	49 ± 3
Couscous	65 ± 7	***Vegetables***	
Sweet corn	52 ± 5	Pumpkin	64
Japonica short-grain brown rice	62 ± 5	Carrots	39 ± 4
Instant white rice	87 ± 2	Baked potato	86 ± 6
Dairy Foods		***Candy***	
Ice cream	57	Marshmallow	62 ± 6
Full-fat milk	41 ± 2	M&M's®, peanut	33 ± 3

* Glycemic response to pure glucose is 100.

Data from Atkinson FS, Foster-Powell K, Brand-Miller. International Tables of Glycemic Index Values: 2008. 2008 Diab Care; 31(12).

Why Do Some Researchers Believe the Glycemic Index Is Useless?

Whether a person is diabetic trying to control blood glucose levels, attempting weight loss, or reducing risk for heart disease, there is no "best way" to improve your diet. Some researchers question the usefulness of conclusions drawn primarily from epidemiological studies, given that these studies can show an association but cannot prove the cause. Additionally, results on the effectiveness of low glycemic index/load diets on health outcomes have been mixed.[m,n]

TABLE B
Sample Substitutions for High-Glycemic-Index Foods*

High-Glycemic-Index Food	Low-Glycemic-Index Alternative
Bread, wheat or white	Oat bran, rye, or pumpernickel bread
Processed breakfast cereal	Unrefined cereal such as oats (either muesli or oatmeal) or bran cereal
Plain cookies and crackers	Cookies made with nuts and whole grains such as oats
Cakes and muffins	Cakes and muffins made with fruit, oats, or whole grains
Bananas	Apples
White potatoes	Sweet potatoes, pastas, or legumes

* Low glycemic index = 55 or less; medium = 56–69; high = 70 or more.

Some believe the glycemic index is too complex for most people to use effectively. A recent study evaluating the reliability of glycemic index values in healthy adults concluded that there are too many factors influencing the accuracy and precision of glycemic index estimates for them to be useful as a basis for making food-based recommendations.[o] The American Diabetes Association has not endorsed widespread adoption of glycemic index diets for those with diabetes.[p]

What's the Bottom Line?

Like many other nutrition issues, the usefulness of the glycemic index as a tool to help make healthier carbohydrate choices continues to be studied. More information is still needed about the influence of processing techniques on the glycemic index, and studies on the reliability of glycemic index values should be replicated. Most researchers also call for prospective, long-term clinical trials to evaluate the effects of low-glycemic-index and low-glycemic-load diets in chronic disease

risk reduction and treatment.[q] Until then, for healthy eating, focus on consuming more whole grains and high-fiber carbohydrates, including minimally refined cereal products. Other low-glycemic-index foods won't hurt, and may help to improve health!

a   Mondazzi L, Arcelli, E. Glycemic index in sport nutrition. *J Am Coll Nutr.* 2009;28(Suppl):455S-463S.
b   Udani J, Singh B, Barrett M, Preuss H. Lowering the glycemic index of white bread using a white bean extract. *Nutr J.* 2009;8:52.
c   Foster-Powell K, Holt SH, Brand-Miller JC. International table of glycemic index and glycemic load values: 2002. *Am J Clin Nutr.* 2002;76:5-56.
d   Pi-Sunyer FX. Glycemic index and disease. *Am J Clin Nutr.* 2002;76(Suppl):290S-298S.
e   Fernandes G, Velangi A, Wolever T. Glycemic index of potatoes commonly consumed in North America. *J Am Diet Assoc.* 2005;105(4):557-562.
f   Franz M, Powers M, Leontos C, et al. The evidence for medical nutrition therapy for type 1 and type 2 diabetes in adults. *J Am Diet Assoc.* 2010;110(12):1852-1889.
g   Finley C, Barlow C, Halton T, Haskell W. Glycemic index, glycemic load, and prevalence of the metabolic syndrome in the Copper Center Longitudinal Study. *J Am Diet Assoc.* 2010;110(12):1820-1829.
h   Lowering the glycemic index of your diet pays health dividends. *Tufts University Health and Nutrition Letter.* September 2013.
i   Hu J, La Vecchia C, Augustin LS, et al. Glycemic index, glycemic load and cancer risk. *Ann Oncol.* 2013;24(1):245-251.
j   Mirrahimi A, Chiavaroli L, Srichaikul K, et al. The role of glycemic index and glycemic load in cardiovascular disease and its risk factors: a review of the recent literature. *Curr Atheroscler Rep.* 2014;16(1):381.
k   Goff LM, Cowland DE, Hooper L, Frost GS. Low glycemic index diets and blood lipids: a systematic review and meta-analysis of randomized controlled trials. *Nutr Metab Cardiovasc Dis.* 2013;23(1):1-10.
l   Cari K. Low-glycemic load diets: How does the evidence for prevention of disease measure up? *J Am Diet Assoc.* 2010;110(12):1818-1819.
m   Kristo AS, Matthan NR, Lichtenstein AH. Effect of diets differing in glycemic index and glycemic load on cardiovascular risk factors: review of randomized controlled-feeding trials. *Nutrients.* 2013;5(4):1071-1080.
n   Esfahani A, Wong JM, Mirrahimi A, Villa CR, Kendall CW. The application of the glycemic index and glycemic load in weight loss: a review of the clinical evidence. *IUBMB Life.* 2011;63(1):7-13.
o   Matthan NR, Ausman LM, Meng H, et al. Estimating the reliability of glycemic index values and potential sources of methodological and biological variability. *Am J Clin Nutr.* 2016;104(4):1004-1013.
p   American Diabetes Association. Nutrition recommendations and interventions for diabetes: a position statement of the American Diabetes Association. *Diabetes Care.* 2007;30(Suppl 1):S48-S65.
q   Ludwig DS, Eckel RH. The glycemic index at 20 y. *Am J Clin Nutr.* 2002;76(Suppl):264S-265S.

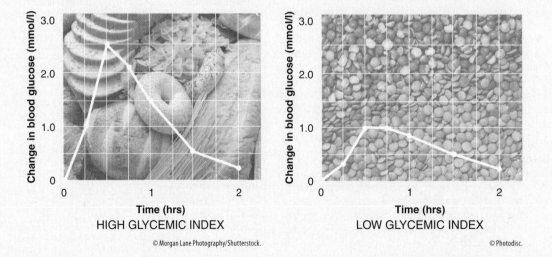

HIGH GLYCEMIC INDEX

LOW GLYCEMIC INDEX

© Morgan Lane Photography/Shutterstock.

© Photodisc.

The **glycemic load** is similar to the glycemic index except it accounts for the amount of carbohydrates in a serving of a particular food, whereas the glycemic index does not. Therefore, glycemic load is thought to be a more useful tool because it provides a more practical assessment of a food's actual impact on blood sugar. Foods with a high glycemic index and/or glycemic load cause a faster and higher rise in blood glucose, whereas foods with a low glycemic index/glycemic load cause a slower rise in blood glucose. Foods rich in simple carbohydrates or starch but low in fat or fiber tend to be digested and absorbed rapidly. This rapid absorption causes a corresponding large and rapid rise in blood glucose levels.[22] The body reacts to this rise by pumping out extra insulin, which rapidly lowers blood glucose levels. Other foods—especially those rich in dietary fiber, resistant starch, or fat—cause a less dramatic blood glucose response accompanied by smaller swings in blood glucose levels. Although some experts disagree on the usefulness of the glycemic index and glycemic load, diets that use glycemic index and load as a guide may offer important health benefits.[23]

The Role of Carbohydrates in Our Diet

🍎 **Why Is This Important?** In the United States, current consumption of carbohydrates does not align with recommended intakes, especially regarding fiber and added sugar. It is important to understand the discrepancies between what we currently eat and what we should be eating for optimal health so that nutrition and public health strategies can be developed to help close this gap.

The minimum amount of carbohydrate required by the body is based on the brain's requirement for glucose. This glucose can come either from dietary carbohydrate or from synthesis of glucose from protein in the body. What foods supply our dietary carbohydrates? **FIGURE 4.11** shows many foods rich in carbohydrates. Plant foods are our main dietary sources of carbohydrates: Grains, legumes, and vegetables provide starches and fibers; fruits provide sugars and fibers. Additional sugar (mainly lactose) is found in dairy foods, and various sugars are found in beverages, jams, jellies, candy, and sweet desserts.

Recommended Intake of Carbohydrate

Because adaptation to using protein for glucose and ketone bodies for energy may be incomplete, relying on protein alone is not recommended.[24] Therefore, a Recommended Dietary Allowance (RDA) for carbohydrate of 130 grams per day has been set for individuals age 1 year or older. The RDA for carbohydrate rises to 175 grams per day during pregnancy and 210 grams per day during lactation. The Acceptable Macronutrient Distribution Range (AMDR) for carbohydrate is 45 to 65 percent of daily energy intake. For an adult who eats about 2,000 kilocalories daily, this represents 225 to 325 grams of carbohydrate. The Daily Value for carbohydrate is 300 grams per day, representing 60 percent of the energy in a 2,000-kilocalorie diet.

It's important that sugar doesn't account for too much of this total. Although the AMDR for added sugars is no more than 25 percent of daily energy intake—a point at which the micronutrient quality of the diet declines—many sources suggest that added sugar intake should be lower. For example, the *2015–2020 Dietary Guidelines for Americans* and the World Health Organization recommend limiting added sugar to less than 10 percent of total energy intake. The *Dietary Guidelines*

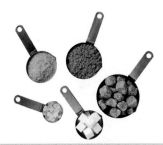

Table sugar, corn syrup, and brown sugar are rich in sucrose, a simple carbohydrate.

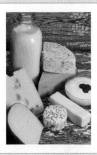

Milk and milk products are rich in lactose, a simple carbohydrate.

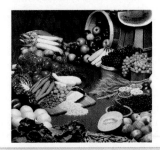

Fruits and vegetables provide simple sugars, starch, and fiber.

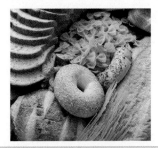

Bread, flour, cornmeal, rice, and pasta are rich in starch and, sometimes, dietary fiber.

FIGURE 4.11 Sources of carbohydrates. Table sugar, corn syrup, and brown sugar are rich in sucrose, a simple carbohydrate. Milk and milk products are rich in lactose, a simple carbohydrate. Fruits and vegetables provide simple sugars, starch, and fiber. Bread, flour, cornmeal, rice, and pasta are rich in starch and, sometimes, dietary fiber.

Measuring cups of sugars: © Photodisc; Milk products: © Comstock/Thinkstock; Fruits and vegetables: Photo by Keith Weller. Courtesy of USDA.; Bread, dried pasta, croissants, etc.: © Morgan Lane Photography/Shutterstock.

further suggests that we "reduce the intake of added sugars in an effort to build healthy eating patterns."[25] One key recommendation is to choose and prepare nutrient-dense foods and beverages with little added sugar.

As far as fiber is concerned, the *2015–2020 Dietary Guidelines for Americans* recommends that we consume a healthy eating pattern that includes a variety of dark green, red, and orange vegetables, as well as legumes (beans and peas) and starchy vegetables, fruits (especially whole fruits), and grains (at least half of which are whole grains).[26] The Adequate Intake (AI) value for total fiber is 38 grams per day for men ages 19 to 50 years and 25 grams per day for women in the same age group. This AI value is based on a level of intake (14 grams per 1,000 kilocalories) that provides the greatest risk reduction for heart disease.[27] The Daily Value for fiber used on food labels is 25 grams.

Current Consumption: How Much Carbohydrate Do You Eat?

Adult Americans currently consume about 49 to 50 percent of their energy intake as carbohydrate; however, this does not account for the quality of the carbohydrate consumed. According to National Health and Nutrition Examination Survey (NHANES) data, approximately 13 percent of adults' total caloric intakes came from added sugars. On average, men had an added sugar intake of about 83 grams per day, while women had an added sugar intake of 60 grams per day.[28] Increased consumption of added sugars has been linked to a decrease in intake of essential micronutrients and an increase in body weight.[29]

About one-third of Americans' added sugar intake comes from sugar-sweetened soft drinks in the form of white sugar and **high-fructose corn syrup (HFCS)**. This is of concern because as soft drink consumption rises, energy intake increases, but milk consumption and the vitamin and mineral quality of the diet decline.[30] Many studies suggest that rising soft drink consumption is a factor in overweight and obesity, even among very young children.[31] Regular soft drinks, sugary sweets, sweetened grains, and regular fruit-flavored beverages comprise 72 percent of the intake of added sugar.[32] Studies also show that consumption of sugar-sweetened beverages is associated with higher concentrations of insulin and leptin, both of which may be early markers of metabolic dysfunction, which can increase the risk of developing cardiovascular disease and diabetes.[33]

Most Americans do not consume enough dietary fiber, with usual intakes for men and women averaging only 18 and 15 grams per day, respectively.[34] With the exception of older women (51 years and older), only 0 to 5 percent of individuals in all other life stage groups have fiber intakes meeting or exceeding the AI—this is a consequence of Americans failing to meet recommendations for fruits, vegetables, and whole grain consumption.[35] The major sources of dietary fiber in the American diet are white flour and potatoes, not because they are concentrated fiber sources but because they are widely consumed.[36]

THINK About It 2

Choosing Carbohydrates Wisely

The *2015–2020 Dietary Guidelines for Americans* encourages a healthy eating pattern that contains fruits, vegetables, legumes, whole grains, and fat-free or low-fat milk, but keeps caloric intake under control. Choosing

▶ **glycemic load** The glycemic index of a food adjusted for the amount of carbohydrate in a serving of a particular food.

▶ **high-fructose corn syrup** Sweetener made from corn commonly added to food products and beverages in the United States. It is composed of either 42 percent or 55 percent fructose, with the remaining sugar being glucose.

Quick Bite

Sugar Overload

Americans consume very large quantities of carbonated soft drinks each year. Soft drink manufacturers produce enough of the sweet beverage to provide 557 12-ounce cans to every man, woman, and child in the United States each year. That equals over 52 gallons of soft drink each year! Today, adults consume nearly twice as many ounces of sugar-sweetened sodas as milk. Children's milk consumption was more than three times their soda consumption in the late 1970s, but today children consume roughly equal amounts of each.

Quick Bite

Low-Carb Diets

Over the last 20 years, low-carbohydrate diets, such as Atkins and the Paleo diet, have become popular weight loss strategies. Although these diets have been shown to be effective in helping people lose weight, and may even improve markers of cardiovascular disease risk and diabetes, there is also a considerable amount of controversy surrounding them. Many critics of low-carbohydrate diets argue that fruit, vegetable, and whole-grain intake is minimized and is insufficient to meet fiber requirements as well as vitamin and mineral needs. It is important to remember that there is no "magic bullet" for weight loss. Current recommendations to achieve and maintain a healthy weight include monitoring your calories consumed versus calories burned while eating a *balanced* diet that meets all nutrient requirements.

a variety of fruits and vegetables, and particularly including choices from all five vegetable subgroups (dark green vegetables, orange vegetables, legumes, starchy vegetables, and other vegetables) provides vitamins such as A, C, and folate; minerals such as potassium; phytochemicals; and fiber, yet little or no fat. **TABLE 4.2** lists various foods that are high in simple and complex carbohydrates.

Fiber in Our Diet

Along with fruits and vegetables, whole grains are important sources of fiber. Whole kernels of grain consist of four parts: germ, endosperm, bran, and husk. (See **FIGURE 4.12.**) The **germ**, the innermost part at the base of the kernel, is the portion that grows into a new plant. It is rich in protein, oils, vitamins, and minerals. The **endosperm** is the middle portion (and largest part) of the grain kernel. It is high in starch and provides food for the growing plant embryo. The **bran** is composed of layers of protective coating around the grain kernel and is rich in dietary fiber. The **husk** is an inedible covering.

When grains are refined—making white flour from wheat, for example, or making white rice from brown rice—the process removes the outer husk and bran layers and sometimes the inner germ of the grain kernel. Because the bran and germ portions of the grain contain much of the dietary fiber, vitamins, and minerals, the nutrient content of whole grains is far superior to that of refined grains. Although food manufacturers add iron, thiamin, riboflavin, folate, and niacin back to white flour through enrichment, they usually do not add back lost dietary fiber and nutrients such as vitamin B_6, calcium, phosphorus, potassium, magnesium, and zinc, which are lost in processing.

Read labels carefully to choose foods that contain whole grains. Terms such as *whole-wheat, whole-grain, rolled oats*, and *brown rice* indicate that the entire grain kernel is included in the food. Even better, look for the words *100 percent whole grain* or *100 percent whole wheat*.

To increase your fiber intake:

- Eat more whole-grain breads, cereals, pasta, and rice as well as more fruits, vegetables, and legumes.
- Incorporate more spiralized vegetables (e.g., zucchini noodles) in place of refined white pasta.
- Eat fruits and vegetables with the peel, if possible. The peel is high in fiber.
- Add fruits to muffins and pancakes.
- Add legumes—such as lentils and pinto, navy, kidney, and black beans—to casseroles and mixed dishes as a meat substitute.
- Substitute whole-grain flour for all-purpose flour in recipes whenever possible.
- Use brown rice or cauliflower rice instead of white rice.
- Substitute oats for flour in crumb toppings.
- Choose high-fiber cereals.
- Choose whole fruits rather than fruit juices.
- Choose whole vegetables rather than vegetable juices.

When increasing your fiber intake, do so gradually, adding just a few grams a day, because sudden or large increases in fiber can lead to

TABLE 4.2 High-Carbohydrate Foods	
High in Complex Carbohydrates	**High in Simple Carbohydrates**
Bagels	Fruits (naturally present)
Tortillas	Fruit juices
Cereals	Skim milk
Crackers	Plain nonfat yogurt
Rice cakes	Vanilla cake
Legumes	Soft drinks
Corn	Sherbet
Potatoes	Syrups
Peas	Sweetened nonfat yogurt
Squash	Candy
Popcorn	Jellies
	Jams
	Gelatin
	High-sugar breakfast cereals
	Cookies
	Frosting

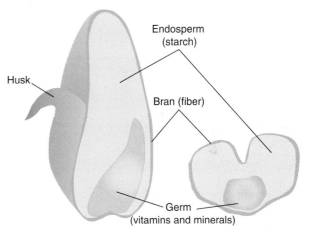

FIGURE 4.12 Anatomy of a kernel of grain. Whole kernels of grains consist of four parts: germ, endosperm, bran, and husk.

▶ **germ** The innermost part of a grain, located at the base of the kernel, that can grow into a new plant. The germ is rich in protein, oils, vitamins, and minerals.

▶ **endosperm** The largest, middle portion of a grain kernel. The endosperm is high in starch to provide food for the growing plant embryo.

▶ **bran** The layers of protective coating around the grain kernel that are rich in dietary fiber and nutrients.

▶ **husk** The inedible covering of a grain kernel. Also known as the *chaff*.

GI distress. Parents and caregivers should also emphasize foods rich in fiber for children older than 2 years, but must take care that these foods do not fill a child up before energy and nutrient needs are met.

Although health food stores, pharmacies, and even grocery stores sell many types of fiber supplements, most experts agree that you should get fiber from food rather than from a supplement.

Moderating Added Sugar Intake

Most of us enjoy the taste of sweet foods, and there's no reason why we should not. But for some individuals, habitually high sugar intake, specifically intake of sugar added during processing of foods, crowds out foods that are higher in fiber, vitamins, and minerals. To reduce added sugars in your diet:

- Use less of all added sugars, including white sugar, brown sugar, honey, agave syrup, and high-fructose corn syrup.
- Limit consumption of soft drinks, high-sugar breakfast cereals, candy, ice cream, and sweet desserts.
- Use fresh or frozen fruits and fruits canned in natural juices or light syrup for dessert and to sweeten waffles, pancakes, muffins, and breads.

Read ingredient lists carefully. Food labels list the total grams of sugar in a food, which includes both sugars naturally present in foods and sugars added to foods. Many terms for added sweeteners appear on food labels. Foods likely to be high in added sugar list some form of sweetener as the first, second, or third ingredient on labels. The updated Nutrition Facts panel (discussed at the end of this chapter) has a separate line for "added sugar" to provide further help for differentiating between the amount of naturally present sugar versus added sugar in a food product. **TABLE 4.3** lists various forms of sugar used in foods.

TABLE 4.3
Forms of Sugar Used in Foods

Agave syrup
Brown sugar
Concentrated fruit juice sweetener
Confectioners' sugar
Corn syrup
Dextrose
Galactose
Glucose
Granulated sugar
High-fructose corn syrup
Honey
Invert sugar
Lactose
Levulose
Maltose
Mannitol
Maple sugar
Molasses
Natural sweeteners
Raw sugar
Sorbitol
Turbinado sugar
White sugar
Xylitol

> **Key Concepts** Current recommendations suggest that Americans consume at least 130 grams of carbohydrate per day. An intake of total carbohydrates representing between 45 and 65 percent of total energy intake and a fiber intake of 14 grams per 1,000 kilocalories are associated with reduced heart disease risk. Added sugar should account for no more than 25 percent of daily energy and ideally should be much less. Americans generally eat too little fiber. An emphasis on a healthy eating pattern containing whole grains, legumes, fruits, and vegetables would help to increase fiber intake.

Nutritive Sweeteners

Nutritive sweeteners are digestible carbohydrates and therefore provide energy. They include monosaccharides, disaccharides, and **sugar alcohols** from either natural or refined sources. White sugar, brown sugar, honey, maple syrup, agave syrup, high-fructose corn syrup (HFCS), glucose, fructose, xylitol, sorbitol, and mannitol are just some of the many nutritive sweeteners used in foods. One slice of vanilla cake, for example, can contain about 5 teaspoons of sugar. Fruit-flavored yogurt contains about 7 teaspoons of sugar. Even two sticks of chewing gum contain about 1 teaspoon of sugar. Whether sweeteners are added to foods or are present naturally, all are broken down in the small intestine and absorbed as monosaccharides and provide energy. Because all these absorbed monosaccharides end up as glucose, the body cannot tell whether they came from honey or table sugar.

THINK About It 3

▶ **nutritive sweeteners** Substances that impart sweetness to foods and that can be absorbed and yield energy in the body. Simple sugars, sugar alcohols, and high-fructose corn syrup are the most common nutritive sweeteners used in food products.

▶ **sugar alcohols** Compounds formed from monosaccharides by replacing a hydrogen atom with a hydroxyl group (−OH); commonly used as nutritive sweeteners. Also called *polyols*.

Quick Bite

Why Is Honey Dangerous for Babies?

Because honey and Karo syrup (corn syrup) can contain spores of the bacterium *Clostridium botulinum*, they should never be fed to infants younger than 1 year of age. Infants do not produce as much stomach acid as older children and adults, so *C. botulinum* spores can germinate in an infant's GI tract and cause botulism, a deadly foodborne illness.

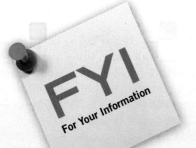

Excessive Sugar in the American Diet

Foods high in sugar are popular in American diets. These empty-calorie foods (e.g., candy, caloric soft drinks, sweetened gelatin, some desserts) provide energy but contain little or no dietary fiber, vitamins, or minerals. Data from the 2005–2010 NHANES study indicate that the average American consumes about 18 teaspoons of added sugars per day. American adults consume about 13 percent of their calories from added sugars; children (ages 2–19) consume about 16 percent of their calories from added sugars.[a,b] Caloric sweetened sodas and fruit drinks (containing less than 100 percent juice by volume) are major sources of added sugars in American diets, contributing an average of 8.78 teaspoons of added sugars each day. Teenagers (ages 12–19) consume 13.88 teaspoons of added sugars from sodas and fruit drinks per day.[c] Soda and other sugar-sweetened beverages are the largest source of added sugar in the diets of both children and adults in the United States. Studies have linked the increasing prevalence of obesity in children to consumption of sugar-sweetened drinks.[d] Consider that one 12-ounce soft drink contains 10 to 12 teaspoons of sugar. Would you add that much sugar to a glass of iced tea?

People with high energy needs, such as active teenagers and young adults, can afford to get a bit more of their calories from high-sugar foods. People with low energy needs, such as some elderly or sedentary people or people trying to lose weight, cannot afford as many calories from high-sugar foods. Most people can include moderate amounts of sugar in their diet and still meet other nutrient needs. But, as the amount of added sugar in the diet increases, intake of vitamins and minerals tends to decrease.[e,f]

a Ervin RB, Ogden CL. Consumption of added sugars among U.S. adults, 2005-2010. *NCHS Data Brief*. 2013;122.

b Ervin RB, Kit BK, Carroll MD, Ogden CL. Consumption of added sugar among U.S. children and adolescents, 2005-2008. *NCHS Data Brief*. 2012;87.

c Ogden CL, Kit BK, Carroll MD, Park S. Consumption of sugar drinks in the United States, 2005-2008. *NCHS Data Brief*. 2011;71.

d Evans AE, Springer AE, Evans MH, et al. A descriptive study of beverage consumption among an ethnically diverse sample of public school students in Texas. *J Am Coll Nutr*. 2010;29(4):387-396.

e Gibson S, Boyd A. Associations between added sugars and micronutrient intakes and status: further analysis of data from the National Diet and Nutrition Survey of Young People ages 4 to 18 years. *Br J Nutr*. 2009;101(1):100-107.

f Marriott BP, Olsho L, Hadden L, Connor P. Intake of added sugars and selected nutrients in the United States, National Health and Nutrition Examination Survey (NHANES) 2003-2006. *Crit Rev Food Sci Nutr*. 2010;50(3):228-258.

The sugar alcohols in sugarless chewing gums and candies are also nutritive sweeteners, but the body does not digest and absorb them fully, so they provide only about 2 kilocalories per gram, compared with the 4 kilocalories per gram that other sugars provide.

Natural Sweeteners   Natural sweeteners such as honey and maple syrup contain monosaccharides and disaccharides that make them taste sweet. Honey contains a mix of fructose and glucose—the same two monosaccharides that make up sucrose. Bees make honey from the sucrose-containing nectar of flowering plants. Real maple syrup contains primarily sucrose and is made by boiling and concentrating the sap from sugar maple trees. Most maple-flavored syrups sold in grocery stores, however, are made from corn syrup with maple flavoring added.

Many fruits also contain sugars that impart a sweet taste. Usually the riper the fruit, the higher its sugar content—a ripe pear tastes sweeter than an unripe one.

Refined Sweeteners   **Refined sweeteners** are monosaccharides and disaccharides that have been extracted from plant foods. White table sugar is sucrose extracted from either sugar beets or sugar cane. Molasses is a by-product of the sugar-refining process. Most brown sugar is really white table sugar with molasses added for coloring and flavor.

▶ **refined sweeteners** Composed of monosaccharides and disaccharides that have been extracted and processed from other foods, such as high-fructose corn syrup and agave syrup.

Quick Bite

▶ **polyols** See *sugar alcohols.*

▶ **nonnutritive sweeteners** Substances that impart sweetness to foods but supply little or no energy to the body. They include acesulfame, aspartame, saccharin, and sucralose. Also called *artificial sweeteners* or *alternative sweeteners.*

▶ **saccharin [SAK-ah-ren]** An artificial sweetener that tastes about 300 to 700 times sweeter than sucrose.

▶ **aspartame [AH-spar-tame]** An artificial sweetener composed of two amino acids. It is 200 times sweeter than sucrose and sold under the trade name NutraSweet.

▶ **acesulfame K [ay-see-SUL-fame]** An artificial sweetener that is 200 times sweeter than common table sugar (sucrose). Because it is not digested and absorbed by the body, acesulfame contributes no calories to the diet and yields no energy when consumed.

▶ **sucralose** An artificial sweetener made from sucrose; it was approved for use in the United States in 1998 and has been used in Canada since 1992. Sucralose is nonnutritive and about 600 times sweeter than sugar.

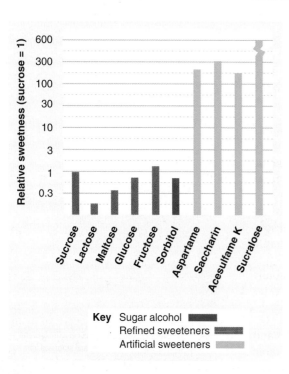

Key Sugar alcohol
Refined sweeteners
Artificial sweeteners

FIGURE 4.13 Comparing the sweetness of sweeteners. Nonnutritive sweeteners are much sweeter than table sugar.

Manufacturers make high-fructose corn syrup (HFCS) by treating cornstarch with acid and enzymes to break down the starch into glucose. Then different enzymes convert about half the glucose to fructose. HFCS has about the same sweetness as table sugar but costs less to produce. On average, Americans consume 118 calories of HFCS each day. Some studies indicate that increased HFCS consumption can contribute to obesity and high triglyceride levels,[37,38] but it remains unclear whether HFCS *causes* obesity. Caution is perhaps the best advice: Individuals should aim to limit their consumption of HFCS, but can enjoy it in moderation as part of an overall healthy eating pattern.

Another popular sweetener is agave syrup. Agave sweeteners are derived from the blue agave plant, which is also used to make tequila. Similar to HFCS, these sweeteners are highly processed and contain more fructose than glucose. Per tablespoon, agave contains more calories than table sugar, but it is 1.5 times sweeter. Therefore, replacing table sugar with agave sweetener can lower calorie intake, but only if smaller amounts are used. Research on potential health benefits of agave sweeteners is limited. The position of the American Diabetes Association is that agave consumption should be limited, just like consumption of sugar, honey, HFCS, and maple syrup.[39,40]

Sugar Alcohols The sugar alcohols sorbitol, xylitol, and mannitol occur naturally in a wide variety of fruits and vegetables and are commercially produced from other carbohydrates such as sucrose, glucose, and starch. Also known as **polyols**, these sweeteners are not as sweet as sucrose, but they do have the advantage of being less likely to cause tooth decay. The body does not digest and absorb sugar alcohols fully, so they provide only 2 kilocalories per gram compared with the 4 kilocalories per gram that other sugars provide. When sugar alcohols are used as the sweetener, the product may be sugar- (sucrose-) free, but it is not calorie-free. Check the label to be sure. Manufacturers use sugar alcohols to sweeten sugar-free products, such as gum and mints, and to add bulk and texture, provide a cooling sensation in the mouth, and retain moisture in foods. An excess intake of sugar alcohols may cause diarrhea.[41]

Nonnutritive (Artificial) Sweeteners

Gram for gram, most **nonnutritive sweeteners** (also called *artificial sweeteners*) are many times sweeter than nutritive sweeteners. As a consequence, food manufacturers can use much less artificial sweetener to sweeten foods. **FIGURE 4.13** compares the sweetness of sweeteners. Although some nonnutritive sweeteners do provide energy, their energy contribution is minimal given the small amount used.

Common nonnutritive sweeteners in the United States are **saccharin, aspartame, acesulfame K**, and **sucralose**. For people who want to decrease their intake of sugar and energy while still enjoying sweet foods, nonnutritive sweeteners offer an alternative. Also, nonnutritive sweeteners do not contribute to tooth decay. In the United States, our consumption of artificial sweeteners in foods and beverages has increased; however, only 15 percent of the population regularly consumes foods

TABLE 4.4
Summary of Nonnutritive Sweeteners

Nonnutritive Sweetener	Relative Sweetness to Sucrose	FDA Approval?	Typical Foods Where It Is Added	Acceptable Daily Intake (mg/kg body weight)
Saccharin	300x	Yes	Tabletop sweetener, beverages, fruit juices, drink mix	15
Aspartame	200x	Yes	Beverages, gelatin desserts, gums, fruit spreads	50*
Acesulfame K	200x	Yes	Gum, powdered drink mixes, nondairy creamers, gelatins, pudding	15
Sucralose	600x	Yes	Baked goods, beverages, gelatin desserts, frozen dairy desserts, tabletop sweetener	5
Neotame	7,000–13,000x	Yes	Tabletop sweetener	0.3
Stevioside (also known as stevia)	300x	No†	Sold as dietary supplement	–

*Set for general population. Individuals with phenylketonuria (PKU) should control phenylalanine intake from all sources, including aspartame.

†Rebaudioside A (a specific steviol glycoside) has been approved by the FDA as a food additive.

Data from U.S. Department of Health and Human Services, U.S. Food and Drug Administration. Additional information about high-intensity sweeteners permitted for use in food in the United States. http://www.fda.gov/food/ingredientspackaginglabeling/foodadditivesingredients/ucm397725.htm. Accessed August 21, 2017.

with artificial sweeteners, and average intakes are consistently below the acceptable daily intakes set by the FDA.[42] Common nonnutritive sweeteners are summarized in **TABLE 4.4**.

Carbohydrates and Health

🍎 **Why Is This Important?** As a nutrition expert, you will be inundated with questions such as, "Should I cut carbs to lose weight?" and "Will eating fiber prevent me from getting heart disease?" To address concerns and misconceptions within the general population, it is important to understand the current scientific evidence regarding the role of carbohydrates in health and disease.

THINK About It 4

Carbohydrates contribute both positively and negatively to health. On the upside, foods rich in fiber help keep the gastrointestinal tract healthy and may reduce the risk of heart disease and cancer. On the downside, excess sugar can contribute to weight gain, poor nutrient intake, and tooth decay.

Fiber and Obesity

Foods rich in fiber usually are low in fat and energy. They offer a greater volume of food for fewer calories, take longer to eat, and are filling. Once eaten, foods high in soluble fiber take longer to leave the stomach and they attract water, adding to the feeling of fullness. Consider, for example, three apple products with the same energy but different fiber content: a large apple (5 grams fiber), 1/2 cup of applesauce (2 grams fiber), and 3/4 cup of apple juice (0.2 grams fiber). Most of us would find the whole apple more filling and satisfying than the applesauce or apple juice.

Studies show that people who consume more fiber weigh less than those who consume less fiber, suggesting that fiber intake has a role in weight control. Although research supports a role for dietary fiber in reducing hunger and promoting satiety, studies on specific types of fiber have produced inconsistent results.[43]

Fiber and Type 2 Diabetes

People who consume plenty of dietary fiber, especially the fiber in whole grains and cereal, have a low incidence of type 2 diabetes.[44] Evidence suggests that the intake of certain fibers may delay glucose uptake and smooth out the blood glucose response, thus providing a protective effect against diabetes.[45] Current dietary recommendations for people with type 2 diabetes advise a high intake of foods rich in dietary fiber.[46]

Fiber and Cardiovascular Disease

High blood cholesterol levels increase the risk for heart disease. Dietary trials using high doses of oat bran, which is high in soluble fiber, show blood cholesterol reductions of 2 percent per gram of intake.[47] Because every 1 percent decrease in blood cholesterol levels decreases the risk of heart disease by 2 percent, high fiber intake can decrease the risk of heart disease substantially. Studies show a 20 to 40 percent difference in heart disease risk between the highest and lowest fiber-intake groups.[48]

Soluble fiber from oat bran, legumes, and psyllium can lower blood cholesterol levels. Your body uses cholesterol to make bile, which is secreted into the intestinal tract to aid fat digestion. Most bile is reabsorbed and recycled. In the gastrointestinal tract, fiber can bind bile and reduce the amount available for reabsorption. With less reabsorbed bile, the body makes up the difference by removing cholesterol from the blood and making new bile. The short-chain fatty acids produced from bacterial breakdown of fiber in the large intestine also may prevent cholesterol formation.[49]

Studies also show a relationship between high intake of whole grains and low risk of heart disease.[50] Whole grains contain fiber as well as antioxidants and other compounds that may protect against cellular damage that promotes heart disease. It is likely that the combination of compounds found in grains, rather than any one component, explains the protective effects against heart disease.[51] Consuming at least three 1-ounce servings of whole grains each day can reduce heart disease risk.[52]

Negative Health Effects of Excess Fiber

Despite its health advantages, high fiber intake can cause problems, especially for people who drastically increase their fiber intake in a short period of time. If you increase your fiber intake, you also need to increase your water intake to prevent the stool from becoming hard and impacted. A sudden increase in fiber intake also can cause increased intestinal gas and bloating. You can prevent these problems both by increasing fiber intake gradually over several weeks and by drinking plenty of fluids.

Fiber can bind small amounts of minerals in the GI tract and prevent them from being absorbed. In particular, fiber binds the minerals zinc, calcium, and iron. For people who get enough of these minerals, however, the recommended amounts of dietary fiber do not affect mineral status significantly.[53]

If the diet contains high amounts of fiber, some people, such as young children and the elderly, can become full before meeting their energy and nutrient needs. Because of a limited stomach capacity, they

Position Statement: Academy of Nutrition and Dietetics

Health Implications of Dietary Fiber

It is the position of the Academy of Nutrition and Dietetics that the public should consume adequate amounts of dietary fiber from a variety of plant foods.

Reprinted from *Journal of the Academy of Nutrition and Dietetics*, 108(10), Position of the American Dietetic Association: Health Implications of Dietary Fiber, Page no. 1716-1731., 2008, with permission from Elsevier.

TABLE 4.5
Summary of the Effects of Fiber in the GI Tract and Health Benefits

Digestive System	Effect on Digestion/Absorption	Health Benefits
Mouth	• Increased chewing	Eating less at a meal promotes calorie control. Reduces risk for *obesity*.
Stomach	• Increased feeling of fullness/satiety • Delayed stomach emptying	Eating less in-between meals promotes calorie control. Reduces risk for *obesity*
Small intestine	• Delays absorption of nutrients by physically blocking digestive enzymes • Decreases glycemic and insulin response • Binds cholesterol/bile and prevents absorption	Reduces risk for *type 2 diabetes* Reduces risk for *cardiovascular disease*
Large intestine	• Promotes growth of healthy bacteria. • Fermentation produces beneficial short-chain fatty acids. • Adds bulk to feces; decreases intestinal transit time.	Reduces risk of *colon cancer, constipation,* and *diverticular disease*

must be careful that fiber intake does not interfere with their ability to consume adequate energy and nutrients.

Because of the bulky nature of fibers, excess consumption is likely to be self-limiting. Although a high fiber intake might cause occasional adverse gastrointestinal symptoms, serious chronic adverse effects have not been observed. As part of an overall healthy diet, a high intake of fiber will not produce significant deleterious effects in healthy people. Therefore, a Tolerable Upper Intake Level (UL) is not set for fiber. A summary of the health benefits of fiber can be found in **TABLE 4.5**.

Key Concepts High intake of foods rich in dietary fiber offers many health benefits, including reduced risk of obesity, type 2 diabetes, cardiovascular disease, and gastrointestinal disorders. Increase fiber intake gradually while drinking plenty of fluids. Children and the elderly with small appetites should take care that energy needs are still met. No UL is set for fiber.

Health Effects of Sugar: Causation or Correlation?

Sugar has become the vehicle used by some diet zealots to create a new crusade. Cut sugar to trim fat! Bust sugar! Break the sugar habit! These battle cries demonize sugar as a dietary villain. But what are the facts?

Sugar and Obesity

Excess energy intake—not sugar intake—is associated with a greater risk of obesity. Take a look at fat. Fat is a more concentrated source of energy because it provides 9 kilocalories per gram compared to the 4 kilocalories per gram provided by carbohydrate. Many foods high in sugar, such as doughnuts and cookies, are also high in fat. Excess energy intake from any source will cause obesity, but sugar by itself is no more likely to cause obesity than starch, fat, or protein.

The increased availability of low-fat and fat-free foods has not reduced obesity rates in the United States, with obesity prevalence holding steady in children and increasing slightly in adults. Some speculate that consumers equate fat-free with calorie-free and eat more of these foods, not realizing that fat-free foods often have a higher sugar content, which makes any calorie savings negligible. Also, increased added sugar intake is associated with increased total calorie intake because foods high in added sugars often have low nutrient value and become "extras" in the diet.

Sugar and Diabetes Mellitus

It was once believed that eating too much carbohydrate or sugar could cause diabetes. However, contrary to popular beliefs, high intake of carbohydrate or sugar does not cause diabetes. It's actually obesity, specifically abdominal obesity, that is the single largest modifiable risk factor in the development of diabetes. If high sugar intake contributes to caloric excess—leading to weight gain, increased body fat, and obesity—then it will raise diabetes risk.

Sugar and Heart Disease

Risk factors for heart disease include a genetic predisposition, smoking, excessive alcohol consumption, physical inactivity, high blood pressure, high blood cholesterol levels, diabetes, and obesity.[54] Sugar by itself does not cause heart disease; however, added sugar intake is correlated with increased risk for cardiovascular disease mortality.[55] For example, when intake of high-sugar foods is part of an unhealthy diet that contributes to obesity, then risk for heart disease increases. In addition, excessive intake of refined sugar can alter blood lipids in carbohydrate-sensitive people, increasing their risk for heart disease. However, a high fat intake can also promote obesity. The take-away message is this: Any calorie imbalance that causes obesity raises the risk of heart disease; sugar should not be singled out as the only cause.

Sugar and ADHD in Children

Many parents and child care professionals will comment that eating sugary foods makes their children hyperactive. Attention-deficit hyperactivity disorder (ADHD) characterized by inattentive, hyperactive, and impulsive behavior is estimated to affect 5 percent of children worldwide.[56] What could be making this relationship so hard to understand? It is important to keep other environmental factors in mind when assessing the relationship between high-sugar foods and behavior. Take, for example, a child's birthday party, where a large dose of high-sugar foods such as cake, ice cream, soda, and goodie bags are all part of the celebration that involves games, prizes, and other exciting activities. A child's hyperactive behavior could be related to the exciting environment and enthusiasm for the special event. Alternatively, a child whose diet is regularly high in sugar is likely eating less nutritious foods overall; therefore, the child's irritable or restless behavior could be attributed to a nutrient deficiency or more generalized malnutrition.

Sugar and Dental Caries

In the previous examples, you learned that sugar intake is associated with potential health problems, but it is unclear whether they actually cause these health conditions. However, there is at least one impact on health where its role is clear: High sugar intake contributes to **dental caries**, or cavities. (See **FIGURE 4.14**.) When bacteria in your mouth feed on sugars, they produce acids that eat away tooth enamel and dental structure, causing dental caries. Although these bacteria quickly metabolize sugars, they feed on any carbohydrate, including starch.

▶ **dental caries [KARE-ees]** Destruction of the enamel surface of teeth caused by acids resulting from bacterial breakdown of sugars in the mouth.

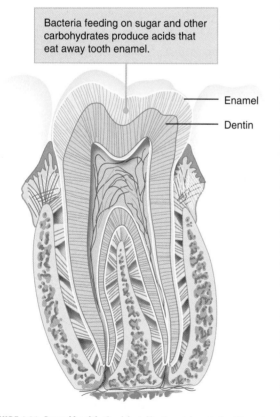

Bacteria feeding on sugar and other carbohydrates produce acids that eat away tooth enamel.

— Enamel

— Dentin

FIGURE 4.14 Dental health. Good dental hygiene, adequate fluoride, and proper nutrition help maintain healthy teeth. A well-balanced diet contains vitamins and minerals crucial for healthy bones and teeth. To help prevent dental caries, avoid continuous snacking on high-sugar foods, especially those that stick to the teeth.

The longer a carbohydrate remains in the mouth, or the more frequently it is consumed, the more likely it is to promote dental caries. Foods that stick to your teeth, such as caramel, licorice, crackers, sugary cereals, and cookies, are more likely to cause dental caries than foods that are quickly washed out of your mouth. High-sugar beverages such as soft drinks are likely to cause dental caries when they are sipped slowly over an extended period of time. A baby should never be put to bed with a bottle, because the warm milk or juice may remain in the mouth for long periods of time, providing a ready source of carbohydrate for bacteria to break down. Snacking on high-sugar foods throughout the day provides a continuous supply of carbohydrates that nourish the bacteria in your mouth, promoting the formation of dental caries. Good dental hygiene, adequate fluoride, and a well-balanced diet for strong tooth formation can help prevent such cavities.[57]

Health Effects of Artificial Sweeteners

Several safety concerns have been raised regarding the regular use of artificial sweeteners. Some groups claim that aspartame, for example, could cause high blood levels of phenylalanine. In reality, high-protein foods such as meats contain much more phenylalanine than foods sweetened with aspartame. The amounts of phenylalanine in aspartame-sweetened foods are not high enough to cause concern for most people. However, people with a genetic disease called **phenylketonuria (PKU)** cannot properly metabolize the amino acid phenylalanine, so they must carefully monitor their phenylalanine intake from all sources, including aspartame.

▶ **phenylketonuria (PKU)** An inherited disorder caused by a lack or deficiency of the enzyme that converts phenylalanine to tyrosine.

Although some people report headaches, dizziness, seizures, nausea, or allergic reactions with aspartame use, scientific studies have failed to confirm these effects, and most experts believe aspartame is safe for healthy people.[58] The FDA sets a maximum allowable daily intake of aspartame of 50 milligrams per kilogram of body weight.[59] This amount of aspartame equals the amount in sixteen 12-ounce diet soft drinks for adults and eight diet soft drinks for children.

Artificial sweeteners can help you lower sugar intake, but foods containing artificial sweeteners may not provide less energy than similar products containing nutritive sweeteners. Rather than sugar, other energy-yielding nutrients, such as fat, are the primary source of the calories in these foods. Also, as use of artificial sweeteners has increased in the United States, so has sugar consumption—an interesting paradox!

Key Concepts Sweeteners add flavor to foods. Nutritive sweeteners provide energy, whereas non-nutritive sweeteners provide little or no energy. The body cannot tell the difference between sugars derived from natural and refined sources.

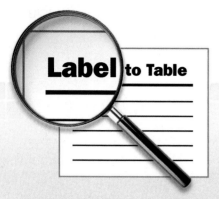

Recent changes to the Nutrition Facts food label have revised how carbohydrate information is presented to consumers. Look at the center of the original Nutrition Facts label (left panel), and you'll see the Total Carbohydrates along with two of the carbohydrate "subgroups"—Dietary Fiber and Sugars. Recall that carbohydrates are classified into simple carbohydrates and the two complex carbohydrates starch and fiber. Using this food label, you can determine all three of these components. There are 37 total grams of carbohydrate, with 1 gram coming from sugars and 4 grams from fiber. This means the remaining 32 grams must be from starch, which is not required to be listed separately on the label. Without even knowing what food this label represents, you can decipher that it contains a high proportion of starch (32 of the 37 grams) and is probably a potato, bread, pasta, or rice food item.

Do you see the "12%" listed to the right of Total Carbohydrate in the original label in the left panel? This doesn't mean that the food item contains 12 percent of its calories from carbohydrate. Instead, it refers to the Daily Value for carbohydrates listed at the bottom of the label. There you can see that a person consuming 2,000 kilocalories per day should consume 300 grams of carbohydrates each day. This product contributes 37 grams per serving, which is 12 percent of the Daily Value of 300 grams per day. Note that the Percent Daily Value for fiber is "16%" and would be considered a "good source" of fiber (defined as 10–19% of the DV).

In May 2016, the FDA introduced a new Nutrition Facts label (right panel) to reflect new scientific evidence on diet and chronic disease. One of the major changes to the label is the addition of "Added Sugars" in grams and percent Daily Value. This change is based on reported evidence that it is difficult to meet nutrient needs within calorie limits if you consume more than 10 percent of total calories from added sugar. Manufacturers have until July 2018 to comply with the new label requirements. Now, in addition to discerning the sugar, starch, and fiber content of foods, you will be able to determine the amount of sugar found naturally in the food versus how much has been added in processing.[a]

Recall that carbohydrates contain 4 kilocalories per gram. Armed with this information and the product's calorie information from the Nutrition Facts label, can you calculate the percentage of calories that come from carbohydrate?

Here's how:

37 g carbohydrate × 4 kcal per g = 148 carbohydrate kcal
148 carbohydrate kcal ÷ 230 total kcal = 0.64, or 64 percent carbohydrate kcal

[a] U.S. Food and Drug Administration. (2016). New Nutrition Facts Label - Side by Side Comparison. Retrieved from, https://www.fda.gov/downloads/Food/GuidanceRegulation/GuidanceDocumentsRegulatoryInformation/LabelingNutrition/UCM501646.pdf.

Original Label

Nutrition Facts

Serving Size 2/3 cup (55g)
Servings Per Container About 8

Amount Per Serving

Calories 230   Calories from Fat 72

	% Daily Value*
Total Fat 8g	**12%**
Saturated Fat 1g	**5%**
Trans Fat 0g	
Cholesterol 0mg	**0%**
Sodium 160mg	**7%**
Total Carbohydrate 37g	**12%**
Dietary Fiber 4g	**16%**
Sugars 1g	
Protein 3g	
Vitamin A	10%
Vitamin C	8%
Calcium	20%
Iron	45%

* Percent Daily Values are based on 2,000 calorie diet. Your daily value may be higher or lower depending on your calorie needs.

	Calories:	2,000	2,500
Total Fat	Less than	65g	80g
Sat Fat	Less than	20g	25g
Cholesterol	Less than	300mg	300mg
Sodium	Less than	2,400mg	2,400mg
Total Carbohydrate		300g	375g
Dietary Fiber		25g	30g

New Label

Nutrition Facts

8 servings per container
Serving size   2/3 cup (55g)

Amount Per Serving
Calories   **230**

	% Daily Value*
Total Fat 8g	**10%**
Saturated Fat 1g	**5%**
Trans Fat 0g	
Cholesterol 0mg	**0%**
Sodium 160mg	**7%**
Total Carbohydrate 37g	**13%**
Dietary Fiber 4g	**14%**
Total Sugars 12g	
Includes 10g Added Sugars	**20%**
Protein 3g	
Vitamin D 2mcg	10%
Calcium 260mg	20%
Iron 8mg	45%
Potassium 235mg	6%

*The % Daily Value (DV) tells you how much a nutrient in a serving of food contributes to a daily diet. 2,000 calories a day is used for general nutrition advice.

Learning Portfolio

Key Terms

Study Points

- Carbohydrates include the simple sugars and complex carbohydrates.
- Monosaccharides are the building blocks of carbohydrates.
- Three monosaccharides are important in human nutrition: glucose, fructose, and galactose.
- The monosaccharides combine to make disaccharides: sucrose, lactose, and maltose.
- Starch, glycogen, and fiber are long chains (polysaccharides) of monosaccharide units; starch and glycogen contain only glucose.
- Fibers are indigestible oligosaccharides and polysaccharides that can be classified as soluble or insoluble.
- Carbohydrates are digested by enzymes from the mouth, pancreas, and small intestine and absorbed as monosaccharides.
- The liver converts the monosaccharides fructose and galactose to glucose.
- Blood glucose levels rise after eating and fall between meals. Two pancreatic hormones, insulin and glucagon, regulate blood glucose levels, preventing extremely high or low levels.
- The main function of carbohydrates in the body is to supply energy. In this role, carbohydrates spare protein for use in making body proteins and allow for the complete breakdown of fat as an additional energy source.
- Carbohydrates are found mainly in plant foods as starch, fiber, and sugar.
- In general, Americans consume more sugar and less whole grains and fiber than is recommended.
- Carbohydrate intake can affect health. Excess sugar can contribute to low nutrient intake, excess energy intake, and dental caries.

Learning Portfolio (continued)

- Diets high in complex carbohydrates, including fiber, have been linked to reduced risk for GI disorders, heart disease, and cancer.

Study Questions

1. What are the differences among a monosaccharide, disaccharide, and polysaccharide?

2. What advantage does the branched-chain structure of glycogen provide compared to a straight chain of glucose?

3. Describe the difference between starch and fiber.

4. Which blood glucose regulation hormone is secreted in the fed state? The fasting state?

5. Which foods contain carbohydrates?

6. What are the most common nonnutritive sweeteners used in the United States?

7. What are potential consequences of habitually high sugar intake?

8. List the benefits of eating more fiber. What are the consequences of eating too much? Too little?

Try This

Banana Basics

Purchase one banana that is covered with brown spots (if necessary, let it sit on the counter for several days). Purchase another banana with a yellow skin, possibly with a greenish tinge, and no brown spots. Note that this may require two trips to the market.

Now it's time for the taste test. Mash each banana separately so both have the same consistency and texture. Taste each one. Which is sweeter?

As ripening begins, starch is converted to sugar. As fruit continues to ripen, sugar content increases. The sugar content of ripe, spotted bananas is higher than that of a green banana—by 20 percent or more!

The Sweetness of Soda

This experiment is to help you understand the amount of sugar found in a can of soda. Take a glass and fill it with 12 ounces (1 1/2 cups) of water. Using a measuring spoon, add 10 to 12 teaspoons of sugar to the water. Stir the sugar water until all the sucrose has dissolved. Now sip the water. Does it taste sweet? It shouldn't taste any sweeter than a can of regular soda. This is the amount of sugar found in one 12-ounce can!

The Fiber-Type Experiment

This experiment is to help you understand the difference between sources of dietary fiber. Go to the store and buy a small amount of raw bran. It is usually sold in a bin at a health food store or neat the hot cereals in a grocery store. Also purchase some pectin (near the baking items) or some Metamucil (in the pharmacy section). Once you're home, fill two glasses with water and put the raw bran in one glass and the pectin or Metamucil in the other. Stir each glass for a minute or two and watch what happens. Describe the differences. What would happen in your GI tract? What type of fiber is pectin? What type of fiber is in bran?

References

1. Biesiekierski JR, Rosella O, Rose R, et al. Quantification of fructans, galactooligosaccharides, and other short-chain carbohydrates in processed grains and cereals. *J Hum Nutr Diet.* 2011;24(2):154-176.

2. Hennet T, Weiss A, Borsig L. Decoding breast milk oligosaccharides. *Swiss Med Wkly.* 2014;144:w13927.

3. Musilova S, Rada V, Vikova E, Bunesova V. Beneficial effects of human milk oligosaccharides on gut microbiota. *Benef Microbes.* 2014;5:273-283.

4. Bruggencate T, Bovee-Oudenhoven IM, Feitsma AL, van Hoffen E, Schoterman MH. Functional role and mechanisms of sialyllactose and other sialylated milk oligosaccharides. *Nutr Rev.* 2014;72(6):377-389.

5. Syahariza ZA, Sar S, Hasjim J, Tizzotti MJ, Gilbert RG. The importance of amylose and amylopectin fine structures for starch digestibility in cooked rice grains. *Food Chem.* 2013;136(2):742-749.

6. Birt DF, Boylston T, Hendrich S, et al. Resistant starch: promise for improving human health. *Adv Nutr.* 2013;4(6):587-601.

7. Meat processing. *Encyclopedia Britannica* [online]. http://www.britannica.com/topic/meat-processing. Accessed August 22, 2017.

8. Rapoport B. Metabolic factors limiting performance in marathon runners. *PLoS Comput Biol.* 2010;6(10). doi: 10.1371/journal.pcbi.1000960.

9. Kerksick C, Harvey T, Stout J, et al. International Society of Sports Nutrition position stand: nutrient timing. *J Int Soc Sports Nutr.* 2008;5:17.

10. Hawley JA, Nutritional strategies to modulate the adaptive response to endurance training. *Nestle Nutr Inst Workshop Ser.* 2013;75:1–14.

11. Schisti C, Richter A, Blandr A, Richt A. Hemicellulose concentration and composition in plant cell walls under extreme carbon source-sink imbalances. *Physiol Plantarum.* 2010;139(3):241-255.

12. Walsh AM, Sweeney T, Bahar B, O'Doherty JV. Multi-functional roles of chitosan as a potential protective agent against obesity. *PLoS One.* 2013;8(1):e53828. doi:10.1371/journal.pome.0053828. Epub 2013 Jan 14.

13. Rodrigues MR, de Oliveira HP. Use of chitosan in the treatment of obesity: evaluation of interaction with vitamin B12. *Int J Food Sci Nutr.* 2012;63(5):548-552.

14. Kaczmarczyk MM, Miller MJ, Freund GG. The health benefits of dietary fiber: beyond the usual suspects of type 2 diabetes mellitus, cardiovascular disease, and colon cancer. *Metabolism.* 2012;61(8):1058-1066.

15. Martini FH. *Fundamentals of Anatomy and Physiology.* 9th ed. San Francisco: Benjamin Cummings; 2011.

16. Ibid.

17. Ibid.

18. Ibid.

19. Position of the Academy of Nutrition and Dietetics: weight management. *J Am Diet Assoc.* 2009;109(2):330-346.

20. Ibid.

21. Franz MJ, Powers MA, Leontos C, et al. The evidence for medical nutrition therapy for type 1 and type 2 diabetes in adults. *J Am Diet Assoc.* 2010;110(12):1852-1889.

22. The National Academy of Medicine, Food and Nutrition Board: Health and Medicine Division. Homepage. https://www.nap.edu/author/FNB/health-and-medicine-division/food-and-nutrition-board/. Accessed September 2017.

23. Burton PM, Monro JA, Alvarez L, Gallagher E. Glycemic impact and health: new horizons in white bread formulations. *Crit Rev Food Sci Nutr.* 2011;51(10):965-982.

24. The National Academy of Medicine, Food and Nutrition Board: Health and Medicine Division. Op. cit.

25. U.S. Department of Health and Human Services, U.S. Department of Agriculture. *2015-2020 Dietary Guidelines for Americans.* 8th ed. December 2015. http://health.gov/dietaryguidelines/2015/guidelines/. Accessed August 22, 2017.

26. Ibid.

27. The National Academy of Medicine, Food and Nutrition Board: Health and Medicine Division. Op. cit.

28. Ervin RB, Ogden CL. *Consumption of Added Sugars Among U.S. Adults, 2005-2010.* NCHS Data Brief No. 122. 2013.

29. Ibid.

30. U.S. Department of Health and Human Services, U.S. Department of Agriculture. *2015-2020 Dietary Guidelines for Americans.* 8th ed. December 2015. http://health.gov/dietaryguidelines/2015/guidelines/. Accessed August 22, 2017.

31. Nayga RM. Childhood obesity and unhappiness: the influence of soft drinks and fast food consumption. *J Happiness Stud.* 2010;11(3):261-275.

32. Marriott BP, Olsho L, Hadden L, Connor P. Intake of added sugars and selected nutrients in the United States, National Health and Nutrition Examination Survey (NHANES) 2003–2006. *Crit Rev Food Sci Nutr.* 2010;50:228-258.

33. Lana A, Rodriguez-Artalejo F, Lopez-Garcia E. Consumption of sugar-sweetened beverages is positively related to insulin resistance and higher plasma leptin concentrations in men and nonoverweight women. *J Nutr.* 2014; 144(7):1099-1105.

34. U.S. Department of Health and Human Services, U.S. Department of Agriculture. *2015-2020 Dietary Guidelines for Americans.* 8th ed. December 2015. http://health.gov/dietaryguidelines/2015/guidelines/. Accessed August 22, 2017.

35. Marriott BP, et al. Intake of added sugars and selected nutrients in the United States, National Health and Nutrition Examination Survey (NHANES) 2003–2006. Op. cit.

36. Slavin JL. Position of the American Dietetic Association: health implications of dietary fiber. *J Am Diet Assoc.* 2008;108(10):1716-1731.

37. Chan TF, Lin WT, Chen YL, et al. Elevated serum triglyceride and retinol-binding protein 4 levels associated with fructose-sweetened beverages in adolescents. *PLoS One.* 2014 Jan 27;9(1).

38. Ferder L, Ferder MD, Inserra F. The role of high-fructose corn syrup in metabolic syndrome and hypertension. *Curr Hypertens Rep.* 2010;12(2):105-112.

39. Horton J. The truth about agave. http://www.webmd.com/diet/features/the-truth-about-agave#1. External link on USDA Food and Nutrition Center *Nutritive and Nonnutritive Sweetener Resources.* Accessed November 3, 2016.

40. Position of the Academy of Nutrition and Dietetics: use of nutritive and non-nutritive sweeteners. *J Am Diet Assoc.* 2012;112(5):739-758.

41. Ibid.

42. U.S. Department of Health and Human Services, National Toxicology Program. *14th Report on Carcinogens, Appendix B: Substances Delisted from Report on Carcinogens.* November 3, 2016. Homepage: https://ntp.niehs.nih.gov/pubhealth/roc/index-1.html. Accessed September 8, 2017.

43. Karczak R, Lindeman K, Thomas W, Slavin JL. Bran fibers and satiety in women who do not exhibit restrained eating. *Appetite.* 2014;80:257-263.

44. Derosa G, Limas CP, Macias PC, et al. Dietary and nutraceutical approach to type 2 diabetes. *Arch Med Sci.* 2014;10(2):336-344.

45. Yu K, Ke MY, Li WH, Zhang SQ, Fang XC. The impact of soluble dietary fiber on gastric emptying, postprandial blood glucose, and insulin in patients with type 2 diabetes. *Asia Pac J Clin Nutr.* 2014;23(2):210-218.

46. American Diabetes Association. Home page. http://www.diabetes.org. Accessed August 22, 2017.

47. The National Academy of Medicine, Food and Nutrition Board: Health and Medicine Division. Op. cit.

48. Ibid.

49. Dalen JE, Devries S. Diets to prevent coronary heart disease 1957–2013: what have we learned? *Am J Med.* 2014;127(5):364-369.

50. Tovar J, Nilsson A, Johansson M, Bjorck I. Combining functional features of whole-grain barley and legumes for dietary reduction of cardiometabolic risk: a randomized cross-over intervention in mature women. *Br J Nutr.* 2014;111(4):706-714.

51. Oties S, Ozgoz S. Health effects of dietary fiber. *Acta Sci Pol Technol Aliment.* 2014;13(2):191-202.

52. The National Academy of Medicine, Food and Nutrition Board. *Dietary Reference Intakes for Energy, Carbohydrate, Fiber, Fat, Fatty Acids, Cholesterol, Protein, and Amino Acids (Macronutrients).* Washington, DC: National Academies Press; 2005. https://www.nap.edu/read/10490/chapter/1. Accessed September 7, 2017.

53. Ibid.

54. Centers for Disease Control and Prevention. Heart disease risk factors. http://www.cdc.gov/heartdisease/risk_factors.htm. Accessed August 22, 2017.

55. Yang Q, Zhang A, Gregg EW. Added sugar intake and cardiovascular diseases mortality among US adults. *JAMA Intern Med.* 2014;174(4):516-524.

56. American Psychiatric Association. *Diagnostic and Statistical Manual of Mental Disorders.* 4th ed., text rev. Washington, DC: American Psychiatric Association; 2000.

57. American Dental Association. *Fluoridation Facts.* Chicago: American Dental Association; 2005. http://www.ada.org/sections/professionalResources/pdfs/fluoridation_facts.pdf. Accessed August 22, 2017.

58. Position of the Academy of Nutrition and Dietetics: Use of Nutritive and Non-nutritive Sweeteners. Op cit.

59. Whitehouse C, Boullata J, McCauley LA. The potential toxicity of artificial sweeteners. *AAOHN J.* 2008;56(6):251-259.

Spotlight on Alcohol

Revised by Carolyn Dunn

THINK About It

1   In a word or two, how would you describe alcohol? Is it a nutrient?

2   What's your impression of the alcohol content of wine compared with that of beer? How about compared with vodka?

3   Have you ever thought of alcohol as a poison?

4   After a night out, which included drinking alcohol, your friend awakens with a splitting headache and asks you for a pain reliever. What would you recommend?

LEARNING Objectives

1 Describe the chemical characteristics of alcohol.

2 Describe the process of alcohol absorption.

3 Explain how differences in ethnicity, age, and gender affect a person's response to alcohol.

4 Describe the effects of alcohol on the nervous system.

5 Discuss the use and abuse of alcohol by college students, and devise strategies to change the culture.

6 Explain the effects of alcohol on the gastrointestinal system.

7 Contrast the health benefits of moderate alcohol consumption with the harmful effects of inappropriate intake.

▶ **alcohol** Common name for ethanol or ethyl alcohol. As a general term, it refers to any organic compound with one or more hydroxyl (–OH) groups.

T hink about **alcohol**. What images come to mind: Champagne toasts? Elegant gourmet dining? Hearty family meals in the European countryside? Or, do you think of wild parties? Sick, out-of-control drunks? Violence? Car accidents? Broken homes? No other food or beverage has the power to elicit such strong, disparate images—images that reflect the healthfulness of alcohol in moderation, the devastation of excess, and the political, social, and moral issues surrounding alcohol.

Alcohol has a long and checkered history. More of a drug than a food, alcoholic beverages produce druglike effects in the body while providing little, if any, nutrient value other than energy. Yet it is still important to consider alcohol in the study of nutrition. Alcohol is common to the diets of many people. In moderation, it may provide health benefits; yet even small quantities can raise risks for birth defects and breast cancer. In large amounts, it interferes with our intake of nutrients as well as the body's ability to use them, and it causes significant damage to every organ system in the body. The *2015–2020 Dietary Guidelines for Americans* advises that, "If alcohol is consumed, it should be in moderation—up to one drink per day for women and up to two drinks per day for men—and only by adults of legal drinking age."[1]

Alcohol in Context

🍎 **Why Is This Important?** Understanding the history of alcohol use will help you better understand how it fits into contemporary society and how our knowledge of its impact on health have changed over time.

For most people, alcohol consumption is a pleasant social activity. Moderate alcohol use generally does no harm. Nonetheless, many people have serious trouble with drinking. Episodes of heavy drinking are common among both adult populations and people under the age of 21. **Binge drinking**—described as a pattern of drinking that brings a person's blood alcohol concentration to 0.08 percent or higher—is the most common pattern of excessive alcohol use in the United States.[2] Binge drinking also can be defined for men as having five or more drinks within about two hours, and for women as having four

▶ **binge drinking** Consuming excessive amounts of alcohol in short periods of time.

Methanol
(wood alcohol)

Ethanol
(EtOH)

Methanol is an alcohol used as an alternative car fuel and in paint strippers, duplicator fluid, and model airplane fuels.

Ethanol is the alcohol in beer, wine, and liquor.

Glycerol

Isopropanol
(rubbing alcohol)

Glycerol is the alcohol that forms the backbone of triglyceride molecules.

Isopropanol is an alcohol that is used as a disinfectant or solvent, and in making many commercial products.

FIGURE SA.1 Alcohols. Ethanol is not the only alcohol people consume. When people eat fat, they consume the alcohol glycerol. Consuming the alcohol methanol or isopropanol can be deadly.

© Photodisc; © Photodisc; © Jones and Bartlett Publishers. Photographed by Kimberly Potvin.

or more drinks within the same time period.[3] According to the Centers for Disease Control and Prevention (CDC), about 90 percent of the alcohol consumed by youth under the age of 21 in the United States is in the form of binge drinking.[3] Binge drinking is associated with many nutrition-related health problems, including high blood pressure, stroke, and other cardiovascular diseases; liver disease; and poor control of diabetes.[4] It can also cause liver cirrhosis, brain damage, and harm to the fetus during pregnancy. In addition, drinking increases the number of deaths from automobile crashes, recreational accidents, on-the-job accidents, homicide, and suicide. Excessive alcohol use is the fourth leading lifestyle-related cause of death for the nation.[5] For teenagers, the leading causes of death are accidents (unintentional injuries), homicide, and suicide,[6] with alcohol being the leading contributor to accidents and injury deaths.[7]

History of Alcohol Use

Alcohol has had a prominent role throughout history. Old religious and medical writings frequently recommend its use, although with warnings for moderation. Thanks to alcohol's antiseptic properties, fermented drinks were safer than water during the centuries before modern sanitation, especially as people moved to towns and villages where water supplies were contaminated. Even mixing alcohol with dirty water afforded some protection from bacteria.[8]

At a time when life was filled with physical and emotional hardships, people valued alcohol for its analgesic and euphoric qualities. People relied on it to lift spirits, ease boredom, numb hunger, and dull the discomfort, even pain, of daily routine. Before the twentieth century, it was one of the few painkillers available in the Western world.[9]

The Character of Alcohol

Although there are many types of alcohol, the term *alcohol* commonly refers to the specific alcohol compound in beer, wine, and spirits. (See **FIGURE SA.1**.) Its technical name is **ethanol**, or **ethyl alcohol**. Ethanol is commonly abbreviated to EtOH, shorthand often preferred by health professionals. In this chapter, when we use the term *alcohol*, we are referring to ethanol.

Other types of alcohol are unsafe to drink. The simplest alcohol is *methanol*, also called methyl alcohol or wood alcohol, a solvent used in paints and for woodworking. Methanol is used in a number of consumer products, including paint strippers, duplicator fluid, model airplane fuel, and dry gas. Most windshield washer fluids are 50 percent methanol. If consumed, methanol can cause blindness or death.[10]

Is Alcohol a Nutrient?

Alcohol eludes easy classification. Like fat, protein, and carbohydrate, it provides energy when metabolized. Laboratory experiments in the nineteenth century demonstrated that upon oxidation, pure alcohol releases 7 kilocalories per gram, but many people doubted it actually produced energy in the body. These doubts were the basis of the controversial conclusion that alcohol was not food—a conclusion used by early Prohibitionists in their fight against alcohol. (See **FIGURE SA.2**.) However, a classic series of experiments by energy researchers Francis Atwater and Wilbur Benedict showed that alcohol did indeed produce

A MORAL AND PHYSICAL THERMOMETER.

A scale of the progress of Temperance and Intemperance.—Liquors with effects to their usual order.

TEMPERANCE.
Health and Wealth.

70	Water,	
60	Milk and Water,	
50	Small Beer,	Serenity of Mind, Reputation, Long Life, and Happiness.
40	Cider and Perry	
30	Wine,	Cheerfulness, Strength, and Nourishment, where taken only in small quantities, and at meals.
20	Porter,	
10	Strong Beer,	
0		

INTEMPERANCE.

		VICES.	DISEASES.	PUNISHMENTS.
0		Idleness,	Sickness,	Debt.
10	Punch	Gaming,	Tremors of the hands in	Jail.
20	Toddy and Egg Rum,	peevishness,	the morning, puking,	
30	Grog-Brandy and Water,	quarreling	bloatedness,	Black eyes,
		Fighting	Inflamed eyes, red nose	and Rags,
40	Flip and Shrub,	Horse-	and face,	Hospital or
50	Bitters infused in Spirits and Cordials.	Racing,	Sore and swelled legs,	Poor house.
		Lying and	jaundice,	
60	Drams of Gin, Brandy and Rum, in the morning,	Swearing,	Pains in the hands, burning in the hands, and feet	Bridewell.
70	The same morning and evening, The same during day and night,	Stealing & Swindling,	Dropsy, Epilepsy, Melancholy, Palsy, Appeplexy, Madness, Despair	State prison do for Life.
		Perjury,		
		Burglary,		
		Murder,		Gallows.

FIGURE SA.2 A moral and physical thermometer of temperance and intemperance. As part of a late eighteenth-century temperance movement, Philadelphian Dr. Benjamin Rush (1745–1813) created the Moral and Physical Thermometer and distributed it to clergy in a campaign against heavy drinking.

Reproduced from Rush B, 1823, *An Inquiry into the Effects of Ardent Spirits upon the Human Body and Mind*, 8th ed. (James Loring: Boston), 2-3.

7 kilocalories per gram in the body—findings that were a great disappointment to the temperance movement, because they showed that alcohol was a food.[11]

But alcohol's status as a nutrient is more questionable. It is certainly different from any other substance in the diet. It provides energy but is not essential, performing no necessary function in the body. Unlike the nutrients, alcohol is not stored in the body. And for no nutrient are the dangers of overconsumption so dramatic and the window of safety so narrow. In the small amounts most people usually consume, alcohol acts as a drug, producing a pleasant euphoria. For some people, it is addictive, with the characteristics of tolerance, dependence, and withdrawal symptoms. Certainly, alcohol is a substance available in the diet, but it does not meet the technical definition of a nutrient.

THINK About It 1

Key Concepts Alcohol, or more specifically the compound ethyl alcohol, has been part of people's diets for thousands of years. Although it provides calories, alcohol performs no essential function in the body and, therefore, is not a nutrient.

▶ **ethanol** Chemical name for drinking alcohol. Also known as *ethyl alcohol*.

▶ **ethyl alcohol** See *ethanol*.

Quick Bite

Nutrients in Beer?

Most of the carbohydrate used in the production of alcohol is converted to ethanol. In beer, however, some carbohydrate remains, along with a little protein and some vitamins. So although it is technically correct to say there are nutrients in beer, the amounts are small when beer is consumed at recommended low levels.

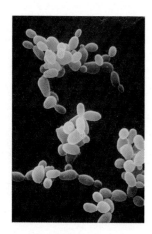

FIGURE SA.3 A micrograph of yeast.
© David M. Phillips/Visuals Unlimited.

▶ **fermentation** The anaerobic conversion of various carbohydrates to carbon dioxide and an alcohol or organic acid.

▶ **congeners** Biologically active compounds in alcoholic beverages that include nonalcoholic ingredients as well as other alcohols such as methanol. Congeners contribute to the distinctive taste and smell of the beverage and may increase intoxicating effects and subsequent hangover.

▶ **standard drink** One serving of alcohol (about 15 grams) is equal to 12 ounces of beer, 4 to 5 ounces of wine, or 1.5 ounces of liquor.

Quick **Bite**

A What?

An oenologist (pronounced EE-nologist) is an expert in the science of wine and wine making. This is different from viticulture, which is the agricultural endeavor of growing grapes for the use of wine making. The word *oenologist* is derived from the Greek (*oinos* meaning "wine," and the suffix *–logy* meaning "the study of").

Quick **Bite**

Energy Drinks + Alcohol = A Recipe for Trouble

Think twice before mixing energy drinks with alcohol. These drinks not only increase the risk of alcohol toxicity, but also increase the risk of serious injury, sexual assault, drunk driving, heart rhythm problems, nervous system problems, impaired judgment, shortness of breath, dizziness, disorientation, and rapid heartbeat. When alcohol is mixed with energy drinks, the high caffeine levels mask the depressant effects of alcohol but have no impact on the actual breakdown of alcohol. This increases the risk of alcohol toxicity.[13] The CDC estimates that people who mix alcohol with energy drinks triple their risk for binge drinking compared to those who don't.[14]

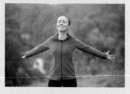
© fizkes/iStock/Getty Images.

Alcohol and Its Sources

When yeast cells metabolize sugar, they produce alcohol and carbon dioxide by a process called **fermentation**. If little oxygen is present, these cells produce more alcohol and less carbon dioxide. **FIGURE SA.3** shows living yeast cells.

Fermentation can occur spontaneously in nature—all that's needed is sugar, water, a warm environment, and yeast (whose spores are present in air and soil). Human experience with alcohol probably began at least 10,000 years ago with spontaneously fermented fruits or honey. Because all humans possess the enzymes to metabolize at least minimal amounts of alcohol,[12] it's reasonable to assume that humans have always had small quantities of alcohol in their diets. Very small amounts of alcohol are even produced by the microorganisms in our intestines.

Humans probably learned to make wine from fruits, mead from honey, and beer from grain about 5,000 years ago. In some areas, people made alcohol-containing dairy products. Using simple yeast fermentation, they could not produce beverages with alcohol levels exceeding 16 percent—the point at which alcohol kills off the yeast, halting alcohol production. Later, seventh-century Egyptian chemists discovered how to use distillation to capture concentrated alcohol, which could be added to drinks to boost alcohol content. Distilled alcoholic beverages (such as rum, gin, and whiskey) are called spirits, liquor, or hard liquor.

Distillation can yield more than just ethanol. Traces of other compounds, such as methanol, evaporate and then condense in the distilled product. Called **congeners**, these biologically active compounds help to create the distinctive taste, smell, and appearance of alcoholic beverages such as whiskey, brandy, and red wine. But congeners are also suspected of causing or contributing to hangovers[15] and may play a role in alcohol's relationship to cancer.

Beer, wine, and liquor have different alcohol levels: Most beer is up to 5 percent alcohol, although some beers exceed 6 percent; wine is 8 to 14 percent alcohol; and hard liquor is typically 35 to 45 percent alcohol. Beer and wine are labeled with the percentage of alcohol, but hard liquor is labeled by "proof," which is twice the alcohol percentage (an 80-proof whiskey is 40 percent alcohol).

THINK About It 2

Pure alcohol—a clear, colorless liquid used in chemistry labs—is 95 percent alcohol. (Even "pure" alcohol contains some water.) The beverage closest to pure alcohol is vodka, which is alcohol, water, and almost nothing else; gin is similar but flavored with juniper berries. Scotch, rum, rye, whiskey, and other liquors have residual flavor traces of the grain from which they were fermented or flavors introduced during storage. All liquors, however, offer little nutritional value besides energy. Beer and wine do contain unfermented carbohydrates and a trace of protein but, like liquor, have negligible minerals. With the exception of niacin in beer (a 12-ounce beer contains 1.8 milligrams of niacin, nearly 10 percent of the Daily Value), alcoholic beverages have negligible vitamins as well. **TABLE SA.1** shows the number of calories in various alcoholic beverages.

One serving of alcohol, or a **standard drink**, is defined as 12 ounces of regular beer, 5 ounces of wine (12 percent alcohol), or 1.5 ounces (a "jigger") of 80-proof liquor.[16] All contain roughly 15 grams (1 measuring tablespoon) of pure alcohol. Most health professionals who speak of "moderate alcohol intake" usually mean no more than one (for women)

TABLE SA.1
Calories in Selected Alcoholic Beverages

Beverage	Serving Size	Approximate Kilocalories
Beer (regular, 4.9% alcohol)	12 fl oz	153
Beer (craft, 6.9% alcohol)	12 fl oz	200
Beer (light)	12 fl oz	103
White wine	5 fl oz	121
Red wine	5 fl oz	125
Sweet dessert wine	3.5 fl oz	165
80-proof distilled spirits (gin, rum, vodka, whiskey)	1.5 fl oz	97

Note: This table is a guide to estimate the caloric intake from various alcoholic beverages. Higher alcohol content and mixing alcohol with other beverages, such as calorically sweetened soft drinks, tonic water, fruit juice, or cream, increases the amount of calories in the beverage. Alcoholic beverages supply calories but provide few essential nutrients.

Modified from U.S. Department of Agriculture, Agricultural Research Service. USDA National Nutrient Database for Standard Reference, release 28. 2015. http://www.ars.usda.gov/ba/bhnrc/ndl. Accessed March 30, 2017.

WHAT IS MODERATE DRINKING?

Women:
No more than **1** drink a day

Men:
No more than **2** drinks a day

COUNT AS ONE DRINK...

12 ounces of regular beer

5 ounces of wine

1.5 ounces of 80-proof distilled spirits

FIGURE SA.4 Moderate drinking.
Reproduced from USDA Center for Nutrition Policy and Promotion; © Photodisc; © Photodisc; © Photodisc.

or two (for men) servings in a day.[17] (See **FIGURE SA.4**.) Moderate intake is not an average of seven drinks per week when there are six days of abstinence followed by seven drinks in one night! That's binge drinking, and it's dangerous.

Key Concepts Alcohol is formed when yeast ferments sugars to yield energy. Distillation methods produce concentrated solutions containing up to 95 percent alcohol. A typical serving of beer, wine, or distilled spirits contains about 15 grams of alcohol.

Alcohol in the Body

Why Is This Important? There are many myths associated with how alcohol is metabolized in the body. Knowing the facts will help you be smarter about consumption of alcohol and better understand the impact it has on your body.

Alcohol Absorption

Alcohol absorption begins immediately in the mouth and esophagus. Although alcohol absorption continues in the stomach, the small intestine efficiently absorbs most of the alcohol a person consumes.[18] (See **FIGURE SA.5**.)

You've heard it before: "Don't drink on an empty stomach." Eating before or with a drink slows down the advance of alcohol into the bloodstream in several ways. Food, especially if it contains fat, delays emptying of the stomach into the small intestine. The delay also provides a longer opportunity for oxidizing stomach enzymes to work. And food dilutes the stomach contents, lowering the concentration of alcohol and its rate of absorption.

About 80 to 95 percent of alcohol is absorbed unchanged. However, some oxidation does take place in the digestive tract, mainly in the stomach, and products of this metabolism join alcohol as it diffuses

Quick Bite

What Ingredients Are in That Beer?

Have you ever wondered why beer and wine do not carry food labels? The alcohol industry is regulated by the U.S. Treasury Department, not the Food and Drug Administration; therefore, the same nutrition food labels are not required on alcohol. Although nutrition labeling is not required on most alcoholic beverages, several large manufacturers include this information due to consumer demand.

▶ **acetaldehyde** A toxic intermediate compound formed by the action of the alcohol dehydrogenase enzyme during the metabolism of alcohol.

into the gut cells.[19] These products travel via the portal vein directly to the liver, where most breakdown of alcohol takes place. When all goes well, metabolism achieves two goals: energy production and protection from the damaging effects of alcohol and its even more toxic metabolite **acetaldehyde**.

Removing Alcohol from Circulation

The body cannot store potentially harmful alcohol, so it works extra hard to get rid of it. To prevent alcohol from accumulating and destroying cells and organs, the body quickly breaks down alcohol and removes it from the blood. Alcohol breakdown (metabolism) always takes priority over the breakdown of carbohydrates, protein, and fats. Liver cells detoxify alcohol and use the products to synthesize fatty acids, which are assembled into fats. The liver can metabolize only a certain amount of alcohol per hour, regardless of the amount in the bloodstream. The rate of alcohol breakdown depends on several factors, including the amount of metabolizing enzymes in the liver, and varies greatly among individuals. In general, the amount of alcohol in the blood (blood alcohol concentration, or BAC) peaks in 30 to 45 minutes. (See **FIGURE SA.6**.) When absorption exceeds the liver's capacity, a bottleneck develops and alcohol enters the general circulation. Alcohol diffuses rapidly, dispersing equally into all body fluids, including cerebrospinal fluid and the brain and, during pregnancy, into the placenta and fetus. About 10 percent of circulating alcohol is lost in urine, through the lungs, and through skin. Consequently, urine tests and breathalyzer tests both reflect concentrations of blood alcohol as well as alcohol levels in the

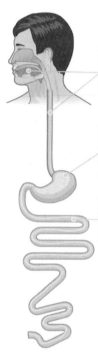

FIGURE SA.5 Alcohol absorption. Alcohol easily diffuses into and out of cells, so most alcohol is absorbed unchanged.

Small amounts of alcohol are absorbed in the mouth and esophagus.

Alcohol is readily absorbed in the stomach, but food will dilute the alcohol and delay gastric emptying.

The primary site of alcohol absorption is the upper small intestine.

Quick Bite

Alcohol Aversion Therapy

In alcohol aversion therapy, the medication disulfiram (Antabuse) deliberately blocks the conversion of toxic acetaldehyde to acetate (acetic acid). Even small amounts of alcohol trigger the highly unpleasant Antabuse–alcohol reaction, which includes a throbbing headache, breathing difficulties, nausea, copious vomiting, flushing, vertigo, confusion, and a drop in blood pressure.

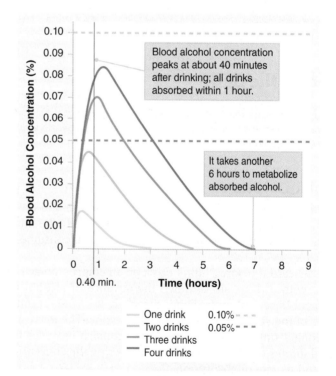

Blood alcohol concentration peaks at about 40 minutes after drinking; all drinks absorbed within 1 hour.

It takes another 6 hours to metabolize absorbed alcohol.

One drink	0.10%
Two drinks	0.05%
Three drinks	
Four drinks	

FIGURE SA.6 Blood alcohol concentration over time. Because the body metabolizes alcohol at a relatively constant rate, it clears small amounts faster than large amounts.

Reproduced from Wilkinson PK, et al. Pharmacokinetics of ethanol after oral administration in the fasting state. *J Pharmacokinet Biopharm*. 1977;5(3):207-224. Reprinted with kind permission from Springer Science + Business Media B.V.

brain and can indicate how much a person's mental and motor functions may be impaired.

Even after a person stops drinking, alcohol in the stomach and small intestine continues to enter the bloodstream and circulate throughout the body. Blood alcohol concentration continues to rise, and it is dangerous to assume the person will be fine by sleeping it off. Rapid binge drinking is especially dangerous, because the victim can ingest a fatal dose of alcohol before becoming unconscious. Excessive alcohol consumption deprives the brain of oxygen. The struggle to deal with an overdose of alcohol and lack of oxygen eventually causes the brain to shut down functions that regulate breathing and heart rate. This shutdown leads to a loss of consciousness and, in some cases, coma and death. When you hear of an **alcohol poisoning** death, it usually is the result of consuming such a large quantity of alcohol in such a short period of time that the brain of the victim is overwhelmed. Heart and lung functions shut down, and the person dies.

THINK
About It
3

The Morning After

After a night of heavy alcohol consumption, the drinker may suffer from a pounding headache, fatigue, muscle aches, nausea, and stomach pain as well as a heightened sensitivity to light and noise—a **hangover** in full force. The sufferer may be dizzy, have a sense that the room is spinning, and be depressed, anxious, and irritable. Usually a hangover begins within several hours after the last drink, when the blood alcohol level is dropping. Symptoms normally peak about the time the alcohol level reaches zero, and they may continue for an entire day.[20]

What causes a hangover? Scientists have identified several causes of the painful symptoms of a hangover. (See **FIGURE SA.7.**) Alcohol causes dehydration, which leads to headache and dry mouth. Alcohol directly irritates the stomach and intestines, contributing to stomach pain and vomiting. The sweating, vomiting, and diarrhea that can accompany a hangover cause additional fluid loss and electrolyte imbalance. Alcohol's hijack of the metabolic process diverts liver activity away from glucose production and can lead to low blood glucose (hypoglycemia), causing light-headedness and lack of energy. Alcohol also disrupts sleep patterns, interfering with the dream state and contributing to fatigue. The symptoms of a hangover are largely due to inflammation. In general, the greater the amount of alcohol consumed, the more likely a hangover will strike. However, some people experience a hangover after only one drink, whereas some heavy drinkers do not experience hangovers at all.[21]

In addition, factors other than alcohol may contribute to the hangover. A person with a family history of alcoholism has increased vulnerability to hangovers. Mixing alcohol and drugs also is suspected of increasing the likelihood of a hangover. The congeners in most alcoholic beverages can contribute to more vicious hangovers.

Treating a Hangover

So what can you do about a hangover? Few treatments have undergone rigorous, scientific investigation. Time is the most effective treatment—symptoms usually disappear in 8 to 24 hours. Eating bland foods that contain complex carbohydrates, such as toast or crackers, can combat low blood glucose and possibly nausea. Sleep can ease fatigue, and drinking nonalcoholic beverages can alleviate dehydration. Limited research suggests that taking vitamin B_6 or an extract from *Opuntia ficus indica* (a type of prickly pear cactus) before drinking may reduce the severity of hangover

▶ **alcohol poisoning** An overdose of alcohol. The body is overwhelmed by the amount of alcohol in the system and cannot metabolize it fast enough.

▶ **hangover** The collection of symptoms experienced by someone who has consumed a large quantity of alcohol. Symptoms can include pounding headache, fatigue, muscle aches, nausea, stomach pain, heightened sensitivity to light and sound, dizziness, and possibly depression, anxiety, and irritability.

Hangover Symptoms

Constitutional—fatigue, weakness, and thirst
Pain—headache and muscle aches
Gastrointestinal—nausea, vomiting, and stomach pains
Sleep and biological rhythms—decreased sleep, decreased dreaming when asleep
Sensory—vertigo and sensitivity to light and sound
Cognitive—decreased attention and concentration
Mood—depression, anxiety, and irritability
Sympathetic hyperactivity—tremor, sweating, increased pulse, and blood pressure

Possible Contributing Factors

Direct effects of alcohol
- Dehydration
- Electrolyte imbalance
- Gastrointestinal disturbances
- Low blood sugar
- Sleep and biological rhythm disturbances

Alcohol withdrawal
Alcohol metabolism (i.e., acetaldehyde toxicity)
Nonalcohol factors
- Compounds other than alcohol in beverages, especially the congener methanol
- Use of other drugs, especially nicotine
- Personality traits such as neuroticism, anger, and defensiveness
- Negative life events and feelings of guilt about drinking
- Family history for alcoholism

FIGURE SA.7 Hangovers. Factors other than just alcohol contribute to the misery of a hangover.

© Scott T. Baxter/Photodisc/Getty Images.

Consequences of Drinking

Youth and young adults who drink alcohol are more likely to experience school problems; social problems; legal problems; physical problems; unwanted, unplanned, and unprotected sexual activity; and physical and sexual assault, and are at a higher risk for suicide and homicide, alcohol-related car crashes and other unintentional injuries, memory problems, abuse of other drugs, changes in brain development, and death from alcohol poisoning.

▶ **alcohol dehydrogenase (ADH)** The enzyme that catalyzes the oxidation of ethanol and other alcohols.

▶ **aldehyde dehydrogenase (ALDH)** The enzyme that catalyzes the conversion of acetaldehyde to acetate, which forms acetyl CoA.

Body composition

Women have a higher percentage of fat than men and thus have less water to dilute alcohol.

Less enzyme activity

Women have 40% less alcohol dehydrogenase than men. Alcohol dehydrogenase is the primary enzyme involved in the metabolism of alcohol.

Body size

Women are smaller on average than men (smaller livers and less total water).

Hormonal fluctuations

Women typically have a heightened response to alcohol that is increased when they are about to have their periods, or when taking birth control pills.

FIGURE SA.8 Women and men respond differently to alcohol. Women tend to have a lower capacity for alcohol than men.

© Edyta Pawlowska/Shutterstock, Inc.

symptoms.[22] The prickly pear cactus extract may reduce three symptoms of hangover—nausea, dry mouth, and loss of appetite.[23] The best way to prevent a hangover, of course, is to abstain from drinking alcohol.

Certain medications also can relieve some symptoms. Antacids, for example, may relieve nausea and stomach pains. Aspirin may reduce headache and muscle aches, but could increase stomach irritation. Avoid acetaminophen, because alcohol breakdown enhances its toxicity to the liver.[24] In fact, people who drink three or more alcoholic beverages per day should avoid all over-the-counter pain relievers and fever reducers. These heavy drinkers may have an increased risk of liver damage and stomach bleeding from medicines that contain aspirin, acetaminophen (Tylenol), ibuprofen (Advil), naproxen sodium (Aleve), or ketoprofen (Orudis KT and Actron).[25]

THINK About It 4

Individual Differences in Alcohol Breakdown

Individuals vary in their ability to metabolize alcohol and acetaldehyde. As a consequence, they differ in their susceptibility to intoxication, hangover, and, in the long term, addiction and organ damage.

The result of individual differences is easiest to see in acute responses to alcohol. For example, when people of Asian descent drink alcohol, about half experience flushing around the face and neck, probably as a result of high blood acetaldehyde levels.[26] These individuals lack gastric **alcohol dehydrogenase**, and their livers have an inefficient form of **aldehyde dehydrogenase**. This may explain why their ancestors depended on boiled water (for teas) as a source of safe liquids. In contrast, Europeans are able to metabolize larger quantities of alcohol and historically have relied on fermentation to produce fluids that were safer to drink.[27]

Elderly people often find their tolerance for alcohol is less than it used to be. Due to decreased tolerance, the effects of alcohol, such as impaired coordination, occur at lower intakes in the elderly than in younger people, whose tolerance increases with increased consumption. This reduced tolerance is compounded by an age-related decrease in body water, so that blood alcohol concentrations in older people are likely to rise higher after drinking.[28]

Women and Alcohol

Men and women respond differently to alcohol. (See **FIGURE SA.8**.) Gender differences in body structure and chemistry cause women to absorb more alcohol and to break it down and metabolize it more slowly compared to men.[29] As a result, the immediate effects of drinking alcohol occur more quickly and last longer.[30] In addition, these differences make women more vulnerable to alcohol's long-term effects on health.[31,32] Let's take a closer look at some factors that are responsible for alcohol's more dominant effect on women.

Body Size and Composition Women, on average, are smaller than men and have smaller livers; thus, they have less capacity for metabolizing alcohol. Women also have lower total body water and higher body fat than men of comparable size. After alcohol is consumed, it diffuses uniformly into all body water, both inside and outside cells. Because of their smaller quantity of body water, women have higher concentrations of alcohol in their blood than men do after drinking equivalent amounts of alcohol.[33]

Less Enzyme Activity   Women also have less alcohol dehydrogenase (the primary enzyme involved in the metabolism of alcohol) activity than men—about 40 percent less.[34] This contributes to higher blood alcohol concentrations and lengthens the time needed to metabolize and eliminate alcohol. The gender difference in blood alcohol levels is due mainly to the significantly lower activity of gastric enzymes in women.[35]

Chronic Alcohol Abuse   Alcoholism and other abuses exact a greater physical toll on women than men. Female alcoholics have death rates 50 to 100 percent higher than those of male alcoholics. Furthermore, a higher percentage of female alcoholics die from suicides, alcohol-related accidents, circulatory disorders, and cirrhosis of the liver.

> **Key Concepts**   Alcohol does not need to be digested prior to absorption and moves easily across the gastrointestinal tract lining into the bloodstream. Once alcohol is absorbed, the liver metabolizes it. The primary metabolic enzymes are alcohol dehydrogenase and aldehyde dehydrogenase. Genetic and gender differences in the amount and activity levels of alcohol-metabolizing enzymes influence a person's response to consuming alcohol.

When Alcohol Becomes a Problem

🍎 **Why Is This Important?**   It is important that you understand when alcohol consumption crosses the line from something that may have health benefits to something that can be harmful or even fatal. Knowing the impact on increased alcohol use will help you make better health decisions.

Alcohol affects every organ system in the body. In the short term, small amounts of alcohol change the levels of neurotransmitters in the brain, reducing inhibitions and physical coordination. In the long term, chronic intake of large amounts of alcohol damages the heart, liver, gastrointestinal (GI) tract, and brain. When a pregnant woman drinks, alcohol can have a devastating effect on the development of her baby.

Alcohol in the Brain and the Nervous System

Alcohol diffuses readily into the brain, and because a small amount is absorbed from the mouth directly into circulating blood, its effects can be almost immediate, reaching the brain in as little as one minute after consumption. Alcohol can produce detectable impairments in memory after only a few drinks and, as the amount of alcohol increases, so does the degree of impairment. Large quantities of alcohol, especially when consumed quickly and on an empty stomach, can produce a blackout, that is, an interval of time for which the intoxicated person cannot recall key details of events, or even entire events. **FIGURE SA.9** shows the effects alcohol has on the brain.

Because alcohol is soluble in fat, it can easily cross the protective fatty membrane of nerve cells. There, it disrupts the brain's complex system for communicating between nerve cells. Neurotransmitters that excite nerve cells and those that inhibit nerve cells are thrown out of balance. Excess of some neurotransmitters produces sleepiness; high levels of others cause a loss of coordination; an imbalance of others impairs judgment and mental ability; and still other neurotransmitters perpetuate the desire to keep drinking, even when it's clearly time to stop. Changes in these messengers are suspected of leading to addiction and symptoms of alcohol withdrawal.[36] In the short run, they probably contribute to a hangover.

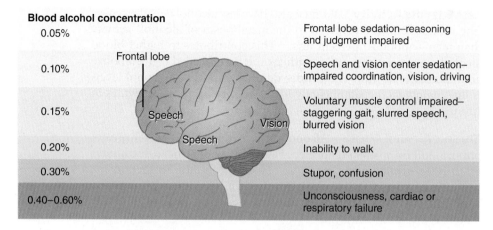

Blood alcohol concentration

BAC	Effect
0.05%	Frontal lobe sedation–reasoning and judgment impaired
0.10%	Speech and vision center sedation–impaired coordination, vision, driving
0.15%	Voluntary muscle control impaired–staggering gait, slurred speech, blurred vision
0.20%	Inability to walk
0.30%	Stupor, confusion
0.40–0.60%	Unconsciousness, cardiac or respiratory failure

FIGURE SA.9 Effects of alcohol on the brain. As blood alcohol concentration rises, different parts of the brain are affected.

Alcohol's short-term effects are related to how much a person drinks. One or two drinks typically bring alcohol blood levels to 0.04 percent and usually cause only mild, pleasant changes in mood and release of inhibitions. With more drinks and rising blood alcohol levels, coordination, judgment, reaction time, and vision are increasingly impaired. In the United States and Canada, it is illegal for a person whose blood level of alcohol has reached or exceeds 0.08 percent to drive a motor vehicle. A review of 112 studies concludes that certain skills required to drive a motor vehicle can become significantly impaired at a blood alcohol concentration as low as 0.05 percent.[37] For commercial drivers, a BAC of 0.04 percent is illegal nationwide. **TABLE SA.2** shows the effects various amounts of alcohol have on mood and behavior.

TABLE SA.2
Alcohol Impairment Chart

	Men								
	Body Weight in Pounds								
	140	160	180	200	220	240	260	280	
Drinks	Approximate Blood Alcohol Percentage								
0	.00	.00	.00	.00	.00	.00	.00	.00	Only Safe Driving Limit
1	.03	.02	.02	.02	.02	.02	.01	.01	Impairment Begins
2	.05	.05	.04	.04	.03	.03	.02	.02	Driving Skills Affected
3	.08	.07	.06	.06	.05	.05	.04	.04	
4	.11	.09	.08	.08	.07	.06	.06	.05	Possible Criminal Penalties
5	.13	.12	.11	.09	.09	.08	.08	.07	
6	.16	.14	.13	.11	.10	.09	.09	.09	
7	.19	.16	.15	.13	.12	.11	.11	.10	Legally Intoxicated
8	.21	.19	.18	.17	.15	.13	.13	.12	
9	.24	.21	.20	.19	.17	.16	.15	.14	Criminal Penalties
10	.27	.23	.21	.19	.17	.16	.16	.15	

(continues)

TABLE SA.2 (*continued*)
Alcohol Impairment Chart

	Women								
	Body Weight in Pounds								
	100	**120**	**140**	**160**	**180**	**200**	**220**	**240**	
Drinks	**Approximate Blood Alcohol Percentage**								
0	.00	.00	.00	.00	.00	.00	.00	.00	Only Safe Driving Limit
1	.05	.04	.03	.03	.03	.02	.02	.02	Impairment Begins
2	.09	.08	.07	.06	.05	.05	.04	.04	Driving Skills Affected
3	.14	.11	.10	.09	.08	.07	.06	.06	Possible Criminal Penalties
4	.18	.15	.13	.11	.10	.09	.08	.08	
5	.23	.19	.16	.14	.13	.11	.10	.09	
6	.27	.23	.19	.17	.15	.14	.12	.11	
7	.32	.27	.23	.20	.18	.16	.14	.13	Legally Intoxicated
8	.36	.30	.26	.23	.20	.18	.17	.15	
9	.41	.34	.29	.26	.23	.20	.19	.17	Criminal Penalties
10	.45	.38	.32	.28	.25	.23	.21	.19	

Note: Your body can get rid of one drink per hour. One drink is 1.25 oz of 80-proof liquor, 12 oz of beer, or 5 oz of table wine.

Data from the National Clearinghouse for Alcohol and Drug Information, Substance Abuse and Mental Health Services Administration.

This chart uses 1.5 oz of 80 proof liquor, 12 oz of beer, or 5 oz of table wine as one drink.

REFERENCES

http://www.alcohol.vt.edu/Students/alcoholEffects/estimatingBAC/index.htm

Tomeo Sills, LLC. Chemical BAC tests. http://www.ctduiattorney.com/dui_information/calculating_bac.html. Accessed August 23, 2017.

Whiting D. How long do breathalyzers detect alcohol? http://www.ehow.com/how_7315381_calculate-estimated-blood-alcohol-content.html. Accessed August 23, 2017.

WikiHow. How to calculate blood alcohol content (Widmark formula). http://www.wikihow.com/Calculate-Blood-Alcohol-Content -(Widmark-Formula). Accessed August 23, 2017.

One possible acute effect of a large alcohol intake is hypoglycemia (low blood glucose), one of the most common and dangerous effects of abusing alcohol.[38] Binge drinking, especially following several days of light eating, also can be deadly. The lack of food depletes glycogen stores, and heavy drinking suppresses gluconeogenesis. The resulting severe hypoglycemia is a medical emergency with the potential for coma and death.

A person who drinks heavily over a long period of time may have brain deficits that persist well after he or she achieves sobriety. Exactly how alcohol affects the brain and the likelihood of reversing the impact of heavy drinking on the brain remain hot topics in alcohol research today.[39] Chronic alcoholism produces many different mental disorders. Malnutrition is a probable factor in most of these, even when diet appears adequate. After years of drinking, brain cells become permanently damaged and are unable to metabolize nutrients properly.

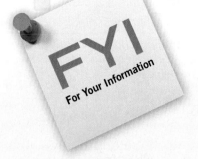

Changing the Culture of Campus Drinking

From car crashes to alcohol poisoning, the culture of drinking on many college campuses puts students at grave risk. Alcohol use is pervasive among college students, many of whom are younger than the legal drinking age.

Excessive alcohol consumption is the third leading preventable cause of death in the United States.[a] College students who drink are more likely to drink and drive, have failing grades, and have medical and legal problems. Increased rates of crime, traffic crashes, rapes and assaults, property damage, and other alcohol-related consequences affect both drinking and nondrinking students, as well as members of the surrounding community.

The Culture of College Drinking

On many campuses, alcohol consumption is a rite of passage, and the influence of peers is an especially powerful force driving college problem drinking.[b] Traditions and beliefs handed down through generations of college drinkers reinforce the perception that alcohol is a necessary component of social success.[c] Many students arrive at college with a history of alcohol consumption and positive expectations about alcohol's effects. The 2015 Youth Risk Behavior Survey found that among high school students, 33 percent had consumed some amount of alcohol and 18 percent engaged in binge drinking.[d]

Rates of excessive alcohol use are highest at colleges and universities where fraternities and sororities are popular, where sports teams have a prominent role, and at schools located in the Northeast.[e] In the local community, tolerance of student drinking may permit alcoholic beverage outlets and advertising to be located near campus. Due to lax enforcement, selling alcohol to students below the legal drinking age often has few consequences. Also, underage students who are caught using fake IDs to obtain alcohol are seldom penalized.[f] Just look at the advertising and sale of alcoholic beverages on or near campuses, and the role of alcohol in college life is evident.

Alcohol Use and Abuse by College Students

According to a national survey, almost 60% of college-age students consumed alcohol within the past month, and almost two out of three engaged in binge drinking during that same time frame.[g,h] Binge drinkers consumed 91 percent of all the alcohol that students reported drinking, and 68 percent of alcohol was consumed by frequent binge drinkers. What happens when these students leave college? Surprisingly, most high-risk student drinkers reduce their consumption of alcohol. However, some continue frequent, excessive drinking, leading to alcoholism or medical problems associated with chronic alcohol abuse.[i]

Binge Drinking

Binge drinking is especially worrisome, and it is widespread on college campuses. Just over two in five students (44 percent) report binge drinking behaviors, and about one in four (23 percent) report bingeing frequently, defined as three or more times in a two-week period. Frequent binge drinkers average more than 14 drinks per week and account for more than 90 percent of the alcohol consumed by college students.[j] Most college binge drinkers drink not for sociability, but solely and purposefully to get drunk.

Binge drinkers often do something they later regret—argue with friends, make fools of themselves, get sick, engage in unplanned (and often unprotected) sexual activity, or drive drunk. Afterward, they may forget where they were or what they did, but the consequences of the binge remain. These consequences may include alienated friends, a hangover, and embarrassment. Or the consequences could be much more serious—sexually transmitted disease, hospitalization, permanent injury, rape, pregnancy, or death. Over 1,800 college students between the ages of 18 and 24 die each year from alcohol-related unintentional injuries, including motor-vehicle crashes.[k] Nearly 700,000 cases of alcohol-related assault and 97,000 cases of alcohol-related sexual assault, including date rape, are reported each year.[l]

Abstaining

Not everyone drinks in college, despite the stereotype. There is a polarizing trend in college drinking, with binge drinkers at one extreme and abstainers at the other. The number of college students who drink no alcohol is rising and now nearly equals the number who binge frequently. About one in five students (19 percent) report consuming no alcohol within the past year.[m] One survey found that one in three college campuses reported banning the use of alcohol on campus by all students, regardless of age.[n]

Prevention Strategies and Changing the Culture of Drinking

Changing the culture of college drinking represents the first step toward an effective prevention strategy, according to a task force of college presidents, alcohol researchers, and students established by the National Institute on Alcohol Abuse and Alcoholism. The report emphasizes the need for collaboration among academic institutions, researchers, and the community to affect lasting change.[o]

The task force strongly supports the use of a "3-in-1 framework" to target three primary audiences simultaneously: (1) individual students, including high-risk drinkers; (2) the student body as a whole; and (3) the surrounding community.[p] The task force reviewed potentially useful preventive interventions, grouping them into tiers according to evidence for their effectiveness.

Tier 1: Strategies Effective Among College Students

Strong evidence supports the following strategies:

1. Simultaneously address alcohol-related attitudes and behaviors (e.g., refuting false beliefs about alcohol's effects while teaching students how to cope with stress without resorting to alcohol).
2. Use survey data to counter students' misperceptions about their fellow students' drinking practices and attitudes toward excessive drinking.
3. Increase student motivation to change drinking habits by providing nonjudgmental advice and progress evaluations.

Programs that combine these three strategies have proved effective in reducing alcohol consumption.[q]

Tier 2: Strategies Effective Among the General Population That Could Be Applied to College Environments

These strategies have proved successful in populations similar to those found on college campuses. Measures include the following:

1. Increase enforcement of minimum legal drinking age laws.[r,s]
2. Implement, enforce, and publicize other laws to reduce alcohol-impaired driving, such as zero-tolerance laws that reduce

the legal blood alcohol concentration for underage drivers to near zero.[t]

3. Increase the prices or taxes on alcoholic beverages.[u]

4. Institute policies and training for servers of alcoholic beverages to prevent sales to underage or intoxicated patrons.[v]

5. Use the secondhand smoke campaign as a model to change the culture of alcohol abuse on campus.[w]

Tier 3: Promising Strategies That Require Research

These strategies make sense intuitively or show theoretical promise, but their usefulness requires further testing. They include more consistent enforcement of campus alcohol regulations and increasing the severity of penalties for violating them, regulating happy hours, enhancing awareness of personal liability for alcohol-related harm to others, establishing alcohol-free dormitories, restricting or eliminating alcohol-industry sponsorship of student events while promoting alcohol-free student activities, and conducting social norms campaigns to correct exaggerated estimates of the overall level of drinking among the student body.

How Can I Say No to Drinking Alcohol and Still Fit in with My Friends?

Drinking alcohol is a personal decision. It is best to make your decision of whether or not to drink based on your own feelings, knowledge, and experiences. You may want to consider the following before you are put in a position where drinking alcohol is encouraged[x]:

- If you choose to abstain, make up your mind to say no before you are ever in the situation.
- Tell people that you feel better when you drink less.
- Stay away from people who give you a hard time about not drinking.

- Learn to hold a glass or beer bottle for a long time, and refill it with whatever you want (such as water or club soda).

a Centers for Disease Control and Prevention. Alcohol and public health: fact sheets—alcohol use and health. http://www.cdc.gov/alcohol/fact-sheets/alcohol-use.htm. Accessed August 25, 2017.

b Ham LS, Hope DA. Incorporating social anxiety into a model of college student problematic drinking. *Addict Behav*. 2005;30(1):127-150.

c National Institute on Alcohol Abuse and Alcoholism (NIAAA). *A Call to Action: Changing the Culture of Drinking at U.S. Colleges*. NIH publication no. 02-5010. Bethesda, MD: NIAAA; 2002.

d Centers for Disease Control and Prevention. Youth Risk Behavior Surveillance—United States, 2015. *MMWR*. 2016;65(6):1-174.

e Centers for Disease Control and Prevention. Alcohol and public health. Fact sheets—underage drinking. http://www.cdc.gov/alcohol/fact-sheets/underage-drinking.htm. Accessed August 25, 2017.

f Carter AC, Brandon KO, Goldman MS. The college and noncollege experience: a review of the factors that influence drinking behavior in young adulthood. *J Stud Alcohol Drugs*. 2010;71(5):742-750.

g Substance Abuse and Mental Health Services Administration. Results from the 2014 National Survey on Drug Use and Health. Table 6.88B—Alcohol use in the past month among persons aged 18 to 22, by college enrollment status and demographic characteristics: percentages, 2013 and 2014. http://www.samhsa.gov/data/sites/default/files/NSDUH-DetTabs2014/NSDUH-DetTabs2014.htm#tab6-88b. Accessed August 25, 2017.

h Substance Abuse and Mental Health Services Administration. Results from the 2014 National Survey on Drug Use and Health. Table 6.89B—Binge alcohol use in the past month among persons aged 18 to 22, by college enrollment status and demographic characteristics: percentages, 2013 to 2014. http://www.samhsa.gov/data/sites/default/files/NSDUH-DetTabs2014/NSDUH-DetTabs2014.htm#tab6-89b. Accessed August 25, 2017.

i Slutske WS. Alcohol use disorders among U.S. college students and their non-college-attending peers. *Arch Gen Psychiatry*. 2005;62:321-327.

j American College Health Association. National college health assessment II. Reference group executive summary. Fall 2010. http://www.achancha.org/docs/ACHA-NCHA-II_ReferenceGroup_ExecutiveSummary_Fall2010.pdf. Accessed August 25, 2017.

k Hingson RW, Zha W, Weitzman ER. Magnitude of and trends in alcohol-related mortality and morbidity among US college students ages 18-24, 1998-2005. *J Stud Alcohol Drugs*. 2009;(suppl 16):12-20.

l Ibid.

m Wechsler H, Nelson TF. What we have learned from the Harvard School of Public Health College Alcohol Study: focusing attention on college student alcohol consumption and the environmental conditions that promote it. *J Stud Alcohol Drugs*. 2008;69(4):481-490.

n McMambridge J, McAlaney J, Rowe R. Adult consequences of late adolescent alcohol consumption: a systematic review of cohort studies. *PLoS Med*. 2011;8(2).

o Wechsler H, Nelson TF. Op. cit.

p Wechsler H, Lee JE, Kuo M, et al. Trends in college binge drinking during a period of increased prevention efforts: findings from 4 Harvard School of Public Health College Alcohol Study Surveys: 1993–2001. *J Am Coll Health*. 2002;50(5):203-217.

q Wechsler H, Seibring M, Liu IC, Ahl M. Colleges respond to student binge drinking: reducing student demand or limiting access. *J Am Coll Health*. 2004;52(4):159-168.

r National Institute on Alcohol Abuse and Alcoholism. Op. cit.

s Hingson RW, Howland J. Comprehensive community interventions to promote health: implications for college-age drinking problems. *J Studies Alcohol*. 2002;(suppl 14):226-240.

t Holder HD, Gruenewald PJ, Ponicki WR, et al. Effect of community-based interventions on high-risk drinking and alcohol-related injuries. *JAMA*. 2000;284:2341-2347.

u Larimer ME, Cronce JM. Identification, prevention, and treatment: a review of individual-focused strategies to reduce problematic alcohol consumption by college students. *J Studies Alcohol*. 2002;(suppl 14):148-163.

v Wagenaar AC, Toomey TL. Effects of minimum drinking age laws: review and analyses of the literature from 1960 to 2000. *J Studies Alcohol*. 2002;(suppl 14):206-225.

w Wagenaar A, O'Malley P, LaFond L. Lowered legal blood alcohol limits for young drivers: effects on drinking, driving, and driving-after-drinking behaviors in 30 states. *Am J Pub Health*. 2001;91(5):801-804.

x Cook PJ, Moore MJ. The economics of alcohol abuse and alcohol-control policies. *Health Affairs*. 2002;21(2):120-133.

Alcohol's Effect on the Gastrointestinal System

Years of heavy drinking and ongoing contact with alcohol and acetaldehyde eventually damage the gastrointestinal system, which in turn discourages eating, affects absorption of protective nutrients, and leaves the digestive lining even more vulnerable to damage as the vicious cycle continues.

Chronic irritation from alcohol and acetaldehyde erodes protective mucosal linings, causing inflammation and release of destructive free radicals. **Esophagitis** (inflammation of the esophagus), esophageal

▶ **esophagitis** Inflammation of the esophagus.

▶ **gastritis** Inflammation of the stomach.

▶ **fatty liver** Accumulation of fat in the liver, a sign of increased fatty acid synthesis.

▶ **fetal alcohol syndrome** A set of physical and mental abnormalities observed in infants born to women who abuse alcohol during pregnancy. Affected infants exhibit poor growth, characteristic abnormal facial features, limited hand–eye coordination, and mental retardation.

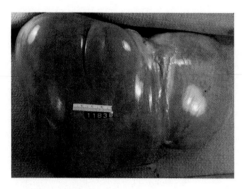

FIGURE SA.10 Fatty liver.
© CNRI / Science Source.

stricture (closing), and swallowing difficulties are common among alcoholics. When the stomach is exposed repeatedly to alcohol at high concentrations, **gastritis** (inflammation of the stomach) often develops. Alcoholics frequently have diarrhea and malabsorption, evidence of intestinal damage. The mouth, throat, esophagus, stomach, and small and large intestines are all at greatly increased risk of cancer.[40]

Alcohol and the Liver

Metabolizing and detoxifying alcohol is almost entirely the responsibility of the liver. So it's not surprising that too much drinking hurts the liver more than any other site in the body. In the United States, heavy alcohol use is considered the most important risk factor for chronic liver disease. According to the Centers for Disease Control and Prevention, over 29,000 people die annually in the United States as a result of chronic liver disease and cirrhosis (nearly 10 deaths per 100,000).[41]

The earliest evidence of liver damage is fat accumulation, which can appear after only a few days of heavy drinking. **Fatty liver** (see **FIGURE SA.10**) recedes with abstinence but persists with continued drinking. Is fatty liver in and of itself harmful? The answer is controversial among liver researchers, with some experts suggesting it's a benign condition. However, studies show that 5 to 15 percent of people with alcoholic fatty liver who continue to drink develop liver fibrosis (excessive fibrous tissue) or cirrhosis (scarring) in only 5 to 10 years.[42] Cirrhosis ultimately kills liver cells by choking off tiny blood vessels that nourish them. About 10 to 20 percent of heavy drinkers develop cirrhosis.[43]

Fat accumulation is one of several factors resulting in alcoholic liver disease. With regular, high intakes of alcohol, alcohol and acetaldehyde continually irritate and inflame the liver, producing alcoholic hepatitis (persistent inflammation of the liver) in 10 to 35 percent of heavy drinkers. The inflammatory process also generates free radicals that batter away at liver cells.[44] The destruction of liver cells becomes self-perpetuating, especially if antioxidant nutrients are unavailable to help break the cycle. If the intestines also have been damaged, toxins, including those produced by the gut's microorganisms, can cross the intestinal barrier into circulation, worsening inflammation.[45] Alcoholic hepatitis may be treatable, but it's often fatal. Alcoholic hepatitis also predisposes a person to liver cancer and cirrhosis, conditions that are usually fatal.

Dietary changes may be helpful in treating liver disease, but abstinence from alcohol is essential. Reducing dietary fats somewhat reduces fat accumulation in the liver. Consuming adequate micronutrients and a healthful balance of macronutrients probably speeds recuperation from liver diseases in their earlier stages.[46] In late-stage liver disease, dietary restrictions, often of proteins, may slow disease progression or improve symptoms.

Fetal Alcohol Syndrome

Fetal alcohol syndrome is a possible result of alcohol consumption during pregnancy. Victims of this syndrome suffer a variety of congenital defects: mental retardation, coordination problems, and heart, eye, and genitourinary malformations, as well as low birth weight and slowed growth rate. Most apparent are characteristic facial abnormalities. Severe cases of fetal alcohol syndrome are rare, but subtle damage with one or two abnormalities, sometimes called "fetal alcohol effects," is probably much more widespread. Symptoms of the syndrome may not emerge until months after birth and are apt to go undiagnosed.[47] This disorder, a major cause of mental retardation in the United States, is preventable.

Alcohol is especially damaging in the early weeks of pregnancy, before a woman may know she's pregnant. Alcohol crosses the placenta into the tiny body of the fetus, where its effects are grossly magnified. Both the congeners in alcoholic beverages and the alcohol itself can interfere with embryonic development by disrupting the body's use of vitamin A and folic acid, nutrients clearly required for fetal growth and development.[48]

Relatively small amounts of alcohol may cause fetal alcohol syndrome. A safe level during pregnancy is not known; therefore, pregnant women should abstain from alcohol consumption. Unlike most other alcohol-related diseases, fetal alcohol damage does not require chronic intake. A binge—even having several drinks at a party—at the wrong moment of pregnancy can cause serious problems. However, population studies show that babies with neurodevelopmental problems are more common among women who drink more frequently during pregnancy.[49]

Official health advisories warn women against drinking alcohol if they are pregnant or considering becoming pregnant. Labels on alcoholic beverages must carry a warning for pregnant women. Centers for Disease Control and Prevention studies have shown that 0.2 to 1.5 cases of fetal alcohol syndrome occur for every 1,000 live births in certain areas of the United States, whereas other studies have estimated rates as high as 0.5 to 2.0 cases per 1,000 live births.[50] **FIGURE SA.11** shows the prevalence of alcohol consumption by women of childbearing age.

Key Concepts Alcohol affects every organ system of the body. In the brain and nervous system, alcohol impairs coordination, judgment, reaction time, and vision. In the GI tract, alcohol damages cells of the esophagus and stomach and increases the risk for GI cancers. The liver is most affected by alcohol consumption, culminating in alcoholic hepatitis and cirrhosis after years of alcohol abuse. Alcohol intake during pregnancy can have devastating effects on fetal development.

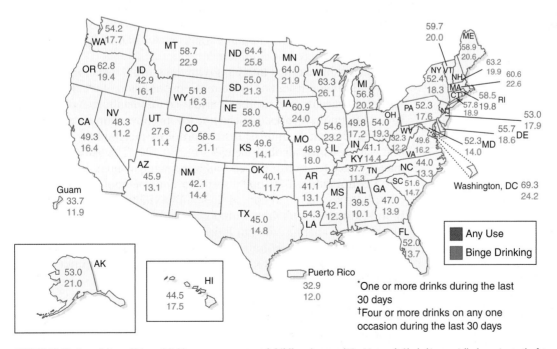

FIGURE SA.11 Prevalence of binge drinking among women of childbearing age (18–44 years). Alcohol is especially damaging to the fetus during the early weeks of pregnancy—before a woman may know she is pregnant.

Courtesy of the Centers for Disease Control and Prevention.

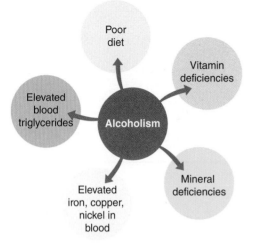

FIGURE SA.12 Alcoholism and malnutrition. Alcoholics' poor diets interact with alcohol's toxicity to worsen their malnutrition.

Alcoholics and Malnutrition

In the United States and Canada, where food is plentiful and fortification of foods with vitamins and minerals is common, overt nutrient deficiencies are rare—except among alcoholics. The results of their poor diet interact with the results of alcohol's toxicity—which include diarrhea, malabsorption, liver malfunction, bleeding, bone marrow changes, and hormonal changes—to worsen malnutrition. (See **FIGURE SA.12**.) In general, the more a person drinks, the worse the malnutrition.

Poor Diet

The quality of an alcoholic's diet correlates to how much and how often he or she drinks. A nationally representative study found that diet quality was poorest among the highest-quantity, lowest-frequency drinkers and best among the lowest-quantity, highest-frequency drinkers.[51] Heavy drinkers who get about half their calories from alcohol cannot eat enough to obtain adequate vitamins and minerals. Severely malnourished alcoholics often have multiple deficiencies.

Vitamin Deficiencies

Inadequate intake, poor absorption, increased vitamin destruction in the body, and urinary losses all contribute to vitamin deficiencies in the alcoholic. Alcohol also interferes with the conversion of vitamin precursors to active forms.

Folate, thiamin, and vitamin A are most often affected by alcoholism. Folate deficiency contributes to malabsorption, anemia, and nerve damage—all of which worsen malnutrition. Vitamin A deficiency also creates a vicious cycle by damaging the gastrointestinal lining and by impairing immunity, leaving the victim susceptible to infections. Thiamin deficiency contributes to classic diseases of alcoholism: the brain damage of Wernicke-Korsakoff syndrome, polyneuropathy (nerve inflammation), and cardiomyopathy (heart inflammation). Alcoholics can have overt scurvy from vitamin C deficiency. Vitamin B_6 and vitamin B_{12} deficiencies are less common.

Alcohol breakdown interferes with the normal metabolism of vitamins and other nutrients. For example, metabolism of ethanol uses up the dehydrogenase enzyme that is also used for metabolism of retinol.[52] Retinol (vitamin A) uses that enzyme for its conversion to other active forms of vitamin A, and the disruption of its metabolism is probably one way in which alcohol increases cancer risk. The same disruption may produce fetal birth defects when pregnant women drink.

Alcohol-induced fat malabsorption and metabolic abnormalities contribute to the depletion of fat-soluble vitamins A, D, E, and K. Blood-clotting factors drop with depleted vitamin K, increasing risk of bleeding and anemia. Vitamin E deficiency is not generally recognized as a complication of alcoholism, but its depletion due to fat malabsorption is possible. Optimal vitamin E status is necessary to quench free radicals generated during alcohol metabolism.[53]

Mineral Deficiencies

Alcoholics are commonly deficient in minerals such as calcium, magnesium, iron, and zinc. Alcohol itself does not seem to affect their absorption; rather, fluid losses and an inadequate diet are the primary culprits. Magnesium deficiency causes "shakes" similar to that seen in alcohol

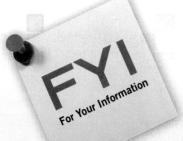

Myths About Alcohol

Myths and misunderstandings just keep circulating about alcohol. Some of these statements are partly true, but most are completely false. You may have heard some of the following:

- *Drinking isn't all that dangerous.* Wrong! One in three 18- to 24-year-olds admitted to emergency rooms for serious injuries is intoxicated. Alcohol use is also associated with homicides, suicides, and drownings.

- *I can manage to drive well enough after a few drinks.* No. It only takes a few drinks to raise your BAC level to 0.08 percent, too high to drive safely. About one-half of all fatal traffic crashes among 18- to 24-year-olds involve alcohol.
- *I can sober up quickly if needed.* No. It takes about three hours to eliminate the alcohol content of two drinks, depending on your weight and other factors. Nothing can speed up this process—not even coffee or cold showers.
- *Alcohol is a stimulant.* No. It's actually a depressant, but its initial depressing effect on inhibitions and judgment may make it seem stimulating.

- *Alcohol keeps you warm.* Partly true. It dilates blood vessels near the body's surface, giving a feeling of warmth. But as body heat escapes, alcohol cools the inner body.
- *Alcohol is an aphrodisiac.* Partly true. By suppressing inhibitions, it may loosen behavior. However, sexual function is often compromised by alcohol.
- *Most alcoholics are homeless.* No. The highly visible homeless alcoholic represents only a minority of alcoholics.
- *Beer is a source of vitamins.* Partly true. Beer does contain a fair amount of niacin. But you'd need about 1 liter to fulfill daily niacin requirements. Levels of other vitamins are much lower.

- *Alcohol helps you sleep.* No. Alcohol disrupts sleep patterns, leading to a restless, unsatisfying sleep.
- *Laboratory animals love to drink.* No. Alcohol is usually given by tube feeding because most animals refuse to drink it willingly.
- *It's good to have a beer before breastfeeding.* No. Alcohol may be relaxing and allow milk to flow more readily, but alcohol concentrations in breast milk are similar to those in the mother's blood. Alcohol in breast milk reduces milk production by reducing the intensity of the infant's suckling.

withdrawal. Chronic diarrhea and loss of epithelial tissue (caused by skin rashes or sloughing off of the digestive lining) may seriously deplete zinc, a mineral needed for immune function. In cases of bleeding, especially gastrointestinal blood loss, iron levels fall.

Not all minerals are lower in heavy drinkers than in nondrinkers. If there is no bleeding, a heavy drinker's iron levels tend to be higher than normal in the blood and liver, potentially contributing to harmful oxidation. Copper and nickel levels also may be elevated in advancing disease, but the reason and the effects are unclear.[54]

Macronutrients

Animal experiments can demonstrate a number of ways that alcohol alters digestion and metabolism of carbohydrate, fat, and protein, but the relevance to humans at usual levels of intake is not certain. Alcohol interferes with amino acid absorption, but its overall effect on protein balance appears minimal. It inhibits gluconeogenesis and lowers blood glucose levels, probably contributing to hangovers and, at the most extreme, causing acute, potentially lethal hypoglycemia if a person who drinks heavily neglects to eat.[55]

Alcohol's most dramatic effect is on fats. You have seen that alcohol causes fatty liver. On the one hand, excess alcohol has the undesirable effect of raising blood triglyceride levels, often significantly. Hyperlipidemia (high blood fats) is common among heavy drinkers. Abstinence and a balanced diet can usually return blood lipids to normal.[56] On the other hand, moderate alcohol use increases protective high-density lipoproteins (HDL, or "good cholesterol"), an important factor in alcohol's relationship to the reduced risk for coronary artery disease.

Body Weight

Although alcoholic beverages provide minimal nutrient value, they do provide calories; alcohol contains 7 kilocalories per gram. Does alcohol consumption contribute to obesity? It appears likely. One reason for weight gain associated with alcohol intake is that the calories in alcohol can easily add up. Some cocktail-type drinks, such as margaritas or piña coladas, can contain more than 500 calories per drink! In addition, food choices that accompany drinking are generally low in nutrient density and high in calories, adding to an overall excess calorie intake. The excess calories promote body fat accumulation and weight gain.

Key Concepts   Alcohol interferes with normal nutrition by reducing the intake of nutrient-dense foods and by affecting the absorption, metabolism, and excretion of many vitamins and minerals. Alcohol contains a significant number of calories (7 kilocalories per gram), and heavy episodic drinkers tend to weigh more than light drinkers.

Does Alcohol Have Benefits?

Why Is This Important?   Understanding the potential health benefits of moderate alcohol consumption can help you make good decisions for your own health.

Can a potentially harmful drink like alcohol play a role in a healthful diet? The consensus of health experts is that it can—but not for everyone. The question continues to arouse much debate, however, and even those supporting alcohol's usefulness often have reservations. Public health statements on alcohol are typically accompanied by plenty of "ifs" and "buts."

Consistent epidemiological evidence suggests that low to moderate drinking reduces mortality among some groups.[57,58] (**TABLE SA.3** gives definitions of different levels of drinking.) Compared with nondrinkers or heavy drinkers, middle-aged and older adults who drink moderate amounts of alcohol have a lower risk of mortality from all causes.[59] This includes people with heart disease,[60] diabetes,[61] high blood pressure,[62] or a prior heart attack.[63] Research also suggests that moderate intake of alcohol can protect against other diseases, such as cancer, diabetes, inflammatory liver disease, and lower extremity arterial disease, as well as have positive effects on bone density in older women.[64] Consistent and growing evidence shows that alcohol reduces insulin resistance and may protect against heart disease by improving "good" cholesterol levels and reducing blood clotting.[65]

No evidence has suggested that moderate drinking harmed the people in the studies. In fact, analysis of data from the Nurses' Health Study, which involves more than 12,000 participants, suggests that in women, up to one drink per day does not impair mental functioning and may actually decrease the risk of mental decline with age.[66]

Tracked against alcohol intake, death rates typically follow what statisticians describe as a "*U*-shaped" curve. Compared with people who rarely or never drink, people who drink slightly or moderately have lower total mortality rates. People who consume two drinks per day have

TABLE SA.3
How Much is Too Much?

Term	Definition
Moderate alcohol consumption	According to the *2015–2020 Dietary Guidelines for Americans*, moderate alcohol consumption is up to one drink per day for women and up to two drinks per day for men.
Low-risk drinking	For women, low-risk drinking is defined as no more than 3 drinks on any single day and no more than 7 drinks per week. For men, it is defined as no more than 4 drinks on any single day and no more than 14 drinks per week. National Institute for Alcohol Abuse and Alcoholism (NIAAA) research shows that only about 2 in 100 people who drink within these limits have an alcohol use disorder (AUD).
Binge drinking	The NIAAA defines binge drinking as a pattern of drinking that brings blood alcohol concentration (BAC) levels to 0.08 g/dL. This typically occurs after four drinks for women and five drinks for men—in about two hours.
	The Substance Abuse and Mental Health Services Administration (SAMHSA), which conducts the annual National Survey on Drug Use and Health (NSDUH), defines binge drinking as drinking 5 or more alcoholic drinks on the same occasion on at least 1 day in the past 30 days.
Heavy drinking	SAMHSA defines heavy drinking as drinking 5 or more drinks on the same occasion on each of 5 or more days in the past 30 days.
Alcohol use disorder (AUD)	AUD is a medical condition that doctors diagnose when a patient's drinking causes distress or harm. The fourth edition of the *Diagnostic and Statistical Manual of Mental Disorders (DSM-IV)*, published by the American Psychiatric Association, described two distinct disorders—alcohol abuse and alcohol dependence—with specific criteria for each. The fifth edition, *DSM-5*, integrates the two *DSM-IV* disorders, alcohol abuse and alcohol dependence, into a single disorder called alcohol use disorder (AUD) with mild, moderate, and severe subclassifications.

Modified from http://www.niaaa.nih.gov/alcohol-health/overview-alcohol-consumption/alcohol-facts-and-statistics.

about the same mortality rate as nondrinkers.[67] Beyond three drinks per day, the death rate rises dramatically.[68] Heavy alcohol consumption increases the risk of stroke, for example, whereas light or moderate drinking appears to reduce that risk.[69] Alcohol's primary benefit is to raise protective HDL cholesterol levels. It may also inhibit formation of blood clots, but this connection is less clear.[70] In addition, alcohol may have subjective benefits such as stress relief and relaxation.

In most studies, wine, beer, and spirits appear equal in offering protection against heart disease. Findings of reduced rates of nonfatal heart attacks among moderate drinkers support the view that protective benefits are due to alcohol itself rather than other substances in alcoholic beverages.[71] However, international comparisons that highlight unexpectedly low rates of heart disease in France, despite a high-fat diet (the **French paradox**), suggest that red wine may have a unique protective effect. Some studies show that moderate consumption of red wine reduces the risk of heart disease, attributing this association to the polyphenols in the wine itself other studies do not support the hypothesis that polyphenols account for the suggested[72] benefits of red wine.[73] The apparent benefits of red wine may result from overall healthier behavior of people who drink red wine. Although a direct connection between red wine and health benefits remains unproven, recognizing that alcohol generally confers moderate protection and noting the possibility that wine has a particular benefit, the Bureau of Alcohol, Tobacco, and Firearms granted permission for wine labels to include one of the following statements[74]:

- "The proud people who made this wine encourage you to consult your family doctor about the health effects of wine consumption."
- "To learn the health effects of wine consumption, send for the Federal Government's *Dietary Guidelines for Americans*."

▶ **French paradox** The phenomenon observed in the French, who have a lower incidence of heart disease than people whose diets contain comparable amounts of fat. Part of the difference has been attributed to the regular and moderate drinking of red wine.

Addiction
Alcohol addiction destroys lives, families, and communities. Researchers are trying to learn why some people, and not others, become addicted.

Accidents and violence
These result from impairment of mental function and coordination.

Birth defects
Fetal alcohol syndrome can occur when pregnant women drink.

Emotional and social
Emotional, social, and economic problems are associated with heavy drinking.

Cardiomyopathy
Inflammation of the heart muscle is much more common in heavy drinkers.

Brain
Acute effect is drunkenness. Long-term effects of chronic alcohol excess are dementia, memory loss, and generalized impairment of mental function.

Liver disease
Heavy drinking can lead to alcoholic fatty liver, alcoholic hepatitis, cirrhosis, and liver cancer.

Gastritis
Continued contact with excess alcohol irritates and inflames the stomach lining.

Pancreatitis
Both chronic and acute pancreatitis are increased by alcoholism.

Anemia
Heavy drinkers often have poor diets and may bleed from the digestive tract.

Cancer
Excess alcohol increases the risk of gastrointestinal, liver, and breast cancers. Smoking further increases these risks.

Osteoporosis
Heavy drinking contributes to bone loss, especially in older women.

Peripheral neuropathy
Painful nerve inflammation in hands, arms, feet, and legs is common in long-time heavy alcohol users.

FIGURE SA.13 Harmful effects of alcohol. Because excess alcohol reaches all parts of the body, it causes a wide array of physical problems. Here are some of the ways alcohol can harm.

Because of the many harmful effects of alcohol (see **FIGURE SA.13**), public health agencies and organizations caution against inappropriate drinking. Although low to moderate alcohol use may offer some benefit, these groups advise people to discuss their alcohol intake with their doctors, and they urge moderation. The U.S. Preventive Services Task Force recommends that primary care doctors routinely screen patients for unhealthy alcohol use and, when appropriate, intervene with a brief counseling session to reduce alcohol misuse.[75,76] Public health officials also point out that numerous groups should not drink any alcohol[77]:

- People who cannot restrict their alcohol intake to moderate levels
- Anyone younger than the legal drinking age

- People taking prescription or over-the-counter medications that can interact with alcohol
- People who have an alcohol-related illness or another illness that will be worsened by alcohol
- People who plan to drive, operate machinery, or take part in other activities that require attention, skill, or coordination or participate in situations where impaired judgment could cause injury or death
- Women who are pregnant or may become pregnant
- Women who are breastfeeding
- People with a personal or strong family history of alcoholism

Key Concepts Although alcohol has the potential to reduce risk for heart disease, most health organizations recommend moderate to no drinking. It is too early in the scientific investigation of alcohol's benefits to recommend alcohol intake for all adults. Some people, such as pregnant women, should not drink any alcohol.

Recommendation: American Heart Association

Alcohol and Heart Health

If you drink alcohol, do so in moderation. This means an average of one to two drinks per day for men and one drink per day for women. Drinking more alcohol increases such dangers as alcoholism, high blood pressure, obesity, stroke, breast cancer, suicide, and accidents. Also, it's not possible to predict in which people alcoholism will become a problem. Given these and other risks, the American Heart Association cautions people NOT to start drinking... if they do not already drink alcohol. Consult your doctor on the benefits and risks of consuming alcohol in moderation.

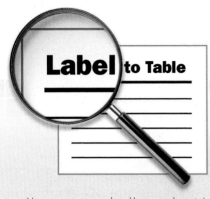

Have you ever wondered how much protein, carbohydrate, and fat are in a can of beer? If you've ever looked at a beer label, you know it's quite different from a food label. Look at the following information from a can of light beer and see if you can calculate the calories from carbohydrate, fat, and protein.

Serving size = 12 fl oz
Calories = 103 (kcal)
Carbohydrate = 5 g
Protein = 1 g
Fat = 0 g

First, to figure out how many calories come from the three macronutrients, multiply the number of grams by their respective calorie contribution per gram:

5 g carbohydrate × 4 kcal/g = 20 kcal from carbohydrate

1 g protein × 4 kcal/g = 4 kcal from protein

0 g fat × 9 kcal/g = 0 kcal from fat

Uh-oh. Is this adding up correctly? So far, we have accounted for only 24 of the 103 kilocalories in this beer. Where are the other 79 kilocalories? Don't forget that many of the calories in beer come from alcohol, and it's easy to calculate just how many grams are in this can of light beer. Remember, alcohol has 7 kilocalories per gram, so the remaining 79 kilocalories come from 11 grams of alcohol (79 ÷ 7 = 11.3).

So, for the 103 kilocalories this beer provides, you get very little (if any) protein, carbohydrate, or fat. Instead, a majority of the calories come from alcohol. This holds true for the micronutrients as well: Beer contains negligible amounts of vitamins or minerals.

This is why people say alcoholic beverages have only "empty calories." They provide calories, but almost no nutrient value!

GOVERNMENT WARNING: (1) ACCORDING TO THE SURGEON GENERAL, WOMEN SHOULD NOT DRINK ALCOHOLIC BEVERAGES DURING PREGNANCY BECAUSE OF THE RISK OF BIRTH DEFECTS. (2) CONSUMPTION OF ALCOHOLIC BEVERAGES IMPAIRS YOUR ABILITY TO DRIVE A CAR OR OPERATE MACHINERY, AND MAY CAUSE HEALTH PROBLEMS. PER 12 FL. OZ. SIZE AVERAGE ANALYSIS: 103 CALORIES, 5.0 GRAMS CARBOHYDRATES, 1.0 GRAMS PROTEIN, 0.0 GRAMS FAT

Learning Portfolio

Key Terms

Study Points

- Alcohol provides 7 kilocalories per gram but no essential function for the body; therefore, alcohol is not a nutrient.

- Alcohol requires no digestion and is absorbed easily all along the gastrointestinal tract.

- Fatty liver is apparent even after one night of binge drinking.

- Different rates of alcohol breakdown can be attributed to different levels of the alcohol-metabolizing enzymes; these differences are due to genetic and gender variations.

- Alcohol affects all organs in the body, but the most obvious effects are in the brain and the nervous system, the GI system, and the liver.

- Malnutrition among alcoholics is common due to poor food choices and alcohol's interference with the absorption, metabolism, and excretion of nutrients.

- Fetal alcohol syndrome is one of the most devastating consequences of alcohol consumption, and it is preventable.

- Moderate alcohol consumption has been linked to reduced risk of heart disease.

- The potential benefits of moderate alcohol consumption may be related to effects on lipoprotein levels and the antioxidant components of beverages such as wine.

- Health organizations recommend moderate to no alcohol consumption.

Study Questions

1. How much alcohol is in beer, wine, and liquor?
2. List the ways food helps to delay or avoid inebriation.
3. Where does the breakdown of alcohol take place?
4. What causes a hangover? Is there any way to relieve one?
5. List some factors that affect our ability to metabolize alcohol.
6. How is alcohol absorption by the GI tract affected by nutrition status?
7. Why do healthcare professionals advise pregnant women not to drink alcohol?
8. List the positive and the negative effects of alcohol.

Try This

Cruising Through the Medicine Cabinet

This exercise will increase your awareness of the amounts of alcohol in over-the-counter medications. Look through your medicine cabinet and check the ingredient lists of all the products there. In particular, take a close look at any mouthwash or cough syrup. Which products contain alcohol? How much? What do you think its purpose is in these products?

References

1. U.S. Department of Agriculture, U.S. Department of Health and Human Services. *2015–2020 Dietary Guidelines for Americans.* 8th ed. Washington, DC: U.S. Government Printing Office; 2015.
2. Centers for Disease Control and Prevention. Fact sheet—binge drinking. http://www.cdc.gov/alcohol/fact-sheets/binge-drinking.htm. Accessed August 25, 2017.
3. Ibid.
4. Ham LS, Hope DA. Incorporating social anxiety into a model of college student problematic drinking. *Addict Behav.* 2005;30(1):127-150.
5. Centers for Disease Control and Prevention. Alcohol-attributable deaths and years of potential life lost—11 states, 2006–2010. MMWR. 2014;63(10):213-216. http://www.cdc.gov/mmwr/preview/mmwrhtml/mm6310a2.htm?s_cid=mm6310a2_w. Accessed August 25, 2017.

Learning Portfolio (continued)

6.   Minino AM. Mortality Among Teenagers Aged 12–19 Years: United States, 1999–2006. Data Brief No. 37. Hyattsville, MD: National Center for Health Statistics; 2010.

7.   National Institute on Alcohol Abuse and Alcoholism. Underage Drinking. https://pubs.niaaa.nih.gov/publications/UnderageDrinking/Underage-Fact.htm. Accessed September 18, 2017.

8.   Roe DA. *Alcohol and the Diet*. Westport, CT: AVI; 1979.

9.   Ibid.

10. Paasma R, Hovda KE, Jacobsen D. Methanol poisoning and long-term sequelae—a six-year follow-up after a large methanol outbreak. *BMC Clin Pharmacol*. 2009;9:5.

11. Roe DA. Op. cit.

12. Haseba T, Ohno Y. A new view of alcohol metabolism and alcoholism—role of the high-Km class III alcohol dehydrogenase (ADH3). *Int J Environ Res Pub Health*. 2010;7(3):1076-1092.

13. Ferreira SE, Tulio de Mello M, Pompei S, Oliveria de Souzza-Formigoni ML. Effects of energy drink ingestion on alcohol intoxication. *Alcohol Clin Exp Res*. 2006;30(4):598-605.

14. O'Brien MC, McCoy TP, Rhode SD, Wagoner A, Wolfson M. Caffeinated cocktails; energy drink consumption, high-risk drinking and alcohol-related consequences among college students. *Acad Emerg Med*. 2008;15(5):453-460.

15. Mitchinson A. Hangovers: uncongenial congeners. *Nature*. 2009;462 (7276):992.

16. U.S. Department of Agriculture, U.S. Department of Health and Human Services. Op. cit.

17. Ibid.

18. Strohle A, Wolters M, Hahn A. [Alcohol intake—a two-edged sword. Part 1: Metabolism and pathogenic effects of alcohol.] *Med Monatsschr Pharm*. 2012;35(8):281-292.

19. Zakhari S. Overview: how is alcohol metabolized by the body? *Alcohol Res Health*. 2006;29(4):245-254.

20. Verster JC, Penning R. Treatment and prevention of alcohol hangover. *Curr Drug Abuse Rev*. 2010;3(2):103-109.

21. Piasecki TM, Robertson BM, Epler AJ. Hangover and risk for alcohol use disorders: existing evidence and potential mechanisms. *Curr Drug Abuse Rev*. 2010;3(2):92-102.

22. Tomczyk M, Zocko-Koncic M, Chrostek L. Phytotherapy of alcoholism. *Nat Prod Commun*. 2012;7(2):273-280.

23. Ibid.

24. Fruchter LL, Alexopoulou I, Lau KK. Acute interstitial nephritis with acetaminophen and alcohol intoxication. *Ital J Pediatr*. 2011;15(37):17.

25. Ibid.

26. Chen YC, Peng GS, Tsao TP, Wang MF, Lu RB, Yin SJ. Pharmacokinetic and pharmacodynamics basis for overcoming acetaldehyde-induced adverse reaction in Asian alcoholics, heterozygous for the variant ALDH2*2gene allele. *Pharmacogenet Genomics*. 2009;19(8):588-599.

27. Vallee BL. Alcohol in the Western world. *Sci Am*. 1998 June;80-85.

28. Buffa R, Floris GU, Putzu PF, Marini E. Body composition variations in ageing. *Coll Anthropol*. 2011;35(1):259-265.

29. Centers for Disease Control and Prevention. Alcohol and public health. Fact sheets—excessive alcohol use and risks to women's health. http://www.cdc.gov/alcohol/fact-sheets/womens-health.htm. Accessed August 25, 2017.

30. Ibid.

31. Ibid.

32. Dufour MC. What is moderate drinking? *Alcohol Res Health*. 1999;23(1):1-14.

33. National Institute on Alcohol Abuse and Alcoholism. Alcohol—An Important Women's Health Issue. Alcohol Alert No. 62. Bethesda, MD: NIAAA; 2004. http://www.niaaa.nih.gov/alcohol-health/alcohols-effects-body. Accessed August 25, 2017.

34. Swift R, Davidson D. Op. cit.

35. Kiechl S, Willeit J. The complex association between alcohol consumption and myocardial infarction: always good for a new paradox. *Circulation*. 2014;

36. Banerjee N. Neurotransmitters in alcoholism: a review of neurobiological and genetic studies. *Indian J Hum Genet*. 2014;20(1):20-31.

37. Friedman TW, Robinson SR, Yelland GW. Impaired perceptual judgment at low blood alcohol concentrations. *Alcohol*. 2011;45(7):711-718.

38. Zasimowicz E, Wolszczak B, Zasimowicz B. Influence of ethyl alcohol on diabetes pathogenesis type. *Pol Merkur Lekarski*. 2014;36(213):212-214.

39. Parada M, Corral M, Caamano-Isorna F, et al. Binge drinking and declarative memory in university students. *Alcohol Clin Exp Res*. 2011;35(8):1475-1484.

40. Hsu WL, Chien YC, Chiang CJ, et al. Lifetime risk of distinct upper aerodigestive tract cancers and consumption of alcohol, betel, and cigarette. *Int J Cancer*. 2014;135(6):1480-1486.

41. Centers for Disease Control and Prevention. FastStats. Chronic liver disease and cirrhosis. http://www.cdc.gov/nchs/fastats/liver-disease.htm. Accessed August 25, 2017.

42. Fujii H, Kawada N. Fibrogenesis in alcoholic liver disease. *World J Gastroenterol*. 2014;20(25):8048-8054.

43. University of Maryland Medical Center. Cirrhosis. http://www.umm.edu/health/medical/altmed/condition/cirrhosis. Accessed October 10, 2017.

44. Ibid.

45. Ibid.

46. Bruha R, Dvorak K, Petrtyl J. Alcoholic liver disease. *World J Hepatol*. 2012;4(3):81-90.

47. Thompson BL, Levitt P, Stanwood GD. Prenatal exposure to drugs: effects on brain development and implications for policy and education. *Neuroscience*. 2009;10(4):303-312.

48. Ibid.

49. Gray R, Mukherjee RA, Rutter M. Alcohol consumption during pregnancy and its effects on neurodevelopment: what is known and what remains uncertain. *Addiction*. 2009;104(8):1270-1273.

50. Centers for Disease Control and Prevention. Fetal alcohol spectrum disorders (FASDs). Data & statistics. http://www.cdc.gov/ncbddd/fasd/data.html. Accessed August 25, 2017.

51. Breslow RA, Guenther PM, Juan W, Graubard B. Alcoholic beverage consumption, nutrient intakes, and diet quality in the U.S. adult population, 1999–2006. *J Am Diet Assoc*. 2010;110(4):551-562.

52. Chase JR, Poolman MG, Fell DA. Contribution of NADH increases to ethanol's inhibition of retinol oxidation by human ADH isoforms. *Alcohol Clin Exp Res*. 2009;33(4):571-580.

53. Lieber CS. Nutrition and diet in alcoholism. In: Shils ME, Olson JA, Shike M, eds. *Modern Nutrition in Health and Disease*. 10th ed. Philadelphia: Lippincott Williams & Wilkins; 2005.

54. Ibid.

55. Ibid.

56. Ibid.

57. Pontes Ferreira M, Weems MKS. Alcohol consumption by aging adults in the United States: health benefits and detriments. *J Am Diet Assoc*. 2008;108(10):1668-1676.

58. MacArthur GJ, Smith MC, Meloti R, et al. Patterns of alcohol use and multiple risk behavior by gender during early and late adolescence: the ALSPAC cohort. *J Public Health* (Oxf). 2012;34(Suppl 1):i20-i30.

59. Pontes Ferreira M, Weems MKS. Op. cit.

60. Shuval K, Barlow CE, Chartier KG, Gabriel KP. Cardiorespiratory fitness, alcohol, and mortality in men: the Copper Center Longitudinal Study. *Am J Prev Med*. 2010;42(5):460-467.

61. Kim SJ, Kim DJ. Alcoholism and diabetes mellitus. *Diabetes Metab J*. 2012;36(2):108-115.

62. Malinski MK, Sesso HD, Lopez-Jimenez F, et al. Alcohol consumption and cardiovascular mortality in hypertensive patients. Paper presented at

41st Annual Conference on Cardiovascular Disease Epidemiology and Prevention; March 2, 2001; San Antonio, TX.

63. Muntwyler J, Hennekens CH, Buring JE, et al. Mortality and light to moderate alcohol consumption after myocardial infarction. *Lancet.* 1998;352:1882-1885.

64. Pontes Ferreira M, Weems MKS. Op. cit.

65. Estruch R. Sacanella E. Mota F, et al. Moderate consumption of red wine, but not gin, decreases erythrocyte superoxide dismutase activity: a randomized cross-over trial. *Nutr Metab Cardiovasc Dis.* 2011;21(1):46-53.

66. Sun Q, Townsend MK, Okereke OI, et al. Alcohol consumption at midlife and successful ageing in women: a prospective cohort analysis in the Nurses' Health Study. *PLoS Med.* 2011;8(9).

67. Gaziano JM, Gaziano TA, Glynn RJ, et al. Light-to-moderate alcohol consumption and mortality in the Physicians' Health Study enrollment cohort. *J Am Coll Cardiol.* 2000;35:96-105.

68. Pearson TA. Alcohol and heart disease. *Circulation.* 1996;94:3023-3025.

69. Stockley CS. Is it merely a myth that alcoholic beverages such as red wine can be cardioprotective? *J Sci Food Agric.* 2012;92(9):1815-1821.

70. Ibid.

71. Ibid.

72. Xiang L, Xiao L, Wang Y, et al. Health benefits of wine: don't expect resveratrol too much. *Food Chem.* 2014;156:258-263.

73. Botden IP, Draijer R, Westerhof BE, et al. Red wine polyphenols do not lower peripheral or central blood pressure in high normal blood pressure and hypertension. *Am J Hypertens.* 2012;25(6):718-723.

74. U.S. Treasury Department, Bureau of Alcohol, Tobacco, and Firearms. Treasury announces actions concerning labeling of alcoholic beverages. Press release. February 5, 1999.

75. Saitz R. Unhealthy alcohol use. *N Engl J Med.* 2005;352:596–607.

76. Moyer V, on behalf of U.S. Preventive Services Task Force. Screening and behavioral counseling interventions in primary care to reduce alcohol misuse: U.S. Preventive Services Task Force recommendation statements. http://www.uspreventiveservicestaskforce.org/uspstf12/alcmisuse/alcmisusefinalrs.pdf. Accessed August 25, 2017.

77. U.S. Department of Health and Human Services, U.S. Department of Agriculture. Op. cit.

Chapter 5

Lipids: Not Just Fat

Revised by Melissa Bernstein

THINK About It

1   How important is fat to the foods you find tasty?

2   What's your view about the value of body fat?

3   What's your take on the differences between fat and cholesterol?

4   What's your understanding of "good" versus "bad" cholesterol?

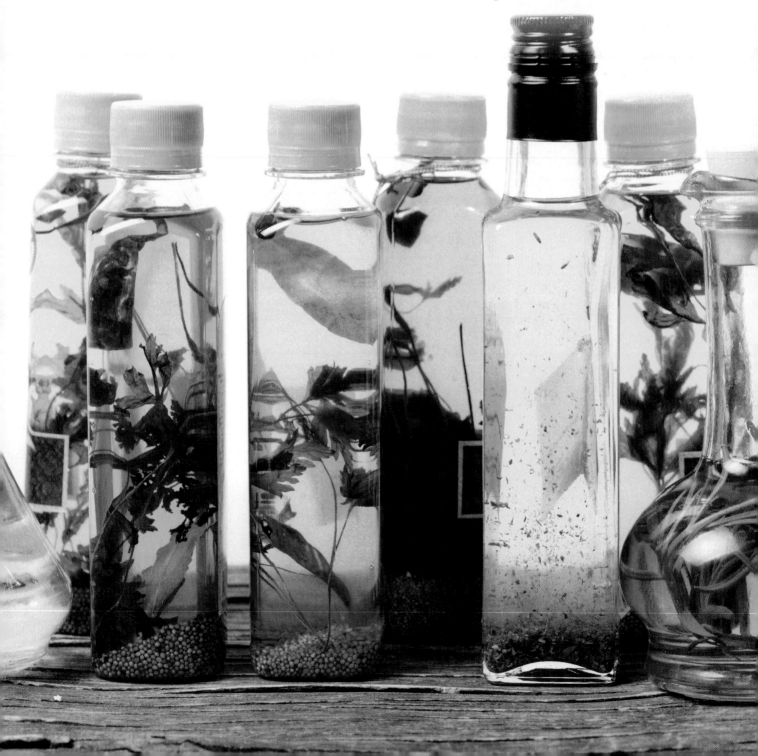

LEARNING Objectives

1 Differentiate between types of fatty acids according to chain length, saturation, location of the double bond, and whether they are essential or nonessential.

2 Explain how lipids are digested, absorbed, and transported in the body.

3 Differentiate between VLDL, LDL, and HDL cholesterol using their key components and their role in the development of atherosclerosis.

4 Suggest dietary fats to include in a healthy eating pattern.

5 List possible health problems associated with a high-fat diet.

Maria and Rachel are trying to lose weight. Maria swears by a new diet program that allows you to eat all the fat you want but no high-carbohydrate, "starchy" foods. Her new diet is working—she's already lost 10 pounds! Then there's Rachel, whose goal is to eat zero grams of fat. She's fat-obsessed—insisting on "fat-free" everything and bothering her friends with information about the number of fat grams in whatever they eat. As you listen to Maria and Rachel compare dieting stories, you wonder which one has the right approach to fat consumption—or even if there *is* a right approach. On the one hand, it seems you hear about U.S. high-fat diets and high rates of obesity and heart disease. On the other hand, can a "no-fat" diet be healthy? Are all low-fat and no-fat products really more nutritious? Is there a way to include dietary fats in a healthy eating pattern?

Fat is an essential nutrient that provides energy and helps transport fat-soluble nutrients to destinations throughout the body. Triglycerides—the fats we associate with fried foods, cream cheese, vegetable oil, and salad dressing—are one type of a larger group of compounds called lipids. Cholesterol, another lipid, is familiar to most Americans, but you may not realize that your body makes cholesterol; the cholesterol you eat contributes only a small portion of the total amount in your body. All lipids have important roles, but at the same time, too many triglycerides or too much cholesterol can increase the risk for chronic disease.

THINK About It
1

Fats contribute greatly to the flavor and texture of foods. When food manufacturers remove fat to produce a low-fat product, they often have to boost the flavor with sugar, sodium, or other additives to create a tasty product. This means that fat-free foods sometimes aren't any lower in calories or sugar than regular food—so Rachel can't eat the whole box of fat-free cookies and still expect to lose weight! Overeating calories, whether they come from fat, carbohydrate, or protein, will lead to energy storage as fat and ultimately increases in body weight.

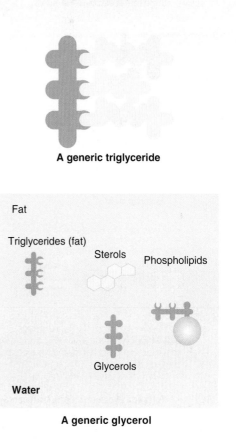

A generic fatty acid

A generic triglyceride

Fat

Triglycerides (fat)

Sterols

Phospholipids

Glycerols

Water

A generic glycerol

What Are Lipids?

🍎 **Why Is This Important?** Once you have an understanding of the role of lipids in the body and in foods, you'll be able to make informed choices when selecting a healthy eating pattern with neither too much nor too little fat.

The term *lipids* applies to a variety of substances, including triglycerides, phospholipids, and sterols. **Triglycerides** are the most abundant lipid. In the body, fat cells store triglycerides in adipose tissue. Triglycerides are the body's main storage form of energy and source of fuel for the body cells, with the exception of the nervous system and red blood cells, which prefer glucose. In foods, we call triglycerides "fats and oils," with fats usually being solid and oils being liquid at room temperature. Overall, however, the choice of terms—fat, triglyceride, oil—is somewhat arbitrary, and these words often are used interchangeably. In this chapter, when we use the word *fat* or *oil*, we are referring to triglycerides.

About 2 percent of dietary lipids are **phospholipids**. They are found in foods of both plant and animal origin, and the body can make them. Unlike other lipids, phospholipids are soluble in both fat and water. This will be important to remember when we talk about the functions of lipids later in this chapter. It is this versatility that enables phospholipid molecules to play crucial roles as major components of cell membranes and in blood and body fluids, where they help keep fats suspended.

Only a small percentage of our dietary lipids are sterols, yet one infamous member, cholesterol, causes much public concern. The body makes cholesterol, which is an important component of cell membranes and a precursor of sex hormones, adrenal hormones (e.g., cortisol), vitamin D, and bile salts.

▶ **triglycerides** Fats composed of three fatty acid chains linked to a glycerol molecule.

▶ **phospholipids** Compounds that consist of a glycerol molecule bonded to two fatty acid molecules and a phosphate group with a nitrogen-containing component. Phospholipids have both water-soluble and fat-soluble regions, which makes them good emulsifiers.

▶ **fatty acids** Compounds containing a long hydrocarbon chain with a carboxyl group (–COOH) at one end and a methyl group (–CH$_3$) at the other end.

▶ **chain length** The number of carbons that a fatty acid contains. Foods contain fatty acids with chain lengths of 4 to 24 carbons, and most have an even number of carbons.

Fatty Acids Are Key Building Blocks

Fatty acids determine the characteristics of a fat, such as whether it is solid or liquid at room temperature. The basic structure of a fatty acid is a chain of carbon atoms with a carboxyl (acid) group (–COOH) at one end and a methyl group (–CH$_3$) at the other end. (See **FIGURE 5.1**.) Fatty acids that are not attached to other compounds are sometimes called free fatty acids. Some free fatty acids have their own distinct flavor. Butyric acid, for example, gives butter its flavor.

Chain Length

Fatty acids differ in **chain length** (the number of carbons in the chain). Foods contain fatty acids with chain lengths of 4 to 24 carbons, and most have an even number of carbons. Fatty acids are grouped as short-chain (fewer than 6 carbons), medium-chain (6 to 10 carbons), and long-chain (12 or more carbons). (See **FIGURE 5.2**.) The shorter carbon chain fatty acids remain liquid at room temperature and even with refrigeration. (See **FIGURE 5.3**.) Shorter fatty acids also are more water-soluble, a property that affects their absorption in the digestive tract.

Saturation

The carbons in a fatty acid chain are attached to each other and to hydrogen atoms. If all the bonds between the carbon atoms in a fatty acid chain are single bonds (C–C), then the fatty acid is called

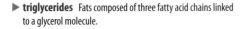

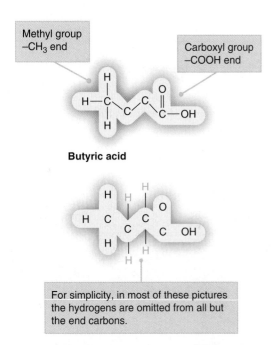

Methyl group –CH$_3$ end

Carboxyl group –COOH end

Butyric acid

For simplicity, in most of these pictures the hydrogens are omitted from all but the end carbons.

FIGURE 5.1 Fatty acid structure. The basic structure of a fatty acid is a carbon chain with a methyl end (–CH$_3$) and an acid (carboxyl) end (–COOH). Butyric acid (shown here) is a fatty acid found in butterfat.

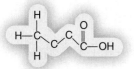

Short-chain fatty acid
(2–4 carbons)

Butyric acid C4:0

Medium-chain fatty acid
(6–10 carbons)

Caprylic acid C8:0

Long-chain fatty acid
(12 or more carbons)

Palmitic acid C16:0

Very-long-chain fatty acid
(20 or more carbons)

FIGURE 5.2 Fatty acid chain lengths. Fatty acids can be classified by their chain length as short-, medium-, and long-chain fatty acids.

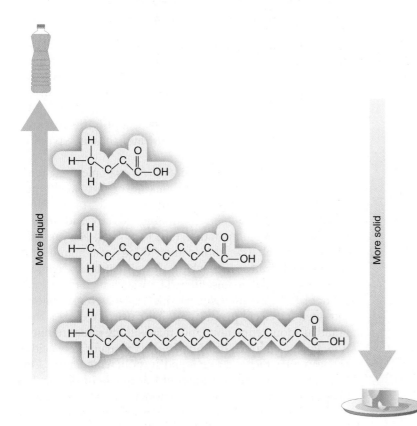

FIGURE 5.3 Fatty acid chain lengths and liquidity. As chain lengths of fatty acids increase, fats tend to become more solid at room temperature.

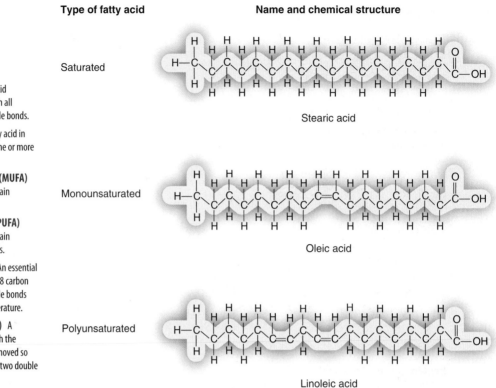

Type of fatty acid | **Name and chemical structure**

Saturated — Stearic acid

Monounsaturated — Oleic acid

Polyunsaturated — Linoleic acid

▶ **saturated fatty acid** A fatty acid completely filled by hydrogen, with all carbons in the chain linked by single bonds.

▶ **unsaturated fatty acid** A fatty acid in which the carbon chain contains one or more double bonds.

▶ **monounsaturated fatty acid (MUFA)** A fatty acid in which the carbon chain contains one double bond.

▶ **polyunsaturated fatty acid (PUFA)** A fatty acid in which the carbon chain contains two or more double bonds.

▶ **linoleic acid [lin-oh-LAY-ik]** An essential omega-6 fatty acid that contains 18 carbon atoms and 2 carbon–carbon double bonds (18:2); a thin liquid at room temperature.

▶ **conjugated linoleic acid (CLA)** A polyunsaturated fatty acid in which the position of the double bonds has moved so that a single bond alternates with two double bonds.

▶ **alpha-linolenic acid [al-fah-lin-oh-LEN-ik]** An essential omega-3 fatty acid that contains 18 carbon atoms and 3 carbon–carbon double bonds (18:3).

FIGURE 5.4 Saturated, monounsaturated, and polyunsaturated fatty acids. All fatty acids have the same basic structure. Hydrogens saturate the carbon chain of a saturated fatty acid. Unsaturated fatty acids have fewer hydrogens and have one (mono) or more (poly) carbon–carbon double bonds.

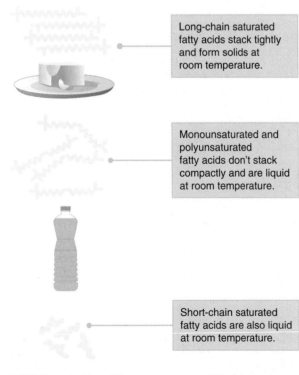

Long-chain saturated fatty acids stack tightly and form solids at room temperature.

Monounsaturated and polyunsaturated fatty acids don't stack compactly and are liquid at room temperature.

Short-chain saturated fatty acids are also liquid at room temperature.

FIGURE 5.5 Liquid or solid at room temperature? Short-chain and unsaturated fatty acids cannot pack tightly together and tend to be more liquid than long-chain saturated fatty acids.

a **saturated fatty acid**. Hydrogen atoms completely fill (saturate) all the other available bonding sites. If one or more bonds between carbon atoms is a double bond (C=C), the fatty acid is an **unsaturated fatty acid**. A fatty acid with one double bond is a **monounsaturated fatty acid (MUFA)**; one with two or more double bonds is a **polyunsaturated fatty acid (PUFA)**. **FIGURE 5.4** illustrates the three types of fatty acids.

Even though we refer to olive oil, for example, as a monounsaturated fat, food fats are a mixture of fatty acid types. Saturation of fatty acids affects the properties of the foods that contain them. Foods rich in saturated fatty acids tend to be solid at room temperature. (See **FIGURE 5.5**.) For example, stearic acid is an 18-carbon saturated fatty acid abundant in chocolate and meat fats, which are solid at room temperature. Food fats rich in unsaturated fatty acids tend to be liquid at room temperature. Oleic acid is an 18-carbon monounsaturated fatty acid plentiful in olive oil. Olive oil is a thick liquid at room temperature but may solidify under refrigeration. Polyunsaturated **linoleic acid** is the major fatty acid of soybean oil, which is a thin liquid at room temperature. One form of linoleic acid, **conjugated linoleic acid (CLA)**, has been shown to have anticancer, antidiabetic, and antiobesity effects.[1] Another polyunsaturated fatty acid, **alpha-linolenic acid** (don't confuse linolenic with linoleic), is abundant in flaxseed oil, a very thin liquid at room temperature.

Key Concepts The term *lipids* refers to a group of substances that includes triglycerides, phospholipids, and sterols. Fatty acids are key building blocks of both triglycerides and phospholipids. Fatty acids are carbon chains of varying lengths. Fatty acids filled with hydrogen are called saturated, and those with missing hydrogen are unsaturated fatty acids.

Cis Versus Trans

Otherwise identical unsaturated fatty acids can have different shapes. The carbon chain of a **cis fatty acid** is bent, whereas the chain of a **trans fatty acid** is straighter. (See **FIGURE 5.6**.) Most naturally occurring unsaturated fatty acids are cis fatty acids. Although there are small amounts of trans fatty acids in meats and dairy products from cows and sheep, a commercial process called **hydrogenation** creates most trans fatty acids in our diets. The process of hydrogenation adds hydrogen to an unsaturated fatty acid, thereby making it more saturated. This process also straightens the fatty acid to a trans configuration. You probably have heard about the health concerns surrounding trans fatty acids. Trans fatty acids have been shown to raise low-density lipoprotein (LDL) cholesterol levels and are also associated with reducing plasma high-density lipoprotein (HDL), and therefore increasing one's risk for heart disease.[2] Dietary trans fatty acids are discussed in more detail later in this chapter.

Omega-3 and Omega-6 Fatty Acids

The body is a good chemist, synthesizing many types of fatty acids as needed. Because it is not essential to have the fatty acids your body can manufacture in your diet, they are called **nonessential fatty acids**. Don't confuse "nonessential" with "unimportant"—you must have an adequate supply of nonessential fatty acids, by either making or eating them.

The body, however, cannot make all the types of fatty acids it needs; some must come from food. These fatty acids are called **essential fatty acids (EFAs)**. (See **FIGURE 5.7**.) There are two families of essential fatty acids: **omega-3** and **omega-6**. These numbers refer to the location of the first double bond in these unsaturated fatty acids, counting from the carbon in the methyl (omega) end. Alpha-linolenic is the major omega-3 fatty acid, and linoleic is the major omega-6 fatty acid. Arachidonic acid, a longer omega-6 fatty acid, was once thought to be essential, but our bodies can make it from linoleic acid. Essential fatty acids deficiency is extremely rare. It typically occurs only with severe fat malabsorption or prolonged intravenous feeding without supplemental fat. A lack of linoleic acid leads to a scaly skin rash and dermatitis, poor growth in children, and a lowered immune response.

Plant foods are generally rich in polyunsaturated fatty acids. **TABLE 5.1** lists the omega fatty acids in some foods. Soybean oil, canola oil, and walnuts contain alpha-linolenic acid, the essential omega-3 fatty acid. However, the most generous source is flaxseed (or linseed) oil, which is more than 50 percent alpha-linolenic acid. Longer-chain omega-3s—eicosapentaenoic acid (EPA) and docosahexaenoic acid (DHA)—are found in fatty fish (e.g., salmon, tuna, and mackerel) and in fish oil supplements. Because fish oil supplements can have potent effects, children, pregnant women, and nursing mothers should not take them without medical supervision.[3] Good sources of the 18-carbon omega-6 fatty acid linoleic acid include seeds and nuts; the richest sources are common vegetable oils such as corn oil. Small amounts of arachidonic acid, a 20-carbon omega-6 fatty acid, are found in meat,

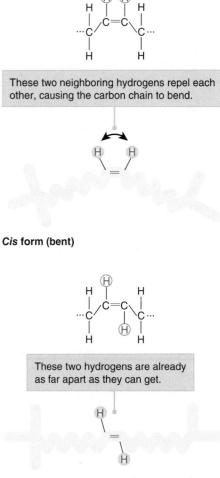

These two neighboring hydrogens repel each other, causing the carbon chain to bend.

Cis form (bent)

These two hydrogens are already as far apart as they can get.

Trans form (straighter)

FIGURE 5.6 Cis and trans fatty acids. Fatty acids with the bent cis form are more common in food than is the trans form. Trans fatty acids most commonly are found in hydrogenated fats, such as those in stick margarine, shortening, and deep-fat-fried foods.

▶ **cis fatty acid** An unsaturated fatty acid with a bent carbon chain. Most naturally occurring unsaturated fatty acids are cis fatty acids.

▶ **trans fatty acid** An unsaturated fatty acid with a straighter chain than a cis fatty acid, usually as a result of hydrogenation; trans fatty acids are more solid than cis fatty acids.

▶ **hydrogenation [high-dro-jen-AY-shun]** A chemical reaction in which hydrogen atoms are added to a fat; hydrogenation produces more saturated fatty acids and converts some unsaturated fatty acids from a cis form to a trans form.

▶ **nonessential fatty acids** Fatty acids that your body can make when they are needed. It is not necessary to consume them in the diet.

▶ **essential fatty acids (EFAs)** Fatty acids that the body needs but cannot synthesize and must obtain from the diet.

▶ **omega-3 fatty acid** An essential fatty acid; alpha-linolenic acid is the primary type.

▶ **omega-6 fatty acid** An essential fatty acid; linoleic acid is the primary type.

TABLE 5.1
Good Food Sources of Omega-3 Fatty Acids

Walnuts and walnut oil
Flaxseeds and flaxseed oil
Chia seeds
Hemp hearts
Canola oil
Salmon
Mackerel
Tuna
Fortified foods such as eggs, milk, margarine, and yogurt
Enriched foods such as breads, cereals, and pastas

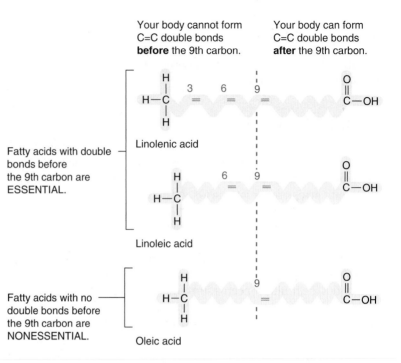

FIGURE 5.7 Essential and nonessential fatty acids. Your body makes some types of fatty acids, but others are essential in your diet.

▶ **eicosanoids** A class of hormone-like substances formed in the body from long-chain essential fatty acids.

▶ **glycerol [GLISS-er-ol]** The backbone of mono-, di-, and triglycerides; alone, it is a thick, smooth liquid.

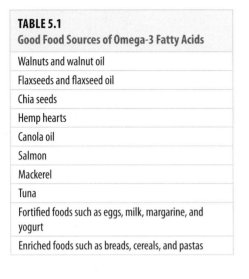

A generic triglyceride

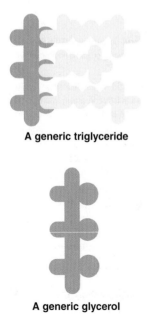

A generic glycerol

poultry, and eggs, but not in plant foods. The FYI feature "Fats on the Health Food Store Shelf" discusses the omega-3 fatty acids in some foods and supplements.

Essential fatty acids are precursors to hormone-like compounds called **eicosanoids**. Eicosanoids formed from the omega-6 fatty acid arachidonic acid play a role in increasing blood pressure, heart rate, blood clotting, immune response, and inflammation. Eicosanoids formed from the omega-3 fatty acid called alpha-linolenic acid have opposing "heart-healthy" effects of dilating blood vessels, discouraging blood clotting, and reducing inflammation. The health effects of omega fatty acids are discussed later in this chapter.

Key Concepts Unsaturated fatty acids can have cis or trans double bonds. The body can make many, but not all, types of the fatty acids it needs. A fatty acid the body can make is a nonessential fatty acid, and one that must come from the diet is an essential fatty acid.

Triglycerides

🍎 **Why Is This Important?** The most abundant lipids found in the diet and stored in the body's adipose tissue are triglycerides; therefore, learning the basic structure and functions of triglycerides will provide a foundation for understanding the relationship between dietary fats and health. Triglycerides add flavor and texture (and calories!) to foods and are an important source of energy.

Triglyceride Structure

Most fatty acids in food and in the body exist as part of a triglyceride molecule. A triglyceride consists of three fatty acids attached to a glycerol backbone. Alone, **glycerol** is a thick, smooth liquid often used by the food industry. **FIGURE 5.8** illustrates the formation of a triglyceride.

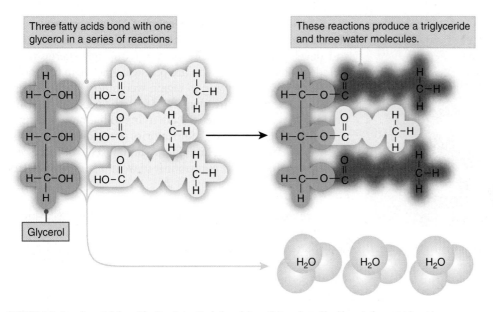

Three fatty acids bond with one glycerol in a series of reactions.

These reactions produce a triglyceride and three water molecules.

Glycerol

FIGURE 5.8 Forming a triglyceride. Reactions attach three fatty acids to a glycerol backbone to form a triglyceride. These reactions release water.

Two fatty acids attached to a glycerol form a **diglyceride**. A **monoglyceride** has one fatty acid attached to glycerol. Our foods contain relatively small amounts of mono- and diglycerides, mostly as food additives used for their emulsifying or blending qualities.

▶ **diglyceride** A molecule of glycerol combined with two fatty acids.

▶ **monoglyceride** A molecule of glycerol combined with one fatty acid.

Triglyceride Functions

Although some of us, like Rachel at the beginning of this chapter, think of fat as something to avoid, fat is a key nutrient with important body functions. Fat serves many essential functions in the body. In addition to providing a valuable source of stored energy, lipids are essential to normal cellular structure and function. **FIGURE 5.9** shows the functions of triglycerides.

Energy Source

Fat is a rich and efficient source of calories. Under normal circumstances, dietary and stored fats supply about 60 percent of the body's resting energy needs. Like carbohydrate, fat is protein-sparing; that is, fat is burned for energy, saving valuable proteins for their important roles as muscle tissue, enzymes, antibodies, and the like. Different body tissues prefer different sources of calories. Whereas muscle tissue at rest prefers to burn fat (see **FIGURE 5.10**), brain cells rely almost exclusively on glucose except during prolonged starvation. During physical activity, glucose and glycogen join fat in supplying energy to muscles.

High-fat foods are higher in calories than either high-protein or high-carbohydrate foods. One gram of fat contains 9 kilocalories, compared with only 4 kilocalories in a gram of carbohydrate or protein, or 7 kilocalories per gram of alcohol. For example, a tablespoon of corn oil (pure fat) has 120 kilocalories, whereas a tablespoon of sugar (pure carbohydrate) has only 50 kilocalories.

The high concentration of calories in fat can be advantageous to good health in some circumstances. An infant, for example, who needs ample energy for fast growth but whose stomach can hold only a limited amount of food, needs the high fat content of breast milk

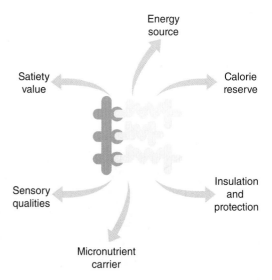

Energy source

Calorie reserve

Satiety value

Insulation and protection

Sensory qualities

Micronutrient carrier

FIGURE 5.9 Functions of triglycerides. Fat performs a number of essential functions in the body.

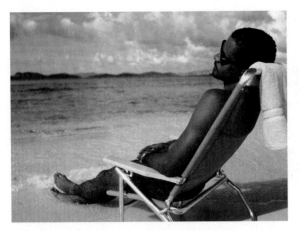

FIGURE 5.10 Fat is an important energy source. When at rest, muscles prefer to use fat for fuel.
© Photodisc.

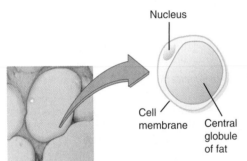

FIGURE 5.11 Adipose cells store fat. Adipocytes (fat cells) in adipose (fat) tissue store fat as an energy reserve. These are simple cells with just a nucleus, cell membrane, and fat droplet.
photo: © Donna Beer Stolz, Ph.D., Center for Biologic Imaging, University of Pittsburgh Medical School.

▶ **adipocytes** Fat cells.

▶ **adipose tissue** Body fat tissue.

▶ **visceral fat** Fat stores that cushion body organs.

▶ **subcutaneous fat** Fat stores under the skin.

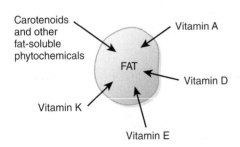

FIGURE 5.12 Fat is a micronutrient carrier. Fat holds more than just energy. It also carries important nutrients, such as fat-soluble vitamins and carotenoids.

or infant formula to get enough calories. When inappropriately put on a low-fat diet, infants and young children do not grow and develop properly. Other people with high energy needs include athletes, people who are physically active in their jobs, and people who are trying to regain weight lost due to illness.

Of course, the caloric density of fat has a negative side, and we do not welcome it when we are trying to maintain a healthy weight. In practical terms, 9 kilocalories per gram makes it easy to eat too many calories, and dietary fat in excess of a person's energy needs is a major contributor to weight gain and obesity.

Energy Reserve

We store excess dietary fat as body fat to hold us over during periods of calorie deficit. It is actually this adaptation of the body that enables us to survive times of food shortage. Because fat is calorie-dense, it can store a lot of energy in a small space.

The fat is stored inside fat cells called **adipocytes**, which form body fat tissue, technically called **adipose tissue**. (See **FIGURE 5.11**.) Hibernating animals have perfected this process; the fat stores they build in autumn can see them through a winter's fast.

The body has complex mechanisms for freeing triglycerides and fatty acids from storage in adipose tissue and delivering them when and where they are needed for energy. Cells throughout the body then break down these lipids to release the energy that is stored in their chemical bonds.

Insulation and Protection

Fat tissue usually accounts for about 15 to 30 percent of body weight. Part of this is **visceral fat**, adipose tissue around organs. Visceral fat cushions and shields delicate organs, especially the kidneys. Women have extra fat, most noticeably in the hips and breasts, to help shield their reproductive organs and to guarantee adequate calories during pregnancy. Other fat tissue is **subcutaneous**, lying under the skin, where it protects and insulates the body. In contrast is ectopic fat, where triglycerides are stored in nonadipose tissue locations. Ectopic fat in vital organs and blood vessels appears to impair their function and disrupt metabolic processes, contributing to insulin resistance and increased risk of type 2 diabetes mellitus and cardiovascular disease.[4]

Perhaps nowhere is fat's structural role more dramatic than in the brain, which is 60 percent fat.[5] Lipids in the brain can fundamentally determine brain function. Lipid homeostasis in the brain is an area of research for prevention and treatment of psychiatric disorders such as depression, anxiety, and schizophrenia.[6]

Can a person have too little body fat? Just ask someone whose body fat has been depleted by illness. It hurts to sit and it hurts to lie down. For people without enough body fat, cool temperatures are intolerable, and even room temperature may be uncomfortably cool. Women stop menstruating and become infertile. Children stop growing. Skin deteriorates from pressure sores or from fatty acid deficiency and may become covered with fine hair called lanugo. Illness, involuntary starvation, and famine can deplete fat to this extent, as can excessive dieting and exercise.

THINK About It

2

Carrier of Fat-Soluble Compounds

Dietary fats dissolve and transport micronutrients, such as fat-soluble vitamins (A, D, E, and K) and fat-soluble phytochemicals (carotenoids, for example). (See **FIGURE 5.12**.) Dietary fats carry fat-soluble substances through the digestive process, improving intestinal absorption and bio-availability. For example, the body absorbs more lycopene, the healthful red-colored phytochemical in tomatoes, if the tomatoes are served with a little oil or salad dressing.

Removing a food's lipid portion—for example, removing butterfat from milk—also removes fat-soluble vitamins. In the case of most dairy products, vitamin A and vitamin D are usually replaced. Refining wheat grain to white flour extends shelf life but removes the lipid-rich germ portion. Vitamin E is lost with the germ and is not replaced, which is another good reason to eat more whole-grain bread products. Processing fats may destroy fat-soluble vitamins; for example, some vitamin E is lost in processing vegetable oils.

Sensory Qualities

Fat contributes greatly to the flavor, odor, and texture of food. Simply put, it makes food taste good. (See **FIGURE 5.13**.) Flavorful chemicals dissolve in the fat of a food; heat sends them into the air, producing mouth-watering odors that perk up appetites. Fats have a rich, satisfying feeling in the mouth. Fats make baked goods tender and moist. And fats can be heated to high temperatures for frying, which seals in flavors and cooks food quickly. These are all good qualities—but too good for many people who find high-fat foods irresistible and eat too much of them. Alas, fat's most appealing attributes also are serious drawbacks to maintaining a healthful diet.

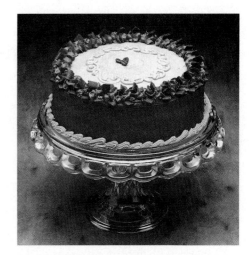

FIGURE 5.13 Sensory decadence. Fat imparts a rich texture and smooth mouth feel to food.
© Photodisc.

> **Key Concepts** Triglycerides are formed when a glycerol molecule combines with three fatty acids. Dietary triglycerides add texture and flavor to food and are a concentrated source of calories. The body stores excess calories as adipose tissue. While storing energy, adipose tissue also insulates the body and cushions its organs. The fats in food carry valuable fat-soluble nutrients into the body and help with their absorption.

Triglycerides in Food

The average American diet contains about 35–40 percent (80–130 g/day) of total calories from fat, and of that more than 90 percent comes from triglycerides.[7] Dietary triglycerides are found in a variety of fats and oils as well as in foods that contain them, such as salad dressing and baked goods. Some food fats are obvious, such as butter, margarine, cooking oil, and the fat along a cut of meat or under the skin of chicken. Baked goods, snack foods, nuts, and seeds also provide fat, but it is less noticeable.

Fats and oils are mixtures of many triglycerides, but we often classify them by their most prevalent type of fatty acid—saturated, monounsaturated, or polyunsaturated. (See **FIGURE 5.14**.) Canola oil, for example, often is classified as a monounsaturated fat because most of the fatty acids in canola oil are the monounsaturated fatty acid oleic acid. Coconut oil, on the other hand, is considered a saturated fat because the most prevalent fatty acids are saturated.

Commercial Processing of Fats

In earlier times, people could obtain concentrated fats and oils only through simple processing: removing fats from meats and poultry, skimming or churning the butterfat from milk, skimming the oil from ground nuts, or pressing

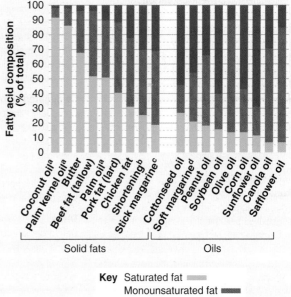

Key Saturated fat ▬
Monounsaturated fat ▬
Polyunsaturated fat ▬

[a]Coconut oil, palm kernel oil, and palm oil are called oils because they come from plants. However, they are semi-solid at room temperature due to their high content of short-chain saturated fatty acids. They are considered solid fats for nutritional purposes.
[b]Partially hydrogenated vegetable oil shortening, which contains *trans* fats.
[c]Most stick margarines contain partially hydrogenated vegetable oil, a source of *trans* fats.
[d]The primary ingredient in soft margarine with no *trans* fats is liquid vegetable oil.

U.S. Department of Agriculture, Agricultural Research Service, Nutrient Data Laboratory. USDA National Nutrient Database for Standard Reference, Release 22, 2009. Available at http://www.ars.usda.gov/ba/bhnrc/ndl. Accessed July 19, 2010.

FIGURE 5.14 The diversity of fats. Fats contain a mix of saturated and unsaturated fatty acids. Depending on which type of fatty acid is most prevalent, the fat is classified as saturated, monounsaturated, or polyunsaturated.
Modified from *Nutrition Today*, May/June 1996;31(3).

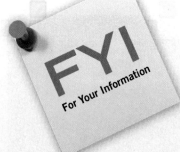

Fats on the Health Food Store Shelf

Many claims made for lipid products sold as supplements may not hold up under scientific scrutiny. You may not even recognize these products as lipids, especially because their long, complicated names are often abbreviated.

EPA and DHA in Fish Oil Capsules
These omega-3 fatty acids are thought to help lower blood pressure, reduce inflammation, reduce blood clotting, and lower high serum triglyceride levels.[a] Some studies indicate that nutrition intake that includes omega-3 fatty acids is a viable treatment alternative in patients with psoriasis.[b] EPA and DHA usually make up only about one-third of the fatty acids in fish oil capsules, and research studies often use multiple doses. These should not be taken without close medical supervision because their blood-thinning properties can cause bleeding. Because fish oil is highly unsaturated, antioxidant vitamins are included to prevent **oxidation**. Another problem, though not health related, is that fish oil capsules often leave a fishy aftertaste. The aftertaste can be avoided by taking the fish oil capsules with meals or at bedtime. A concentrated, purified Food and Drug Administration–approved prescription form of omega-3 fatty acids has been developed that has a minimal aftertaste.[c] Findings from an analysis of randomized trials, however, do not suggest that fish oil supplements provide any cardiovascular benefits.[d]

Flaxseed Oil Capsules
Flaxseed oil is an unusually good source of omega-3 alpha-linolenic acid, which accounts for about 55 percent of its fatty acids. Like fish oil, flaxseed oil is highly unsaturated and thus very susceptible to rancidity. Capsules protect the oil from oxygen, but limit the dose. A half-tablespoon of canola oil has about as much omega-3 as a capsule of flaxseed oil but adds more calories.

GLA in Borage, Evening Primrose, or Black Currant Seed Oil Capsules
These oils contain 9 to 24 percent gamma-linolenic acid (GLA), an omega-6 derivative of linoleic acid. Studies of GLA's effects on skin diseases and heart conditions have been disappointing, and research on potential benefits of GLA supplements in rheumatoid arthritis has been conflicting.[e]

Medium-Chain Triglycerides
Medium-chain triglycerides (MCTs) can be purchased as such or found as ingredients in "sports" drinks and foods. Because MCTs are absorbed easily, they are marketed to athletes as a noncarbohydrate source of quick, concentrated energy. However, they have no specific performance benefits. A tablespoon of MCT contains about 100 kilocalories.

Lecithin Oil or Granules
Lecithin supplements are a mixture of phospholipids derived from soybeans. They often are promoted as emulsifiers that lower cholesterol, but because dietary phospholipids are broken down in the small intestine, it is unlikely that supplemental lecithin will be effective. They may be useful as a source of choline. Because choline is the precursor of acetylcholine (a neurotransmitter), lecithin is promoted for treating Parkinson's and Alzheimer's diseases, which are associated with low levels of acetylcholine in the brain. Unfortunately, these claims have little scientific support.[f]

Conjugated Linoleic Acid
Conjugated linoleic acid (CLA) is linoleic acid with a different pattern of chemical bonds. It is promoted as an aid for reducing body fat and has been suggested to have anticancer properties. Studies show promising results, but more work is needed to identify specific functions of CLA and evaluate its long-term safety.[g]

DHEA
Dehydroepiandrosterone (DHEA) is a testosterone precursor formed from cholesterol. It is present in the body in large quantities during adolescence, peaks in the 20s, and gradually declines with age. Many elderly people have low levels, and levels also dip during serious illnesses. With only a few exceptions, attempts to use DHEA for illnesses or to slow aging have been disappointing. Researchers generally use doses many times greater than those in over-the-counter supplements—levels that may cause hairiness in women and, more seriously, a risk of liver problems.[h]

Squalene Capsules and Shark Liver Oil
Squalene, an intermediary compound in the synthesis of cholesterol in the body, and shark liver oil, which contains squalene, are said to help liver, skin, and immune function. The basis for these claims is unclear.

Coconut Oil
The health claims for coconut oil tout the benefits of this dietary "super-food" for everything from promoting weight loss to protecting against cancer, dissolving kidney stones, promoting oral health, curing thyroid disease, boosting immune function, and warding off Alzheimer's disease. In addition to being labeled a dietary super-food, coconut oil has been used as a natural moisturizer and personal hair care product.

There are three common types of dietary coconut oil.

- *Virgin or cold pressed:* This is considered unrefined because the oil is extracted from the fruit of fresh mature coconuts without using high temperatures or chemicals. The extra-virgin type has some antioxidant properties from phenolic compounds.
- *Refined:* Also called conventional, this type of coconut oil is made from dried coconut meat that is often chemically bleached and deodorized.
- *Partially hydrogenated coconut oil:* Some food manufacturers may use yet another form of coconut oil that's further processed, transforming some of the unsaturated fats into trans fats found in foods such as commercial baked goods.

One tablespoon of coconut oil provides 117 calories, 14 g total fat (12 g saturated fat, 0.8 g monounsaturated fat, 0.2 g polyunsaturated fat), no protein or carbohydrates, and only trace amounts of iron and vitamins E and K. Coconut oil is 92 percent saturated fat, the highest amount of saturated fat of any fat, but like all other plant-based fats it has benefits from phytochemicals and does not contain cholesterol or trans fat unless it has been commercially hydrogenated.

The unfortunate truth is that there isn't yet enough scientific evidence to support any of the claims about coconut oil's potential health benefits.[i] And despite the public hype, the American Heart Association recommends consumers stay away from tropical oils such as coconut oil.[j]

Grapeseed Oil
A relative newcomer in the specialty oil market, grapeseed oil is made from extracting

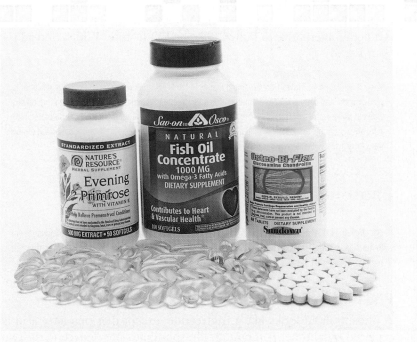

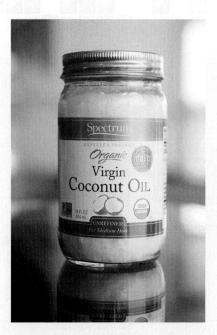

FYI 1 Lipid products found on store shelves. Products make health claims but scientific evidence may be limited.

FYI 2 Coconut oil products are now easily found at health food and local grocery stores.

the oil from the seeds of grapes that are left over in wine production. Grapeseed oils and extracts contain antioxidants and omega fatty acids, and therefore producers claim it is good for your health. Although the benefits of consuming grapes and moderate amounts of wine have been proven, the evidence of the health effects of grapeseed oil and grapeseed extract requires further investigation.[k]

a Meyer BJ. Are we consuming enough long-chain omega-3 polyunsaturated fatty acids for optimal health? *Prostaglandins Leukot Essent Fatty Acids*. 2011;85(5):275-280.

b Ricketts JR, Rothe MJ, Grant-Kels JM. Nutrition and psoriasis. *Clin Dermatol*. 2010;28(6):615-626.

c Abete P, Testa G, Galizia G, et al. PUFA for human health: diet or supplementation? *Curr Pharm Des*. 2009;15(36):4186-4190.

d Chowdhury R, Warnakula S, Kunutsor S, et al. Association of dietary, circulating, and supplement fatty acids with coronary risk: a systematic review and meta-analysis. *Ann Intern Med*. 2014;160(6):398-406. doi: 10.7326/M13-1788

e Cameron M, Gagnier JJ, Crubasik S. Herbal therapy for treating rheumatoid arthritis. *Cochrane Database Syst Rev*. 2011;(2):CD002948.

f Sarubin Fragakis A, Tomson CA. *The Health Professional's Guide to Popular Dietary Supplements*. 3rd ed. Chicago: Academy of Nutrition and Dietetics; 2006.

g Racine NM, Watras AC, Carrel AL, et al. Effect of conjugated linoleic acid on body fat accretion in overweight or obese children. *Am J Clin Nutr*. 2010;91(5):1157-1164.

h Christensen JJ, Bruun JM, Christiansen JS, et al. Long-term dehydroepiandrosterone substitution in female adrenocortical failure, body composition, muscle function, and bone metabolism—a randomized trial. *Eur J Endocrinol*. 2011;165(2):293-300.

i Center for Science in the Public Interest. Coconut oil myths persist in face of the facts. June 22, 2016. http://www.cspinet.org/nah/articles/coconut-oil.html. Accessed September 5, 2017.

j American Heart Association. Fats and oils: AHA recommendation. http://www.heart.org/HEARTORG/GettingHealthy/FatsAndOils/Fats101/Fats-and-Oils-AHA-Recommendation_UCM_316375_Article.jsp. Accessed September 5, 2017.

k University of Maryland Medical Center. Grape seed. http://umm.edu/health/medical/altmed/herb/grape-seed. Accessed September 5, 2017.

a few oil-rich plant parts such as coconuts or olives. In the 1920s, new technology began producing pure vegetable oils. Processing vegetable oils reduces waste and prevents spoilage during normal use. Processing removes damaging free fatty acids and certain destructive enzymes and also adds antioxidants such as vitamin E to delay rancidity and extend shelf life.

Unfortunately, processing has a negative side. To achieve stability and uniform taste, processing removes potentially healthful phospholipids, plant sterols, and other phytochemicals; a significant portion of the natural vitamin E also is lost. Oils have become so familiar that we often forget they are highly processed, highly refined foods. Further processing of oils into solid fats, such as margarine or shortening, also

▶ **oxidation** Occurs when oxygen attaches to the double bonds of unsaturated fatty acids. It causes fats to become rancid.

Quick **Bite**

The Marvelous Storage Efficiency of Fat

Why do you think we don't store all our extra energy as readily available glycogen? It would take more than 6 pounds of glycogen to store the same energy as 1 pound of fat. Just imagine how much bulkier we would be! How cumbersome it would be to move about! That's why only a very small portion of the body's energy reserve is glycogen.

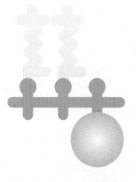

A generic phospholipid

A generic phospholipid. Like triglycerides, phospholipids contain glycerol and fatty acids; however, phospholipids also contain other substances that give them entirely different properties and functions. Our bodies can make phospholipids, so we do not need them in our diets.

produces some undesirable changes, such as increasing the proportion of trans fatty acids. This might lead you to wonder whether margarine is a better alternative to butter. (See the FYI feature "Which Spread for Your Bread?")

> **Key Concepts** Triglycerides are found mainly in foods we think of as fats and oils but also in nuts, seeds, meats, and dairy products. Saturated fatty acids are found mainly in animal foods and tropical oils, whereas polyunsaturated fatty acids are found in vegetable oils and other plant foods. Unsaturated fatty acids are susceptible to spoilage by oxidation. Hydrogenation of oils protects fats from oxidation but creates trans fatty acids, which increase the risk for heart disease.

Phospholipids

🍎 **Why Is This Important?** Phospholipids are soluble in both fat and water, allowing them to function in critical roles both in cell membranes and in the blood or other body fluids where they can keep fats suspended.

Phospholipid Structure

A phospholipid looks like a triglyceride, except that one fatty acid is replaced by another compound. Phospholipids are diglycerides—two fatty acids attached to a glycerol backbone. A **phosphate group** with a nitrogen-containing component occupies the third attachment site. **FIGURE 5.15** shows the structure of a phospholipid.

The phosphate–nitrogen component of phospholipids is soluble in water, so a phospholipid is compatible with both fat and water. The fatty acids in the diglyceride area attract fats, and the phosphate–nitrogen component attracts water-soluble substances.

Phospholipid Functions

Because phospholipids have both water-soluble and fat-soluble parts, they are ideal emulsifiers (compounds that help keep fats suspended in a watery environment). In foods, phospholipids can keep oil and water mixed. This same property makes phospholipids a perfect structural element for cell membranes—able to communicate with the watery environments of blood and cell fluids, yet with a lipid portion that allows other lipids to enter and exit cells.

Cell Membranes

Phospholipids are major components of cell membranes. Cell membranes are a double layer of phospholipids that selectively allow both fatty and water-soluble substances into the cell. (See **FIGURE 5.16**.) They also store fatty acids temporarily, donating them when the body has short-term energy needs or must make regulatory chemicals (e.g., eicosanoids). One phospholipid, phosphatidylcholine, whose **choline** component eventually becomes part of the major neurotransmitter acetylcholine, plays an especially important role in nerve cells. By keeping fatty acids, choline, and other biologically active substances bound in phospholipids and freeing them only as needed, the body can regulate them closely.

Lipid Transport

The ability of phospholipids to combine both fatty and watery substances comes in handy throughout the body. In the stomach, dietary phospholipids help break fats into tiny particles for easier digestion.

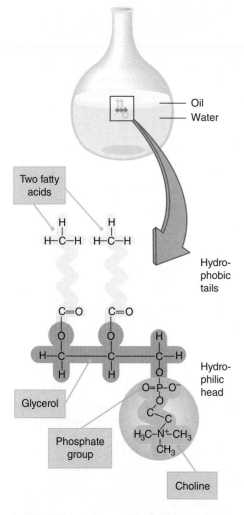

FIGURE 5.15 Phospholipid. Phospholipids are molecules of two fatty acids attached to a glycerol molecule with a phosphate group and a nitrogen-containing component. A phospholipid is compatible with both oil and water. This is a useful property for transporting fatty substances in the body's watery fluids.

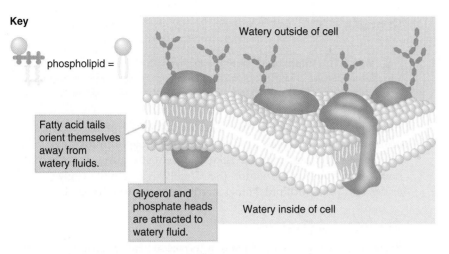

Key

phospholipid =

Fatty acid tails orient themselves away from watery fluids.

Watery outside of cell

Glycerol and phosphate heads are attracted to watery fluid.

Watery inside of cell

FIGURE 5.16 Cell membranes are phospholipid bilayers. Although proteins and other substances are embedded in cell membranes, these membranes primarily consist of phospholipids.

▶ **phosphate group** A chemical group that contains phosphate (–PO₄) attached to a larger molecule. Attaching a phosphate group, along with two fatty acids, to a glycerol backbone forms a phospholipid.

▶ **choline** A nitrogen-containing compound that is part of phosphatidylcholine, a phospholipid. Choline also is part of the neurotransmitter acetylcholine. The body can synthesize choline from the amino acid methionine.

▶ **lecithin** In the body, a phospholipid with the nitrogen-containing component choline. In foods, lecithin is a blend of phospholipids with different nitrogen-containing components.

In the small intestine, phospholipids from bile continue emulsifying. In the watery environment of blood, phospholipids coat the surface of the lipoproteins that carry lipid particles to their destinations in the body.

Emulsifiers (Lecithin)

In the body and in foods of animal origin, phosphatidylcholine also is called **lecithin**. However, for food additives or supplements, the term *lecithin* is used for a mix of phospholipids derived from plants (usually soybeans). Understandably, this inconsistent terminology has caused confusion.

The food industry uses lecithin as an emulsifier to combine two ingredients that don't ordinarily mix, such as oil and water. (See **FIGURE 5.17**.) In high-fat powdered products (e.g., dry milk, milk replacers, coffee creamers), lecithin helps mix fatty compounds with water. Lecithin in salad dressing, for example, allows the ingredients to mix well and remain mixed, avoiding separation. Lecithin is even added to chewing gum to increase shelf life, prolong flavor release, and prevent the gum from sticking to teeth and dental work.

Phospholipids in Food

Phospholipids occur naturally throughout the plant and animal worlds, but in much smaller amounts than triglycerides. They are most abundant in egg yolks, liver, soybeans, and peanuts. Although food processing often removes some phospholipids, other phospholipids are common food additives. Overall, a typical diet contains only about 2 grams per day. Because your body can make phospholipids, they are not a dietary essential.

> **Key Concepts** Phospholipids are diglycerides (glycerol plus two fatty acids) with a phosphate–nitrogen compound attached at the third attachment point of glycerol. This structure makes phospholipids compatible with both fat and water. Phospholipids are major components of cell membranes and act as emulsifiers. They also store fatty acids for release into the cell and serve as a source of choline. Because the body can make phospholipids, they are not needed in the diet.

Quick **Bite**

The Power of the Yolk

A single raw egg yolk is capable of emulsifying many cups of oil. Cooks take advantage of the natural emulsifying ability of egg yolk phospholipids to emulsify and stabilize preparations such as mayonnaise (oil and vinegar emulsion) and hollandaise sauce (butter and lemon juice emulsion). Food producers use phospholipid emulsifiers in processed foods, which today provide much of our intake.

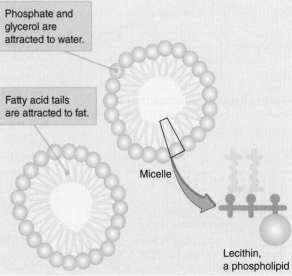

Phosphate and glycerol are attracted to water.

Fatty acid tails are attracted to fat.

Micelle

Lecithin, a phospholipid

FIGURE 5.17 Lecithin and emulsification. Lecithin, a phospholipid, forms water-soluble packages called micelles that suspend fat-soluble compounds in watery mediums. In a micelle, the lecithin molecules form into a water-soluble ball with a fatty core. The water-soluble head of each lecithin molecule points outward in contact with the watery medium, whereas the fat-soluble tail points inward in contact with the fatty core.

Sterols

▶ **sterols** A category of lipids that includes cholesterol. Sterols are hydrocarbons with several rings in their structures.

▶ **cholesterol [ko-LES-te-rol]** A waxy lipid (sterol) whose chemical structure contains multiple hydrocarbon rings.

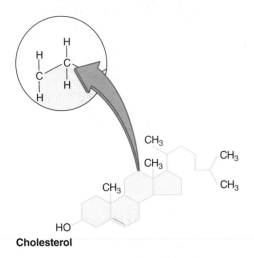

Cholesterol

FIGURE 5.18 Sterols. Sterols are a group of lipids that are multiple-ring structures. Because of its role in heart disease, cholesterol has become the best-known sterol.

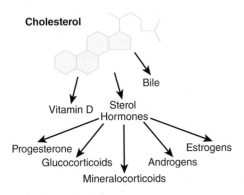

FIGURE 5.19 Cholesterol has important roles. Cholesterol is a precursor of vitamin D and steroid hormones. The liver uses cholesterol to make bile.

Quick Bite

Would You Pay More for Cholesterol-Free Mushrooms?

Several years ago, some plant foods were promoted with labels claiming they were "cholesterol free." As you might expect, the FDA found this misleading, because plant foods never contain cholesterol unless an animal product such as butter or egg has been added. Regulations no longer allow the implication that cholesterol has been removed from a naturally cholesterol-free food. Rather than saying "cholesterol-free mushrooms," labels must now say "mushrooms, a cholesterol-free food."

Why Is This Important? Sterols are a category of lipids, of which probably the most famous is cholesterol. Cholesterol is a precursor to hormones, Vitamin D, and bile salts; it is also a key component of cell membranes. Cholesterol has an important role in lipid transport and cardiovascular health.

Although sterols are lipids, they are quite different from triglycerides and phospholipids. Whereas triglycerides and phospholipids have a glycerol backbone and fingerlike fatty acid structures, **sterols** have a multiple-ring structure. (See **FIGURE 5.18.**) Unlike triglycerides and phospholipids, most sterols contain no fatty acids.

THINK About It **3**

Cholesterol Functions

Because of the publicity generated by its role in heart disease, **cholesterol** is the best-known sterol. But cholesterol is necessary and important in your body; it becomes a problem only when excessive amounts accumulate in your blood. Like phospholipids, it is a major structural component of all cell membranes and is especially abundant in nerve and brain tissue. In fact, most cholesterol resides in body tissue, not in the blood serum or plasma that is routinely tested for cholesterol levels.

Cholesterol is a precursor of important substances. For example, your body can use cholesterol to make vitamin D. Cholesterol also is the precursor of five major classes of sterol hormones: progesterone, glucocorticoids, mineralocorticoids, androgens, and estrogens. (See **FIGURE 5.19.**) When making testosterone (an androgen) from cholesterol, our bodies form an intermediate compound called dehydroepiandrosterone (DHEA). DHEA has become a popular nutritional supplement, marketed with the largely unfulfilled promise that it will boost potency and restore youth.

The liver uses cholesterol to manufacture bile salts, which are secreted in bile. The gallbladder stores and concentrates the bile. On demand, the gallbladder releases the bile into the small intestine, where bile salts emulsify dietary fats.

Cholesterol Synthesis

Because your body can make cholesterol, you do not need cholesterol in your diet. Although researchers believe that all cells synthesize at least some cholesterol, the liver is the primary cholesterol-manufacturing site, and the intestines contribute appreciable amounts. In fact, your body produces approximately 1,000 milligrams of cholesterol per day, far more than is found in the average diet. This production level attests to cholesterol's biological importance. In the lens of the eye, which has a high concentration of cholesterol, on-site cholesterol synthesis may be essential for preventing cataracts.[8]

Sterols in Food

Only foods of animal origin contain cholesterol. The brain has the highest cholesterol content, liver and other organ meats are high, and muscle tissue contains moderate amounts. Egg yolks are high in cholesterol, with about 212 milligrams per large egg. (The egg white contains no cholesterol.) Breast milk is moderately high, suggesting the importance of cholesterol during early growth and development, including its importance for an infant's self-control of feeding.[9] Dairy products

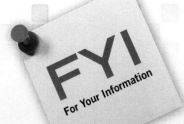

Which Spread for Your Bread?

Okay, it's time to see if you can put some of your new knowledge about lipids to work. You're standing in front of the dairy case ready to pick out the best spread. But, wow! So many choices. Of course, there's butter, which has been around for thousands of years—wholesome, natural, and creamy; sometimes there's just no substitute for the real thing. Margarine, the more recent choice of many, has come to be more familiar than butter to some consumers. Then what's this "vegetable oil spread"? The one that says it "helps promote healthy cholesterol levels."

Butter

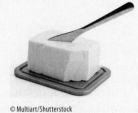

© Multiart/Shutterstock

When it comes to spreads, butter is the most traditional choice; however, it has some disadvantages: (1) Butter is high in saturated fat; (2) it contains cholesterol; and (3) like other fats, it's high in calories.

Here are the facts: one tablespoon of salted butter provides the following:

- 100 kcal
- 11 g fat
- 7 g saturated fat
- 0 g trans fat
- 30 mg cholesterol
- 85 mg sodium
- 8 percent of the Daily Value for vitamin A

The ingredients are usually simple: "cream, salt, annatto (added seasonally)." Annatto is a natural coloring (a carotenoid) that is used to keep the color of butter consistent, despite what dairy cows might have been grazing on.

If you like the taste of butter, but want a bit less saturated fat and cholesterol, you can buy "whipped butter." The ingredients are the same, but the incorporation of air reduces calories, fat, saturated fat, cholesterol, and sodium by 30 to 40 percent.

Margarine

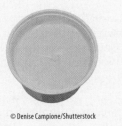

© Denise Campione/Shutterstock

Margarine was developed to be a substitute for butter. Made from vegetable oils, it appears to be more healthful; as a plant-derived food, it's certainly cholesterol-free, and vegetable oils contain more unsaturated fatty acids than butter. Inconveniently, though, unsaturated oils are liquid, and without extra processing, margarine would run right off any slice of bread. Many margarines contain hydrogenated oils to produce a spreadable consistency. But, as you know, hydrogenation increases the number of saturated and trans fatty acids in a fat, and both of these are associated with higher blood cholesterol levels.

Looking at the label of a standard stick of margarine, you'll find the following per tablespoon:

- 100 kcal
- 11 g fat
- 2 g saturated fat
- 2 g trans fat
- 3.5 g polyunsaturated fat
- 3.5 g monounsaturated fat
- 0 mg cholesterol
- 115 mg sodium
- 10 percent of the Daily Value for vitamin A

Compared with butter, margarine has the same amount of calories and fat (a fact unknown to many consumers), less saturated fat and cholesterol, and a bit more sodium and vitamin A. The PUFA and MUFA content of butter are not listed because these are not required elements of the Nutrition Facts label.

Turning to the list of ingredients, we find "liquid soybean oil, partially hydrogenated soybean oil, water, whey, salt, soy lecithin, vegetable mono- and diglycerides (emulsifiers), sodium benzoate (a preservative), vitamin A palmitate, beta carotene (color)." Nothing terribly unusual, especially now that you know what lecithin and mono- and diglycerides are.

Spreads and Other Butter Imitators

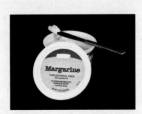

Beyond the traditional stick margarine, there are a growing number of "light," "soft," "whipped," "squeeze," "spray," and "spread" products. These items do not fit the legal definition of "margarine," and so the term *vegetable oil spread* is generally used. In terms of ingredients, these products have more liquid oil and water and less partially hydrogenated oil. More emulsifiers may be needed, along with flavors (including salt) and colors. The result typically is fewer calories, less saturated fat, and still no cholesterol.

Some products tout the inclusion of canola or olive oil for more healthful MUFA. Others indicate "no trans fatty acids" and have no hydrogenated oils on the list. Several spreads contain plant sterols or stanols that reduce intestinal absorption of cholesterol.[a]

Cholesterol-Lowering Margarines

Stanols are plant sterols similar in structure to cholesterol. Ingested plant sterols compete with and inhibit cholesterol absorption. Studies show that consumption of stanols produces favorable lipoprotein lipid changes in men and women with hypercholesterolemia.[b] The "cholesterol-lowering" margarines Benecol and Take Control contain plant stanol esters and plant sterols. Research on the extent of the ability for products such as Benecol and Take Control to improve cholesterol levels is split. Although some studies show a benefit secondary to their use, others have found that the agents have a modest ability to lower LDL cholesterol and are not effective in all conditions, nor do they have an effect on HDL cholesterol or triglyceride levels.[c] People who choose to use stanol- or sterol-ester-containing margarines in an effort to improve cholesterol levels should use caution and talk about their choice with their physician.

Making Choices

The spread you choose may depend on your purpose. There are times, and foods, where nothing but real butter will do. If you've ever tried baking cookies with a soft, reduced-fat spread, you know the outcome … and probably will use butter, margarine, or vegetable shortening next time.

Remember, your overall goal is to limit total fats; in particular, saturated fats and *especially* trans fatty acids. Using less butter or margarine on the whole will do that. Choosing a margarine or spread with liquid vegetable oil as the first ingredient (meaning that the amount of hydrogenated oil is less) will reduce not only saturated fat, but also trans fat. Although the latest scientific research on the topic found no evidence of dangers from saturated fat, it did confirm the link between trans fats and heart disease; these findings should not be seen as a "green light" to eat more butter and other foods rich in saturated fat.[d] Most important, you should not lose sight of the bigger picture,

which is the part all fats play in your total diet. Moderation is the key—making choices that consider your whole diet will help you stay in line with heart-healthy recommendations.

a Clifton P. Lowering cholesterol—a review on the role of plant sterols. *Aust Fam Physician*. 2009;38(4):218-221.
b Maki KC, Lawless AL, Reeves MS, et al. Lipid-altering effects of a dietary supplement tablet containing free plant sterols and stanols in men and women with primary hypercholesterolaemia: a randomized, placebo-controlled crossover trial. *Int J Food Sci Nutr.* 2012;63(4):476-482.
c Doggrell SA. Lowering LDL cholesterol with margarine containing plant stanol/sterol esters: is it still relevant in 2011? *Complement Ther Med.* 2011;19(1):37–46.
d Chowdhury R, Warnakula S, Kunutsor S, et al. Association of dietary, circulating, and supplement fatty acids with coronary risk: a systematic review and meta-analysis. *Ann Intern Med.* 2014;160(6):398-406. doi: 10.7326/M13-1788

▶ **squalene** A cholesterol precursor found in whale liver and plants.

▶ **phytosterols** Sterols found in plants. Phytosterols are poorly absorbed by humans and reduce intestinal absorption of cholesterol. They recently have been introduced as a cholesterol-lowering food ingredient.

TABLE 5.2
Common Foods that Contain Cholesterol
Food
cheddar cheese
cottage cheese (4 percent fat)
whole milk
whipping cream
butter
lard
lean meat
lean pork
ground beef
chicken breast
flounder
salmon
crabmeat (Alaskan King)
lobster meat
egg (high)
beef kidney (very high)
beef liver (very high)
beef brain (exceptionally high)

Data from US Department of Agriculture, Agricultural Research Service. USDA National Nutrient Database for Standard Reference, Release 25. 2012. http://www.ars.usda.gov/ba/bhnrc/ndl. Accessed 12/20/12.

also contain cholesterol, which is found in the butterfat portion.[10] As the fat content of dairy foods drops, so do cholesterol levels. The typical American consumes between 250 and 700 milligrams of cholesterol and 250 milligrams of plant sterols each day.[11] **TABLE 5.2** lists some common foods that contain cholesterol.

Aside from cholesterol and vitamin D, few dietary sterols have been found to have nutritional significance. Whale liver and plants contain the cholesterol precursor **squalene**, an intermediary compound in the synthesis of cholesterol. Although whale liver is not a common item in grocery stores, squalene capsules are sold as dietary supplements with the unproved claim that squalene speeds healing and helps liver, skin, and immune function. The basis for these claims is unclear. Plants contain a number of other sterols (**phytosterols**) that are poorly absorbed. Because phytosterols reduce intestinal absorption of cholesterol, they have attracted much interest and are used as a cholesterol-lowering food ingredient in certain vegetable oil spreads.

Key Concepts Sterols have ring structures and contain no fatty acids. Cholesterol is the best-known sterol; other sterols are hormones or hormone precursors. Cholesterol is an important precursor compound and is a key component of cell membranes. High levels of blood cholesterol increase the risk of heart disease. Cholesterol is found only in foods of animal origin; because the body can make all it needs, cholesterol is not a dietary essential.

Lipid Digestion and Absorption

Why Is This Important? There are unique features to fat digestion, absorption, and transport. Like carbohydrates and proteins, lipids get broken down into smaller parts for digestion and absorption. Also similar is that majority of fat digestion occurs in the small intestine, where intestinal cells absorb fatty acids and glycerol. However, unlike amino acids and glucose, fatty acids are packaged for travel for transport by the lymph system to the bloodstream.

Like the other macronutrients (carbohydrates and proteins), most lipids are broken into smaller compounds for absorption. (See **FIGURE 5.20**.) However, because lipids generally are not water-soluble, and digestive secretions are all water-based, the body must treat lipids a bit differently in order to digest and transport them.

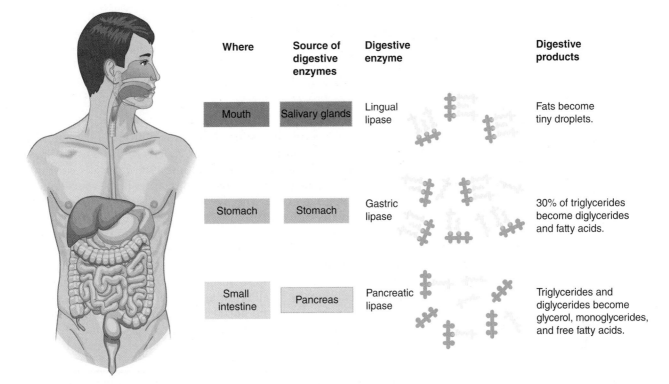

Where	Source of digestive enzymes	Digestive enzyme		Digestive products
Mouth	Salivary glands	Lingual lipase		Fats become tiny droplets.
Stomach	Stomach	Gastric lipase		30% of triglycerides become diglycerides and fatty acids.
Small intestine	Pancreas	Pancreatic lipase		Triglycerides and diglycerides become glycerol, monoglycerides, and free fatty acids.

FIGURE 5.20 Triglyceride digestion. Most triglyceride digestion takes place in the small intestine.

Lipid Digestion

Triglycerides are not soluble in water, but the enzymes that digest them are found only in a watery environment. Don't worry! Your digestive system is equal to the task. Physical actions (e.g., chewing, peristalsis, segmentation), combined with various emulsifiers, allow digestive enzymes to do their work and change dietary fat into molecules that can be digested and absorbed. The digestion of triglycerides and phospholipids is similar; these molecules get broken down to their component parts—fatty acids, glycerol, and, in the case of phospholipids, a component containing phosphate and nitrogen.

Beginning in the mouth, a combination of chewing and the work of lingual lipase starts the digestive process rolling, with the small amount of dietary phospholipid providing emulsification. In the stomach, gastric lipase joins in, and the stomach's churning and contractions keep the fat dispersed. Diglycerides that form in the breakdown process become emulsifiers, too. After two to four hours in the stomach, digestion has broken down about 30 percent of dietary triglycerides to diglycerides and free fatty acids.[12]

Fat in the small intestine stimulates the gallbladder to contract, sending bile down the bile duct to the small intestine. The pancreas releases pancreatic juice rich in pancreatic lipase, which joins bile in the bile duct just before it reaches the small intestine.

Bile contains a large quantity of bile salts and the phospholipid lecithin. These key elements emulsify fat, breaking globules into smaller pieces so water-soluble pancreatic lipase can attack the surface. Emulsification significantly increases the total surface area of fats to aid digestion. Many common household detergents use emulsification to remove grease from dishes or clothing. As bile breaks up clumps of triglycerides into small pieces and keeps them suspended in solution, pancreatic lipase breaks off one fatty acid at a time. Pancreatic juice contains enormous amounts of pancreatic lipase, which rapidly breaks down nearly all accessible triglycerides to monoglycerides and free fatty acids. (See **FIGURE 5.21**.)

Lipid Absorption

Normally, triglyceride digestion and absorption are very efficient. It is abnormal to find more than 6 or 7 percent of ingested lipids still intact in fecal matter. In the small intestine, bile salts surround monoglycerides and free fatty acids, forming **micelles**—water-soluble globules with a fatty core. Micelles carry monoglycerides and long-chain fatty acids through the watery intestinal environment to the surfaces of the microvilli, even penetrating the recesses between individual microvilli. Here, the monoglycerides and long-chain fatty acids immediately diffuse into the intestinal cells, and the bile salts return to the interior of the small intestine to form another micelle. The last section of the small intestine absorbs bile salts for recycling. The bile salts return via the portal vein to the liver, where they are once again secreted as part of bile. This bile recycling pathway—the liver to the intestine and the intestine to the liver—is called *enterohepatic circulation*.

▶ **micelles** Tiny emulsified fat packets. They are composed of emulsifier molecules (phospholipids) oriented with their fat-soluble part facing inward and their water-soluble part facing outward toward the surrounding aqueous environment.

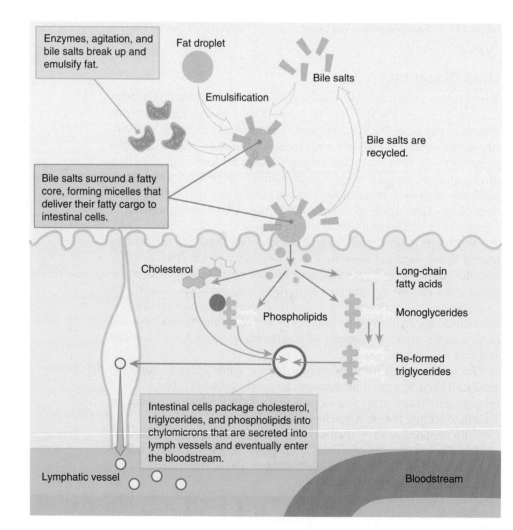

Enzymes, agitation, and bile salts break up and emulsify fat.

Fat droplet

Emulsification

Bile salts

Bile salts are recycled.

Bile salts surround a fatty core, forming micelles that deliver their fatty cargo to intestinal cells.

Cholesterol

Long-chain fatty acids

Phospholipids

Monoglycerides

Re-formed triglycerides

Intestinal cells package cholesterol, triglycerides, and phospholipids into chylomicrons that are secreted into lymph vessels and eventually enter the bloodstream.

Lymphatic vessel

Bloodstream

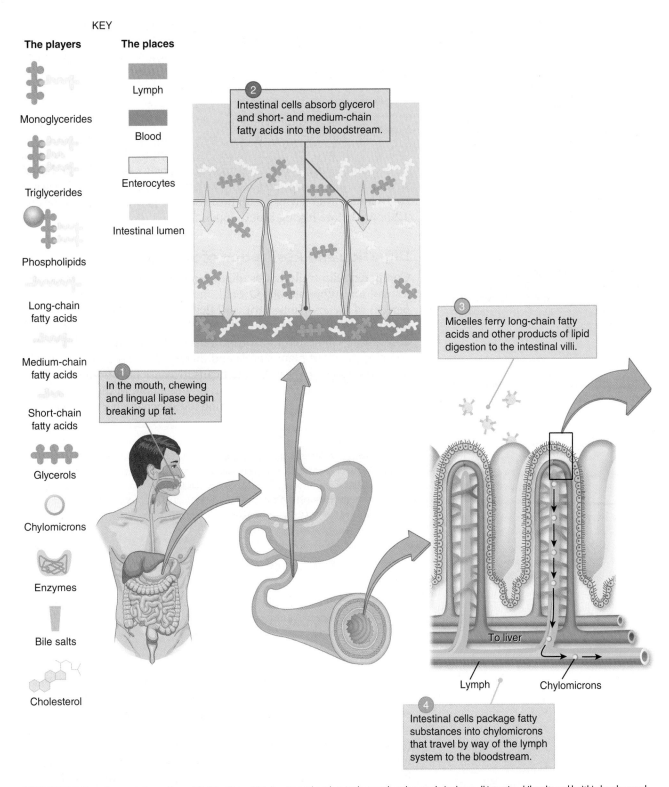

KEY

The players

Monoglycerides

Triglycerides

Phospholipids

Long-chain fatty acids

Medium-chain fatty acids

Short-chain fatty acids

Glycerols

Chylomicrons

Enzymes

Bile salts

Cholesterol

The places

Lymph

Blood

Enterocytes

Intestinal lumen

2 Intestinal cells absorb glycerol and short- and medium-chain fatty acids into the bloodstream.

1 In the mouth, chewing and lingual lipase begin breaking up fat.

3 Micelles ferry long-chain fatty acids and other products of lipid digestion to the intestinal villi.

To liver

Lymph

Chylomicrons

4 Intestinal cells package fatty substances into chylomicrons that travel by way of the lymph system to the bloodstream.

FIGURE 5.21 Digestion and absorption of lipids. Minimal fat digestion takes place in the mouth and stomach. In the small intestine, bile salts and lecithin break up and disperse fatty lipids in tiny globules. Enzymes attack these globules, breaking down triglycerides and phospholipids to fatty acids and other component parts. Glycerol and short- and medium-chain fatty acids are absorbed directly into the bloodstream. Bile salts surround the remaining products of fat digestion, forming water-soluble micelles that carry fat to intestinal cells, where it is absorbed and repackaged for transport by the lymphatic system.

▶ **lipoprotein** A complex that transports lipids in the lymph and blood. Lipoproteins consist of a central core of triglycerides and cholesterol surrounded by a shell composed of proteins, cholesterol, and phospholipids. The various types of lipoproteins differ in size, composition, and density.

▶ **chylomicron [kye-lo-MY-kron]** A large lipoprotein formed in intestinal cells following the absorption of dietary fats. A chylomicron has a central core of triglycerides and cholesterol surrounded by phospholipids and proteins.

Quick Bite

How Do Cholesterol-Lowering Medications Work?

One class of cholesterol-lowering medications, the "bile-acid sequestrants," works by combining bile acid and cholesterol in the intestines to form compounds that the body cannot absorb. Because this cholesterol is then lost in the feces, cholesterol must be taken from the blood to make more bile, thus lowering the blood cholesterol level.

Inside intestinal cells, monoglycerides and fatty acids re-form triglycerides. These triglycerides, as well as cholesterol and phospholipids, join protein carriers to form a **lipoprotein**. When this assemblage leaves the intestinal cell, it is called a **chylomicron**. Chylomicrons make their way to the interior of the villi, where they enter the lymph system, which eventually empties into veins in the neck.

Short- and medium-chain fatty acids are more water-soluble than long-chain fatty acids. Intestinal cells absorb them, along with glycerol, directly into the bloodstream, bypassing the lymph system. One or two hours after you eat, dietary fat begins to appear in the bloodstream. Fat levels peak after 3 to 5 hours, and fats are generally cleared by 10 hours. That's why health professionals instruct people to fast for 12 hours before having blood drawn for lipid testing.

Digestion and Absorption of Sterols

Compared with triglycerides, digestion does little to break down cholesterol and other sterols. Overall, our bodies absorb only about 50 percent of dietary cholesterol, and that proportion falls as cholesterol intake increases. Dietary fat in the small intestine increases cholesterol absorption. Cholesterol absorption declines when the small intestine contains plenty of plant sterols and dietary fiber, especially fiber from fruits, vegetables, oats, peas, and beans. Because fiber from these foods binds bile salts and cholesterol, carrying them out of the colon, health professionals often recommend eating foods rich in fiber to lower blood cholesterol.

Key Concepts Digestion breaks most lipids down into glycerol, free fatty acids, monoglycerides, and, in the case of phospholipids, a compound containing phosphate and nitrogen. In the small intestine, long-chain fatty acids and monoglycerides are absorbed primarily into the lymphatic system while glycerol and short- and medium-chain fatty acids are absorbed directly into the blood. Sterols are mostly unchanged by digestion, and their absorption is relatively poor.

Transportation of Lipids in the Body

🍎 **Why Is This Important?** Lipids are able to travel throughout the body despite their aversion to water (including aqueous solutions such as blood) by traveling on lipoprotein carriers. You will discover that the composition of each type of carrier affects its properties and determines its effects on overall health.

The digestive tract is not the only place where lipids need special handling to move in a water-based environment. To travel in the bloodstream, lipids must be specially packaged into lipoprotein carriers.

Lipoproteins have a lipid core of triglycerides and cholesterol esters (cholesterol linked to fatty acids) surrounded by a shell of phospholipids with embedded proteins and cholesterol. They can carry water-insoluble lipids through the watery environment of the bloodstream. Lipoproteins differ mainly by size, density, and the composition of their lipid cores. (See **FIGURE 5.22**.) In general, as the percentage of triglyceride drops, the density increases. A lipoprotein with a small core that contains few triglycerides is much denser than a lipoprotein with a large core composed mostly of triglycerides. The protein shell portion of the lipoproteins contains apolipoproteins (labeled apo A-E) that assist the lipoprotein in its function.

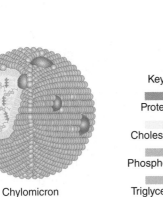

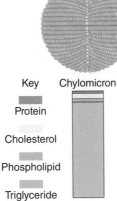

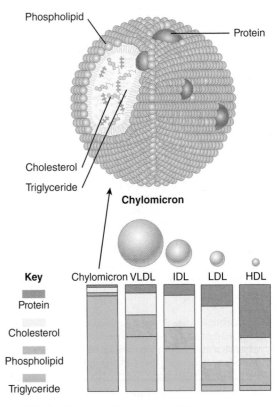

FIGURE 5.22 Lipoprotein sizes and composition. Lipoproteins become less dense as they increase in size. LDL is about double the size of HDL. VLDL is about 60 times larger than HDL. Chylomicrons range from 500 to 1,000 times larger than HDL.

Chylomicrons

Chylomicrons formed in the intestinal tract enter the lymphatic system, which empties into the bloodstream at the jugular veins of the neck. When chylomicrons enter the bloodstream, they are large, fatty lipoproteins. Chylomicrons are about 90 percent fat, but as they circulate through the capillaries, they gradually give up their triglycerides.

An enzyme located on the capillary walls, called **lipoprotein lipase**, breaks apart the chylomicrons and removes triglyceride, breaking it into free fatty acids and glycerol. These components enter adipose cells as needed, where they are reassembled into triglycerides. Alternatively, fatty acids may be taken up by muscle and oxidized for energy or may remain in circulation and return to the liver.[13] After about 10 hours, little is left of a circulating chylomicron except cholesterol-rich remnants. The liver picks up these chylomicron remnants and uses them as raw material to build very-low-density lipoproteins.

▶ **lipoprotein lipase** The major enzyme responsible for the breakdown of lipoproteins and triglycerides in the blood.

▶ **very-low-density lipoproteins (VLDLs)** The triglyceride-rich lipoproteins formed in the liver. VLDL enters the bloodstream and is gradually acted upon by lipoprotein lipase, releasing triglyceride to body cells.

▶ **intermediate-density lipoproteins (IDLs)** The lipoproteins formed when lipoprotein lipase strips some of the triglycerides from VLDL.

Very-Low-Density Lipoproteins

The liver and intestines assemble **very-low-density lipoproteins (VLDLs)** with a triglyceride-rich core. VLDL has a very low density because it is nearly two-thirds triglycerides. As with chylomicrons, lipoprotein lipase splits off and breaks down triglycerides as VLDL circulates through the bloodstream. As VLDL loses triglycerides, it becomes smaller and denser, gradually becoming an intermediate-density lipoprotein.

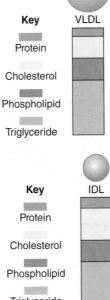

Intermediate-Density Lipoproteins

Intermediate-density lipoproteins (IDLs) are about 40 percent triglyceride. As IDL travels through the bloodstream, it acquires cholesterol from another lipoprotein (HDL; see the "High-Density Lipoproteins" section), and circulating enzymes remove some phospholipids. IDL returns to the liver, where liver cells convert it to low-density lipoprotein.

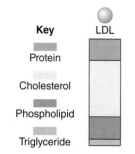

Key   LDL

Protein

Cholesterol

Phospholipid

Triglyceride

▶ **low-density lipoproteins (LDLs)** The cholesterol-rich lipoproteins that result from the breakdown and removal of triglycerides from intermediate-density lipoprotein. LDL cholesterol sometimes is called "bad cholesterol."

▶ **atherosclerosis** A type of "hardening of the arteries" in which cholesterol and other substances in the blood build up in the walls of arteries. As the process continues, the arteries to the heart may narrow, cutting down the flow of oxygen-rich blood and nutrients to the heart.

▶ **high-density lipoproteins (HDLs)** The blood lipoproteins that contain high levels of protein and low levels of triglycerides. Synthesized primarily in the liver and small intestine, HDL picks up cholesterol released from dying cells and other sources and transfers it to other lipoproteins. HDL cholesterol sometimes is called "good cholesterol."

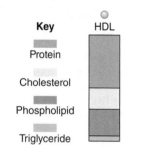

Key   HDL

Protein

Cholesterol

Phospholipid

Triglyceride

Low-Density Lipoproteins

Elevated levels of **low-density lipoproteins (LDLs)** in the blood increase the risk of artery and heart disease, earning this group of lipoprotein molecules the nickname "bad cholesterol." LDLs deliver cholesterol to body cells, which use it to synthesize membranes, hormones, and other vital compounds. LDL is more than half cholesterol and cholesterol esters; triglycerides make up only 6 percent.

Unique receptors on the cell walls bind low-density lipoproteins, which the cell engulfs and ingests. Once inside, the cell breaks down LDL, releasing LDL's load of cholesterol. When the LDL receptors on liver cells bind LDL, they help control blood cholesterol levels. About 70 percent of circulating LDL is removed by the liver; the remaining 30 percent is removed by all the other tissues combined.[14] A lack of LDL receptors reduces the uptake of cholesterol, forcing it to remain in circulation at dangerously high levels. The process by which LDL affects the blood vessels takes place over a number of years. When smoking, diabetes, high blood pressure, or infections injure blood vessel walls, the body's emergency repair team swings into action. It mobilizes white blood cells, which travel to the site of the injury, where they bury themselves in the blood vessel wall. Certain white blood cells bind and ingest LDL, especially altered (oxidized) LDL, which degrades and releases cholesterol. Over time, cholesterol accumulates as plaque thickens and narrows the artery, a condition known as **atherosclerosis**.

High-Density Lipoproteins

High-density lipoproteins (HDLs) are a group of lipoproteins that appear to protect against atherosclerosis, earning HDL cholesterol the nickname "good cholesterol." The liver and intestines make HDL, which is about 5 percent triglyceride, a fat content similar to LDL. On the other hand, HDL is only about 20 percent cholesterol, much less than LDL, which is more than 50 percent cholesterol. HDL has a higher protein content than any other lipoprotein.

In the bloodstream, HDL picks up cholesterol from arterial plaques, reducing their accumulation. HDL also picks up cholesterol released by dying cells and from cell membranes as they are renewed. HDL hands off cholesterol to other lipoproteins, especially IDL, which return cholesterol to the liver for recycling. Low HDL levels are thought to increase risk for atherosclerotic heart disease, whereas high HDL levels have a protective effect.[15]

THINK
About It

4

Key Concepts Lipoprotein carriers transport lipids in the blood. Chylomicrons, formed in the intestinal mucosal cells, transport lipids from the digestive tract into circulation. VLDL carries lipids from the liver to the other body tissues, delivering triglycerides and gradually becoming IDL. The liver takes up IDL and assembles LDL, the main carrier of cholesterol. High blood levels of LDL, the "bad cholesterol," have been shown to be a risk factor for heart disease. Circulating HDL picks up cholesterol and sends it back to the liver for recycling or excretion. A relatively high level of HDL, the "good cholesterol," reduces risk for heart disease.

Recommendations for Fat Intake

🍎 **Why Is This Important?** Knowing how fat is digested, absorbed, and transported in the body will allow you to understand how the type and amount of fat you eat can be included in a healthy eating pattern.

Now that you know something about lipids and their importance in the body, you can see that Rachel's no-fat approach to life has serious flaws. However, consumption of too much dietary fat can contribute unwanted calories and obesity. A high-fat, low-carbohydrate diet tends to contribute extra calories that lead to weight gain. When dietary patterns are high in total fat, saturated fat, and trans fat, there is a higher heart disease risk.[16] In contrast, a low-fat, high-carbohydrate diet that contains a lot of sugar and refined grains is also associated with increased heart disease risk.[17] A whole-diet approach such as balancing calories from fat and carbohydrate, rather than just targeting a reduction in fat alone, has become the focus of healthy eating and heart-protective dietary research.[18] Read on for a discussion of the recommended amounts and balance of lipids in a healthful diet.

As interest in the relationship between fat intake and health grew in the 1970s and 1980s, the American Heart Association (AHA), the National Cholesterol Education Program (NCEP) of the National Institutes of Health, and the *Dietary Guidelines for Americans* established intake guidelines for lipids. These guidelines set limits on total fat and saturated fat intake as a percentage of calories and on the total amount of cholesterol in the diet.

The AHA Diet and Lifestyle Recommendations are designed to assist individuals in reducing **cardiovascular disease (CVD)** risk.[19] (See **TABLE 5.3**.) Goals of the AHA also include improving cardiovascular health and reducing stroke risk at the community level.[20] Consuming an overall healthy diet and aiming for a healthy body weight are two of the AHA's goals.

In 2002, the National Academy of Sciences published its report on Dietary Reference Intakes (DRIs) for the macronutrients.[21] This report recommends an Acceptable Macronutrient Distribution Range (AMDR) for fat of 20 to 35 percent of calories for adults. This is balanced with 45 to 65 percent of calories from carbohydrates and 10 to 35 percent of calories from protein. Because children have higher energy needs, the AMDR for younger ages is more liberal: 30 to 40 percent of calories from fat for children ages 1 to 3 years and 25 to 35 percent of calories from fat for those ages 4 to 18 years. For infants, the Adequate Intake (AI) for fat is 31 grams per day for birth to 6 months of age and 30 grams per day for ages 7 to 12 months. AIs and Recommended Dietary Allowances (RDAs) were not set for older children and adults because there is no defined fat intake level that promotes optimal growth, maintains fat balance, or reduces chronic disease risk. In short, humans can adapt to a wide range of fat intakes. By keeping total fat intake within the AMDR and getting most of our fat from vegetable oils, fish, and nuts, we can move closer to meeting recommendations.

Many nutritionists were surprised to find that the DRI committee did not set a Tolerable Upper Intake Level (UL) for fat, trans fat, or cholesterol. Because it would be virtually impossible to completely exclude lipids from the diet, the committee recommended that saturated fat, trans fat, and cholesterol intake be minimized. Substituting monounsaturated and polyunsaturated sources improves blood lipid values, with the most favorable results produced by replacing saturated fat with monounsaturated fat.[22]

The *2015–2020 Dietary Guidelines for Americans* aligns with the recommendations from the DRI committee and with those of the

---

2015–2020 Dietary Guidelines for Americans

Limit calories from added sugars and saturated fats and reduce sodium intake. Consume an eating pattern low in added sugars, saturated fats, and sodium. Cut back on foods and beverages higher in these components to amounts that fit within healthy eating patterns.

Key Recommendations

A healthy eating pattern includes:

- Fat-free or low-fat dairy, including milk, yogurt, cheese, and/or fortified soy beverages
- A variety of protein foods, including seafood, lean meats and poultry, eggs, legumes (beans and peas), nuts, seeds, and soy products
- Oils

A healthy eating pattern limits:

- Saturated fats and trans fats, added sugars, and sodium

Key recommendations that are quantitative are provided for several components of the diet that should be limited. These components are of particular public health concern in the United States, and the specified limits can help individuals achieve healthy eating patterns within calorie limits:

- Consume less than 10 percent of calories per day from saturated fats

U.S. Department of Health and Human Services and U.S. Department of Agriculture. *2015–2020 Dietary Guidelines for Americans.* 8th Edition. December 2015. Available at http://health.gov/dietaryguidelines/2015/guidelines/.

▶ **cardiovascular disease (CVD)** Any abnormal condition characterized by dysfunction of the heart and blood vessels. CVD includes atherosclerosis (especially coronary heart disease, which can lead to heart attacks), cerebrovascular disease (e.g., stroke), and hypertension (high blood pressure).

TABLE 5.3

AHA Dietary Guidelines

The 2017 American Heart Association Diet and Lifestyle Recommendations are designed to assist individuals in reducing cardiovascular disease risk.

Use up at least as many calories as you take in.

- Start by knowing how many calories you should be eating and drinking to maintain your weight. Nutrition and calorie information on food labels is typically based on a 2,000 calorie diet. You may need fewer or more calories depending on several factors including age, gender, and level of physical activity.
- If you are trying not to gain weight, don't eat more calories than you know you can burn up every day.
- Increase the amount and intensity of your physical activity to match the number of calories you take in.
- Aim for at least 150 minutes of moderate physical activity or 75 minutes of vigorous physical activity—or an equal combination of both—each week.

Regular physical activity can help you maintain your weight, keep off weight that you lose and help you reach physical and cardiovascular fitness. If it's hard to schedule regular exercise sessions, try aiming for sessions of at last 10 minutes spread throughout the week.

If you would benefit from lowering your blood pressure or cholesterol, the American Heart Association recommends 40 minutes of aerobic exercise of moderate to vigorous intensity three to four times a week.

Eat a variety of nutritious foods from all the food groups.

You may be eating plenty of food, but your body may not be getting the nutrients it needs to be healthy. Nutrient-rich foods have minerals, protein, whole grains and other nutrients but are lower in calories. They may help you control your weight, cholesterol and blood pressure.

Eat an overall healthy dietary pattern that emphasizes:

- a variety of fruits and vegetables,
- whole grains,
- low-fat dairy products,
- skinless poultry and fish
- nuts and legumes
- non-tropical vegetable oils

Limit saturated fat, *trans* fat, sodium, red meat, sweets and sugar-sweetened beverages. If you choose to eat red meat, compare labels and select the leanest cuts available.

One of the diets that fits this pattern is the Dietary Approaches to Stop Hypertension (DASH) eating plan. Most healthy eating patterns can be adapted based on calorie requirements and personal and cultural food preferences.

Eat less of the nutrient-poor foods.

The right number of calories to eat each day is based on your age and physical activity level and whether you're trying to gain, lose or maintain your weight. You could use your daily allotment of calories on a few high-calorie foods and beverages, but you probably wouldn't get the nutrients your body needs to be healthy. Limit foods and beverages high in calories but low in nutrients. Also limit the amount of saturated fat, *trans* fat and sodium you eat. Read Nutrition Facts labels carefully — the Nutrition Facts panel tells you the amount of healthy and unhealthy nutrients in a food or beverage.

As you make daily food choices, base your eating pattern on these recommendations:

- Eat a variety of fresh, frozen and canned vegetables and fruits without high-calorie sauces or added salt and sugars. Replace high-calorie foods with fruits and vegetables.
- Choose fiber-rich whole grains for most grain servings.
- Choose poultry and fish without skin and prepare them in healthy ways without added saturated and *trans* fat. If you choose to eat meat, look for the leanest cuts available and prepare them in healthy and delicious ways.
- Eat a variety of fish at least twice a week, especially fish containing omega-3 fatty acids (for example, salmon, trout and herring).
- Select fat-free (skim) and low-fat (1%) dairy products.
- Avoid foods containing partially hydrogenated vegetable oils to reduce *trans* fat in your diet.
- Limit saturated fat and trans fat and replace them with the better fats, monounsaturated and polyunsaturated. If you need to lower your blood cholesterol, reduce saturated fat to no more than 5 to 6 percent of total calories. For someone eating 2,000 calories a day, that's about 13 grams of saturated fat.
- Cut back on beverages and foods with added sugars.
- Choose foods with less sodium and prepare foods with little or no salt. To lower blood pressure, aim to eat no more than 2,400 milligrams of sodium per day. Reducing daily intake to 1,500 mg is desirable because it can lower blood pressure even further. If you can't meet these goals right now, even reducing sodium intake by 1,000 mg per day can benefit blood pressure.
- If you drink alcohol, drink in moderation. That means no more than one drink per day if you're a woman and no more than two drinks per day if you're a man.
- Follow the American Heart Association recommendations when you eat out, and keep an eye on your portion sizes.

Also, don't smoke tobacco—and avoid secondhand smoke.

American Heart Association. (See **FIGURE 5.23**.) Saturated fat and trans fat should be limited and replaced with healthier fats, such as monounsaturated and polyunsaturated fats. For those who need to lower their blood cholesterol, saturated fat should be reduced to no more than 5 or 6 percent of total calories.[23] The *Dietary Guidelines* and American Heart Association recommendations also suggest that trans fat intake be kept as low as possible. The Daily Values on food labels are 65 grams of total fat (29 percent of the calories in a 2,000-kilocalorie diet), 20 grams of saturated fat (9 percent of calories), and 300 milligrams of cholesterol. Since 2006, food manufacturers have been required by the FDA to list trans fats on the Nutrition Facts panel.[24] Additionally, partially hydrogenated oils, the major source of dietary trans fat in processed foods, are no longer Generally Recognized as Safe (GRAS). Although no Daily Value has been set, consumers can use this information to choose foods to minimize trans fat intake. In 2015, the FDA began taking steps to remove artificial trans fat from the food supply in an effort to reduce coronary heart disease.[25]

Recommendations for Omega Fatty Acid Intake

Fat is a critical nutrient, and although too much fat in the diet is not healthful, certain types of fat, such as omega-3s and omega-6s, are essential for good health.[26] On average, Americans consume approximately 1.6 grams of omega-3 fatty acids and almost 10 times more omega-6 fatty acids on a daily basis.[27] The omega-3 and omega-6 fatty acids work together to promote health. Omega-6 fatty acid intake is often adequate when eating a typical American diet; however, recommendations for omega-3 fatty acids are not as easy to meet. Omega-3 fatty acids help reduce inflammation, whereas omega-6 fatty acids tend to promote inflammation. A favorable balance between these two essential fatty acids helps to maintain, and even improve, health; insufficient omega-3 fatty acids may contribute to the development of disease.

Because essential fatty acid deficiency is virtually nonexistent in the United States and Canada, the DRI committee relied on median intake levels of essential fatty acids to set AI levels. For adults ages 19 to 50, the AI for linoleic acid is 17 grams per day for men and 12 grams per day for women. The AI for alpha-linolenic acid is 1.6 grams per day for men and 1.1 grams per day for women. To fulfill our need for omega-6 fatty acids, linoleic acid should provide about 2 percent of our calories. Average U.S. consumption is much more than that. Two teaspoons of corn oil, which is a little more than half linoleic acid, would supply more than 2 percent of the calories in a 2,000-kilocalorie diet.

To meet these recommendations, most people need to eat more fish in place of some poultry and meat.[28] The *2015–2020 Dietary Guidelines for Americans* encourages a diet rich in omega-3 fatty acids as provided by seafood, which is a good source of polyunsaturated omega-3 fatty acids, eicosapentaenoic acid (EPA), and docosahexaenoic acid (DHA). A specific recommendation to consume 8 or more ounces of seafood per week is included to supply dietary EPA and DHA at levels associated with reduced cardiac deaths among individuals with and without pre-existing cardiovascular disease.[29] Because shark, swordfish, king mackerel, and tilefish contain high levels of mercury, in the past the FDA and EPA recommended that women who may become pregnant, pregnant women, nursing mothers, and young children avoid eating these fish.[30] Then, in 2017, in agreement with the *Dietary Guidelines*, the two agencies issued final recommendations,[31] advising that these populations eat types of

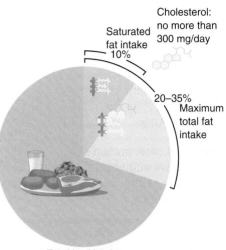

FIGURE 5.23 Recommended fat intake. The *Dietary Guidelines for Americans* recommends a maximum fat intake of 20 to 35 percent of total calories. Saturated fat should supply no more than 10 percent of our total calories, or about one-third of our fat calories. Dietary trans fatty acids should be limited as much as possible.

U.S. Department of Agriculture, Agricultural Research Service. USDA National Nutrient Database for Standard Reference, Release 26. http://www.ars.usda.gov/ba/bhnrc/ndl. Accessed September 5, 2017.

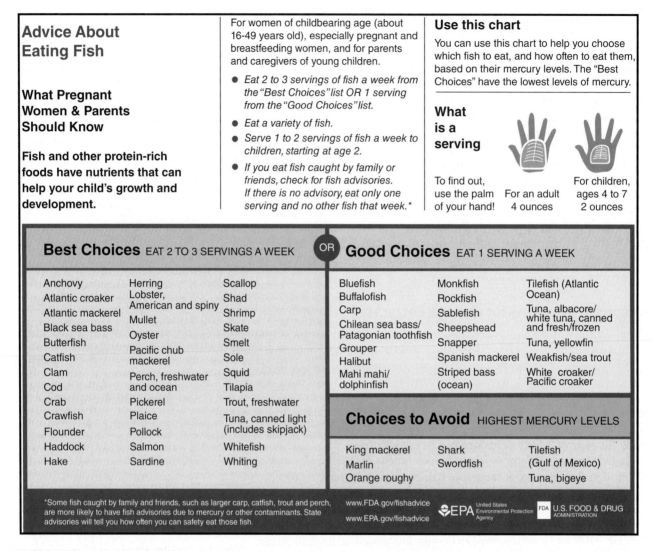

FIGURE 5.24 Choose healthy and safe fish options. Women who are pregnant or may become pregnant, breastfeeding mothers, and parents of young children should make informed choices and select fish that is healthy and safe to eat.

U.S. Department of Health and Human Services, U.S. Food and Drug Administration. Eating Fish: What Pregnant Women and Parents Should Know. http://www.fda.gov/Food/FoodborneIllnessContaminants/Metals/ucm393070.htm. Page updated 1/18/17. Accessed 1/24/17.

Quick Bite

Just the Flax

Flax is nature's richest plant source of omega-3 fatty acids. Ounce for ounce, flaxseed oil has more alpha-linolenic acid than any other food. The oils in flaxseed are more than 50 percent alpha-linolenic acid (ALA). Two tablespoons of ground flax has 2,800 milligrams of ALA omega-3, 850 milligrams of linoleic acid (omega-6), 120 milligrams of lignans (phytoestrogens), and 4 grams of dietary fiber.

fish that have the lowest mercury levels, called "Best Choices," in order to gain desirable developmental and health benefits. (See **FIGURE 5.24**.) The recommendations caution against eating types of fish that typically have high mercury levels, labeling them "Choices to Avoid."[32]

It's important to try to get both enough and the right balance of essential fatty acids in our diets. Remember that consuming too much of the omega-3 fatty acids can have undesirable effects such as suppressing immune function and prolonging bleeding time, so we should be cautious about the high levels of these fatty acids found in some supplements. The DRI committee set an AMDR for omega-6 fatty acids of 5 to 10 percent of energy, and an AMDR for alpha-linolenic acid of 0.6 to 1.2 percent of energy.

Current Dietary Intakes

Fat intake as a percentage of calories is down from 36 percent in the early 1970s, and down markedly from 45 percent in 1965. Currently,

Americans are eating about 34 percent of their total calories each day from fat.[33] Although this value is within the recommended AMDR of 20–35 percent of total calories, about a quarter of the population has a fat intake greater than 35 percent of calories.

Although the percentage of calories from fat dropped, average calorie intake increased, which means Americans are actually consuming more total grams of fat, largely due to snacking on food mixtures (e.g., prepared and convenience foods), processed grain snacks, and pastries.[34] Although intake of whole milk and fats and oils has declined in recent decades, intake of fat from food mixtures is higher.[35] Food mixtures and snacks contribute a significant percentage of daily calories. Frequently consumed snacks include cookies, candies, crackers, popcorn, and potato chips, all generally high in fat.

Current intake of saturated fat is about 11 percent of calories, a little higher than recommended.[36] Major sources of saturated fatty acids in the U.S. diet include regular cheese; pizza; grain-based desserts; chicken and chicken mixed dishes; and sausage, hot dogs, bacon, and ribs. The typical American diet contains 14 to 25 times more omega-6 fatty acids than omega-3 fatty acids.[37] Intake of linoleic acid is estimated to be 6 percent of calories, with alpha-linolenic acid providing 0.75 percent of calories and EPA plus DHA another 0.1 percent of calories. The amount of trans fat in the U.S. diet has been declining over the past decades; however, it still appears to be in the range of 0.6 to 2.9 percent of total energy intake, which for some people is still higher than the AHA recommendations to limit trans fat to less than 1 percent of energy.[38,39] **FIGURE 5.25** provides an overview of the dietary sources of fatty acids. By keeping total fat intake within the AMDR and getting most of our fat from vegetable oils, fish, and nuts, we can move closer to meeting recommendations.

Fat Replacers: What Are They? Are They Safe? Do They Save Calories?

The food industry responded to the public health challenge of the 1990s to lower fat intake by making low-fat, low-calorie goodies that still taste good. Many different types of **fat replacers** have been developed, and over the years thousands of fat-free, low-fat, and reduced-fat foods have hit grocery shelves.

Some fat replacers are carbohydrates: generally starches and fibers such as vegetable gums, cellulose, maltodextrins, and Oatrim (a fat replacer made from oats). Some are more digestible than others, but all provide far fewer than 9 kilocalories per gram. With their moist, thick textures, they mimic fat's richness and smooth "mouth feel."

Proteins provide the raw ingredients of other fat replacers. Food manufacturers can modify egg whites and whey from milk so they become thick and smooth and hold water. Because this protein and water combination has fewer calories per gram than fat, it cuts calories.

The most high-tech fat replacers—and the most controversial—are the "fat-based" replacers also called artificial fats. Digestive enzymes do not recognize the fatty acid arrangement so the fat replacement is not broken down and absorbed; therefore, fat-based fat replacers provide about half the calories of fat. (See **FIGURE 5.26**.) One advantage of fat-based fat replacers is their ability to withstand the heat applied during baking, frying, or other manufacturing processes. However, a disadvantage is that the GI tract does not absorb fat-based fat replacers, leading to fat malabsorption symptoms in some people—diarrhea, gas, and cramps.

BASIC FATTY ACIDS

Saturated
Animal products (including dairy products), palm and coconut oils, and cocoa butter.

Polyunsaturated
Sunflower, corn, soybean, and cottonseed oils.

Monounsaturated
Most nuts and olive, canola, peanut, and safflower oils.

TRANS FATTY ACIDS
Stick margarine (not soft or liquid margarine) and many fast foods and baked goods.

ESSENTIAL FATTY ACIDS

Omega-3 fatty acids
Alpha-linolenic acid
Canola oil, soybeans, olive oil, many nuts (e.g., walnuts, peanuts, filberts, pistachios, pecans, almonds), seeds, and purslane (a green, leafy vegetable).

DHA and EPA
Fish such as mackerel, tuna, salmon, herring, trout, and cod liver oil. The fish with the lowest amount of total fat include Atlantic cod, haddock, and pink salmon. Other fish high in omega-3 but also high in total fat are sardines and bluefish. Human milk.

Omega-6 fatty acids
Linoleic acid
Plants (flax) and some vegetable oils (soybean and canola oil).

FIGURE 5.25   Overview of dietary sources of fatty acids.
Modified from Cancer smart. *Scientific American.* 1998;4(3):9.
© Photodisc; © Photodisc; © Kirsta Mackey/Shutterstock, Inc.; © Photodisc; © John A. Rizzo/Photodisc/Getty Images.

▶ **fat replacers** Compounds that imitate the functional and sensory properties of fats but contain less available energy than fats.

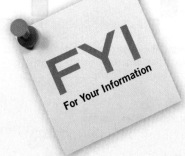

Does Reduced Fat Reduce Calories? Don't Count on It!

Experts often tell us to reduce fat in our diets to help reduce risk for heart disease, cancer, and obesity. Given that fat is our most concentrated source of calories, we would expect a reduced-fat or low-fat food to have fewer calories than its unmodified counterpart. But is this always true?

Many reduced-fat products contain added sugar. Although sugar has fewer calories per gram than fat, the amount added can negate any difference in calories. If fat is your concern, low-fat or fat-free makes sense. But if you're trying to reduce fat and calories, modified products might not be a big help. So, be a smart shopper—check the label before you check out with a cartload of reduced-fat foods.

Sometimes low-fat and fat-free foods make a big difference in calories.

Food	Calories
1 slice American cheese	50
1 slice nonfat American cheese	24
1 slice bologna	90
1 slice fat-free bologna	22
1 tablespoon mayonnaise	103
1 tablespoon fat-free mayonnaise/dressing	11

But sometimes they make almost no difference at all.

Food	Calories
1 cup canned chicken vegetable soup	84
1 cup reduced-fat chicken vegetable soup	96
3 chocolate chip cookies (30 g)	144
3 reduced-fat chocolate chip cookies (30 g)	153
2 tablespoons peanut butter	188
2 tablespoons reduced-fat peanut butter	187
1 oz potato chips	154
1 oz reduced-fat potato chips	134

And don't forget to check the labels and ingredient list for added sugars. Many nutrition experts now believe that the highly refined carbohydrate and sugary foods in our diet are the primary culprits for increasing our risk of chronic conditions such as heart disease, obesity, type 2 diabetes, and cancer. Processed foods such as baked goods, sugar-sweetened beverages, and savory snacks should be the focus of dietary reform. You can improve your diet by eating these foods less often and instead choose wholesome, minimally processed foods as part of a healthy eating pattern.

U.S. Department of Agriculture, Agricultural Research Service, Nutrient Data Laboratory. USDA National Nutrient Database for Standard Reference, Release 28. Version Current: September 2015. Internet: http://www.ars.usda.gov/nea /bhnrc/ndl. Accessed February 4, 2016.

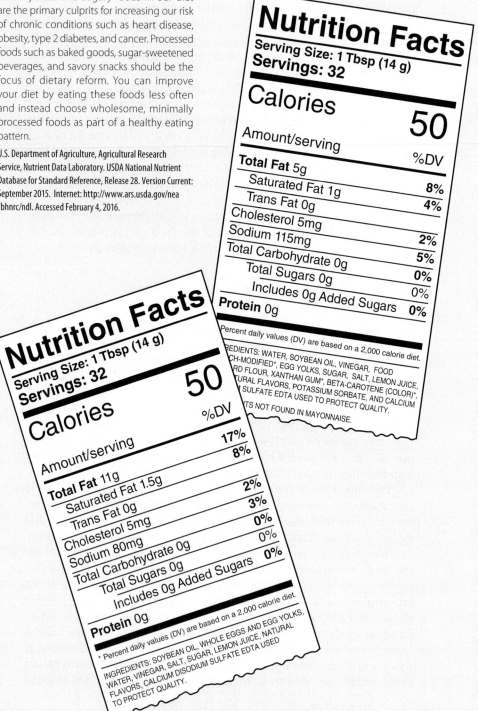

Nutrition Facts
Serving Size: 1 Tbsp (14 g)
Servings: 32

Calories   50

Amount/serving	%DV
Total Fat 5g	
Saturated Fat 1g	8%
Trans Fat 0g	4%
Cholesterol 5mg	
Sodium 115mg	2%
Total Carbohydrate 0g	5%
Total Sugars 0g	0%
Includes 0g Added Sugars	0%
Protein 0g	0%

Percent daily values (DV) are based on a 2,000 calorie diet.

REDIENTS: WATER, SOYBEAN OIL, VINEGAR, FOOD CH-MODIFIED*, EGG YOLKS, SUGAR, SALT, LEMON JUICE, RD FLOUR, XANTHAN GUM*, BETA-CAROTENE (COLOR)*, TURAL FLAVORS, POTASSIUM SORBATE, AND CALCIUM SULFATE EDTA USED TO PROTECT QUALITY.
TS NOT FOUND IN MAYONNAISE.

Nutrition Facts
Serving Size: 1 Tbsp (14 g)
Servings: 32

Calories   50

Amount/serving	%DV
	17%
	8%
Total Fat 11g	
Saturated Fat 1.5g	2%
Trans Fat 0g	3%
Cholesterol 5mg	0%
Sodium 80mg	0%
Total Carbohydrate 0g	0%
Total Sugars 0g	
Includes 0g Added Sugars	
Protein 0g	

* Percent daily values (DV) are based on a 2,000 calorie diet.

INGREDIENTS: SOYBEAN OIL, WHOLE EGGS AND EGG YOLKS, WATER, VINEGAR, SALT, SUGAR, LEMON JUICE, NATURAL FLAVORS, CALCIUM DISODIUM SULFATE EDTA USED TO PROTECT QUALITY.

Americans' fat and calorie intakes have not declined with the growth in the fat-replacer market. It is clear that fat replacers won't help if people treat them simply as an excuse to eat more. Nor should "low-fat foods," which can have added sugar, be confused with "low-calorie foods." In general, eating less "fake" processed foods and instead eating more "real" foods—ones that have stood the test of time, those that are farmed or grown and harvested, not made in a factory—is good practice.

Lipids and Health

🍎 **Why Is This Important?** Lipids can have dramatic effects on health, both positive and negative. Understanding which kinds of dietary fats improve well-being or contribute to chronic, degenerative conditions is key to making food choices that are part of a healthy eating pattern.

If your diet is consistently high in fat, you may be putting yourself at risk for numerous health problems. High-fat diets are typically high in calories and contribute to weight gain and obesity. For decades, health officials have warned that high intakes of saturated fat and trans fat increase the risk for heart disease, and high-fat diets have been linked to several types of cancer. Results from a large study, however, did not find evidence that people who ate higher levels of saturated fat had more heart disease than those who ate less saturated fat, nor did it find that those who ate relatively higher amounts of unsaturated fat or polyunsaturated fats benefitted.[40] That said, it is important to caution that looking at individual nutrient groups such as dietary fats in isolation could be misleading. For example, people who change their diet to eat less saturated fat may replace it with other foods, such as refined carbohydrates, that are detrimental to cardiovascular health.

In addition, poly- and monounsaturated fatty acids in appropriate proportions, soluble fiber (oats and psyllium, in particular), phytosterols, soy protein, oilseeds, and nuts have in general been found to exert a positive impact on human health.[41] A diet should contain plenty of fruits, vegetables, and other antioxidant sources because they play a role in protection against LDL cholesterol oxidation. So, where does that leave you? Rather than embracing strategies that emphasize exclusively one nutrient, such as dietary fat to reduce cardiovascular risk, focus instead on a "whole diet approach" with increasing intake of fruits, vegetables, nuts, and fish.[42,43] It is the combined effect of certain nutrients and food components *and* their cumulative effect on your lipid profile that provides the basis for healthy eating pattern recommendations.[44] There is evidence that this approach reduces cardiovascular risk as well as other degenerative conditions.

Health Effects of Omega Fatty Acids

Omega-3 fatty acids have attracted interest as potential factors in reducing risk for vascular disease. Additional health benefits that have been associated with omega-3 fatty acids include the secondary prevention of chronic diseases such as inflammatory conditions, GI disorders,

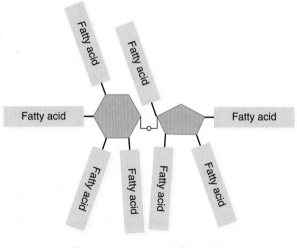

A triglyceride has three fatty acids attached to a glycerol backbone.

Olestra has six to eight fatty acids attached to a sucrose backbone.

FIGURE 5.26 Fat-based fat replacer's structure. The structure of fat-based fat replacers are unlike the structure of a triglyceride. Although fat-based fat replacers impart triglyceride-like qualities to food, your digestive enzymes cannot break them down.

Position Statement: Academy of Nutrition and Dietetics

Dietary Fatty Acids for Healthy Adults
It is the position of the Academy of Nutrition and Dietetics (the Academy) that dietary fat for the healthy adult population should provide 20 to 35 percent of energy, with an increased consumption of omega-3 polyunsaturated fatty acids and limited intake of saturated and trans fats. The Academy recommends a food-based approach through a diet that includes regular consumption of fatty fish, nuts and seeds, lean meats and poultry, low-fat dairy products, vegetables, fruits, whole grains, and legumes.

Reprinted from *Journal of the Academy of Nutrition and Dietetics*,114(1), Gretchen Vannice,Heather Rasmussen, Position of the Academy of Nutrition and Dietetics: Dietary Fatty Acids for Healthy Adults, Page no. 136-153, 2014, with permission from Elsevier.

TABLE 5.4
Health Effects of Omega-3 Fatty Acids

Condition	Health Benefit
Inflammatory conditions	Improves rheumatoid arthritis, psoriasis, asthma, and some skin conditions.
Ulcerative colitis and Crohn's disease	Reduces the severity of symptoms.
Cardiovascular disease	Lowers triglycerides and raises HDL cholesterol levels, improves blood circulation, reduces clotting, improves vascular function, and lowers blood pressure.
Type 2 diabetes mellitus	Reduces high insulin levels and insulin resistance.
Renal (kidney) disease	Maintains kidney function, helps maintain a healthy vein access in dialysis patients, and is cardioprotective.
Mental function	Reduces severity of several mental conditions such as Alzheimer's disease, depression, and bipolar disorder; improvement in children with attention deficit hyperactivity disorder and dyslexia has also been noted.
Growth and development	Neurodevelopment and function of the brain and also the retina of the eye where visual function is affected.

Rigby A. Omega-3 choices: fish or flax? *Today's Dietitian.* 2004;6(1):37; Deckelbaum RJ, Torrejon C. The omega-3 fatty acid nutritional landscape: health benefits and sources. *J Nutr.* 2012;142(3):587S-591S; Position of the Academy of Nutrition and Dietetics: dietary fatty acids for healthy adults. *J Acad Nutr Diet.* 2014;114:136-153.

and type 2 diabetes, as discussed in **TABLE 5.4**. As a result of findings on infant growth and development, DHA (along with omega-6 arachidonic acid) is now being added to some infant formulas. The major advances in understanding the mechanisms of action of dietary fatty acids on lipoprotein metabolism have focused on omega-3 fatty acids; more research is needed to better understand the cardioprotective effects of other dietary fatty acids.[45]

The American Heart Association recommends eating fish (particularly fatty fish) at least two times a week to reduce the risk of cardiovascular disease.[46] Fish is a good source of protein and isn't high in saturated fat, in contrast to fatty meats. Fatty fish such as mackerel, lake trout, herring, sardines, albacore tuna, and salmon are high in two kinds of omega-3 fatty acids: EPA and DHA. Some people with high triglycerides and patients with cardiovascular disease may benefit from more omega-3 fatty acids than they can easily get from diet alone. These people should talk to their doctor about taking supplements to reduce heart disease risk. EPA and DHA in fish oil capsules are thought to help lower blood pressure, reduce inflammation, reduce blood clotting, and lower high serum triglyceride levels.[47] In high doses, fish oil supplements may have harmful effects, such as increased bleeding risk, higher levels of LDL cholesterol, and blood sugar control problems. A "fishy" odor is also a common side effect that deters people from continued use of the supplements.[48] Because fish oil supplements can have potent effects, children, pregnant women, and nursing mothers should not take them without medical supervision.[49]

Heart Disease

Heart disease and stroke are the principal types of cardiovascular disease (CVD), which is the leading cause of death in the United States and Canada. Heart disease claims one life every 40 seconds, accounting for 1 out of every 3 deaths in the United States alone.[50] In the past 50 years, however, lifestyle changes and medical advances have led to significant progress in the fight against CVD.

Elevated triglyceride levels are associated with cardiovascular disease. During 2009–2012, about one-quarter of the American adult population age 20 and older had elevated triglyceride levels. Factors that increase triglyceride levels include sedentary lifestyle, overweight and obesity, cigarette smoking, dietary simple sugars, trans fatty acids, and alcohol.[51] Eating more wholesome foods such as antioxidant-rich fresh fruits, vegetables, and whole grains; consuming smaller amounts of meat and poultry; and replacing trans and saturated fats with monounsaturated or omega-3 polyunsaturated fatty acids are widely accepted as important dietary patterns for heart protection. Because of the complexity of diet and nutrient interactions, more research is needed to better understand the heart-protective effects of dietary fatty acids, including the effects of diets such as the Mediterranean eating pattern recommended by the *Dietary Guidelines for Americans*.[52]

Obesity

Obesity is defined as the excessive accumulation of body fat leading to a body weight in relation to height that is substantially greater than the accepted standard. More than one-third of U.S. adults are obese.[53] Seventeen percent of U.S. children and adolescents ages 2–19 years are obese.[54] The increased prevalence of obesity is a concern for children and adolescents. The prevalence of obesity has significantly increased over the past 30 years, and eating large amounts of dietary fat and added sugars contributes to this obesity epidemic.

Fat is a dense source of calories, it makes food taste good, and it's often unnoticed or "hidden" in restaurant and convenience foods. **TABLE 5.5** shows how fat increases the calorie content of foods. Standard advice to Americans trying to attain or maintain normal weight usually includes cutting back on fats and fatty foods, along with increasing physical activity and eating fewer calories.

Quick **Bite**

NCEP Tips for Healthful Eating Out

- Choose restaurants that have low-fat, low-cholesterol menu items.
- Don't be afraid to ask for foods that follow your eating pattern.
- Select poultry, fish, or meat that is broiled, grilled, baked, steamed, or poached rather than fried.
- Choose lean deli meats like fresh turkey or lean roast beef instead of higher-fat cuts like salami or bologna.
- Look for vegetables seasoned with herbs or spices rather than butter, sour cream, or cheese. Ask for sauces on the side.
- Order a low-fat dessert like sherbet, fruit ice, sorbet, or low-fat frozen yogurt.
- Control serving sizes by asking for a small serving, sharing a dish, or taking some home.
- At fast-food restaurants, go for grilled chicken and lean roast beef sandwiches or lean plain hamburgers (but remember to hold the fatty sauces), salads with low-fat salad dressing, low-fat milk, and low-fat frozen yogurt. Pizza topped with vegetables and minimal cheese is another good choice.

▶ **obesity** Excessive accumulation of body fat leading to a body weight in relation to height that is substantially greater than some accepted standard. A BMI at or above 30 kg/m².

TABLE 5.5
Fat Can Markedly Increase Calories in Food

	Approximate Calories	Approximate Fat (g)
1 small/medium serving (100 g) french-fried potatoes	312	15
100 g boiled potatoes	98	0.1
½ cup creamed cottage cheese	103	4.5
½ cup 1 percent low-fat cottage cheese	82	1.2
½ cup green beans with 1 teaspoon butter	56	4.0
½ cup green beans without butter	22	0.2
3 oz T-bone steak, untrimmed	225	14.9
3 oz T-bone steak, trimmed	161	7.4
½ cup vanilla ice cream	137	7.23
½ cup fat-free vanilla ice cream	92	0

Based on data from U.S. Department of Agriculture, Agricultural Research Service, Nutrient Data Laboratory. USDA National Nutrient Database for Standard Reference, Release 28. Version Current: September 2015. https://ndb.nal.usda.gov/ndb/search/list.

▶ **metabolic syndrome** A cluster of at least three of the following risk factors for heart disease: hypertriglyceridemia (high blood triglycerides), low HDL cholesterol, hyperglycemia (high blood glucose), hypertension (high blood pressure), and excess abdominal fat.

▶ **cancer** A term for diseases in which abnormal cells divide without control. Cancer cells can invade nearby tissues and can spread through the bloodstream and lymphatic system to other parts of the body.

Quick Bite

What Does the Color of Beef Fat Reveal?
Yellow-tinged fat indicates that a steer was fed grass. White fat suggests that the animal was fed corn or cereal grain, at least during its final months.

Metabolic Syndrome

The prevalence of **metabolic syndrome** has increased in the United States from 32.9 in 2002–2004 to 34.7 percent in 2011–2012.[55] Metabolic syndrome is a cluster of at least three of the following[56,57]:

- *Excess abdominal fat:* For most men, a 40-inch waist or greater; for women, a waist of 35 inches or greater
- *High blood glucose:* At least 100 mg/dL after fasting
- *High serum triglycerides:* At least 150 mg/dL
- *Low HDL cholesterol:* Less than 40 mg/dL for men; less than 50 mg/dL for women
- *High blood pressure:* 130/85 mm Hg or higher

Taken individually, each risk factor may not look particularly serious. When you put them together, however, health risks rise dramatically—people with metabolic syndrome have the greatest risk of death from heart attack.

Cancer

Cancer usually develops over time. It results from a complex mix of factors related to lifestyle, heredity, and environment. Researchers have identified a number of factors that increase a person's chance of developing cancer. Although evidence suggests that between 30 and 40 percent of cancers are due to poor food choices and physical inactivity, the role of nutrition and diet in cancer development is complex. Some dietary factors may act as promoters; many others may have protective roles, blocking the cellular changes in one of the developmental stages. The evidence linking dietary fat to cancer is inconclusive.

Putting It All Together

Healthy People 2020 objectives target reducing deaths from heart disease, stroke, cancer, and obesity-related comorbidities.[58] To accomplish these goals, dietitians and health professionals recommend lowering total fat intake, lowering saturated and trans fat intake, maintaining a healthy body weight, and exercising on a regular basis. Eating fruits, vegetables, legumes, and grains that contain fiber helps lower cholesterol levels, too. These foods contain antioxidants and B vitamins, such as B_6 and folate, that may also reduce the risk of heart disease. Substituting fish or soy foods for high-fat meats and cheeses can be beneficial as well.

Key Concepts To reduce your risk of heart disease, don't smoke, get regular exercise, and control your weight. Dietary changes you can make to reduce your heart disease risk include eating less fat, saturated and trans fat, and cholesterol while increasing intake of fruits, vegetables, and whole grains. Look for sources of omega-3 fatty acids and fiber in your food choices. Metabolic syndrome is a cluster of risk factors that dramatically elevates heart disease risk. Although the evidence linking dietary fats with cancer is contradictory, many other dietary factors play key roles in reducing risk. Strategies for reducing cancer risk include eating more fruits, vegetables, and whole grains; increasing physical activity; maintaining a healthy weight; and limiting alcohol consumption.

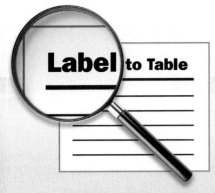

Label to Table

The Nutrition Facts panel shown here highlights all of the lipid-related information you can find on a food label. Look at the label, where it states that this product contains 4 grams of total fat. Do you know how you can estimate the number of calories from fat using information from another part of the label? Recall (or look at the bottom of the label) that each gram of fat contains 9 kilocalories. If this food item has 4 grams of fat, then it should make sense that there are approximately 36 kilocalories provided by fat. "Calories from Fat" will no longer appear on the new Nutrition Facts label because research shows that the type of fat is more important than the amount.

Total fat is the second thing you'll see, along with saturated and trans fat. Manufacturers are required to list only saturated and trans fat content on the label, but they can voluntarily list monounsaturated and polyunsaturated fat. Using this food label, you can estimate the amount of unsaturated fat by simply looking at the highlighted sections. There are 4 total grams of fat: 2.5 of them are saturated and 0.5 are trans. That means the remaining 1.0 gram is either polyunsaturated, monounsaturated, or a mix of both. Without even knowing what food item this label represents, you can see that it contains more saturated and trans fat than unsaturated fat (3.0 grams versus 1.0 gram).

Do you see the "6%" to the right of "Total Fat"? It does not mean that the food item contains 6 percent of its calories from fat. In fact, this food item contains 23 percent of its calories from fat (35 fat kilocalories ÷ 154 total kilocalories = 0.23, or 23% fat kilocalories). The 6% refers to the Daily Values, found below. You can see that a person who consumes 2,000 kilocalories per day could consume up to 65 grams of fat per day. This product contributes just 4 grams per serving, which is 6 percent of that amount (4 ÷ 65 = 0.06, or 6%). Note that the % Daily Value for saturated fat is 12 percent, which means that just a few servings of this food can contribute quite a bit of saturated fat to your diet. There is no DV for trans fat, but intake should be kept as low as possible. Cholesterol also is highlighted on this label (20 mg), along with its Daily Value contribution (7%).

Nutrition Facts

4 servings per container

Serving size — 1 cup (248 g)

Amount per serving

Calories — 150

	% Daily Value*
Total Fat 4g	6%
Saturated Fat 2.5g	12%
Trans Fat 0.5g	
Cholesterol 20mg	7%
Sodium 170mg	7%
Total Carbohydrate 19g	6%
Dietary Fiber 0g	0%
Total Sugars 14g	
Includes 5g Added Sugars	10%
Protein 11g	
Vitamin D 0mcg	0%
Calcium 400mg	40%
Iron 0mg	0%
Potassium 265mg	8%

*The % Daily Value (DV) tells you how much a nutrient in a serving of food contributes to a daily diet. 2,000 calories a day is used for general nutrition advice.

Learning Portfolio

Key Terms

Study Points

- There are three main classes of lipids: triglycerides, phospholipids, and sterols.
- Fatty acids are components of both triglycerides and phospholipids.
- Saturated fatty acids have no double bonds between carbon atoms in their carbon chains, monounsaturated fatty acids have one double bond, and polyunsaturated fatty acids have more than one double bond in their carbon chains.
- Two polyunsaturated fatty acids, linoleic acid and alpha-linolenic acid, are essential and must be supplied in the diet. Phospholipids and sterols are made in the body and do not have to be supplied in the diet.
- Essential fatty acids are precursors of hormone-like compounds called eicosanoids. These compounds regulate many body functions, including blood pressure, heart rate, inflammation, and immune response.
- Triglycerides are food fats and storage fats. They are composed of glycerol and three fatty acids.
- In the body, triglycerides are an important source of energy. Stored fat provides an energy reserve.
- Phospholipids are made of glycerol, two fatty acids, and a compound containing phosphate and nitrogen.
- Phospholipids are components of cell membranes and lipoproteins. Having both fat- and water-soluble components allows them to be effective emulsifiers in foods and in the body.
- Cholesterol is found in cell membranes and is used to synthesize vitamin D, bile salts, and steroid hormones. High levels of blood cholesterol are associated with increased heart disease risk.
- For adults, the Acceptable Macronutrient Distribution Range (AMDR) for fat is 20 to 35 percent of calories.
- Diets high in fat and saturated fat tend to increase blood levels of LDL cholesterol and increase risk for heart disease.
- Excess fat in the diet is linked to obesity, heart disease, and possibly some types of cancer.

Study Questions

1. What do the terms *saturated, monounsaturated,* and *polyunsaturated* mean with regard to fatty acids?
2. What does the hardness or softness of a fat typically signify?
3. Name the two essential fatty acids.
4. What is the most common form of lipid found in food?
5. List the many functions of triglycerides.
6. What are the positive and negative consequences of hydrogenating a fat?
7. Which foods contain cholesterol?
8. Describe the difference between LDL and HDL in terms of cholesterol and protein composition.
9. List the recommendations for intake of total fat, saturated fat, and cholesterol.

Try This

The Fat = Fullness Challenge

The goal of this experiment is to see whether fat affects your desire to eat between meals. Do this experiment for two consecutive breakfasts. Each meal is to include only the foods listed below. Try to eat normally for the other meals of the day and eat around the same time of day. Each of these breakfasts has approximately the same calories, but one has a high percentage of them from fat, the other from carbohydrate. After each breakfast, take note of how many hours pass before you feel hungry again.

Day 1 (~420 kcal; 1.5 grams of fat)	Day 2 (~425 kcal; 18 grams of fat)
1 3-oz bagel with 3 tablespoons of jelly	1 medium blueberry muffin

The Salad Dressing Experiment

You can learn a lot from oil-and-vinegar dressing. The purpose of this experiment is twofold. First, you will understand better what it means to say that lipids are insoluble (or not water-soluble). Second, you will be able to experience how fat acts based on its density. Go to your local grocery store and purchase a seasoning packet for Italian (oil and vinegar) dressing. Make sure you also purchase the amount of oil (any type is fine) and vinegar (any type is fine) you need based on the directions. Once home, prepare the dressing. Shake the dressing as if you were to pour it on a salad and then let it stand. What happens to the dressing? What explains this action? Once the dressing settles, which ingredient is found on top—the oil or the vinegar? What property of fat explains this?

Getting Personal

List all of the foods and drinks that you consume in a 24-hour period, ideally a day where your schedule is fairly predictable and you are eating what is considered normal for you.

1. Let's take a look at your fat intake.
   - What percentage of your calories came from fat?
   - What percentage of your calories came from saturated and unsaturated fat?
   - How about your cholesterol intake? Was it above or below the guidelines?
2. Review your day of eating and make a list of the foods you know contain fat.
   - What foods could you substitute to lower your fat intake?
   - What changes can you make to lower your saturated fat intake?
   - What would these substitutions do to the total calories in your diet?
3. Now look at your essential fatty acids.
   - Does your intake of omega-3 and omega-6 fatty acids meet the recommendations?
   - What foods contributed essential fatty acids to your diet?
   - Make a list of foods that would help increase your essential fatty acids intake.
4. Make a list of two or three cooking techniques you could use to lower your fat intake
5. Make a list of three to five suggestions you would consider following when eating at a restaurant that could lower your fat intake.

Learning Portfolio (continued)

References

1. Koba K, Yanagita T. Health benefits of conjugated linoleic acid (CLA). *Obes Res Clin Pract*. 2014;8(6):e525-e532.

2. Brouwer IA, Wanders AJ, Katan MB. Effect of animal and industrial trans fatty acids on HDL and LDL cholesterol levels in humans—a quantitative review. *PLoS One*. 2010;5(3):e9434.

3. American Heart Association. Fish and omega-3 fatty acids. http://www.heart.org/HEARTORG/HealthyLiving/HealthyEating/HealthyDiet-Goals/Fish-and-Omega-3-Fatty-Acids_UCM_303248_Article.jsp#.WIJpAFPysdV. Accessed September 6, 2017.

4. Shulman GI. Ectopic fat in insulin resistance, dyslipidemia, and cardio-metabolic disease. *N Engl J Med*. 2014;371:1131-1141. doi: 10.1056/NEJMra1011035

5. Chang CY, Ke DS, Chen JY. Essential fatty acids and human brain. *Acta Neurol Taiwan*. 2009;18(4):231-241.

6. Schneider M, Levant B, Reichel M, Gulbins E, Kornhuber J, Müller CP. Lipids in psychiatric disorders and preventive medicine. *Neurosci Biobehav Rev*. 2017 May;76(Pt B):336-362.

7. Jones PJH, Rideout P. Lipids, sterols, and their metabolites. In: Ross AC, Caballero B, Cousins B, Tucker KL, Ziegler TR, eds. *Modern Nutrition in Health and Disease*. 11th ed. Philadelphia: Lippincott Williams & Wilkins; 2014:65–87.

8. Vejux A, Samadi M, Lizard G. Contribution of cholesterol and oxysterols in the physiopathology of cataract: implication for the development of pharmacological treatments. *Journal of Ophthalmology*. 2011. https://www.hindawi.com/journals/joph/2011/471947/. Accessed October 10, 2017.

9. Karatas Z, Durmus Aydogdu S, Dinleyici EC, Colak O, Dogruel N. Breastmilk ghrelin, leptin, and fat levels changing foremilk to hindmilk: is that important for self-control of feeding? *Eur J Pediatr*. 2011;170(10):1273-1280.

10. Ohlsson L. Dairy products and plasma cholesterol levels. *Food Nutr Res*. 2010;19:54.

11. Jones PJH, Rideout P. Lipids, sterols, and their metabolites. In: Ross AC, Caballero B, Cousins B, Tucker KL, Ziegler TR, eds. *Modern Nutrition in Health and Disease*. 11th ed. Philadelphia: Lippincott Williams & Wilkins; 2014:65-87.

12. Ibid.

13. Medeiros DM, Wildman REC. *Advanced Human Nutrition*. 3rd ed. Burlington, MA: Jones and Bartlett Learning; 2015.

14. Ibid.

15. American Heart Association. HDL (good), LDL (bad) cholesterol and triglycerides. http://www.heart.org/HEARTORG/Conditions/Cholesterol/AboutCholesterol/Good-vs-Bad-Cholesterol_UCM_305561_Article.jsp#.WIeTBlMrK00. Accessed September 6, 2017.

16. U.S. Department of Health and Human Services, U.S. Department of Agriculture. *2015–2020 Dietary Guidelines for Americans*. 8th ed. December 2015. Available at http://health.gov/dietaryguidelines/2015/guidelines/. Accessed September 6, 2017.

17. Ibid.

18. Position of the Academy of Nutrition and Dietetics: total diet approach to healthy eating. *J Acad Nutr Diet*. 2013;113:307-317.

19. American Heart Association. The American Heart Association's diet and lifestyle recommendations. 2014. http://www.heart.org/HEARTORG/GettingHealthy/NutritionCenter/HealthyEating/The-American-Heart-Associations-Diet-and-Lifestyle-Recommendations_UCM_305855_Article.jsp. Accessed September 6, 2017.

20. Pearson TA, Palaniappan LP, Artinian NT, et al.; on behalf of the American Heart Association Council on Epidemiology and Prevention. American Heart Association guide for improving cardiovascular health at the community level, 2013 update: a scientific statement for public health practitioners, healthcare providers, and health policy makers. *Circulation*. 2013; Apr 23;127(16):1730-53.

21. Institute of Medicine, Food and Nutrition Board. *Dietary Reference Intakes for Energy, Carbohydrate, Fiber, Fat, Fatty Acids, Cholesterol, Protein, and Amino Acids*. Washington, DC: National Academies Press; 2005.

22. Ibid.

23. American Heart Association. The American Heart Association's diet and lifestyle recommendations. Op. cit.

24. U.S. Food and Drug Administration. Changes to the Nutrition Facts label. http://www.fda.gov/Food/GuidanceRegulation/GuidanceDocuments-RegulatoryInformation/LabelingNutrition/ucm385663.htm. Accessed September 6, 2017.

25. U.S. Food and Drug Administration. FDA cuts trans fat in processed foods. http://www.fda.gov/ForConsumers/ConsumerUpdates/ucm372915.htm. Accessed September 6, 2017.

26. Position of the Academy of Nutrition and Dietetics: dietary fatty acids for healthy adults. *J Acad Nutr Diet*. 2014;114:136-153.

27. Mayo Clinic. Omega-3 fatty acids, fish oil, alpha-linolenic acid. http://www.mayoclinic.org/drugs-supplements/omega-3-fatty-acids-fish-oil-alpha-linolenic-acid/background/hrb-20059372. Accessed September 6, 2017.

28. American Heart Association. Making healthy choices. http://www.heart.org/HEARTORG/HealthyLiving/HealthyEating/Nutrition/Making-Healthy-Choices_UCM_461295_Article.jsp#.WIgt8FMrK00. Accessed September 6, 2017.

29. U.S. Department of Health and Human Services, U.S. Department of Agriculture. Op. cit.

30. U.S. Food and Drug Administration and the U.S. Environmental Protection Agency. Eating fish: what pregnant women and parents should know. https://www.fda.gov/downloads/Food/FoodborneIllnessContaminants/Metals/UCM537120.pdf. Accessed September 26, 2017

31. Environmental Protection Agency. FDA and EPA issue updated draft advice for fish consumption/advice encourages pregnant women and breastfeeding mothers to eat more fish that are lower in mercury. June 9, 2014. http://yosemite.epa.gov/opa/admpress.nsf/596e17d7cac720848525781f0043629e/b8edc480d8cfe29b85257cf20065f826!OpenDocument. Accessed September 6, 2017.

32. U.S. Department of Health and Human Services, U.S. Food and Drug Administration. Eating fish: what pregnant women and parents should know. http://www.fda.gov/Food/FoodborneIllnessContaminants/Metals/ucm393070.htm. Accessed September 6, 2017.

33. U.S. Department of Agriculture, Agricultural Research Service. What we eat in America, NHANES 2013-2014. http://www.ars.usda.gov/nea/bhnrc/fsrg. Accessed January 26, 2017.

34. Office of Disease Prevention and Health Promotion. Scientific report of the 2015 Dietary Guidelines Advisory Committee. Part A. Executive summary. http://www.health.gov/dietaryguidelines/2015-scientific-report/02-executive-summary.asp. Accessed September 6, 2017.

35. Position of the Academy of Nutrition and Dietetics: dietary fatty acids for healthy adults. Op. cit.

36. Ibid.

37. de Batle J, Sauleda J, Balcells E, et al. Association between omega-3 and omega-6 fatty acid intakes and serum inflammatory markers in COPD. *J Nutr Biochem*. 2012;23(7):817-821.

38. Doell D, Folmer D, Lee H, Honigfort M, Carberry S. Updated estimate of trans fat intake in the U.S. population. *Food Add Contamin: Part A*. 2012;29(6):861-874.

39. Wang Q, Afshin A, Yakoob MY, et al. Impact of nonoptimal intakes of saturated, polyunsaturated, and trans fat on global burdens of coronary heart disease. *J Am Heart Assoc*. 2016;5:e002076. http://jaha.ahajournals.org/content/5/1/e002891. Accessed September 6, 2017.

40. Chowdhury R, Warnakula S, Kunutsor S, et al. Association of dietary, circulating, and supplement fatty acids with coronary risk: a systematic review and meta-analysis. *Ann Intern Med*. 2014;160(6):398-406. doi: 10.7326/M13-1788

41. Rosa COB, Dos Santos CA, Leite JI, Caldas AP, Bressan J. Impact of nutrients and food components on dyslipidemias: what is the evidence? *Adv Nutr*. 2015;6(6):703-711. doi: 10.3945/an.115.009480 https://www.ncbi.nlm.nih.gov/pmc/articles/PMC4642424/pdf/an009480.pdf. Accessed September 6, 2017.

42. Dalen JE, Devries S. Diets to prevent coronary heart disease 1957–2013: what have we learned? *Am J Med*. 2014;127(5):364-369.

43. Position of the Academy of Nutrition and Dietetics: dietary fatty acids for healthy adults. Op. cit.

44. Rosa COB, Dos Santos CA, Leite JI, Caldas AP, Bressan J. Op. cit.

45. Ooi EM, Watts GF, Ng TW, Barrett PH. Effect of dietary fatty acids on human lipoprotein metabolism: a comprehensive update. *Nutrients*. 2015;7(6):4416-4425. doi: 10.3390/nu7064416

46. American Heart Association. Fish and omega-3 fatty acids. Op. cit.

47. Meyer BJ. Are we consuming enough long chain omega-3 polyunsaturated fatty acids for optimal health? *Prostaglandins Leukot Essent Fatty Acids*. 2011;85(5):275-280.

48. Mayo Clinic. Omega-3 fatty acids, fish oil, alpha-linolenic acid. Op. cit.

49. American Heart Association. Fish and omega-3 fatty acids. Op. cit.

50. American Heart Association. American Stroke Association. Heart Disease and Stroke Statistics 2017 At-a-Glance. https://www.heart.org/idc/groups/ahamah-public/@wcm/@sop/@smd/documents/downloadable/ucm_491265.pdf. Accessed September 26, 2017.

51. National Center for Health Statistics. Trends in elevated triglyceride in adults: United States, 2001–2012. NCHS Data Brief No. 198. May 2015. http://www.cdc.gov/nchs/data/databriefs/db198.htm. Accessed September 6, 2017.

52. Ooi EM, Watts GF, Ng TW, Barrett PH. Op. cit.

53. Centers for Disease Control and Prevention. Overweight and obesity. Adult obesity facts. http://www.cdc.gov/obesity/data/adult.html. Accessed September 6, 2017.

54. Centers for Disease Control and Prevention. Overweight and obesity. Childhood obesity facts. http://www.cdc.gov/obesity/data/childhood.html. Accessed September 6, 2017.

55. Aguilar M, Bhuket T, Torres S, Liu B, Wong RJ. Prevalence of the metabolic syndrome in the United States, 2003-2012. *JAMA*. 2015;313(19):1973-1974. doi: 10.1001/jama.2015.4260

56. Finley CE, Barlow CE, Halton TL, Haskell WL. Glycemic index, glycemic load, and prevalence of the metabolic syndrome in the Copper Center Longitudinal Study. *J Am Diet Assoc*. 2010;110(12):1820-1829.

57. National Heart, Lung, and Blood Institute. What is metabolic syndrome. https://www.nhlbi.nih.gov/health/health-topics/topics/ms. Accessed January 29, 2017.

58. Office of Disease Prevention and Health Promotion. Healthy people 2020. http://www.healthypeople.gov/2020/default.aspx. Accessed September 6, 2017.

Chapter 6

Proteins and Amino Acids: Function Follows Form

Revised by Melissa Bernstein

THINK About It

1   What's your understanding of the term *protein-sparing*?

2   What percentage of your energy intake do you think comes from protein?

3   Do you take any protein or amino acid supplements? If so, why?

4   Do you follow a vegetarian-type diet, or have you ever considered it?

LEARNING Objectives

1. Describe the structure, functions, and denaturation of amino acids.
2. Identify and describe the structure, functions, and denaturation of proteins.
3. Describe the processes of digesting and absorbing proteins, amino acids, and peptides.
4. Differentiate between essential amino acids and nonessential amino acids.
5. Contrast complete and incomplete proteins, and discuss their relationship to protein quality.
6. Interpret nitrogen balance in terms of protein status and nitrogen excretion.
7. Make appropriate protein intake recommendations using AMDR guidelines and the AI or RDA for different age groups.
8. Discuss the consequences of over- and underconsumption of protein in relation to health and disease.
9. List the health benefits and risks of vegetarian diets.

Think of your favorite meal—perhaps a holiday feast, the foods you always ask for on your birthday, or something from a special restaurant. Is the meal you're conjuring up something along the lines of steak and baked potato, lobster and corn on the cob, or roast turkey with mashed potatoes and all the trimmings, or is it maybe something simpler—a juicy hamburger and fries? What do all these meals have in common? In each case, you imagined a meat or fish item as the focus of the meal, surrounded by various grain or vegetable accompaniments. In contrast, maybe your favorite meal is a tofu stir fry surrounded with crisp vegetables, a platter of red beans and rice with fresh tomato salsa, or a steaming platter of chana palak—a chickpea and spinach stew served with tomatoes, onions, and a hot tandoori naan. In these vegetarian meals, as in the meat- or fish-based meals, protein is a critical component, but it's provided by plant products.

From the body's perspective, protein is critically important. Protein is part of every cell, is needed in thousands of chemical reactions, and keeps us "together" structurally. But, as you are about to learn, the human body is so good at using the protein we feed it that our actual needs for dietary protein are relatively small. All foods made from meat, poultry, seafood, beans and peas, eggs, soy, nuts, and seeds are considered "protein foods." Meat itself doesn't need to be at the center of the plate to keep you healthy! Overemphasizing meat can lead to neglecting other important plant-based proteins and nutrient-rich foods.

Why Is Protein Important?

🍎 **Why Is This Important?** Proteins are essential for building numerous tissues, conducting multiple cellular functions, and producing energy in your body.

The word *protein* was coined by the Dutch chemist Gerardus Mulder in 1838 and comes from the Greek word *protos*, meaning "of prime importance." Second only to water, Mulder discovered that proteins are a major component of all plant and animal tissues. Today, we know

Quick Bite

A Bugburger Anyone?
Did you know that bugs provide 10 percent of the protein consumed worldwide? What creepy crawler would you choose for your dinner plate? A grasshopper is 15 to 60 percent protein. Pound for pound, spiders have more protein than any other bug.

that these intricately constructed molecules are vital to many aspects of health and play an essential role in every living cell. Our bodies use protein for functions such as replacing skin cells that slough off over time, producing antibodies to fight infections, and assisting in the essential body processes of water balance, nutrition transport, and muscle contractions.[1] Proteins are a source of energy and help keep skin, hair, and nails healthy.[2] Protein is absolutely critical for overall good health. Our bodies constantly assemble, break down, and use proteins, so we count on our diet to provide enough protein each day to replace what is being used. When we eat more protein than we need, the excess is either used to make energy or stored as fat.

Most people associate protein with animal foods such as beef, chicken, fish, or milk. However, plant foods such as dried beans and peas, grains, nuts, seeds, and vegetables also provide protein. Many protein-rich plant foods are also rich in vitamins and minerals. These plant foods usually are low in fat and calories.

People living in poverty may suffer from a shortage of both protein and energy in the diet. When the diet lacks protein, the body breaks down tissue such as muscle and uses it as a protein source. This causes loss, or **wasting**, of muscles, organs, and other tissues. Protein deficiency also affects the immune system, making people more vulnerable to infection, and impairs digestion and absorption of nutrients. In the United States and other industrialized countries, most people are able to get more than enough protein to meet the body's needs. In fact, a more common problem in these areas is excess intake of protein.

Amino Acids Are the Building Blocks of Proteins

🍎 **Why Is This Important?** Identifying and describing the functions of proteins in the body begins with understanding the shape and building blocks of proteins themselves. Individual amino acids in combination with others amino acids contribute to the properties of each unique protein, determining its role in the body.

Just as glucose is the basic building block of carbohydrates, **amino acids** are the basic building blocks of proteins. Proteins are sequences of amino acids. When building these sequences, your body has 20 different amino acids from which to choose. Nine of these amino acids are called **essential amino acids** because your body cannot make them and must get them through diet. Your body can manufacture the remaining 11 amino acids, called **nonessential amino acids**, when enough nitrogen, carbon, hydrogen, and oxygen are supplied in the diet. Nonessential amino acids do not need to be provided by your diet.

Some nonessential amino acids may become **conditionally essential amino acids** if the body cannot make them because of illness or in certain circumstances where the body lacks the necessary precursors or enzymes to make them. Tyrosine and cysteine, for example, are both considered conditionally essential amino acids. Under normal circumstances, your body makes tyrosine from the essential amino acid phenylalanine and cysteine from either methionine or serine. However, if a disease or condition interferes with the body's ability to synthesize tyrosine or cysteine from their amino acid precursors, then it will need tyrosine or cysteine from the diet. **TABLE 6.1** lists the essential and nonessential amino acids.

▶ **wasting** The breakdown of body tissue, such as muscle and organ, for use as a protein source when the diet lacks protein.

▶ **amino acids** Compounds that function as the building blocks of protein.

▶ **essential amino acids** Amino acids that the body cannot make at all or cannot make enough of to meet physiological needs. Essential amino acids must be supplied in the diet.

▶ **nonessential amino acids** Amino acids that the body can make if supplied with adequate nitrogen. Nonessential amino acids do not need to be supplied in the diet.

▶ **conditionally essential amino acids** Amino acids that are normally made in the body (nonessential) but become essential under certain circumstances, such as during critical illness.

TABLE 6.1
Essential and Nonessential Amino Acids

Essential	Nonessential
Histidine	Alanine
Isoleucine	Arginine*
Leucine	Asparagine
Lysine	Aspartic acid
Methionine	Cysteine*
Phenylalanine	Glutamic acid
Threonine	Glutamine*
Tryptophan	Glycine
Valine	Proline*
	Serine
	Tyrosine*

* Conditionally essential amino acids

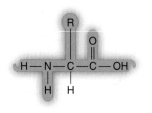

Tyrosine becomes an essential amino acid for individuals with the rare genetic disorder phenylketonuria (PKU). Because people with PKU lack sufficient amounts of an enzyme needed to convert phenylalanine to tyrosine, tyrosine must be supplied in their diets. Phenylalanine intake must be carefully controlled because excess phenylalanine can build up and contribute to permanent intellectual disability and other serious health problems.[3] When babies with PKU receive treatment starting at birth, their IQ development is unaffected. Without treatment, however, they suffer severe mental retardation.

Other amino acids can become essential under certain circumstances. The amino acid glutamine is the main fuel for rapidly dividing cells and plays a key role in transporting nitrogen between organs.[4] Although normally considered nonessential, glutamine can become essential if the body's need for it increases substantially, such as when a person suffers trauma or becomes critically ill.[5] The amino acid arginine can become essential when a person is ill or experiencing severe physiological stress.[6]

Amino Acids Are Identified by Their Side Groups

Amino acids (with the exception of proline) have a central carbon atom attached to one hydrogen atom (H), one carboxylic acid (carboxyl) group (–COOH), one amino (nitrogen-containing) group (–NH$_2$), and one side group unique to each amino acid (R). The side group gives each amino acid its identity. It can vary from a simple hydrogen atom, as in glycine, to a complex ring of carbon and hydrogen atoms, as in phenylalanine. The variations in side groups mean that individual amino acids differ in shape, size, composition, electrical charge, and pH. When amino acids link together to form a protein, these characteristics work together to determine that protein's specific function. **FIGURE 6.1** shows the structure of an amino acid.

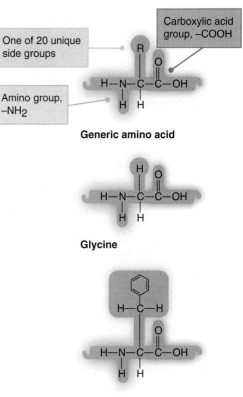

FIGURE 6.1 Structure of an amino acid. All amino acids have a similar structure. Attached to a carbon atom is a hydrogen (H), an amino group (–NH$_2$), an acid group (–COOH), and a side group (R). The side group gives each amino acid its unique identity.

> **Key Concepts** Amino acids, which consist of a central carbon atom bonded to a hydrogen atom, a carboxyl group, an amino group, and a side group, are the building blocks of proteins. Essential amino acids cannot be made by the body and must be supplied in the diet. Nonessential amino acids can be made by the body, given an adequate supply of nitrogen, carbon, hydrogen, and oxygen. Conditionally essential amino acids are normally nonessential but become essential under certain physiological conditions.

Protein Structure: Unique Three-Dimensional Shapes and Functions

Proteins are very large molecules. Just as we combine letters of the alphabet in different sequences to form a nearly infinite variety of words, the body combines amino acids in different sequences to form a nearly infinite variety of proteins. For this reason, protein molecules are more varied than those of either carbohydrates or lipids. (See the FYI feature "Scrabble Anyone?")

Amino Acid Sequence

Amino acids link in specific sequences to form strands of protein (often called *peptides*) up to hundreds of amino acids long. Each amino acid is joined to the next by a **peptide bond**. (See **FIGURE 6.2**.) A **dipeptide** is two amino acids joined by a peptide bond, and a **tripeptide** is three amino acids joined by peptide bonds. The term **oligopeptide** refers to a chain of 4 to 10 amino acids, and a **polypeptide** contains more

▶ **peptide bond** The bond between two amino acids formed when a carboxyl (–COOH) group of one amino acid joins an amino (–NH$_2$) group of another amino acid, releasing water in the process.

▶ **dipeptide** Two amino acids joined by a peptide bond.

▶ **tripeptide** Three amino acids joined by peptide bonds.

▶ **oligopeptide** Four to 10 amino acids joined by peptide bonds.

▶ **polypeptide** More than 10 amino acids joined by peptide bonds.

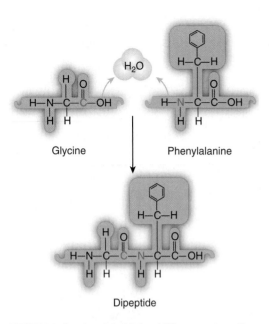

Glycine

Phenylalanine

Dipeptide

FIGURE 6.2 Forming a peptide bond. When two amino acids join together, the acid group of one amino acid is matched with the amino group of another. When amino acids are joined, the reaction forms a peptide bond and releases water.

▶ **hemoglobin [HEEM-oh-glow-bin]** The oxygen-carrying protein in red blood cells that consists of four heme groups and four globin polypeptide chains. The presence of hemoglobin gives blood its red color.

than 10 amino acids.[7] A chain with more than 50 amino acids is called a protein. Proteins in the body and in the diet are long polypeptides, most with hundreds or even thousands of linked amino acids.

Protein Shape

As a cell assembles amino acids into a protein, the protein assumes a unique three-dimensional shape that stems from the sequence and properties of its amino acids. This three-dimensional shape determines the protein's function and the way it interacts with other molecules. As an example, **FIGURE 6.3** illustrates the unique folded and twisted shape of **hemoglobin**, the iron-carrying protein in red blood cells. In the lungs, hemoglobin binds oxygen and releases carbon dioxide. It then travels throughout the body, delivering oxygen to other tissues and picking up carbon dioxide for the return trip to the lungs.

Protein Denaturation: Destabilizing a Protein's Shape

The chemical links that hold a protein's three-dimensional shape can be disrupted. Changes in the acidity or alkalinity of the protein's environment, high temperatures, alcohol, oxidation, and agitation can all cause a protein to unfold and lose its shape (denature), as shown in **FIGURE 6.4**. Because a protein's shape determines its function, denatured proteins lose their ability to function properly.

Amino acid sequence

A simple illustration of a protein just shows the sequence of amino acids that form one or more polypeptide chains.

aa_1 aa_2 aa_3 aa_4 aa_5 aa_6 aa_7 — Amino acids

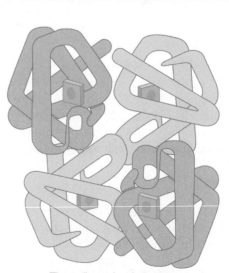

A more complex illustration of a protein shows its three-dimensional structure. This molecule of hemoglobin is composed of four polypeptide chains. The square plates represent nonprotein portions of the molecule (heme) that carry oxygen.

Three-dimensional structure

FIGURE 6.3 Protein structure. The simplest depiction of a protein reveals its unique sequence of amino acids. Each protein becomes folded, twisted, and coiled into a shape all its own. This shape defines how a protein functions in your body.

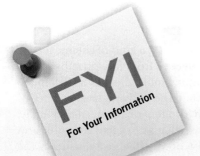

Scrabble Anyone?

Making a meaningful word from available Scrabble tiles is a good analogy for making a functional protein chain from available amino acids. Just as we can make many different words from the same tiles, cells can make many different proteins from the same amino acids.

If your cells have all 20 amino acids at their disposal, these can be arranged in a bewildering number of combinations to create an estimated 250,000–1 million different proteins, just as all the letters of the alphabet can be used to make an almost unlimited number of words.

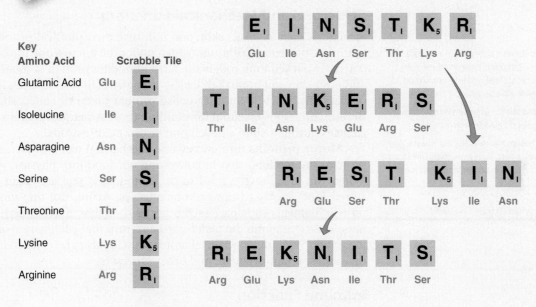

Key Amino Acid	Scrabble Tile
Glutamic Acid	Glu
Isoleucine	Ile
Asparagine	Asn
Serine	Ser
Threonine	Thr
Lysine	Lys
Arginine	Arg

If you've ever cooked an egg, you've witnessed protein **denaturation**. As the egg cooks, some of its protein bonds break. As these proteins unfold, they bump into and bind to each other. Eventually, as these interconnections increase, the liquid egg coagulates to form a solid. Raw egg white proteins denature and stiffen as they are whipped, and milk proteins denature and curdle when acid is added. Denaturation is the first step in breaking down protein for digestion. Stomach acids denature protein, uncoiling the structure into a simple amino acid chain that digestive enzymes can start breaking apart.

▶ **denaturation** A change in the three-dimensional structure of a protein resulting in an unfolded polypeptide chain that cannot fulfill the protein's function. Treatment with heat, acid, alkali, or extreme agitation can denature most proteins.

> **Key Concepts** Proteins are large molecules made up of amino acids joined in various sequences. Amino acids are joined by peptide bonds. Each protein assumes a unique three-dimensional shape depending on the sequence of its amino acids and the properties of their side groups. Acidity, alkalinity, heat, alcohol, and agitation can disrupt chemical forces that stabilize proteins, causing the proteins to denature, or lose their shape.

Functions of Body Proteins

🍎 **Why Is This Important?** Understanding the variety of different roles that proteins play serves as the foundation for knowing how proteins ensure our survival. Proteins have structural and mechanical roles, work as hormones and enzymes to regulate body processes, aid in fluid and acid–base balance, and are important for the body's immune functions.

Each of the human body's thousands of different proteins has a specific function determined by its unique shape. Some act as enzymes, speeding

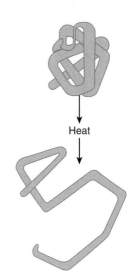

FIGURE 6.4 Denaturation. Heat, pH, oxidation, and mechanical agitation are some of the forces that can denature a protein, causing it to unfold and lose its functional shape.

up chemical reactions. Others act as hormones, a kind of chemical messenger. Antibodies made of protein protect us from foreign substances. Proteins maintain fluid balance by pumping molecules across cell membranes and attracting water. They maintain the acid and base balance of body fluids by taking up or giving off hydrogen ions as needed. Finally, proteins transport many key substances, such as oxygen, vitamins, and minerals, to target cells throughout the body. **FIGURE 6.5** illustrates the functions of proteins in the human body.

Structural and Mechanical Functions

Structures such as bone, skin, and hair owe their physical properties to unique proteins. **Collagen**, which under the microscope looks like a densely packed long rod, is the most abundant protein in mammals and gives skin and bone their elastic strength. Hair and nails are made of **keratin**, which is another dense protein made of coiled shapes. Because protein is essential for building these structures, protein deficiencies during a child's development can be disastrous.

Motor proteins turn energy into mechanical work. In fact, these proteins are the final step in converting our food into physical work. When you bike down a road or up a mountain, you are using your stored food energy to power your muscles. Acting like tiny motors, protein filaments slide past each other as they shorten (contract) your muscle. As you pump the pedals, proteins turn that energy bar you ate into work. Similarly, specialized motor proteins also are involved in cell division, sperm movement, and other processes.

Immune Function

Proteins play an important role in the immune system, which is responsible for fighting invasion and infection by foreign substances.

▶ **collagen** The most abundant fibrous protein in the body. Collagen is the major constituent of connective tissue, forms the foundation for bones and teeth, and helps maintain the structure of blood vessels and other tissues.

▶ **keratin** A water-insoluble fibrous protein that is the primary constituent of hair, nails, and the outer layer of the skin.

▶ **motor proteins** Proteins that use energy and convert it into some form of mechanical work. Motor proteins are active in processes such as cell division, muscle contraction, and sperm movement.

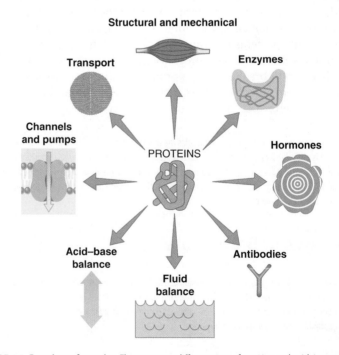

FIGURE 6.5 Functions of proteins. There are many different types of proteins, each with its particular role in the body.

Antibodies are blood proteins that attack and inactivate bacteria and viruses that cause infection. When your diet does not contain enough protein, your body cannot make as many antibodies as it needs. Your **immune response** is weakened, and your risk of infection and illness increases. Each protein antibody has a specific shape that allows it to attack and destroy a specific foreign invader. Once your immune system learns how to make a certain kind of antibody, your body can protect itself by quickly making that antibody the next time the same germ invades.

▶ **antibodies [AN-tih-bod-eez]** Infection-fighting protein molecules in blood or secretory fluids that tag, neutralize, and help destroy pathogenic microorganisms (e.g., bacteria, viruses) or toxins.

▶ **immune response** A coordinated set of steps, including production of antibodies, that the immune system takes in response to an antigen.

Enzymes

Enzymes are proteins that catalyze, or speed up, chemical reactions without being destroyed in the process. (See **FIGURE 6.6a** and **6.6b**.) Every

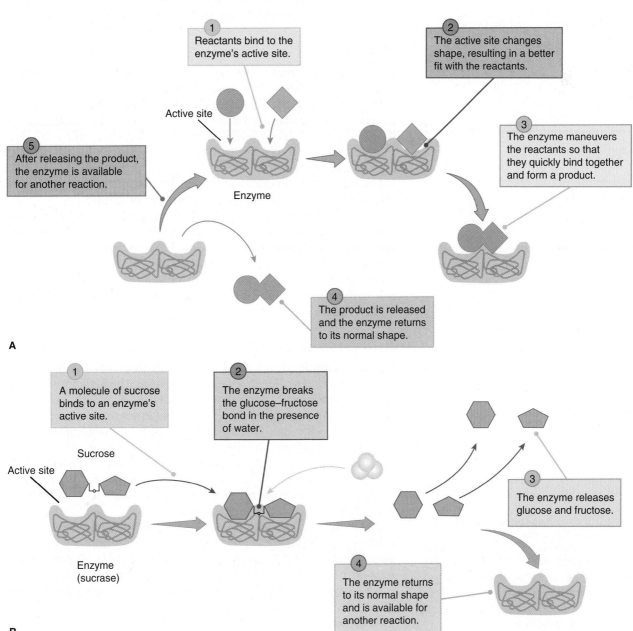

FIGURE 6.6A and **6.6B**   a. Enzymes catalyze (speed up) reactions that make or change substances (reactants). b. Enzymes catalyze reactions that break down molecules.

cell contains thousands of types of enzymes, each with its own purpose. During digestion, for example, enzymes help break down carbohydrates, proteins, and fats into monosaccharides, amino acids, and fatty acids so the body can absorb them. Cellular enzymes release energy from these nutrients to fuel thousands of body processes. Enzymes also trigger the reactions that build muscle and tissue.

Our foods also contain enzymes, but these are inactivated (denatured) by cooking. Stomach acid denatures the enzymes in raw foods. You may notice special purified enzymes being sold as supplements to enhance digestion. Most of the time, stomach acid denatures these enzymes, so they are unable to function in the intestinal tract. However, some enzyme supplements are coated with a special substance to protect them from stomach acid. For example, a specially coated tablet form of the enzyme lactase can help people with lactose intolerance. Such coated enzymes temporarily help break down foods in the small intestine, but eventually are digested themselves.

Hormones

Hormones are chemical messengers that are made in one part of the body but act on cells in other parts of the body. Protein hormones perform many important regulatory functions. Insulin, for example, is a protein hormone that plays a key role in regulating the amount of glucose in the blood. It is released from the pancreas in response to a rise in blood glucose levels and works to lower those levels. People with type 1 diabetes must take insulin injections to control blood glucose levels. Inhaled insulin and insulin pills are currently being studied for effectiveness in the prevention and treatment of diabetes.[8]

Thyroid-stimulating hormone (TSH) and leptin are two other examples of protein hormones. The pituitary gland produces TSH, which stimulates the thyroid gland to produce the hormone thyroxine. Thyroxine, a modified form of the amino acid tyrosine, increases the body's metabolic rate. Leptin is produced by fat cells and plays an important role in the control of food intake, energy expenditure, metabolism, and body weight.[9]

Acid–Base Balance

Measurements on the pH scale (which range from 0 to 14) indicate the concentration of hydrogen ions in a substance. The higher the concentration of hydrogen ions, the lower the pH. Acids, which have a high concentration of hydrogen ions, have a pH lower than 7; bases, which have a low concentration of hydrogen ions, have a pH higher than 7. The lower the pH, the stronger the acid. The higher the pH, the stronger the base. The body works hard to keep the pH of the blood near 7.4, or nearly neutral. We can tolerate only small blood pH fluctuations without disastrous consequences. Only a few hours with a blood pH above 8.0 or below 6.8 will cause death.

Proteins help maintain stable pH levels in body fluids by serving as **buffers**; they pick up extra hydrogen ions when conditions are acidic, and they donate hydrogen ions when conditions are alkaline. If proteins are not available to buffer acidic or alkaline substances, the blood can become too acidic or too alkaline, resulting in either **acidosis** or **alkalosis**. Both conditions can be serious—either can cause proteins to denature, which can lead to coma or death.

▶ **buffers** Compounds that can take up and release hydrogen ions to keep the pH of a solution constant. The buffering action of proteins and bicarbonate in the bloodstream plays a major role in maintaining the blood pH at 7.35 to 7.45.

▶ **acidosis** An abnormally low blood pH (below about 7.35) resulting from increased acidity.

▶ **alkalosis** An abnormally high blood pH (above about 7.45) resulting from increased alkalinity.

Transport Functions

Many substances pass into and out of cells through proteins that cross cell membranes and act as channels and pumps. Some protein channels allow substances to flow rapidly through the membranes without an input of energy. Other channels are protein pumps that use energy to drive substances across membranes.

Proteins also act as carriers, transporting many important substances in the bloodstream for delivery throughout the body. Lipoproteins, for example, package proteins with lipids so lipid particles can be carried in the blood. Other proteins carry fat-soluble vitamins, such as vitamin A and certain other vitamins and minerals. Because protein carries vitamin A in the blood, protein deficiency contributes to vitamin A deficiency. The protein transferrin carries iron in the blood; another protein (ferritin) stores iron in the liver.

Fluid Balance

Fluids in the body are found inside cells (**intracellular fluid**) or outside cells (**extracellular fluid**). There are two types of extracellular fluid—fluid between cells (called *intercellular fluid* or **interstitial fluid**) and fluid in the blood (**intravascular fluid**). Whereas fluid within cells is usually high in potassium and phosphate, fluid between cells is usually high in sodium and chloride. These interior and exterior fluid levels must stay in balance for body processes to work properly.

Proteins in the blood help to maintain appropriate fluid levels in the vascular system. (See **FIGURE 6.7**.) When your heart beats, the force pushes fluid and nutrients from the capillaries out into the fluid

▶ **intracellular fluid**   The fluid in the body's cells. It usually is high in potassium and phosphate and low in sodium and chloride. It constitutes about two-thirds of total body water.

▶ **extracellular fluid**   The fluid located outside of cells. It is composed largely of the liquid portion (plasma) of the blood and the fluid between cells in tissues (interstitial fluid), with fluid in the GI tract, eyes, joints, and spinal cord contributing a small amount. It constitutes about one-third of body water.

▶ **interstitial fluid [in-ter-STISH-ul]**   The fluid between cells in tissues, usually high in sodium and chloride. Also called *intercellular fluid*.

▶ **intravascular fluid**   The fluid portion (plasma) of the blood contained in arteries, veins, and capillaries. It accounts for about 15 percent of the extracellular fluid.

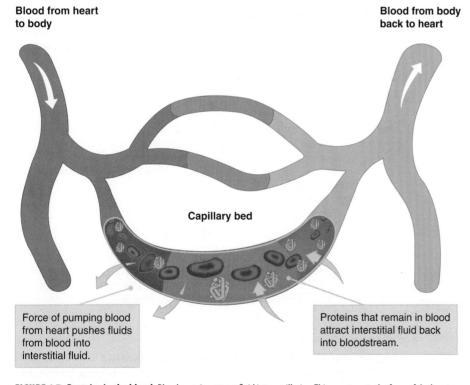

Blood from heart to body

Blood from body back to heart

Capillary bed

Force of pumping blood from heart pushes fluids from blood into interstitial fluid.

Proteins that remain in blood attract interstitial fluid back into bloodstream.

FIGURE 6.7 Proteins in the blood. Blood proteins attract fluid into capillaries. This counteracts the force of the heart beating, which pushes fluid out of capillaries.

▶ **edema** Swelling caused by the buildup of fluid between cells.

▶ **deamination** The removal of the amino group ($-NH_2$) from an amino acid.

surrounding the cells. But blood proteins such as albumin and globulin are too large to leave the capillary beds. These proteins remain in the capillaries, where they attract fluid to replace what has been pushed out. This system maintains a balance of fluids in the vascular system.

If the diet severely lacks protein, and does not include enough to maintain normal levels of blood proteins, fluid will leak into the surrounding tissue and cause swelling, also called **edema**. Children with protein malnutrition often suffer from severe edema. Reestablishing a diet adequate in protein and energy will allow the edema to subside.

Source of Energy and Glucose

Protein, like carbohydrate, when completely metabolized in the body yields 4 kilocalories of energy for every gram consumed. Although your body prefers to burn carbohydrate and fat for energy, if necessary it can use protein for energy or to make glucose. Thus, carbohydrate and fat are protein-sparing, meaning they spare amino acids from being burned for energy and allow them to be used for protein synthesis.

THINK About It **1**

If the diet does not provide enough energy for vital functions, the body will sacrifice its own protein from enzymes, muscle, and other tissues to make energy and glucose for use by the brain, lungs, and heart. This is what happens in cases of starvation.

When the body uses protein for energy, it first breaks the protein into individual amino acids. A process called **deamination** removes the nitrogen group, which is released in urine, and also reduces the amino acid to its carbon skeleton. This carbon skeleton can then be used for energy, and most amino acids yield carbon skeletons that can be used to make glucose.

If your diet contains more protein than you need for protein synthesis, your body cannot store the excess amino acids. Instead your body converts the excess amino acids into energy, makes glucose for storage as glycogen, or converts the amino acids into fatty acids for storage as energy. This is why taking protein supplements or eating high-protein diets as a means of increasing muscle mass may instead add to body fat.

> **Key Concepts** In the body, proteins perform numerous vital functions that are determined by each protein's shape. Protein antibodies protect the body from infection and illness. As enzymes, proteins speed up chemical reactions; as hormones, they are chemical messengers. Proteins also maintain fluid balance and acid–base balance and transport substances throughout the body. If needed, protein can also be used as a source of energy or glucose.

Protein Digestion and Absorption

🍎 **Why Is This Important?** The proteins from the food we eat must be digested into their component amino acids for absorption into the body. Once absorbed, the amino acids are then put back together in new configurations, creating proteins that meet the body's needs.

Protein Digestion

The first step in using dietary protein is breaking down its long polypeptide chains into amino acids. As with the other energy-yielding nutrients, digestion of protein requires enzymes from a number of sources. Digestion of protein begins in the stomach. **FIGURE 6.8** shows the process of protein digestion and absorption.

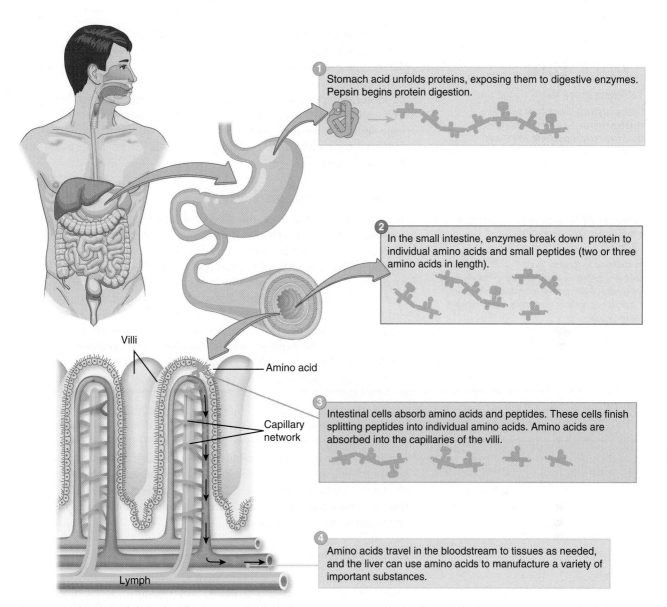

FIGURE 6.8 Digestion and absorption of protein. Digestion breaks down protein to amino acids and small peptides for absorption. Amino acids are absorbed into the capillaries of the villi and transported in the bloodstream.

In the Stomach

In the stomach, hydrochloric acid (HCl) denatures a protein by unfolding it. This makes the amino acid chain more accessible to the action of enzymes. Glands in the stomach lining produce the **proenzyme** pepsinogen, the inactive **precursor** of the enzyme pepsin. When pepsinogen comes in contact with hydrochloric acid, it is converted to the active enzyme pepsin. The acidity of gastric juices is necessary for this enzyme to be active. By the time dietary protein leaves the stomach, pepsin has broken it down into individual amino acids and shorter polypeptides of various lengths that then travel to the small intestine for further digestion.

In the Small Intestine

From the stomach, amino acids and polypeptides pass into the small intestine, where most protein digestion takes place. In the small intestine,

▶ **proenzymes** Inactive precursors of enzymes.

▶ **precursor** A substance that is converted into another active substance. Enzyme precursors also are called *proenzymes*.

Quick Bite

Softening Tough Meat
Cooking tough cuts of meat in liquid over several hours helps dissolve the fibrous connective tissue, the proteins responsible for meat's tough texture.

▶ **proteases [PRO-tea-aces]** Enzymes that break down protein into peptides and amino acids.

▶ **celiac disease [SEA-lee-ak]** A disease that involves an inability to digest gluten, a protein found in wheat, rye, and barley. If untreated, it causes flattening of the villi in the intestine, leading to severe malabsorption of nutrients. Symptoms include diarrhea, fatty stools, swollen belly, and extreme fatigue.

activated **proteases** from the pancreas and intestinal lining cells break down large peptides into smaller peptides. Pancreatic enzymes completely digest only a small percentage of proteins into individual amino acids; enzymes on the surface of the small intestine split the remaining larger polypeptides into tripeptides and dipeptides, and some are even split all the way into amino acids. The intestinal cells absorb these smaller units and break down virtually all the remaining dipeptides and tripeptides into individual amino acids for absorption into the bloodstream.

Undigested Protein

Any parts of proteins not digested and absorbed in the small intestine continue through the large intestine and pass out of the body in the feces. Normally, the body efficiently digests and absorbs protein. Diseases of the intestinal tract, however, decrease the efficiency of absorption and increase protein losses in the feces. People with the autoimmune disorder **celiac disease**, for example, cannot tolerate gluten—a protein found in wheat, rye, and barley. Unless treated with a gluten-free diet, the intestinal villi become damaged; people with celiac disease show poor growth, weight loss, and poor absorption of nutrients.[10] Eliminating gluten from the diet helps people with celiac disease get necessary protein and nutrients so they can maintain a healthy body weight.

Gluten-free diets, such as those used to treat individuals with celiac disease, have recently gained the attention of many people without celiac disease who are trying to lose weight.[11] However, this tactic is considered by experts to be another "get-thin-quick" fad that is not based on sound science. Despite celebrity endorsements, flashy advertising claims, and an estimated $15.6 billion in product sales in 2016, there has been no experimental evidence to support claims that gluten-free eating promotes weight loss.[12,13]

Amino Acid and Peptide Absorption

The end products of protein digestion are amino acids and small peptides. Peptides are rarely absorbed, and whole proteins that escape digestion are almost never absorbed. More than 99 percent of protein enters the bloodstream as individual amino acids. Some amino acids remain in the intestinal cells and are used to synthesize intestinal enzymes and new cells.

Most protein absorption takes place in the cells that line the duodenum and jejunum. Approximately 11 different transport mechanisms for amino acids have been identified within the absorptive cells of the small intestine.[14] Absorption of some amino acids requires active transport, whereas other amino acids are absorbed via facilitated diffusion. There are several active transport mechanisms, and similar amino acids share the same active transport system. Normally, proteins in foods supply a mix of many amino acids, so amino acids that share the same transport system are absorbed fairly equally. When a person consumes a large amount of one particular amino acid, however, absorption of other amino acids that share the same transport system will be deficient. Thus, if you take a supplement of one amino acid, you may be interfering with the absorption of another amino acid from your diet. (See the FYI feature "Do Athletes Need More Protein?") Once absorbed, most amino acids and the few absorbed peptides travel via the portal vein to

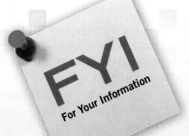

Celiac Disease and Gluten Sensitivity

Unexplained iron-deficiency anemia, fatigue, bone or joint pain, depression or anxiety, seizures or migraines, canker sores inside the mouth, and an itchy skin rash—these are some of the symptoms that adults may experience if they have celiac disease. For children, common symptoms include abdominal bloating and pain, chronic diarrhea, vomiting, constipation, weight loss, fatigue, dental enamel defects of the permanent teeth, and attention deficit hyperactivity disorder (ADHD).

Celiac disease is a hereditary autoimmune disorder affecting about 1 in 100 people worldwide. Is there any treatment? Fortunately, yes. A gluten-free diet greatly reduces the symptoms listed above. Gluten is a protein in grains such as wheat, rye, barley, and triticale (a cross between wheat and rye). It's also present in many processed foods, such as pasta, cereals, pastries, crackers, beer, candies, and condiments, such as soy sauce, malt vinegar, dressings, and marinades. Left untreated, celiac disease can lead to long-term health conditions such as iron-deficiency anemia, early osteoporosis, infertility, vitamin and mineral deficiencies, disorders of the nervous system, conditions affecting the pancreas and gallbladder, and cancerous growths.

Symptoms of celiac disease are not the same for everyone, making the condition sometimes difficult to diagnose. Some people with this disease have no symptoms at all, whereas others experience a variety of digestive symptoms.

Gluten sensitivity is a condition with symptoms similar to those of celiac disease. Like those with the disease, individuals with sensitivity see their symptoms improve when they eliminate gluten from the diet. One important difference between gluten sensitivity and celiac disease is that those with gluten sensitivity do not experience small intestine damage or develop the antibodies found in celiac disease.

It is important not to self-diagnose and self-treat gluten sensitivity or celiac disease. Foods that contain gluten can also be good sources of other nutrients, so eliminating them unnecessarily may compromise your diet. If you think you have celiac disease or gluten sensitivity, talk to your doctor about testing before you start a gluten-free diet. Pharmaceutical companies are racing to develop drugs that will cure or treat celiac disease.

Celiac Disease. Celiac Disease Foundation. http://celiac.org/celiac-disease/. Accessed 1/8/17; National Institute of Health (NIH) Celiac Disease Awareness Campaign. http://celiac.nih.gov. Accessed 1/8/17.

---

the liver, which releases them into general circulation. Intestinal cells retain some amino acids to synthesize enzymes and make new cells.

> **Key Concepts** Protein digestion begins in the stomach, where hydrochloric acid (HCl) denatures protein, and then the enzyme pepsin breaks proteins into smaller peptides. Digestion continues in the small intestine, where proteases break polypeptides into smaller peptide units, which are then absorbed into cells where additional enzymes complete digestion to amino acids.

Proteins in the Body

🍎 **Why Is This Important?** Amino acids from protein in the diet are reassembled into new proteins based on the body's needs. For example, proteins strengthen hair, skin, and nails; they also serve as antibodies to fight infections and enzymes that facilitate chemical reactions.

Once in the bloodstream, amino acids are transported throughout the body and are available for synthesizing cellular proteins. To build proteins, cells use peptide bonds to link amino acids.

Protein Synthesis

Genetic material in the nucleus of every cell provides the blueprint for the thousands of proteins needed to perform life functions. To synthesize a protein, cells assemble amino acids in a specific sequence.

Just as one missing part of a car can stop an entire auto assembly line, one missing amino acid can stop synthesis of an entire protein in the cell. If a nonessential amino acid is missing during protein synthesis, the cell will either make that amino acid or obtain it from the liver via the bloodstream, and protein synthesis will continue. If an essential amino acid is missing, the body may break its own protein down to supply the missing amino acid. If a missing essential amino acid is unavailable, protein synthesis halts, and the partially completed protein is broken down into individual amino acids for use elsewhere in the body.

Genetic defects can cause problems in protein synthesis. People who have sickle cell anemia, for example, cannot construct the correct amino acid sequence to form the protein hemoglobin. A genetic error causes the amino acid valine to be substituted for glutamic acid in two locations in the protein chain. This simple error causes the shape of hemoglobin to change so much that the red blood cell becomes stiff and sickle-shaped instead of soft and disk-shaped. Because this faulty protein cannot carry oxygen efficiently, it causes serious medical problems.

The Amino Acid Pool and Protein Turnover

Cells throughout the body constantly and simultaneously synthesize and break down protein. When cells break down protein, the protein's amino acids return to circulation. (See **FIGURE 6.9**.) These available amino acids, found throughout body tissues and fluids, are collectively referred to as the **amino acid pool**. Some of these amino acids may be used for protein synthesis; others may have their amino group removed and be used to produce energy or nonprotein substances such as glucose.

The constant recycling of proteins in the body is known as **protein turnover**. Each day, more amino acids in your body are recycled than are supplied in your diet. Of the approximately 300 grams of protein synthesized by the body each day, 200 grams are made from recycled amino acids.[15] The protein in the intestine and the liver, which are two tissue types with rapid rates of degradation and resynthesis, account for as much as 50 percent of this protein turnover.[16] This remarkable recycling capacity is the reason we need so little protein in our diet. Although our requirements are small, dietary protein is extremely important. When dietary protein is inadequate, body protein is broken down faster to replenish the amino acid pool. This can lead to the loss of essential body tissue.

Synthesis of Nonprotein Molecules

Amino acids do more than help build peptides and proteins; they are precursors of many molecules with important biological roles. Your body makes nonprotein molecules from amino acids and the nitrogen they contain. The vitamin niacin, for example, is made from the amino acid tryptophan. Precursors of DNA, RNA, and many coenzymes are formed in part from amino acids. Your body also uses amino acids to make **neurotransmitters**, chemicals that send signals from nerve cells to other parts of the body. The neurotransmitter serotonin, which helps regulate mood, is made from tryptophan. Norepinephrine and epinephrine (also called *noradrenaline* and *adrenaline*, respectively), which get the body ready for action, are neurotransmitters made from tyrosine. The simple amino acid glycine combines with many toxic substances to make less harmful substances that the body can eliminate. Your body uses the amino acid histidine to make histamine, which dilates blood vessels and is a culprit in allergic reactions.

▶ **amino acid pool** The amino acids in body tissues and fluids that are available for new protein synthesis.

▶ **protein turnover** Constant breakdown and synthesis of proteins in the body.

▶ **neurotransmitters** Substances released at the end of a stimulated nerve cell that diffuse across a small gap and bind to another nerve cell or muscle cell, stimulating or inhibiting it.

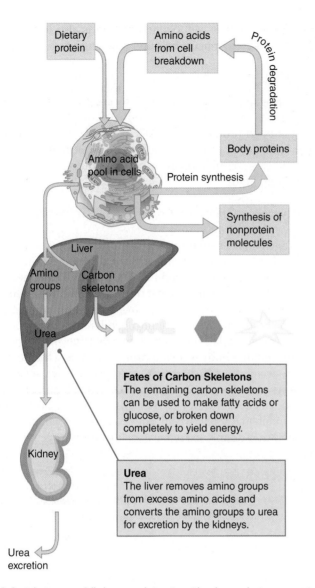

FIGURE 6.9 Protein turnover. Cells draw upon their amino acid pools to synthesize new proteins. These small pools turn over quickly and must be replenished by amino acids from dietary protein and the degradation (breakdown) of body protein. Dietary protein supplies about one-third and the breakdown of body protein supplies about two-thirds of the amino acids needed to synthesize roughly 300 grams of body protein daily. When dietary protein is inadequate, increased degradation of body protein replenishes the amino acid pool. This can lead to the breakdown of essential body tissue.

Protein and Nitrogen Excretion

Cells are constantly breaking down and recycling amino acids. Breakdown of an amino acid yields an amino group ($-NH_2$). This NH_2 molecule is unstable and is quickly converted to ammonia (NH_3). However, ammonia is toxic to cells, so it is expelled into the bloodstream as a waste product and is carried to the liver. In the liver, an amino group and an ammonia group react with carbon dioxide through a series of reactions known collectively as the urea cycle to produce **urea** and water. The nitrogen-rich urea is transported from the liver by way of the bloodstream to the kidneys, where it is filtered from the blood and sent to the bladder for excretion in the urine. Small amounts of other nitrogen-containing compounds, such as ammonia, uric acid, and creatinine, are

▶ **urea** The main nitrogen-containing waste product in mammals. Formed in liver cells from ammonia and carbon dioxide, urea is carried via the bloodstream to the kidneys, where it is excreted in urine.

excreted in the urine as well. Some nitrogen is also lost through skin, sloughed-off GI cells, mucus, hair and nail cuttings, and body fluids.

Nitrogen Balance

Because nitrogen is excreted as proteins are recycled or used, we can use the balance of nitrogen in the body to evaluate whether the body is getting enough protein. (See **FIGURE 6.10**.) To estimate the balance of nitrogen, and therefore protein, in the body, nitrogen intake is compared to the sum of all sources of nitrogen output (urine, feces, skin, hair, and body fluids).[17]

Nitrogen balance = Grams of nitrogen intake – Grams of nitrogen output

If nitrogen intake equals nitrogen output, **nitrogen balance** is zero and the body is in **nitrogen equilibrium**. If nitrogen intake exceeds nitrogen output, the body is said to be in **positive nitrogen balance**. Positive nitrogen balance means that the body is adding protein; growing children, pregnant women, or people recovering from protein deficiency or illnesses should be in positive nitrogen balance. If nitrogen output exceeds nitrogen intake, the body is in **negative nitrogen balance**. This means that the body is losing protein. People who are starving or on extreme weight-loss diets or who suffer from fever, severe illnesses, or infections are in a state of negative nitrogen balance. Healthy adults are in nitrogen equilibrium, which means that they take in enough protein to maintain and repair tissue. They have no net gain or loss of body protein, and they simply excrete excess dietary nitrogen.

Key Concepts Cells throughout the body constantly synthesize and break down protein simultaneously, a process known as protein turnover. Nitrogen-containing end products of protein metabolism are excreted in urine via the kidneys. Comparison of nitrogen intake (from dietary protein) to nitrogen excretion gives a measure of nitrogen balance and indicates protein status in the body.

▶ **nitrogen balance** Intake minus the sum of all sources of nitrogen excretion.

▶ **nitrogen equilibrium** Nitrogen intake equals the sum of all sources of nitrogen excretion; nitrogen balance equals zero.

▶ **positive nitrogen balance** Nitrogen intake exceeds the sum of all sources of nitrogen excretion.

▶ **negative nitrogen balance** Nitrogen intake is less than the sum of all sources of nitrogen excretion.

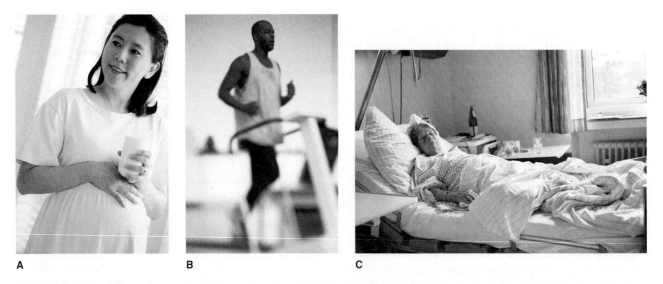

A   B   C

FIGURE 6.10 Nitrogen balance. Nitrogen balance reflects whether a person is gaining or losing protein. a. A pregnant woman is adding protein, so she has a positive nitrogen balance. b. A healthy person who is neither gaining nor losing protein is in nitrogen equilibrium (zero balance). c. A person who is severely ill and losing protein has a negative nitrogen balance.
a. © EyeWire; b. © Photodisc; c. © iStockphoto/SilviaJansen.

Proteins in the Diet

🍎 **Why Is This Important?** For proteins to perform all their essential functions, the diet must provide adequate amounts of the various amino acids. The body gets high-quality proteins from foods such as meats, eggs, fish and dairy.

Many government and health organizations have made recommendations about the amount of protein in a healthful diet, just as they have for other nutrients. Meat, eggs, milk, legumes, grains, and vegetables are all sources of protein. Fruits contain minimal amounts and, along with fats, are not considered protein sources. **FIGURE 6.11** shows some good sources of protein.

Recommended Intakes of Protein

In the United States and Canada, the Recommended Dietary Allowance (RDA) is the accepted dietary standard for protein. RDAs are set to meet the nutritional needs of most healthy people, so most of us actually require somewhat less protein than the RDA. RDA values also assume we are consuming adequate energy and other nutrients to allow our bodies to use dietary protein for protein synthesis, rather than for energy.

THINK About It 2 Based on evidence of increased heart disease risk when diets are low in fat and high in carbohydrate, and increased risk of obesity and heart disease when diets are high in fat, the Food and Nutrition Board developed Acceptable Macronutrient Distribution Ranges (AMDRs) for the energy-yielding nutrients.[18] For adults, the AMDR for fat is 20 to 35 percent of energy intake, and the AMDR for carbohydrate is 45 to 65 percent of energy intake. This leaves about 10 to 35 percent of energy intake from protein, a level that is typically higher than the RDA.

Adults

For adults, the RDA for protein intake is 0.8 gram per kilogram of body weight.[19] Using a reference body weight of 57 kilograms (125 pounds) for adult women and 70 kilograms (154 pounds) for adult men, this translates into a daily protein recommendation of 46 grams for women and 56 grams for men. When calculated as a percentage of average energy intake, the protein RDA for adults provides about 8 to 11 percent of energy intake for adults, staying within the recommended energy levels.

Other Life Stages

Both pregnancy and breastfeeding increase a woman's need for protein. The RDA for pregnant and lactating women is 1.1 grams per kilogram. This is an increase of about 25 grams per day over the female RDA for protein. Most American women already consume more than enough protein to support pregnancy and breastfeeding.

Infants have the highest protein needs relative to body weight of any time of life. (See **TABLE 6.2**.) Protein is needed to support rapid growth during infancy. The Adequate Intake (AI) value for infants 0 to 6 months of age is based on the protein content of human milk and the average milk consumption of breastfed babies. Protein requirements per kilogram body weight gradually fall throughout childhood and adolescence until a person reaches adulthood. (See **FIGURE 6.12**.)

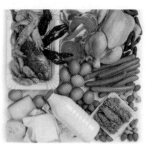

Rich sources of protein include meats, fish, poultry, eggs, dairy products, legumes, and nuts.

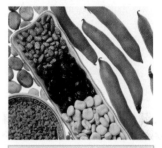

Legumes and nuts are important sources of protein for vegetarians.

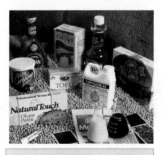

Soybeans and soy products are plant sources of complete protein.

FIGURE 6.11 Protein sources. Meat, fish, eggs, dairy products, and soy are excellent protein sources. Legumes, grain products, starchy vegetables, nuts, and seeds also are good sources.

Top: © iStockphoto/Thinkstock; Middle: Photo by Keith Weller. Courtesy of USDA; Bottom: Photo by Scott Bauer. Courtesy of USDA.

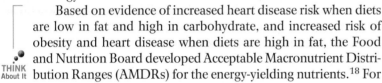

Calculating Your Protein RDA

Convert weight to kg
(pounds ÷ 2.2)
Multiply kg by 0.8 = Protein RDA in g

Examples:

Male, 19-24 years old, 70 kg (154 lb)
70 kg × 0.8 g/kg = 56 g protein

Female, 19-24 years old, 57 kg (125 lb)
57 kg × 0.8 g/kg = 46 g protein

TABLE 6.2
Protein AI or RDA for Infants, Children, and Teens

Age	Protein AI or RDA (g/kg Body Weight)
0 to 6 months	1.52
7 to 12 months	1.5
1 to 3 years	1.1
4 to 8 years	0.95
9 to 13 years	0.95
14 to 18 years	0.85

Data from Institute of Medicine, Food and Nutrition Board. *Dietary Reference Intakes for Energy, Carbohydrate, Fiber, Fat, Fatty Acids, Cholesterol, Protein, and Amino Acids (Macronutrients)*. Washington, DC: National Academies Press; 2005.

The RDA for protein for all adults, regardless of age, is set at 0.8 gram of protein per kilogram of body weight. Although elderly people, on average, have less lean body mass to maintain than younger people, some experts believe that the protein requirement for people over the age of 50 should be higher than 0.8 g/kg/day.[20] Evidence indicates that protein intake greater than the RDA may improve muscle mass, strength, and function in this population.[21] Immune status, wound healing, blood pressure, and bone health may also be improved by meeting protein needs in this group. Because energy needs decline with age, protein should provide a larger percentage of energy intake. An intake of 1.0–1.6 grams of protein per kilogram per day is a reasonable target for individuals older than 50 years.[22] To maximize protein utilization efficiency, older adults should try to eat 25–30 grams of high-quality protein at each meal throughout the day.[23] Choosing a healthy diet has many challenges in old age, making it hard to meet recommended levels for protein and other nutrients.

Physical Stress

Severe physical stress can increase your body's need for protein. Infections, burns, fevers, and surgery all increase protein losses, and the diet must replace that lost protein. A severe infection can increase protein

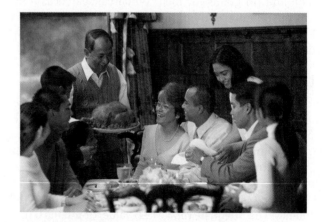

FIGURE 6.12 Protein needs change as we age. Growing children have higher protein needs (as grams per kilogram body weight) than older adults.
© Ariel Skelly/Blend Images/age fotostock.

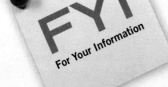

Do Athletes Need More Protein?

Athletes don't just pump iron these days—they also pump protein supplements in hopes of building muscle and improving performance. Look inside many sports magazines, and you'll see ads for protein or amino acid supplements aimed at athletes. You cannot force your body to build muscle by pumping in more protein than you need, any more than you can make your car run faster by adding more gas to a full tank. Extra protein does not build muscles; only regular workouts fueled by a mix of nutrients can do that.

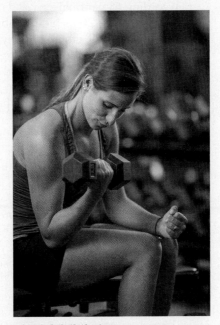

© Christopher Futcher/ E+/ Getty Images.

Protein Requirements for Athletes

Many people assume that because muscle fibers are protein, building muscle must require protein. This is only partially true. The heavy resistance–type exercise that is needed to stimulate muscle growth must first be fueled by glucose and fatty acids. (Glucose will be the predominant fuel.) Little protein is used as a fuel source in resistance-type exercise. Some studies have shown that men who consume the RDA for protein (0.8 gram per kilogram body weight) and engage in heavy resistance exercise go into negative nitrogen balance. However, other studies have shown positive nitrogen balance and muscle hypertrophy during resistance training with intake at the RDA.[a] The DRI committee reviewing evidence on macronutrients concluded that a higher RDA was not warranted for healthy adults doing resistance or endurance exercise.[b] More recent evidence, however, recommends protein in amounts higher than the RDA to maximize training benefits and optimize athletic performance.[c] According to the Academy of Nutrition and Dietetics, athletes may need protein intakes in excess of the RDA.[d] A range of 1.2–2.0 g/kg/day is recommended by the Academy of Nutrition and Dietetics, Dietitians of Canada, the American College of Sports Medicine, and the International Society of Sports Nutrition as necessary to support metabolic adaptations to exercise, repair and remodeling of tissue, and protein turnover. During periods of intensive training or if energy intakes are low, even higher amounts may be needed.[e]

Every effort should be made to meet an athlete's protein requirements with careful meal and snack planning that spreads protein sources throughout the day and provides a variety of high quality dietary choices. Because Americans, on average, consume much more protein than they actually need, any increased need for athletes most likely is being met already. A male athlete in training (let's make him 70 kilograms [154 pounds]) might consume as many as 5,000 kilocalories per day. Even if his diet contained only 10 percent of calories as protein (the low side of the AMDR for protein, and lower than average), he would be getting about 126 grams of protein daily—about 1.8 grams per kilogram. It is unlikely that an athlete would not be able to meet his or her protein needs from a normal, mixed diet. Adequate intake and appropriate timing of protein ingestion have been shown to be beneficial in multiple exercise modes, including endurance, anaerobic, and strength exercise.[f]

Risks of Supplements

Maybe there's no benefit to taking protein or amino acid supplements, but there's no harm either, right? Not necessarily. If excess protein means excess calories, it could lead to added weight as fat, not muscle, which can slow down your performance. Purified protein supplements can contribute to calcium losses, thereby harming bone health. Excess protein means excess nitrogen that must be excreted. This can place an extra burden on kidneys and pose a risk for dehydration if fluid intake is inadequate. Supplements of single amino acids can interfere with the absorption of other amino acids and can affect neurotransmitter activity. The bottom line is that protein or amino acid supplementation has not been shown to positively influence athletic performance, and therefore should not be universally recommended.[g]

If you are a "weekend warrior" there's probably no need to increase the protein in your diet, and little reason to expect that doing so will help your performance. If you are a competitive athlete, choosing adequate calories from a wide variety of foods will ensure an adequate protein intake. Supplements are unnecessary and expensive, and they may disrupt normal protein balance in the body. Play it safe—choose a healthful diet to fuel your exercise.

a Vieillevoye S, Poortmans JR, Duchateau J, Carpentier A. Effects of a combined essential amino acid/carbohydrate supplementation on muscle mass, architecture, and maximal strength following heavy-load training. *Eur J Appl Physiol*. 2010;110(3):479-488.

b Institute of Medicine, Food and Nutrition Board. *Dietary Reference Intakes for Energy, Carbohydrate, Fiber, Fat, Fatty Acids, Cholesterol, Protein, and Amino Acids (Macronutrients)*. Washington, DC: National Academies Press; 2005. https://www.nap.edu/catalog/10490/dietary-reference-intakes-for-energy-carbohydrate-fiber-fat-fatty-acids-cholesterol-protein-and-amino-acids. Accessed September 29, 2017.

c Position of the Academy of Nutrition and Dietetics, Dietitians of Canada, and the American College of Sports Medicine: nutrition and athletic performance. *J Acad Nutr Diet*. 2016;116(3):501-528.

d Ibid.

e Campbell B, Kreider RB, Ziegenfuss T, et al. International Society of Sports Nutrition position stand: protein and exercise. *J Int Soc Sports Nutr*. 2007;4:8.

f Kreider RB, Campbell B. Protein for exercise and recovery. *Phys Sports Med*. 2009;37(2):12-21.

g Position of the American Dietetic Association, Dietitians of Canada, and the American College of Sports Medicine: nutrition and athletic performance. Op. cit.

Quick Bite

Mother's Milk
Because it contains less protein, and in particular less casein protein, infants digest human milk more readily than cows' milk. Milks high in casein protein tend to form curds (clumps) in the stomach upon exposure to stomach acid. These tough curds are hard for digestive enzymes to break apart.

requirements by one-third. Severe burns can increase requirements two to four times. Less severe physical stressors, such as a viral illness with a mild fever lasting only a few days, rarely increase protein requirements. Muscle-building activities, such as intense weight training, increase protein needs much less than most people think. In fact, the typical U.S. diet supplies an ample amount of protein for most people, even for bodybuilders. (See the FYI feature "Do Athletes Need More Protein?")

Protein Consumption

According to national survey data, the median daily intake of protein for women age 20 or older is about 68 grams of protein daily and for men is about 99 grams per day.[24] Individual intake of protein has a large range, but, based on average intake data, Americans are generally eating within the recommended range of 10 to 35 percent of calories from protein.

Does eating more protein help you to build more muscle? No. If dietary intake of protein is greater than the body's protein requirements, the excess amino acids can be converted to glucose for energy or to fatty acids and stored as adipose tissue.[25] Currently under investigation are other detrimental health effects of excess dietary protein, including increased renal stress, bone loss, and increased incidence of colon cancer.[26] On the other hand, if your protein intake is insufficient, the body may break down stored protein in the muscles and transport the amino acids to more vital organs.[27] If energy intake falls dangerously low, protein amino acids can be taken from the muscles and sent to the liver to be converted into glucose to help meet energy needs.

> **Key Concepts**   Infants, who are growing rapidly, have the highest protein needs in proportion to body weight. The recommended intakes, AIs or RDAs, decline from 1.52 grams per kilogram for infants under 6 months old to 0.8 gram per kilogram for adults. Pregnancy, lactation, and severe physical stress all can alter protein requirements. Adults currently consume about 16 percent of their energy as protein, a level that provides ample protein for most people.

Protein Quality

Although both animal and plant foods contain protein, the quality of protein in these foods differs. Foods that supply all the essential amino acids in the proportions needed by the body are called *high-quality proteins*, or **complete proteins**. Foods that lack adequate amounts of one or more essential amino acids are called *low-quality proteins*, or **incomplete proteins**.

Because we typically eat a variety of foods that provide ample dietary protein, we don't ordinarily worry about protein quality. But for people with marginal protein or energy intake and for people who use only one or a few plant foods as their main dietary protein source, protein quality is a critical issue.

Complete Proteins

Animal foods generally provide complete protein; that is, they provide all the essential amino acids in approximately the right proportions. One exception is gelatin, a protein derived from animal collagen that lacks the essential amino acid tryptophan. Red meats, poultry, fish, eggs, milk, and milk products (all animal foods) contain complete protein. Protein supplies more than 20 percent of the energy content of these foods. In water-packed tuna, protein provides about 80 percent of the energy.

▶ **complete proteins**   Proteins that supply all of the indispensable amino acids in the proportions the body needs. Also known as *high-quality proteins*.

▶ **incomplete proteins**   Proteins that lack one or more indispensable amino acids. Also called *low-quality proteins*.

TABLE 6.3
Top 10 Sources of Protein for Children and Adolescents (Ages 2–18) in the United States

Rank	Food	Grams of Protein Consumed[a]
1	Chicken and chicken mixed dishes	9.1
2	Pizza	5.6
3	Reduced fat milk	5.5
4	Beef and beef mixed dishes	3.9
5	Burgers	3.8
6	Yeast breads	3.8
7	Pasta and pasta dishes	3.7
8	Whole milk	2.9
9	Mexican mixed dishes	2.7
10	Regular cheese	2.6

[a] Mean intake of protein = 70 grams

Modified from National Cancer Institute. Sources of protein among US children & adolescents, 2005–06. http://appliedresearch.cancer.gov/diet/foodsources/protein/. Accessed Feb 14, 2017.

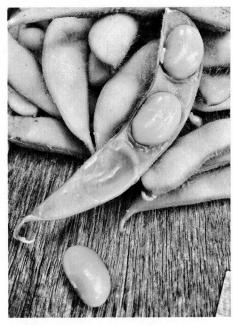

© successo images/Shutterstock.

There is also good news for vegetarians (discussed later in this chapter.) The protein in quinoa is a notable exception to the rule that most plant proteins are incomplete. Also, soybeans provide a good source of protein that has health benefits.[28] (See the FYI feature "High-Protein Plant Foods.")

Americans, on average, get about 63 percent of their protein intake from animal foods.[29] (See **TABLE 6.3**.) In other parts of the world, animal proteins play a smaller role. In Africa and East Asia, for example, animal foods provide only 20 percent of protein intake.[30] Despite national nutrition recommendations to eat a plant-based diet, the United States is a nation of meat-eaters. Beef, chicken, and pork top the list of animal protein sources, with total consumption of beef averaging 67 pounds per person per year.[31] The amount of beef purchased by U.S. consumers in 2016 was almost 26 billion pounds.[32]

Incomplete and Complementary Proteins

With few exceptions, the protein in plant foods is incomplete; that is, it lacks or has only a short supply of one or more essential amino acids and does not match the body's amino acid needs as closely as animal foods do. Although the protein in one plant food may lack certain amino acids, the protein in another plant food may be a **complementary protein** that completes the amino acid pattern. The protein of one plant food can provide the essential amino acid(s) that the other plant food is missing. **TABLE 6.4** lists some examples of complementary food combinations.

Generally, when you combine grains with legumes, or legumes with nuts or seeds, you will get complete, high-quality protein. For example, grain products such as pasta are low in the essential amino acid lysine but high in the essential amino acids methionine and cysteine. Legumes such as kidney beans are low in methionine and cysteine but high in lysine. In a dish that combines these foods, such as a pasta–kidney bean

▶ **complementary protein** An incomplete food protein whose assortment of amino acids makes up for, or complements, another food protein's lack of specific essential amino acids so that the combination of the two proteins provides sufficient amounts of all the essential amino acids.

TABLE 6.4
Examples of Complementary Food Combinations

Beans and corn or wheat tortilla
Rice and lentils
Rice and black-eyed peas
Pea soup with bread or crackers
Hummus (garbanzo beans [chickpeas] with sesame paste [tahini])
Pasta with beans
Peanut butter on bread

salad, the protein from pasta complements the protein from kidney beans, so together they provide a complete protein.

Small amounts of animal foods can also complement the protein in plant foods. For example, Asians often flavor rice with small amounts of beef, chicken, or fish, complementing the protein in the rice. Americans eat breakfast cereal with milk, which complements the protein in the cereal.

If you consume little or no animal protein, you should pay attention to complementary proteins. Consuming a wide variety of plant protein sources is the key to obtaining adequate amounts of all the essential amino acids. When protein and energy intakes are adequate, there is no need to plan complementary proteins at each meal.[33] In the past, it was mistakenly believed that complementary proteins needed to be eaten at the same meal for your body to use them together. Now studies show that your body can combine complementary proteins that are eaten within the same day.[34]

Boosting your intake of plant protein foods can provide additional excellent health benefits. High-protein plant foods are usually rich in vitamins, minerals, dietary fiber, and other health-promoting phytochemicals. Plant foods contain no cholesterol and little fat, and they usually cost less than animal foods high in protein.

Evaluating Protein Quality and Digestibility

A high-quality protein (1) provides all the essential amino acids in the amounts the body needs, (2) provides enough other amino acids to serve as nitrogen sources for making nonessential amino acids, and (3) is easy to digest. If a food protein contains the right proportion of amino acids but cannot be digested and absorbed, it is useless to the body. Protein quality might be assessed to plan a special diet or develop a new product, such as infant formula.

A simple way to determine a food's protein quality is to compare its amino acid composition to that of a reference pattern of amino acids. The reference pattern closely reflects the amounts and proportions of amino acids humans need. The **protein digestibility-corrected amino acid score (PDCAAS)** accounts for both the amino acid composition of a food and the digestibility of the protein. The amino acid present in the smallest amount relative to biological need is called the **limiting amino acid**.

The U.S. Food and Drug Administration (FDA) recognizes the PDCAAS as the official method for determining the protein quality of most food.[35] If the percent Daily Value (%DV) for protein is listed on a food label, it must be based on the food's PDCAAS. It would be misleading to say that, for example, 8 grams of protein from tuna and 8 grams of protein from kidney beans would contribute equally to amino acid needs. Consequently, even though the number of grams of protein per serving might be the same, the %DV would be different for these two foods.

Proteins and Amino Acids as Additives and Supplements

Proteins contribute to the structure, texture, and taste of food. They often are added to foods to enhance these properties. The milk protein casein, for example, is added to frozen dessert toppings. **Protein hydrolysates**—proteins that have been broken down into amino acids

▶ **protein digestibility-corrected amino acid score (PDCAAS)** A measure of protein quality that takes into account the amino acid composition of the food and the digestibility of the protein.

▶ **limiting amino acid** The amino acid in shortest supply during protein synthesis. Also the amino acid in the lowest quantity when evaluating protein quality.

▶ **protein hydrolysates** Proteins that have been treated with enzymes to break them down into amino acids and shorter peptides.

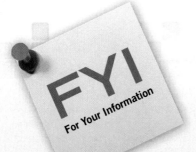

High-Protein Plant Foods

Of the top 10 sources of protein in the U.S. diet, only two—yeast breads and pasta—are plant-based. (See Table 6.3.) Lentils, a dense source of plant protein, don't even make the list. Yet look at the comparison between the nutritional profile of lentils and the profile of beef in **TABLE A**.

TABLE A
How Do Lentils Stack Up Against Beef?

	Cooked Lentils	Lean, Broiled Sirloin
Amount	1 cup	6 oz
Energy	230 kcal	290 kcal
Protein	18 grams	48 grams
Fat	< 1 gram	10 grams
Cholesterol	0	146 milligrams
Carbohydrate	40 grams	0
Dietary fiber	16 grams	0
Percentage of calories from fat	3%	31%

Based on data from U.S. Department of Agriculture, Agricultural Research Service. 2012. USDA National Nutrient Database for Standard Reference,. Nutrient Data Laboratory Home Page, Release 28. September 2015. http://www.ars.usda.gov/nea/bhnrc/ndl. Accessed September 6, 2017.

When we consider these two foods in light of recommendations to eat a more plant-based diet, it's no contest. To reduce dietary fat, saturated fat, and cholesterol while increasing fiber, the lentils win hands down! With all that lentils have going for them, you'd think more Americans would be eating them. Yet dried beans, peas, and lentils combined contribute less than 1 percent of the daily protein intake of Americans, whereas beef contributes 17.7 percent.

High-protein plant foods also contribute complex carbohydrates, dietary fiber, vitamins, and minerals. Because these plant foods contain little fat, they are nutrient dense; that is, they provide a high amount of protein and nutrients in proportion to their energy contribution.

Sources of Plant Protein

Grains and grain products, legumes (lentils and dried beans and peas such as kidney beans or chickpeas), starchy vegetables, and nuts and seeds all provide protein (see **TABLE B**). A serving of a grain product or starchy vegetable provides about 5 grams of protein, a serving of legumes provides 10 to 20 grams of protein, and a serving of vegetables provides about 3 grams of protein. Although a serving of these foods contains less protein than a serving of meat, you can eat more plant protein foods for fewer calories.

Complementing Plant Proteins

It's important to remember that most plant proteins lack one or more of the essential amino acids needed to build body proteins, so individual plant proteins need to complement each other. A simple rule to remember in complementing plant proteins is that combining grains and legumes or combining legumes and nuts or seeds provides complete, high-quality protein.

TABLE B
Plant Sources of Protein

Plant Protein Source	Grams of Protein	Calories
Grain Products		
1 oat bran bagel (3 inch)	7	176
1 whole English muffin, mixed grain	6	155
1 large flour tortilla (10 inch)	6	217
1 cup cooked spaghetti	8	221
1 cup cooked brown rice	5	216
1 cup cooked oatmeal	6	166
2 slices whole wheat bread	7	138
½ cup low-fat granola	4	191
1 cup quinoa	8	222
1 cup amaranth	9	251
Starchy Vegetables		
1 cup cooked corn	5	143
1 cup baked winter squash	2	76
1 medium baked potato with skin	4	161
Legumes		
½ cup tofu	8	92
1 cup cooked lentils	18	230
1 cup cooked kidney beans	15	225
Vegetables		
1 cup cooked broccoli	4	55
1 cup cooked cauliflower	2	29
1 cup cooked Brussels sprouts	4	56
Nuts and Seeds		
2 tablespoons peanut butter	8	188
¼ cup peanuts	9	207
¼ cup sunflower seeds	7	204
1 ounce chia seeds	5	138

Based on data from U.S. Department of Agriculture, Agricultural Research Service. 2012. USDA National Nutrient Database for Standard Reference, Release 28. Nutrient Data Laboratory Home Page, http://www.ars.usda.gov/ba/bhnrc/ndl. Accessed January 14, 2017.

Soy Protein

The protein in soybeans is a notable exception to the rule that most plants are not a good source of protein. Soy provides high-quality protein comparable to that in animal foods.

Soy also contains isoflavonoids, which act as antioxidants, protecting cells and tissues from damage. Isoflavonoids protect low-density lipoprotein (LDL) cholesterol (the kind of cholesterol associated with greater risk of heart disease) from oxidation. Oxidized LDL cholesterol contributes to the plaque buildup in arteries. The isoflavonoids in soybeans also act as phytoestrogens, helping to protect older women from cardiovascular disease and osteoporosis. Soy foods that contain most or all of the bean, such as soy milk, sprouts, flour, and tofu, are the best sources of these phytochemicals. It is easy to incorporate a variety of soy foods into your diet. Tofu, tempeh, ground soy, soy milk, soy flour, and textured soy protein are soy-based products that can be included in many meals and snacks (see **TABLE C**).

The nutritional benefits of plant protein sources such as soy foods and other legumes, grains, and vegetables deserve a closer look. Most Americans would benefit from emphasizing plant protein foods in their diet. Next time you plan to make a meatloaf, try a lentil loaf instead.

TABLE C
Soy Food Products and Suggested Uses

Food	Description
Tofu	A solid cake of curdled soy milk, similar to soft cheese. Tofu comes in hard and soft varieties. It absorbs the flavors of the foods it is mixed with. Soft tofu can be substituted for cheese in pasta dishes, stuffed in large shell pasta, blended with fruit, or used to make pie filling. Hard tofu can be used in salads and shish kebabs and can replace meat in stir-fry or mixed dishes.
Tempeh	A flat cake made from fermented soybeans. It has a mild flavor and chewy texture. Tempeh can be grilled, included in sandwiches, or combined in casseroles such as vegetarian chili.
Meat analogs	Meat alternatives made primarily of soy protein. Flavored and textured to resemble chicken, beef, and pork, they can be substituted for meat in mixed dishes, pizza, tacos, or sloppy joes.
Soy milk	The liquid of the soybean. It comes in regular and low-fat versions and in different flavors. Soy milk can be used plain or substituted for regular milk on cereals or in hot cocoa, puddings, or desserts. Soy milk can be substituted in cooking or baking when a recipe calls for regular milk.
Soy flour	Made from roasted soybeans ground into flour. Soy flour can replace up to one-quarter of the regular flour in a recipe.
Textured soy protein	Textured soy protein resembles ground beef. It can be rehydrated and substituted for ground beef in any recipe.

and shorter peptides—are added to many foods as thickeners, stabilizers, or flavor enhancers.

Amino acids also are used as additives. Monosodium glutamate (sodium bound to the amino acid glutamic acid) is a flavor enhancer added to many foods. The artificial sweetener aspartame is a dipeptide composed of aspartic acid and phenylalanine.

Protein and amino acid supplements are sold to dieters, athletes, and people who suffer from certain diseases. Some protein powders and amino acid supplements are marketed with the claim that they enhance muscle building and exercise performance. Although the anecdotal evidence (stories from friends and health food store clerks) for these products may be convincing, there are limited reliable scientific studies to back up these claims for those who are already eating enough protein from foods. Remember, muscle work builds muscle strength and size, and muscles prefer carbohydrate to fuel this type of work.

THINK
About It

3

Consuming large amounts of individual amino acids has not been shown to be beneficial. An excess of a single amino acid in the digestive tract can impair absorption of certain other amino acids. This could cause a deficiency of one or more amino acids and an unhealthy excess of the supplemented amino acid.

Key Concepts In general, animal foods provide complete protein that contains the right mix of all the essential amino acids. With only a few exceptions, plant foods contain incomplete protein; that is, protein lacking one or more essential amino acids. Plant foods can be combined to complement each other's amino acid patterns. The FDA uses the protein digestibility-corrected amino acid score (PDCAAS) as the official method for determining protein quality. Supplements of protein or amino acids are rarely necessary and might even be harmful.

Vegetarian Eating Patterns

🍎 **Why Is This Important?** National nutrition recommendations emphasize the benefits of a plant-based diet for health benefits such as reducing overweight and obesity and the risk of heart disease, diabetes, and cancer. Even if you do not plan on going completely vegan or even vegetarian, shifting your dietary choices to include more plant foods is a healthy decision.

What did Socrates, Plato, Albert Einstein, Leonardo da Vinci, William Shakespeare, Charles Darwin, and Mahatma Gandhi have in common? They all advocated a vegetarian lifestyle.[36,37] George Bernard Shaw, vegetarian, famous writer, and political analyst of the early 1900s, wrote, "A man fed on whiskey and dead bodies cannot do the finest work of which he is capable."[38]

Meat-eaters often argue that vegetarian diets don't provide enough protein and other essential nutrients, but this isn't necessarily so. With careful planning, a diet that contains limited or even no animal products can be nutritionally complete and offer many health benefits. However, just like a diet that contains animal products, a poorly planned vegetarian diet can be nutritionally inadequate and pose health risks.

Why People Become Vegetarians

In some parts of the world where food is scarce, vegetarianism is not a choice but a necessity. Where food is abundant, people choose vegetarianism for many reasons such as religious beliefs, concern for the environment, a desire to reduce world hunger and to make better use of scarce resources, an aversion to eating another living creature, or concerns about cruelty to animals. Still others become vegetarians because they believe it is healthier. **TABLE 6.5** shows the vegetarian practices of four religious groups. In 2016, about 3.3 percent of U.S. adults considered themselves vegetarian, and almost half of vegetarians are vegan; that is, they eat no animal products at all.[39] Over one-third of Americans make dietary choices to limit their meat intake, and sales of meat alternative products reached $553 million in 2012.[40,41]

THINK About It
4

Quick **Bite**

Eating Lower on the Food Chain Is Good for the Planet

Eating less meat and more plant-based foods is one way to reduce your carbon footprint. Efforts to align diet with global sustainability point to vegetarian diets as an environmentally friendly way to eat. Diets that contain animal proteins require almost 3 times more water, 2.5 times more energy, 13 times more fertilizer, and almost 1.5 times more pesticides than vegetarian diets.

TABLE 6.5
Religions with Vegetarian Dietary Practices

Religion	Dietary Practices
Buddhism	Some sects are lacto-vegetarian; other sects are vegan.
Hinduism	Generally lacto-vegetarian, but mutton or pork are eaten occasionally.
Jainism	Majority lacto-vegetarian, some vegan. Strict Jains will avoid root vegetables, honey, and some fruits and green vegetables.
Seventh-Day Adventism	Lacto-ovo-vegetarian emphasizing whole-grain foods; avoid alcohol, tobacco, and caffeine.

Types of Vegetarian Diets

Although all vegetarians share the common practice of limiting animal products, they differ greatly in specific dietary practices. Some vegetarians avoid red meat but eat small amounts of chicken or fish. Lacto-ovo-vegetarians consume animal products such as milk, cheese, and eggs, but don't eat the flesh of animals. Vegans eat no animal-based foods, including additives derived from animals or insects, and sweeteners such as honey; vegans may also avoid cosmetics and medications containing animal-based ingredients. A "raw vegan" eats only raw fruit, nuts, and green foliage.

The Mediterranean diet, known for reducing the risk of heart disease, is a vegetarian diet rich in grains, pasta, vegetables, cheeses, and olive oil, supplemented with small amounts of chicken and fish. Macrobiotic diets are mostly vegan and stress whole grains, locally grown vegetables, beans, sea vegetables, and soups. Extreme macrobiotic diets can be very limited. **TABLE 6.6** lists different types of vegetarian diets and the foods typically included and excluded.

Health Benefits of Vegetarian Diets

A carefully planned vegetarian eating pattern can be an important contributor to good health. A vegetarian diet that is high in fiber and phytochemicals from whole foods, while at the same time low in processed foods, provides tremendous benefits for prevention and treatment of chronic health conditions.[42] Vegetarian-style diet patterns are associated with lower death from all causes. Vegetarian diets reduce the risk of heart disease—because they usually contain less total fat, saturated fat, trans fat, and cholesterol, but more fiber than nonvegetarian diets.

Vegetarians have a reduced incidence of diabetes and lower rates of cancer, particularly gastrointestinal cancer, than do nonvegetarians.[43,44] Eating red meat, for example, has been linked to a higher risk of colorectal cancer. Vegetarian diets that emphasize fresh fruits and vegetables contain high amounts of antioxidants such as beta-carotene and vitamins C and E, which protect the body's cells and tissues from damage. Fruits and vegetables also contain dietary fiber and phytochemicals; although

TABLE 6.6
Common Types of Vegetarian Diets

Type	Animal Foods Included	Foods Excluded
Vegetarian	Dairy products, eggs, chicken, and fish	Red meats (beef, pork)
Pesco-vegetarian	Dairy products, eggs, and fish	Beef, pork, and poultry
Lacto-ovo-vegetarian	Dairy products and eggs	All animal flesh
Lacto-vegetarian	Dairy products	Eggs and all animal flesh
Ovo-vegetarian	Eggs	Dairy products and all animal flesh
Vegan	None	All animal products
Raw vegan	None	All cooked foods

Modified from Position of the Academy of Nutrition and Dietetics: Vegetarian diets. Academy of Nutrition and Dietetics. Position of the Academy of Nutrition and Dietetics: Vegetarian diets. *J Acad Nutr Diet*. 2016;116:1970-1980.

these substances are not essential in the diet, they can have important health effects.[45]

Vegetarians usually weigh less for their height than nonvegetarians, partly because their diets provide less energy and partly because of other correlated healthful lifestyle factors, such as regular exercise.[46] There is overwhelming evidence of health benefits from following a vegetarian-style eating pattern for the prevention and dietary treatment of numerous chronic conditions, including overweight and obesity, cardiovascular disease, diabetes, cancer, and osteoporosis.[47,48] Vegetarian diets are also good for environmental sustainability. Plant-based diets use fewer natural resources and place less burden on the environment.[49]

Health Risks of Vegetarian Diets

Although vegetarian diets offer many health benefits, certain types of vegetarian diets pose some unique nutritional risks. Vegetarians who simply avoid animal foods or include lots of processed meat-free products while not eating a variety of natural foods, fruits, vegetables, and whole grains may miss out on essential nutrients and therefore compromise their health. The more limited the vegetarian diet, the more likely it is to cause nutritional problems. Some individuals who adopt a vegetarian diet may have unhealthy or disordered eating patterns; elimination of animal foods as a method of weight management can precede an eating disorder.

Vegetarian diets must be planned especially carefully for anyone with special dietary needs or underlying health conditions, the elderly, and anyone experiencing rapid growth, including children and women who are pregnant or breastfeeding.

The nutritional areas of concern for vegetarian children include:

- Providing sufficient energy and nutrients for normal growth
- Providing an adequate iron intake to prevent iron-deficiency anemia
- Identifying adequate sources of vitamin B_{12} to prevent deficiency
- Obtaining sufficient vitamin D and calcium to prevent rickets
- Ensuring a plentiful supply of omega-3 fatty acids from nonmeat sources and fortified foods
- Having food in an appropriate form and combination to ensure that nutrients can be digested and absorbed by the child

Dietary Recommendations for Vegetarians

The *2015–2020 Dietary Guidelines for Americans* and MyPlate dietary guidelines include recommendations and an eating plan for vegetarian diets.[50,51] Vegetarians who include milk, milk products, and eggs in their diet can easily meet their nutritional needs for protein and other essential nutrients, but like meat-eaters they should take care to choose low-fat milk products and limit eggs to avoid excess saturated fat and cholesterol. **TABLE 6.7** lists healthy tips for vegetarians.

Because grains, vegetables, and legumes (soybeans, dried beans, and peas) all provide protein, vegans who eat a variety of foods also can meet their protein needs easily. Although most plant foods do not contain complete protein, eating complementary plant protein sources during the same day adequately meets the body's needs for protein production.

Poorly planned vegetarian diets can be low in zinc, iron, calcium, vitamin D, vitamin B_{12}, and omega-3 fatty acids. The best sources of these nutrients are animal foods—red meat for iron and zinc, milk for

---

TABLE 6.7

Healthy Tips for Vegetarians

A vegetarian eating pattern can be a healthy option. The key is to consume a variety of foods and the right amount of foods to meet your calorie and nutrient needs.

1. **Think about protein.**
   Your protein needs can easily be met by eating a variety of plant foods. Sources of protein for vegetarians include beans and peas, nuts, and soy products (such as tofu and tempeh). Lacto-ovo vegetarians also get protein from eggs and dairy foods.

2. **Bone up on sources of calcium.**
   Calcium is used for building bones and teeth. Some vegetarians consume dairy products, which are excellent sources of calcium. Other sources of calcium for vegetarians include calcium-fortified soymilk (soy beverage), tofu made with calcium sulfate, calcium-fortified breakfast cereals and orange juice, and some dark-green leafy vegetables (collard, turnip, and mustard greens; and bok choy).

3. **Make simple changes.**
   Many popular main dishes are or can be vegetarian, such as pasta primavera, pasta with marinara or pesto sauce, veggie pizza, vegetable lasagna, tofu-vegetable stir-fry, and bean burritos.

4. **Enjoy a cookout.**
   For barbecues, try veggie or soy burgers, soy hot dogs, marinated tofu or tempeh, and fruit kabobs. Grilled veggies are great, too!

5. **Include beans and peas.**
   Because of their high nutrient content, consuming beans and peas is recommended for everyone, vegetarians and nonvegetarians alike. Enjoy some vegetarian chili, three-bean salad, split pea soup or a hummus-filled pita sandwich.

6. **Try different veggie versions.**
   A variety of vegetarian products look—and taste—like their nonvegetarian counterparts but are usually lower in saturated fat and contain no cholesterol. For breakfast, try soy-based sausage patties or links. For dinner, rather than hamburgers, try bean burgers or falafel (chickpea patties).

7. **Make some small changes at restaurants.**
   Most restaurants can make vegetarian modifications to menu items by substituting meatless sauces or nonmeat items, such as tofu and beans for meat, and adding vegetables or pasta in place of meat. Ask about available vegetarian options.

8. **Nuts make great snacks.**
   Choose unsalted nuts as a snack and use them in salads or main dishes. Add almonds, walnuts, or pecans instead of cheese or meat to a green salad.

9. **Get your vitamin B$_{12}$.**
   Vitamin B$_{12}$ is naturally found only in animal products. Vegetarians should choose fortified foods such as cereals or soy products, or take a vitamin B$_{12}$ supplement if they do not consume any animal products. Check the Nutrition Facts label for vitamin B$_{12}$ in fortified products.

10. **Find a vegetarian pattern for you.**
    Go to the *Dietary Guidelines for Americans* and check the appendices for vegetarian (and vegan) adaptations of the USDA food patterns at different calorie levels.

Adapted from U.S. Department of Agriculture. ChooseMyPlate.gov. 10 Tips: Healthy Eating for Vegetarians. http://www.choosemyplate.gov/healthy-eating-tips/tips-for-vegetarian.html. Accessed Feb 15, 2017.

Quick Bite

Paleolithic Protein

How does the fad diet known as "Paleo" stack up to the actual diet of our Paleolithic ancestors? Researchers estimate that ancient hunter-gatherers had diets that were about one-third meat and two-thirds vegetable. The meat from wild game, however, averages only one-seventh the fat of domesticated beef (about 4 grams of fat per 100 grams of wild meat, compared with 29 grams of fat per 100 grams of domestic meat). In addition, compared with the meat at your local supermarket, the fat contained in game animals that graze on the free range has five times as much polyunsaturated fat.

---

calcium and vitamin D, fish for omega-3 fatty acids, and animal foods (fish, meat, poultry, eggs, milk, and milk products) for vitamin B$_{12}$. Because plant foods contain a form of iron that is not as well absorbed as the iron in animal foods, vegetarians need to include more iron in their diets, preferably with a source of vitamin C (from fruits and vegetables), which aids iron absorption into the body. Supplemental and fortified foods are useful to supply missing nutrients and help ensure nutritional adequacy.

Vegans who avoid all animal products must supplement their diets with a reliable source of vitamin B_{12}, such as fortified soy milk. Although bacteria in some fermented foods and in the knobby growths of some seaweeds produce vitamin B_{12}, most vegans do not eat enough seaweeds and fermented foods to meet their vitamin B_{12} needs. Vegans also need a dietary source of vitamin D when sun exposure is limited, either due to SPF sunscreen use or infrequent time spent outdoors.

> **Key Concepts** Vegetarian diets eliminate animal products to various degrees. For example, lacto-ovo-vegetarians include milk and eggs in their diets, whereas vegans eat no animal foods. Vegetarian diets tend to be low in fat and high in fiber and phytochemicals, which may help reduce chronic disease risks. Careful diet planning is necessary for vegans and growing children to ensure that all nutrient needs are met.

The Health Effects of Too Little or Too Much Protein

🍎 **Why Is This Important?** Because protein plays such a vital role in so many body processes, protein deficiency can wreak havoc in numerous body systems. If your body doesn't have enough available protein, it will not have the essential amino acids needed to synthesize body proteins. Too much protein, on the other hand, could contribute to kidney problems, osteoporosis, heart disease, and cancer.

Protein deficiency occurs when energy and/or protein intake is inadequate. Adequate energy intake spares dietary and body proteins so they can be used for protein synthesis. Without adequate energy intake, the body burns dietary protein for energy rather than using it to make body proteins. Protein deficiency can occur even in people who eat seemingly adequate amounts of protein if the protein they eat is of poor quality or cannot be absorbed.

Although protein deficiency is widespread in poverty-stricken communities and in some nonindustrialized countries, most people in industrialized countries face the opposite problem—protein excess. The RDA for a 70-kilogram (154-pound) person is 56 grams, but the average American man (age 20 or older) consumes approximately 100 grams of protein daily, and the average woman (age 20 or older) about 70 grams.[52] Some research suggests that high protein intake contributes to risk for heart disease, cancer, and osteoporosis. However, because high protein intake often goes hand in hand with high intakes of saturated fat and cholesterol, the independent effects of high protein intake are difficult to determine. (See the FYI feature "High-Protein Diets and Supplements.")

Protein-Energy Malnutrition

Hunger and malnutrition are problems worldwide. In the United States, millions of families and individuals with food insecurity worry about where their food will come from and struggle to meet their basic nutritional needs. Malnutrition is a debilitating and widespread problem that leaves individuals vulnerable to disease and death. Worldwide, 1 out of 9 people go to bed hungry, and even worse, 1 in 3 suffer from some form of malnutrition.[53] In children under 5 years of age, nearly half of all deaths are attributable to undernutrition.[54] Fatal cases of undernutrition are caused by a condition called **protein-energy malnutrition (PEM)**, which is a deficiency of protein, energy, or both.

📎 *Position Statement: Academy of Nutrition and Dietetics*

Vegetarian Diets

It is the position of the Academy of Nutrition and Dietetics that appropriately planned vegetarian, including vegan, diets are healthful, nutritionally adequate, and may provide health benefits in the prevention and treatment of certain diseases. These diets are appropriate for all stages of the life cycle, including pregnancy, lactation, infancy, childhood, adolescence, older adulthood, and for athletes. Plant-based diets are more environmentally sustainable than diets rich in animal products because they use fewer natural resources and are associated with much less environmental damage.

Reprinted from Academy of Nutrition and Dietetics. Position of the Academy of Nutrition and Dietetics: Vegetarian diets. *J Acad Nutr Diet.* 2016; 116:1970-1980.

▶ **protein-energy malnutrition (PEM)** A condition resulting from long-term inadequate intakes of energy and protein that can lead to wasting of body tissues and increased susceptibility to infection.

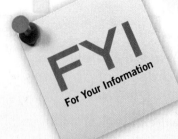

High-Protein Diets and Supplements

One trend popular in sports nutrition is the use of protein and amino acid supplements to build muscle. The theory is straightforward: Muscle mass is predominantly protein, so eating more dietary protein must lead to building bigger muscles. In the 1990s, high-protein diets also became popular, not just for athletes but for those wanting to lose weight. Diets that contained very little fat and carbohydrate unscientifically recommended high amounts of dietary protein as the key to weight loss and peak athletic performance. Do you need more protein to lose weight or gain a competitive edge? Let's take a look at the evidence.

Search the Web for weight loss plans and you'll find programs such as the Paleo diet, Whole 30, and the Protein Power diet, along with older programs such as the Atkins diet plan and the Zone diet. All of these plans promote various high-protein diets for weight loss. These diets revisit the idea, popular in the 1970s (and with historical roots dating back nearly 200 years), that carbohydrates (starches and sugars) make us fat. Proponents of high-protein diets point to the fact that throughout the high-carb, low-fat 1980s and early 1990s and with the explosion of fat-free foods, Americans got fatter. They fail to note that although the percentage of calories from fat in U.S. diets has decreased, Americans are eating more total fat and total

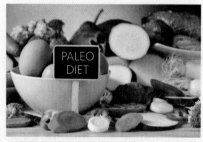

Nito/Shutterstock.

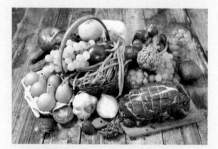

© margouillat photo/Shutterstock.

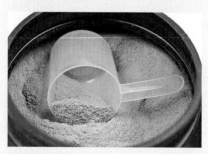

DeymosHR/Shutterstock.

calories (and therefore more total grams of fat) and exercising less—a recipe for weight gain.

Do High-Protein, Low-Carbohydrate Diets Work?

The Atkins diet made headlines in November 2002 when researchers from Duke University presented results of a study comparing the Atkins diet to the American Heart Association's (AHA's) low-fat diet at the AHA's annual scientific meeting. However, skeptics argued that the study, funded by the Atkins Center for Complementary Medicine, included too few people and failed to monitor participants' actual food intake and exercise levels.

Since this report, numerous studies of low-carbohydrate diets have been published, some of which were funded by government sources. An early review of published studies concluded that participant weight loss on low-carbohydrate diets was mainly associated with decreased calorie intake rather than reduced carbohydrate content.[a] A study that compared four different types of popular weight-loss diets also confirmed that overall weight loss at one year was similar regardless of diet.[b] More recently, a systematic review of the effects of high-protein versus low-protein diets on health outcomes found that higher-protein diets may improve risk factors for heart disease and diabetes, but the benefits were minimal and potential for harm should be considered.[c] High-protein diets do seem to influence metabolic pathways leading to satiety, and long-term adherence appears to lead to reduced food intake and lower body fat and body weight.[d]

So what explains reports of dramatic weight loss and no hunger while eating pork rinds, bacon, sausage, and steak? In the short term, removing carbohydrates from the diet causes the body to deplete glycogen stores, which results in a rapid loss of water. The ketosis that results from low carbohydrate intake can also enhance fluid loss. High protein intake tends to be satiating, and the monotony of the diet also blunts the appetite. However, findings seem to all be pointing at one key feature: reducing calories leads to weight loss.

Are High-Protein, Low-Carbohydrate Diets Safe?

Serious health concerns regarding high-protein, low-carbohydrate diets include accumulation of ketone bodies, abnormal insulin metabolism, impaired liver and kidney function, salt and water depletion, impaired kidney function, and high lipid levels resulting from high fat intake. But because such diets are hard to stick with over time, many people fortunately do not develop serious complications. In the short term, constipation, nausea, weakness, dehydration, and fatigue are common side effects. Like many weight loss programs, a high-protein diet may not be dangerous for most healthy people, but those with high risk for bone loss or kidney disease should proceed with caution and seek medical guidance.

If there was one best diet, we wouldn't have so many diet plans vying for our attention and money! What we know about our nutrient needs still points to the *Dietary Guidelines for Americans* for guidance: the best diet emphasizes fruits, vegetables, and whole grains, with a variety of protein foods. It is very difficult for individuals to stick to a particular diet, especially those diets that are most restrictive. The most successful diet is the one a person can stay with over time.[e] For a diet to produce meaningful weight loss, the priority should be on reducing calories, not proportions of protein, carbohydrate, or fat.[f] Successful weight management requires permanent changes to eating habits and, more importantly, increased physical activity.

a Bravata DM, Sanders L, Huang J, et al. Efficacy and safety of low-carbohydrate diets: a systematic review. *JAMA*. 2003;289(14):1837-1850.

b Dansinger ML, Gleason JA, Griffith JL, et al. Comparison of the Atkins, Ornish, Weight Watchers, and Zone diets for weight loss and heart disease risk reduction: a randomized trial. *JAMA*. 2005;293:43-53.

c Santesso N, Akl EA, Bianchi M, et al. Effects of higher- versus lower-protein diets on health outcomes: a systematic review and meta-analysis. *Eur J Clin Nutr*. 2012;66(7):780-788.

d Cuenca-Sánchez M, Navas-Carrillo D, Orenes-Piñero E. Controversies surrounding high-protein diet intake: satiating effect and kidney and bone health. *Adv Nutr*. 2015;6(3):260-266.

e Makris A, Foster GD. Dietary approaches to the treatment of obesity. *Psychiatr Clin North Am*. 2011;34(4):813-827.

f Sacks FM, Bray GA, Carey VJ, et al. Comparison of weight-loss diets with different compositions of fat, protein, and carbohydrates. *N Engl J Med*. 2009;360(9):859-873.

Protein and energy intakes are difficult to separate because diets adequate in energy usually are adequate in protein, and diets inadequate in energy inhibit the body's use of dietary protein for protein synthesis. When both calories and protein are inadequate, dietary protein is used for energy rather than for other necessary functions, forcing the body to break down its own protein to be used as needed. Because protein is a key component for so many different functions in the body, chronic protein deficiency can lead to a number of health problems.

Many situations contribute to PEM, including poverty, insufficient food intake, poor food quality, unsanitary living conditions, and improper feeding of infants and young children.[55] Although it can occur at all stages of life, PEM is most common during childhood, when protein is needed to support rapid growth. Symptoms of PEM can be mild or severe and exist in either acute or chronic forms.

Protein-energy malnutrition occurs in all parts of the world but is most common in Africa, South and Central America, East and Southeast Asia, and the Middle East. Malnutrition is a serious problem, not only in developing countries, but also in the United States. In industrialized countries, PEM occurs most often among people living in poverty, in the elderly, and in hospitalized patients with other conditions such as anorexia nervosa, AIDS, and cancer.

There are two forms of severe malnutrition: **kwashiorkor** and **marasmus**. In some instances, either calorie or protein deficiency exists without the other. Severe protein deficiency is called kwashiorkor, whereas severe calorie and protein deficiency is called marasmus. In general, marasmus is an insufficient energy intake that does not meet the body's requirements. As a result, the body draws on its own stores, resulting in emaciation. In kwashiorkor, adequate carbohydrate consumption and decreased protein intake lead to decreased synthesis of visceral proteins. Children will often have fluid accumulation and the characteristic appearance of a bloated or enlarged abdomen.[56] See **FIGURE 6.13** for signs and symptoms of kwashiorkor and marasmus.

Kwashiorkor

The term *kwashiorkor* is a Ghanaian word that describes the "illness of the first child when the second child is born." In many cultures, babies are breastfed until the next baby comes along. When the new baby arrives, the first baby is weaned from nutritious breast milk and placed on a watered-down version of the family's diet. In areas of poverty, this diet is often low in protein, or the consumed protein is not digested and absorbed easily.

One symptom of kwashiorkor that sets it apart from marasmus is edema, or swelling of body tissue, usually in the feet and legs. Lack of blood proteins reduces the force that keeps fluid in the bloodstream, allowing fluid to leak out into the tissues. Because proteins are unavailable to transport fat, it accumulates in the liver. Combined with edema, this accumulation produces a bloated belly. Other features of kwashiorkor include stunted weight and height; increased susceptibility to infection; dry and flaky skin, and sometimes skin sores; dry, brittle, and unnaturally blond hair; and changes in skin color. Because the energy deficit is usually not as severe (or as long-standing) in kwashiorkor as in marasmus, people with kwashiorkor may still have some body fat stores left.

Kwashiorkor usually develops in children between 18 and 24 months of age, about the time weaning occurs. Its onset can be rapid and is often triggered by an infection or illness that increases the child's

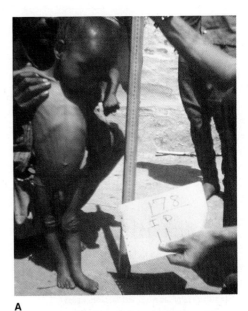

A

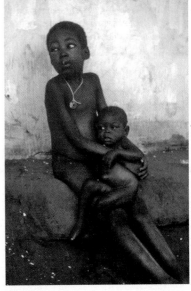

B

FIGURE 6.13 Kwashiorkor and marasmus. a. Edema in the feet and legs and a bloated belly are symptoms of kwashiorkor. b. Children with marasmus are short and thin for their age and can appear frail and wrinkled.

a. Courtesy of CDC/ Dr. Lyle Conrad; b. Courtesy of CDC/Dr. Edward Brink.

▶ **kwashiorkor** A type of malnutrition that occurs primarily in young children who have an infectious disease and whose diets supply marginal amounts of energy and very little protein. Common symptoms include poor growth, edema, apathy, weakness, and susceptibility to infections.

▶ **marasmus** A type of malnutrition resulting from chronic inadequate consumption of protein and energy that is characterized by wasting of muscle, fat, and other body tissue.

protein needs. In hospital settings, kwashiorkor can develop in situations where protein needs are extremely high (e.g., trauma, infection, burns) but dietary intake is poor. Kwashiorkor is associated with extreme poverty in developing countries and, except for people with chronic illness, is rarely seen in affluent countries.

Marasmus

Marasmus is derived from the Greek word *marasmos*, which means "withering" or "to waste away." It develops more slowly than kwashiorkor and results from chronic PEM. Protein, energy, and nutrient intakes are all grossly inadequate, depleting body fat reserves and severely wasting muscle tissue, including vital organs like the heart. Growth slows or stops, and children are both short and very thin for their age. Metabolism slows and body temperature drops as the body tries to conserve energy. Children with marasmus are apathetic, often not even crying in an effort to conserve energy. Their hair is sparse and falls out easily. Because muscle and fat are used up, a child with marasmus often looks like a frail, wrinkled, elderly person.

Marasmus occurs most often in infants and children 6 to 18 months of age who are fed diluted or improperly mixed formulas. Because this is a time of rapid brain growth, marasmus can permanently stunt brain development and lead to learning disabilities. Marasmus also occurs in adults who have cancer or are experiencing starvation, including the self-imposed starvation of the eating disorder known as anorexia nervosa.

Health Effects of Excess Dietary Protein

In industrialized countries, an excess of protein and energy is more common than a deficiency. Generally, self-selected diets do not contain more than 40 percent of calories from protein.[57] Although high protein intake has been suggested to contribute to kidney problems, osteoporosis, heart disease, and cancer (see **FIGURE 6.14**), the Food and Nutrition Board decided that evidence to support these links was not strong enough to set a UL for protein.[58]

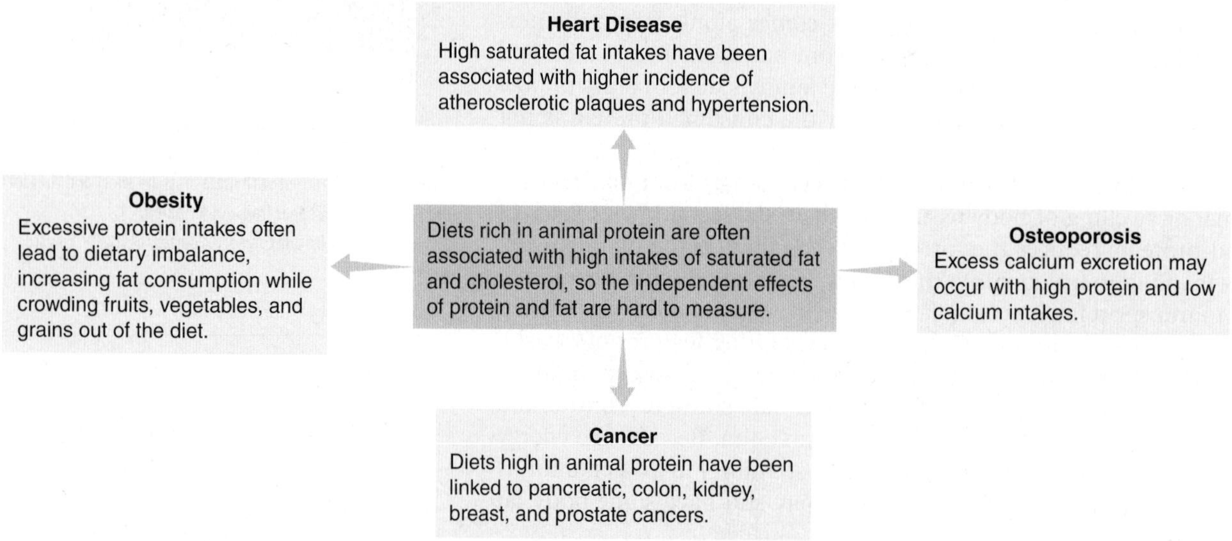

Quick Bite

The Source of Salisbury Steak

Dr. James Salisbury, a London physician who lived in the late 1800s, believed humans to be two-thirds carnivorous and one-third herbivorous. He recommended a diet low in starch and high in lean meat, with lots of hot water to rinse out the products of fermentation. His diet regimen included broiled, lean, minced beef three times a day. Although we call it Salisbury steak as a courtesy to Dr. Salisbury's heritage, minced beef patties are really more like hamburgers.

Heart Disease
High saturated fat intakes have been associated with higher incidence of atherosclerotic plaques and hypertension.

Obesity
Excessive protein intakes often lead to dietary imbalance, increasing fat consumption while crowding fruits, vegetables, and grains out of the diet.

Diets rich in animal protein are often associated with high intakes of saturated fat and cholesterol, so the independent effects of protein and fat are hard to measure.

Osteoporosis
Excess calcium excretion may occur with high protein and low calcium intakes.

Cancer
Diets high in animal protein have been linked to pancreatic, colon, kidney, breast, and prostate cancers.

FIGURE 6.14 Excess protein. In developed countries, excess protein and energy are a more common problem than protein deficiency and may lead to undesirable health consequences.

Kidney Function

Because the kidneys must excrete the products of protein breakdown, there is concern that a high protein intake can strain kidney function and is especially harmful for people with kidney disease or diabetes. A diet with a higher proportion of calories coming from protein increases kidney filtration rate in healthy adults, suggesting that a high-protein diet may have a long-term adverse consequence on kidney function.[59]

To prevent dehydration, it is important to drink plenty of fluids to dilute the byproducts of protein breakdown for excretion. Human infants should not be fed unmodified cow's milk until they are at least 1 year of age because the high protein concentration in cow's milk combined with an immature kidney system can cause excessive fluid losses and dehydration.

Mineral Losses

The impact of dietary protein on calcium and bone health is controversial. It was once widely thought that high intakes of protein from animal sources would lead to bone loss and increases in fractures. The link between high-protein diets and osteoporosis is based on studies showing that a high protein intake increases calcium excretion, which could then contribute to bone mineral losses. However, these studies generally used purified proteins rather than food proteins. Other studies have found favorable effects on bone mineral density from increasing intake of protein, as long as the diet contains adequate dietary calcium.[60] A review of research using various study designs suggests that dietary protein improves the retention of calcium and promotes bone metabolism.[61]

Obesity

Some epidemiological studies have shown a correlation between high protein intake and body fatness.[62] High-protein foods can be high in fat, and a diet high in fat and protein may provide too much energy, contributing to obesity. Additionally, eating large amounts of high-protein foods displaces fruits, vegetables, and grains—foods that contain fewer calories. Despite this, however, higher protein intakes (1.2 g/kg body weight) have been shown to be beneficial to both body weight and blood pressure.[63,64] Currently, protein is being studied for the role it plays in satiety and energy expenditure.[65]

Heart Disease

Research has linked high intake of foods rich in animal protein, especially processed meats, to high blood cholesterol levels and increased risk of heart disease, stroke, cancer, and diabetes.[66-71] Foods high in animal protein are also high in saturated fat and cholesterol. Whether protein alone—independent of fat—plays a role in the development of heart disease is less clear. Soy protein foods contain no saturated fat or cholesterol, and the FDA approved a health claim saying that soy protein is beneficial in reducing the risk of heart disease. Some epidemiological studies, however, found that consuming soy protein has little or no effect on the risk factors for heart disease.[72] The researchers suggested that consuming soy protein products, such as tofu, soy butter, soy nuts, and some soy burgers, should be beneficial because of their low saturated fat content and high content of polyunsaturated fats, fiber, vitamins, and minerals. Using these and other soy foods to replace foods high in animal protein can reduce intake of saturated fat and cholesterol.[73] Choosing less red meat, and processed meat in particular, could have beneficial effects toward reducing the risk of type 2 diabetes and cardiovascular disease.[74]

Cancer

Studies suggest a correlation between a diet high in certain animal proteins and an increased risk for certain types of cancers. For example, prolonged high intake of both red meat (e.g., beef, pork) and processed meat (e.g., ham, smoked meats, sausage, bacon) has been convincingly linked to increased colon cancer risk and cancer mortality.[75-79]

Key Concepts Protein-energy malnutrition (PEM) is a common form of malnutrition in the developing world, with potentially devastating effects for children. PEM can take two forms: kwashiorkor and marasmus. Among other symptoms, kwashiorkor is characterized by edema, or swelling of the tissues. Marasmus results from chronic PEM and is characterized by severe wasting of body fat and muscles. Intake of too much protein may contribute to obesity, heart disease, and certain forms of cancer. These links, however, may be attributed to the high fat intake that often accompanies high protein intake.

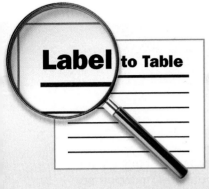
Have you ever visited a health food store and noticed all the protein powders, amino acid supplements, and high-protein bars? Do you believe claims like "protein boosts your energy level" or "amino acid *x* helps you build muscle" or "protein shakes are the best preworkout fuel"? You know from this text that protein is an important nutrient and it's used to build and repair tissue. But do you need one of these supplements? Before reaching into your wallet, check out the Nutrition Facts of this protein powder and determine whether it's a good buy.

Look at this label and note how far down protein is on the list of nutrients. This placement is intentional and attempts to encourage consumers to de-emphasize protein in their diets. You may recall that most Americans eat more protein than they need, and because much of that protein comes from animal foods, they are also getting excess saturated fat. Although there is a DV for protein (50 grams), manufacturers must first determine a food protein's quality before they can determine %DV. Manufacturers are not required to give the %DV for protein on food labels.

Do protein and amino acid supplements do what they claim to do? In terms of building muscle, exercise physiologists agree that it takes consistent muscle work (i.e., weight lifting) and a healthful diet that meets the body's calorie needs. Building muscle does not depend on extra protein. In fact, muscles mainly use carbohydrate and fat for fuel, not protein, so these other nutrients are more important for effective workouts.

In terms of protein's ability to boost your energy level, recall that anything with calories (carbohydrates, proteins, and fats) provides the body with "energy." In fact, unlike carbohydrates and fats, only a small amount of protein is used for energy expenditure. Research shows that the best thing to eat before a workout is carbohydrate, not protein, because carbohydrate provides glucose to the muscle cells. Review this label again. What percentage of this protein powder's calories comes from protein?

154 kilocalories

11 grams protein × 4 kilocalories per gram = 44 protein kilocalories

44 ÷ 154 = 0.28, or 28% protein kilocalories

Surprise, surprise! Only about one-quarter of the powder's calories are protein anyway, so it's okay as a preworkout fuel, not because of its protein content but because of its ample carbohydrate!

Nutrition Facts

18 servings per container

Servings size	2 scoops

Amount per serving

Calories	150

	% Daily Value*
Total Fat 4g	
Saturated Fat 2.5g	6%
Trans Fat 0g	12%
Cholesterol 20mg	
Sodium 170mg	7%
Total Carbohydrate 17g	7%
Dietary Fiber 0g	6%
Total Sugars 14g	0%
Includes 10g Added Sugars	20%
Protein 11g	
Vitamin D 0mcg	0%
Calcium 400mg	40%
Iron 0mg	0%
Potassium 185mg	5%

*The % Daily Value (DV) tells you how much a nutrient in a serving of food contributes to a daily diet. 2,000 calories a day is used for general nutrition advice.

Learning Portfolio

Key Terms

Study Points

- Many vital molecules in the human body are proteins, including enzymes, hormones, transport proteins, and regulators of both acid–base and fluid balance.
- Amino acids are composed of a central carbon atom bonded to a hydrogen atom, carboxyl and amino groups, and side groups.
- Twenty amino acids are important in human nutrition; 9 of these amino acids are considered essential (must come from the diet), whereas the body can make the other 11 nonessential amino acids.
- Proteins are long chains of amino acids.
- The amino acid sequence of a protein determines its shape and function.
- Denaturing proteins changes their shape and therefore their functional properties.
- Hydrochloric acid in the stomach denatures proteins so the enzyme pepsin can begin their digestion.
- Proteins are completely digested in the small intestine and, after absorption, are carried to the liver.
- Dietary protein is found in meats, dairy products, legumes, nuts, seeds, grains, and vegetables.
- In general, animal foods contain higher-quality protein than is found in plant foods.
- Protein needs are highest when growth is rapid, such as during infancy, childhood, adolescence, and pregnancy.
- The protein intake of most Americans exceeds their RDA.
- Protein deficiency is most common in developing countries and often results in marasmus and kwashiorkor.
- Protein excess is also harmful and may affect risk for heart disease and cancer.

Study Questions

1. Describe the differences among essential, nonessential, and conditionally essential amino acids.
2. List the functions of body proteins.
3. How is protein related to immune function?
4. What is meant by nitrogen balance? Give examples of conditions associated with positive and negative nitrogen balance.

5. What are complementary proteins? List three examples of food combinations that contain complementary proteins.

6. Describe a vegan diet.

7. List the potential health benefits of a vegetarian diet.

8. What health effects occur if you are protein deficient?

9. What health effects can occur over time from consuming too much protein?

Try This

The Sweetness of NutraSweet

The purpose of this experiment is to see the effect of high temperatures on the dipeptide known as NutraSweet (aspartame). Make a cup of hot tea (or coffee) and add one packet of Equal (one brand of aspartame). Stir and taste the tea; note its sweetness. Reheat the tea (via a microwave or stovetop) so it boils for 30 to 60 seconds. After the tea cools, taste it. Does it still taste sweet? Why or why not?

The Vegetarian Challenge

The purpose of this activity is to eat a completely vegan diet for a few days. Begin by making a list of your typical meals and snacks. Once the list is complete, review each food item and determine whether it contains animal products. Cross off items that contain animal products, and circle the remaining vegan-friendly options. Double-check the circled list with a friend or roommate. You may have missed something! Create a full day's worth of meals and snacks using your circled foods as well as additional vegan options. Make sure your menu looks complete and nutritionally balanced. Try to stick to this menu for at least three days. Pay attention to deviations you make, and determine whether these are vegan food choices.

Getting Personal

General instructions: List all of the foods and drinks that you consume in a 24-hour period, ideally on a day where your schedule is fairly predictable and you are eating what you consider normal for you.

Take a minute to review your food intake, focusing especially on protein.

Part A: Compare your intake to the recommendations:

1. How do you think you did? Do you think you're lower or higher than the RDA?

2. Calculate your RDA. Your protein RDA is calculated as follows:

___ (your weight in pounds) ÷ 2.2 pounds = ___ kilograms × 0.8 g/kg/day = ___ g protein daily

3. Compare your protein RDA with your protein intake. Are you surprised by the results? Are you eating too much protein or just the right amount? How many more or fewer grams should you consume?

4. Another way to evaluate your protein intake is in terms of calories. What was your total kilocalorie intake? If your total protein intake is ___ grams (× 4 kcal/gram) = __ kilocalories come from protein.

   a. For example: 96 g protein × 4 kcal/g = 384 kcal from protein. Assuming a 2,300-kcal diet, this amount is 17 percent of calories from protein. This falls within the recommended AMDR of 10–35 percent calories from protein.

5. What percentage of your total calories comes from protein? How does this compare to the AMDR for your caloric intake? (See sample calculation above.) Does the percentage of protein in your diet fall within the recommended range?

6. Compare the two numbers (your RDA calculation vs. your AMDR) for recommended protein intake. Do you meet the guidelines for protein intake using both recommendations? What could be the reason?

Part B: Now look at the protein-containing foods in your diet:

1. What foods contribute most to the protein in your diet?

2. **Activity:** Meatless Monday planning: Try to increase your plant-based choices. For each animal product on your list, suggest a plant-based substitute for that food. Then, compare the amount of protein in the plant-based food to the animal product.

   a. What happens to your protein intake when you go meatless? What effect does this have on your total calorie and fat intake?

   b. What other nutrients could these changes affect?

   c. What would be some challenges to eating a diet that is more plant-based?

   d. List three plant-based foods that would be a good source of protein that you are willing to try.

Learning Portfolio (continued)

References

1. Matthews DE. Proteins and amino acids. In Ross AC, Caballero B, Cousins RJ, Tucker KL, Ziegler TR, eds. *Modern Nutrition in Health and Disease.* 11th ed. Baltimore, MD: Lippincott Williams and Wilkins; 2014:3–35.

2. Ibid.

3. National Institutes of Health, U.S. National Library of Medicine. Genetics home reference: phenylketonuria. July 2017. https://ghr.nlm.nih.gov /condition/phenylketonuria. Accessed September 29, 2017.

4. Ziegler TR. Glutamine. In Ross AC, Caballero B, Cousins RJ, Tucker KL, Ziegler TR, eds. *Modern Nutrition in Health and Disease.* 11th ed. Baltimore, MD: Lippincott Williams and Wilkins; 2014:464–476.

5. Ibid.

6. Luiking YC, Castillo L, Deutz NEP. Arginine, citrulline, and nitric oxide. In Ross AC, Caballero B, Cousins RJ, Tucker KL, Ziegler TR, eds. *Modern Nutrition in Health and Disease.* 11th ed. Baltimore, MD: Lippincott Williams and Wilkins; 2014.

7. Gropper SG, Smith JL, Carr TP. *Advanced Nutrition and Human Metabolism.* 7th ed. Boston MA: Cengage Learning; 2017.

8. Nathan DM. Diabetes: advances in diagnosis and treatment. *JAMA.* 2015;314(10):1052-1062. doi:10.1001/jama.2015.9536

9. Marroqui L, Gonzalez A, Neco P, et al. Role of leptin in the pancreatic beta-cell: effects and signaling pathways. *J Mol Endocrinol.* 2012;49(1): R9-R17. doi: 10.1530/JME-12-0025

10. Pietzak M. Celiac disease, wheat allergy, and gluten sensitivity: when gluten free is not a fad. *J Parenter Enteral Nutr.* 2012;36(1 Suppl):68S-75S. doi: 10.1177/0148607111426276

11. Ibid.

12. Gaesser GA, Angadi SS. Navigating the gluten-free boom. *J Am Acad Physician Assist.* 2015;28(8). doi: 10.1097/01.JAA.0000469434.67572.a4

13. Hartman LR. Gluten-free products are going gangbusters. *Food Process.* July 29, 2015. http://www.foodprocessing.com/articles/2015/gluten-free-products-are-going-gangbusters/?show=all. Accessed September 7, 2017.

14. Matthews DE. Op. cit.

15. Medeiros DM, Wildman RC. *Advanced Human Nutrition.* 3rd ed. Burlington, MA: Jones & Bartlett Learning; 2015.

16. Institute of Medicine, Food and Nutrition Board. *Dietary Reference Intakes for Energy, Carbohydrate, Fiber, Fat, Fatty Acids, Cholesterol, Protein, and Amino Acids.* Washington, DC: National Academies Press; 2005.

17. Gropper SG, Smith JL, Carr TP. Op. cit.

18. Institute of Medicine, Food and Nutrition Board. *Dietary Reference Intakes for Energy, Carbohydrate, Fiber, Fat, Fatty Acids, Cholesterol, Protein, and Amino Acids (Macronutrients).* Washington, DC: National Academies Press; 2005. https://www.nap.edu/catalog/10490 /dietary-reference-intakes-for-energy-carbohydrate-fiber-fat-fatty-acids -cholesterol-protein-and-amino-acids. Accessed September 29, 2017.

19. Ibid.

20. Bernstein MA, Munoz N. Position of the Academy of Nutrition and Dietetics: food and nutrition for older adults: promoting health and wellness. *J Acad Nutr Diet.* 2012;112:1255-1277.

21. Ibid.

22. Ibid.

23. Paddon-Jones D, Rasmussen B. Dietary protein recommendations and the prevention of sarcopenia. *Curr Opin Clin Nutr Metab Care.* 2009;12(1):86-90.

24. U.S. Department of Agriculture. What we eat in America. NHANES 2011-2012. http://www.ars.usda.gov/Services/docs.htm?docid=18349. Accessed September 7, 2017.

25. Hall J. *Guton and Hall Textbook of Medical Physiology.* 12th ed. Philadelphia: Saunders/Elsevier; 2011.

26. Medeiros DM, Wildman RC. Op. cit.

27. Mahan LK, Raymond J, Escott-Stump S. *Krause's Food and Nutrition Therapy.* 13th ed. St. Louis, MO: Saunders Elsevier; 2011.

28. Tuso PJ, Ismail MH, Ha BP, Bartolotto C. Nutrition update for physicians: plant-based diets. *Perm J.* 2013;17(2):61-66.

29. U.S. Department of Agriculture. Nutrient content of the U.S. food supply. http://www.cnpp.usda.gov/USfoodsupply. Accessed September 7, 2017.

30. Ibid.

31. Davis CG, Biing-Hwan L. Factors affecting U.S. beef consumption. U.S. Department of Agriculture, Economic Research Service. October 2005. https://wayback.archive-it.org/5923/20111209010403/http://www.ers .usda.gov/Publications/LDP/Oct05/LDPM13502/. Accessed September 7, 2017.

32. National Cattlemen's Beef Association. Beef Industry Statistics http:// www.beefusa.org/beefindustrystatistics.aspx. Accessed September 28, 2017.

33. Position of the Academy of Nutrition and Dietetics: Vegetarian diets. *J Acad Nutr Diet.* 2016;116:1970-1980.

34. Ibid.

35. U.S. Food and Drug Administration. Guidance for industry: a food labeling guide. January 2013. http://www.fda.gov/Food/GuidanceRegulation/GuidanceDocumentsRegulatoryInformation/LabelingNutrition /ucm2006828.htm. Accessed September 7, 2017.

36. Ballentine R. *Transition to Vegetarianism: An Evolutionary Step.* Honesdale, PA: Himalayan International Institute of Yoga Science and Philosophy; 1987.

37. Null G. *The Vegetarian Handbook: Eating Right for Total Health.* New York: St. Martin's Press; 1987.

38. Ibid.

39. Vegetarian Resource Group. How many adults in the U.S. are vegetarian and vegan? How many adults eat vegetarian and vegan meals when eating out? http://www.vrg.org/nutshell/Polls/2016_adults_veg.htm. Accessed September 7, 2017.

40. Ibid.

41. Position of the Academy of Nutrition and Dietetics: vegetarian diets. Op. cit.

42. Physicians Committee for Responsible Medicine. Vegetarian foods: powerful for health. http://www.pcrm.org/health/diets/vegdiets/vegetarian-foods-powerful-for-health. Accessed September 7, 2017.

43. Tonstad S, Stewart K, Oda K, Batech M, Herring RP, Fraser GE. Vegetarian diets and incidence of diabetes in the Adventist Health Study-2. *Nutr Metab Cardiovasc Dis.* 2013;23(4):292-299. doi:10.1016/ j.numecd.2011.07.004. Epub October 7, 2011.

44. Tantamango-Bartley Y, Jaceldo-Siegl K, Fan J, Fraser G. Vegetarian diets and the incidence of cancer in a low-risk population. *Cancer Epidemiol Biomarkers Prev.* 2013;22(2):286-294. doi: 10.1158/1055-9965.EPI-12-1060. Epub November 20, 2012.

45. McEvoy CT, Temple N, Woodside JV. Vegetarian diets, low-meat diets and health: a review. *Public Health Nutr.* 2012;15(12):2287-2294. doi: 10.1017/S1368980012000936. Epub April 3, 2012.

46. Orlich MJ, Singh PN, Sabaté J, et al. Vegetarian dietary patterns and mortality in Adventist Health Study 2. *JAMA Intern Med.* 2013;173(13):1230-1238. doi: 10.1001/jamainternmed.2013.6473

47. U.S. Department of Health and Human Services, U.S. Department of Agriculture. *2015–2020 Dietary Guidelines for Americans.* 8th ed. December 2015. http://health.gov/dietaryguidelines/2015/guidelines/. Accessed September 7, 2017.

48. Position of the Academy of Nutrition and Dietetics: vegetarian diets. Op. cit.

49. Nelson ME, Hamm MW, Hu FB, Abrams SA, Griffin TS. Alignment of healthy dietary patterns and environmental sustainability: a systematic review. *Adv Nutr.* 2016;7(6):1005-1025.

50. U.S. Department of Agriculture. 10 tips: healthy eating for vegetarians. ChooseMyPlate.gov. http://www.choosemyplate.gov/healthy-eating-tips/tips-for-vegetarian.html. Accessed September 7, 2017.

51. U.S. Department of Agriculture, U.S. Department of Health and Human Services. *2015–2020 Dietary Guidelines for Americans*. Op. cit.

52. U.S. Department of Agriculture, Agriculture Research Service. What we eat in America, NHANES 2013-2014. https://www.ars.usda.gov/ARSUserFiles/80400530/pdf/1314/Table_1_NIN_GEN_13.pdf. Accessed September 7, 2017.

53. World Food Programme. Zero hunger. http://www1.wfp.org/zero-hunger. Accessed September 7, 2017.

54. UNICEF. Undernutrition contributes to nearly half of all deaths in children under 5 and is widespread in Asia and Africa. http://data.unicef.org/topic/nutrition/malnutrition/. Accessed September 7, 2017.

55. World Health Organization. WHO global database on child growth and malnutrition. http://www.who.int/nutgrowthdb/en. Accessed September 7, 2017.

56. Scheinfeld N. Protein-energy malnutrition. http://emedicine.medscape.com/article/1104623-overview#a0104. Accessed September 7, 2017.

57. Institute of Medicine, Food and Nutrition Board. *Dietary Reference Intakes for Energy, Carbohydrate, Fiber, Fat, Fatty Acids, Cholesterol, Protein, and Amino Acids*. Op. cit.

58. Ibid.

59. Juraschek SP, Appel LJ, Anderson CA, Miller ER 3rd. Effect of a high-protein diet on kidney function in healthy adults: results from the Omni-Heart trial. *Am J Kidney Dis*. 2013;61(4):547-554. doi: 10.1053/j.ajkd.2012.10.017. Epub December 4, 2012.

60. Mangano KM, Sahni S, Kerstetter JE. Dietary protein is beneficial to bone health under conditions of adequate calcium intake: an update on clinical research. *Curr Opin Clin Nutr Metab Care*. 2014;17(1):69-74.

61. Kerstetter JE, Kenny AM, Insogna KL. Dietary protein and skeletal health: a review of recent human research. *Curr Opin Lipidol*. 2011;22(1):16-20.

62. Hall KD. Predicting metabolic adaptation, body weight change, and energy intake in humans. *Am J Physiol Endocrin Metab*. 2010;298(3):E449-E466.

63. Westerterp-Plantenga MS, Lemmens SG, Westerterp KR. Dietary protein—its role in satiety, energetics, weight loss and health. *Br J Nutr*. 2012;108(Suppl 2):S105-S112.

64. Soenen S, Martens EA, Hochstenbach-Waelen A, Lemmens SG, Westerterp-Plantenga MS. Normal protein intake is required for body weight loss and weight maintenance, and elevated protein intake for additional preservation of resting energy expenditure and fat free mass. *J Nutr*. 2013;143(5):591-596.

65. Tremblay A, Bellisle F. Nutrients, satiety and control of energy intake. *Appl Physiol Nutr Metabol*. 2015;40(10):971-979.

66. Bernstein AM, Pan A, Rexrode KM, et al. Dietary protein sources and the risk of stroke in men and women. *Stroke*. 2012;43(3):637-644. doi: 10.1161/STROKEAHA.111.633404. Epub December 29, 2011.

67. Pan A, Sun Q, Bernstein AM, et al. Red meat consumption and mortality: results from 2 prospective cohort studies. *Arch Intern Med*. 2012;172(7):555-563. doi: 10.1001/archinternmed.2011.2287. Epub March 12, 2012.

68. Micha R, Michas G, Mozaffarian D. Unprocessed red and processed meats and risk of coronary artery disease and type 2 diabetes—an updated review of the evidence. *Curr Atheroscler Rep*. 2012;14(6):515-524. doi: 10.1007/s11883-012-0282-8

69. Feskens EJ, Sluik D, van Woudenbergh GJ. Meat consumption, diabetes, and its complications. *Curr Diab Rep*. 2013;13(2):298-306. doi: 10.1007/s11892-013-0365-0

70. Pan A, Sun Q, Bernstein AM, et al. Op. cit.

71. Feskens EJ, Sluik D, van Woudenbergh GJ. Op cit.

72. Messina M. Insights gained from 20 years of soy research. *J Nutr*. 2010;140(12):2289S-2295S.

73. Patisaul HB, Jefferson W. The pros and cons of phytoestrogens. *Front Neuroendocrinol*. 2010;31(4):400-419.

74. Micha R, Michas G, Mozaffarian D. Op. cit.

75. Tuan J, Chen YX. Dietary and lifestyle factors associated with colorectal cancer risk and interactions with microbiota: fiber, red or processed meat and alcoholic drinks. *Gastrointest Tumors*. 2016;3:17-24.

76. Corpet DE. Red meat and colon cancer: should we become vegetarians, or can we make meat safer? *Meat Sci*. 2011;89(3):310-316.

77. Hu J, La Vecchia C, Morrison H, et al. Salt, processed meat, and the risk of cancer. *Eur J Cancer Prev*. 2011;20(2):132-139.

78. Pan A, Sun Q, Bernstein AM, et al. Op. cit.

79. Carr PR, Walter V, Brenner H, Hoffmeister M. Meat subtypes and their association with colorectal cancer: systematic review and meta-analysis. *Int J Cancer*. 2016 138(2):293-302. doi: 10.1002/ijc.29423. Epub February 24, 2015.

Chapter 7

Vitamins: Vital Keys to Health

Revised by Feon Cheng and Fabio Giallongo

THINK About It

1   What food group, if any, supplies most of your vitamin needs?

2   When cooking vegetables, do you think about vitamin loss?

3   You decide to follow a strict vegan lifestyle. What vitamin deficiencies should you watch out for?

4   Do you know anyone who takes vitamin supplements to increase their energy levels? What do you think of this strategy?

LEARNING Objectives

1 Describe the key features of the fat-soluble and water-soluble vitamins.
2 List the major functions of each vitamin.
3 Identify the major food sources of each vitamin.
4 Specify the major symptoms and diseases associated with deficiency and toxicity of different vitamins.
5 Discuss why fat-soluble vitamins have greater toxicity than water-soluble vitamins.
6 Discuss the reasons behind enrichment and fortification programs for the prevention of neural tube defects, anemia, and vitamin deficiencies.
7 List ways to select, prepare, and store foods to maximize vitamin content.

Feeling tired, run down, stressed out? You've heard that vitamins give you energy. So a lack of energy must be a signal that you need more vitamins, right? Well, probably not. Although many people like to think of vitamins as energy boosters, in truth, vitamins do not supply calories for the body—a fact that distinguishes them from fat, carbohydrate, and protein. However, you do need certain vitamins to obtain energy from those nutrients, and vitamins can aid the body's healing process during times of physical stress, such as injury or illness.

What about if you're a serious athlete—surely then you should take a vitamin supplement, right? Again, not necessarily. Physical activity requires energy and vitamins to aid metabolism. But the extra food you eat to meet your greater energy needs already contains vitamins—unless your diet consists mostly of chips, sodas, and the like. In most cases, adding fruits, vegetables, and grains will provide all the vitamins and energy you need. So, check out the vitamin content of your diet before you check out the vitamin supplements! This chapter will help you understand the facts about vitamins—what they are, what they do in the body, and which foods contain them—as well as explore some of the implications of too much or too little of each type of vitamin in the diet.

Understanding Vitamins

🍎 **Why Is This Important?** Vitamins are nutrients that play important roles in our body. Understanding the different types of vitamins, which foods contain them, and how they are affected by food preparation can help you make wise decisions for good health.

Vitamins differ from fat, protein, and carbohydrate in many important ways. For one, the body requires large amounts of carbohydrate, protein, and fat—amounts measured in grams. By comparison, the daily needs for vitamins are small—a mere microgram or two in some cases. In addition, unlike fat, protein, and carbohydrate, vitamins are not a source of energy. However, many vitamins play crucial roles in the chemical

Quick Bite

Over a Third of Americans Take Multivitamins

Multivitamin/mineral supplements are the most commonly used dietary supplements in the United States. The first multivitamin/mineral formula was introduced in the 1930s, and now more than one-third of adults in the United States report regular use.

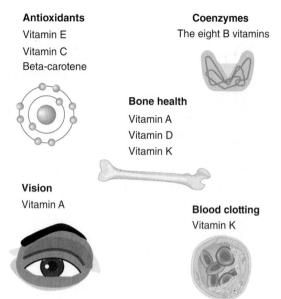

Antioxidants
Vitamin E
Vitamin C
Beta-carotene

Coenzymes
The eight B vitamins

Bone health
Vitamin A
Vitamin D
Vitamin K

Vision
Vitamin A

Blood clotting
Vitamin K

FIGURE 7.1 Major roles of vitamins and carotenoids. Vitamins are crucial for normal functioning, growth, and maintenance of body tissues. Compared with carbohydrate, fat, and protein, the body needs tiny amounts of vitamins.

reactions that extract energy from those nutrients. Another difference is structural: Vitamins are individual units rather than long chains of smaller units.

Like fat, carbohydrate, and protein, however, vitamins are organic (carbon-containing) compounds essential for normal functioning, growth, and maintenance of the body. The functions of vitamins can be interrelated (see **FIGURE 7.1**), so a deficiency of just one can cause profound health problems.

Fat-Soluble Versus Water-Soluble Vitamins

Scientists classify vitamins as *fat-soluble* and *water-soluble*. Vitamins A, D, E, and K are fat-soluble vitamins. The B vitamins and vitamin C, in contrast, dissolve in water. A general comparison of fat-soluble and water-soluble vitamins can be found in **TABLE 7.1**. This difference in solubility affects the way our body absorbs, transports, and stores vitamins. (See **FIGURE 7.2**.)

Intestinal cells absorb fat-soluble vitamins along with dietary fat and package them into lipoproteins, which are released to the lymph system. Fat-soluble vitamins travel through the lymph system, and eventually the bloodstream, until they reach the liver, where they are stored or repackaged for delivery to other tissues.

Suppose you eat more fat-soluble vitamins than you need. As vitamin intake rises above the body's needs, the amount absorbed generally falls. Excess fat-soluble vitamins accumulate in your liver and fatty tissues, building up reserves that can tide you over for weeks or months.

Water-soluble vitamins are dissolved in the watery compartments of foods, and intestinal cells absorb water-soluble vitamins directly into the bloodstream. Although small variations in daily intake of water-soluble vitamins typically do not cause problems, they should be part of your daily diet. Because your body does not store most water-soluble vitamins in appreciable amounts, it needs a regular supply from your

TABLE 7.1

A Comparison of Fat-Soluble and Water-Soluble Vitamins

	Fat-Soluble Vitamins (Vitamins A, D, E, and K)	Water-Soluble Vitamins (B Vitamins and Vitamin C)
Solubility	Soluble in fat.	Soluble in water.
Digestion	Digestion begins in the mouth to break foods into small pieces, helping to release vitamins. In the stomach, digestive enzymes work to release vitamins from food. Bile is required to emulsify fat and aid digestion and absorption.	Digestion begins in the mouth to break foods into small pieces, helping to release vitamins. In the stomach, digestive enzymes work to release vitamins from food.
Absorption	Absorption occurs in the small intestine and is similar to that of dietary fats, with incorporation into micelles. Inside the intestinal cells, fat-soluble vitamins are packaged in chylomicrons and move to lymphatic circulation before being transported to the blood.	Absorption from the small intestine is similar to that of glucose and amino acids, directly into the blood.
Transport	Transported by protein carriers (lipoproteins) through watery compartments in the body.	Travel freely in the watery compartments of the body.
Storage	Liver or fatty tissue such as adipose tissue.	Not stored in the body, with the exception of vitamin B_{12} in the liver.
Excretion	Tend to build up in tissues because they are not readily excreted.	Readily excreted in urine.
Dietary requirement	Daily intake is not required because of body storage.	Regular intake is required and varies by vitamin because the body does not usually store appreciative amounts.

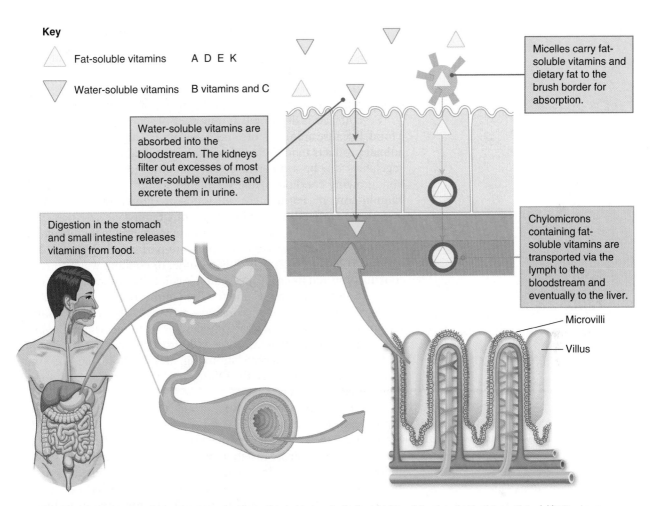

Key

△ Fat-soluble vitamins   A D E K

▽ Water-soluble vitamins   B vitamins and C

Micelles carry fat-soluble vitamins and dietary fat to the brush border for absorption.

Water-soluble vitamins are absorbed into the bloodstream. The kidneys filter out excesses of most water-soluble vitamins and excrete them in urine.

Digestion in the stomach and small intestine releases vitamins from food.

Chylomicrons containing fat-soluble vitamins are transported via the lymph to the bloodstream and eventually to the liver.

Microvilli

Villus

FIGURE 7.2 Absorption of vitamins. Water-soluble vitamins are absorbed by intestinal cells and delivered directly to the bloodstream. Fat-soluble vitamins are absorbed with fat into the lymphatic system.

diet. After 20 to 40 days of a diet deficient in vitamin C, for example, symptoms of vitamin C deficiency will emerge.

In general, excess fat-soluble vitamins, which tend to be stored in the body, are more likely to cause adverse effects than excess water-soluble vitamins. The kidneys filter out excess amounts of most water-soluble vitamins and excrete them in urine. But there are exceptions; for example, vitamin B_{12} is stored in the liver in large amounts. Vitamin K is excreted more readily than the other fat-soluble vitamins, making it less likely to reach toxic levels. And large amounts of some water-soluble vitamins—vitamin B_6, folate, niacin, even vitamin C—can be problematic.

Vitamin toxicity is rarely linked to high vitamin intakes from food or to the use of supplements that contain even 100 to 150 percent of the recommended amounts. However, people who take megadoses of one or more vitamins run the risk of consuming toxic amounts.

Key Concepts Vitamins are organic substances needed in minuscule amounts to help regulate body processes. Vitamins can be classified as fat-soluble (vitamins A, D, E, and K) or water-soluble (the B vitamins and vitamin C). Fat-soluble vitamins, which are stored in the liver and fatty tissues of the body, are excreted more slowly than water-soluble vitamins, and reserves last longer. Fat-soluble vitamins, when consumed in excess, generally pose a greater risk of toxicity than excess water-soluble vitamins.

Quick **Bite**

Is It a Fruit or a Vegetable?
In the eighteenth century, botanists defined fruits as the organ surrounding the seeds. This definition considers tomatoes, cucumbers, egg-plants, peppers, pea pods, and corn kernels as fruits. Legally, though, these are all vegetables. In the late 1800s, the U.S. Supreme Court, while trying the case of a tomato importer, established a definition based on linguistic custom and usage. The importer had to pay the vegetable tax.

Food Preparation Affects Vitamins in Foods

Vitamins are found in every food, including the fats and oils that many of us are trying to reduce in our diets. This is one more reason to eat a variety of foods. No single food group or single choice within a food group is a good source of all vitamins.

THINK
About It
1

Several factors determine the amounts of specific vitamins in a food. Because animals store and concentrate vitamins in their tissues, animal products tend to have fairly constant vitamin levels. Fruits and vegetables can be a different story. Sunlight, moisture, soil composition, growing conditions, and the plant's maturity at harvest all affect vitamin content. Fortunately, our foods are grown in diverse locales, so eating a varied diet supplies plenty of vitamins.

In general, water-soluble vitamins are more fragile than fat-soluble vitamins, and some cooking practices are particularly harmful. Many cooks add baking soda, which is alkaline, to cooking water to reduce cooking time and intensify a vegetable's color; however, both alkalinity and heat destroy vitamin C and the B vitamins thiamin and riboflavin. When vegetables are boiled, cooking water easily leaches water-soluble vitamins. Yet cooking only partially destroys a food's vitamin content, and some cooking methods are less destructive than others. The best cooking methods—steaming, stir-frying, and microwaving—use minimal amounts of water. (See the FYI feature "Fresh, Frozen, or Canned? Raw, Dried, or Cooked?")

Packaging and storage also can affect a food's vitamin content. Exposure to light damages vitamin A, the B vitamin riboflavin, and vitamin C. Exposure to air and heat has damaging effects on fat- and water-soluble vitamins. Most food processing (e.g., refining oils, milling grains, canning vegetables, drying fruit) reduces vitamin content. The more a food is processed or refined, the more it tends to lose vitamins. Eating a variety of foods and using different preparation techniques helps to ensure that your diet supplies plenty of vitamins. Varied diets contain significant amounts of many vitamins, and vitamins often are added to foods such as cereals and other grain products.

Enrichment and Fortification

In the 1940s, the U.S. government mandated enrichment of bread and cereal products made from milled grains. Milling or refining grains removes the bran and germ to make white flour, white rice, refined cornmeal, flour for pasta, and most breakfast cereals. Processing grains also removes most B vitamins, vitamin E, and minerals such as iron, magnesium, and zinc. The loss of these nutrients from such staple foods could be devastating. In fact, during the nineteenth and early twentieth centuries, widespread adoption of these milling techniques left a wake of vitamin deficiency diseases like beriberi (thiamin) and pellagra (niacin).

To prevent overt deficiencies, food manufacturers now return iron and B vitamins to the grains they process. Replacing lost nutrients is called *enrichment*. Most countries now require enrichment of staple grain products.

Food manufacturers also "fortify" foods. Fortification is the process of adding extra nutrients to foods where they wouldn't be found naturally in consistently significant amounts. Iodized table salt (salt with added iodine) is a fortified food. Read the labels on some breakfast cereals—the ones with the long list of added vitamins and minerals are fortified foods. Because most breakfast cereals are fortified, they usually are good sources of vitamins and minerals. Fortification is sometimes

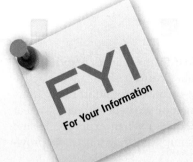

Fresh, Frozen, or Canned? Raw, Dried, or Cooked?

Selecting and Preparing Foods to Maximize Vitamin Content

Wouldn't it be great if we could all shop daily for fresh fruits and vegetables? When picked at their prime ripeness, fresh fruits and vegetables taste the best and contain peak amounts of different vitamins and phytochemicals. Remember that light, heat, air, acid, and alkali can destroy many vitamins, and cooking liquids can leach them out. Even if you can't buy fresh foods daily, you can

still minimize nutrient loss after purchase. Start by choosing clean, undamaged produce on your regular shopping trips. Then store foods with minimal exposure to light and air. Many fruits, most vegetables, and all animal products require refrigeration. Get them cold right away, and keep them cold. Because vitamin content can decrease with time, plan on using fruits and vegetables soon after purchase. The vitamin C of fresh green beans, for example, drops by half after six days at home.

What about frozen and canned foods? Their vitamin content is much better than you might guess. When vegetables are frozen immediately after they are picked, their nutritional value and flavor are preserved.[a] Although canning uses destructive heat, the processor typically uses fresh-picked produce, which is higher in vitamins than fresh food transported to faraway markets. When using canned vegetables, incorporate the liquid in soups and stews to get the benefit of any vitamins that may have leached out. Recipes prepared with canned foods and no added salt have similar nutritional values to those prepared with fresh or frozen ingredients.[b]

Carotenoids are stable during the canning process. In fact, research suggests the lycopene in processed tomato products is better absorbed into the body than that from raw tomatoes.[c] Vitamins are lost from fresh produce during transport and storage. Processing fruits minimizes postharvest damage, yet chemical and temperature processing cause nutrient losses. One exception to this is vitamin

C—there is not a significant difference in the vitamin C content of fresh fruits and vegetables and those that have been frozen, canned, or juiced.[d]

Dried fruits also are a good way to eat your daily fruit. The biggest concern is portion size, because when fruits are dried their nutrient, calorie, and sugar content become concentrated, and it is easy to eat too much. Dried fruits have a low to moderate glycemic index and a glycemic response that's comparable to that of fresh fruits. They are a good source of nutrients such as potassium and fiber.[e] Data from the National Health and Nutrition Examination Survey (NHANES) showed that dried fruit consumption is associated with lower body mass index (BMI), reduced waist circumference, reduced abdominal obesity, improved nutrient intake (higher vitamin A, vitamin K, potassium, iron, magnesium, and fiber intake), more fruit servings per day, and healthier overall diets for both adults and children.[f,g]

What is the best way to cook fruits and vegetables? To maximize vitamin content, think minimal—minimal heat, minimal cooking water, and minimal exposure to air. Try also to minimize handling the food before and during cooking. Dicing a food such as a potato reduces cooking time but also exposes more surface area to vitamin destruction. So, cut if you must, but not too small.

Because steaming, stir-frying, and microwaving minimize cooking time and water use, they are the best cooking methods for preserving vitamin content. If you boil foods, use the

cooking water for sauces, stews, or soups to salvage lost water-soluble vitamins. And do not add baking soda to beans or vegetables (some folks do that to intensify color and tenderize); baking soda destroys some vitamins.

Remember, to retain the most vitamins in your food, choose seasonal freshly picked produce and be gentle with storage and handling, kind with cooking, and "minimize (heat, water, and air exposure) to maximize"!

a Fruit and Veggies—More Matters. Fresh, frozen, canned, dried and 100% juice: all forms of fruits and vegetables matter! http://www.fruitsandveggiesmorematters.org/?page_id=47. Accessed September 7, 2017.

b Fruit and Veggies—More Matters. Facts about canned foods. http://www.fruitsandveggiesmorematters.org/5-facts-about-canned-foods. Accessed September 7, 2017.

c Carlsen MH, Halvorsen BL, Holte K, et al. The total antioxidant content of more than 3,100 foods, beverages, spices, herbs, and supplements used worldwide. *Nutr J.* 2010;9:3.

d Kyureghian G, Flores R. Meta-analysis of studies on vitamin C contents of fresh and processed fruits and vegetables. *J Food Nutr Disor.* 2012;1:2. doi.org/10.4172/2324-9323.1000101

e Fruit and Veggies—More Matters. About the buzz: fresh fruit is much healthier than dried fruit? http://www.fruitsandveggiesmorematters.org/?page_id=18744. Accessed September 7, 2017.

f Ibid.

g Keast D, Jones J. Dried fruit consumption associated with reduced improved overweight or obesity in adults: NHANES, 1999–2004. *Fed Am Soc Exp Bio J.* 2009;23:LB511.

required by law, as in the addition of vitamins A and D to milk and the addition of folic acid to enriched flour, cereal, and grain products.

Enrichment and mandatory fortification programs helped eliminate most overt deficiency diseases in the United States and many other countries. However, mandatory enrichment replaces only some of the many nutrients lost in milling. During the production of highly refined grain products, processing also removes vitamin B_6, magnesium, and zinc. To ensure a good balance of nutrients, experts recommend that people regularly eat whole-grain products such as whole-wheat bread, brown rice, and oatmeal.

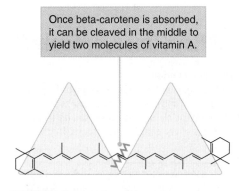

Once beta-carotene is absorbed, it can be cleaved in the middle to yield two molecules of vitamin A.

FIGURE 7.3 Beta-carotene. Beta-carotene may be cleaved at different locations, so it may yield less than two molecules of vitamin A. Other provitamin A carotenoids yield less vitamin A than beta-carotene does.

▶ **provitamins** Inactive forms of vitamins that the body can convert into active usable forms. Also referred to as *vitamin precursors*.

▶ **vitamin precursors** See *provitamins*.

▶ **retinol** The alcohol form of vitamin A; one of the retinoids; the main physiologically active form of vitamin A; interconvertible with retinal.

▶ **retinal** The aldehyde form of vitamin A; one of the retinoids; the active form of vitamin A in the retina; interconvertible with retinol.

▶ **retinoic acid** The acid form of vitamin A; one of the retinoids; formed from retinal but not interconvertible; helps growth, cell differentiation, and the immune system; does not have a role in vision or reproduction.

▶ **retinoids** Compounds in foods that have chemical structures similar to vitamin A. Retinoids include the active forms of vitamin A (retinol, retinal, and retinoic acid) and the main storage forms of retinol (retinyl esters).

▶ **carotenoids** A group of yellow, orange, and red pigments in plants. Many of these compounds are precursors of vitamin A.

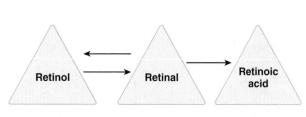

| Retinol | Retinal | Retinoic acid |

FIGURE 7.4 Forms of vitamin A. Whereas retinol and retinal are interconvertible, the reaction that forms retinoic acid is irreversible.

Provitamins

Some vitamins in foods are in inactive forms, called **provitamins** or **vitamin precursors**. The body must convert them to the active forms. One familiar provitamin is beta-carotene, found in many fruits and vegetables. Your body converts much of the beta-carotene you eat to its active form, vitamin A. (See **FIGURE 7.3**.) When experts calculate vitamin requirements or monitor consumption, they must take provitamins into account.

Key Concepts Growing conditions, storage, processing, and cooking affect the amounts of vitamins in foods. Enrichment and fortification programs replace some vitamins and minerals lost in processing and add other nutrients to foods. Provitamins are vitamin precursors that can be converted to the active vitamin forms.

The Fat-Soluble Vitamins

🍎 **Why Is This Important?** Understanding the different forms, functions, requirements, and food sources of each fat-soluble vitamin is important to preventing deficiency and toxicity.

Despite their common property of dissolving in fat, the fat-soluble vitamins have diverse roles. Vitamin A is crucial for vision and renewing cells. Vitamin D helps regulate blood levels of calcium and is essential for bone health. Vitamin E and carotenoids are antioxidants that help protect cells from damage. Vitamin K is known for its role in blood clotting, but it also is crucial for bone health along with vitamin D.

Vitamin A and Carotenoids

Vitamin A's best known effects are in the eye. You need vitamin A to change incoming light to visual images and to keep the eye's surface healthy. Vitamin A also helps direct development of the body's cells—how and when they grow and divide and what form they take. As such, this vitamin is essential to proper growth and reproduction. It plays a role in immune function, both as a cell regulator and by helping maintain the skin and mucous membranes. In fact, vitamin A plays a crucial role in maintaining or regulating many tissues throughout the body.

The liver stores over 90 percent of the vitamin A in the body, with the rest found in fatty tissues, lungs, and kidneys.[1] A healthy liver can store up to a year's supply of vitamin A, releasing it in just the right amounts to maintain normal vitamin A blood levels—a nice benefit, but one with a drawback: Large doses of vitamin A can exceed storage capacity and cause toxicity.

Forms of Vitamin A

The body uses three active forms of vitamin A—**retinol**, **retinal**, and **retinoic acid**—known collectively as the **retinoids**. (See **FIGURE 7.4**.) Although all three forms are essential, retinol is the key player in the vitamin A family.[2]

Colorful plant pigments called **carotenoids** are precursors of vitamin A. There are several hundred carotenoids found in nature, and the body converts some of them to vitamin A. Of the carotenoids, beta-carotene supplies the most vitamin A.

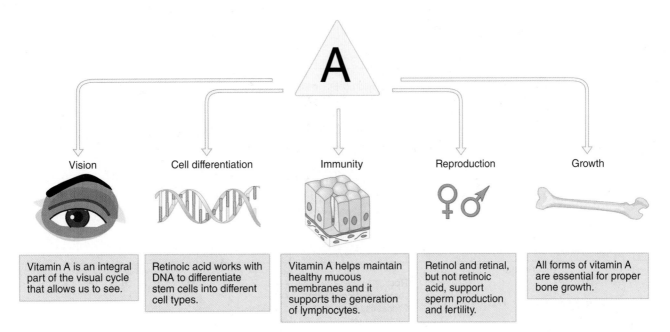

FIGURE 7.5 Major functions of vitamin A. Vitamin A plays a crucial role in vision and is essential for proper cell synthesis, immunity, reproduction, and bone growth.

Functions of Vitamin A

Vitamin A is crucial for vision, for maintaining healthy cells (particularly skin cells), for fighting infections and bolstering immune function, and for promoting growth and development. (See **FIGURE 7.5**.)

Vision: Night and Day

Vitamin A is needed to change incoming light to visual images and to keep the eye's surface healthy. Vitamin A allows night vision and color vision by actually becoming a functioning part of the retina. The **retina** is the paper-thin tissue lining the back of the eye, where light images are received and relayed to the brain, resulting in vision. **Rod cells**, the cells in the retina that react to dim light, are rich in a purple pigment called **rhodopsin**, or "visual purple." Rhodopsin is composed of a protein, **opsin**, plus vitamin A.

Light entering the eye and striking the retina splits rhodopsin, causing it to lose color as it releases opsin and vitamin A (retinal) (See **FIGURE 7.6**.) This **bleaching process** triggers electric impulses that the brain interprets as black-and-white visual images. In well-nourished people, vitamin A recombines with opsin, forming new rhodopsin that again can respond to light. If vitamin A levels are low, the body cannot re-form rhodopsin, and **night blindness** results. Although the eyes contain only 0.01 percent of the body's vitamin A, they are so sensitive to vitamin A levels that one injection of the vitamin can relieve this type of night blindness within minutes.[3]

If you awaken in the middle of the night and turn on a bright light, the light level is blinding until your eyes adjust. Rhodopsin breaks down quickly in bright light, and the reduced supply makes the rod cells less light sensitive. Conversely, when you enter a dark room, your eyes not only dilate, but also produce rhodopsin to increase their sensitivity to light. Known as **dark adaptation**, the speed of adjustment to dim light is related directly to the amount of

THiNK
About It
2

▶ **retina** A paper-thin tissue that lines the back of the eye and contains cells called rods and cones.

▶ **rod cells** Light-sensitive cells in the retina that react to dim light and transmit black-and-white images.

▶ **rhodopsin** Found in rod cells, this light-sensitive pigment molecule consists of a protein called opsin combined with retinal.

▶ **opsin** A protein that combines with retinal to form rhodopsin in rod cells.

▶ **bleaching process** A complex light-stimulated reaction in which rod cells lose color as rhodopsin is split into retinal and opsin.

▶ **night blindness** The inability of the eyes to adjust to dim light or to regain vision quickly after exposure to a flash of bright light.

▶ **dark adaptation** The process that increases the rhodopsin concentration in your eyes, allowing them to detect images in the dark better.

STRUCTURE OF RETINA   VISUAL CYCLE IN RETINA

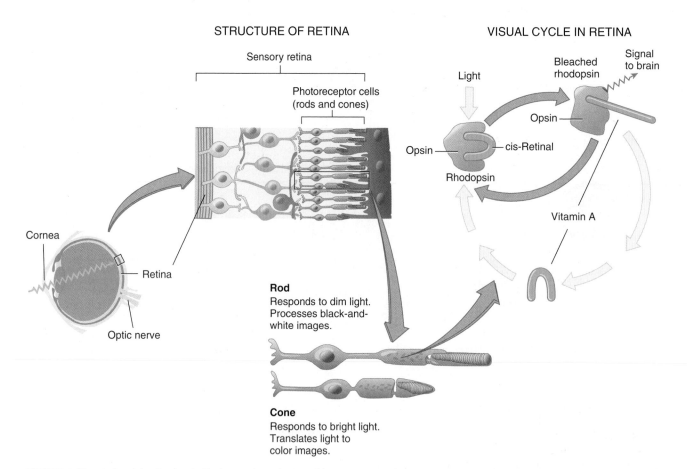

FIGURE 7.6 Vitamin A and the visual cycle. Rhodopsin is the combination of the protein opsin and vitamin A (retinal). When stimulated by light, both opsin and vitamin A change shape. This sends a signal to the brain, and you see an image in black and white. A similar process using a different protein called iodopsin provides color.

vitamin A available to regenerate rhodopsin. People with night blindness cannot adjust to dim light or regain vision quickly after exposure to a flash of bright light.

Color vision also requires vitamin A. **Cone cells**, which are responsible for color vision, are rich in the pigment **iodopsin**. The iodopsin cycle is similar to the rhodopsin cycle, with vitamin A playing a crucial role. A prolonged lack of vitamin A impairs color vision, but because it affects rod cells before cone cells, night blindness emerges first.

Vitamin A in Cell Production and Differentiation

When your body needs to make the proteins that form new cells or other protein compounds, vitamin A plays a role in directing protein production. It helps regulate production of enzymes, blood carrier proteins, structural proteins such as those in skin, and more.

Vitamin A works in cell differentiation, the process that causes immature, characterless cells (undifferentiated cells called **stem cells**) to mature into specific types of cells with unique functions. For example, if you cut your hand, the new cells produced to repair the cut are specifically suited to the job; stomach cells or lung cells would not do.

With these very basic, crucially important biological functions, vitamin A plays a role in building and maintaining tissues throughout the body.

▶ **cone cells** Cells in the retina that are sensitive to bright light and translate it into color images.

▶ **iodopsin** Color-sensitive pigment molecules in cone cells that consist of opsin-like proteins combined with retinal.

▶ **stem cells** A formative cell whose daughter cells can differentiate into other cell types.

Vitamin A and Skin

Skin, mucous membranes, and other lining materials in the body are all **epithelial tissues**. Together they cover us on the outside, act as a lining or covering on the inside, and provide lubrication where it's needed—for example, along bronchial tubes and the digestive tract. **Epithelial cells** are on the front line protecting your body, and they are destroyed and replaced relatively quickly. Replacing these cells, as well as maintaining normal structure and function, requires vitamin A. Because the turnover of skin cells is rapid, signs of vitamin A deficiency show up early in the skin and mucous membranes.

Vitamin A and Immune Function

Vitamin A influences the immune system in important ways. Epithelial tissues, which include the skin and mucous membranes, are your body's first line of defense against bacterial, parasitic, and viral attack. By helping to maintain the health of these tissues, vitamin A plays an important role in the integrity of the immune system. But if dangerous microorganisms successfully breach these barriers, your body's defense system mobilizes immune cells to attack the invaders. To produce these immune cells, your body needs vitamin A.

Vitamin A and Reproduction

Although the exact biochemical mechanism is unclear, vitamin A affects both male and female reproductive processes. Vitamin A aids reproduction, probably by keeping the secretion-producing linings of the reproductive tract healthy. In women, vitamin A helps maintain fertility. In men, it is needed for sperm production. Vitamin A's role in cell production and differentiation also makes it crucial to the proper development of an embryo.

Vitamin A and Bones

Vitamin A helps produce bone cells needed for growth and is required for bone remodeling. As children grow, their bones get longer. But simply adding length would produce some strange-looking bones. Therefore, during normal growth the bone ends are actually broken down and then lengthened; that is, they are remodeled. A lack of vitamin A in the growing child disrupts bone remodeling and interferes with the development of immature bone cells. The result is weak, poorly formed bones. On the other end of the spectrum, too much vitamin A has been linked to bone loss and an increased risk of fracture. Excessive amounts of vitamin A can interfere with the ability of vitamin D to promote calcium absorption and can trigger an increase in cellular activity that breaks down bone.[4]

Dietary Recommendations for Vitamin A

Remember, vitamin A includes retinoids—retinol, retinoic acid, and retinal—and is formed from precursor carotenoids. Similar amounts of dietary retinoids and carotenoids do not provide the same amount of vitamin A. To reconcile the differences, scientists use a measure called **retinol activity equivalent (RAE)**. One RAE equals the activity of 1 microgram (1/1,000,000 of a gram) of retinol. On average, 12 micrograms of beta-carotene from food produce 1 microgram of retinol. Other provitamin carotenoids like alpha-carotene are converted even less efficiently: It takes 24 micrograms to produce 1 microgram of retinol.[5] (See **FIGURE 7.7**.)

▶ **epithelial tissues** Closely packed layers of epithelial cells that cover the body and line its cavities.

▶ **epithelial cells** The millions of cells that line and protect the external and internal surfaces of the body. Epithelial cells form epithelial tissues such as skin and mucous membranes.

▶ **retinol activity equivalent (RAE)** A unit of measurement of the vitamin A content of a food. One RAE equals 1 microgram of retinol.

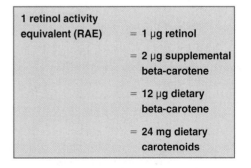

1 retinol activity equivalent (RAE)	= 1 µg retinol
	= 2 µg supplemental beta-carotene
	= 12 µg dietary beta-carotene
	= 24 mg dietary carotenoids

FIGURE 7.7 Retinol activity equivalent conversion.

Most Americans take in adequate amounts of vitamin A and have large stores of the vitamin in their livers. The RDA for vitamin A for males age 14 years or older is 900 micrograms RAE per day. For females age 14 years or older, the vitamin A RDA is 700 micrograms RAE per day. Pregnant women should consume slightly more vitamin A (770 micrograms), and women who are breastfeeding their children are advised to consume 1,300 micrograms RAE per day.[6]

Sources of Vitamin A

Most dietary vitamin A comes from animal food sources as **preformed vitamin A**, known as the retinoids (including retinyl esters, which are the main storage form of vitamin A). Only foods of animal origin contain retinoids. Plant foods, especially yellow-orange vegetables and fruits, contain **provitamin A** carotenoids such as beta-carotene. (Read more under "The Carotenoids" later in this chapter.) On average, we get about one-quarter to one-third of our dietary vitamin A as carotenoids, mainly beta-carotene, but that figure varies widely.[7]

Liver (e.g., beef) and fish oils (e.g., cod liver oil) are the richest sources of vitamin A, as you would expect; just as the human liver stores vitamin A, other animals' livers do, too. Other good sources include milk fat (as in whole milk, butter, and other dairy products) and egg yolk. (See **FIGURE 7.8**.)

Because low-fat milk is fortified, it is a good vitamin A source, despite having little or no butterfat. Producers also fortify some foods

▶ **preformed vitamin A** Retinyl esters, the main storage form of vitamin A. About 90 percent of dietary retinol is in the form of esters, mostly found in foods from animal sources.

▶ **provitamin A** Carotenoid precursors of vitamin A in foods of plant origin, primarily deeply colored fruits and vegetables.

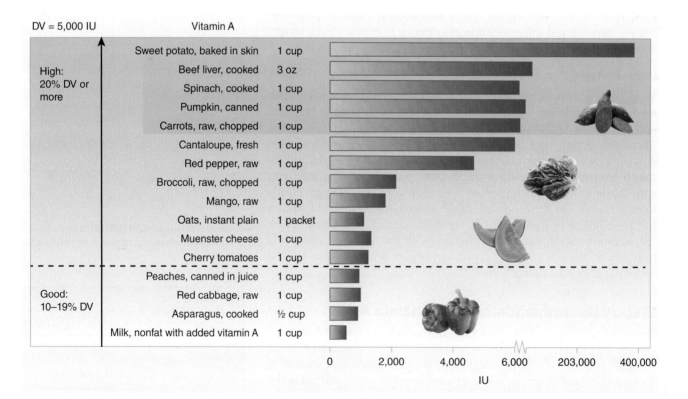

FIGURE 7.8 Food sources of vitamin A. Vitamin A is found as retinol in animal foods and as beta-carotene and other carotenoids in plant foods. Some of the best sources are liver, orange and deep-yellow vegetables, and dark-green leafy vegetables.

Data from U.S. Department of Agriculture, Agricultural Research Service, Nutrient Data Laboratory. USDA National Nutrient Database for Standard Reference, Release 28. Version Current: September 2015. Internet: http://www.ars.usda.gov/nea/bhnrc/ndl.

Red pepper: © Nattika/Shutterstock, Inc.; Sweet potatoes: © Kroeger/Gross/Getty Images, Cantaloupe: © Ursula Alter/Getty Images, Inc.; Spinach leaves: © dionisvero/Getty Images Inc.

of plant origin, including margarine, some breakfast cereals, and some special dietary foods like "nutrition bars."

> **Key Concepts**   Vitamin A occurs in three forms in the body: retinol, retinal, and retinoic acid. Retinol is found in a few animal-derived foods. Vitamin A is also formed from precursors called carotenoids. Intake recommendations for vitamin A are expressed in RAEs (retinol activity equivalents) to account for differences between retinoids and carotenoids. Most vitamin A is processed and stored in the liver and is released as needed. Vitamin A in the cells of the retina plays a crucial role in vision. It is also involved in cell differentiation, reproduction, maintaining epithelial tissues, immune function, and bone health.

Vitamin A Deficiency

Although dietary deficiency of vitamin A is rare in North America and Western Europe, it is the leading cause of childhood blindness worldwide, especially in Southeast Asia, parts of Africa, India, and Central and South America. In these regions, vitamin A deficiency typically occurs alongside general protein-energy malnutrition in infants and young children. Protein deficiency reduces levels of retinol-binding protein, the carrier protein that transports vitamin A in the blood. Vitamin A deficiency interacts with other nutrient deficiencies and with infection, worsening respiratory infections or diarrhea and causing countless deaths. (See **FIGURE 7.9**.)

Certain North American groups are at risk for vitamin A deficiency. Newborns, especially premature infants, do not have vitamin A reserves in their livers. People with alcoholism or liver disease may have damaged livers that cannot store much vitamin A. Cystic fibrosis, Crohn's disease, pancreatic disease, fat malabsorption diseases, or medicines that inhibit fat absorption also impair vitamin A absorption. Because the body needs zinc to use vitamin A efficiently, inadequate zinc intake can cause vitamin A deficiency symptoms.

The Eyes

Early treatment can rapidly correct night blindness, an early symptom of vitamin A deficiency. But a worsening and prolonged deficiency threatens eyesight. Cells in the **cornea** (part of the eye's covering) stop reproducing, and the deficiency damages mucous membranes that provide lubrication. Without adequate mucus, dirt and bacteria accumulate as the eye dries out. As the cornea deteriorates, foamy white patches called Bitot's spots appear on the eye. In extreme cases, the cornea eventually develops scars and ulcers and may even liquefy, causing total blindness.

The Skin and Other Epithelial Cells

Hard, bumpy, scaly skin—"goose flesh" that doesn't go away—is an early symptom of vitamin A deficiency. The deficiency disrupts epithelial cell production, and the skin's hair follicles become plugged with **keratin**. Vitamin A deficiency also impairs normal secretions, blocking perspiration and mucus. The lack of mucus damages the linings of the mouth, respiratory tract, and urinary and genital tracts. In men, a vitamin A deficiency reduces the production of sperm, and in women it can cause infertility by disrupting the production of reproductive tract secretions, which can impede the movement of sperm in the genital tract.

Because vitamin A is essential to cell growth and differentiation, a deficiency can cause a variety of problems, including growth retardation, bone deformities, and defective teeth. An excessive buildup of keratin near sensory receptors causes a loss of taste and smell, which in turn can cause loss of appetite and weight.

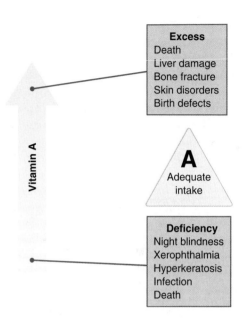

FIGURE 7.9 Vitamin A deficiency and toxicity. A broad range of vitamin A intake is adequate and provides for normal function. Too little or too much vitamin A can have serious consequences.

▶ **cornea**   The transparent outer surface of the eye.

▶ **keratin**   A water-insoluble fibrous protein that is the primary constituent of hair, nails, and the outer layer of the skin.

Immune Function

Vitamin A deficiency leaves a person especially vulnerable to infection. Damaged epithelium allows microorganisms to breach this first line of defense. Under ordinary circumstances, entry of these enemy invaders would then trigger protective immune cells to quickly multiply. But immune cells need vitamin A to multiply. With too few immune cells to mount an effective attack, the invading microorganisms can cause severe, even fatal, diarrhea or respiratory infection. When a child is deficient in vitamin A, a relatively harmless infection such as measles can be fatal.[8]

Vitamin A Toxicity

Vitamin A toxicity occurs infrequently; however, the enthusiasm for megadoses of vitamin supplements has increased the potential for toxic dosing. With the exception of a sustained diet of large amounts of liver or fish oils, food alone generally cannot supply massive amounts of vitamin A. Children are more vulnerable to toxicity, and overenthusiastic supplementation of vitamin A is dangerous and can be fatal. Consumption of large amounts of fish liver has been found to cause vitamin A toxicity in children.[9]

Vitamin A toxicity has a wide range of symptoms, both subtle and overt, including fatigue, vomiting, abdominal pain, bone and joint pain, loss of appetite, skin disorders, headache, blurred or double vision, hip fracture, and liver damage. (See Figure 7.9.) Vitamin A toxicity can be acute, but more often it develops gradually over months or years. Toxicity symptoms can often be corrected when intake levels are lowered.

Excess preformed vitamin A is a known **teratogen** (it causes birth defects). The birth defects it causes include cleft palate, heart abnormalities, and brain malfunction.[10] It is most dangerous during the two weeks prior to conception and the first two months of pregnancy, when cell differentiation is most intense. Pregnant women should get the approval of their doctor before taking preformed vitamin A supplements. For adults, including adult women who are pregnant or breast-feeding, the Tolerable Upper Intake Level (UL) for vitamin A is 3,000 micrograms RAE as retinol.

Acne Treatment

Some close cousins (or analogs) of vitamin A are given in therapeutic doses to treat skin problems. Two commercially available forms of retinoic acid, Retin-A and Accutane, are widely used for acne. But, like vitamin A, these retinoids can cause birth defects. Any woman who may become pregnant should not use these medicines. In fact, because these medications accumulate in fat stores, even when applied on the skin, women should discontinue them at least two years before pregnancy.

▶ **teratogen** Any substance that causes birth defects.

Key Concepts Vitamin A deficiency causes blindness; damages skin, bone, and other tissues; and limits immune function, leaving a person vulnerable to infection. Excessive vitamin A supplementation can cause toxicity, even with doses just a few times higher than the RDA. Vitamin A toxicity during pregnancy could be devastating; pregnant women should be wary of retinol-containing supplements and avoid retinoid-containing medicines.

The Carotenoids

Carotenoids are plant pigments that give the deep yellow, orange, and red colors to fruits and vegetables such as apricots, carrots, and tomatoes.

The major carotenoids are alpha-carotene, beta-carotene, lutein, zeaxanthin, cryptoxanthin, and lycopene. Among them, beta-carotene, the yellow-orange pigment in cantaloupe, carrots, and squash, is the most common. Alpha-carotene, beta-carotene, and beta-cryptoxanthin can be converted to vitamin A. Other carotenoids such as lycopene, zeaxanthin, and lutein have no vitamin A activity. (See **TABLE 7.2**.)

Functions of Carotenoids

Aside from conversion to vitamin A, the carotenoids do not appear to be essential in the technical sense; a carotenoid-free diet does not cause deficiency disease. Therefore, the Food and Nutrition Board has not established Dietary Reference Intakes (DRIs) for them.[11] Yet people who eat generous amounts of foods rich in carotenoids reduce their risk of many major degenerative diseases. Beta-carotene and other carotenoids function as potent antioxidants—substances that can interfere with the damaging effects of free radicals—highly unstable, reactive compounds—which may explain their beneficial effects. (See **FIGURE 7.10**.) There is an ongoing demand for dietary antioxidants to prevent and reduce the oxidative damage from free radicals.[12] This damage may form the biological basis of several diseases. People who eat generous amounts of foods rich in carotenoids reduce their risk of many major degenerative conditions such as premature aging, cancer, atherosclerosis, cataracts, age-related macular degeneration, bone loss, and diabetes.[13]

Carotenoids and Vision

Higher intakes of carotenoids, especially lutein and zeaxanthin, from foods or supplements may play an important role in protecting vision.[14]

Quick **Bite**

Help the Vitamins Go Down
Pink and red grapefruits are a great source of lycopene. If you find grapefruit too sour for your taste, try sprinkling on a little sugar or a low-calorie sweetener before eating one to bring out the rich natural sweetness.

TABLE 7.2
Common Carotenoids

Class/Components	Source[a]	Potential Benefit	Tips for Including Carotenoids in the Diet
Beta-carotene	Carrots, pumpkins, sweet potatoes, cantaloupes	Neutralizes free radicals, which may damage cells; bolsters cellular antioxidant defenses; can be made into vitamin A in the body	For beta-carotene–rich french fries: thinly slice sweet potatoes and coat with olive oil or fat-free cooking spray, and add spices to taste (pepper, rosemary, thyme). Bake in a 425°F oven until golden brown on both sides (10–15 minutes). Time-saver: buy precut sweet potatoes in the frozen foods section.
Lutein, zeaxanthin	Kale, collards, spinach, corn, eggs, citrus	May contribute to maintenance of healthy vision	Freezing kale can bring out a sweeter, more flavorful taste. For an easy sautéed side dish, try this simple recipe: add kale to a skillet with oil and garlic, slivered almonds, and red pepper flakes. If kale doesn't top your list of food preferences, spinach, which provides the same health benefits, can be an easy substitute. Many multivitamin/mineral dietary supplements include lutein.
Lycopene	Tomatoes and processed tomato products, watermelons, red/pink grapefruit	May contribute to maintenance of prostate health	Research shows lycopene is best absorbed by the body when consumed from tomatoes that have been cooked using a small amount of oil. This includes products such as tomato sauce and tomato paste. Try adding 1 cup tomato sauce to sautéed zucchini for a colorful side dish.

[a] Examples are not an all-inclusive list.

Note: Preformed vitamin A is found in foods that come from animals. Provitamin A carotenoids are found in many darkly colored fruits and vegetables and are a major source of vitamin A for vegetarians.

Adapted from International Food Information Council Foundation. Functional foods component chart. 2009. http://www.foodinsight.org/Content/6/FINAL-IFIC-Fndtn-Functional-Foods-Backgrounder-with-Tips-and-changes-03-11-09.pdf. Accessed September 7, 2017.

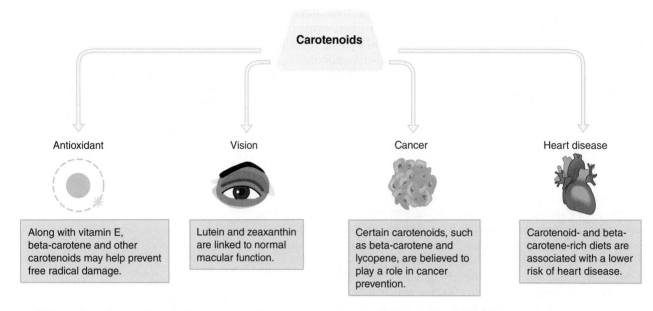

FIGURE 7.10 Major functions of carotenoids. Independent of vitamin A activity, carotenoids can function as antioxidants and may be involved in normal macular function and reduced risk of cancer and heart disease.

Lutein and zeaxanthin are found in the macula of the eye, the central portion of the retina responsible for sharp, detailed vision. Scientists believe that carotenoids may protect the eyes by inhibiting the oxidative damage that contributes to age-related blindness.[15] Macular degeneration is the leading cause of age-related blindness, affecting approximately 50 million people worldwide.[16] Research has demonstrated that a supplement containing carotenoids and other antioxidants can slow the progression of age-related macular degeneration.[17] People with the highest intakes of lutein and zeaxanthin also have a decreased risk of cataracts.[18]

Carotenoids and Cancer

People with the highest intakes of carotenoid-rich fruits and vegetables and/or high blood levels of specific carotenoids tend to have the lowest risk for certain cancers. Tomato products, for example are excellent sources of lycopene, and research suggests that a diet rich in tomato products reduces the risk of heart disease, osteoporosis, and several cancers.[19]

The beneficial effects of carotenoids on health generally reflect food intake, not supplement use. To date, trials of beta-carotene supplements for cancer prevention have been disappointing; paradoxically, megadose supplements are associated with increased lung cancer among smokers or those exposed to asbestos.[20]

Food Sources and Absorption of Carotenoids

Orange and yellow fruits and vegetables generally contain beta-carotene, alpha-carotene, and cryptoxanthin. Good sources of beta-carotene include carrots, pumpkins, winter squash, sweet potatoes, and some orange-colored fruits like cantaloupe, apricots, and mango. Dark-green vegetables also contain abundant carotenoids, but the carotenoid colors are hidden by the plentiful green pigment chlorophyll. Carotenoids from

Quick Bite

And They Called It Cantaloupe
The word *cantaloupe* comes from a papal garden in a small town near Rome named Cantaloupo. One-half of a medium cantaloupe has 466 RAE as beta-carotene.

dark-green leafy vegetables, however, produce less vitamin A than those from ripe orange-colored fruit.[21]

Surprisingly, oranges and tangerines have little beta-carotene, but they are rich in cryptoxanthin. Cryptoxanthin also is found in mangos, nectarines, and papaya. Lycopene has a more reddish color; you will see it in tomatoes, pink grapefruit, guava, and watermelon. Lutein and zeaxanthin are in leafy green vegetables, pumpkin, and red pepper.[22] Because all major carotenoids are important, and they are difficult to identify in food just by looking, you should eat a wide variety of fruits and vegetables to ensure a good intake.

Your body generally absorbs only 20 to 40 percent of the carotenoids you eat; however, this proportion drops to 10 percent or less as the amount of carotenoids you eat increases. Dietary fat, protein, and vitamin E increase absorption. Factors that limit fat absorption limit carotenoid absorption as well. It's now known that the cell walls of carotenoid-rich plants inhibit absorption. Cooking vegetables for a few minutes breaks the cell walls, releasing the carotenoids and improving their absorption.

Carotenoid Supplementation

Eating carotenoid-rich fruits and vegetables is clearly linked to reduced disease rates. Eating even extremely large amounts of carotenoid-rich foods has not been associated with toxic effects. However, the use of carotenoid supplements, which has become popular in recent years, can cause more harm than good. Carotenoid supplements should not be taken without careful oversight by a healthcare provider. Beta-carotene supplementation can actually harm some individuals such as smokers, by increasing their risk of lung cancer. The Food and Nutrition Board advises against carotenoid supplementation use for the general population, recommending that people eat more carotenoid-rich fruits and vegetables instead.[23] A UL has not been set for the carotenoids.

Vitamin D

This fat-soluble nutrient is called the sunshine vitamin. When the ultraviolet rays of the sun strike your skin, they convert cholesterol to vitamin D. Vitamin D is unique because, given sufficient sunlight, your body can make all that it needs—dietary vitamin D is unnecessary. However, when coupled with too little sun exposure, a lack of dietary vitamin D does cause a vitamin deficiency.

Vitamin D is essential for bone health, and it protects against certain cancers, heart disease, and other chronic diseases. In children, it promotes bone development and growth. In adults, it is necessary for bone maintenance. In older adults, vitamin D and calcium supplementation helps prevent bone loss and fractures.[24] Desirable blood levels of vitamin D are currently under investigation for its role in the prevention of cardiovascular disease, type 2 diabetes, and cancer, as well as immunity and muscular disorders.[25,26] Vitamin D may even help to reduce the risk of death in elderly people.[27]

Forms and Formation of Vitamin D

Vitamin D is a group of about 10 related compounds. The most important of these are vitamin D_2 (ergocalciferol) and vitamin D_3 (cholecalciferol). Ergocalciferol is found exclusively in plant foods.

Quick Bite

A Yellowish-Orange Hue

You may know light-skinned people who consumed so much carrot juice that their skin acquired a yellowish-orange cast. This phenomenon is common in infants whose introduction to solid foods includes a lot of strained carrots and sweet potatoes! Dark-skinned people may notice a yellowing of the palms and soles of their feet. In this example, the accumulation of excess beta-carotene in the blood is responsible for this harmless condition.

Quick Bite

Pizza Versus Tomato Juice

One U.S. study linked intake of tomato sauce, tomatoes, and pizza to lowered risk of prostate cancer. Tomato juice, however, was not protective. That's not surprising. According to John Erdman, PhD, of the University of Illinois at Urbana–Champaign, the cancer-fighting carotenoid found in tomatoes (lycopene) is a fat-soluble substance, so it needs some fat like that found in pizza and most pasta sauces to be absorbed.

Quick Bite

The Production Continues

Compared to freshly picked fruit, watermelon stored for 14 days at 70°F gained up to 40 percent more lycopene and 50 to 139 percent more beta-carotene. Study findings showed watermelons continue to produce these nutrients after they are picked, and that chilling slows this process.

▶ **calcitriol** The active form of vitamin D; an important regulator of blood calcium levels.

▶ **parathyroid hormone (PTH)** A hormone secreted by the parathyroid glands in response to low blood calcium. It stimulates calcium release from bone and calcium absorption by the intestines, while decreasing calcium excretion by the kidneys. It acts in conjunction with 1,25(OH)$_2$D$_3$ to raise blood calcium. Also called *parathormone.*

▶ **calcitonin** A hormone secreted by the thyroid gland in response to elevated blood calcium. It stimulates calcium deposition in bone and calcium excretion by the kidneys, thus reducing blood calcium.

Cholecalciferol is found in certain animal foods, but most is synthesized in the skin.

In the skin, ultraviolet (UV) radiation from the sun converts a form of cholesterol to cholecalciferol. Both the cholecalciferol synthesized in the skin and that consumed from the diet travel to the liver. The liver converts both synthesized and dietary vitamin D to an intermediate form (25-hydroxyvitamin D$_3$), which it sends to the kidneys. The kidneys perform the final step—conversion to the active form of vitamin D, known as 1,25-dihydroxyvitamin D$_3$ or **calcitriol**.[28]

Functions of Vitamin D

Vitamin D is considered both a vitamin and a hormone. Many simply regard vitamin D as a vitamin that keeps bones healthy, but it is first and foremost a regulator. (See **FIGURE 7.11**.) Because vitamin D made in one part of the body regulates activities in other parts, scientists consider it a hormone. Vitamin D has a role in preventing cancer cells from dividing and has anti-inflammatory properties; as such it may play a role in preventing cancer and cardiovascular disease, an area of considerable research activity.[29,30] Vitamin D also is involved in the regulation of insulin formation and secretion, which suggests a role in blood sugar maintenance and the development of type 2 diabetes mellitus—another area of current research interest.[31]

Regulation of Blood Calcium Levels

The primary regulatory role of vitamin D$_3$ is to maintain blood calcium and phosphorus levels within a normal range. Vitamin D$_3$ acts in concert with two other hormones: **parathyroid hormone (PTH)** from the parathyroid glands and **calcitonin** from the thyroid gland. Together,

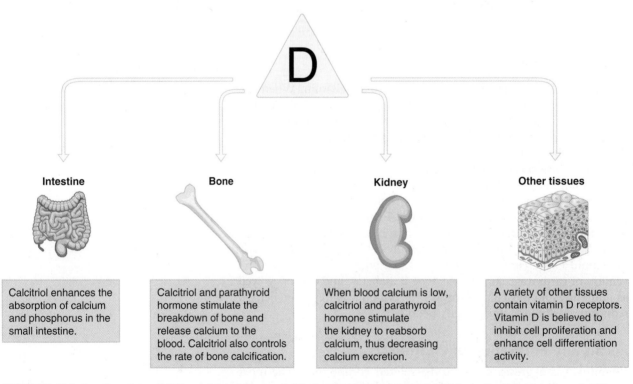

Intestine

Calcitriol enhances the absorption of calcium and phosphorus in the small intestine.

Bone

Calcitriol and parathyroid hormone stimulate the breakdown of bone and release calcium to the blood. Calcitriol also controls the rate of bone calcification.

Kidney

When blood calcium is low, calcitriol and parathyroid hormone stimulate the kidney to reabsorb calcium, thus decreasing calcium excretion.

Other tissues

A variety of other tissues contain vitamin D receptors. Vitamin D is believed to inhibit cell proliferation and enhance cell differentiation activity.

FIGURE 7.11 **Major functions of vitamin D.** Vitamin D and calcium are essential to bone health. To regulate blood calcium levels, vitamin D works with parathyroid hormone (PTH) to stimulate the body to move calcium back and forth between the blood and the reservoir of calcium in bone.

levels of these three hormones continually rise and fall, adjusting blood calcium levels by changing urinary calcium excretion, intestinal calcium absorption, and the flow of calcium into and out of bone.

Here's how it works. Much like a thermostat monitoring temperature, the parathyroid glands monitor blood calcium levels, releasing PTH when calcium levels drop. PTH signals specific bone cells to break down bone tissue and release calcium into the bloodstream. In addition, PTH signals the kidneys to slow calcium excretion and increase vitamin D_3 production. In turn, vitamin D_3 stimulates the small intestine to absorb more calcium from food, thereby raising blood calcium levels further.

When blood calcium levels become too high, the thyroid gland releases calcitonin and the parathyroid glands slow their release of PTH. Calcitonin inhibits factors causing bone breakdown, allowing bone-forming activities to prevail. Bone-forming cells remove calcium from the blood and deposit it in bone. Lower PTH levels allow the kidneys to continue excreting calcium and decrease vitamin D_3 production. In turn, low vitamin D_3 levels cause the small intestine to reduce calcium absorption from food, thereby lowering blood calcium levels further.

Dietary Recommendations for Vitamin D

Despite our ability to synthesize vitamin D, it is an essential nutrient. The updated Dietary Reference Intakes for vitamin D are based on skeletal health and assume only minimal sunlight exposure. When updating the recommendations, the Food and Nutrition Board recognized that sunlight availability varies throughout the year and that some people have limited exposure.[32] The expert panel considered the role of vitamin D in conditions such as cancer, cardiovascular disease, diabetes, infections, and autoimmune disorders, but the evidence was insufficient to make additional intake recommendations.[33] The panel also cautioned against exceeding recommendations for calcium and vitamin D: "Higher levels of both nutrients have not been shown to confer greater benefits, and in fact, they have been linked to other health problems, challenging the concept that 'more is better.'"[34]

Because infants and children have inadequate vitamin D intakes and limited direct sun exposure, the panel recommended that all infants, children, and adolescents consume a minimum of 400 IU of daily vitamin D beginning soon after birth.[35] For people between the ages of 1 and 70 years, the RDA for vitamin D is 600 IU per day.[36] Because vitamin D skin synthesis decreases markedly with age, RDA recommendations increase to 800 IU per day for men and women over the age of 70 years.[37]

Sources of Vitamin D

We get vitamin D from exposure to sunlight, our diets, and dietary supplements. Sensible sun exposure can provide an adequate amount of vitamin D, which is stored in body fat during the winter, when vitamin D production is low. How much exposure to the sun is needed for an adequate supply of vitamin D? Short exposure to direct sunlight, as little as 15 minutes for a fair-skinned person to a few hours for a person with darker skin, can produce as much vitamin D as your body can make in a day.[38] The exact amount of sun exposure depends on several factors, including time of day, season, location, sunscreen use, and skin type. The sun's rays are more intense at latitudes closer to the equator and during midday and summertime. Topical sunscreens (those with a

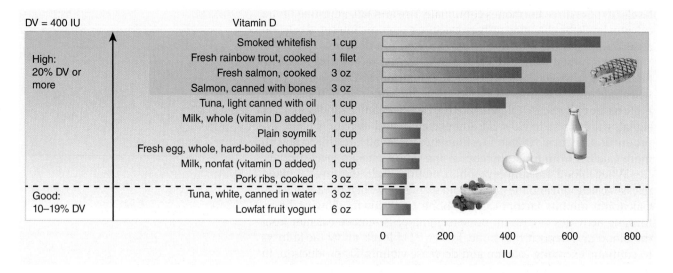

FIGURE 7.12 Sources of vitamin D. Given sufficient sunlight, your body can make all the vitamin D it needs. Only a few foods are naturally good sources of vitamin D. Therefore, fortified foods such as milk and ready-to-eat cereals are important dietary sources, especially for people with limited exposure to the sun.

Data from U.S. Department of Agriculture, Agricultural Research Service, Nutrient Data Laboratory. USDA National Nutrient Database for Standard Reference, Release 28. Version Current: September 2015. Internet: http://www.ars.usda.gov/nea/bhnrc/ndl.

Grilled salmon steak: © indigolotos/Shutterstock, Inc.; Quart bottle of milk: © pjohnson1/Getty Images, Inc.; Yogurt: © Volosina/Getty Images; Boiled eggs: © eventina/Getty Images, Inc.

sun protection factor [SPF] of 8 or greater) block ultraviolet (UV) light. People with dark skin do not absorb UV rays as well as light-skinned people do. Pollution and smog also can reduce UV rays.

The major dietary sources of vitamin D are fortified foods, mainly fortified milk and fortified breakfast cereals. Other fortified foods, such as orange juice, margarine, yogurt, grains, and breads, have become available in the United States. The few foods that naturally contain vitamin D include oily fish (e.g., herring, salmon, sardines), egg yolk, butter, and liver, with amounts dependent on the animal's diet. (See **FIGURE 7.12.**) A diet high in oily fish prevents vitamin D deficiency. More concentrated vitamin D is available in cod liver or other fish liver oils. Plants are poor sources, so strict vegetarians must get their vitamin D through exposure to sunlight, fortified foods, or supplements. Among older adults, usual dietary intake from food alone is approximately one-third of the AI for vitamin D.[39]

Vitamin D Deficiency

Approximately 1 billion people worldwide in all age and ethnic groups have inadequate levels of vitamin D in their blood, including an estimated 20 percent to 80 percent of U.S., Canadian, and European men and women.[40-42] Experts believe that an increase in the incidence of obesity, a decrease in milk consumption, and an increase in sun protection are major contributors to the high number of children and adults in the United States with low vitamin D levels.[43]

Vitamin D deficiency damages bones and contributes to a wide range of acute and chronic conditions. Babies with vitamin D deficiency have soft, weak bones that bend and bow under their weight as they start to walk. The condition is called **rickets**, and is characterized by "bow legs," "knock-knees," and other skeletal deformities. In the United States and Canada, nutritional rickets was all but eliminated by vitamin D–fortified milk, infant formula and vitamin supplements, and vitamin supplements for children with fat malabsorption conditions. Still, rickets from inadequate vitamin D intake and decreased sunlight

▶ **rickets** A bone disease in children that results from vitamin D deficiency.

Quick Bite

"Children's Disease of the English"

In the seventeenth century, vitamin D deficiency was so common in British children that rickets was called the "children's disease of the English." Diets provided little vitamin D, and the lack of sun during many months of the year inhibited vitamin D synthesis in the skin.

exposure continues to occur in infants who are exclusively breastfed and infants with darker skin.[44,45]

Cases of rickets caused by a nutritional deficiency of vitamin D also have been reported in children and adolescents.[46] In a large, nationally representative sample, about 9 percent of U.S. children and adolescents (7.6 million) were found to be vitamin D deficient, which predisposes them to the development of rickets. Lower vitamin D levels were found more often in older children, girls, non-Hispanic African Americans, Mexican Americans, those living in low-income households, obese children, and those who spent more time watching television, playing video games, or using computers. In comparison, children who drank milk daily and/or took vitamin D supplements were less likely to be deficient.[47]

In adults, vitamin D deficiency causes **osteomalacia**, or "soft bones." The condition reduces calcium absorption and increases calcium loss from bone, increasing the risk of bone fractures. People with diseases that affect organs responsible for absorption or activation of vitamin D have a high risk of osteomalacia. Vitamin D deficiency worsens **osteoporosis**, a disease closely related to osteomalacia, with similar symptoms of bone loss and increased risk of fractures. Vitamin D deficiency causes muscle weakness and increases the risk of bone fractures.

Unless a person frequently eats oily fish, it is difficult to obtain sufficient vitamin D from the diet, and increased sun exposure increases the risk of cancer. Factors contributing to low levels of vitamin D include excessive use of sunscreen, living in northern latitudes (see **FIGURE 7.13**), old age, and diets that exclude milk or other fortified foods.

Vitamin D and Other Conditions

Researchers are currently investigating vitamin D's role in the prevention of numerous cancers, including colorectal cancer. They are also examining the potential role of vitamin D in the prevention and treatment of autoimmune diseases, such as diabetes, multiple sclerosis, and rheumatoid arthritis, as well as hypertension and other medical conditions.[48]

Vitamin D Toxicity

Although sun exposure does not cause vitamin D toxicity, supplement megadoses are highly toxic. The daily UL for adults over 19 years of age is 4,000 IU.[49] Because some people are adversely affected by elevated levels of vitamin D, high-dose supplementation should be used only after careful consideration and consultation with a knowledgeable medical professional.[50]

The hallmark of vitamin D toxicity is a high concentration of calcium in the blood. If prolonged, the body deposits excess calcium in soft tissues, including the kidneys, blood vessels, heart, and lungs. Other symptoms include severe depression, nausea, vomiting, and loss of appetite. Ironically, excess vitamin D also causes loss of bone mass.

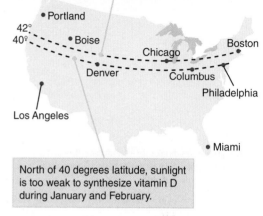

North of 42 degrees latitude, sunlight is too weak to synthesize vitamin D from late October through early March. The same effect occurs during the winter in the southern hemisphere south of 42 degrees latitude.

North of 40 degrees latitude, sunlight is too weak to synthesize vitamin D during January and February.

FIGURE 7.13 Mapping vitamin D synthesis. Vitamin D synthesis halts for part of the winter if sunlight is too weak. In Los Angeles and Miami, the sunlight is strong enough to synthesize vitamin D year round, even in January.

▶ **osteomalacia**   A disease in adults that results from vitamin D deficiency; it is marked by softening of the bones, leading to bending of the spine, bowing of the legs, and increased risk for fractures.

▶ **osteoporosis**   A bone disease characterized by a decrease in bone mineral density and the appearance of small holes in bones due to loss of minerals.

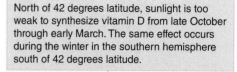

A Fishy Cure

Cod liver oil was well known in the early nineteenth century as a treatment for rickets, a bone disease common in children. It wasn't until the early 1900s, however, that vitamin D was identified as the "antirachitic" (antirickets) substance in cod liver oil.

Key Concepts   Some vitamin D is consumed in the diet, but it is primarily synthesized from cholesterol when the skin is exposed to sunlight. Vitamin D's best-understood function is regulation of blood calcium levels. Along with two other hormones, it regulates urinary calcium excretion, intestinal calcium absorption, and the amount of calcium in bone. Dietary needs increase with age, as the ability of skin to synthesize vitamin D declines. Most dietary vitamin D is from fortified milk and other fortified foods. Vitamin D deficiency in children causes rickets; in adults it leads to osteomalacia and contributes to osteoporosis. In excess, vitamin D causes loss of bone and deposits of calcium in soft tissue.

Vitamin E

Consumers have long embraced the practice of taking large amounts of vitamin E. Since its discovery in 1922 and the finding that its deficiency made laboratory rats sterile, vitamin E has been a reputed aphrodisiac. Vitamin E supplements also have been promoted for "antiaging," with the ability to prevent everything from gray hair and wrinkles to cancer and heart disease. Although science does not support most rumored benefits, a growing body of research suggests vitamin E may be important in defending against chronic diseases associated with aging.

Forms of Vitamin E

▶ **tocopherol** The chemical name for vitamin E. There are four tocopherols (alpha, beta, gamma, and delta), but only alpha-tocopherol is active in the body.

In 1922, researchers discovered that an unknown substance in vegetable oils was necessary for reproduction in rats. It was given the chemical name **tocopherol**, from the Greek word *tokos*, meaning "childbirth," added to the verb *phero*, meaning "to bring forth." The ending *ol* reflects the alcohol nature of the molecule. It was a full 40 years after discovery, however, before scientists gathered evidence showing that humans also need this substance, which they labeled vitamin E. Vitamin E is actually a family of eight similar compounds. Although all are absorbed, only one, called alpha-tocopherol, is considered for the human vitamin E requirement, and milligrams of alpha-tocopherol are the standard measure of vitamin E.

Unlike the fat-soluble vitamins A and D, vitamin E is not stored primarily in the liver. Body fat holds about 90 percent of the vitamin E reserves. Virtually every tissue has some vitamin E, providing protection within every cell membrane.

Functions of Vitamin E

Vitamin E's most well-known function is as an antioxidant. It protects vulnerable polyunsaturated lipids in cell membranes, in the blood, and elsewhere throughout the body. (See **FIGURE 7.14**.) Like carotenoids, it works by countering, or "scavenging," free radicals.

Numerous studies have suggested that dietary factors such as high intakes of antioxidant vitamins, including vitamin E, may lower the risk of some chronic diseases, especially heart disease.[51] However, results from large clinical trials generally do not support routine use of vitamin E supplementation for the prevention of cardiovascular disease or reduction in related morbidity and mortality.[52] Although antioxidant food sources, especially plant foods, whole grains, and vegetable oils, are recommended, current evidence is insufficient to recommend supplemental vitamin E for heart disease prevention in the general population.[53]

What about other age-related diseases? Nutritionists have investigated a possible preventive role for vitamin E and have found promising results in numerous conditions, including cancer; eye disorders, such as age-related macular degeneration and cataracts; immune function; cognitive declines; and Alzheimer's disease. In general, however, research does not support large-scale supplementation with vitamin E for the prevention or treatment of these conditions.[54] See **FIGURE 7.15** for the major functions of vitamin E.

Dietary Recommendations for Vitamin E

Vitamin E needs are related to body size and the intake of polyunsaturated fatty acids (PUFAs), which are especially vulnerable to destructive oxidation. When you eat minimal amounts of PUFAs, you need

Key

◉ Free radical

△ Vitamin E

● Neutralized free radical

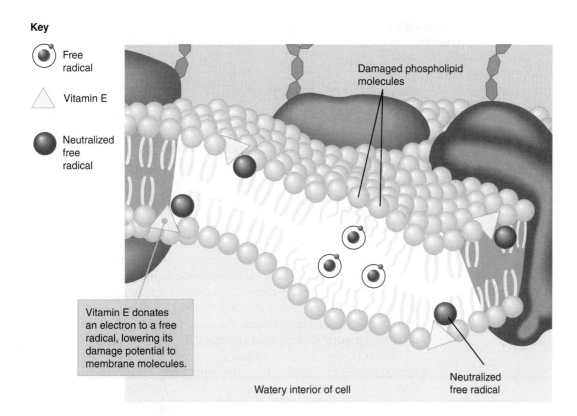

Damaged phospholipid molecules

Vitamin E donates an electron to a free radical, lowering its damage potential to membrane molecules.

Watery interior of cell

Neutralized free radical

FIGURE 7.14 Free radical damage. Vitamin E helps prevent free radical damage to polyunsaturated fatty acids in cell membranes.

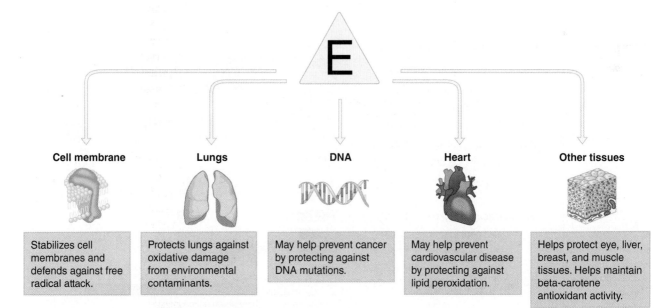

Cell membrane

Stabilizes cell membranes and defends against free radical attack.

Lungs

Protects lungs against oxidative damage from environmental contaminants.

DNA

May help prevent cancer by protecting against DNA mutations.

Heart

May help prevent cardiovascular disease by protecting against lipid peroxidation.

Other tissues

Helps protect eye, liver, breast, and muscle tissues. Helps maintain beta-carotene antioxidant activity.

FIGURE 7.15 Major functions of vitamin E. The antioxidant activity of vitamin E helps stabilize cell membranes, protects tissues from oxidative damage, and may reduce the risk of cancer and heart disease.

smaller amounts of protective vitamin E. When you eat more vegetable oils, the major PUFA source, you need more vitamin E. Because the vitamin E in vegetable oils tends to be proportional to their PUFA content, to some extent these oils help provide extra vitamin E as needed. The RDA for vitamin E accommodates generous PUFA intake. It is set at 15 milligrams per day of alpha-tocopherol for adults (including pregnant women) and 19 milligrams per day for women who are breastfeeding.

Sources of Vitamin E

Alpha-tocopherol is present in appreciable amounts only in foods such as nuts (e.g., almonds), some seeds (e.g., sunflower), and vegetable oils (e.g., soybean, safflower, corn, canola). Whole-grain products provide vitamin E, and wheat germ oil has one of the highest vitamin E concentrations. Most fruits and vegetables contribute only small amounts, and animal-derived products are inconsistent sources, depending on the animal's diet. (See **FIGURE 7.16**.)

Although most Americans eat a diet relatively rich in soybean and corn oils, only about 10 percent is alpha-tocopherol, the active form of vitamin E.[55] Foods made from vegetable oils, such as margarine and salad dressings, also are good sources. Cooking, processing, and storage can reduce the vitamin E content of foods substantially. (See **TABLE 7.3**.) Light and heat accelerate vitamin E's destruction. Safflower oils stored at room temperature for three months lose more than half of their vitamin E. Roasting destroys 80 percent of the vitamin E in almonds. Consuming sufficient vitamin E to meet requirements appears to be challenging for most Americans. NHANES III data suggest that American adults consume 8 to 12 milligrams of vitamin E per day from foods with about 20 percent coming from salad oils, margarine, and shortening.[56] However, this value is likely to be less than actual consumption due to typical underreporting of total fat and energy intake.[57]

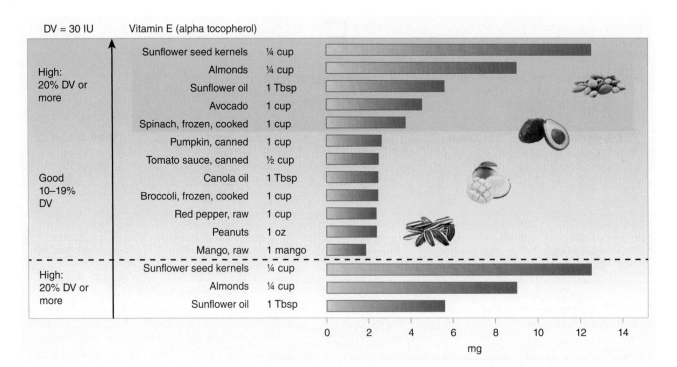

FIGURE 7.16 Food sources of vitamin E. Nuts, seeds, vegetable oils, and products made from vegetable oil are among the best sources of vitamin E.

Data from U.S. Department of Agriculture, Agricultural Research Service, Nutrient Data Laboratory. USDA National Nutrient Database for Standard Reference, Release 28. Version Current: September 2015. Internet: http://www.ars.usda.gov/nea/bhnrc/ndl.

Almonds: © Africa Studio/Shutterstock, Inc.; Avocados: © masa44/Shutterstock ,Inc.; Mango: © Maks Narodenko/Shutterstock, Inc.; Sunflower seeds: © JIANG HONGYAN/Shutterstock, Inc.

TABLE 7.3
Reported Storage and Processing Losses of Vitamin E

Food	Test Conditions	Vitamin E Losses
Peanut oil	Frying at 347°F (175°C), 30 minutes	32%
Safflower oil	Storing at room temperature, 3 months	55%
Tortillas	Storing at room temperature, 12 months	95%
Almonds	Roasting	80%
Wheat germ	Storing at 39°F (4°C), 6 months	10%
Wheat	Processing to white flour	92%
Bread	Baking	5–50%

Vitamin E Factbook. LaGrange, IL: VERIS; 1999. Reprinted with permission from Veris Research Information Services.

Vitamin E Deficiency

Overt vitamin E deficiency is so rare in humans that the Food and Nutrition Board could not use signs of deficiency (e.g., neurological abnormalities) as a basis for estimating dietary requirements. Vitamin E deficiency occurs mostly in people with fat malabsorption or rare genetic disorders. In adults, it takes 5 to 10 years of a deficiency before symptoms emerge.

Vitamin E Toxicity

For a fat-soluble vitamin, vitamin E is surprisingly nontoxic, and adverse effects have not been found from consuming foods rich in vitamin E. However, it is not totally safe, and large supplement amounts may cause an increased risk of bleeding, especially in people with vitamin K deficiency and in those taking anticoagulant medication or aspirin.[58] For adults, therefore, the UL is 1,000 milligrams per day of supplemental alpha-tocopherol. Despite some large studies that found that vitamin E supplementation led to a small increase in the risk of death, other evidence does not support those findings.[59]

> **Key Concepts** Alpha-tocopherol is the only form of vitamin E that meets the vitamin E requirements. It is an antioxidant, protecting cell membranes from the damaging effects of oxidation. Some evidence suggests that vitamin E might delay degenerative diseases such as heart disease and cancer. Vitamin E is found mainly in vegetable and seed oils and products made from them. Considerable vitamin E is lost in food processing, cooking, and storage. Vitamin E deficiency is rare. Vitamin E is relatively nontoxic, though large doses interfere with blood clotting.

Vitamin K

Vitamin K was named for the Danish word *koagulation*. The name says it all. Vitamin K is essential for blood clotting (also called coagulation). Although most people give little thought to consuming enough of this nutrient, vitamin K stands between life and death. Without it, you would bleed to death from a single cut. Vitamin K is actually a family of compounds known as quinones. It includes **phylloquinone** (K$_1$) from plant sources, **menaquinones** (collectively known as K$_2$) from animal sources and synthesized by our intestinal bacteria, and **menadione (K$_3$)**, a synthetic form. Phylloquinone is the major form

▶ **phylloquinone** The form of vitamin K that comes from plant sources. Also known as *vitamin K$_1$*.

▶ **menaquinones** The form of vitamin K that comes from animal sources or is produced by intestinal bacteria. Also known as *vitamin K$_2$*.

▶ **menadione** A medicinal form of vitamin K. Also known as *vitamin K$_3$*.

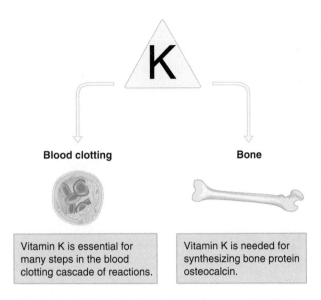

Blood clotting

Vitamin K is essential for many steps in the blood clotting cascade of reactions.

Bone

Vitamin K is needed for synthesizing bone protein osteocalcin.

FIGURE 7.17 Major functions of vitamin K. Without vitamin K, our blood would not clot and our bones would become weak.

in the diet and the most biologically active. Vitamin K is stored primarily in the liver and is also found in bone. Unlike other fat-soluble vitamins, the liver rapidly breaks down vitamin K and eliminates it, and thus reserves can be depleted quickly.

Functions of Vitamin K

When you bleed from a cut, your body starts a chain of reactions that forms a clot and stops the flow of blood. Many reactions in this coagulation cascade require vitamin K and calcium. Vitamin K also helps with bone formation, increases bone strength, and decreases fractures.[60, 61] (See **FIGURE 7.17**.) Low levels of vitamin K are associated with age-related bone loss.[62] Other vitamin K–dependent proteins have been isolated in bone, underscoring the vitamin's importance to bone health.

Dietary Recommendations for Vitamin K

Dietary intake of vitamin K varies with age; however, typical diets easily meet the dietary recommendations for vitamin K. The AI for vitamin K for adult men is 120 micrograms daily, and for women, including those pregnant or breastfeeding, it is 90 micrograms.[63] As with other fat-soluble vitamins, vitamin K absorption depends on normal consumption and digestion of dietary fat. Even under normal conditions, absorption of dietary vitamin K may be as low as 40 percent.

Sources of Vitamin K

We obtain vitamin K from two sources: food (mostly plant food) and bacteria living in our colons. Dietary vitamin K is absorbed in the small intestine, and vitamin K produced by bacteria is absorbed in the colon. Plant foods, especially green leafy vegetables, such as spinach, turnip greens, broccoli, and Brussels sprouts, are our primary sources of vitamin K, as phylloquinone. Certain plant oils (soybean, cottonseed, canola, and olive) also are important sources.[64] (See **FIGURE 7.18**.) In general, animal products contain limited amounts of vitamin K.

Vitamin K Deficiency

In adults, vitamin K deficiency is rare and usually occurs in people with fat malabsorption problems. However, newborn babies lack vitamin K–producing intestinal bacteria, so they are at risk of vitamin K deficiency. Because breast milk has little vitamin K, breastfed babies are especially vulnerable. Physicians routinely give newborns a vitamin K injection. This usually meets the infant's needs for several weeks, until vitamin K–producing bacteria establish themselves in the intestine. People who suffer fat-malabsorption syndromes, such as celiac disease, cystic fibrosis, ulcerative colitis, and Crohn's disease, can develop vitamin K deficiency. Prolonged use of antibiotics may cause a deficiency because the drugs can destroy the intestinal bacteria that produce vitamin K. Megadoses of vitamins A and E interfere with the actions of vitamin K. People who take some anticoagulants such as warfarin should maintain a consistent pattern of vitamin K consumption,

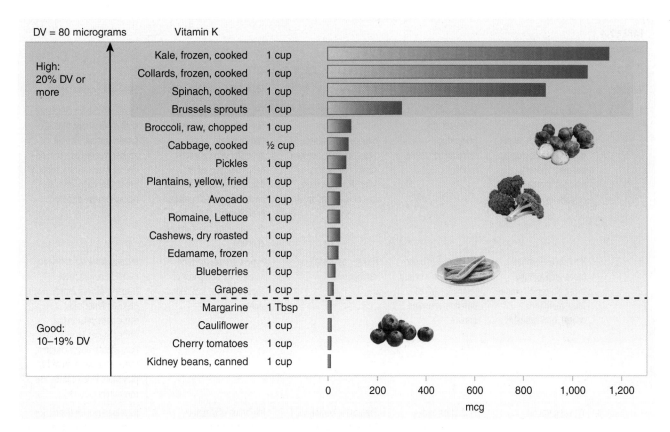

FIGURE 7.18 Food sources of vitamin K. The best sources of vitamin K are vegetables, especially leafy greens and those in the cabbage family.

Data from U.S. Department of Agriculture, Agricultural Research Service, Nutrient Data Laboratory. USDA National Nutrient Database for Standard Reference, Release 28. Version Current: September 2015. Internet: http://www.ars.usda.gov/nea/bhnrc/ndl.

Fried plantain banana: © bonchan/Getty Images, Inc.; Brussels sprouts: © Brigitte Sporrer/Getty Images, Inc.; Broccoli florets: © Antonova Anna/Shutterstock, Inc; Blueberries: © photastic/Shutterstock, Inc.

because large fluctuations can interfere with the effectiveness of these drugs.[65] Some newer blood thinning medications do not require dietary restrictions of vitamin K.

Although vitamin K has a crucial role in blood clotting, the body needs only small amounts. This makes vitamin K deficiency rare in healthy adults. On the other hand, preliminary research suggests that typical diets are supplying less than optimal amounts for bone health.

Vitamin K Toxicity

Because the body excretes vitamin K much more rapidly than other fat-soluble vitamins, vitamin K toxicity from food is rare. The Food and Nutrition Board has not set a UL for vitamin K.

TABLE 7.4 provides a review of the key features for the fat-soluble vitamins A, D, E, and K.

> **Key Concepts** Vitamin K is required for blood clotting and bone health. It is found primarily in green vegetables and in some vegetable oils. Newborns are routinely given injections of vitamin K. Deficiencies are very rare. Because vitamin K is readily excreted, especially compared with other fat-soluble vitamins, toxicity also is rare.

Quick Bite

Does Blocking Vitamin K Cure or Kill?

The medication warfarin (Coumadin) prevents undesired blood clotting by blocking vitamin K. Warfarin in very large amounts also is used in common rat poison to cause internal hemorrhage and death.

TABLE 7.4
Summary of Fat-Soluble Vitamins

Vitamin	Important Dietary Sources	Major Functions	Signs/Symptoms of Deficiency	Toxic Effects of Megadoses	Special Considerations
A	Liver, fish liver oil, milk fat, carrots, spinach, broccoli, squash, sweet potatoes, cantaloupes, peaches, apricots, mangos, margarine, cereals, low-fat milk	Vision, cell differentiation, immunity, reproduction, bone health	Growth retardation, vision loss/night blindness/blindness, excess keratin, reduced sperm production, infertility in women, loss of taste and smell	Fatigue, vomiting, abdominal pain, bone and joint pain, loss of appetite, skin disorders, headache, blurred or double vision, liver damage, birth defects (cleft palate, heart abnormalities, brain malfunction), spontaneous abortion	Increased risk for deficiency with medications that alter fat absorption, alcohol abuse/liver disease, protein-energy malnutrition, infancy/premature birth, and fat-malabsorptive disorders
D	Vitamin D–fortified foods such as milk, breakfast cereal, orange juice, margarine, yogurt, grains/breads	Regulation of blood calcium, bone health, regulation of cell differentiation and growth	Rickets, osteomalacia, osteoporosis	Hypercalcemia (causing nausea, vomiting, loss of appetite), bone loss, kidney stones	Increased risk for deficiency in children, girls, non-Hispanic African Americans, Mexican Americans, those born outside the United States, low-income households, obese children, those who watch more TV/play more video games/use computers
E	Wheat germ oil, safflower oil, cottonseed oil, sunflower seed oil, foods made from oils (margarine, salad dressing), sunflower seeds, almonds, spinach, fortified cereals	Protection and maintenance of cellular membranes through antioxidant capacity	Premature hemolysis, hemolytic anemia, neurological problems	Inhibition of platelet adhesion and countering vitamin K's blood clotting mechanism	Increased risk for deficiency with fat-malabsorptive disorders
K	Spinach, greens, broccoli, Brussels sprouts, vegetable oils (soybean, cottonseed, canola, olive)	Blood clotting, bone health/sustaining bone mineral density	Reduced bone density, bone fractures, bleeding	Hemolytic anemia	Increased risk for deficiency with fat-malabsorptive disorders and long-term antibiotic use (due to antibiotics destroying the intestinal bacteria that produce vitamin K)

The Water-Soluble Vitamins: Eight Bs and a C

🍎 **Why Is This Important?** Water-soluble vitamins consist of the eight B vitamins and vitamin C. Knowing the different water-soluble vitamins—their functions, requirements, and food sources—is important to understanding their roles in sustaining energy production and maintaining health.

The scientists who first discovered vitamin B believed "it" was a single compound. As they learned more, they discovered "it" was actually several vitamins. In fact, there are eight B vitamins. Initially, to differentiate them, numbers were added to the letter B. Today, with the exception of B_6 and B_{12}, we usually refer to the B vitamins by their names: thiamin, riboflavin, niacin, pantothenic acid, biotin, and folate.

B vitamins act primarily in energy metabolism as coenzymes (or parts of coenzymes)—the keys that unlock the action of enzymes. Enzymes regulate countless life-sustaining chemical reactions. They hurry reactions along or slow them down, as needed, even allowing them to proceed when it would otherwise be impossible. But many enzymes cannot work until the body supplies a missing component—a coenzyme.

Let's use an analogy to clarify how vitamins function as coenzymes. Suppose you had an appointment in 15 minutes that was 10 miles away. You could walk there, but you would be too late. You could drive your car, but you cannot find your key. Now you find your key (the coenzyme), turn on your car (the enzyme), and quickly drive to your destination (the reaction taking place in your body). (See **FIGURE 7.19**.)

Vitamin C is an antioxidant, but unlike the antioxidant vitamin E, it is water-soluble. Despite differences in solubility, vitamin C and vitamin E work together. When vitamin E quenches a free radical, vitamin E in turn becomes a free radical, although a less reactive one. Vitamin C can stabilize it, restoring vitamin E's antioxidant abilities.

Thiamin

The thiamin-deficiency disease **beriberi** was first described in Chinese writings over 4,000 years ago, but it was not widespread until the nineteenth century, when highly milled or "polished" white rice became popular. In 1885, Dr. K. Takaki of the Japanese Naval Medical Services first demonstrated beriberi's dietary origins. He cured sailors sick with beriberi by adding meat, milk, and whole grains to their diets.[66] Years later, Christian Eijkman, a Dutch medical officer, fed birds only white rice until they had beriberi and then cured them by adding bran to their diet.[67] This led to the discovery of an "anti-beriberi" factor—thiamin.

Functions of Thiamin

Thiamin works as a coenzyme in reactions that produce energy. Deprive your body of thiamin, and you deprive every cell of its ability to use energy. As the vitamin component of the coenzyme **thiamin pyrophosphate (TPP)**, thiamin helps reactions that break down glucose, make RNA and DNA, or produce energy-rich molecules that power protein synthesis. TPP also helps synthesize and regulate neurotransmitters—chemicals that act as messengers between nerve cells.[68]

Dietary Recommendations and Sources of Thiamin

Because thiamin needs are related to energy requirements and carbohydrate intake, they are slightly greater for men than for women. The RDA for adult men age 19 years or older is 1.2 milligrams per day; for adult women, it is 1.1 milligrams. Pregnancy and breastfeeding increase energy requirements, so thiamin RDA rises to 1.4 milligrams per day during pregnancy and 1.4 milligrams when a woman is breastfeeding.[69] If a person's diet supplies adequate energy and includes thiamin-rich foods, it generally contains enough thiamin.

Because thiamin is found in small amounts throughout the food supply, eating a wide variety of foods is the best way to ensure a good intake. Pork is one of the richest sources. Legumes (mature beans and peas), some nuts and seeds (e.g., sunflower seeds), and some types of fish and seafood are good sources. (See **FIGURE 7.20**.) Other meats, dairy

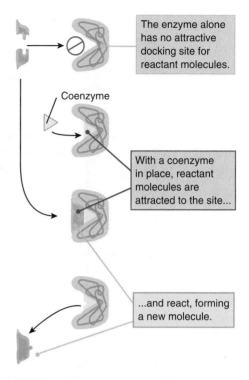

The enzyme alone has no attractive docking site for reactant molecules.

Coenzyme

With a coenzyme in place, reactant molecules are attracted to the site...

...and react, forming a new molecule.

FIGURE 7.19 The coenzyme–enzyme partnership. The B vitamins form coenzymes that enable specific enzymes to catalyze reactions.

▶ **beriberi** Thiamin-deficiency disease. Symptoms include muscle weakness, loss of appetite, nerve degeneration, and edema in some cases.

▶ **thiamin pyrophosphate (TPP)** A coenzyme of which the vitamin thiamin is a part. It plays a key role in removing carboxyl groups in chemical reactions and helps drive the reaction that forms acetyl CoA from pyruvate during metabolism.

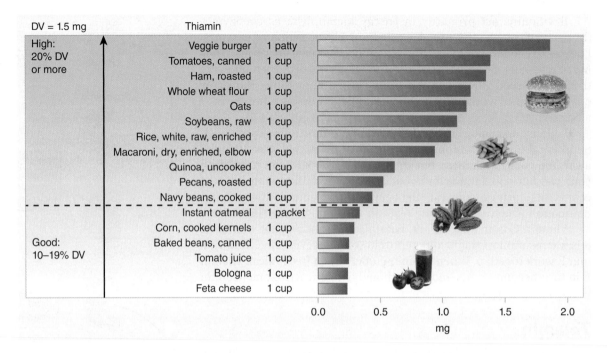

FIGURE 7.20 **Food sources of thiamin.** Pork, whole and enriched grains, and fortified cereals are rich in thiamin. Most animal foods contain little thiamin.

Data from U.S. Department of Agriculture, Agricultural Research Service, Nutrient Data Laboratory. USDA National Nutrient Database for Standard Reference, Release 28. Version Current: September 2015. Internet: http://www.ars.usda.gov/nea/bhnrc/ndl.

Veggie burger: © Lew Robertson/Getty Images, Inc.; Soy beans: © Roger Dixon/Shutterstock, Inc.; Tomato juice: © gbrundin/Getty Images, Inc.; Brown pecans: © nanka/ Shutterstock, Inc.

products, and most fruits contain little thiamin. Most thiamin we eat comes from enriched grain products: bread, pasta, rice, and ready-to-eat cereals.[70] Heat and alkaline cooking water easily destroy thiamin, so cooking reduces a food's thiamin content.

Thiamin Deficiency

Beriberi means "I can't, I can't," in one of the languages of Southeast Asia. The phrase describes how doctors long ago diagnosed the disease: Their patients were unable to rise from a squatting position. In fact, overall profound muscle weakness combined with nerve destruction ultimately leaves the victim of beriberi almost unable to move.

Milder symptoms of thiamin deficiency can appear after only 10 days on a thiamin-free diet. These include headache, irritability, fatigue, depression, and loss of appetite—signs of nervous system disturbance—and contribute to a worsening food intake, causing further muscle weakness and nerve degeneration.

Those body systems with high energy needs deteriorate first. Digestive damage causes diarrhea, muscle damage causes muscle wasting and pain, and nerve damage disrupts coordination and causes "pins and needles" sensations in hands and feet. Death, however, most often comes from damage to the heart. As the heart muscle fails, feet and legs fill with fluid (edema), the so-called wet beriberi. (See **FIGURE 7.21**.) Outbreaks of beriberi commonly occur in refugee and displaced populations dependent on international food aid. They often must subsist on milled white cereals, including polished rice and white flour, all poor sources of thiamin when not enriched. Because many B vitamins are in the same foods as thiamin, thiamin deficiency and other B vitamin deficiencies often go hand in hand.

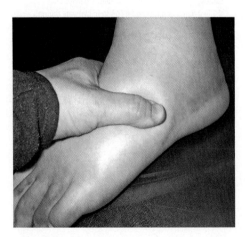

FIGURE 7.21 **Edema, especially in the feet and legs, is a symptom of wet beriberi.**

Courtesy of Scott Landis, Bryan College.

The poor and the elderly may be at risk of deficiency due to inadequate energy intake or consumption of nutrient-poor foods. In industrialized countries, thiamin deficiency usually is related to heavy alcohol consumption combined with limited food consumption. Alcoholics are at risk for thiamin deficiency for two reasons: (1) alcohol contributes calories without contributing nutrients, and (2) alcohol interferes with absorption of thiamin and many other vitamins. Alcohol-induced malnutrition is the most common cause of Wernicke–Korsakoff syndrome, another thiamin-deficiency disease. Symptoms include mental confusion, staggering, and constant rapid eye movements or paralysis of the eye muscles. Although the syndrome most often is associated with the stereotypical alcoholic, it can occur in any heavy drinker, especially an elderly one. Recently, a genetic defect that affects thiamin's transport and metabolism has been described in patients with other inborn errors of metabolism, which can often be overcome with high concentrations of thiamin.[71]

Thiamin Toxicity

Thiamin supplements, which are cheap to produce, often include up to 200 times the Daily Value for thiamin, but, to date, there have been no reports of thiamin toxicity. The Food and Nutrition Board has not set a Tolerated Upper Intake Level (UL) for this nutrient. The kidneys quickly excrete excess thiamin in urine.[72]

Riboflavin

At first, riboflavin and thiamin were considered the same vitamin. When riboflavin was finally isolated from the "anti-beriberi factor," it was dubbed vitamin B_2, and later riboflavin for its yellow color (*flavin* means "yellow" in Latin). In foods, though, it may give a green or bluish cast. You'll notice the color in uncooked egg whites and some brands of fat-free milk.

Functions of Riboflavin

Riboflavin is a part of two coenzymes, flavin mononucleotide and flavin adenine dinucleotide. Both coenzymes are required in reactions that extract energy from glucose, fatty acids, and amino acids. Riboflavin also supports the antioxidant activity of the enzyme **glutathione peroxidase**. Riboflavin-containing coenzymes also participate in reactions that remove ammonia during the deamination of some amino acids.[73]

▶ **glutathione peroxidase** A selenium-containing enzyme that reduces toxic hydrogen peroxide formed within cells; works with vitamin E to reduce free radical damage.

Dietary Recommendations and Sources of Riboflavin

As with thiamin, riboflavin requirements increase along with increasing energy needs. For adults age 19 or older, the RDA is 1.3 milligrams per day for men and 1.1 milligrams for women, reflecting the higher energy needs of men. Pregnancy increases the riboflavin RDA to 1.4 milligrams per day; breastfeeding increases it to 1.6 milligrams.[74]

Milk and milk-containing beverages, cottage cheese, and yogurt are excellent riboflavin sources. Enriched grain products, eggs, and organ meats also are good sources. (See **FIGURE 7.22.**) Riboflavin absorption from food is good, and it generally is more stable than thiamin and resistant to acid, heat, and oxidation; however, light can destroy it. Riboflavin-rich foods should be stored in opaque packages. For example,

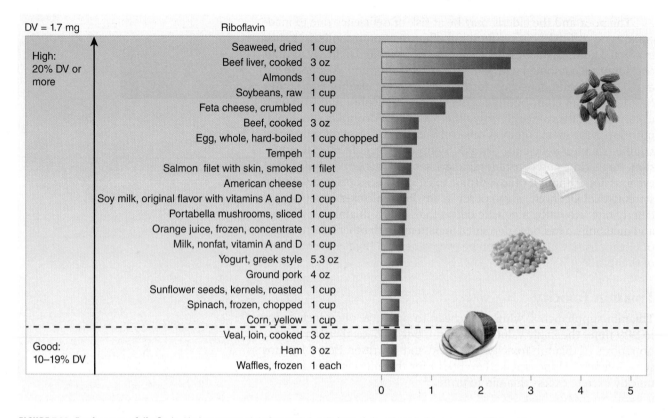

DV = 1.7 mg   Riboflavin

High: 20% DV or more

Good: 10–19% DV

Food	Amount
Seaweed, dried	1 cup
Beef liver, cooked	3 oz
Almonds	1 cup
Soybeans, raw	1 cup
Feta cheese, crumbled	1 cup
Beef, cooked	3 oz
Egg, whole, hard-boiled	1 cup chopped
Tempeh	1 cup
Salmon filet with skin, smoked	1 filet
American cheese	1 cup
Soy milk, original flavor with vitamins A and D	1 cup
Portabella mushrooms, sliced	1 cup
Orange juice, frozen, concentrate	1 cup
Milk, nonfat, vitamin A and D	1 cup
Yogurt, greek style	5.3 oz
Ground pork	4 oz
Sunflower seeds, kernels, roasted	1 cup
Spinach, frozen, chopped	1 cup
Corn, yellow	1 cup
Veal, loin, cooked	3 oz
Ham	3 oz
Waffles, frozen	1 each

0   1   2   3   4   5

FIGURE 7.22 Food sources of riboflavin. The best sources of riboflavin include milk, liver, whole and enriched grains, and fortified cereals.

Data from U.S. Department of Agriculture, Agricultural Research Service, Nutrient Data Laboratory. USDA National Nutrient Database for Standard Reference, Release 28. Version Current: September 2015. Internet: http://www.ars.usda.gov/nea/bhnrc/ndl. Accessed January 29, 2016.

Almonds: © vkbhat/Getty Images, Inc.; Ham: © Paul Poplis/Getty Images; Cheese slices: © Binh Thanh Bui/Shutterstock, Inc.; Corn kernels: © Renee Comet Photography/Getty Images, Inc.

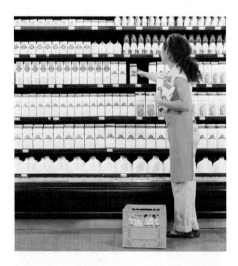

FIGURE 7.23 Packaging affects riboflavin content in milk. Light breaks down riboflavin easily, so foods high in riboflavin (e.g., milk) are best stored in opaque containers.

© Paul Burns /Getty Images Inc.

▶ **anemia** Abnormally low concentration of hemoglobin in the bloodstream; can be caused by impaired synthesis of red blood cells, increased destruction of red blood cells, or significant loss of blood.

packaging milk in paper or plastic cartons rather than clear glass better protects milk's riboflavin content.[75] (See **FIGURE 7.23**.)

Riboflavin Deficiency

Overt riboflavin deficiency is now rare, and like thiamin deficiency occurs most often in chronic alcoholism. Long-term use of sedatives and other barbiturates accelerates liver breakdown of riboflavin and contributes to deficiency.

Riboflavin deficiency shows up first around the mouth. The tongue gets shiny, smooth, and inflamed; the mouth becomes painful and sore; the skin at the corners of the mouth cracks; and the lips become inflamed and split. The oil-producing glands of the skin become clogged, and as the deficiency becomes severe, a characteristic **anemia** develops. Riboflavin deficiency usually exists along with other nutrient deficiencies. In fact, because riboflavin is involved in the metabolism of other B vitamins, such as vitamin B_6, folate, and niacin, severe riboflavin deficiency may even make other deficiencies worse.

Riboflavin Toxicity

Excess riboflavin is readily excreted, and even large doses don't appear harmful. There are no reported cases of toxicity. A UL has not been set for riboflavin.

Niacin

Niacin is the name for two similar compounds: nicotinic acid and nicotinamide (also known as niacinamide). Ironically, this healthful substance got its name from a singularly unhealthful substance. In 1867, nicotinic acid was produced from nicotine in tobacco. Understand clearly, though, that nicotinic acid is not the same as or even closely related to nicotine. In the early 1940s, with its role as a vitamin established, it was renamed "niacin" so people wouldn't confuse it with nicotine.

Functions of Niacin

Niacin forms a part of crucially important coenzymes that participate in at least 200 metabolic pathways. As such, it plays a key role in energy metabolism, both under normal conditions and during times of vigorous activity when energy use swings into high gear. The body also needs niacin to synthesize fatty acids.

Dietary Recommendations and Sources of Niacin

Niacin is unique among the B vitamins—your body can make it from the amino acid **tryptophan** as well as obtain it from foods. Intake recommendations are expressed as **niacin equivalents (NEs)**, a measure that includes both niacin and tryptophan. The RDA is 16 milligrams of NE per day for adult men and 14 milligrams per day for adult women, increasing to 18 milligrams during pregnancy and 17 milligrams during breastfeeding.[76]

Most niacin in the U.S. diet comes from meat, poultry, fish, and enriched and whole-grain products and fortified ready-to-eat cereals. (See **FIGURE 7.24**.) Niacin is stable when heated, so little is lost during cooking. In a typical U.S. diet, beef and processed meats are substantial contributors. Other good sources of niacin include mushrooms, peanuts, liver, and seafood.[77]

> *Quick* **Bite**
>
> **Are You Smoking That Bread?**
> In the 1940s, antitobacco forces were confused about the differences between niacin and nicotine. They mistakenly warned that niacin-enriched bread could cause an addiction to cigarettes!

▶ **tryptophan** An amino acid that serves as a niacin precursor in the body. In the body, 60 milligrams of tryptophan yield about one milligram of niacin, or 1 niacin equivalent (NE).

▶ **niacin equivalents (NEs)** A measure that includes preformed dietary niacin as well as niacin derived from tryptophan; 60 milligrams of tryptophan yield about 1 milligram of niacin.

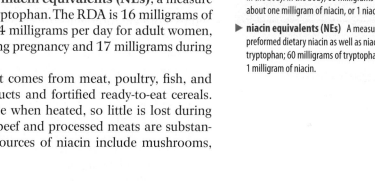

DV = 20 mg Niacin

	Food	Serving	
High: 20% DV or more	Turkey breast, cooked	1 breast	
	Salmon, alaska with skin	1 filet	
	Peanuts, roasted	1 cup	
	Tuna, light, canned in oil	1 cup	
	Rice, white, enriched, raw	1 cup	
	Veal, loin cooked	3 oz	
	Chicken, thigh meat, cooked	1 thigh	
	Ground pork	4 oz	
	Corn, yellow	1 cup	
	Ham,	3 oz	
	Beef, rib-eye	3 oz	
Good: 10–19% DV	Peanut butter	1 Tbsp	
	Spinach, frozen, chopped	1 cup	
	Yogurt, greek style	5.3 oz	
	Milk, nonfat	1 cup	

(scale: 0 20 40 60 80 100 120)

FIGURE 7.24 Food sources of niacin. Niacin is found mainly in meats and grains. Enrichment adds niacin as well as thiamin, riboflavin, folic acid, and iron to processed grains.

Data from U.S. Department of Agriculture, Agricultural Research Service, Nutrient Data Laboratory. USDA National Nutrient Database for Standard Reference, Release 28. Version Current: September 2015. Internet: http://www.ars.usda.gov/nea/bhnrc/ndl. Accessed January 29, 2016.

Jar of Peanut Butter: © Andrea Bricco/Getty Images Inc.; Lone rib eye steak: © JoeGough/Getty Images, Inc.; Dried peanuts: © Hong Vo/Shutterstock, Inc.; Grilled chicken thighs: © Yury Smelov/ Shutterstock, Inc.

The niacin precursor tryptophan supplies about half of our niacin intake. Tryptophan is an essential amino acid and is an integral part of dietary protein. It is in almost all protein foods but is notably low in the protein of corn. Sixty milligrams of tryptophan yield about 1 milligram of niacin, or 1 niacin equivalent (NE). Because the body needs other nutrients (riboflavin, vitamin B_6, and iron) to convert tryptophan to niacin, a deficit of any of them can worsen a niacin deficiency.

Niacin Deficiency

Pellagra is the disease of severe niacin deficiency. The word *pellagra* means "rough skin" in Italian and describes the dermatitis—a rough, darkened rash—that occurs where the victim's skin is exposed to sunlight. However, because niacin coenzymes are involved in just about every metabolic pathway, deficiency devastates the entire body. The hallmarks of pellagra are "the four Ds": dermatitis, diarrhea, dementia, and, ultimately, death. Deficiencies of other nutrients such as iron, riboflavin, and vitamin B_6 can contribute to the damage.

Descriptions of pellagra were first documented in 1735, but the great pellagra epidemic in America's South did not emerge until the early twentieth century. The rural poor began subsisting on a diet of corn (maize), molasses, and fatty salt pork, all poor sources of niacin and tryptophan. Although corn contains niacin, the niacin is bound to a protein, which impairs absorption. We now know that soaking corn in a solution of lime (calcium hydroxide) helps release niacin, which much improves absorption. (See **FIGURE 7.25**.)

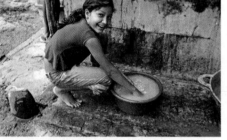

FIGURE 7.25 Soaking corn in a solution of lime (calcium hydroxide) releases bound niacin.

© Tina Manley/Alamy Images.

Widespread pellagra began to decline during World War II after the federal government mandated enrichment of bread flour and other cereal grains with niacin. Today, pellagra has virtually disappeared in industrialized countries, except in some people with chronic alcoholism or disorders that disrupt synthesis from tryptophan. Pellagra continues to plague people living in Southeast Asia and Africa, however, whose diets lack sufficient niacin and protein.

Niacin Toxicity and Medicinal Uses of Niacin

For adults, the UL for niacin is 35 milligrams per day from fortified foods, supplements, and medications. Although niacin has shown little severe toxicity, its side effects discourage widespread use. The principal side effects are flushing (a feeling of prickly heat on the face and upper body), related itching, and tingling. Niacin's side effects usually are reversible with drug discontinuation or dose reduction. Niacin supplements containing more than the RDA should be taken only under medical supervision.

Because megadoses of niacin lower LDL cholesterol and raise HDL cholesterol, physicians may prescribe it. Still, the evidence for lowering heart attack and stroke risk is not entirely consistent. A study by the National Institutes of Health was stopped early when the high-dose, extended-release niacin plus statin treatment in people with heart and vascular disease did not reduce the risk of cardiovascular events, including heart attacks and stroke, and even found a small and unexplained increase in stroke rates.[78] These results, however, cannot be applied to everyone. Niacin supplementation has been investigated for its possible effectiveness in treating other conditions such as osteoarthritis, Alzheimer's disease, atherosclerosis, diabetes, and cataracts.[79] People considering or currently taking niacin supplementation should seek the advice of their physician.

Quick Bite

Disputing Conventional Wisdom

Early 1900s medical theory wrongly held that bacterial infection due to poor sanitation caused pellagra. Dr. Joseph Goldberg of the U.S. Public Health Service suffered much social criticism as he fought conventional wisdom to prove the crucial link between poor nutrition and the scourge pellagra. About 10 years later, Conrad A. Elvehjem at the University of Wisconsin identified the "pellagra preventive factor" as niacin.

Vitamin B$_6$

Vitamin B$_6$ (also known as pyridoxine) is a group of six compounds, three with a phosphate group and three without. Digestion strips the phosphate group and sends the remaining compounds to the liver, which converts them to pyridoxal phosphate (PLP), the primary active coenzyme form.[80]

Functions of Vitamin B$_6$

PLP is a coenzyme for more than 100 different enzymes. Its better-known roles involve protein and amino acid metabolism. Enzymes that require PLP help change one amino acid into another and enable us to make the nonessential amino acids. Without adequate vitamin B$_6$, all amino acids become essential—the body cannot make them and must get them from food. Vitamin B$_6$ also helps make glucose from amino acids (a process called gluconeogenesis) and helps release glucose from glycogen.

PLP supports white blood cell synthesis and a healthy immune system. Healthy red blood cells also need PLP. The coenzyme helps synthesize their oxygen-carrying hemoglobin and helps bind oxygen. PLP also helps produce a number of major neurotransmitters.

Vitamin B$_6$, folate, and vitamin B$_{12}$ work in concert to lower blood levels of the amino acid homocysteine. Each vitamin forms a coenzyme that helps convert homocysteine to other amino acids—cysteine and methionine. (See **FIGURE 7.26**.) Low intake of B$_6$ or folate can increase homocysteine levels, and high homocysteine levels may be a marker for heart disease.[81]

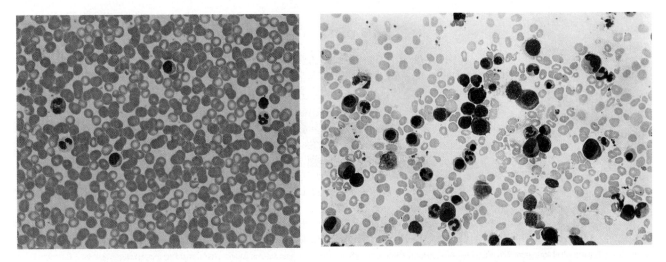

FIGURE 7.26 Homocysteine and heart disease. Elevated homocysteine levels are linked to an increased risk of heart disease. Enzymes dependent on B$_6$, B$_{12}$, and folate help lower the amount of homocysteine by converting it to cysteine and methionine.

© Donna Beer Stolz, Ph.D., Center for Biologic Imaging, University of Pittsburgh Medical School; © John Durham/Science Source.

Dietary Recommendations and Sources of Vitamin B_6

The vitamin B_6 RDA for men and women 19 to 50 years old is 1.3 milligrams per day. Because requirements appear to increase with age, the RDA is set at 1.7 milligrams for older men and 1.5 milligrams for older women.[82]

Good sources of vitamin B_6 include meat (especially organ meats like liver), fish, or poultry; potatoes and other starchy vegetables; and fortified soy-based meat substitutes.[83] Although whole grains naturally contain vitamin B_6, refining removes B_6 and enrichment does not replace it; however, it is added to some fortified breakfast cereals. Vitamin B_6 also pops up in unexpected places, like bananas and sunflower seeds. (See **FIGURE 7.27**.)

Vitamin B_6 is not particularly stable and is especially sensitive to temperature. Heat can destroy up to half of a food's vitamin B_6.

Vitamin B_6 Deficiency

Overt vitamin B_6 deficiency is rare, although some medications used for Parkinson's disease and asthma, for example, can cause deficiency. Excessive alcohol interferes with the vitamin's absorption and its coenzyme activities, worsening B_6 deficits created by the alcoholic's typically poor diet.

Overt vitamin B_6 deficiency produces a skin rash and anemia and also disrupts nervous system activity. Inadequate vitamin B_6 disrupts the synthesis of red blood cells and their oxygen-binding ability, causing a type of anemia in which red blood cells are small and pale. The pale color reflects their lack of adequate hemoglobin to carry sufficient

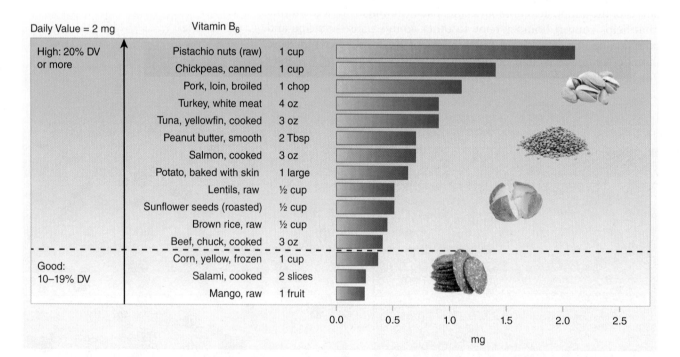

FIGURE 7.27   Food sources of vitamin B_6. Meats are generally good sources of vitamin B_6, along with certain fruits (e.g., bananas) and vegetables (e.g., potatoes).

Data from U.S. Department of Agriculture, Agricultural Research Service, Nutrient Data Laboratory. USDA National Nutrient Database for Standard Reference, Release 28. Version Current: September 2015. Internet: http://www.ars.usda.gov/nea/bhnrc/ndl.

Salami: © Sergiy Kuzmin/Shuttterstock, Inc.; Dried pistachio: © Dionisvera/Shutterstock, Inc.; Pile of lentils: © Imageman/Shutterstock, Inc.; Baked potato: © Joe Gough/Shutterstock, Inc.

oxygen. Vitamin B_6 deficiency also damages the nervous system, causing depression, headaches, confusion, and convulsions.

Even subtle deficits of vitamin B_6 disrupt homocysteine metabolism, leading to increased levels of homocysteine, a marker for vascular disease.

Vitamin B_6 Toxicity and Medicinal Uses of Vitamin B_6

Vitamin B_6 megadoses are not without risk and can cause subtle neurological damage. Other side effects include upset stomach, headache, sleepiness, and a tingling, prickling, or burning sensation. Some women self-prescribe large doses of vitamin B_6 as an antidote to treat premenstrual syndrome (PMS)—the headache, bloating, irritability, and depression that may occur during the week or so before the onset of menstruation.

Women have taken vitamin B_6 for PMS and to reduce symptoms of morning sickness during pregnancy with promising results; however, current scientific evidence of these benefits is unclear, and additional research is needed to confirm its safety and effectiveness. Women should not take supplemental vitamin B_6 without consulting their physician.[84]

High-dose vitamin B_6 has also been used for carpal tunnel syndrome—a wrist injury that causes painful tingling in hands and fingers. Most well-designed scientific studies have found no evidence that vitamin B_6 improves carpal tunnel syndrome.[85] The UL for vitamin B_6 intake is 100 milligrams per day. Unfortunately, over-the-counter supplements often contain this amount or more. Doses above the UL should be taken only under medical supervision.

Folate

Folate is named for its best natural source: green leafy vegetables (foliage). The term *folate* actually refers to a group of several closely related folate forms. Folic acid is the most stable form and is used for supplementation and fortification.

Functions of Folate

As a coenzyme, folate is crucial to DNA synthesis and cell division, amino acid metabolism, and the maturation of red blood cells and other cells. This involvement in basic cell reproduction and growth makes folate essential for healthy embryonic development. Good folate status in early pregnancy greatly reduces the risk of birth defects called **neural tube defects (NTDs)**.[86] However, many women do not realize they have become pregnant or don't seek prenatal care until it's too late. That is why experts recommend folic acid supplements before pregnancy to all women who may become pregnant—and it is why the U.S. government mandated folic acid fortification. Folate functions in close cooperation with vitamins B_6 and B_{12}. All three support red blood cell synthesis and help control homocysteine levels.

▶ **neural tube defects (NTDs)** Birth defects resulting from failure of the neural tube to develop properly during early fetal development.

Dietary Recommendations and Sources of Folate

The body absorbs nearly 100 percent of folic acid in supplements and fortified foods, but depending on stomach contents only about half to two-thirds of the folate naturally present in food.[87] To account for these differences, RDA values are expressed as **dietary folate equivalents (DFEs)**. For men and women age 19 years or older, the RDA for folate

▶ **dietary folate equivalents (DFEs)** A measure of folate intake used to account for the high bioavailability of folic acid taken as a supplement compared with the lower bioavailability of the folate found in foods.

is 400 micrograms of DFE per day. Requirements increase to 600 micrograms during pregnancy and 500 micrograms while breastfeeding.

Poor folate status during the early stages of pregnancy is strongly linked with birth defects, specifically neural tube defects. Since 1998, folic acid fortification of enriched flour (including that used by commercial bakers) and enriched grain products has been mandatory in the United States and Canada.[88] Scientists estimate that folate fortification increases folic acid intake by about 100 micrograms per day (an amount provided by slightly more than one-half cup of enriched pasta or one slice of bread), with the goal being to boost daily consumption by women of childbearing age to 400 micrograms of folic acid.

According to the Centers for Disease Control and Prevention, 50 to 70 percent of NTDs could be prevented by taking 400 micrograms of folate daily before and during pregnancy.[89] Because most U.S. women still are not eating enough foods fortified with folic acid to optimally reduce the risk of birth defects, the U.S. Preventive Services Task Force recommends that all women who are capable of becoming pregnant take a daily supplement containing 400–800 micrograms of folic acid.[90]

Fortified breakfast cereals supply dietary folate. Some provide 400 micrograms in a moderate-size serving. A serving of enriched pasta, for example, typically provides 30 percent of the RDA for folate. Dark-green leafy vegetables, asparagus, broccoli, orange juice, wheat germ, liver, sunflower seeds, and legumes are other good sources. (See **FIGURE 7.28**.)

Similar to other water-soluble vitamins, folate is extremely vulnerable to heat, ultraviolet light, and oxygen. Cooking and other food-processing and preparation techniques can destroy up to 90 percent

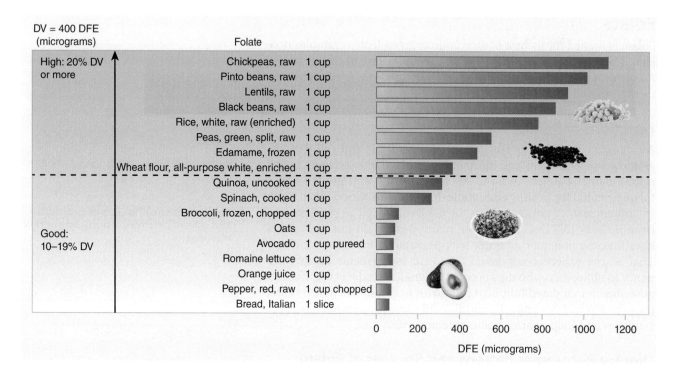

FIGURE 7.28 Food sources of folate. Good sources of folate are a diverse collection of foods: liver, legumes, leafy greens, and orange juice. Enriched grains and fortified cereals are other ways to include folic acid in the diet.

Data from U.S. Department of Agriculture, Agricultural Research Service, Nutrient Data Laboratory. USDA National Nutrient Database for Standard Reference, Release 28. Version Current: September 2015. Internet: http://www.ars.usda.gov/nea/bhnrc/ndl.

of a food's folate. Experts recommend eating folate-rich fruits and vegetables raw or cooking them quickly in minimal amounts of water via steaming, stir-frying, or microwaving. Vitamin C in foods also helps protect folate from oxidation.

Folate Deficiency

Approximately 10 percent of the U.S. population may have insufficient folate stores. Many scientists believe that folate deficiency is the most prevalent of all vitamin deficiencies. Our understanding of the role of folate in human health and disease has been expanding rapidly. Folate deficiency appears to play an important role in the development of anemia, atherosclerosis, neural tube defects, adverse pregnancy outcomes, and neuropsychiatric disorders.

In developed countries, folate deficiency has been associated with people who have poor nutrition, such as the elderly or those with alcoholism. Others may have increased risk due to intestinal malabsorption, certain anemias, and the use of medications that interfere with folate absorption or activity.

When your folate reserves are good, your body normally can store enough folate to last two to four months without additional intake. Abnormal cell reproduction due to folate deficiency can be corrected within 24 hours by vitamin replacement.

Anemia

Both folate and vitamin B_{12} are required for DNA synthesis and normal cell growth. A deficiency shows up soonest in cells that are reproducing the fastest, such as rapidly dividing red blood cells. Immature red blood cells cannot grow or mature normally, and instead grow into large bizarre shapes and have greatly shortened life spans. These abnormal cells replace normal red blood cells, leading to a type of anemia called **megaloblastic anemia**. (See **FIGURE 7.29**.) The blood's ability to carry oxygen drops, causing weakness and fatigue. Folate-deficiency anemia commonly causes depression, irritability, forgetfulness, and disturbed sleep. A lack of folate also impairs the synthesis of white blood cells, which are vital to the immune response.

Birth Defects

Poor folate status during the early stages of pregnancy is linked to an increased risk of a birth defect known as a neural tube defect (NTD). These defects in the central nervous system occur within the first 30 days after conception.[91] Most common is **spina bifida**, in which a protective covering fails to form over part or all of the fragile spinal cord. (See **FIGURE 7.30**.) Other neural tube defects include an abnormally small brain (**microencephaly**) or no brain at all (**anencephaly**). Folate may also be important in the prevention of other undesirable birth outcomes such as low-birth-weight babies, premature deliveries, and congenital birth defects such as cleft lip and palate.[92]

Heart Disease

Folate has an important role in preventing heart disease. Folate works with vitamins B_{12} and B_6 to reduce elevated homocysteine, which is a risk factor for cardiovascular disease. Meeting the RDA for folate intake helps maintain homocysteine at reduced levels. The role of folate in

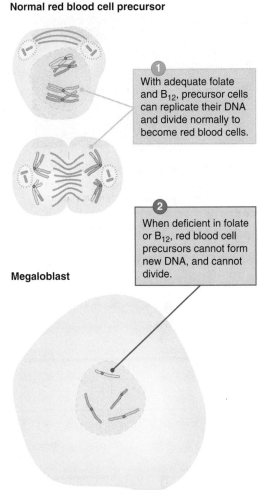

Normal red blood cell precursor

1 With adequate folate and B_{12}, precursor cells can replicate their DNA and divide normally to become red blood cells.

2 When deficient in folate or B_{12}, red blood cell precursors cannot form new DNA, and cannot divide.

Megaloblast

FIGURE 7.29 Megaloblastic anemia. When red blood cell precursors in the bone marrow cannot form new DNA, they cannot divide normally. These precursor cells continue to grow and become large, fragile, immature cells called megaloblasts. Megaloblasts displace red blood cells, resulting in megaloblastic anemia.

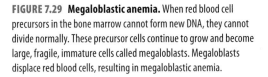

▶ **megaloblastic anemia** Excess amounts of megaloblasts (immature red blood cells) in the blood caused by deficiency of folate or vitamin B_{12}.

▶ **spina bifida** A type of neural tube birth defect.

▶ **microencephaly** A type of neural tube birth defect in which the brain is abnormally small.

▶ **anencephaly** A type of neural tube birth defect in which part or all of the brain is missing.

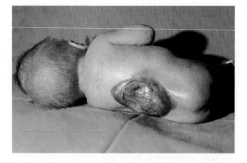

FIGURE 7.30 Neural tube defects. Poor folate status during the early stages of pregnancy, even before a woman may realize she is pregnant, increases the risk of a neural tube defect.
Courtesy of Leonard V. Crowley, MD, Century College.

protecting against heart disease contributed to the FDA decision to fortify grain products, which has successfully increased blood folate levels and decreased homocysteine levels in the United States.[93] The role of folate supplementation for the prevention or treatment of cardiovascular disease, stroke, and all-cause mortality is currently under investigation. Recommended folate intakes help maintain homocysteine at reduced levels.

Folate and Cancer

Folate's role in the synthesis, repair, and function of DNA and RNA has led researchers to investigate DNA damage that may lead to cancer as a result of deficiency of this vitamin. Although not uniformly consistent, a large body of epidemiological studies generally indicates that a diet high in folate offers protection against various forms of cancer, particularly colorectal cancer.[94,95] However, the precise roles of folate and the effects of folate supplementation in cancer prevention remain unclear.[96]

Folate Toxicity

Deficiency of either folate or vitamin B_{12} produces the same type of anemia, but B_{12} deficiency also causes nerve damage. Taking folate supplements can mask the symptoms of B_{12}-deficiency anemia until nerve damage becomes irreversible. (See the section "Vitamin B_{12} Deficiency.") Although rare, hypersensitive people who take folic acid supplements may suffer hives or respiratory distress. The UL for adults is 1,000 micrograms per day of folic acid from supplements and fortified foods.

Vitamin B_{12}

Vitamin B_{12} is unlike other B vitamins. Plants do not provide it, and your body stores large amounts. Vitamin B_{12} is a group of cobalt-containing compounds, known collectively as cobalamin. In the United States, cyanocobalamin, hydroxocobalamin, and methylcobalamin are forms of vitamin B_{12} commercially available in supplements.

Functions of Vitamin B_{12}

Vitamin B_{12} is essential to the conversion of folate to an activated form. Without vitamin B_{12}, folate cannot function in DNA synthesis or blood cell synthesis, nor can it metabolize homocysteine. All folate functions are blocked. Thus, a deficiency of vitamin B_{12} will produce folate deficiency symptoms, even though folate levels might be adequate.

Vitamin B_{12} has another essential job. It helps maintain the **myelin sheath**, a protective coating that surrounds nerve fibers. A vitamin B_{12} deficiency ultimately destroys nerve cells, which can increase the risk of falls.

▶ **myelin sheath** The protective coating that surrounds nerve fibers.

Dietary Recommendations and Sources of Vitamin B_{12}

The RDA for vitamin B_{12} for men and women ages 19 to 50 is 2.4 micrograms per day. Although the value for adults 51 years and older is the same, up to 30 percent of older adults have a condition that decreases the bioavailability of vitamin B_{12} naturally found in animal foods; they are advised to increase their intake of B_{12} by consuming B_{12}-fortified foods or supplements.

Our bodies efficiently absorb vitamin B_{12} from these sources.[97] All naturally occurring vitamin B_{12} originates with bacteria. Bacteria produce it, and animals obtain it from bacteria on their food or from

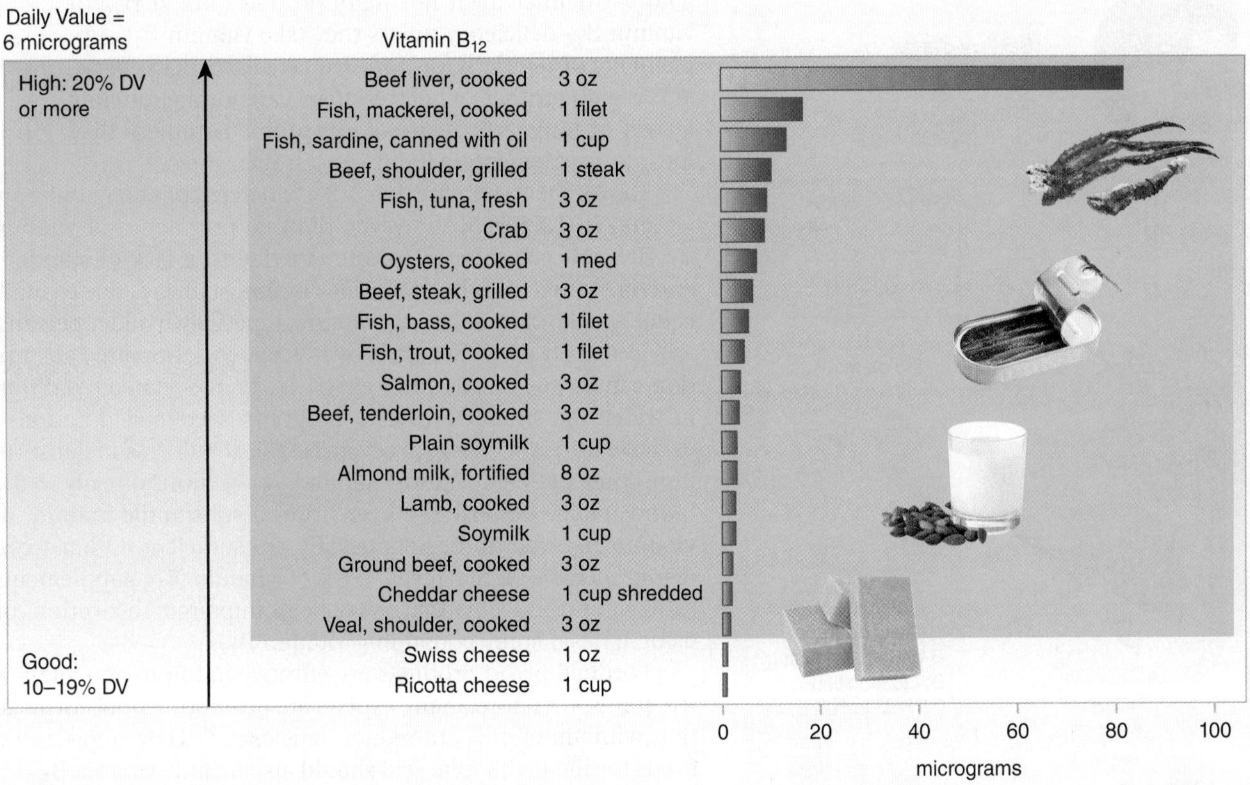

Daily Value =
6 micrograms

Vitamin B$_{12}$

High: 20% DV or more		
Beef liver, cooked	3 oz	
Fish, mackerel, cooked	1 filet	
Fish, sardine, canned with oil	1 cup	
Beef, shoulder, grilled	1 steak	
Fish, tuna, fresh	3 oz	
Crab	3 oz	
Oysters, cooked	1 med	
Beef, steak, grilled	3 oz	
Fish, bass, cooked	1 filet	
Fish, trout, cooked	1 filet	
Salmon, cooked	3 oz	
Beef, tenderloin, cooked	3 oz	
Plain soymilk	1 cup	
Almond milk, fortified	8 oz	
Lamb, cooked	3 oz	
Soymilk	1 cup	
Ground beef, cooked	3 oz	
Cheddar cheese	1 cup shredded	
Veal, shoulder, cooked	3 oz	
Good: 10–19% DV	Swiss cheese	1 oz
	Ricotta cheese	1 cup

0   20   40   60   80   100
micrograms

FIGURE 7.31 Food sources of vitamin B$_{12}$. Vitamin B$_{12}$ is found naturally only in foods of animal origin, such as liver, meats, and milk. Some cereals are fortified with vitamin B$_{12}$.

Data from U.S. Department of Agriculture, Agricultural Research Service, Nutrient Data Laboratory. USDA National Nutrient Database for Standard Reference, Release 28. Version Current: September 2015. Internet: http://www.ars.usda.gov/nea/bhnrc/ndl

King crab legs: © supermimicry/Getty Images; Anchovies fillets in tin can: Jiri Hera/Shutterstock, Inc.; Almond milk: 5 second Studio/Shutterstock, Inc.; Piece of cheese: Binh Thanh Bui/Shutterstock, Inc.

their intestinal bacteria. Animals concentrate and store B$_{12}$, mainly in the liver. Consequently, animal-derived foods are our only good natural source of vitamin B$_{12}$, and liver is the richest source.

Blue-green algae (cyanobacteria) are sometimes promoted as a B$_{12}$ plant source, but their cobalamin is an inactive and unavailable form. For vegans (vegetarians who avoid eggs and dairy, as well as meats), the most reliable food sources are fortified breakfast cereals, fortified soy products, and other foods fortified with B$_{12}$. (See **FIGURE 7.31**.)

Absorption of Vitamin B$_{12}$

Unless you're a vegan, it's easy to get enough vitamin B$_{12}$ from your diet. But absorbing it is another matter. Readying vitamin B$_{12}$ for absorption is a complex, multistep digestive process, starting in the mouth and ending with absorption in the small intestine. The process requires production of adequate stomach acid and a substance called intrinsic factor. (See **FIGURE 7.32**.) A defect in any step can cause B$_{12}$ deficiency.

Vitamin B$_{12}$ Deficiency

We can store enough vitamin B$_{12}$ in the liver to last more than 2 years, and symptoms of deficiency may not appear for up to 12 years. Vegetarians

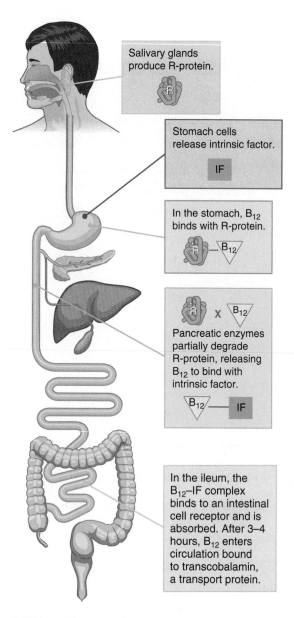

Salivary glands produce R-protein.

Stomach cells release intrinsic factor.

IF

In the stomach, B_{12} binds with R-protein.

Pancreatic enzymes partially degrade R-protein, releasing B_{12} to bind with intrinsic factor.

In the ileum, the B_{12}–IF complex binds to an intestinal cell receptor and is absorbed. After 3–4 hours, B_{12} enters circulation bound to transcobalamin, a transport protein.

FIGURE 7.32 **Absorption of vitamin B_{12}.** Absorption of vitamin B_{12} is a complex process that involves many factors and sites in the GI tract. Defects in this process, especially a lack of intrinsic factor, impair B_{12} absorption and can lead to B_{12} deficiency.

▶ **atrophic gastritis** An age-related condition in which the stomach loses its ability to secrete acid. In severe cases, ability to make intrinsic factor is also impaired.

▶ **pernicious anemia** A form of anemia that results from an autoimmune disorder that damages cells lining the stomach and inhibits vitamin B_{12} absorption; causes vitamin B_{12} deficiency.

who eat neither meat nor dairy products are at risk of vitamin B_{12} deficiency unless they take vitamin B_{12} supplements or regularly eat fortified cereals. Strict vegetarian (vegan) mothers who breastfeed can put their infants at risk of long-term neurological problems unless they include supplemental vitamin B_{12} in their diets.

THINK About It 3

Researchers estimate that 3.2–12 percent of older adults are vitamin B_{12} deficient; however, the true prevalence of vitamin B_{12} deficiency is difficult to estimate due to a lack of standard criteria.[98] A vitamin B_{12} deficiency is almost always due to inadequate intake or impaired absorption, especially in older persons, and is also observed in gastric bypass patients. Impaired absorption can be due to **atrophic gastritis**, an age-related condition in which the stomach loses its ability to secrete acid and also to make intrinsic factor (in severe cases). To address malabsorption, some patients require vitamin B_{12} injections directly to the bloodstream. Because the liver stores a substantial amount of vitamin B_{12}, monthly shots usually are sufficient. Other treatments include taking megadoses of vitamin B_{12} supplements (300 times the RDA) that overwhelm impaired absorption, or using a nasal spray containing vitamin B_{12}.

Fortified bread products are effective in improving vitamin B_{12} status; therefore, many experts are promoting flour fortification with vitamin B_{12} to reduce deficiency.[99] They suggest that foods fortified with folic acid should also include vitamin B_{12}.[100]

Pernicious anemia is a major cause of vitamin B_{12} deficiency that can affect people of all ages, races, and ethnic origins. In this disease, an inappropriate immune response may attack and destroy certain cells lining the stomach. This, in turn, reduces the production of intrinsic factor that is needed for B_{12} absorption, and deficiency develops. In this type of anemia, red blood cells are large, fragile, and strangely shaped, just like in folate-deficiency anemia. But, when a B_{12} deficiency causes the anemia, nerve cells can be irreversibly destroyed. This is the crucial difference between B_{12}-deficiency anemia and folate-deficiency anemia—folate deficiency does not destroy nerves. If B_{12}-deficiency anemia is incorrectly treated with folic acid, anemia symptoms may disappear as nerve degeneration continues. The mistake may not become apparent until the damage is irreversible. Proper treatment of B_{12}-deficiency anemia includes B_{12} injections, nasal spray, or megadose supplement.

Vitamin B_{12} Toxicity

High levels of vitamin B_{12} from food or supplements have not been shown to cause harmful side effects in healthy people. Large vitamin B_{12} doses routinely used to treat pernicious anemia have no apparent ill effect. Doses of 1,000 micrograms monthly are used routinely in medical situations. A UL for vitamin B_{12} has not been determined.

Key Concepts Vitamin B_6, folate, and vitamin B_{12} work closely together. Deficiency of folate increases risk for birth defects. Deficiency of B_{12} causes irreversible nerve damage. All three deficiencies cause anemia. All three deficiencies compromise homocysteine metabolism. Fortified grains have become an important folate source. Only animal-derived or fortified foods contain significant amounts of vitamin B_{12}. Megadoses of vitamin B_6 can cause nerve damage.

Pantothenic Acid

Pantothenic acid is widespread in the food supply; in fact, its name comes from the Greek word *pantothen*, meaning "from every side." Although marketers have promoted pantothenic acid supplements for a long list of uses, in most cases there is not enough scientific evidence to determine its effectiveness.[101]

Functions of Pantothenic Acid

Pantothenic acid is a component of coenzyme A (CoA), which in turn is part of acetyl CoA, a compound that sits at the crossroads of energy-generating and biosynthetic pathways. (See **FIGURE 7.33**.) It is critical for extracting energy from nutrients and for building new fatty acids.

Dietary Recommendations and Sources of Pantothenic Acid

There are few data upon which to base dietary recommendations (RDA) for pantothenic acid, so an Adequate Intake (AI) level has been set instead. For adults ages 19 to 50, the AI is 5 milligrams per day.[102] Mother Nature must have known the importance of this vitamin because it is found throughout the food supply. Pantothenic acid is in foods as diverse as meat (e.g., chicken, beef, liver, kidney), mushrooms, potatoes, oats, tomato products, yeast, egg yolk, broccoli, and whole grains.[103] Pantothenic acid is easily damaged. Freezing and canning appear to decrease the pantothenic acid content of vegetables, meat, fish, and dairy products. Processing and refining grains destroys nearly 75 percent.[104]

Pantothenic Acid Deficiency

Pantothenic acid deficiencies are virtually nonexistent in the general population. In research settings, deficiency-induced symptoms include irritability and restlessness, fatigue, digestive disturbance, sleep disturbance, numbness and tingling, muscle cramps, staggered gait, and low blood glucose levels.

Pantothenic Acid Toxicity

High intakes of pantothenic acid have no apparent adverse effects. Therefore, a UL has not been established.

Biotin

In 1924, researchers thought they had identified three growth factors—"bios II," "vitamin H," and "coenzyme R." But it soon became clear that there was only one substance at work—the B vitamin biotin.

Functions of Biotin

Like the other B vitamins, biotin acts as a coenzyme in dozens of reactions. Among these reactions are amino acid metabolism, including the conversion of amino acids to glucose (gluconeogenesis), fatty acid synthesis, release of energy from fatty acids, and DNA synthesis.

Dietary Recommendations and Sources of Biotin

We know so little about biotin requirements that there are not enough data on biotin to establish an EAR or an RDA. The AI for adults

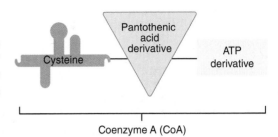

FIGURE 7.33 Pantothenic acid and coenzyme A. Pantothenic acid forms part of coenzyme A, which in turn is a component of acetyl CoA. Through coenzyme A, pantothenic acid is involved in many metabolic reactions that extract energy from nutrients and other reactions that build fatty acids.

Quick Bite

Busy Bacteria

You may be aware that bacteria in the colon synthesize vitamin K, but did you know that these bacteria also make some biotin? However, in synthesizing this B vitamin, these busy microbes may be undertaking a futile effort. Because the colon is downstream from the small intestine, the site of most biotin absorption, the bacteria's biotin may not be absorbed efficiently. Bacterial synthesis of biotin probably does not make an important contribution to your body's supply of biotin.

avidin A protein in raw egg whites that binds biotin, preventing its absorption. Avidin is denatured by heat.

is mathematically determined from the infant AI, which in turn is based on the biotin levels of human milk. The AI for biotin for adults is 30 micrograms daily.[105] Good sources of biotin include cauliflower, liver, peanuts, and cheese, whereas most fruits and meats are poor sources.

In raw egg white, a protein called **avidin** binds biotin and prevents its absorption from raw eggs. Cooking denatures avidin, preventing it from binding to biotin. Therefore, egg yolks are a good biotin source, as long as eggs are cooked. Of course, you should avoid eating anything that contains raw eggs anyway, because they might harbor *Salmonella* bacteria and cause foodborne illness.

Biotin Deficiency

Deficiency is rare, but it can occur. Eating raw egg whites—about a dozen or more daily over months or years—could produce biotin deficiency, but this scenario is unlikely. Some anticonvulsant drugs break down biotin, increasing risk of deficiency.

A rare genetic defect can lead to biotin depletion in infants. Symptoms progress from initial hair loss, rash, and delayed growth and development to convulsions and other neurological problems. Early diagnosis and daily biotin supplements usually clear up symptoms. If untreated, biotin deficiency can lead to coma and death.

Biotin Toxicity

High doses of biotin do not appear toxic, and no UL for biotin has been established.

Choline: A Vitamin-Like Substance

Choline is a vitamin-like nutrient, but differs from a true vitamin. You can make the majority of choline you need from the amino acids serine and methionine, but synthesis alone is insufficient to meet the body's requirements. For this reason, dietary recommendations are made for choline.

Along with vitamins B_{12}, B_6, and folate, choline helps metabolize homocysteine. But unlike most vitamins, choline is more than a catalyst or coenzyme. Most choline in your body is actually a component of other substances, such as the neurotransmitter acetylcholine. It is also a component of phospholipids. You may recall that a phospholipid has two fatty acids (responsible for solubility in fat) and a phosphate–nitrogen group (responsible for solubility in water). Choline is the phosphate–nitrogen group in many phospholipids. In cell membranes, phospholipids help protect the cell, allowing only certain substances to enter and leave, and they help maintain the cell's shape. Throughout the body, phospholipids act as emulsifiers, enabling fatty substances to mix with water-soluble ones.

The AI for choline is 550 milligrams per day for adult men and 425 milligrams for adult women.[106] Overall, choline is abundant in the food supply—the risk of a deficiency is minimal in healthy people. Milk, liver, egg yolk, beef, cauliflower, and peanuts are good sources; so is lecithin, a common food additive. A deficiency produces fat accumulation in the liver and then liver damage, but is unlikely in healthy people. High doses of choline can cause diarrhea, falling blood pressure, and a disconcerting fishy body odor. The UL for choline is 3,500 milligrams per day.

Key Concepts Pantothenic acid and biotin are widespread in the food supply, and deficiencies are rare. Like the other B vitamins, they are parts of coenzymes involved in the metabolism of fat, carbohydrate, and protein. Choline is an essential nutrient that is a component of phospholipids and neurotransmitters.

Vitamin C

For centuries, the treacherous disease scurvy dogged humankind. Explorers and seafaring men especially feared this mysterious ailment that inflicted aching pain and made each journey a gamble with death. Writings dating back as far as 1500 BCE describe their suffering in detail. In 1747, James Lind, a 30-year-old Scottish physician who was a ship surgeon in the British navy, proved that eating lemons and oranges cured the disease. But scientists did not isolate the substance responsible for curing scurvy and name it vitamin C until 1930.[107] The chemical name for vitamin C is ascorbic acid. This name comes from the fact that vitamin C is antiscorbutic (antiscurvy).

Most animals manufacture their own vitamin C, but humans cannot, sharing this dubious distinction with fruit-eating bats, guinea pigs, and a few other isolated species.

Functions of Vitamin C

Unlike the B vitamins, vitamin C does not act as a coenzyme, yet it is an important participant in many reactions and is known for its antioxidant activities.

Antioxidant Activity

Like vitamin E, vitamin C is an antioxidant and helps protect cells from oxidative damage. But unlike vitamin E, vitamin C is water-soluble rather than fat-soluble. Eating foods rich in vitamin C may promote bone health and reduce the risk of chronic diseases such as heart disease, certain forms of cancer, and macular degeneration. Studies investigating vitamin C supplements have contradictory findings, and it remains unclear whether the protective effects are due to vitamin C or to fruit and vegetable consumption in general.[108]

Collagen Synthesis

We need vitamin C to form collagen, a fibrous protein that helps reinforce the **connective tissues** that hold together the structures of the body. Collagen is made up of individual, linear proteins that wrap around one another like a cord of rope, forming a triple helix that imparts strength and flexibility. It is the most abundant protein in our bodies and the main fibrous component of skin, bone, tendons, cartilage, and teeth.

▶ **connective tissues** Tissues composed primarily of fibrous proteins, such as collagen, and that contain few cells. Their primary function is to bind together and support various body structures.

Other Vital Roles

Your body needs vitamin C to make many other essential compounds, among them thyroid hormone, steroid hormones, bile salts, the neurotransmitter serotonin, and parts of the DNA molecule. Also, vitamin C enhances the absorption of iron from plant foods.

THINK About It
4

Vitamin C enables cells in our immune system to function effectively. Based in part on the vitamin's importance to immunity, vitamin C has been reputed to prevent or cure the common cold. Regular supplementation with vitamin C has been found to have a modest effect on shortening the duration of the common cold in the general population; however, it is particularly beneficial in individuals exposed to extreme physical stress.[109]

Quick Bite

Chili Peppers Are Hot Stuff

An estimated one-quarter of the world's adults eat chili peppers every day. By weight, chili peppers are one of the richest sources of vitamins A and C. In addition, capsaicin, the substance that causes your mouth to burn, jump-starts the digestive process by stimulating salivation, gastric secretions, and gut motility.

Dietary Recommendations and Sources of Vitamin C

The RDA for vitamin C is 90 milligrams per day for men and 75 milligrams per day for women, increasing to 85 milligrams per day during pregnancy and 120 milligrams during breastfeeding (levels far above the 5 or 10 milligrams required daily to prevent scurvy). Cigarette smoking increases the need for vitamin C by 35 milligrams per day.[110]

Many, but not all, fruits and vegetables are high in vitamin C. Good sources include citrus fruits, tomatoes, fortified juice drinks, broccoli, strawberries, kiwifruit, cabbage, leafy greens, peppers, and potatoes. (See **FIGURE 7.34**.) Because vitamin C is highly vulnerable to heat and oxygen, fresh fruits and vegetables are the best sources. Frozen orange juice concentrate preserves vitamin C content better than cartons of ready-to-drink orange juice. For more information about frozen foods, see the FYI feature "Fresh, Frozen, or Canned? Raw, Dried, or Cooked?"

The more vitamin C you consume, the less efficiently your intestines absorb the vitamin. If your intake is under 30 milligrams daily, you absorb nearly all of it. Between 30 and 120 milligrams, you absorb about 80 to 90 percent. As intake increases further, the efficiency of absorption continues to decline, falling to about 20 percent at 6,000 milligrams. Any excess vitamin C that is absorbed is excreted in urine.

Vitamin C Deficiency

After about a month on a diet without vitamin C, symptoms of scurvy start to surface. As the body loses its ability to synthesize collagen,

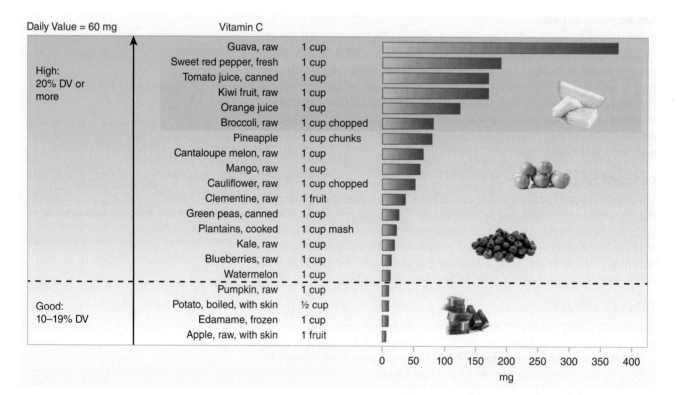

FIGURE 7.34 Food sources of vitamin C. Vitamin C is found mainly in fruits and vegetables. Although citrus fruits are notoriously good sources, many other popular fruits and vegetables are rich in vitamin C.

Data from U.S. Department of Agriculture, Agricultural Research Service, Nutrient Data Laboratory. USDA National Nutrient Database for Standard Reference, Release 28. Version Current: September 2015. Internet: http://www.ars.usda.gov/nea/bhnrc/ndl.

connective tissue starts breaking down. Gums and joints begin to bleed. Small blood vessels break, and tiny hemorrhages appear just under the skin. Mild bruising produces exaggerated black-and-blue marks. As the disease progresses, previously healed wounds reopen. Teeth are lost. Bone pain, fractures, diarrhea, and psychological problems such as depression appear. Left untreated, scurvy is fatal.

Scurvy is rare in developed countries, except among alcoholics or those on severely restricted diets.[111] Marginal vitamin C deficiency is more common; its symptoms include sore, inflamed gums and fatigue.

Vitamin C Toxicity

High vitamin C increases iron absorption—useful for some people, but problematic for those who already have too much body iron. Excess vitamin C may cause abdominal cramps, diarrhea, nausea, nosebleeds, and kidney stones in people with certain kidney conditions. At megadose levels, greater than 2,000 milligrams daily, vitamin C may switch from its antioxidant role to a pro-oxidant role, encouraging oxidation.[112] The UL for vitamin C is 2,000 milligrams per day.[113]

TABLE 7.5 provides a review of the key features for the water-soluble vitamins.

Key Concepts Vitamin C is found in many fruits and vegetables. It functions in collagen synthesis, acts as an antioxidant, helps boost iron absorption, plays a role in immunity, and helps synthesize many essential substances. Deficiency causes scurvy. Megadoses can cause digestive disturbance.

TABLE 7.5
Summary of Water-Soluble Vitamins

Vitamin	Important Dietary Sources	Major Functions	Signs/Symptoms of Deficiency	Toxic Effects of Megadoses	Special Considerations
Thiamin	Pork, legumes, types of nuts and seeds, types of fish and seafood, fortified foods including bread, pasta, rice, and ready-to-eat cereals	Important participant in energy-yielding reactions (as part of the coenzyme thiamin pyrophosphate), nerve function	Beriberi (symptoms include muscle wasting, mental confusion, anorexia, enlarged heart, nerve changes), and Wernicke–Korsakoff syndrome (alcohol-induced deficiency with symptoms including mental confusion, staggering, rapid eye movements, paralysis of the eye muscles)	n/a	Increased risk for deficiency with alcohol abuse and for the poor and the elderly (due to consumption of inadequate energy and nutrient-poor foods)
Riboflavin	Milk, milk drinks, yogurt, fortified bread products, and ready-to-eat cereals	Energy metabolism, maintenance of the integrity of skin, mucous membranes, and nervous system structures	Shiny, smooth, inflamed tongue, painful mouth, cracks at the corners of the mouth, inflamed lips	n/a	Increased risk for deficiency with alcohol abuse, long-term barbiturate use, cancer, heart disease, diabetes
Niacin	Meat, poultry, fish, seafood, peanuts, liver, mushrooms, enriched and whole grain breads, grain products, and ready-to-eat cereal	Transformation of carbohydrates, fats, and protein into usable forms of energy	Redness around the neck, dermatitis, dementia, diarrhea	Flushing of the face and upper body, itching and tingling, liver toxicity	Increased risk for deficiency with diets primarily consisting of corn, and for people with limited protein in their diet

(continues)

TABLE 7.5 *(continued)*
Summary of Water-Soluble Vitamins

Vitamin	Important Dietary Sources	Major Functions	Signs/Symptoms of Deficiency	Toxic Effects of Megadoses	Special Considerations
B$_6$	Fortified and ready-to-eat cereals; mixed foods that contain primarily meat, fish, or poultry; white potatoes and other starchy vegetables; noncitrus fruits; organ meats; soy-based meat substitutes; bananas; sunflower seeds	Supports protein metabolism, blood cell synthesis, carbohydrate metabolism, and neurotransmitter synthesis	Small and pale red blood cells, clogged oil glands of the skin, depression, confusion, convulsions	Irreversible nerve damage affecting the ability to walk and causing numbness in the extremities	Increased risk for deficiency with alcohol abuse
Folate	Fortified cereals, flour, and grain products; dark green leafy vegetables; asparagus; broccoli; orange juice; wheat germ; liver; sunflower seeds; legumes	Supports DNA synthesis and cell division, amino acid metabolism, maturation of red blood cells and other cells, and embryonic development	Anemia, atherosclerosis development, neural tube defects, adverse pregnancy outcomes, neuropsychiatric disorders	Masks B$_{12}$ deficiency; hives and/or respiratory distress	Increased risk for deficiency with poor nutrition status, advanced age, alcohol abuse, intestinal malabsorption, medications that interfere with folate metabolism, certain types of anemia, pregnancy, leukemia, lymphoma, psoriasis, and with prolonged diarrhea
B$_{12}$	Mixed foods with the main ingredient of fish, meat, or poultry; liver; crab; fortified cereals; milk/milk products; beef	Plays a key role in folate metabolism, the conversion of homocysteine to methionine, maintaining the myelin sheath, and preparation of fatty acid chains for entry into the citric acid cycle	Anemia, brain abnormalities and spinal cord degeneration, neurological symptoms including tingling and numbness in the extremities, abnormal gait, and cognitive changes	n/a	Increased risk for deficiency with pernicious anemia, strict vegetarianism, advanced age, and impaired absorption (e.g., after gastric bypass surgery)
Pantothenic acid	Chicken, beef, potatoes, oats, tomato products, liver, kidney, yeast, egg yolk, broccoli, whole grains	Metabolism of fats, carbohydrate, and protein	Irritability, restlessness, fatigue, apathy, malaise, sleep disruption, nausea/vomiting, numbness, tingling, muscle cramps, staggering gait, hypoglycemia	n/a	Increased risk for deficiency with administration of substances that prevent pantothenic acid metabolism
Biotin	Cauliflower, liver, peanuts, cheese	Coenzyme for dozens of reactions including the reactions of gluconeogenesis, fatty acid synthesis, release of energy from fatty acids, and DNA synthesis	Hair loss, rash, neurologic disorders (convulsions), delay of growth and development	n/a	Increased risk for deficiency with the consumption of raw egg whites over a long period of time (months to years), long-term anticonvulsant drug therapy, and in infants born with biotinidase deficiency

TABLE 7.5 (*continued*)
Summary of Water-Soluble Vitamins

Vitamin	Important Dietary Sources	Major Functions	Signs/Symptoms of Deficiency	Toxic Effects of Megadoses	Special Considerations
Vitamin C	Potatoes, citrus fruits, tomatoes, fortified juice drinks, broccoli, strawberries, kiwi, cabbage, spinach, leafy greens, green peppers	Antioxidant activity; the synthesis of collagen, carnitine, norepinephrine, epinephrine, serotonin, thyroxine, bile acids, steroid hormone, and purine bases; the absorption of nonheme iron; participant in immune function	Connective tissue breakdown, inflammation/bleeding of the gums and joints, fatigue/weakness, hemorrhage, bone pain and fracture, diarrhea, depression	Nausea, abdominal cramping, diarrhea, nose bleeds, formation of oxalate-containing kidney stones, possible free radical damage	Increased risk for deficiency with alcohol/drug abuse, limited fruit and vegetable consumption, and restrictive diets

Conditional Nutrients

Relatively speaking, there are few substances we need for life that our bodies cannot make. These substances are nutrients such as vitamins that we must get from food. Our bodies routinely make countless other essential substances. However, under some circumstances—such as during illness or because of inherited metabolic errors—we cannot make enough, so we must obtain them from our diets. These substances are "conditional nutrients." Inositol, carnitine, taurine, and lipoic acid are examples of conditional nutrients. Inositol helps form cell membrane phospholipids and precursors of eicosanoids, substances that work like hormones. Carnitine transports fatty acids to sites in the cell where your body can break them down. Taurine, derived from the amino acids methionine and cysteine, seems to play a role in such diverse functions as vision, insulin activity, and cell growth. Lipoic acid is a potent antioxidant and a necessary cofactor in many energy-releasing reactions. You may see conditional nutrients in dietary supplements, and they may be prescribed medically.

Key Concepts A conditional nutrient is not ordinarily required from our diet. People with certain medical conditions may benefit from supplements of some conditional nutrients.

Quick **Bite**

Bogus Vitamins

Some supplements contain unnecessary substances, yet savvy promoters will often call them "vitamins" and tout their supposed benefits: "health boosters," "youth-enhancers," "physical performance enhancers," and the like. Other products are subtly and unethically promoted to cure disease, despite ample scientific evidence to the contrary. The Internet is full of websites representing themselves as "nutrition sites" that endorse nutritional supplements to prevent or cure almost any condition, despite ample scientific evidence to the contrary. Consumers should be wary of anything that sounds "too good to be true" and investigate the claims using reputable websites and resources.

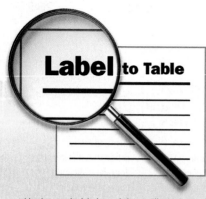

Label to Table

You've probably heard that milk is an excellent source of calcium, but did you know that milk also contains three of the four fat-soluble vitamins and contains a significant amount of some of the water-soluble vitamins? Let's take a look at the Nutrition Facts from a carton of nonfat milk.

Milk contains the fat-soluble vitamins A and D. Vitamin A is found naturally in whole milk, but all milk is fortified with this vitamin. That includes whole, reduced-fat, evaporated, powdered, lactose-free, and fat-free milks. (But yogurt, cheese, and ice cream generally are not fortified.) Fortification provides 10 percent of the Daily Value for vitamin A in 1 cup. Drink 3 cups in a day, and you'll get about one-third of your recommended vitamin A. That's good news because dietary vitamin A is not always easy to obtain. Keep in mind when selecting milk that nonfat (skim) milk contains vitamins A and D just like whole milk.

Vitamin D is important for bone health because it helps with absorption of calcium and phosphorus. Fortifying milk with vitamin D ensures that growing children will have the vitamin D they need, even if they don't get much sunlight or eat foods naturally rich in vitamin D such as sardines. As shown on the nutrition label here, just 1 cup of milk gives you one-quarter of the vitamin D Daily Value, or 2.5 micrograms.

The new food label includes a declaration of Vitamin D with the actual gram amount, in addition to the %DV. Vitamin D is a nutrient that some people are not getting enough of, which puts them at higher risk for chronic disease. The %DV for calcium continues to be required, along with the actual gram amount. Vitamins A and C are no longer required because deficiencies of these vitamins are rare, but these nutrients can be included on a voluntary basis.

When thinking about water-soluble vitamins, milk is a good source of those, too. Riboflavin and vitamins B_6 and B_{12} are not always required on the food labels. One cup of milk contributes 15 percent of your vitamin B_{12} and 18 percent of your riboflavin needs for the day. Vitamins C and B_6 are also found in milk at 4 percent and 5 percent of their Daily Value, respectively. In terms of health benefits, drinking milk not only helps you grow and maintain a healthy skeleton, but also helps to reduce your risk of osteoporosis, cardiovascular disease, and type 2 diabetes; lower blood pressure; and maintain a healthy body weight.

Nutrition Facts

8 servings per container

Serving size 1 cup (124g)

Amount per serving

Calories 200

	% Daily Value*
Total Fat 1g	2%
Saturated Fat 0g	
Trans Fat 0g	
Cholesterol 0mg	0%
Sodium 0mg	0%
Total Carbohydrate 41g	0%
Dietary Fiber 2g	14%
Total Sugars 1g	
Includes 0g Added Sugars	8%
Protein 7g	
Vitamin D 0mcg	0%
Calcium 0mg	0%
Iron 2mg	0%
Potassium 55mg	0%
Thiamin 1mg	10%
Riboflavin .26mg	?%
Niacin 4mg	35%
Folate 120mcg	15%
	20%
	30%

* The % Daily Value (DV) tells you how much a nutrient in a serving of food contributes to a daily diet. 2,000 calories a day is used for general nutrition advice.

Learning Portfolio

Key Terms

Study Points

- There are two classes of vitamins: fat-soluble vitamins (A, D, E, and K) and water-soluble vitamins (eight B vitamins and vitamin C).

- Vitamin A comes from preformed retinoids and the precursor carotenoids. Sources include butterfat, liver, green leafy and yellow-orange vegetables, and yellow-orange fruits.

- Vitamin A is essential to vision, cell differentiation, growth and development, and immune function. Night blindness is an early symptom of vitamin A deficiency that, if not treated, can result in permanent blindness.

- In large doses, vitamin A is toxic. When taken during pregnancy, excess vitamin A may cause birth defects.

- Because UV light hitting the skin converts a cholesterol precursor to vitamin D, vitamin D is known as the "sunshine vitamin." Ultimately, the kidneys convert this to the active form of vitamin D.

- Vitamin D in foods is available mainly from fortified milk and other fortified products.

- The primary function of vitamin D is the regulation of blood levels of calcium. Vitamin D deficiency contributes to skeletal problems. High supplement doses can be toxic.

- Vitamin E is an important antioxidant in the body and may help reduce the risk of chronic diseases such as heart disease and cancer.

- Vitamin E is found in vegetable oils and foods made from those oils. Deficiency and toxicity of vitamin E are relatively rare.

- Vitamin K is an important factor in blood coagulation and bone health.

- Although synthesized by intestinal bacteria, most of the vitamin K in the body comes from dietary sources, especially green vegetables. Vitamin K deficiency is rare, but newborns are susceptible if not given an injection of vitamin K at birth. Because the body excretes vitamin K easily, toxicity is unlikely.

Learning Portfolio (continued)

- The B vitamins function as coenzymes.

- Thiamin deficiency results in the classic disease beriberi. In industrialized countries, thiamin deficiency most often is associated with alcoholism. High doses of thiamin do not appear to be toxic.

- Riboflavin forms part of the coenzymes that function in energy metabolism. Milk is a good source of riboflavin, but light can destroy the vitamin. Packaging milk in paper or plastic cartons rather than in clear glass better protects milk's riboflavin content.

- Niacin deficiency results in pellagra, a disease characterized by diarrhea, dermatitis, dementia, and death. High doses of niacin, such as in the treatment of high blood cholesterol, can have toxic side effects, including liver damage.

- Vitamin B_6, folate, and vitamin B_{12} work together to control blood levels of homocysteine.

- A deficiency of vitamin B_6 can lead to a type of anemia marked by small, pale red blood cells.

- Poor folate status is associated with development of neural tube defects during pregnancy. Therefore, women of childbearing age need folic acid from supplements in addition to fortified foods and other dietary folate.

- Deficiency of either folate or vitamin B_{12} can lead to megaloblastic anemia, but vitamin B_{12} deficiency also causes irreversible nerve damage.

- Pantothenic acid is widespread in the food supply, and deficiency is virtually nonexistent. In the body, pantothenic acid is part of coenzyme A.

- Biotin-containing enzymes are important in many pathways involving energy-yielding nutrients. Biotin deficiency is rare but may be induced by regularly consuming large quantities of raw egg whites.

- Choline is a vitamin-like substance that the body makes but that, under some circumstances, must be supplied by diet.

- Vitamin C (ascorbic acid) functions in the synthesis of collagen and other vital compounds and also works as an antioxidant. Vitamin C deficiency can cause scurvy.

Study Questions

1. Describe two differences between fat-soluble and water-soluble vitamins.

2. What are the main roles of vitamin A in the body? What is an early sign of vitamin A deficiency?

3. What is vitamin D's nickname? Why? Why is vitamin D also considered a hormone?

4. What is vitamin E's primary function? What are the best sources of vitamin E?

5. What is the best-known function of vitamin K?

6. Which two fat-soluble vitamins potentially are the most toxic? Which two are the least toxic?

7. List the nine water-soluble vitamins and one main function for each.

8. Name the diseases and/or characteristic symptoms of deficiencies of each water-soluble vitamin.

9. List the water-soluble vitamins demonstrated to be toxic in large doses. What signs indicate toxic levels of each vitamin?

Try This

The PUFA Protection Challenge: Vitamin E vs. Oxygen

The object of this experiment is to see if vitamin E protects polyunsaturated fats (PUFAs) from oxidation. You'll need two glasses, one bottle of either safflower or corn oil, and some liquid vitamin E gel caps (which can be purchased at any pharmacy). Pour equal amounts of oil into each glass. Bite a hole in 10 of the vitamin E gel caps, squeeze their contents into one of the glasses, and stir. Mark this glass with tape and write the letter E on it. Let the glasses sit uncovered on a countertop for several days or weeks. Check the freshness or rancidity of the oils by smelling them and noting whether they look clear or cloudy. Over time, one will become more rancid than the other. Which glass container won the challenge—the one with or without vitamin E? Why?

Supplemental Income

The object of this exercise is to critically review vitamin supplements. Search the Internet to look for a few multivitamin supplements and "stress" formulas. Start by looking at the advertised benefits of the supplement. Is there peer-reviewed scientific evidence to support the claimed benefits for taking the supplement? Next, look at the %DV for the water-soluble vitamins. Do you see any that have more than 1,000 percent of the DV? Compare prices. Is it more expensive to buy supplements with more of these vitamins? Considering what you learned in this chapter, would it benefit you to take supplements that contain such a high amount of these vitamins? Why do you think supplements contain such large quantities of these vitamins? Are there warnings about toxicity or exceeding the UL?

Getting Personal

Select one day this week to evaluate your intake of fat-soluble and water-soluble vitamins. Ideally, choose a day where your schedule is predictable and you are eating what is considered normal for you. Using the table below, list all of the foods and drinks that you consume in a 24-hour period.

Time	Food or Drink	Amount

Let's review your intake of the fat-soluble and water-soluble vitamins.

1. Which foods or drinks provided you with high amounts of fat-soluble vitamins, and which ones provided high amounts of water-soluble vitamins?

2. Which foods or drinks provided you with low amounts of fat-soluble vitamins, and which ones provided low amounts of water-soluble vitamins?

3. Is your intake meeting your needs of fat-soluble vitamins? What about water-soluble vitamins?

   Select two fat-soluble vitamins:

   - What are your best sources of these two fat-soluble vitamins?

   - How can you improve your intakes of these two fat-soluble vitamins?

   Select two water-soluble vitamins:

   - What are your best sources of these two water-soluble vitamins?

   - How can you improve your intakes of these two water-soluble vitamins?

4. Which foods could you add to your diet to help increase your intake of fat-soluble vitamins, and which ones could you add to boost your intake of water-soluble vitamins?

5. Select two processed foods from your diet and substitute them with fruits or vegetables. How will this change the overall vitamin content of your diet? Explain.

References

1. Mahan KL, Escott-Stump S, Raymond JL, eds. *Krause's Food and the Nutrition Care Process*. 13th ed. Philadelphia: WB Saunders; 2011.
2. Institute of Medicine, Food and Nutrition Board. *Dietary Reference Intakes for Vitamin A, Vitamin K, Arsenic, Boron, Chromium, Copper, Iron, Manganese, Molybdenum, Nickel, Silicon, Vanadium, and Zinc*. Washington, DC: National Academies Press; 2001.
3. Guyton AC, Hall JE. *Textbook of Medical Physiology*. 13th ed. Philadelphia: Saunders; 2013.
4. National Institutes of Health. Osteoporosis and related bone diseases national resource center. Vitamin A and bone health. http://www.niams.nih.gov/Health_Info/Bone/Bone_Health/Nutrition/vitamin_a.asp. Accessed September 8, 2017.
5. Institute of Medicine, Food and Nutrition Board. Op. cit.
6. Ibid.
7. Institute of Medicine, Food and Nutrition Board. Op. cit.
8. Gropper SS, Smith JL, Carr TP. *Advanced Nutrition and Human Metabolism*. 7th ed. Belmont, CA: Cengage Learning; 2017.
9. Hayman RM, Dalziel SR. Acute vitamin A toxicity: a report of three paediatric cases. *J Paediatr Child Health*. 2012:48(3):E98-E100.
10. Institute of Medicine, Food and Nutrition Board. Op. cit.
11. Institute of Medicine, Food and Nutrition Board. *Dietary Reference Intakes for Vitamin C, Vitamin E, Selenium, and Carotenoids*. Washington, DC: National Academies Press; 2000.
12. Bouayed J, Bohn T. Exogenous antioxidants—double-edged swords in cellular redox state: health beneficial effects at physiologic doses versus deleterious effects at high doses. *Oxid Med Cell Longev*. 2010;3(4):228-237.
13. Liu RH. Health-promoting components of fruits and vegetables in the diet. *Adv Nutr*. 2013;4:384S-392S.
14. Linus Pauling Institute. Carotenoids: alpha-carotene, beta-carotene, beta-cryptoxanthin, lycopene, lutein, and zeaxanthin. http://lpi.oregonstate.edu/infocenter/phytochemicals/carotenoids/. Accessed September 8, 2017.
15. Gropper SS, Smith JL, Carr TP. Op. cit.
16. Weikel KA, Chiu CJ, Taylor A. Nutritional modulation of age-related macular degeneration. *Mol Aspects Med*. 2012;33(4):318-375.
17. Olson JH, Erie JC, Bakri SJ. Nutritional supplementation and age-related macular degeneration. *Semin Ophthalmol*. 2011;26(3):131-136.
18. Liu XH, Yu RB, Liu R, Hao ZX, Han CC, Zhu ZH, Ma L. Association between lutein and zeaxanthin status and the risk of cataract: a meta-analysis. *Nutrients*. 2014;6(1):452-465. doi: 10.3390/nu6010452
19. Raiola A, Rigano MM, Calafiore R, Frusciante L, Barone A. Enhancing the health-promoting effects of tomato fruit for biofortified food. *Mediators Inflamm*. 2014;2014:139873. doi:10.1155/2014/139873.
20. Institute of Medicine, Food and Nutrition Board. *Dietary Reference Intakes for Vitamin A, Vitamin K, Arsenic, Boron, Chromium, Copper, Iron, Manganese, Molybdenum, Nickel, Silicon, Vanadium, and Zinc*. Op. cit.
21. Ibid.

Learning Portfolio (continued)

22. U.S. Department of Agriculture, Agricultural Research Service. USDA national nutrient database for standard reference, release 26. 2013. http://www.ars.usda.gov/ba/bhnrc/ndl. Accessed September 8, 2017.

23. Institute of Medicine, Food and Nutrition Board. *Dietary Reference Intakes for Vitamin A, Vitamin K, Arsenic, Boron, Chromium, Copper, Iron, Manganese, Molybdenum, Nickel, Silicon, Vanadium, and Zinc.* Op. cit.

24. Avenell A, Mak JC, O'Connell D. Vitamin D and vitamin D analogues for preventing fractures in post-menopausal women and older men. *Cochrane Database Syst Rev.* 2014;4:CD000227. doi: 10.1002/14651858.CD000227.pub4

25. Wacker M, Holick MF. Vitamin D—effects on skeletal and extraskeletal health and the need for supplementation. *Nutrients.* 2013;5(1):111-148. doi: 10.3390/nu5010111

26. Battault S, Whiting SJ, Peltier SL, Sadrin S, Gerber G, Maixent JM. Vitamin D metabolism, functions, and needs: from science to health claims. *Eur J Nutr.* 2013;52(2):429-441. Epub August 12, 2012.

27. Bjelakovic G, Gluud LL, Nikolova D, et al. Vitamin D supplementation for prevention of mortality in adults. *Cochrane Database Syst Rev.* 2014;1:CD007470. doi: 10.1002/14651858.CD007470.pub3.

28. Gropper SS, Smith JL, Carr TP. Op. cit.

29. Manson JE, Mayne ST, Clinton SK. Vitamin D and prevention of cancer—ready for prime time? *N Engl J Med.* 2011;364(15):1385-1387.

30. Toner CD, Davis CD, Milner JA. The vitamin D and cancer conundrum: aiming at a moving target. *J Am Diet Assoc.* 2010;110(10):1492-1500.

31. Shapses SA, Manson JE. Vitamin D and prevention of cardiovascular disease and diabetes: why the evidence falls short. *JAMA.* 2011;305(24):2565-2566.

32. Institute of Medicine, Food and Nutrition Board. *Dietary Reference Intakes for Calcium and Vitamin D.* Washington, DC: National Academies Press; 2010.

33. Ibid.

34. Institute of Medicine of the National Academies of Science. *Dietary Reference Intakes for Calcium and Vitamin D.* March 2011. https://www.ncbi.nlm.nih.gov/books/NBK56070/. Accessed September 8, 2017.

35. Wagner CL, Greer FR, and the Section on Breastfeeding and Committee on Nutrition Clinical Report. Prevention of rickets and vitamin D deficiency in infants, children, and adolescents. *Pediatrics.* 2008;122(5):1142-1152.

36. Institute of Medicine, Food and Nutrition Board. *Dietary Reference Intakes for Calcium and Vitamin D.* Op. cit.

37. Ibid.

38. Vitamin D Council. How do I get the vitamin D my body needs? http://www.vitamindcouncil.org/about-vitamin-d/how-do-i-get-the-vitamin-d-my-body-needs/. Accessed September 8, 2017.

39. Bailey RL, Dodd KW, Goldman JA, et al. Estimation of total usual calcium and vitamin D intakes in the United States. *J Nutr.* 2010;140:817-822.

40. Lips P. Worldwide status of vitamin D nutrition. *J Steroid Biochem Mol Biol.* 2010;121:297-300.

41. Holick MF. Vitamin D deficiency. *N Engl J Med.* 2007;357:266-281.

42. Hossein-nezhad A, Holick MF. Vitamin D for health: a global perspective. *Mayo Clin Proc.* 2013;88(7):720-755. http://www.mayoclinicproceedings.org/article/S0025-6196(13)00404-7/pdf. Accessed September 8, 2017.

43. Ibid.

44. Institute of Medicine, Food and Nutrition Board. *Dietary Reference Intakes for Calcium and Vitamin D.* Op. cit.

45. Wagner CL, Greer FR, and the Section on Breastfeeding and Committee on Nutrition Clinical Report. Op. cit.

46. Ibid.

47. Kumar J, Muntner P, Kaskel FJ, et al. Prevalence and associations of 25-hydroxyvitamin D deficiency in U.S. children: NHANES 2001–2004. *Pediatrics.* 2009;124(3):e362-370. Epub August 3, 2009. doi: 10.1542/peds.2009-0051

48. National Institutes of Health, Office of Dietary Supplements. Vitamin D: fact sheet for health professionals. http://ods.od.nih.gov/factsheets/VitaminD-HealthProfessional/. Accessed September 8, 2017.

49. Institute of Medicine, Food and Nutrition Board. *Dietary Reference Intakes for Calcium and Vitamin D.* Op. cit.

50. Toner CD, Davis CD, Milner JA. Op. cit.

51. Mente A, de Koning L, Shannon HS, Anand SS. A systematic review of the evidence supporting a causal link between dietary factors and coronary heart disease. *Arch Intern Med.* 2009;13:169(7):659-669.

52. National Institutes of Health, Office of Dietary Supplements. Vitamin E: fact sheet for health professionals. http://ods.od.nih.gov/factsheets/vitamine. Accessed September 8, 2017.

53. American Heart Association. Vitamin supplements: hype or help for healthy eating. http://www.heart.org/HEARTORG/GettingHealthy/NutritionCenter/Vitamin-and-Mineral-Supplements_UCM_306033_Article.jsp. Accessed September 8, 2017.

54. Traber MG. Vitamin E. In: Ross AC, Caballero B, Cousins RJ, Tucker KL, Ziegler TR, eds. *Modern Nutrition in Health and Disease.* 11th ed. Philadelphia: Lippincott Williams & Wilkins; 2014:293-304.

55. Institute of Medicine, Food and Nutrition Board. *Dietary Reference Intakes for Vitamin C, Vitamin E, Selenium, and Carotenoids.* Op. cit.

56. Ibid.

57. Ibid.

58. Mayo Clinic. Drugs and supplements: vitamin E. http://www.mayoclinic.org/drugs-supplements/vitamin-e/background/hrb-20060476. Accessed September 8, 2017.

59. National Institutes of Health, Office of Dietary Supplements. Vitamin E: fact sheet for health professionals. Op. cit.

60. Devlin TM, ed. *Textbook of Biochemistry with Clinical Correlations.* 7th ed. Hoboken, NJ: John Wiley & Sons; 2011.

61. Iwamoto J, Sato Y, Takeda T, Matsumoto H. High-dose vitamin K supplementation reduces fracture incidence in postmenopausal women: a review of the literature. *Nutr Res.* 2009;29(4):221-228.

62. Gundberg CM, Lian JB, Booth SL. Vitamin K-dependent carboxylation of osteocalcin: friend or foe? *Adv Nutr.* 2012;3(2):149-157.

63. Institute of Medicine, Food and Nutrition Board. *Dietary Reference Intakes for Vitamin A, Vitamin K, Arsenic, Boron, Chromium, Copper, Iron, Manganese, Molybdenum, Nickel, Silicon, Vanadium, and Zinc.* Op. cit.

64. U.S. Department of Agriculture, Agricultural Research Service. USDA national nutrient database for standard reference, release 26. Op. cit.

65. Fiumara K, Goldhaber SZ. A patient's guide to taking Coumadin/warfarin. *Circulation.* 2009;119:e22-e222. doi: 10.1161/CIRCULATIONAHA.108.803957

66. Carpenter KJ. A short history of nutritional science: part 2 (1885–1912). *J Nutr.* 2003;133:975-984.

67. Ibid.

68. Manzetti S, Zhang J, van der Spoel D. Thiamin function, metabolism, uptake, and transport. *Biochemistry.* 2014;53(5):821-835. doi: 10.1021/bi401618y. Epub January 31, 2014.

69. Institute of Medicine, Food and Nutrition Board. *Dietary Reference Intakes for Thiamin, Riboflavin, Niacin, Vitamin B₆, Folate, Vitamin B₁₂, Pantothenic Acid, Biotin, and Choline.* Washington, DC: National Academies Press; 1998.

70. Larson Duyff R. *The American Dietetic Association Complete Food and Nutrition Guide.* 4th ed. Hoboken, NJ: John Wiley and Sons; 2012.

71. Brown G. Defects of thiamine transport and metabolism. *J Inherit Metab Dis.* 2014;37(4):577-585.

72. Institute of Medicine, Food and Nutrition Board. *Dietary Reference Intakes for Thiamin, Riboflavin, Niacin, Vitamin B₆, Folate, Vitamin B₁₂, Pantothenic Acid, Biotin, and Choline.* Op. cit.

73. Rodwell VW, Bender D, Botham KM, et al. *Harper's Illustrated Biochemistry.* 30th ed. New York: McGraw-Hill Education/Medical; 2015.

74. Institute of Medicine, Food and Nutrition Board. *Dietary Reference Intakes for Thiamin, Riboflavin, Niacin, Vitamin B$_6$, Folate, Vitamin B$_{12}$, Pantothenic Acid, Biotin, and Choline*. Op. cit.

75. Mestdagh F, DeMeulenaer B, De Clippeleer J, et al. Protective influence of several packaging materials on light oxidation of milk. *J Dairy Sci*. 2005;88:499-510.

76. Institute of Medicine, Food and Nutrition Board. 1998 Op. cit.

77. U.S. Department of Agriculture, Agricultural Research Service. USDA national nutrient database for standard reference, release 26. Op. cit.

78. National Institutes of Health. NIH stops clinical trial on combination cholesterol treatment. May 26, 2011. http://www.nhlbi.nih.gov/news/press-releases/2011/nih-stops-clinical-trial-on-combination-cholesterol-treatment.html. Accessed September 8, 2017.

79. U.S. National Library of Medicine, National Institutes of Health. Niacin and niacinamide (vitamin B$_3$). http://www.nlm.nih.gov/medlineplus/druginfo/natural/924.html. Accessed September 8, 2017.

80. Gropper SS, Smith JL, Carr TP. Op. cit.

81. Ciaccio M, Bellia C. Hyperhomocysteinemia and cardiovascular risk: effect of vitamin supplementation in risk reduction. *Curr Clin Pharmacol*. 2010;5(1):30-36.

82. Institute of Medicine, Food and Nutrition Board. 1998. Op. cit.

83. U.S. Department of Agriculture, Agricultural Research Service. USDA national nutrient database for standard reference, release 26. Op. cit.

84. National Institutes of Health, Office of Dietary Supplements. Vitamin B$_6$: dietary supplement fact sheet. http://ods.od.nih.gov/factsheets/VitaminB6-HealthProfessional/. Accessed September 8, 2017.

85. LeBlanc KE, Cestia W. Carpal tunnel syndrome. *Am Fam Physician*. 2011;83(8):952-958.

86. Centers for Disease Control and Prevention. Folic acid. http://www.cdc.gov/ncbddd/folicacid/index.html. Accessed September 8, 2017.

87. Institute of Medicine, Food and Nutrition Board. 1998. Op. cit.

88. Crider KS, Bailey LB, Berry RJ. Folic acid food fortification: its history, effect, concerns, and future directions. *Nutrients*. 2011;3:370-384.

89. Centers for Disease Control and Prevention. Folic acid: data and statistics. http://www.cdc.gov/ncbddd/folicacid/data.html. Accessed September 8, 2017.

90. U.S. Preventive Services Task Force. Folic acid for the prevention of neural tube defects. U.S. Preventive Services Task Force recommendation statement. *Ann Intern Med*. 2009;150(9):626-631.

91. National Institute of Neurological Disorders and Stroke. Spina bifida fact sheet. http://www.ninds.nih.gov/disorders/spina_bifida/detail_spina_bifida.htm. Accessed September 8, 2017.

92. Greenberg JA, Bell SJ, Guan Y, Yu Y-H. Folic acid supplementation and pregnancy: more than just neural tube defect prevention. *Rev Obstet Gynecol*. 2011;4(2):52-59.

93. Ganji V, Kafai MR. Demographic, lifestyle, and health characteristics and serum B vitamin status are determinants of plasma total homocysteine concentration in the post-folic acid fortification period, 1999–2004. *J Nutr*. 2009;139(2):345-352.

94. Lee JE, Willett WC, Fuchs CS, et al. Folate intake and risk of colorectal cancer and adenoma: modification by time. *Am J Clin Nutr*. 2011;93(4):817-825.

95. Kennedy DA, Stern SJ, Moretti M, et al. Folate intake and the risk of colorectal cancer: a systematic review and meta-analysis. *Cancer Epidemiol*. 2011;35(1):2-10.

96. Mason JB. Folate, cancer risk, and the Greek god, Proteus: a tale of two chameleons. *Nutr Rev*. 2009;67(4):206-212.

97. National Institutes of Health. Vitamin B$_{12}$: dietary supplement fact sheet. http://ods.od.nih.gov/factsheets/VitaminB12-HealthProfessional/. Accessed September 8, 2017.

98. Langan RC, Zawistoski KJ. Update on vitamin B$_{12}$ deficiency. *Am Fam Physician*. 2011;83(12):1425-1430. http://www.aafp.org/afp/2011/0615/p1425.html. Accessed September 8, 2017.

99. Allen LH, Rosenberg IH, Oakley GP, Omenn GS. Considering the case for vitamin B$_{12}$ fortification of flour. *Food Nutr Bull*. 2010;31(1 Suppl):S36-S46.

100. Selhub J, Paul L. Folic acid fortification: why not vitamin B$_{12}$ also? *Biofactors*. 2011;37(4):269-271. doi: 10.1002/biof.173. Epub June 14, 2011.

101. U.S. National Library of Medicine. Pantothenic acid (vitamin B$_5$). http://www.nlm.nih.gov/medlineplus/druginfo/natural/853.html. Accessed September 8, 2017.

102. Institute of Medicine, Food and Nutrition Board. *Dietary Reference Intakes for Thiamin, Riboflavin, Niacin, Vitamin B$_6$, Folate, Vitamin B$_{12}$, Pantothenic Acid, Biotin, and Choline*. Op. cit.

103. U.S. Department of Agriculture, Agricultural Research Service. USDA national nutrient database for standard reference, release 26. Op. cit.

104. Institute of Medicine, Food and Nutrition Board. *Dietary Reference Intakes for Thiamin, Riboflavin, Niacin, Vitamin B$_6$, Folate, Vitamin B$_{12}$, Pantothenic Acid, Biotin, and Choline*. Op. cit.

105. Ibid.

106. Ibid.

107. Carpenter KJ. A short history of nutritional science: part 1 (1785–1885). *J Nutr*. 2003;133:638-645.

108. Lykkesfeldt J, Poulsen HE. Is vitamin C supplementation beneficial? Lessons learned from randomized controlled trials. *Br J Nutr*. 2010;103(9):1251-1259.

109. Hemilä H, Chalker E. Vitamin C for preventing and treating the common cold. *Cochrane Database Syst Rev*. 2013;1:CD000980. doi: 10.1002/14651858. CD000980.pub4.

110. Institute of Medicine, Food and Nutrition Board. *Dietary Reference Intakes for Vitamin C, Vitamin E, Selenium, and Carotenoids*. Op. cit.

111. Ibid.

112. Gropper SS, Smith JL, Carr TP. Op. cit.

113. Institute of Medicine, Food and Nutrition Board. *Dietary Reference Intakes for Vitamin C, Vitamin E, Selenium, and Carotenoids*. Op. cit.

Spotlight on Dietary Supplements and Functional Foods

Revised by Melissa Bernstein

CHAPTER Menu

- Dietary Supplements: Vitamins and Minerals
- Dietary Supplements: Natural Health Products
- Dietary Supplements in the Marketplace
- Functional Foods

LEARNING Objectives

1. Describe how dietary supplements are regulated in the food supply.

2. Discuss the potential benefits and harmful effects of dietary supplements and herbal supplements.

3. List individuals for whom dietary supplements would be considered appropriate.

4. Discuss functional foods and give three to five examples including the food source and potential benefit.

5. Define phytochemicals.

W hen she feels down, Jana takes the herb St. John's wort to give her a lift. Whenever she has the option, Sherina chooses calcium-fortified foods. Carlos swears by creatine in his muscle-building regimen. Jason tries a new energy bar with added ginkgo biloba, hoping it will improve his memory. Others in search of better health turn to massage therapy, meditation, organic diets, homeopathy, acupuncture, and many other practices.

Any trip to the grocery store will tell you that a new era in product development is here—one in which food products are more often touted for what they contain (e.g., soy **isoflavones**, vitamins and minerals, herbal ingredients) than for what they lack (e.g., sugar, fat, cholesterol). Beverages, energy bars, food products, and teas marketed as functional foods with special health benefits sit side by side on the shelves with traditional foods. The market for **dietary supplements**—which are much more than the simple vitamins and minerals our parents knew—continues to grow.

This spotlight looks at dietary supplements, functional foods, and the role of nutrition in **complementary and integrative health care**. We will discuss not only the claims made for products and therapies in terms of current scientific knowledge, but also the regulatory and safety issues. Making decisions about nutrition and health requires both consumers and professionals to stay informed and consult reliable sources before trying a new product or embarking on a new health regimen.

▶ **isoflavones** Plant chemicals that include genistein and daidzein and may have positive effects against cancer and heart disease. Also called *phytoestrogens*.

▶ **dietary supplements** Products taken by mouth in tablet, capsule, powder, gelcap, or other nonfood form that contain one or more of the following: vitamins, minerals, amino acids, herbs, enzymes, metabolites, or concentrates.

▶ **complementary and integrative health care** A broad range of healing philosophies, approaches, and therapies that include treatments and healthcare practices not taught widely in medical schools, not generally used in hospitals, and not usually reimbursed by medical insurance companies.

Dietary Supplements: Vitamins and Minerals

🍎 **Why Is This Important?** Consumers spend billions of dollars each year on dietary supplements for many reasons. Individuals with health conditions such as osteoporosis or those who follow restrictive diet patterns such as vegetarianism may require additional help in meeting their nutrient requirements. Dietary supplements can provide a valuable source of nutrients when diet alone just isn't enough.

Dietary supplements come in various forms—vitamins, minerals, amino acids, herbs, extracts, enzymes, and many others. The marketplace includes a wide variety of products claiming to do everything from enhancing immune function to improving memory and mood. Dietary supplement use is common in the United States among adults, with over half the population using at least one, the most common of which

Position Statement: Academy of Nutrition and Dietetics

Nutrient Supplementation

It is the position of the Academy of Nutrition and Dietetics that the best nutrition-based strategy for promoting optimal health and reducing the risk of chronic disease is to wisely choose a wide variety of foods. Additional nutrients from supplements can help some people meet their nutrition needs as specified by science-based nutrition standards such as the Dietary Reference Intakes.

Reproduced from Marra MV, Boyar AP. Position of the American Dietetic Association: nutrient supplementation. *J Am Diet Assoc.* 2009;109(12):2073-2085.

▶ **megadoses**   Doses of a nutrient that are 10 or more times the recommended amount.

are multivitamin/mineral dietary supplements.[1,2] **TABLE SF.1** lists many popular supplements, claims, and important cautions. Despite the enticing claims made for many nonnutrient supplements, scientific evidence has confirmed health benefits for some dietary supplements but not others. It is always important to look for reliable sources of information on dietary supplements and evaluate the claims made about them.[3]

"Should I take a vitamin (or mineral) supplement?" Apparently many people already have answered that question for themselves. (See **FIGURE SF.1**.) Multivitamin/mineral supplements and other single-vitamin or -mineral supplements are popular and are taken by a substantial percentage of Americans.[4] Dietary supplement use generally falls into two categories: (1) moderate doses that are in the range of the Daily Values (DVs) or levels you might eat in a nutrient-rich diet and (2) **megadoses**, or high levels that are typically multiples of the DVs and much greater amounts than diet alone could supply.

Moderate Supplementation

The most common reasons people use supplements are to improve or maintain health, yet less than a quarter of adults who take dietary supplements do so based on a recommendation from a healthcare provider.[5]

TABLE SF.1

Some Commonly Used Dietary Supplements and Their Claims

Supplement	Claimed Benefit	What Does the Science Say?
Beta-carotene	Prevents cancer and heart disease, boosts immunity, improves eye health	Diets rich in beta-carotene–containing fruits and vegetables reduce heart disease and cancer risk. Supplements have not been shown to be beneficial. Taking supplements may increase lung cancer risk in smokers. In combination with vitamin C, vitamin E, and zinc, it may slow progression of age-related macular degeneration.
Chromium picolinate	Builds muscle, helps with blood glucose control in diabetes, promotes weight loss, reduces cholesterol	No solid evidence that chromium picolinate supplements perform as claimed or benefit healthy people. Some evidence that supplements may harm cells.

TABLE SF.1 (*continued*)
Some Commonly Used Dietary Supplements and Their Claims

Supplement	Claimed Benefit	What Does the Science Say?
Coenzyme Q_{10}	Prevents heart disease, improves health of people with heart disease and hypertension, cure-all	May have value in preexisting heart disease, but benefits for healthy people are unproved.
Cranberry	Prevents and treats urinary tract infections (UTIs)	There is some evidence that cranberry can help to *prevent* urinary tract infections; however, the evidence is not definitive, and more research is needed. Cranberry has not been shown to be effective as a *treatment* for an existing urinary tract infection.
Creatine	Increases muscle strength and size, improves athletic performance	May enhance power and strength for some athletes, but is ineffective for casual exercisers and distance athletes.
Echinacea	Protects against and cures colds, boosts immunity	Study results are mixed on whether echinacea can *prevent* or effectively *treat* upper respiratory tract infections such as the common cold. Other studies have shown that echinacea may be beneficial in treating upper respiratory infections.
Ephedra	Weight control, herbal "high," decongestant	Ephedra raises heart rate and blood pressure, causes gastrointestinal problems, and is dangerous for people with diabetes, hypertension, or heart disease. According to the Food and Drug Administration (FDA), there is little evidence of ephedra's effectiveness, except for short-term weight loss—and the increased risk of heart problems and stroke outweighs any benefits. The FDA has prohibited sales of ephedra-containing supplements.

(continued)

TABLE SF.1 (*continued*)
Some Commonly Used Dietary Supplements and Their Claims

Supplement	Claimed Benefit	What Does the Science Say?
Feverfew	Prevents migraines	Some evidence of reduced severity and frequency of migraines, but high dropout rates in studies. Study results are mixed, and there is not enough evidence available to assess whether feverfew is beneficial for other uses.
Flaxseed and flaxseed oil	Laxative, lowers cholesterol levels, prevents cancer	Studies of flaxseed preparations to lower cholesterol levels show mixed results. Some studies suggest that alpha-linolenic acid found in flaxseed and flaxseed oil may benefit people with heart disease. Flaxseed might reduce the risk of certain cancers; however, research does not yet support a recommendation for this use.
Garlic	Lowers blood pressure and blood cholesterol, reduces cancer risk	There is some evidence that garlic reduces cholesterol and blood pressure. Dietary garlic may reduce cancer risk; however, results are conflicting.
Ginkgo biloba	Improves blood flow and circulatory disorders; prevents or cures absentmindedness, memory loss, dementia	Studies on ginkgo biloba found it to be ineffective in lowering the overall incidence of dementia and Alzheimer's disease in older adults, improving memory, slowing cognitive decline, lowering blood pressure, or reducing the incidence of hypertension; there is conflicting evidence on the efficacy of ginkgo for tinnitus.
Ginseng	Improves athletic performance, fights fatigue, helps control blood glucose in people with diabetes, reduces cancer risk	There is no evidence that ginseng has any beneficial effects. Many products on the market contain no ginseng.
Glucosamine and chondroitin sulfate	Relieve arthritis pain, slow progression of arthritis	Some evidence of reduced pain and improved symptoms, although more studies are needed. Does not reverse arthritis. Variable amounts in products.

TABLE SF.1 (*continued*)
Some Commonly Used Dietary Supplements and Their Claims

Supplement	Claimed Benefit	What Does the Science Say?
Kava	Promotes relaxation and relieves anxiety	The FDA has issued a warning that using kava supplements has been linked to a risk of severe liver damage. Banned in Switzerland, Germany, and Canada.
Melatonin	Promotes sleep, counters jet lag, improves sex life, prevents migraine	May be effective for jet lag; studies are contradictory relative to sleep. No evidence for anti-aging or sex-drive claims. No data on long-term safety.
Milk thistle	Reduces liver damage in alcoholic liver disease, promotes general liver health	Previous studies suggested that milk thistle may benefit the liver by protecting and promoting the growth of liver cells, fighting oxidation, and inhibiting inflammation. However, results from small clinical trials of milk thistle for liver diseases have been mixed or found no benefit.
Saw palmetto	Shrinks prostate, reduces symptoms of benign prostatic hyperplasia, prevents prostate cancer	Several small studies suggest that saw palmetto may be effective for treating benign prostatic hyperplasia (BPH) symptoms. However, another study found saw palmetto did not reduce the urinary symptoms associated with BPH more than a placebo.
St. John's wort	Alleviates depression, promotes emotional well-being	Some studies of St. John's wort have reported benefits for depression; however, others have not. St John's wort has not been found to be any more effective than a placebo in treating depression.
Valerian	Enhances sleep, reduces stress and anxiety	Valerian may be helpful for insomnia. Results are inconclusive to date; more research is needed.

Data from National Center for Complementary and Integrative Health (NCCIH) . Herbs at a glance. http://nccih.nih.gov/health/herbsataglance .htm Accessed March 28, 2017; National Institutes of Health, Office of Dietary Supplements. Dietary supplement fact sheets. http://ods.od.nih .gov/factsheets/list-all. Accessed March 28, 2017.

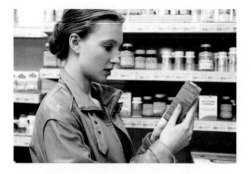

FIGURE SF.1 Increasing popularity of dietary supplements. Over half of adult Americans regularly purchase dietary supplements.

Healthcare practitioners often recommend moderate nutrient supplementation for people with elevated nutrient needs and for people who may not always eat a well-balanced diet.[6] **TABLE SF.2** lists some examples of people for whom nutritional supplementation may be recommended.

In addition to those listed in Table SF.2, other groups may also be vulnerable to nutrient inadequacies, such as individuals who are food insecure, are alcohol/drug dependent, or have altered nutritional needs due to an illness or medication use. Many people take nutrient supplements to ensure they meet their nutritional needs. However, taking supplements to "fix" a poor diet is not a perfect solution. Experts advocate achieving healthy dietary patterns through healthy, nutrient-dense food and beverage choices rather than nutrient or dietary supplements, except when needed.[7] According to the Academy of Nutrition and Dietetics, "focusing on variety, moderation, and proportionality in the context of a healthy lifestyle, rather than targeting specific nutrients or foods, can help reduce consumer confusion

TABLE SF.2

People for Whom Nutrition Supplementation May Be Recommended

Women of childbearing age who may become pregnant as well as pregnant and breastfeeding women: Taking supplemental folic acid prior to and during pregnancy can reduce the incidence of birth defects. During pregnancy, it's hard to meet the increased needs for iron and other nutrients through diet alone. Morning sickness makes it even harder. When a woman breastfeeds, some of her nutrient needs are even higher than they were in pregnancy.	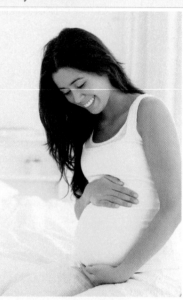 © wavebreakmedia ltd/Shutterstock.
Women with heavy menstrual bleeding: Women with high iron losses may need a supplement, but they should not take high doses of iron without a doctor's recommendation. Lab tests can show whether a woman gets enough blood-building nutrients or whether she needs supplements.	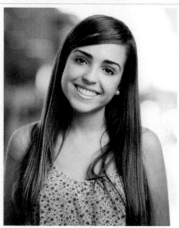 © Asier Romero/Shutterstock.

TABLE SF.2   *(continued)*
People for Whom Nutrition Supplementation May Be Recommended

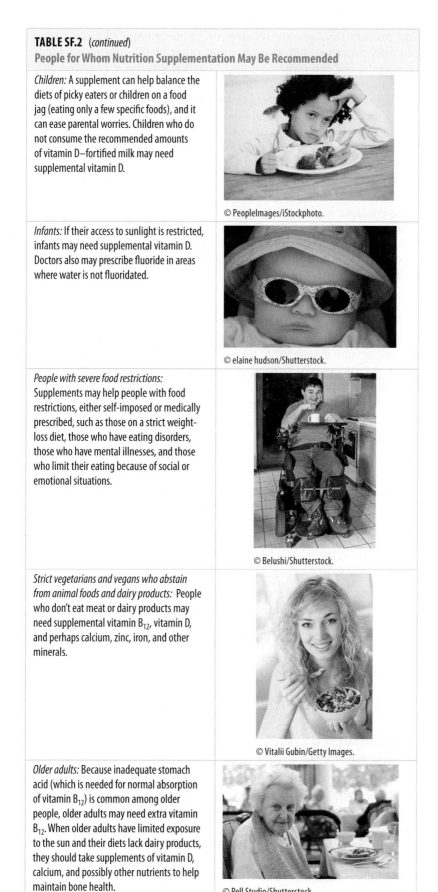

Children: A supplement can help balance the diets of picky eaters or children on a food jag (eating only a few specific foods), and it can ease parental worries. Children who do not consume the recommended amounts of vitamin D–fortified milk may need supplemental vitamin D.

© PeopleImages/iStockphoto.

Infants: If their access to sunlight is restricted, infants may need supplemental vitamin D. Doctors also may prescribe fluoride in areas where water is not fluoridated.

© elaine hudson/Shutterstock.

People with severe food restrictions: Supplements may help people with food restrictions, either self-imposed or medically prescribed, such as those on a strict weight-loss diet, those who have eating disorders, those who have mental illnesses, and those who limit their eating because of social or emotional situations.

© Belushi/Shutterstock.

Strict vegetarians and vegans who abstain from animal foods and dairy products: People who don't eat meat or dairy products may need supplemental vitamin B_{12}, vitamin D, and perhaps calcium, zinc, iron, and other minerals.

© Vitalii Gubin/Getty Images.

Older adults: Because inadequate stomach acid (which is needed for normal absorption of vitamin B_{12}) is common among older people, older adults may need extra vitamin B_{12}. When older adults have limited exposure to the sun and their diets lack dairy products, they should take supplements of vitamin D, calcium, and possibly other nutrients to help maintain bone health.

© Pell Studio/Shutterstock.

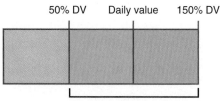

FIGURE SF.2 Moderate supplementation. Healthcare practitioners often recommend moderate nutrient supplementation for people with elevated nutrient needs and for people who have consistently poor diets.

▶ **malabsorption syndromes** Conditions that result in imperfect, inadequate, or otherwise disordered gastrointestinal absorption.

▶ **orthomolecular medicine** The preventive or therapeutic use of high-dose vitamins to treat disease.

American Heart Association

Vitamin and Mineral Supplements

The American Heart Association recommends that healthy people get adequate nutrients by eating a variety of foods in moderation, rather than by taking supplements.

"The Dietary Recommended Intakes (DRIs) published by the Institute of Medicine are the best available estimates of safe and adequate dietary intakes," says the AHA. "There aren't sufficient data to suggest that healthy people benefit by taking certain vitamin or mineral supplements in excess of the DRIs." Moreover, "vitamin or mineral supplements aren't a substitute for a balanced, nutritious diet that limits excess calories, saturated fat, trans fat, sodium, and dietary cholesterol. This dietary approach has been shown to reduce coronary heart disease risk in both healthy people and those with coronary disease."

Reprinted with permission, www.heart.org,
© 2017 American Heart Association, Inc.

and prevent unnecessary reliance on supplements."[8] Foods provide not only nutrients, but also fiber and other health-promoting phytochemicals. For the most healthful benefits, whenever possible, meet your nutritional needs with food.

If you are one of those people who should take multivitamin/mineral supplements, look for brands that contain no more than 100 percent of the Daily Value unless otherwise instructed by your doctor. (See **FIGURE SF.2.**) Although many products have appropriate nutrient levels, some formulas are irrational and unbalanced, with less than 10 percent of the Daily Value of some nutrients and more than 1,000 percent of others.

Key Concepts Vitamin and mineral supplements are popular; however, it is better to obtain nutrients from food. Some conditions and circumstances make it difficult to meet nutritional needs through food alone or to consume enough food to accommodate increases in nutrient needs. Multivitamin/mineral supplements should be well balanced, with doses no greater than about 100 percent of the Daily Value of each nutrient.

Megadoses in Conventional Medical Management

High doses of vitamins and minerals have become so much a part of treating certain illnesses that when physicians prescribe these nutrients, many see themselves as following "standard medical practice" rather than as "practicing nutrition." Here are some situations in which physicians may prescribe a vitamin or mineral at megadose levels:

- When a medication dramatically depletes or destroys the stores or blocks the functions of vitamins or minerals, megadosing can overcome these effects. For example, folic acid and vitamin B_6 are used during long-term treatment with some tuberculosis drugs.
- People with **malabsorption syndromes** such as cystic fibrosis often take large nutrient doses to compensate for nutritive losses and to override intestinal barriers to absorption.
- Megadoses of vitamin B_{12} can overcome the malabsorption seen in pernicious anemia, a condition in which a key substance needed for vitamin B_{12} absorption is lacking.

A vitamin at megadose levels can have *pharmacological activity*—that is, it acts as a drug. Nicotinic acid (niacin) is a good example. At usual levels (around 10 or 20 milligrams), it functions as a vitamin, but at levels 50 or 100 times higher it acts as a drug to lower blood lipid levels. Niacin has been used since the 1950s as a lipid-altering drug for low-density lipoprotein (LDL) cholesterol and is currently an effective agent available for raising high-density lipoprotein (HDL) cholesterol.[9] Like any drug, though, it can have serious side effects.

Megadosing Beyond Conventional Medicine: Orthomolecular Nutrition

In 1968, Linus Pauling, the best-known advocate of megadosing, coined the term **orthomolecular medicine**. To him, *orthomolecular* meant achieving the optimal nutrient levels in the body.[10] Few nutritionists argue with the importance of optimum nutrition. In fact, some nutritionists share Pauling's concerns that the typical diet is too refined to provide adequate nutrients and that intake equal to RDA values may not be high enough to achieve optimal body levels.

Most nutritionists would argue, however, with the high doses Pauling recommended to attain those optimal body levels and with the therapeutic value he and his followers attributed to those doses. Most notably, Pauling suggested in the early 1970s that an optimal daily intake of vitamin C was 2,000 milligrams—more than 30 times the current Daily Value. (See **FIGURE SF.3**.) Dr. Pauling claimed megadoses of vitamin C prevented or cured the common cold. Although many researchers have attempted to confirm this theory, studies do not support the idea that vitamin C prevents colds. A few studies found that colds were slightly less severe or less frequent in those who took high doses of vitamin C, but most studies found no beneficial effect.[11]

Drawbacks of Megadoses

THINK About It 1

Megadose vitamins and minerals remain popular, but when taken without recommendation or prescription from a qualified health professional they can cause problems. Because high doses of a nutrient can act as a drug, with a drug's risk of adverse side effects, people who choose to take megadoses should always check first with their doctors.

Excesses of some nutrients can create deficits of other nutrients. High doses of supplemental minerals, especially calcium, iron, zinc, and copper, can interfere with absorption of the others.[12] If you use high doses of the fat-soluble vitamin A, it is easy to reach toxic levels. Even megadoses of water-soluble vitamins can be problematic; for example, nerve damage can result from vitamin B_6 at 50 to 100 times the DV. **FIGURE SF.4** lists some more examples of medical side effects that can occur from megadose supplementation. It is good practice to review the DRI tables for tolerable upper intake levels (ULs) before taking any vitamin and mineral supplement.

> **Key Concepts** High doses (megadoses) of vitamins or minerals turn nutrients into drugs—chemicals with pharmacological activity. Although there may be medical reasons for prescribing high-dose supplements, they should be taken under a physician's supervision. Many claims for high-dose supplements are not supported by clinical studies.

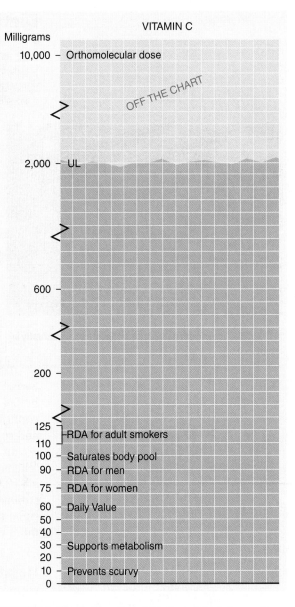

FIGURE SF.3 **Vitamin C megadoses.** Megadoses of vitamin C are much higher intakes than currently recommended.

Supplement	Common Side Effect of Megadoses
Iron	Constipation
Vitamin C	Diarrhea
Folic acid	Breakthrough seizures for those on antiseizure medication
Vitamin K	Disrupts balance of blood-clotting medication
Vitamin E	Bleeding problems during surgery
Antioxidant formulas	Counteract some chemotherapy and radiation treatments

FIGURE SF.4 **Dietary supplement megadoses.** Megadoses of vitamins and minerals can cause medical side effects and complications.

Dietary Supplements: Natural Health Products

🍎 **Why Is This Important?**   Natural medicines and herbal supplements are no longer relegated to the fringes of modern medicine. Americans are spending billions of dollars on natural product supplements, and government agencies are supporting research and clinical trials to scientifically test effectiveness and safety. Still, taking a critical approach to herbal and natural products is wise.

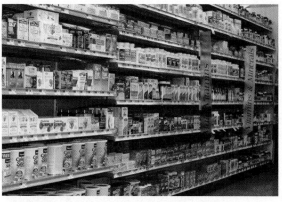

FIGURE SF.5   Use of herbal supplements has grown significantly in recent years.

Supplementation with herbal and other "natural" products is a popular form of integrative medicine. (See **FIGURE SF.5**.) The first decade of this century saw a dramatic rise in the popularity of dietary supplements—a trend that continues today. Currently in the United States, more than 150 million people use dietary supplements, accounting for $36.7 billion in annual sales.[13] Health Canada estimates that 71 percent of Canadians have consumed natural health products: herbs, vitamins and minerals, and homeopathic products.[14] **Herbal therapy (phytotherapy)** is nothing new, however. Most cultures have long traditions of using plants (and some animal products) to treat illness or sustain health. For centuries there were no other medicines. Even now, most of the world's people depend primarily on plants for medications; in some remote areas, modern medicines are just not obtainable.

Traditional herbalists know their patients and individualize their herbal remedies accordingly. Those who turn to the mass market for herbal supplements rarely receive such attention and are likely to be confused by nutrition and health-related claims that surround foods and supplements.

In the Western world, the assumption that "natural" is better than "chemical" or "synthetic" has launched the market for "natural" foods to a $12.9 billion industry, with "all natural" becoming the second most common claim to be found on new food labels in recent years.[15] Consumers interpret claims such as "100% natural" to mean the product is more wholesome, nutritious, and healthy.

Quick Bite

Culinary Herbs Are Not Medicinal Herbs—Or Are They?

Herbs used in cooking are called *culinary herbs* to distinguish them from medicinal herbs. But culinary herbs are also rich in phytochemicals. Some examples are beta-carotene in paprika, the antioxidants in rosemary, the mild antibiotic allicin in garlic, and the mild antiviral curcumin in turmeric.

Helpful Herbs, Harmful Herbs

Until recently, most research on herbs was published in obscure or foreign-language journals that were hard to locate or read. Traditional herbal medical practices are difficult to study in a controlled manner because they use plants to make teas or soups, a far cry from the purified extracts and herbal blends sold in a supermarket. Nevertheless, for some herbs, researchers have enough data to plan carefully controlled studies.

In 1998, Congress established the National Center for Complementary and Alternative Medicine at the **National Institutes of Health (NIH)** to stimulate, develop, and support research on complementary and alternative medicine for the benefit of the public. At the end of 2014, the NIH agency with primary responsibility for research on promising health approaches that already are in use by the American public was renamed the **National Center for Complementary and Integrative Health (NCCIH)**.[16] The NCCIH is an advocate for quality science, rigorous and relevant research, and encouraging objective inquiry into which complementary and alternative medicine (CAM) practices work, which do not, and why. The mission of the NCCIH "is to define, through rigorous scientific investigation, the usefulness and safety of complementary

▶ **herbal therapy (phytotherapy)**   The therapeutic use of herbs and other plants to promote health and treat disease.

▶ **National Institutes of Health (NIH)**   A U.S. Department of Health and Human Services agency composed of 27 separate institutes and centers with a mission to advance knowledge and improve human health.

▶ **National Center for Complementary and Integrative Health (NCCIH)**   An NIH organization established to stimulate, develop, and support objective scientific research on complementary and integrative health for the benefit of the public.

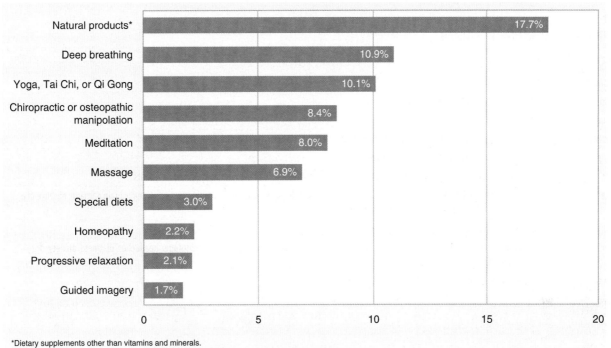

*Dietary supplements other than vitamins and minerals.

FIGURE SF.6 Ten most common complementary health approaches among adults.

Reproduced from Clark TC, Black LI, Stussman BJ, Barnes PM, Nahin RL. Trends in the use of complementary health approaches among adults: United States, 2002-2012. National Health Statistics reports; no 79. Hyattsville, MD: National Center for Health Statistics, 2015.

and integrative health approaches and their roles in improving health and health care."[17] (For more information about how to define CAM, see the FYI feature "Where Does Nutrition Fit?") According to the NCCIH, natural products are the most common type used in a complementary approach, as shown in **FIGURE SF.6**. Approximately 59 million Americans spend $30.2 billion a year on complementary health practices, almost 10 percent of out-of-pocket spending on health care.[18]

Almost 18 percent of American adults have used a nonvitamin/nonmineral natural product in recent years; fish oil/omega-3s were the most commonly used natural products among adults.[19] Some natural products have been studied in large, scientific trials, and although there are indications that some may be helpful, many have failed to show anticipated effects. (See Table SF.1 earlier in this text.) The suggested benefits of other herbs are based not on scientific study but on years of informal observation: Mint helps indigestion; ginger helps nausea and motion sickness; lemon perks appetite; chamomile helps insomnia. More research is still needed about the effects of these products in the human body and about their safety and potential interactions with medicines and with other natural products.

THINK About It 2

If you're considering using an herb, remember this important rule of thumb: Any herb that is strong enough to help you can be strong enough to hurt you. Like any medicine, herbs can have side effects, and herbs can be contraindicated. Herbs can interfere with standard medicines. They can affect the way the body processes both over-the-counter and prescription medications, causing the medications to not work the way they should, and therefore can make people with underlying health problems quite sick.[20] Herbal products and supplements may not be safe if you have certain health problems or take certain medications.

Quick Bite

Office of Dietary Supplements

The Office of Dietary Supplements (ODS) is a Congressionally mandated office in the National Institutes of Health (NIH). The mission of the ODS is to strengthen knowledge and understanding of dietary supplements by evaluating scientific information, stimulating and supporting research, disseminating research results, and educating the public to foster an enhanced quality of life and health for the U.S. population.

TABLE SF.3

Potential Adverse Effects of Selected Herbs

Herb	Adverse Effects
Chamomile (tea)	Allergic reaction
Echinacea	Allergic reaction; gastrointestinal side effects
Ephedra	Stroke, heart attack, sudden death, seizures
Ginkgo biloba	Headache, nausea, gastrointestinal upset, diarrhea, dizziness, allergic skin reactions, increased bleeding risk
Ginseng	Headaches, insomnia, diarrhea, itching, nervousness
Kava	Liver damage including hepatitis and liver failure, abnormal muscle spasm or involuntary muscle movements
Licorice	Headaches; fluid retention; increased blood pressure; electrolyte imbalance; weakness, paralysis, and occasionally brain damage; absence of a menstrual period in women, decreased sexual interest and function in men
Senna	Laxative dependency, diarrhea, cramps, electrolyte disturbances
St. John's wort	Adverse interactions with many medications, increased sensitivity to light, gastrointestinal symptoms, headaches, dizziness, anxiety, dry mouth, fatigue, sexual dysfunction
Valerian	Drowsiness; withdrawal symptoms if abruptly discontinued

Data from Medline Plus. Herbs and supplements. http://www.nlm.nih.gov/medlineplus/druginfo/herb_All.html. Accessed March 28, 2017 .

▶ **bioflavonoids** Naturally occurring plant chemicals, especially from citrus fruits, that reduce the permeability and fragility of capillaries.

▶ **nucleic acids** A family of more than 25,000 molecules found in chromosomes, nucleoli, mitochondria, and the cytoplasm of cells.

Some herbs and herbalist treatments are downright dangerous. (See **TABLE SF.3**.) Some hazardous therapies even use lead or arsenic, known poisons. St. John's wort, ginseng, ginkgo biloba, garlic, grapefruit juice, hawthorn, saw palmetto, danshen, echinacea, yohimbe, licorice, and black cohosh are examples of common herbal remedies known to be potentially dangerous for people taking medications for cardiovascular disease.[21] Other herbs, such as ephedra (ma huang), chaparral, and comfrey, have also been shown to be dangerous.

Quality control is a big issue in herbal medicines. In 2007, the FDA issued final regulations requiring Current Good Manufacturing Practices (CGMPs) for the manufacturing, packaging, labeling, and storage of dietary supplements. Under the regulations, manufacturers are required to evaluate the identity, purity, strength, and composition of their products and ensure proper labeling.[22]

Other Dietary Supplements

The supplement market used to include only vitamins, minerals, and a handful of other products, such as brewer's yeast and sea salt. Today there are thousands more products, with new ones continuously popping up.

Supplement categories, for example, now include protein powders, amino acids, carotenoids, **bioflavonoids**, digestive aids, fatty acid formulas and special fats, lecithin and phospholipids, probiotics, products from sharks and other sea animals, algae, metabolites such as coenzyme Q_{10} and **nucleic acids**, glandular extracts, garlic products, and fibers such as guar gum. Supplement producers also blend these products with herbs and nutrients, resulting in the countless array of individual and combination supplements sold today. In many cases, labeling and advertising claims extend beyond current knowledge about these products. Although some supplements are useful, many are of dubious benefit. Wise consumers look for scientific evidence and reliable medical guidance before wasting their money or, worse, risking their health.

Key Concepts Herbal products are among the many dietary supplements available today. Herbal medicine has a long history in many cultures. Although there is anecdotal support for the use of many herbal products, there is little scientific evidence to back it up. The FDA has set standards for production and sale of herbal supplements. It is important to remember that any herb that is strong enough to help you can also be strong enough to hurt you. Before taking any supplements, it's a good idea to consult your healthcare practitioner.

Dietary Supplements in the Marketplace

🍎 **Why Is This Important?** There are lots of important things to consider before you start taking a dietary supplement. Does the supplement actually do what it says it can? How much is safe to take? What is the potential for serious side effects? Before you spend a dime, it is important that you are an informed consumer!

There are more than 50,000 dietary supplements on the market, including vitamins and minerals, herbs, botanicals, and other products, such as fish oils and probiotics. Although some dietary supplements have drug-like actions (e.g., reducing cholesterol levels), government agencies regulate supplements differently from drugs. Manufacturers are allowed to make a wide variety of claims for product effects without having to provide scientific evidence to support those claims. The freedoms of speech and press prevail; in practical terms, almost anything goes. Promotional books, infomercials, magazine articles, CDs and DVDs, lectures, staged interviews, podcasts, and web pages—all are protected by the First Amendment, and their authors have the freedom to inform or to deceive. It's up to the listener or reader to distinguish fact from fiction. (See **FIGURE SF.7**.)

The FTC and Supplement Advertising

The Federal Trade Commission (FTC) in the U.S. Department of Commerce is responsible for ensuring that advertisements and commercials are truthful and do not mislead. The agency depends on and encourages voluntary self-monitoring by the supplement industry. In pursuing deceptive companies, the FTC prioritizes cases that put people's health and safety at serious risk or that affect sick and vulnerable consumers. Unfortunately, this means many products escape notice and are falsely marketed without repercussions. The supplements industry is creative in its advertising campaigns (exaggerating the benefits of many supplements), and it is resourceful in finding loopholes in federal regulations to continue selling products.

The FDA and Supplement Regulation

The Food and Drug Administration has primary responsibility for regulating labeling and content of dietary supplements under the Federal Food, Drug, and Cosmetic Act, as amended by the 1994 **Dietary Supplement Health and Education Act (DSHEA)**.[23] How do you know a product is a "dietary supplement"? Simple. The law defines *dietary supplements*, in part, as products that are taken by mouth that contain a "dietary ingredient."[24] Dietary supplements include vitamins, minerals, herbs or botanicals, and amino acids as well as other substances such as enzymes, organ tissues, metabolites, extracts, or concentrates, used to supplement the diet.

Dietary supplements are *not* drugs. A drug is intended to diagnose, cure, mitigate, treat, or prevent disease. Before marketing, drugs must undergo extensive studies of effectiveness, safety, interactions

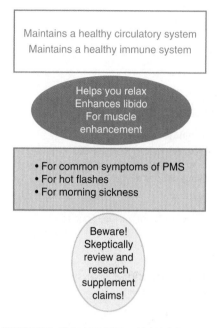

FIGURE SF.7 Dietary supplement label claims. Although claims such as these appear on dietary supplement labels, they do not have to be approved by the FDA. All should be viewed with skepticism.

▶ **Dietary Supplement Health and Education Act (DSHEA)** Legislation that regulates dietary supplements.

Quick Bite

Pronouncing the Acronym

The Dietary Supplement Health and Education Act of 1994 is better known by its acronym DSHEA, pronounced "da-shay."

▶ **Supplement Facts panel** Content label that must appear on all dietary supplements.

with other substances, and dosing. The FDA gives formal premarket approval to a drug and monitors its safety after the drug is on the market. If a drug is subsequently shown to be dangerous, the FDA can act quickly to have it removed from the market. None of this is true for dietary supplements. The current law gives the FDA only limited authority over supplements, making it difficult for the government to remove unsafe supplements from the marketplace. The FDA does not evaluate the safety and effectiveness of supplements before they hit the marketplace. There are some legislators in Congress who want to improve the law by requiring supplement makers to put safer products on the shelves and label products more clearly. The objective is to ensure that consumers can tell the difference between dietary supplements that are safe and those that have potentially serious side effects or drug interactions.

Supplement Labels

Like food labels, supplement labels have mandatory and optional information. All labels on dietary supplements must include ingredient information and a **Supplement Facts panel**.[25] You'll notice in **FIGURE SF.8** that the format is similar to the Nutrition Facts panel on food labels. Supplements that contain *proprietary blends*—products or techniques exclusive to the manufacturer—are not required to list specific amounts of each ingredient.[26]

Supplement labels, like food labels, may contain health claims, structure/function claims, and nutrient content claims. (See **FIGURE SF.9**.) Qualified health claims may also apply to dietary supplements.

Manufacturers can use structure/function claims without FDA authorization and can base their claims on their own review and interpretation of the scientific literature. Structure/function claims are easy to spot because they are accompanied by the following disclaimer: "This statement has not been evaluated by the Food and Drug Administration. This product is not intended to diagnose, treat, cure, or prevent any disease."[27] A dietary supplement with a label claiming to cure or treat a specific condition is considered an unapproved drug.[28]

Canadian Regulations

Beginning January 1, 2004, all natural health products sold in Canada have been subject to Health Canada's Natural Health Products Regulations.[29] By definition, natural health products include vitamins, minerals, herbal remedies, and homeopathic medicines. Health Canada has developed a product approval system whereby each product must meet the requirements of the Natural Health Products Regulations to acquire a license and be legally sold in Canada. Authorization requires evidence of safety and efficacy. The regulations also include provisions for on-site licensing, good manufacturing practices, labeling and packaging requirements, and adverse reaction reporting. The Canadian regulations go further than DSHEA in terms of ensuring the safety and efficacy of supplements.

Key Concepts Dietary supplements are neither foods nor drugs, and the government regulates their manufacture and sale differently than it does for foods, additives, and drugs. The FTC and FDA monitor advertising and labeling of dietary supplements. A Supplement Facts panel is now required on labels. Canada's regulations for natural health products require premarket approval and product licensing.

Serving size is the manufacturer's suggested serving expressed in the appropriate unit (tablet, capsule, softgel, packet, teaspoonful).

Each tablet contains heads the listing of dietary ingredients contained in the supplement.

Each dietary ingredient is followed by the quantity in a serving. For proprietary blends, total weight of the blend is listed, with components listed in descending order by weight.

Dietary ingredients that have no daily value are listed below this line.

Botanical supplements must list the part of plant present and its common name (latin name if common name not listed in *herbs of commerce*).

Supplement Facts

Serving Size 1 Tablet

Each tablet contains		%DV
Vitamin A 5,000 IU		100%
50% as Beta-carotene		
Vitamin C	90 mg	150%
Vitamin D	400 IU	100%
Vitamin E	45 IU	150%
Thiamine	1.5 mg	100%
Riboflavin	1.7 mg	100%
Niacin	20 mg	100%
Vitamin B$_6$	2 mg	100%
Folate	400 mcg	100%
Vitamin B$_{12}$	6 mcg	100%
Calcium	100 mg	10%
Iron	18 mg	100%
Iodine	150 mcg	100%
Magnesium	100 mg	25%
Zinc	15 mg	100%
Ginseng root (*Panax ginseng*)	25 mg	*
Ginkgo biloba Leaf (*Ginkgo biloba*)	25 mg	*
Citrus bioflavonoids Complex	10 mg	*
Lecithin (Glycine max) (bean)	10 mg	*
Nickel	5 mcg	*
Silicon	2 mcg	*
Boron	60 mcg	*

* Daily Value (%DV) not established

%DV indicates the percentage of the daily value of each nutrient that a serving provides.

An **asterisk** under %dv indicates that a daily value is not established for that ingredient.

List of ingredients shows the nutrients and other ingredients used to formulate the supplement, in decreasing order by weight.

INGREDIENTS: Dicalcium phosphate, magnesium oxide, ascorbic acid, cellulose, vitamin A acetate, beta-carotene, vitamin D, Dl-alpha tocopherol acetate, ginseng root (*Panax ginseng*), gelatin, ginkgo biloba leaf (*Ginkgo biloba*), ferrous fumarate, niacinamide, zinc oxide, silicon dioxide, lecithin, citrus bioflavonoids complex, pyridoxine hydrochloride, riboflavin, thiamin mononitrate, folic acid, potassium iodine, boron, cyanocobalamin, nickelous sulfate

Contact information shows the manufacturer's or distributor's name, address, and zip code.

DISTRIBUTED BY COMPANY NAME
P.O. BOX XXX
CITY, STATE 00000-0000

FIGURE SF.8 Supplement Facts panel. Similar to the Nutrition Facts panel on food labels, the Supplement Facts panel required on dietary supplement labels shows the product composition.

Choosing Dietary Supplements

Knowledge of nutrition science is your most valuable tool for evaluating a supplement. Read each label and judge each implied claim in light of what you know. For tips on choosing supplements, see the

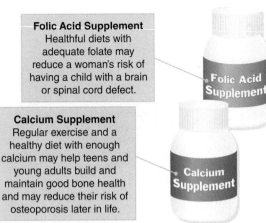

Folic Acid Supplement
Healthful diets with adequate folate may reduce a woman's risk of having a child with a brain or spinal cord defect.

Calcium Supplement
Regular exercise and a healthy diet with enough calcium may help teens and young adults build and maintain good bone health and may reduce their risk of osteoporosis later in life.

FIGURE SF.9 Health claims for supplements. Calcium and folic acid supplements may carry health claims similar to these model statements. Data from U.S. Food and Drug Administration.

▶ **bioavailability** A measure of the extent to which a nutrient becomes available to the body after ingestion and thus is available to the tissues.

▶ **U.S. Pharmacopeia (USP)** Established in 1820, the USP is a nonprofit healthcare organization that sets quality standards for a range of healthcare products.

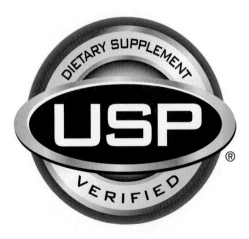

FIGURE SF.10 U.S. Pharmacopeia verification mark. Dietary supplements can earn the USP-Verified mark through a comprehensive testing and evaluation process.
Registered trademark of The United States Pharmacopeial Convention. Used with permission.

FYI feature "Shopping for Supplements." Ask the following questions:

- *Is the quantity enough to have an effect or is it trivial?* What will happen if you take more than you need?
- *Is the product new to you?* Learn about it from the many reliable resources available. Evaluate the product in light of scientific research.
- *Can the supplement cross the intestine and travel to its presumed site of action in the body?* There are little data on the absorption and **bioavailability** of herbal preparations and other types of nonnutrient supplements.
- *Can this supplement interact with any prescription or over-the-counter medications?* Some combinations of supplements or using some supplements together with either prescription or OTC medications could produce potentially harmful adverse effects.
- *Does the product promise too much?* A product touted to control high blood cholesterol, hangnails, psoriasis, and insomnia is unlikely to do much of anything.
- *Who is selling the product?* Alternative practitioners, dietitians, and even physicians sometimes sell the supplements they recommend—which is a possible conflict of interest that could compromise their objectivity. The Academy of Nutrition and Dietetics has issued guidelines for practitioners' recommendations and sales of supplements.[30]
- *What is the evidence?* Carefully evaluate the reliable scientific evidence to support the use of the dietary supplement for the intended purpose. Good places to start your research for current and accurate information are the NIH websites for the NCCIH (http://nccih.nih.gov) and the Office of Dietary Supplements (http://ods.od.nih.gov).

Even the best-intentioned, most carefully considered supplement can prove ineffective or even risky. A good indicator of quality is the voluntary **U.S. Pharmacopeia (USP)** verification mark (see **FIGURE SF.10**), which verifies that the product meets the U.S. Pharmacopeia's standards for product purity, accuracy of ingredient labeling, and proper manufacturing practices.[31] The USP verification mark helps assure consumers, healthcare professionals, and supplement retailers that a product has passed USP's rigorous program and does the following:

- Contains the ingredients declared on the product label
- Contains the amount or strength of ingredients declared on the product label
- Meets requirements for limits on potential contaminants
- Has been manufactured properly by complying with USP and FDA standards for current good manufacturing practices (cGMPs)

Fraudulent Products

Some health advocates consider the burgeoning market of dietary supplements an unwelcome return to the "snake oil" era of the late nineteenth and early twentieth centuries, when "magic" potions and cures were sold door to door and at county fairs and markets. Most

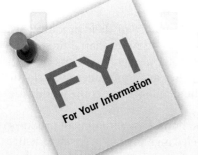

Shopping for Supplements

Thinking about buying a dietary supplement? Before you do, ask yourself, "Why do I need this supplement?" and "Is it suitable for me?" Think about your typical diet and what it may be lacking. Remember, the word *supplement* means just that—a product meant to supplement your food. A well-chosen supplement can be beneficial under some circumstances, especially if your diet is limited. However, if you're healthy and eat a good balance of healthful foods, supplements probably won't help you much.

It's a good idea to let your doctor know your supplement plans. Some supplements are contraindicated during pregnancy or lactation; others should not be used with certain chronic illnesses. Supplements sometimes interfere with the action of medicines. Some slow blood clotting, which is a concern if surgery is planned.

To a great extent, you will need to rely on your own understanding of diet and nutrition to make your selection. And, you must rely on the supplement manufacturer for the product's safety, its purity and cleanliness, and the label's accuracy. If you are concerned about potential side effects or contraindications, you will probably need to contact the manufacturer or distributor.

Choose Quality

In 2010, the FDA finalized guidelines for current good manufacturing practices by supplement manufacturers.[a] Additionally, you should also use tip-offs to judge a quality company—the kind you would expect to have good quality control procedures and to manufacture, store, and transport products safely and carefully.

A quality company will not promise miracles on its website, in catalogues, in commercials or advertisements, or in in-store promotions. A quality company will not manipulate statistics or distort research findings in an attempt to mislead you. And a quality company will take care with its labels, print materials, and Web information.

Confirm Supplement Ingredients

Use resources that analyze and confirm supplement content, dose, and purity. Consumer-Lab.com is one such service. Pharmaceutical researchers also report findings on supplement label accuracy; a search on PubMed can lead you to this information.

Look for the U.S. Pharmacopeia (USP) logo (USP verification mark) on supplement labels. The mark certifies that the USP has found the ingredients consistent with those stated on the label; that the supplement has been manufactured in a safe, sanitary, controlled facility; and that the product dissolves or disintegrates to release nutrients in the body. However, the USP does not test the supplement's efficacy.

Choose Freshness

Finding the freshest supplement is often easier if you shop in a retail store. Choose a store where turnover is likely to be quick, and check expiration dates. Supplements should be displayed away from direct sunlight, bright lights, or nearby heat sources, because heat ages many supplements.

Expect Accountability

How easily can you obtain information about the product? Look for a phone number on the label so you can call with questions or to report side effects. On websites, look for a domestic address and phone number, in addition to an email contact. Does a knowledgeable company representative respond to your questions, or is the only person available one who reads a scripted response?

If you're shopping online but are uncertain whether the supplement is right for you, check the Web retailer's return policy. A Web retailer that also has a brick-and-mortar outlet near your locale may be preferable.

a Data from Food and Drug Administration. Guidance for industry: current good manufacturing practice in manufacturing, packaging, labeling, or holding operations for dietary supplements; small entity compliance guide. December 2010. http://www.fda.gov/Food/GuidanceRegulation/GuidanceDocumentsRegulatoryInformation/DietarySupplements/ucm238182.htm . Accessed March 29, 2017.

Be a Safe and Informed Consumer

When buying supplements, follow this advice from the Food and Drug Administration:

- Let your healthcare professional advise you on sorting reliable information from questionable information.
- Contact the manufacturer for information about the product you intend to use.
- Be aware that some supplement ingredients, including nutrients and plant components, can be toxic. Also, some ingredients and products can be harmful when consumed in high amounts, when taken for a long time, or when used in combination with certain other drugs, substances, or foods.
- Do not self-diagnose any health condition. Work with healthcare professionals to determine how best to achieve optimal health.
- Do not substitute a dietary supplement for a prescription medicine or therapy, or for the variety of foods important to a healthful diet.
- Do not assume that the term *natural* in relation to a product ensures that the product is wholesome or safe.
- Be wary of hype and headlines. Sound health advice is generally based on research over time, not a single study.
- Learn to spot false claims. If something sounds too good to be true, it probably is.
- Subscribe by email to the FDA's rapid public notification feed to quickly receive warnings about tainted products.

Food and Drug Administration. FDA 101: Dietary supplements. Updated July 15, 2015. http://www.fda.gov/ForConsumers/ConsumerUpdates/ucm050803.htm. Accessed March 30, 2017; Food and Drug Administration. FDA Tainted Products Marketed as Dietary Supplements. Page updated 3/17/2017. https://www.fda.gov/ForConsumers/ConsumerUpdates/ucm236774.htm Accessed March 30, 2017.

manufacturers work hard to ensure the quality of their products, yet some supplements on the market are nothing more than a mixture of ineffective ingredients. The Internet and social media network marketing are changing the industry because they are a prominent vehicle for promoting and selling products, reaching millions of people worldwide instantly at any time.

In recent years, the FDA has found hundreds of fraudulent products that contain hidden or deceptively labeled ingredients.[32] Most frequently recalled products with potentially harmful ingredients are those that are promoted for weight loss, sexual enhancement, and bodybuilding. When considering the use of dietary supplements, do your homework—make sure the product is safe and effective. It's always a good idea to ask your healthcare professional for help in distinguishing between reliable and questionable information.

Key Concepts When considering a dietary supplement, it is important to consider the product and its claims carefully. Be aware that some products may promise more than they can deliver. A good indicator of quality is the USP verification mark, but this does not guarantee that a product will fulfill its claims.

Functional Foods

🍎 **Why Is This Important?**   What if you could choose between two seemingly equivalent foods or beverages after discovering that one may benefit your health whereas the other may not. Indeed, many such choices exist. Read on to find out what properties boost foods to provide more than just nourishment.

What do garlic, tomato sauce, tofu, and oatmeal all have in common? They aren't in the same food group, nor do they have the same nutrient composition. Instead, all of these foods could be considered "functional foods." Although there is not yet a legal definition for the term, a **functional food** is widely considered to be a food or food component that provides a health benefit beyond basic nutrition.[33] Garlic contains sulfur compounds that may reduce heart disease risk, and tomato sauce is rich in **lycopene**, a compound that may reduce prostate cancer risk. The soy protein in tofu and the fiber in oatmeal can help reduce the risk of heart disease. (See **FIGURE SF.11**.)

THINK About It

3

The functional food industry has grown rapidly since its birth in Japan in the late 1980s; in 2014, it reached almost $177 billion in sales worldwide. In the United States, functional food and beverage sales account for 5 percent of the overall food market.[34]

Phytochemicals Make Foods Functional

Many functional foods get their health-promoting properties from naturally occurring compounds in plants that are not considered nutrients, which you recall are called **phytochemicals**. Although the word *phytochemical* may sound intimidating, its meaning is simple: "plant chemical." A vitamin is a food substance essential for life. Phytochemicals, in contrast, are substances in plants that may affect health, even though they are not essential for life.

Phytochemicals are complex chemicals that vary from plant to plant. They include pigments, antioxidants, and thousands of other

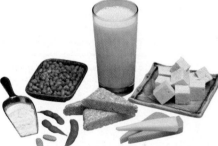

FIGURE SF.11 Soy is rich in phytochemicals. Soybeans contain phytochemicals called isoflavones. High intake of soy products such as tofu is linked to a lower incidence of heart disease and cancer.

© Photodisc.

▶ **functional food** A food that may provide a health benefit beyond basic nutrition.

▶ **lycopene** One of a family of plant chemicals, the carotenoids. Others in this big family include alpha-carotene and beta-carotene.

▶ **phytochemicals** Substances in plants that may possess health-protective effects, even though they are not essential for life.

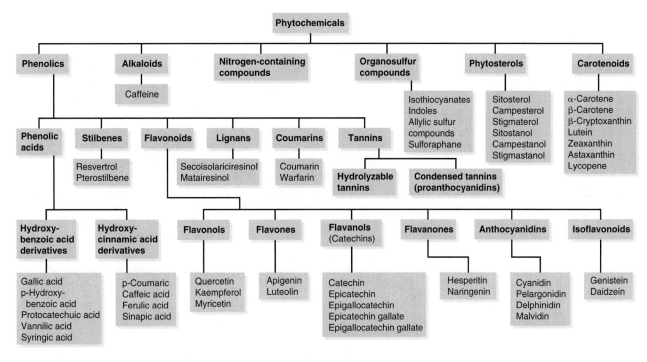

FIGURE SF.12 **The classifications of the most well-known dietary phytochemicals that affect human health.**

Reproduced from *Adv Nutr.* May 2013; 4(3): 384S–392S. Published online May 6, 2013. Copyright © 2013 American Society for Nutrition.

compounds, many of which have been associated with protection from heart disease, vision loss, hypertension, cancer, and diabetes. The flow chart in **FIGURE SF.12** shows the classifications of the most well-known dietary phytochemicals that affect human health. **TABLE SF.4** lists many examples of phytochemicals and their potential benefits.

Plants contain phytochemicals in abundance because these substances are of benefit to the plant itself. For example, an orange has at least 170 distinct phytochemicals. Individually and together, these compounds help plants resist the attacks of bacteria and fungi, the ravages of free radicals, and high levels of ultraviolet light from the sun. When we eat these plants, the phytochemicals end up in our tissues and provide many of the same protections that benefit plants.

Phytochemicals are part of the reason why the *Dietary Guidelines for Americans* recommends that we eat a variety of fruits and vegetables each day, especially dark-green, red, and orange vegetables and beans and peas.[35] The emphasis also can literally be seen in the MyPlate food plan, which encourages you to make half your plate fruits and vegetables.[36] Fruits and vegetables are naturally low in fat and calories and tend to be rich in fiber, potassium, and vitamins. In addition, studies consistently show that people who consume more fruits and vegetables tend to have lower rates of common chronic diseases.

Benefits of Phytochemicals

What are some of the specific benefits of phytochemicals? People who eat tomatoes and processed tomato products take in lycopene, which is associated with a decreased risk of chronic diseases, such as cancer and cardiovascular diseases.[37] Scientists believe that the high

Quick Bite

Functional Food Decisions

Are you a health-conscious consumer who seeks out functional foods? More than half of consumers "strongly agree" that functional foods offer health benefits. The top functional foods named by consumers included fruits and vegetables, fish and seafood, dairy, meat and poultry, herbs/spices, fiber, tea/green tea, nuts, whole grains, water, cereal, and oat products. The top three food components people look for when choosing foods and beverages for themselves and their children are fiber, whole grains, and protein.

TABLE SF.4
Examples of Functional Components in Foods

Class/Components	Sources[a]	Potential Benefits	Tips for Including Healthful Components in the Diet
Carotenoids			
Beta-carotene	Carrots, pumpkin, sweet potato, cantaloupe	Neutralizes free radicals that may damage cells; bolsters cellular antioxidant defenses; can be made into vitamin A in the body	For beta-carotene–rich french fries, try sweet potatoes coated lightly with olive oil or fat-free cooking spray, and add spices to taste (e.g., pepper, rosemary, thyme).
Lutein, zeaxanthin	Kale, collards, spinach, corn, eggs, citrus	May contribute to maintenance of healthy vision	For a simple way to enjoy kale, purchase a prewashed and destemmed ready-to-eat bag. Toss lightly with olive or peanut oil and salt, and then roast for 10–12 minutes at 425 degrees.
Lycopene	Tomatoes and processed tomato products, watermelon, red/pink grapefruit	May contribute to maintenance of prostate health	Try adding 1 cup tomato sauce to sautéed zucchini for a colorful side dish.
Dietary (Functional and Total) Fiber			
Insoluble fiber	Wheat bran, corn bran, fruit skins	May contribute to maintenance of a healthy digestive tract; may reduce the risk of some types of cancer	Try adding a little dry wheat bran when making smoothies or muffins to bulk up the fiber content; this may help keep you full longer.
Beta-glucan[b]	Oat bran, oatmeal, oat flour, barley, rye	May reduce risk of coronary heart disease (CHD)	Instant oatmeal packets are easily stored in your backpack or desk drawer to have on hand when you missed breakfast or need a hearty afternoon snack.
Soluble fiber[b]	Psyllium seed husk, peas, beans, apples, citrus fruit	May reduce risk of CHD and some types of cancer	Try adding canned beans (black, pinto, or garbanzo) to a quesadilla or an omelet, or enjoy them cold in a mixed green salad.
Whole grains[b]	Cereal grains, whole wheat bread, oatmeal, brown rice	May reduce risk of CHD and some types of cancer; may contribute to maintenance of healthy blood glucose levels	Did you know that air-popped popcorn is a great low-fat source of whole grains? Try spicing up your popcorn with garlic powder and cinnamon or rosemary and parmesan cheese.
Fatty Acids			
Monounsaturated fatty acids (MUFAs)[b]	Tree nuts, olive oil, canola oil	May reduce risk of CHD	For a quick and healthy on-the-go snack with heart-healthy fats make snack bags of mixed nuts (e.g., almonds, pecans). Throw in some dried fruit for an antioxidant boost.
Polyunsaturated fatty acids (PUFAs): omega-3 fatty acids, alpha-linolenic acid (ALA)	Walnuts, flax	May contribute to maintenance of heart health; may contribute to maintenance of mental and visual function	When cooking, try substituting a tablespoon of flaxseed oil in a recipe that calls for canola or olive oil, once or twice a week. Add ground flax to baked products, smoothies, yogurt, and hot cereal.
PUFAs: omega-3 fatty acids, docosahexaenoic acid (DHA)/ eicosapentaenoic acid (EPA)[b]	Salmon, tuna, and other fish oils	May reduce risk of CHD; may contribute to maintenance of mental and visual function	Salmon or tuna that is canned in water or in a shelf-stable pouch can make easy and affordable meals.
Conjugated linoleic acid (CLA)	Beef and lamb; some cheese	May contribute to maintenance of desirable body composition and healthy immune function	Try something fun at your next cookout by preparing kebabs for the grill by alternating beef and vegetables.

TABLE SF.4 *(continued)*
Examples of Functional Components in Foods

Class/Components	Sources[a]	Potential Benefits	Tips for Including Healthful Components in the Diet
Flavonoids			
Anthocyanins: cyanidin, delphinidin, malvidin	Berries, cherries, red grapes	Bolster cellular antioxidant defenses; may contribute to maintenance of brain function	For a cold treat, try frozen berries. They are also tasty additions to any yogurt and can help to cool and flavor your oatmeal in the morning.
Flavanols: catechins, epicatechins, epigallocatechin, procyanidins	Tea, cocoa, chocolate, apples, grapes	May contribute to maintenance of heart health	Go ahead and indulge in an occasional piece of chocolate.
Flavanones: hesperetin, naringenin	Citrus fruits	Neutralize free radicals, which may damage cells; bolster cellular antioxidant defenses	Squeeze half an orange and half a lemon into a small dish; add olive or flax oil and dashes of salt, pepper, and basil for a perfectly refreshing salad dressing.
Flavonols: quercetin, kaempferol, isorhamnetin, myricetin	Onions, apples, tea, broccoli	Neutralize free radicals, which may damage cells; bolster cellular antioxidant defenses	Caramelized onions make a sweet and tasty garnish to many main dishes. Sautee onions over low heat in oil until a deep gold color; add on top of prepared steak, chicken, fish, or whole grain.
Proanthocyanidins	Cranberries, cocoa, apples, strawberries, grapes, wine, peanuts, cinnamon	May contribute to maintenance of urinary tract health and heart health	Grab an apple or a bunch of grapes for a snack—what could be easier than that?
Isothiocyanates			
Sulforaphane	Cauliflower, broccoli, broccoli sprouts, cabbage, kale, horseradish	May enhance detoxification of undesirable compounds; bolsters cellular antioxidant defenses	Keep frozen broccoli and cauliflower on hand for an easy dinner side dish.
Phenolic Acids			
Caffeic acid, ferulic acid	Apples, pears, citrus fruits, some vegetables, coffee	May bolster cellular antioxidant defenses; may contribute to maintenance of healthy vision and heart health	Love your morning coffee? Good news—coffee is a powerful source of antioxidants.
Plant Stanols/Sterols			
Free stanols/sterols[b]	Corn, soy, wheat, wood oils, fortified foods and beverages	May reduce risk of CHD	Get your free stanols/sterols from fortified foods such as bread containing whole-wheat flour, low-fat yogurt, and some cereals.
Stanol/sterol esters[b]	Stanol ester dietary supplements, fortified foods and beverages, including table spreads	May reduce risk of CHD	Many table spreads (butter or margarine alternatives) are now fortified with stanol and/or sterol esters. Check labels for other commercial products now commonly fortified with stanols and sterols including orange juices, yogurt beverages, chocolate, and granola bars.
Polyols			
Sugar alcohols[b]: xylitol, sorbitol, mannitol, lactitol	Some chewing gums and diet candies	May reduce risk of dental caries	Reduce your risk for dental caries and curb your appetite by chewing gum containing xylitol after eating.
Prebiotics			
Inulin, fructo-oligosaccharides (FOS), polydextrose	Whole grains, onions, some fruits, garlic, honey, leeks, fortified foods and beverages	May improve gastrointestinal health; may improve calcium absorption	You can get prebiotics by simply adding honey to some of your routine meals. Try honey in your oatmeal or yogurt, or use in place of sugar as a sweetener.

(continues)

TABLE SF.4 *(continued)*

Examples of Functional Components in Foods

Class/Components	Sources[a]	Potential Benefits	Tips for Including Healthful Components in the Diet
Probiotics			
Yeast, *Lactobacilli*, *Bifidobacteria*, and other specific strains of beneficial bacteria	Certain yogurts and other cultured dairy and nondairy products	May improve gastrointestinal health and systemic immunity; benefits are strain-specific	For an easy way to add probiotics into your diet, choose from a variety of flavored yogurts with probiotics.
Phytoestrogens			
Isoflavones: daidzein, genistein	Soybeans and soy-based foods	May contribute to maintenance of bone health, healthy brain, and immune function; for women, may contribute to maintenance of menopausal health	Get your isoflavones by getting soft, silken tofu and adding it to the cheese sauce mixture used to make lasagna.
Lignans	Flax, rye, some vegetables	May contribute to maintenance of heart health and healthy immune function	Add ground flaxseeds to a smoothie or a recipe for baked goods to pack a lignan punch!
Soy Protein			
Soy protein	Soybeans and soy-based foods	May reduce risk of CHD	Soybeans are also called edamame. Look for edamame in the frozen section to easily prepare as a healthy snack or party sampler. Edamame that has been cooked and removed from the pod adds great flavor and extra protein to any salad.
Sulfides/Thiols			
Diallyl disulfide, allyl methyl trisulfide	Garlic, onions, leeks, scallions	May enhance detoxification of undesirable compounds; may contribute to maintenance of heart health and healthy immune function	Scallions, or green onions, are milder than traditional onions and are commonly added at the last minute to salads or cooked sauces as a garnish. Leeks can also be an easy substitute, but are more commonly used in soups.
Dithiolethiones	Cruciferous vegetables, varieties of cabbage, bok choy, Brussels sprouts, kale	May enhance detoxification of undesirable compounds; may contribute to maintenance of healthy immune function	Use cabbage to make a variety of slaws and add to fresh salads. Bok choy is great in any stir-fry or raw in a salad with Asian dressing.

[a] Examples are not an all-inclusive list.

[b] FDA-approved health claim established for component.

Modified from the International Food Information Council Foundation. Functional foods. July 2011. http://www.foodinsight.org/Content/3842/Final%20Functional%20Foods%20Backgrounder.pdf. Accessed December 20, 2015.

consumption of soy products in Asian countries contributes to lower rates of colon, prostate, uterine and breast cancers.[38] Depending on the source of the isoflavones, the kind of cancer, and the study population, the outcomes of these studies are occasionally conflicting.[39] The foods and herbs with the highest anticancer activity include garlic, soybeans, cabbage, ginger, and licorice as well as the family of vegetables that includes celery, carrots, and parsley. The benefits of phytochemicals seem to be as varied as the phytochemicals themselves, with ongoing and exciting health-promoting perks being discovered by nutrition scientists even today.

How do phytochemicals work to prevent chronic disease? A number of phytochemicals, including those from soybeans and from the cabbage family, are able to modify estrogen metabolism or block the effect of estrogen on cell growth. Such compounds are known as **phytoestrogens**. Other phytochemicals neutralize **free radicals**. Free radicals (active oxidants) are continually produced in our cells and over time can result in damage to DNA and important cell structures. Eventually, this damage can promote both cancer and cell aging. Many different plant chemicals, such as the pigments in grapes and red wine (see **FIGURE SF.13**), are able to neutralize or reduce concentrations of free radicals, thus protecting us against the development of both cancer and heart disease. Phytochemicals in fruits and vegetables have a number of other potential benefits. Lutein and zeaxanthin are carotenoids (plant pigments) found in dark-green leafy vegetables, corn, and egg yolks. Increased consumption of these compounds is associated with a lower incidence and slower progression of age-related macular degeneration, the leading cause of blindness in older people.[40,41]

Adding Phytochemicals to Your Diet

After learning about all the powerful health-protecting effects of phytochemicals, you are likely wondering how you can simply and quickly change your own food choices to include more. Before you reach for your next slice of bread, it is worth remembering that refined wheat, the source of white flour, has lost more than 99 percent of its phytochemical content. Because phytochemicals are so beneficial, why can't we just purify the important ones and add them to our diet as supplements, the way we put vitamins back into white flour after processing? The short answer is that we don't know enough about how phytochemicals function. There are numerous known and still unidentified bioactive compounds in foods, such as phytochemicals, that have potential health benefits; however, the precise role, requirement, interactions, and toxicity levels of many of these substances remain unclear. Furthermore, whole foods might contain additional nutritional substances that have not yet been elucidated, and their health benefits might not be maintained when components are isolated and consumed as supplements or fortification ingredients.[42] Thus, appropriate food choices, rather than supplements, should be the foundation for achieving nutritional adequacy. Table SF.4 has some practical suggestions that require minimal effort.

Many phytochemicals appear to act synergistically, both fighting free radicals and blocking the negative effects of hormones. Yet there is no doubt that consumption of plant foods containing multiple antioxidants is strongly associated with health benefits. The weight of evidence and experience strongly favors finding a place for more fruits and vegetables in the diet. (See **FIGURE SF.14**.) The MyPlate graphic and the Fruits & Veggies—More Matters logo both encourage fruit and vegetable consumption. In addition, MyPlate's advice to "Make at least half your grains whole grains" helps promote intake of disease-fighting phytochemicals naturally found in whole grains. Changing your diet to include more functional foods and fewer empty calories needn't be painful. Sometimes you can have

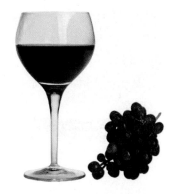

FIGURE SF.13 Grapes, red wine, and heart disease. Grapes and red wine contain phytochemicals that appear to reduce the risk of heart disease. Studies show that moderate consumption of alcohol independently reduces heart disease risk.
© Photodisc.

▶ **phytoestrogens** Compounds that have weak estrogen activity in the body.

▶ **free radicals** Short-lived, highly reactive chemicals often derived from oxygen-containing compounds, which can have detrimental effects on cells, especially DNA and cell membranes.

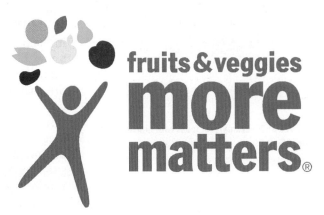

FIGURE SF.14 The National Fruit and Vegetable Program. This program encourages Americans to increase their consumption of fruits and vegetables for better health. It is a public–private partnership, consisting of government agencies, nonprofit groups, and industry. For more information, visit www .fruitsandveggiesmorematters.org.
Courtesy of FruitsandVeggiesMatter.gov.

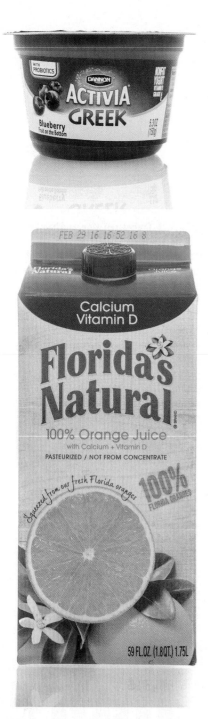

FIGURE SF.15 Examples of foods with functional ingredients.
© Keith Homan/Shutterstock, Inc.

your pizza and eat it, too. Next time, ask for your pizza loaded with vegetables. Whole-wheat crust would be a plus. The combination of lycopene from tomato sauce, quercetin from onions, and carotenoids and glucarates from colored peppers can turn your pizza into a phyto-chemical cornucopia.

Foods Enhanced with Functional Ingredients and Additives

Phytochemicals are not the only substances that make foods functional. Another type of functional food is one that gets its health-promoting properties from what has been added during processing. Calcium-fortified orange juice, breakfast cereals fortified with folic acid, yogurt with live active cultures, and margarines with added plant sterol and plant stanol esters are examples. (See **FIGURE SF.15**.) Health properties come from added nutrients, bacteria, fiber, or other substances. Some are foods and beverages that contain added herbal compounds, such as those sold in pill form as dietary supplements. The result is a wide variety of products making an often confusing array of label statements and health claims. There are instances where functional foods do not deliver the health benefit they claim; consumers should be skeptical of products that sound too good to be true.

Using additives to create functional foods raises questions of how much should be used and how much is safe. In addition, although there are guidelines for the use of vitamins and minerals in the fortification of food and for the use of approved food additives, not much is known about what happens to many novel ingredients, such as botanical extracts, when they are put into a food. Prebiotics and probiotics added to yogurt, for example, are common examples of additives in functional foods with intended health benefits.

Regulatory Issues for Functional Foods

Food labeling is required for most prepared foods, such as breads, cereals, canned and frozen foods, snacks, desserts, drinks, and so on. Nutrition labeling for raw produce such as fruits and vegetables and fish is voluntary. The FDA refers to these products as *conventional* foods. The terms *functional foods* and *nutraceuticals* are widely used in the marketplace and media. Such foods are regulated by the FDA under the authority of the Federal Food, Drug, and Cosmetic Act, even though they are not specifically defined by law.[43] Although this may sound a little confusing, a *food* is a product that we eat or drink as well as all the components of that product. This definition distinguishes a food from a *drug*, which is a substance intended to diagnose, cure, mitigate, treat, or prevent disease. Foods also are distinct from *dietary supplements*, which are products intended to supplement the diet but that do not represent themselves as a conventional food, meal, or diet.

Although some manufacturers have tried to market functional products as dietary supplements rather than foods to take advantage of broader allowances for label claims, the FDA's position is that products that are conventional foods and beverages are subject to the regulations for food and not for dietary supplements. A substance added to a food for health benefits must still conform to

FDA regulations for food. Any food containing an unapproved food additive is considered adulterated and cannot legally be marketed in the United States.

> **Key Concepts** Functional foods provide health benefits beyond basic nutrition. Phytochemicals are "plant chemicals" that include thousands of compounds, pigments, and natural antioxidants, many of which are associated with protection from heart disease, hypertension, cancer, and diabetes. Just like conventional foods, functional foods are subject to FDA regulations for claims and safety.

Health Claims for Functional Foods

As consumer choices continue to expand and the abundance of functional foods and supplements increases, products that make exaggerated health claims will continue to mislead consumers about their benefits. Although many foods and products have legitimate functional benefits, many people put their money and hopes for good health into unneeded functional foods and supplement products that make misleading health claims with little or no scientific evidence of effectiveness.[44] To avoid wasting money on unnecessary products, be an informed consumer (see the FYI feature "Shopping for Supplements").

When a functional food meets the appropriate FDA guidelines, it may make a nutrient content claim or health claim on the label.[45] For example, tofu containing at least 6.25 grams of soy protein per serving may make a health claim about the role of soy protein in reducing the risk of heart disease. Oatmeal with an adequate amount of beta-glucan fiber can highlight its benefit in reducing the risk of heart disease. Another health claim applies to a functional food created through the addition of plant sterol or plant stanol esters to a vegetable-oil–based spread. The Benecol and Take Control product lines (spreads and salad dressings) contain these plant esters, which have been shown to reduce cholesterol levels when consumed daily in adequate amounts. (See **FIGURE SF.16**.)

Structure/Function Claims for Functional Foods

Structure/function claims on conventional or functional foods must be based on the food's nutritive value. An example is orange juice with added vitamin C, vitamin E, and zinc to "support your natural defenses." However, structure/function claims are not as stringently regulated by the FDA as health claims. So, at present, many manufacturers are making claims about non-nutrients in foods and their effects on body structure or function. For example, a cereal with added St. John's wort and kava extract is "accented with herbs to support emotional and mental balance," and a bottled tea is "infused with memory-enhancing ginkgo biloba and Panax ginseng." Consumers should beware; many companies continue to deliberately confuse consumers by exaggerating the health effects or ingredients of their products, despite the FDA sending warning letters to food manufacturers about misleading labeling.[46]

THINK About It 4

> **Key Concepts** Under FDA guidelines, a functional food's label may have a nutrient content claim, health claim, or structure/function claim. A structure/function claim promotes a substance's effect on the structure or function of the body. For foods, the claimed effect must be based on the food's "nutritive value." Currently, many manufacturers make structure/function claims about nonnutrients in foods.

Quick Bite
Early Food Laws
In 1202, King John of England proclaimed the first English food law, the Assize of Bread, which prohibited adulteration of bread with such ingredients as ground peas or beans.

Quick Bite
Old Concept, New Frontier
Functional foods are a new frontier of nutrition and food science, but the idea has been around for centuries. Hippocrates, the father of modern medicine, proclaimed, "Let food be your medicine, and medicine be your food."

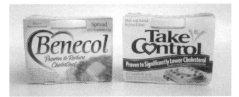

FIGURE SF.16 Some functional foods can make health claims. Manufacturers have obtained approval from the FDA to make health claims for these margarine products.

Quick Bite

Mayonnaise Protects Against Strokes

Is this claim science or snake oil? Studies show that foods rich in vitamin E help protect against heart disease and stroke. In one study of stroke reduction in postmenopausal women, mayonnaise was the most concentrated food source of vitamin E. But to claim that mayonnaise prevents strokes is unwarranted and overstates the evidence.

Strategies for Functional Food Use

So, should you run out and fill your shopping cart with functional foods? Which ones would you buy? The best course of action is to stick with what scientists have agreed upon so far. First, fruits and vegetables promote health and reduce disease risk through a whole host of natural phytochemicals. Use the list of foods and phytochemicals in Table SF.4 to enhance your shopping list with nature's functional foods. Second, consider nutrient-fortified products when a particular nutrient is lacking in your diet and you either don't like or can't eat good food sources of that nutrient. For example, if you are allergic to milk and dairy products, consider calcium-fortified orange juice as a nutritious way to get the calcium you need. Third, *read, read, read* about functional foods, and be skeptical when you evaluate what's on the Internet. **FIGURE SF.17** lists some questions to ask when assessing the credibility of websites. For more tips on how to evaluate health information on the Internet, visit the Office of Dietary Supplements website.[47] Do your homework by looking at scientific articles—your instructor can help you find and interpret studies of functional food components. Finally, be critical of advertising and hype that sound too good to be true.

Questions to Ask to Assess the Credibility of Websites

Checking Out a Health Website: Five Quick Questions
Many online health resources are useful, but others may present information that is inaccurate or misleading, so it's important to find sources you can trust and to know how to evaluate their content.

If you're visiting a health website for the first time, these five quick questions can help you decide whether the site is a helpful resource.
Who? Who runs the website? Can you trust them?
What? What does the site say? Do its claims seem too good to be true?
When? When was the information posted or reviewed? Is it up-to-date?
Where? Where did the information come from? Is it based on scientific research?
Why? Why does the site exist? Is it selling something?

FIGURE SF.17 Establishing credibility. Here are some quick questions to ask when determining the credibility of a complementary health website.

NIH National Center for Complementary and Integrative Health. Finding and evaluating online resources on complementary health approaches. https://nccih.nih.gov/health/webresources#ask. Accessed March 30, 2017.

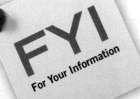

Defining Complementary and Integrative Health: How Does Nutrition Fit?

Alternative approaches to health care are therapies and treatments outside the medical mainstream. Historically, they tended to be based mainly or solely on observation or anecdotal evidence rather than controlled research. According to the NCCIH, "Large population-based surveys have found that the use of alternative medicine—unproven practices used in place of conventional medicine—is rare. Integrative health care, defined as a comprehensive, often interdisciplinary approach to treatment, prevention and health promotion that brings together complementary and conventional therapies, is more common."[a]

The term *alternative* suggests practices that replace conventional ones. *Complementary* implies practices that are used *in addition to* conventional ones. A practice that combines both conventional and complementary treatments for which there is evidence of safety and effectiveness is referred to as *integrative*. For example, using only herbs and megavitamins to treat AIDS would be alternative, whereas using herbs to combat diarrhea caused by conventional AIDS medications and taking supplements to replace lost vitamins would be complementary or integrative. Complementary and integrative health care includes a broad range of healing therapies and philosophies. Several among them involve nutrition, including special diet therapies, phytotherapy (herbalism), orthomolecular medicine, and other biologic interventions. The use of an integrative approach to health and wellness has grown within care settings across the United States, including hospitals, hospices, and military health facilities.

More than 30 percent of adults and about 12 percent of children in the United States use some form of complementary therapy.[b] Commonly used complementary therapies include a variety of natural products and diet-based therapies, as well as mind–body practices such as deep breathing exercises, prayer, and relaxation techniques such as guided imagery, meditation, spinal manipulation (chiropractic care), Tai chi and yoga, acupuncture, massage therapy, and movement therapies. People seek out complementary therapies for numerous reasons, including fear of aging, personal beliefs, and distrust of institutional medicine.

Where Does Nutrition Fit?

A number of alternative therapies involve nutrition, and sometimes the line between standard and alternative nutrition is not clear. A variety of health conditions, such as diabetes, gastrointestinal disorders, and kidney disease, require special diets. Alternative nutrition practices include diets to prevent and treat diseases not shown to be diet-related. (See **FIGURE 1.**) What often makes these practices "alternative" is the limited nature of the diet, the lack of rigorous scientific evidence showing effectiveness, and the divergence from science-based healthy

eating patterns such as the Mediterranean diet, DASH diet, or MyPlate. Other practices outside the nutritional mainstream have gained recent popularity, such as reliance on only raw foods and the extensive use of herbal and botanical supplements as well as megadoses of vitamin/mineral supplements, which we have already discussed. Most nutritionists consider vegetarianism a routine variation of a normal diet, particularly if the vegetarian's motivation is religious or philosophical, the result of a concern for animals, or an aversion to animal products. When a meat eater goes vegetarian in an attempt to prevent or cure disease, that's alternative.

Food Restrictions and Food Prescriptions

Societies throughout the world commonly use dietary changes to treat or prevent illness. The specifics vary from place to place, however, which suggests that they are based on cultural factors rather than science.

In recent years, we have seen yeast-free diets, dairy-free diets, sugar-free diets, white-flour–free diets, cleansing diets, raw food diets, both low-carbohydrate and high-carbohydrate diets, both low-red-meat and high-red-meat diets, caffeine-free diets, salicylate-free diets, and more. People with subjective symptoms such as headaches, fatigue, or back pain have been instructed to avoid irrational lists of

"allergenic foods" based on "blood screening." We've also seen illogical instructions on how to combine foods or what foods not to combine. For weight loss, we've had grapefruit diets, hard-boiled-egg diets, cottage-cheese diets, water diets, high-fat diets, low-fat diets, and blue-foods–only diets; the list goes on and on.

Many types of diets can be described as alternative. Their origins and claims vary, and their proponents often cannot show that they improve health; some alternative diets can actually be harmful by restricting foods and thereby lowering the body's intake of necessary nutrients. Such fad diets come and go. Most often they are not based on science and eventually fail to interest people when they don't work. Those few that prove effective and have a scientific basis become *integrated* into conventional nutrition and diet therapy. (See **FIGURE 2.**)

a   National Institutes of Health, National Center for Complementary and Integrative Health. NIH complementary and integrative health agency gets new name. https://nccih.nih.gov/news/press/12172014. Accessed March 30, 2017.

b   National Institutes of Health, National Center for Complementary and Integrative Health. Complementary, alternative, or integrative health: what's in a name? https://nccih.nih.gov/health/integrative-health. Accessed August 30, 2017.

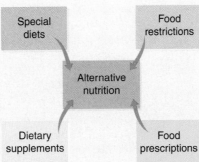

FIGURE 1 Alternative nutrition practices. Although many mainstream medical practices may involve special dietary regimens, alternative nutrition practices often are overly restrictive, depart from established dietary guidelines, and lack rigorous scientific evidence.

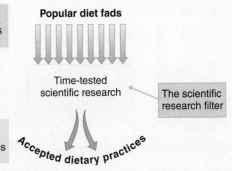

FIGURE 2 Many apply but few are chosen. Dietary practices with a scientific basis and proven efficacy are incorporated into conventional nutrition and diet therapy.

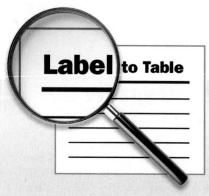

Label to Table

If you picked up a multivitamin/mineral container from your drugstore shelf, would you know how to read the label? Look at this Supplement Facts panel from a basic multivitamin/mineral supplement. Here are some questions that you might have:

1. If you were a 20-year-old woman who knew she wasn't consuming enough calcium, would this supplement allow you to get your recommended intake?

2. If 25 percent of the vitamin A in this supplement comes from beta-carotene, where does the rest come from?
3. What trend do you see in the amounts of B vitamins?
4. What trend do you see in the amounts of bone minerals?
5. What trend do you see in the amounts of antioxidant vitamins?

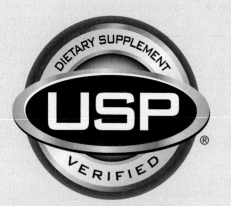

Registered trademark of The United States Pharmacopeial Convention. Used with permission.

Supplement Facts
Daily multivitamin/mineral dietary supplement

USP USP has tested and verified ingredients, potency, and manufacturing process. USP sets official standards for Dietary Supplements. For more information, go to www.uspverified.org.

Serving Size 1 tablet

Each tablet contains	%DV	Each tablet contains	
Vitamin A 10,000 I.U.	200%	Iodine 150 mcg	100%
25% as beta-carotene		Magnesium 100 mg	25%
Vitamin C 120 mg	200%	Zinc 22.5 mg	150%
Vitamin D 400 IU	100%	Selenium 45 mcg	64%
Vitamin E 60 IU	200%	Copper 3 mg	150%
Vitamin K 25 mcg	31%	Manganese 2.5 mg	125%
Thiamine (vit. B_1) 1.5 mg	100%	Chromium 100 mcg	83%
Riboflavin (vit. B_2) 1.7 mg	100%	Molybdenum 25 mcg	33%
Niacin 20 mg	100%	Chloride 36.3 mg	1%
Vitamin B_6 2 mg	100%	Sodium less than 5 mg	less than 1%
Folate (folic acid) 400 mcg	100%	Potassium 40 mg	1%
Vitamin B_{12} 6 mcg	100%	Nickel 5 mcg	*
Biotin 30 mcg	10%	Tin 10 mg	*
Pantothenic acid 10 mg	100%	Silicon 2 mg	*
Calcium 162 mg	16%	Vanadium 10 mcg	*
Iron 9 mg	50%	Boron 150 mcg	*
Phosphorus 109 mg	11%		

* Daily Value (%DV) not established

Learning Portfolio

Key Terms

	page
bioavailability	308
bioflavonoids	304
complementary and integrative health care	293
Dietary Supplement Health and Education Act (DSHEA)	305
dietary supplements	293
free radicals	315
functional food	310
herbal therapy (phytotherapy)	302
isoflavones	293
lycopene	310
malabsorption syndromes	300
megadoses	294
National Center for Complementary and Integrative Health (NCCIH)	302
National Institutes of Health (NIH)	302
nucleic acids	304
orthomolecular medicine	300
phytochemicals	310
phytoestrogens	315
Supplement Facts panel	306
U.S. Pharmacopeia (USP)	308

Study Points

- Dietary supplements encompass vitamins, minerals, herbal products, amino acids, glandular extracts, enzymes, and many other products.
- Vitamin and mineral supplements may be warranted in certain circumstances, although the preferred mode of obtaining adequate nutrition is through foods.
- Megadose vitamin or mineral therapy has not been proved effective in the treatment of cancer, colds, or heart disease. Moreover, such megadoses act more like drugs than nutrients in the body and should be approached with caution.
- Herbal medicine is a traditional form of healing in many cultures. Some herbal medicines have shown enough promise to warrant large-scale clinical studies involving supplements. However, herbal products can have side effects and can interfere with prescription medications.

- Dietary supplements are regulated according to the provisions of the Dietary Supplement Health and Education Act of 1994 (DSHEA). Unlike drugs and additives, dietary supplements do not need premarket approval.
- Claims for dietary supplements can include health claims, structure/function claims, and nutrient content claims.
- Dietary supplements must have a Supplement Facts panel on the label.
- Consumers should carefully evaluate claims and evidence for dietary supplements and consult their physician before taking a supplement.
- A functional food is considered to be a food that may provide a health benefit beyond basic nutrition.
- Phytochemicals are plant chemicals responsible for the health-promoting properties of many functional foods.
- Consumption of plant foods containing multiple antioxidants is strongly associated with health benefits. Scientific evidence strongly supports eating at least five servings of fruits and vegetables daily and emphasizing whole grains.
- Complementary and integrative health care comprises practices outside the medical mainstream that are becoming increasingly popular and that include a broad range of therapies, many of which include nutrition. People seek complementary and integrative health care for a variety of reasons, including environmental concerns and a fear of aging.

Study Questions

1. How do you know a product is a dietary supplement?
2. If a dietary supplement product label contains the words "High in vitamin E," what type of claim is it making? What other claims can a supplement make?
3. What things should someone do before purchasing supplements?
4. What are phytochemicals, and how do they benefit plants and humans?
5. Name three conditions that consuming functional foods may help prevent.

Learning Portfolio (continued)

6. What are some of the possible complications involved in using herbal medicines?

7. What role does nutrition have in complementary and integrative health care?

Try This

Finding Functional Beverages

This exercise will familiarize you with the many beverages that contain functional ingredients now available to consumers. Take a trip to your grocery store and spend some time in the beverage aisles. You may want to check out the chilled juice section in addition to the bottled teas and juice beverages. Pick out about 10 different products that have either a nutrient or herbal compound added and try to identify how many have nutrient content claims, health claims, and structure/function claims. Note the prices of these products. How does their nutritional content compare to a 100-percent fruit juice like orange juice? How does it compare to soda?

Take a Walk on the "Web Side"

This exercise will familiarize you with various websites that promote and sell supplements. Do an Internet search with keywords affiliated with supplements. Try *vitamins, minerals, supplements, herbs*, and even some specific terms like *chromium picolinate* and *ginseng*. On the websites you visit, how is the nutrition information presented? Do the supplement's benefits sound too good to be true? See if you can spot a fraud. Use the information in the "Fraudulent Products" section of this chapter to identify the accuracy of the product information you find.

Getting Personal

Are you or is someone you know taking a dietary supplement because of a desirable health or performance benefit?

Let's investigate this choice.

1. List the supplements you or your friend have taken or are still taking.

2. What research was done prior to using the dietary supplement to determine if the claimed benefits are accurate and the supplement is safe?

3. How does the dosage compare to the RDI-recommended Tolerable Upper Intake Level (UL)?

4. How much does the supplement cost?

5. Was the supplement use discussed with a health-care provider or primary care physician?

6. Are there any known side effects of the dietary supplement?

7. Have there been any reports of adverse effects of the dietary supplement?

8. What reliable, evidence-based scientific research can you find that supports the claimed benefits of the dietary supplement?

References

1. Gahche J, Bailey R, Burt V, et al. Dietary supplement use among U.S. adults has increased since NHANES III (1988–1994). NCHS Data Brief No. 61. April 2011. http://www.cdc.gov/nchs/data/databriefs/db61.pdf. Accessed August 30, 2017.

2. Bailey RL, Gahche JJ, Miller PE, Thomas PR, Dwyer JT. Why U.S. adults use dietary supplements. *JAMA Intern Med.* 2013;173(5):355-361. doi: 10.1001/jamainternmed.2013.2299.

3. National Center for Complementary and Integrative Health. Using dietary supplements wisely. https://nccih.nih.gov/health/supplements/wiseuse.htm. Accessed August 30, 2017.

4. Position of the Academy of Nutrition and Dietetics: nutrient supplementation. *J Am Diet Assoc.* 2009;109:2073-2085.

5. Bailey RL, Gahche JJ, Miller PE, Thomas PR, Dwyer JT. Op. cit.

6. Position of the Academy of Nutrition and Dietetics: nutrient supplementation. Op. cit.

7. National Institutes of Health, Office of Dietary Supplements. A compilation of dietary supplement statements from the scientific report of the 2015 Dietary Guidelines Advisory Committee. February 2015. http://ods.od.nih.gov/pubs/2015_DGAC_Scientific_Report_ODS_Compiled_DS_Statements.pdf. Accessed August 30, 2017.

8. Position of the Academy of Nutrition and Dietetics: functional foods. *J Acad Nutr Diet.* 2013;113:1096-1103.

9. Hochholzer W, Berg DD, Giugliano RP. The facts behind niacin. *Ther Adv Cardiovasc Dis.* 2011;5(5):227-240. doi: 10.1177/1753944711419197. Epub September 5, 2011.

10. Pauling L. Orthomolecular psychiatry. Varying the concentrations of substances normally present in the human body may control mental disease. *Science.* 1968;160(3825):265-271.

11. Institute of Medicine, Food and Nutrition Board. *Dietary Reference Intakes for Vitamin C, Vitamin E, Selenium, and Carotenoids.* Washington, DC: National Academies Press; 2000.

12. Institute of Medicine, Food and Nutrition Board. *Dietary Reference Intakes for Vitamin A, Vitamin K, Arsenic, Boron, Chromium, Copper, Iron, Manganese, Molybdenum, Nickel, Silicon, Vanadium, and Zinc.* Washington, DC: National Academies Press; 2001.

13. Council for Responsible Nutrition. Dietary supplements—safe, beneficial, and regulated. http://www.crnusa.org/CRNRegQandA.html. Accessed August 30, 2017.

14. Health Canada. About natural health products. https://www.canada.ca/en/health-canada/services/drugs-health-products/natural-non-prescription/regulation/about-products.html. Accessed August 30, 2017.

15. Silverglade B, Ringel Heller I. Food labeling chaos. The case for reform. 2010. Center for Science in the Public Interest. http://cspinet.org/new/pdf/food_labeling_chaos_report.pdf. Accessed August 30, 2017.

16. National Institutes of Health, National Center for Complementary and Integrative Health. NIH complementary and integrative health agency gets new name. https://nccih.nih.gov/news/press/12172014. Accessed August 30, 2017.

17. National Institutes of Health, National Center for Complementary and Integrative Health. Complementary, alternative, or integrative health: what's in a name? https://nccih.nih.gov/health/integrative-health#vision. Accessed August 30, 2017.

18. Nahin RL, Barnes PM, Stussman BJ. *Expenditures on Complementary Health Approaches: United States, 2012*. National Health Statistics Reports. Hyattsville, MD: National Center for Health Statistics; 2016.

19. National Institutes of Health, National Center for Complementary and Integrative Health. Use of complementary health approaches in the U.S. What complementary and integrative approaches do Americans use? Key findings from the 2012 National Health Interview Survey. https://nccih.nih.gov/research/statistics/NHIS/2012/key-findings. Accessed August 30, 2017.

20. Kennedy DA, Seely D. Clinically based evidence of drug–herb interactions: a systematic review. *Expert Opin Drug Saf*. 2010;9(1):79-124.

21. Tachjian A, Maria V, Jahangir A. Use of herbal products and potential interactions in patients with cardiovascular diseases. *J Am Coll Cardiol*. 2010;55(6):515-525.

22. U.S. Food and Drug Administration. FDA issues dietary supplements final rule. FDA press release. June 22, 2007.

23. U.S. Food and Drug Administration. Dietary supplements. https://www.fda.gov/Food/DietarySupplements/. Accessed August 30, 2017.

24. U.S. Food and Drug Administration. FDA 101: dietary supplements. http://www.fda.gov/ForConsumers/ConsumerUpdates/ucm050803.htm. Accessed August 30, 2017.

25. U.S. Food and Drug Administration. Dietary supplement labeling guide. Guidance for industry. http://www.fda.gov/food/guidanceregulation/guidancedocumentsregulatoryinformation/dietarysupplements/ucm2006823.htm. Accessed August 30, 2017.

26. National Institutes of Health, Office of Dietary Supplements. Dietary supplements. Background information. https://ods.od.nih.gov/factsheets/DietarySupplements-HealthProfessional/. Accessed August 30, 2017.

27. U.S. Food and Drug Administration. Structure/function claims. http://www.fda.gov/Food/IngredientsPackagingLabeling/LabelingNutrition/ucm2006881.htm. Accessed August 30, 2017.

28. U.S. Food and Drug Administration. Dietary supplements. http://www.fda.gov/Food/Dietarysupplements/default.htm. Accessed August 30, 2017.

29. Health Canada. About natural health product regulation in Canada. https://www.canada.ca/en/health-canada/services/drugs-health-products/natural-non-prescription/regulation.html. Accessed August 30, 2017.

30. Academy of Nutrition and Dietetics. Guidelines regarding the recommendation and sale of dietary supplements: full text. http://www.eatrightpro.org/resource/career/code-of-ethics/ethics-education-resources/guidelines-regarding-the-recommendation-and-sale-of-dietary-supplements-full-text. Accessed August 30, 2017.

31. U.S. Pharmacopeial Convention. Home page. http://www.usp.org. Accessed August 30, 2017.

32. U.S. Food and Drug Administration. Beware of fraudulent dietary supplements. http://www.fda.gov/forconsumers/consumerupdates/ucm246744.htm. Accessed August 30, 2017.

33. Position of the Academy of Nutrition and Dietetics: functional foods. Op. cit.

34. Daniells S. What's driving functional food and beverage growth? Snacking, convenience, and customer behavior. November 20, 2014. http://www.nutraingredients-usa.com/Markets/What-s-driving-functional-food-and-beverage-growth-Snacking-convenience-and-consumer-behavior. Accessed August 30, 2017.

35. U.S. Department of Agriculture, U.S. Department of Health and Human Services. *2015–2020 Dietary Guidelines for Americans*. 8th ed. http://health.gov/dietaryguidelines/2015/guidelines/. Accessed August 30, 2017.

36. U.S. Department of Agriculture. MyPlate. http://www.choosemyplate.gov. Accessed August 30, 2017.

37. Mordente A, Guantario B, Meucci E, et al. Lycopene and cardiovascular diseases: an update. *Curr Med Chem*. 2011;18(8):1146-1163.

38. Andres S, Abraham K, Appel KE, Lampen A. Risks and benefits of dietary isoflavones for cancer. *Crit Rev Toxicol*. 2011;41(6):463-506.

39. Ibid.

40. Wong IY, Koo SC, Chan CW. Prevention of age-related macular degeneration. *Int Ophthalmol*. 2011;31(1):73-82.

41. Gorusupudi A, Nelson K, Bernstein PS. The age-related eye disease study: micronutrients in the treatment of macular degeneration. *Adv Nutr*. 2017;8:40-53.

42. Position of the Academy of Nutrition and Dietetics: functional foods. Op. cit.

43. U.S. Food and Drug Administration. Labeling and nutrition. http://www.fda.gov/food/ingredientspackaginglabeling/labelingnutrition/default.htm. Accessed August 30, 2017.

44. Position of the Academy of Nutrition and Dietetics: functional foods. Op. cit.

45. U.S. Food and Drug Administration. Guidance for industry: a food labeling guide. Appendix C: health claims. January 2013. http://www.fda.gov/food/guidanceregulation/guidancedocumentsregulatoryinformation/labelingnutrition/ucm064919.htm. Accessed August 30, 2017.

46. Silverglade B, Ringel Heller I. Op. cit.

47. National Institutes of Health, Office of Dietary Supplements. How to evaluate health information on the Internet: questions and answers. http://ods.od.nih.gov/Health_Information/How_To_Evaluate_Health_Information_on_the_Internet_Questions_and_Answers.aspx. Accessed August 30, 2017.

Chapter 8

Water and Minerals: The Ocean Within

Revised by Carolyn Dunn

THINK About It

1 Do you ever feel dehydrated?

2 How often do you salt your food before tasting it?

3 You disclose to a friend that you tend to be low in iron. She knows you are a vegetarian and suggests you drink milk. What false assumption might she be making?

4 Some people argue that fluoridation is overdone. What is your position? Would you vote for fluoridating all water supplies?

LEARNING Objectives

1. State the functions of water.
2. Identify the factors that affect mineral bioavailability.
3. Describe the absorption, storage, and transport of minerals.
4. List the major functions of each mineral.
5. Identify major food sources for each mineral.
6. Specify the major symptoms and diseases associated with mineral deficiency and toxicity.
7. Discuss the risks and benefits of mineral supplementation.
8. Discuss the role of minerals in health and disease.

On a coast-to-coast flight with your father and your older brother, you observe your father drinking water frequently throughout the flight, while your brother rejects the beverages offered. When you arrive at your destination, your brother complains of feeling utterly exhausted. In contrast, your father is lively and ready for a "night on the town." How could you explain this?

First, it's important to know that the familiar beverage cart is not a random gesture of kindness by the airlines: regular fluid intake on flights is necessary for health. Although you may be unaware of it, water evaporates from the skin faster than usual in the low-humidity, high-altitude, pressurized cabin of an airplane, so drinking fluids during the flight helps prevent dehydration. But you must choose fluids carefully. Caffeine has a diuretic effect and thus increases fluid loss in urine. It is much better to consume water to replace fluids lost during flight.

Your brother's lack of energy may be a symptom of mild dehydration. Dad had the right idea—plenty of water along the way.

Water: Crucial to Life

🍎 **Why Is This Important?** Water is absolutely essential. You could most likely survive weeks without food, but you can live only a few days without water. Unlike storage of energy in your body, you have no capacity to store extra water, so you must continually replace water that is lost.

Overall, water makes up between 45 and 75 percent of a person's weight. (See **FIGURE 8.1**.) About two-thirds of body water is intracellular fluid, the fluid inside cells. The remaining one-third is extracellular fluid, which is mainly between cells (interstitial) and in blood (the **plasma** portion). (See **FIGURE 8.2**.)

Electrolytes and Water: A Delicate Balance

When minerals or **salts** dissolve in water, they form **ions** (**electrolytes**). Sodium and potassium, for example, form **cations** (positively charged ions), whereas chloride and phosphate form **anions** (negatively charged ions).

▶ **plasma** The fluid portion of the blood that contains blood cells and other components.

▶ **salts** Compounds that result when the hydrogen of an acid is replaced with a metal or a group that acts like a metal.

▶ **ions** Atoms or groups of atoms with an electrical charge resulting from the loss or gain of one or more electrons.

▶ **electrolytes [ih-LEK-tro-lites]** Substances that separate into charged particles (ions) when dissolved in water or other solvents and thus become capable of conducting an electrical current. The terms *electrolyte* and *ion* often are used interchangeably.

▶ **cations** Ions that carry a positive charge.

▶ **anions** Ions that carry a negative charge.

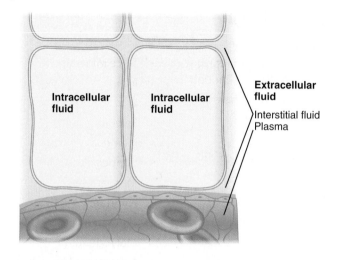

FIGURE 8.2 **Intracellular and extracellular fluid.** Extracellular fluids and their dissolved substances (except for proteins) move across capillary membranes easily. Plasma (the fluid portion of the blood) has a higher concentration of proteins than does interstitial fluid. Excluding protein, their compositions are roughly the same.

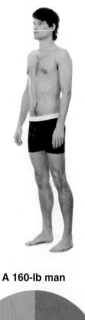

A 160-lb man

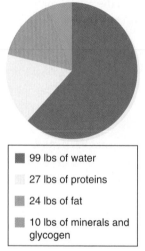

■ 99 lbs of water

□ 27 lbs of proteins

■ 24 lbs of fat

□ 10 lbs of minerals and glycogen

FIGURE 8.1 **Body composition.** The main constituent of the body is water. Generally, adult males have more lean tissue (and therefore more water) and less fat than adult females.
Adult man: © Piotr Marcinski/Shutterstock, Inc.

▶ **osmosis** The movement of a solvent, such as water, through a semi-permeable membrane from the dilute to the concentrated side until the concentrations on both sides of the membrane are equal.

▶ **heat capacity** The amount of energy required to raise the temperature of a substance 1°C.

Your body precisely controls and balances the concentration of electrolytes dissolved in its watery fluids—there must be just the right mix of water and electrolytes, both within and outside of each cell. Cells use pumps embedded in their membranes to move electrolytes in and out. In sync with the movement of electrolytes, water flows back and forth through the cell membrane, a process called **osmosis**. When electrolytes are more concentrated on one side of the membrane, osmosis moves water from the dilute side to the concentrated side to equalize the concentrations. (See **FIGURE 8.3**.)

Cells must contain just the right amount of water. Too little and the cell will shrink and die. Too much and the cell will burst. Too much water in spaces surrounding cells causes swelling (edema).

Functions of Water

Water is the highway that moves nutrients and wastes between cells and organs. It carries food through your digestive system, transports nutrients to your cells and tissues, and carries waste out of your body in urine. (See **FIGURE 8.4**.) What about nutrients and wastes that are not water-soluble? Your body either modifies them chemically so they dissolve in water or packages them with proteins (e.g., lipoproteins). Your body's watery fluids, such as the bloodstream, can easily transport these protein packages throughout the body.

Watery fluids also have mechanical functions. They act as shock absorbers, lubricators, and cleansing agents. For example, amniotic fluid cushions and protects the fetus, synovial fluid allows joints to move smoothly, tears lubricate and cleanse the eyes, and saliva moistens food and makes swallowing possible.

Water is an essential part of your body's chemistry. It helps break apart substances and is a by-product in many anabolic reactions (reactions that combine substances). Reactions involving water also help maintain the body's acid–base (pH) balance in the narrow range required for life.

Water has a high **heat capacity**, meaning a large amount of energy must be added or removed to raise or lower its temperature. When microwaving food, for example, you may have noticed that watery foods like soup heat much more slowly than foods like pizza that contain little water. Because your body is nearly two-thirds water, your body temperature remains relatively stable. Plus, water is the prime component of your body's cooling system. If you get too warm, blood vessels dilate and you begin to sweat. The perspiration on your skin evaporates and cools you off.

> **Key Concepts** Water is so essential that we cannot survive without it for more than a few days. We need water for temperature regulation, acid–base balance, lubrication, and protection. Water dissolves or carries vital substances throughout the body and participates in chemical reactions.

Intake Recommendations: How Much Water Is Enough?

There is no one answer to this question. We each need a different amount, depending on our size, body composition, and activity level, as well as the temperature and humidity of the environment.

The Adequate Intake (AI) for total water is 3.7 liters (approximately 4 quarts) per day for men and 2.7 liters (approximately 3 quarts) per day for women.[1] Intake recommendations are higher during pregnancy (3.0 liters per day) and lactation (3.8 liters per day). Activity and sweating increase water needs, so athletes and active people need much more water, especially if they work and train in warm, humid climates.

Water intake comes from a combination of drinking water and beverages, and the water in foods. Survey data suggest that about 75 to 80 percent of our total water intake comes from beverages, with the remaining 20 to 25 percent from foods. Some foods, such as fruits and vegetables, contain a substantial amount of water whereas others—grain products, for example—provide very little. (See **FIGURE 8.5**.) Our bodies also produce a small amount of water (about 250 to 350 milliliters per day) in metabolic reactions.

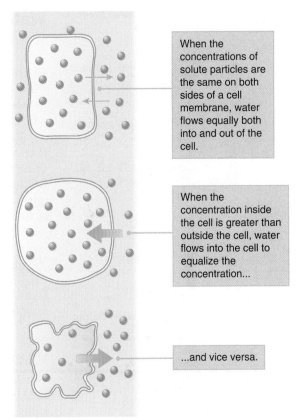

FIGURE 8.3 Osmosis. Water moves across cell membranes to equalize concentrations of dissolved particles.

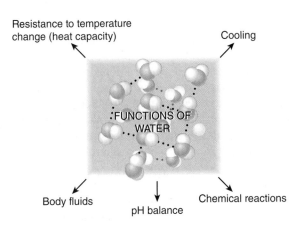

FIGURE 8.4 Functions of water. Water is so critical to human body functioning that we can live only a few days without it.

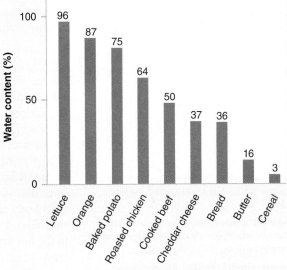

FIGURE 8.5 Water content of various foods. As you might expect, crunchy vegetables contain more water than dry cereal. But did you know that potatoes contain a high percentage of water?

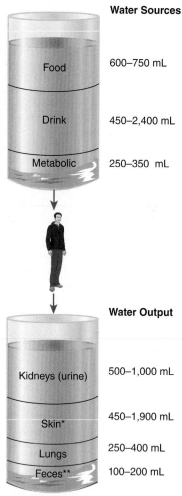

Water Sources

Food   600–750 mL

Drink   450–2,400 mL

Metabolic   250–350 mL

Water Output

Kidneys (urine)   500–1,000 mL

Skin*   450–1,900 mL

Lungs   250–400 mL

Feces**   100–200 mL

* (Insensible and perspiration)
The volume of perspiration is normally about 100 mL per day. In very hot weather or during heavy exercise, a person may lose 1 to 2 liters per hour.

** People with severe diarrhea can lose several liters of water per day in feces.

FIGURE 8.6 Typical daily water intake and output. To maintain water balance, your body regulates its fluid intake and output.

Adult male: © Piotr Marcinski/Shutterstock, Inc.

▶ **insensible water loss** The continual loss of body water by evaporation from the respiratory tract and diffusion through the skin.

▶ **antidiuretic hormone (ADH)** A hormone secreted by the pituitary gland that increases blood pressure and prevents fluid excretion by the kidneys. Also called *vasopressin*.

▶ **aldosterone [al-DOS-ter-own]** A hormone secreted from the adrenal glands that acts on the kidneys to regulate electrolyte and water balance. It raises blood pressure by promoting retention of sodium (and thus water) and excretion of potassium.

Water Excretion: Where Does the Water Go?

We continuously lose water through various routes—exhaled air, perspiration, feces, and urine. (See water sources and water output in **FIGURE 8.6**.) **Insensible water loss**—the continuous evaporation of water from the lungs and skin—typically accounts for about one-fourth to one-half of daily fluid loss. These losses increase at high altitudes and during low humidity.

Each day, we typically lose about 1 to 2 liters of water in urine. If we eat the typical U.S. diet containing excess protein and salt, our urine production increases to eliminate surplus urea (a breakdown product from protein) and sodium. Fever, coughing, rapid breathing, and watery nasal secretions all increase water loss significantly. This is one reason why doctors recommend increasing your fluid intake when you are sick.

> **Key Concepts** The AI for fluid intake is 3.7 liters per day for men and 2.7 liters per day for women. Water intake comes from a combination of foods, fluids, and water produced in normal metabolism. Fluid is lost mainly by urination. Additional losses occur through the skin and lungs and in feces. Water is critical in eliminating the body's waste products.

Water Balance

Our bodies carefully maintain water balance by manipulating water intake and output. When water intake is low, the kidneys conserve water and only excrete a small volume of concentrated urine. When the body has an excess of water, the kidneys excrete a large volume of dilute urine.

How do the kidneys know when to conserve water? Special cells in the brain sense rising sodium levels in the body. These cells signal the pituitary gland to release **antidiuretic hormone (ADH)**, which in turn signals the kidneys to conserve water—effectively diluting sodium levels. Sensors in the kidneys themselves can detect a rapid loss of fluid through a drop in blood pressure. They trigger a complex process that includes the release of the hormone **aldosterone** by the adrenal glands. Aldosterone signals the kidneys to retain sodium. When sodium is retained, water follows to avoid an increased concentration of sodium.

Thirst

Although taste, availability, cultural patterns, and personal habits influence our consumption of fluids, thirst remains our most important stimulus for drinking fluids. Yet thirst is not always a reliable guide to avoiding dehydration. In older adults, for example, sensitivity to thirst declines, placing them at higher risk for dehydration. Under normal circumstances, water losses in adults can range from 0.3 liters per hour in sedentary conditions to 2.0 liters per hour during high activity in the heat.[2] And, after you drink water, your body can take 30 to 60 minutes to absorb and distribute it throughout the body. For example, imagine you are rollerblading in the hot sun and after an hour you pause momentarily to quench your thirst with a half-liter bottle of water. That's not enough! You still have a deficit of 1/2 to 1 1/2 liters of water, and you'll continue to lose water while your body absorbs and distributes the water you just drank. To avoid dehydration in hot weather or when exercising, you need to drink fluids early and often.

THINK About It 1

Key Concepts The body uses complex mechanisms to precisely regulate water balance. Antidiuretic hormone (ADH) stimulates water reabsorption in the kidneys, and aldosterone stimulates the kidneys to reabsorb sodium and water. Although our sense of thirst usually reminds us to drink enough so that we don't become dehydrated, it is an unreliable signal during hot weather or heavy exercise, when fluid losses are high.

Alcohol, Caffeine, and Common Medications Affect Fluid Balance

Anyone who regularly consumes alcohol probably realizes that it is a diuretic—a substance that increases fluid loss through increased urination. Alcohol suppresses ADH production, and excessive alcohol consumption can cause dehydration with symptoms of thirst, weakness, dryness of mucous membranes, dizziness, and light-headedness—all common effects of a hangover.

A cup of coffee can provide a morning pick-me-up, but the caffeine is a diuretic. A typical pattern of many busy Americans is a few cups of coffee in the morning, a caffeinated soda with lunch, another in the afternoon, and maybe a glass of wine or a beer with dinner. Studies of the effects of caffeinated beverages on overall hydration status have produced inconsistent results, however.[3] Although some suggest that a fondness for caffeinated beverages can cause chronic mild dehydration, the Dietary Reference Intake (DRI) committee examining water and electrolyte requirements concluded that caffeinated beverages contribute to the total water intake in a manner similar to noncaffeinated beverages.[4] Most Americans seem to consume a sufficient quantity and variety of fluids from foods and beverages to maintain fluid balance.[5]

Doctors often prescribe diuretic medications to help lower blood pressure or decrease swelling caused by fluid retention. Because these medications can disrupt sodium and potassium balance, doctors typically monitor the patient's blood electrolyte levels and may prescribe potassium supplements to maintain a proper balance.

Dehydration

Any condition causing rapid water loss is dangerous: burns in which damaged skin cannot control water evaporation, the heat of fever, extreme environmental heat, or exertion without replenishing water. Early signs of dehydration include fatigue, dry mucous membranes, headache, and dark urine with a strong odor. Physical and mental performance slip. A water loss of 20 percent of body weight can cause coma and death. (See **FIGURE 8.7**.)

Chronic mild dehydration—a fluid deficit of as little as 1 to 2 percent of body weight—can cause declines in alertness and the ability to concentrate while increasing feelings of tiredness, reducing physical performance, and causing headache.[6] Such low levels of dehydration also impair decision making and reaction times. This may be important for tasks that involve judgment and skill, such as driving a car. Chronic underconsumption of water may play a role in many conditions such as constipation, asthma, cardiovascular disease, some forms of cancer, and complications of diabetes.[7] For some people, increased water consumption may reduce caloric intake, thereby aiding in the prevention of obesity and diabetes.[8] One good rule of thumb to test hydration levels is to look at the color of your urine in the

Quick **Bite**

How Do Desert-Dwelling Animals Avoid Dehydration?
Some desert animals can concentrate their urine to nearly 100 times the maximum concentration of human urine. This allows such animals to survive on water obtained from food and their own metabolic reactions. In contrast, some animals that live in freshwater minimally concentrate their urine. Beavers concentrate their urine to only about half that of humans.

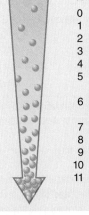

% Body weight loss	
0	
1	Thirst
2	Increased thirst, loss of appetite, discomfort
3	Impatience, decreased blood volume
4	Nausea, slowing of physical work
5	Difficulty concentrating, apathy, tingling extremities
6	Increasing body temperature, pulse and respiration rate
7	Stumbling, headache
8	Dizziness, labored breathing
9	Weakness, mental confusion
10	Muscle spasms, indistinct speech
11	Kidney failure, poor circulation due to decreased blood volume

FIGURE 8.7 Effects of progressive dehydration. Dehydration quickly diminishes physical and mental performance. Severe dehydration can be fatal.

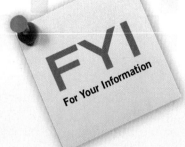

Tap, Filtered, or Bottled: Which Water Is Best?

Everywhere you look, it seems like more and more people are carrying and sipping on bottles of water. Theme parks even sell shoulder holsters for you to carry your bottle around with you. What's with the water craze? And what's wrong with the good old water fountain?

During the mid-to-late 1980s, the growth in use of bottled water began. Initially, bottled mineral waters, such as Perrier, were associated with wealth and glamour. But like many trends adopted by the wealthy (white bread, for instance), bottled water soon became desirable to a wider range of people. It is estimated that Americans drink approximately 11 billion gallons of bottled water each year.[a] In 2014, the U.S. per capita consumption of bottled water was 34.2 gallons.[b] U.S. residents now drink more bottled water annually than any other beverage except carbonated soft drinks. Soft drink consumption, at 12.6 billion gallons in 2014, is just a little more than bottled water consumption.[c] Soft drink consumption has been declining steadily over the last seven years and is predicted to be less than bottled water by 2017 if the decline continues.[d] Major soft drink companies, such as Coca-Cola and PepsiCo, sell their own brands of bottled water.

Several factors are fueling the growth of the bottled-water industry. Baby boomers are seeking natural, low-calorie beverages, and fitness consciousness has reemphasized the importance of hydration. Media reports of contamination of tap water in major metropolitan areas sparked concerns about the safety and quality of tap water, with the lead contamination crisis in Flint, Michigan, being one of the most recent examples. Most Americans choose bottled water for what they think is *not* in it rather than for what it contains.

Some bottled water companies now add dietary supplements such as vitamins to their water. Other companies make powdered dietary supplements that are designed to be added to your water. In addition to vitamins and minerals, these products may contain other ingredients such as herbs. Being aware of the ingredients and the effect they can have on your body can help you make informed decisions about what to drink.

When choosing among vitamin waters, powdered supplements, or plain water, consider the following[e]:

- *Sugar and calories:* Look at the Nutrition Facts or ingredient label to know if the product has added sugar. Sugar adds calories to water, which can lead to unwanted weight gain. Remember, plain water has zero calories.
- *Vitamins at 100% DV:* The best way to get your daily value of vitamins and minerals is by eating a variety of foods in the appropriate amounts. Vitamins and minerals from food are much better absorbed.
- *Herbals and botanicals:* Many bottled waters advertise that they contain plant extracts like echinacea or ginseng; however, most of these extracts are in relatively small amounts in the water and have little to no effect on your body.

From a nutritional perspective, it's important to drink plenty of fluids. Water is one of the best ways to replace lost fluids, and, at the simplest level, the source of the water doesn't really matter. Standards for municipal water systems are enforced by the Environmental Protection Agency (EPA), which requires regular testing and monitoring. In most places, tap water can be considered a safe, clean source of water. Many municipal water systems add fluoride to tap water, an important weapon in the prevention of tooth decay. However, home-installed filtration systems for removing chlorine might also remove added fluoride, and most bottled waters do not contain fluoride. Some people don't like the taste of their local water supply and don't want to bother with maintaining a filtration system. In this case, or if you want your water "to go," bottled water can be the choice. The bottled-water industry offers:

- High-volume, returnable containers from suppliers who stock the water coolers for offices or supermarkets
- The familiar brands (e.g., Evian, Dasani, Aquafina) that are sold as alternatives to soft drinks
- Bottled water in vending machines

The bottled-water industry is regulated by the Food and Drug Administration (FDA), which, in 1995, published Standards of Identity for bottled water, set maximum allowable standards for contaminants, and established Current Good Manufacturing Practices (CGMPs) for bottling plants. Keep in mind that the FDA regulates bottled waters that are sold interstate, and not those sold only in a particular area or state. Individual states can have their own quality standards for locally distributed waters.

Look beyond terms such as *artesian, mineral, spring,* or *purified* (see **TABLE A**). The labels

---

TABLE A
Definitions of Bottled Water Terms

Mineral water must contain at least 250 parts per million (ppm) of dissolved minerals and come from a geologically and physically protected underground water source.

Purified water is tap or ground water that has been treated by distillation, deionization, or reverse osmosis. This may be labeled "distilled water" if produced by steam distillation and condensation.

Spring water comes from an underground formation from which water flows naturally to the surface; it is collected either at the spring or from a borehole to the underground formation.

Artesian water comes from tapping a confined underground aquifer that is below the natural water table. Generally, the artesian well is located in a depression where the water table of the surrounding hills is higher. The "head" of pressure from the water table forces the water up through the tap line.

Ground water comes from a subsurface saturated zone and is not under the direct influence of surface water.

Well water comes from a drilled hole that taps the water of an aquifer and is pumped to the surface.

Data from International Bottled Water Association. Labeling. www.bottledwater.org/content/labeling-0. Accessed September 8, 2017.

on most bottled water list the source of the water. Some consumers are surprised to find that their favorite brand of water is really from a municipal source, not an underground spring! Nutrition Facts labels are required if the manufacturer makes a claim (e.g., sodium free) or adds minerals. These labels often do not show the natural mineral content of the water, which is really the only other nutritional aspect that could be expected.

The Academy of Nutrition and Dietetics suggests the following five factors be considered when choosing between bottled and tap water: the environment, safety, cost, taste, and fluoride.[f] The bottom line, according to the Academy, is that both tap and bottled water are safe, and that bottled water offers no nutritional advantage unless it is fortified. Bottled water might encourage fluid consumption by making water more accessible; however, this can come at an environmental cost by contributing to additional waste.[g] Drinking sufficient water is the primary objective, especially when it replaces high-calorie, low-nutrient beverages. The amount of water needed daily depends on gender, size, and physical activity level.[h]

Ultimately, the choice is up to the consumer—there is no clearly best choice of water.

a International Bottled Water Association. Bottled water market. http://www.bottledwater.org/economics/bottled-water-market. Accessed September 8, 2017.

b International Bottled Water Association. Bottled water sales and consumption projected to increase in 2014. http://www.bottledwater.org/bottled-water-sales-and-consumption-projected-increase-2014-expected-be-number-one-packaged-drink. Accessed September 8, 2017.

c Esterl M. Soft drinks hit 10th year of decline. *The Wall Street Journal.* March 26, 2015. http://www.wsj.com/articles/pepsi-cola-replaces-diet-coke-as-no-2-soda-1427388559. Accessed September 8, 2017.

d Sanger-Katz M. The decline of 'big soda.' *The New York Times.* October 2, 2015. http://www.nytimes.com/2015/10/04/upshot/soda-industry-struggles-as-consumer-tastes-change.html. Accessed September 8, 2017.

e Oates VJ. Vitamin water and powdered multivitamin supplements in water. January 5, 2011. http://www.extension.org/pages/32335/vitamin-water-and-powdered-multivitamin-supplements-in-water#.VdKzLINViko. Accessed September 8, 2017.

f Academy of Nutrition and Dietetics. Bottled water: is bottled water a better choice than tap water? May 2008. http://www.eatright.org/cps/rde/xchg/ada/hsxsl/nutrition_17382_ENU_HTML.htm. Accessed May 24, 2012.

g Ibid.

h Academy of Nutrition and Dietetics. Rethink your drinks and hydrate right this summer with tips from the Academy of Nutrition and Dietetics. June 24, 2014. http://www.eatrightpro.org/resource/media/press-releases/new-in-food-nutrition-and-health/rethink-your-drinks-and-hydrate-right-this-summer-with-tips-from-the-academy. Accessed January 29, 2016.

toilet. It should be the color of pale lemonade. Darker urine is a sign that you are not fully hydrated.

Seniors and infants are particularly vulnerable to dehydration. The sense of thirst often diminishes with age, and seniors often take diuretic medications. For a variety of reasons, seniors may eat and drink less. The resulting physical and mental deterioration creates a vicious cycle, with food and fluid intake continuing to worsen.

Because infants can lose water rapidly through their skin, they need ample fluid relative to their size. Breast milk or infant formula generally provides all the fluid a baby needs. Severe diarrhea can cause swift and deadly dehydration, especially in seniors and infants. Normally, the intestines reabsorb nearly all the fluid secreted by digestive organs. But when intestinal disease causes diarrhea or prolonged vomiting, dehydration can occur. Worldwide, dehydration is a major killer of babies and young children, with infection being the underlying culprit.

Water consumption, of course, is the primary treatment for dehydration. (See the FYI feature "Tap, Filtered, or Bottled: Which Water Is Best?") Often electrolytes also must be replaced, particularly in cases of diarrhea and vomiting. For moderate to severe dehydration, intravenous fluids and hospitalization may be necessary. In remote areas or developing countries, rehydration packets—a mix of potassium and sodium salts and sugar—dissolved in boiled water have saved countless lives.

Water Intoxication

Because drinking fluids temporarily alleviates thirst, we rarely drink to the point of overhydration and dilution of body fluids. Overhydration first causes headaches and confusion, and then seizures and can be fatal. Replacement of fluid losses following intensive or prolonged exercise with plain water (and no electrolytes) can result in overhydration and hyponatremia (low blood sodium) in athletes.[9] Acute water toxicity has

Quick Bite

Water, Water Everywhere and Not a Drop to Drink!

When shipwrecked sailors drink seawater, they quickly become severely dehydrated. This is because the concentration of salt in seawater is about double the maximum concentration of salt in urine. Thus, it takes 2 liters of urine to rid the body of the solutes ingested by drinking 1 liter of seawater.

▶ **major minerals** Minerals that are required in the diet and are present in the body in large amounts compared with trace minerals. Also known as *macrominerals.*

▶ **trace minerals** Minerals present in the body and required in the diet in relatively small amounts compared with major minerals. Also known as *microminerals.*

been reported due to rapid consumption of large quantities of fluids that greatly exceeded the kidney's maximal excretion rate of approximately 0.7 to 1.0 liters per hour.[10] A fraternity hazing ritual, for example, caused fatal water intoxication in a California State University student who was forced to drink large quantities of water while exercising vigorously.[11]

Key Concepts Diuretic medications increase urinary fluid losses. Dehydration is a potential consequence of gastrointestinal disease, burns, and heavy sweating. Treatment involves replacing fluids, along with electrolytes if the condition is severe. Although unlikely, water intoxication is possible.

Minerals

🍎 **Why Is This Important?** Minerals, like vitamins, are essential for a number of vital functions in the body. Minerals are involved in literally thousands of processes in the body, from turning food into energy to building tissue to producing enzymes upon which every cell in the body depends.

What distinguishes minerals from vitamins, carbohydrates, proteins, and fats? Minerals are elemental atoms or ions rather than organic compounds. Unlike vitamins, minerals are not destroyed by heat, light, acidity, or alkalinity. Calcium, for example, remains calcium, whether in seashells, milk, or bones. Iron remains iron, whether it is part of a cast-iron skillet or part of hemoglobin.

Like vitamins, however, minerals are micronutrients. Compared with carbohydrates, proteins, and fats, they are needed in relatively small amounts—at most a few grams per day.

Minerals often are grouped as **major minerals** (or *macrominerals*) and **trace minerals** (or *microminerals*). This classification of minerals is unrelated to the mineral's biological importance and is arbitrarily based on the amount you need in your diet and the amount present in your body. You need more than 100 milligrams per day of each major mineral and less than 100 milligrams daily of each trace mineral. (See **FIGURE 8.8**.) Compared with the major minerals, the total amount of each trace mineral present in your body is small. For example, your total body iron, a trace mineral, is 2 to 4 grams, or about the amount of iron in a small nail, but it plays a critical role in many major metabolic reactions. Contrast that with your total body calcium, a major mineral and the most abundant mineral in the human body. Approximately 40 percent of the mineral mass in the body and about 1.5 percent of total body mass are calcium.[12] Despite the amounts found in the body or required from diet, both major and trace minerals are important. (See **TABLE 8.4** at the end of this chapter for a summary of macrominerals and microminerals.)

Often a single mineral has several quite diverse functions. Some minerals, such as iodine, are components of hormones. Many are components of enzymes or enzyme cofactors. Others serve a structural function; for example, calcium and phosphorus are among the minerals that make bones hard.

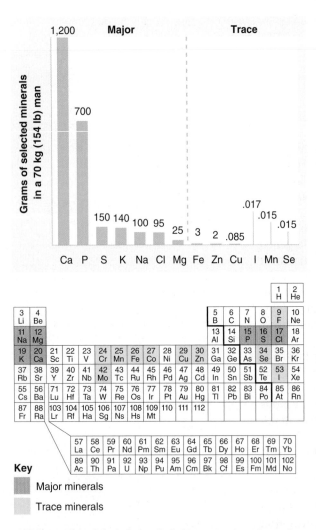

Key

▮ Major minerals

▮ Trace minerals

FIGURE 8.8 Minerals in the human body. Dietary minerals are elements in the periodic table. Based on the amount of a mineral needed in the diet and the amount in the body, nutritionists categorize a mineral as major or trace.

Data from Gropper SS. Smith JL, Groff JL. *Advanced Nutrition and Human Metabolism.* 5th ed. Belmont, CA: Wadsworth/ Cengage Learning; 2009; and Stipanuk MH. *Biochemical and Physiological Aspects of Human Nutrition.* 2nd ed. Philadelphia: WB Saunders; 2006.

Minerals in Foods

Foods from both plants and animals are sources of minerals. Generally speaking, animal tissue contains minerals in the proportion that the animal needs, so animal-derived foods are more reliable mineral sources.

Plant foods can be excellent sources of several minerals, but the mineral content of plants can vary dramatically depending on the minerals, such as selenium, in the soil where the plants are found. (See **FIGURE 8.9**.) Even the maturity of a vegetable, fruit, or grain can influence its mineral content. Like plant foods, drinking water has variable mineral content, and it sometimes can be a significant source of minerals, such as sodium, magnesium, and fluoride.

Bioavailability

Our gastrointestinal (GI) tracts absorb a much smaller proportion of minerals than vitamins—and probably for good reason. Once absorbed, excess minerals often are difficult for the body to flush out. In many cases, the body adjusts mineral absorption to our needs; for example, a calcium-deficient person absorbs calcium more readily than does a person with normal calcium levels.

Megadosing with single-mineral supplements can hamper the absorption of other minerals. Minerals such as calcium, iron, zinc, and magnesium, for example, all have similar chemical properties and compete for absorption.

Fiber and other components of food also affect mineral bioavailability. (See **FIGURE 8.10**.) High-fiber diets reduce absorption of iron, calcium, zinc, and magnesium. **Phytate** (a component of whole grains) binds minerals and carries them out of the intestine unabsorbed. **Oxalate** (found in spinach and rhubarb) binds calcium, markedly reducing calcium absorption.

> **Key Concepts** Minerals are essential inorganic elements. They are found in a wide variety of foods, but their bioavailability is affected by several factors, among them our physiological need, presence of competing minerals, and presence of other dietary components.

Major Minerals and Health

The seven major minerals, sometimes called macrominerals—sodium, potassium, chloride, calcium, phosphorus, magnesium, and sulfur—have significant roles, and when mineral status goes awry, your health can suffer. Two disorders in which major minerals play critical parts are **hypertension** and osteoporosis.

Sodium

You probably know sodium best as a component of table salt. Table salt, or sodium chloride, is 40 percent sodium. And you've probably heard that we eat too much sodium. The *2015–2020 Dietary Guidelines for Americans* tells us to "Reduce daily sodium intake to less than 2,300 milligrams (mg)." The new guidelines also state that for individuals with prehypertension and hypertension "further reduction to 1,500 mg per day can result in even greater blood pressure reduction."[13]

Excess sodium in the human diet is a relatively recent problem. For centuries in many regions, salt was highly prized and hard to come by. Our language reflects that: "He's worth his salt" means he's a valuable

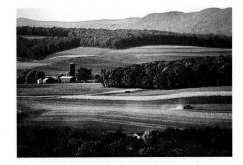

FIGURE 8.9 Growing conditions influence mineral content. The mineral content of plants reflects the mineral content of the soil in which they are grown.

Courtesy of Scott Bauer/ARS Photo Library/USDA.

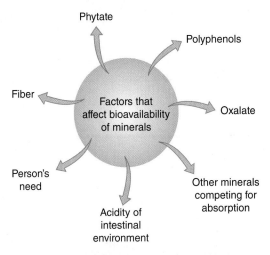

FIGURE 8.10 Factors that affect the bioavailability of minerals. A person's need and the dietary components of a meal can enhance or inhibit the absorption of a mineral.

▶ **phytate (phytic acid)** A phosphorus-containing compound in the outer husks of cereal grains that binds with minerals and inhibits their absorption.

▶ **oxalate (oxalic acid)** An organic acid in some leafy green vegetables, such as spinach, that binds to calcium to form calcium oxalate, an insoluble compound the body cannot absorb.

▶ **hypertension** Condition in which resting blood pressure persistently exceeds 140 mm Hg systolic or 90 mm Hg diastolic.

Quick Bite

Is Airline Drinking Water Tainted?

The tap water on airplanes may become unsanitary. This prompted the Environmental Protection Agency to launch the Airline Drinking Water Rule (ADWR) in 2009 to ensure that safe and reliable drinking water is available on aircraft. The rule provides protection for the public against disease-causing organisms that are sometimes found in the tap water on airplanes. The ADWR requires airlines to sample for bacteria, follow best management practices, take corrective action, notify the public, train operators, and follow guidelines for reporting and record-keeping to improve public health protection.

Quick Bite

Why Do Salty Foods Make You Thirsty?

The thirst mechanism is highly sensitive to extracellular sodium concentration. Even a tiny rise in sodium crosses the thirst threshold and triggers the desire to drink.

Quick Bite

Processed Foods and Salt

Salt has been used for centuries to preserve foods. Salt removes water from food and acts to dry the food. Dried (or salt-cured) food is too dry to support the growth of harmful bacteria or mold and will keep for long periods of time without refrigeration. Salt cod and salt-cured meat are examples of this. Salt is also used in many processed foods; however, in this case it acts as a flavor enhancer as opposed to a preservative. Below are examples of the amounts of salt used in processing. It is easy to see how processed foods contribute so heavily to the overall sodium content of the diet.

person; the word *salary* is derived from the Latin word for salt. Sodium is, in fact, an essential nutrient of great importance.

Sodium is critical for regulating both cellular fluid and total body fluid. Although most sodium is in extracellular fluid, it acts together with other electrolytes both within and outside of cells to regulate fluid levels, blood pressure, and pH (acidity and alkalinity). The movement of sodium back and forth across cell membranes helps regulate the transit of other substances that tag along or travel in the opposite direction. Sodium, as well as other electrolytes, helps transmit nerve impulses and other electrical messages.

Dietary Recommendations and Sources of Sodium

Although sodium is required for optimal health, getting enough of this mineral is rarely an issue; in fact, most of us eat substantially more than we need. Actual sodium requirements by the body are relatively small—only a few hundred milligrams daily. To make sure that the diet contains adequate amounts of all nutrients, however, the Food and Nutrition Board set the AI for sodium for adults at 1,500 milligrams per day (the amount in about 2/3 teaspoon of table salt).[14] This suggested AI level is similar to the American Heart Association's recommendation to "Choose and prepare foods with little or no salt." The recommendation for Americans to reduce sodium from the typical intake of 3,000–6,000 mg per day is strongly supported in the scientific literature. Lowering sodium intake to 2,300 mg per day is associated with a decreased risk of chronic illness, specifically heart disease and hypertention.[15] To lower blood pressure, aim to eat no more than 2,400 milligrams of sodium per day. Reducing daily intake to 1,500 mg is desirable because it can lower blood pressure even further.[16] Further, the Tolerable Upper Intake Level (UL) for sodium is 2,300 milligrams per day (the amount in about 1 teaspoon of table salt), which all Americans, regardless of risk factors, should try to stay below. The typical American diet contains 3,000 to 6,000 milligrams of sodium daily. Surprisingly, processed foods—not table salt—contribute the most sodium. **TABLE 8.1** shows the effects processing has on the sodium content of various foods.

The suggestion by the American Heart Association and the *2015–2020 Dietary Guidelines for Americans* to further reduce sodium to 1,500 mg for some groups is, however, not without controversy. An Institute of Medicine report indicates that recommending sodium intake below 2,300 mg is not strongly grounded in science and that more controlled studies are needed before this recommendation should be made.[17] Simultaneous to this debate is the fact that typical intake in most people is well above even the 2,300 mg level, let alone approaching 1,500 mg. With the current food supply (i.e., processed foods containing large amounts of sodium even in "low-sodium" versions of products), it may not be possible to reach dietary guidelines of even 2,300 mg per day.[18] More research is needed to identify optimal sodium levels for all populations to decrease risk of chronic illness. Work with food manufacturers is needed to decrease levels of sodium found in foods commonly consumed.

Dealing with Excess Sodium

Although some illnesses can drive down blood sodium to dangerously low levels, our bodies usually must deal with an excess of sodium.

THINK About It 2

TABLE 8.1
Sodium Content of Various Foods

Food	Serving Size	Sodium (mg)
Cucumber, with peel, raw	1 large (301 g)	6
Pickles, cucumber, dill	1 large (135 g)	1,092
Pork, loin, roasted	3 oz (85 g)	42
Ham, cured	3 oz (85 g)	1,128
Whole-wheat bread	1 slice (28 g)	146
Biscuit from recipe	4" biscuit (101 g)	586
Tomatoes, fresh	1 (123 g)	6
Spaghetti sauce, ready-to-serve	1/2 cup (132 g)	577
Milk, 2% milkfat	1 cup (244 g)	145
American cheese	1 oz (28.35 g)	468
Baked potato	1 (156 g)	8
Potato chips	1 oz (28.35 g)	148

Note: As food becomes more processed, the sodium content increases.

Data from US Department of Agriculture, Agricultural Research Service. USDA National Nutrient Database for Standard Reference, Release 28. 2015. http://www.ars.usda.gov/Services/docs.htm?docid=8964. Accessed September 8, 2017.

In some people, eating too much sodium over a long period of time can contribute to hypertension. Your intestinal tract absorbs nearly all dietary sodium, which travels throughout the body in the bloodstream. Your kidneys, those remarkable organs, retain the exact amount of sodium the body needs and excrete the excess sodium in the urine along with water.

Key Concepts Sodium in the extracellular fluid plays a critical role in regulating water distribution and blood pressure. The American diet contains an overabundance of sodium—3,000 to 6,000 milligrams daily. The AI for sodium is 1,500 milligrams per day (the amount in about 2/3 teaspoon of table salt), and the UL is 2,300 milligrams (the amount in about 1 teaspoon of table salt). Processed foods supply most of the sodium in our diets. Extreme sodium restriction is unwise and may reduce the availability of some vitamins and minerals.

Potassium

Nearly all the body's potassium resides within cells, with the highest amount in muscle cells. The flow of potassium into and out of cells is coupled to the flow of sodium. Together, potassium and sodium help contract muscles, transmit nerve impulses, and regulate blood pressure and heartbeat. The central nervous system protects its potassium, maintaining constant levels even when muscle and blood levels drop.

Like sodium, potassium affects blood pressure, but in a different way. When people with hypertension eat a diet low in sodium and rich in high-potassium foods (such as fruits and vegetables), their blood pressure and risk of coronary heart disease often improves.[19]

2015–2020 Dietary Guidelines for Americans

Key Recommendations
- Reduce daily sodium intake to less than 2,300 milligrams (mg); further reduction to 1,500 mg per day *can* [emphasis added] result in even greater blood pressure reduction.
- Limit consumption of foods that contain refined grains, especially refined grain foods that contain solid fats, added sugars, and sodium.

U.S. Department of Agriculture and U.S. Department of Health and Human Services. *Dietary Guidelines for Americans, 2010*. 7th Edition, Washington, DC: U.S. Government Printing Office, December 2010.

Dietary Recommendations and Sources of Potassium

Based on studies showing that potassium blunts the blood-pressure-raising effects of salt, the DRI committee suggested a target intake level (AI) of 4,700 milligrams of potassium per day for adults.[20] This amount is higher than the current Daily Value of 3,500 milligrams and substantially more than most Americans eat (2,000 to 3,000 milligrams per day).

Vegetables and fruits, especially potatoes, spinach, melons, and bananas, are important dietary potassium sources. Meat, fish, poultry, and dairy products are also good sources. (See **FIGURE 8.11**.) Many, but not all, salt substitutes contain potassium chloride. Generous intakes of fruits and vegetables, as recommended by the MyPlate food guidance system, will help increase potassium intake. African Americans may especially benefit from increased potassium intake—this population group typically has a low intake of potassium and a high prevalence of hypertension and salt sensitivity.[21] Although food manufacturers often add sodium to processed foods, they do not routinely add potassium. So if a person's diet includes a lot of processed foods, it may fail to meet the potassium recommendations.

When Potassium Balance Goes Awry

Moderate potassium deficiency is a likely factor in hypertension risk, especially when coupled with high sodium intakes. Results from a recent study suggest that U.S. adults who were eating more sodium and less potassium had a 50 percent higher risk of dying from any cause and more than twice the likelihood of dying from a heart attack than adults who ate less sodium and more potassium.[22] These findings further emphasize current dietary recommendations to reduce sodium intake and eat more fruits and vegetables.

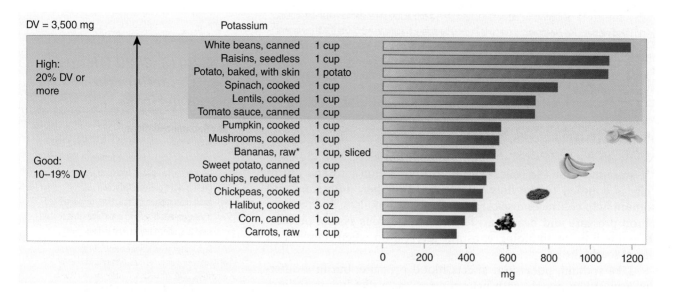

FIGURE 8.11 Food sources of potassium. The best food sources of potassium are fresh fruits and vegetables, certain dairy products, and fish.

Data from US Department of Agriculture, Agricultural Research Service, Nutrient Data Laboratory. USDA National Nutrient Database for Standard Reference, Release 28. Version Current: September 2015. Internet: http://www.ars.usda.gov/nea/bhnrc/ndl.
Raisins: © Kekyalyaynen/ Shutterstock, Inc; A bowl with cooked lentils: © nito/ Shutterstock, Inc.; Bananas: © Maks Narodenko/Shutterstock; Heap of potato chips: © Pavlo_K/ Shutterstock, Inc.

Low potassium intake can also disrupt acid–base balance in the body and contribute to bone loss and kidney stones.[23] Severe potassium deficiency usually results from excessive losses. Prolonged vomiting, chronic diarrhea, laxative abuse, and use of diuretics are the most common causes of low blood potassium. Physicians monitor electrolyte blood levels of patients taking diuretics and recommend potassium supplements if needed. Symptoms of low blood potassium include muscle weakness, loss of appetite, and confusion. If potassium depletion is severe or rapid, heart rhythms may be disrupted—a potentially fatal problem.

Because the kidneys effectively remove excess potassium, in healthy people the risk of toxicity from dietary intake is low. Potassium supplements, available over the counter and sold in health food stores, should be taken only when recommended by a physician. Extremely high blood potassium levels can slow and eventually stop the heart.

> **Key Concepts** Potassium is found mainly in intracellular fluid. Along with sodium, it regulates muscle contractions and nerve impulse transmissions. For healthy adults, the AI for potassium is 4,700 milligrams per day, substantially more than most Americans consume. Vegetables and fruits are good potassium sources and are low in sodium. Extremely high or low blood potassium can cause heartbeat irregularities and death.

Chloride

Chloride is a component of table salt and other salts. (Do not confuse chloride with chlorine gas, Cl_2, a highly reactive gas used in water treatment plants and swimming pools to kill germs.)

Both sodium and chloride help maintain the body's fluid balance. You have probably noticed the salty taste that sodium chloride (NaCl) imparts to blood, sweat, and tears. Although chloride readily moves into and out of cells, it resides mainly in extracellular fluid. Chloride is crucial to transmitting nerve impulses and to maintaining acid–base balance. It also is a component of hydrochloric acid produced by the stomach. Hydrochloric acid is required for digestion; it also kills disease-causing bacteria ingested in food.

Dietary Recommendations and Sources of Chloride

Most of us consume much more chloride than the 2,300 milligrams per day that is the adult AI.[24] The Daily Value for chloride is 3,400 milligrams, just under the adult UL, which is 3,600 milligrams per day. Most of our chloride intake comes from salt. (For dietary sources, see the "Sodium" section earlier in this chapter.) You usually can estimate the chloride content of processed foods from the sodium content with this simple formula:

$$\text{Chloride content} = 1.5 \times \text{Sodium content}$$

The average intake of chloride from salt alone is 4,500 milligrams per day (7.5 grams of salt), which is much more than recommended. Reducing the use of salt, as recommended in the *2015–2020 Dietary Guidelines for Americans*, will reduce chloride intake. The kidneys excrete excess chloride, and some chloride also is lost in sweat. Severe dehydration is the only known cause of high blood chloride levels.

Quick **Bite**

Versatile Potassium

During the Middle Ages, saltpeter (potassium nitrate) was discovered to be a useful substance. It was used as a means of extracting other minerals from rock, as a fertilizer, and as an ingredient in gunpowder. It wasn't used to cure meat until the sixteenth or seventeenth century. Saltpeter was a major ingredient in the curing mixture until 1940, about the time that refrigeration emerged. Today, food manufacturers use small amounts of nitrites rather than saltpeter to preserve foods such as bacon, ham, and some sausages.

Quick **Bite**

Low-Calorie Chlorine?

Sucralose is a low-calorie sweetener made from sugar. During manufacture, a multistep process substitutes three chlorine atoms for three hydrogen–oxygen groups on the sugar molecule. This creates an exceptionally stable molecular structure that is 600 times sweeter than sugar. The sucralose molecule is chemically and biologically inert, so it passes through the body without being digested and is eliminated after consumption.

Who Risks Chloride Deficiency?

Excessive chloride loss is the most common cause of chloride deficiency. Vomiting expels stomach acid (hydrochloric acid), which contains a lot of chloride. People with bulimia nervosa often use self-induced vomiting as a way to compensate for binge eating and thus may have low chloride levels. Low blood chloride slows blood flow to the brain and oxygen delivery to tissues. It also disrupts the body's acid–base balance and causes heartbeat irregularities. Untreated low blood chloride levels can be life threatening.

Key Concepts In addition to its role as an electrolyte, chloride is a component of hydrochloric acid. The minimum chloride requirement for healthy adults is 750 milligrams per day, far below average intakes. Most dietary chloride comes from salt intake. People who frequently induce vomiting risk chloride deficiency.

Calcium

Although only 1.5 to 2 percent of our body weight, calcium is the most abundant mineral in our bodies. It's important to have adequate calcium throughout life so that bones and teeth can remain strong into old age. Getting enough calcium in your diet also may help prevent hypertension, decrease your odds of getting colon or breast cancer, improve weight control, and reduce the risk of developing kidney stones.

Functions of Calcium

Over 99 percent of your body's calcium is found in bones and teeth, making them hard and strong. Although less than 1 percent of body calcium is in blood and soft tissue, that tiny amount has vitally important roles in muscle contraction, nerve impulse transmission, blood clotting, and cell metabolism. (See **FIGURE 8.12**.)

Bone Structure

Think of bone as living tissue that responds to physical stresses. Most of the time, bone is able to withstand tremendous force without breaking. By weight, bone is two-thirds mineral and one-third water and protein, primarily collagen. Most bone calcium is part of **hydroxyapatite**—a hard, crystalline complex of calcium and phosphorus that surrounds collagen fibers.

Our bones undergo constant remodeling by two types of bone cells—**osteoblasts** and **osteoclasts**. Osteoblasts are the construction team, and osteoclasts are the demolition team. Together they determine how bones grow and change over time. Bone **mineralization** is greatest while children are growing taller and for 5 to 10 years thereafter. Although we usually achieve our peak bone mass at around age 30, bone responds to physical activities throughout our lives. In areas under repeated stress, bone thickens and becomes denser. Even older adults can strengthen and rebuild their bones through weight-bearing exercise such as walking or weight lifting.[25]

Bone also is a reservoir of calcium and phosphorus. When needed, blood and soft tissues can draw upon this reserve. Blood calcium levels must be kept constant at all costs, even at the expense of bone

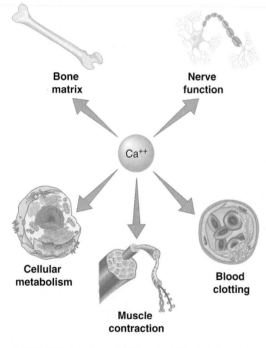

FIGURE 8.12 **Functions of calcium.** In addition to its key role in bone health, calcium in blood and soft tissues is essential for such diverse functions as blood clotting, muscle contractions, and nerve impulse transmission.

▶ **hydroxyapatite** A crystalline mineral compound of calcium and phosphorus that makes up bone.

▶ **osteoblasts** Bone cells that synthesize and excrete the extracellular matrix that forms the structure of bone.

▶ **osteoclasts** Bone cells that break down bone structure and release calcium and phosphate into the blood.

▶ **mineralization** The addition of minerals, such as calcium and phosphate, to bones and teeth.

strength, so that calcium's roles in nerve function, blood clotting, muscle contraction, and cellular metabolism can proceed without a hitch.

Calcium, Muscles, and Metabolism

Calcium has a central role in muscle contractions, because the flow of calcium ions inside muscle cells causes muscles to contract or relax. During exercise, one cause of muscle fatigue is the impaired activity of calcium in muscle cells.

Calmodulin is a calcium-sensing protein found throughout the body. When it binds calcium, calmodulin helps regulate a number of cellular processes, including cell division, cell proliferation, **ciliary action**, and cell secretions.

Other Functions of Calcium

Blood cannot clot without calcium, but blood calcium levels seldom fall this low. Calcium participates in nearly every step in the production of **fibrin**, the protein that gives structure to blood clots. Nerve cells need calcium to transmit signals. In fact, the strength of a nerve signal is in direct proportion to the number of calcium ions crossing the nerve cell membrane.

Regulation of Blood Calcium Levels

To prevent even minor dips in blood calcium levels, your body will demineralize bone. Even if calcium intake is very low, blood calcium levels remain steady. Three hormones—calcitriol (the active form of vitamin D), parathyroid hormone (PTH), and calcitonin—regulate calcium status.

When blood calcium levels are low, calcitriol increases intestinal absorption of calcium. PTH from the parathyroid glands activates osteoclasts that release bone calcium. PTH also signals the kidneys to conserve more calcium and to produce more calcitriol. When calcium levels become too high, the thyroid gland secretes calcitonin, which acts in opposition to PTH and causes blood calcium levels to return to normal.

Dietary Recommendations for Calcium

During every life stage, optimal calcium intake is critical. If children and young adults fail to take in enough calcium, they are more likely to develop osteoporosis later in life. As we age, optimal calcium intake slows bone loss, helping preserve bone density.

Calcium recommendations are aimed at minimizing osteoporosis risk. The RDAs are 1,000 milligrams calcium per day for adults ages 19 to 50 years and men to age 70. For women 51 years or older and adults over the age of 70 years, this increases to 1,200 milligrams per day. For children and teens ages 9 to 18 years, the RDA is 1,300 milligrams per day, a level meant to maximize peak bone mass.[26] Unfortunately, many of us fall far short of recommended calcium intakes. Most children and adolescents worldwide fail to meet calcium recommendations, making it difficult for them to achieve peak bone mass and leaving them vulnerable to osteoporosis as they age.[27] Excessive caffeine, alcohol, and sodium intake and misuse of diuretics—factors that increase urinary calcium—make bone loss worse.[28]

▶ **calmodulin** A calcium-binding protein that regulates a variety of cellular activities, such as cell division and proliferation.

▶ **ciliary action** Wave-like motion of small hair-like projections on some cells.

▶ **fibrin** A stringy, insoluble protein that is the final product of the blood-clotting process.

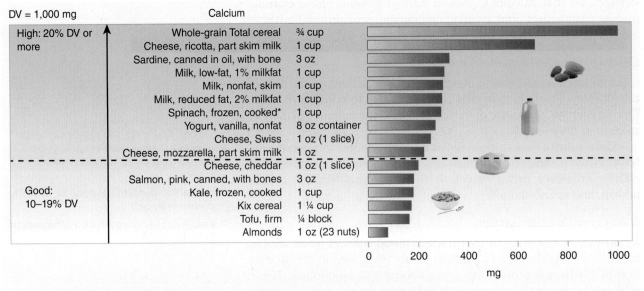

DV = 1,000 mg   Calcium

		mg
High: 20% DV or more	Whole-grain Total cereal	¾ cup
	Cheese, ricotta, part skim milk	1 cup
	Sardine, canned in oil, with bone	3 oz
	Milk, low-fat, 1% milkfat	1 cup
	Milk, nonfat, skim	1 cup
	Milk, reduced fat, 2% milkfat	1 cup
	Spinach, frozen, cooked*	1 cup
	Yogurt, vanilla, nonfat	8 oz container
	Cheese, Swiss	1 oz (1 slice)
	Cheese, mozzarella, part skim milk	1 oz
Good: 10–19% DV	Cheese, cheddar	1 oz (1 slice)
	Salmon, pink, canned, with bones	3 oz
	Kale, frozen, cooked	1 cup
	Kix cereal	1 ¼ cup
	Tofu, firm	¼ block
	Almonds	1 oz (23 nuts)

0   200   400   600   800   1000
mg

* In spinach, oxalate binds calcium and prevents absorption of all but about 5 percent of the plant's calcium.

FIGURE 8.13 **Food sources of calcium.** Calcium is found in milk and dairy products, certain green leafy vegetables, and canned fish with bones.

Data from US Department of Agriculture, Agricultural Research Service, Nutrient Data Laboratory. USDA National Nutrient Database for Standard Reference, Release 28. Version Current: September 2015. Internet: http://www.ars.usda.gov/nea/bhnrc/ndl.

Bowl of sugar-coated corn flakes and spoon: © Oliver Hoffmann/Shutterstock, Inc.; Ripe white Mozzarella di Bufala, Italian water buffalo milk cheese: © Dorling Kindersley/ Getty Images; Milk Bottle with Red Cap: © Mega Pixel/ Shutterstock, Inc.; Dried almonds: © Dionisvera/Shutterstock, Inc.

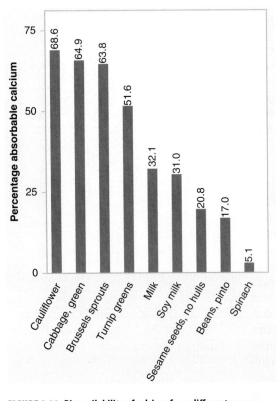

FIGURE 8.14 **Bioavailability of calcium from different sources.** Your body can absorb more than two-thirds of the calcium in cauliflower, but only about 5 percent of the calcium in spinach. Oxalate in spinach binds to calcium and inhibits its bioavailability.

Modified from Weaver CM, Plawecki KL. Dietary calcium: adequacy of a vegetarian diet. *Am J Clin Nutr.* 1994;59(suppl):1238S–1241S.

Sources of Calcium

Dairy products are the best source of calcium in the American diet.[29] (See **FIGURE 8.13**.) Nonfat milk and yogurt are especially good, providing high calcium with minimal calories and little or no fat. Although ice cream and cheese are good sources, they are also high in fat. Among dairy foods, cottage cheese and cream cheese contain the least calcium.

Other significant sources are green vegetables such as broccoli, Chinese cabbage, turnip greens and other "greens," and tofu processed with calcium. However, leafy vegetables in the spinach family are high in the mineral oxalate, which binds to calcium, thus limiting intestinal absorption. (See **FIGURE 8.14**.) If you eat the bones, canned fish with bones, such as sardines, provide lots of calcium.

Certain brands of soy milk, fruit juice, breakfast cereal, and bread are now fortified with calcium. These are convenient calcium sources for people who don't eat dairy foods. Check labels carefully because only a few products are fortified with calcium. Some dairies also add extra calcium or calcium-containing milk solids to their products.

People with limited dairy intake may need calcium supplements to ensure adequate intake. Flavored chewable calcium supplements that also contain vitamins D and K are an easy-to-take source of extra calcium. (See the FYI feature "Calcium Supplements: Are They Right for You?")

Calcium Absorption

Calcium absorption is relatively inefficient; we usually absorb only about 25–35 percent of the calcium we eat, and the efficiency of absorption decreases as calcium intake increases.[30]

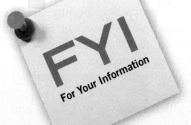

Calcium Supplements: Are They Right for You?

After reading the section on calcium, you may be wondering whether you need a calcium supplement. After all, calcium is critical for so many bodily functions, and getting enough calcium reduces the risk of osteoporosis later in life.

Before you head to the supplement aisle at the grocery store, take a critical look at your diet, especially your intake of milk and other dairy products. In the United States and Canada, dairy foods are the major sources of dietary calcium; without them, it may be difficult to reach the RDA for calcium. People who exclude dairy products, such as vegans and those with milk allergy, must choose foods carefully to find rich calcium sources.

Calcium sources vary widely in their bioavailability. Although labels are required to list the %DV for calcium, they don't indicate how much of that calcium the body will absorb. For example, 1/2 cup of spinach contains about 120 milligrams of calcium, but also contains oxalate, which binds to calcium in the gut; therefore, the body will absorb only 5 percent of that calcium. Intake recommendations are based on the mix of sources in the typical American diet. Other cultures manage on much lower intakes, in part because they do not consume the many food constituents that deplete calcium or reduce its absorption. Vegetarians may, in fact, need less calcium than meat eaters. If you are considering spinach as your sole source of calcium, however, you will need to eat almost 8 cups to equal the calcium available from 1 cup of milk. (About 30 percent of the 300 milligrams of calcium in 1 cup of milk is bioavailable.)

The amount of bioavailable calcium varies quite a bit among green leafy vegetables. The calcium in kale, Chinese cabbage, and mustard greens, for example, is significantly more bioavailable than spinach. Tofu can be a good vegetarian source of bioavailable calcium. If your diet is low in calcium, try adding some of the foods that are higher in calcium. Incorporating calcium-rich and calcium-fortified foods into the diet adds other important vitamins and minerals.

Even armed with more information about calcium in the diet, you may decide to investigate the supplement market. Again, you have a variety of choices: calcium carbonate, calcium citrate, calcium lactate, calcium phosphate, coral calcium … how to decide? First, it's important to know that the absorption of calcium from most supplements is about equal—roughly 30 percent. The calcium citrate malate that is used in some brands of fortified juice and a limited number of supplements is absorbed a little better—35 percent. However, a typical calcium citrate malate tablet has less calcium than a tablet of another type such as calcium carbonate. Calcium carbonate is usually the most concentrated per tablet, so taking fewer pills per day will supply enough; also, this type of supplement tends to be less expensive. Chelated calcium supplements can improve absorption a bit, but the extra expense probably is not worth it.

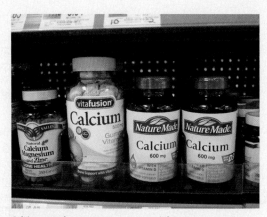

Calcium supplements are a common sight on grocery store shelves.
© picturelibrary/Alamy.

Other factors to consider are that, because minerals compete with each other for absorption, calcium supplements may be absorbed better if taken between meals. Calcium carbonate has been shown to cause constipation in some, especially in high dosage. Also, you need to get plenty of vitamin D, either through casual exposure to the sun, in fortified milk, or as part of a supplement (many calcium supplements have added vitamin D). Vitamin D is important for the absorption of calcium. In addition, bones get stronger with regular, weight-bearing exercise, such as walking, so make sure to include that in your healthful lifestyle.

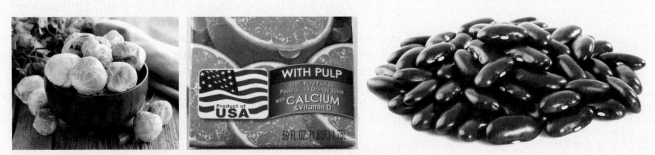

Foods that provide the calcium equivalent of 1 cup (8 fl oz) of milk.
4 cups of brussels sprouts: © Dream79/Shutterstock; Orange juice carton: © Jones & Bartlett Learning. Photo by Amy Rathburn; 7 cups of red beans: © jeehyun/Shutterstock.

Other dietary factors also affect absorption. Wheat bran, phytate (in whole grains, nuts, and seeds), and oxalate (in foods such as spinach) reduce calcium absorption. High supplement doses of phosphorus and magnesium may also interfere with calcium absorption. Because calcium depends on vitamin D to enter intestinal cells, calcium absorption drops dramatically if vitamin D status is poor.

Calcium absorption is particularly efficient during pregnancy and infancy and is least efficient in old age. If both a healthy child and a healthy adult eat exactly the same meal, all other things being equal, the growing child will absorb a much greater proportion of the dietary calcium than the adult. Low estrogen levels in postmenopausal women can lower calcium absorption to about 20 percent. Older women may take estrogen supplements, as well as calcium supplements and vitamin D, to help boost calcium absorption.

When Calcium Balance Goes Awry

Because the body uses bone calcium to maintain normal blood calcium levels, low blood calcium is relatively uncommon in the absence of illness or vitamin D deficiency. Chronically low calcium intake can overtax this reserve and lead to suboptimal bone growth in childhood and adolescence or increased rate of bone loss after menopause. Studies also link low calcium intake to an increased risk of cardiovascular disease, hypertension, colon cancer, and obesity.[31]

Although certain illnesses can cause high blood calcium, dietary calcium intake does not. Of greater dietary concern is the interaction of calcium supplements with the absorption of iron, zinc, magnesium, and phosphorus. Although calcium supplements can dramatically affect absorption of other minerals, dietary calcium intake has not been shown to cause a deficiency for any of these minerals.[32] The Food and Nutrition Board has established a UL for calcium of 2,500 milligrams per day for adults ages 19 to 50 years.

> **Key Concepts** Calcium is a major component of bones and teeth. It is also required for muscle contraction, nerve impulse transmission, blood clotting, and regulation of cell metabolism. The body ensures adequate blood calcium levels by withdrawing it from bone if needed. Dairy foods and fortified foods are major dietary sources of calcium. Optimal calcium intake throughout life reduces chances of osteoporosis.

Phosphorus

Phosphorus, along with calcium, is a component of the mineral complex hydroxyapatite in bone. Bones are the major storehouse of phosphorus, holding nearly 85 percent of our supply. The remaining phosphorus is found in cells of soft tissues, with a little bit in extracellular fluid. Most of the body's phosphorus is in the form of phosphate ion (phosphorus joined to oxygen), our most abundant anion.

Phosphorus helps activate and deactivate enzymes during the final steps in the extraction of energy from carbohydrate, fat, and protein. It also is a component of ATP, the universal energy source, and of DNA and RNA. Phosphorus is also a component of phospholipids, found in cell membranes and lipoproteins.

Dietary Recommendations and Sources of Phosphorus

The phosphorus RDA for adolescents is 1,250 milligrams per day to support growth. Although adults need only 700 milligrams per day, the average adult consumes much more, about 1,000 to 1,500 milligrams per day.[33]

Phosphorus is abundant in our food supply. Foods rich in protein (milk, meat, and eggs) generally are rich in phosphorus. (See **FIGURE 8.15**.) Food additives, especially those in processed meat and soft drinks, supply up to 30 percent of our phosphorus. To improve moisture retention and smoothness, food processors often add phosphate salts to processed foods.

Soft drinks often contain phosphoric acid, although the phosphorus level is not high—about 50 milligrams in a 12-ounce cola, compared with 370 milligrams in 12 ounces of fat-free milk. However, among heavy cola drinkers, soda is an important contributor to phosphorus intake.[34] Dairy products have phosphorus plus calcium (460 milligrams in 12 ounces), whereas sodas have phosphorus but virtually no calcium (10 milligrams or less in a 12-ounce can)—an important distinction.

We absorb about 55 to 70 percent of the phosphorus we eat. Unlike calcium absorption, phosphorus absorption does not increase as dietary intake decreases.[35] Although phosphorus is part of phytate in plant seeds (beans, peas, cereals, and nuts), we can still absorb about 50 percent. Two familiar hormones, PTH (parathyroid hormone) and calcitriol (activated vitamin D), regulate intestinal absorption of phosphorus. When phosphorus levels are low, calcitriol enhances intestinal absorption of both calcium and phosphorus. When levels are high, PTH greatly increases urinary excretion of phosphorus.

When Phosphate Balance Goes Awry

Phosphorus is so common in foods that only near total starvation causes deficiency. Some medical disorders, however, can cause low blood phosphate. Kidney disease is the most common cause of high blood phosphate. Other causes include overuse of vitamin D supplements, overuse

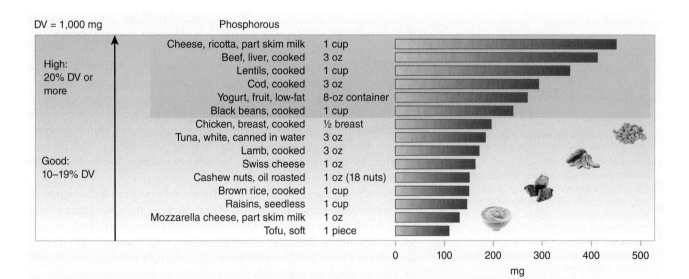

FIGURE 8.15 Food sources of phosphorus. Phosphorus is abundant in the food supply. Meats, legumes, nuts, dairy products, and grains tend to have more phosphorus than fruits and vegetables.

Data from US Department of Agriculture, Agricultural Research Service, Nutrient Data Laboratory. USDA National Nutrient Database for Standard Reference, Release 28. Version Current: September 2015. Internet: http://www.ars.usda.gov/nea/bhnrc/ndl.

Bowl of pink yogurt: © MaraZe/Shutterstock, Inc.; Beef liver: © nadi555/ Shutterstock,Inc.; Chicken breasts: © Viktor1/Shutterstock, Inc.; Cashew nuts: © SOMMAI/ Shutterstock, Inc.

Quick **Bite**

The Double Helix Depends on Phosphorus
The backbone of DNA's twisting ladder-like structure contains alternating molecules of phosphoric acid and deoxyribose.

of phosphate-containing laxatives, and diseases of the parathyroid gland. At the extreme, symptoms include muscle spasms and convulsions.

In the short term, high phosphorus intake is unlikely to produce problems in healthy people.[36] But over the long run, eating too much phosphorus, together with too little calcium, may increase bone loss. People who replace milk with cola increase their ratio of dietary phosphorus to calcium, possibly increasing their risk of osteoporosis later in life. The UL for phosphorus is 4,000 milligrams per day for people ages 9 to 70.

> **Key Concepts** Phosphorus is a component of bone, ATP, phospholipids, and genetic material. It acts as an electrolyte regulator as well. Milk, meat, and food additives are major sources of dietary phosphorus. Diets high in phosphorus and low in calcium can contribute to bone loss.

Magnesium

Magnesium is the fourth most abundant cation in our bodies. Bone holds about half the magnesium in our bodies, with the remainder distributed equally between muscle and other soft tissue. Like bone calcium, bone magnesium is a large reservoir that soft tissue can draw upon when needed. Most magnesium resides in cells, with only 1 percent in extracellular fluid.

Magnesium participates in more than 300 types of enzyme-driven reactions, including those in DNA and protein synthesis, blood clotting, muscle contraction, and ATP production. Because ATP is the universal energy source, an absence of magnesium would halt all cellular activity.

Dietary Recommendations and Sources of Magnesium

The magnesium RDA is 400 milligrams per day for men ages 19 to 30 years and 310 milligrams per day for women of the same age. The RDA rises for those 31 or older, to 420 milligrams for men and 320 milligrams for women. The average American gets only about three-fourths of this level, yet overt symptoms of low magnesium are relatively uncommon in healthy people.[37]

Magnesium is found throughout the food supply. Our main sources are plant foods. Whole grains, many vegetables, legumes, tofu, and some seafood are good sources, and chocolate contains modest amounts. (See **FIGURE 8.16**.) In some communities, "hard" tap water has significant amounts of magnesium. Unfortunately, processing and refining remove a great deal of magnesium—up to 80 percent in refined grains—and enrichment does not replace it. In general, refined foods are low in magnesium.

We absorb about 50 percent of dietary magnesium. Although high-fiber diets often have a negative effect on mineral absorption, some high-fiber foods actually improve magnesium absorption. High calcium intake, usually in the form of supplements, can interfere with magnesium absorption. People who must take calcium supplements should be sure to regularly eat foods with high magnesium content.

When Magnesium Balance Goes Awry

Magnesium deficiency is often associated with alcoholism because alcohol increases urinary magnesium excretion. Low magnesium intake typically goes hand in hand with poor intake of other nutrients, and

Quick **Bite**

Lost in Space
Knowing that stress on bones maintains their strength, what would you guess happens in the gravity-free environment of outer space? Experience with prolonged space travel has made it clear that extensive bone and mineral loss is one health hazard of living without gravity's constant pull. Interestingly, changes in non-weight-bearing bones were not seen in studies of space travelers. As humans spend longer periods in space, scientists will be challenged to discover how to preserve bone strength without the constant stimulation of gravity on weight-bearing bones.

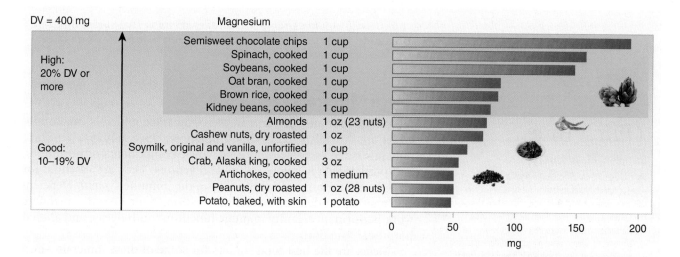

DV = 400 mg

Magnesium

High: 20% DV or more	Semisweet chocolate chips	1 cup
	Spinach, cooked	1 cup
	Soybeans, cooked	1 cup
	Oat bran, cooked	1 cup
	Brown rice, cooked	1 cup
	Kidney beans, cooked	1 cup
Good: 10–19% DV	Almonds	1 oz (23 nuts)
	Cashew nuts, dry roasted	1 oz
	Soymilk, original and vanilla, unfortified	1 cup
	Crab, Alaska king, cooked	3 oz
	Artichokes, cooked	1 medium
	Peanuts, dry roasted	1 oz (28 nuts)
	Potato, baked, with skin	1 potato

FIGURE 8.16 Food sources of magnesium. Most of the magnesium in the diet comes from plant foods such as grains, vegetables, and legumes.

Data from US Department of Agriculture, Agricultural Research Service, Nutrient Data Laboratory. USDA National Nutrient Database for Standard Reference, Release 28. Version Current: September 2015. Internet: http://www.ars.usda.gov/nea/bhnrc/ndl.

Chocolate chips: © masa44/ Shutterstock, Inc.; Dish of steamed spinach: © Smneedham/ iStockphoto; King Crab Legs: © Jason Lugo/ iStock / Getty Images Plus; Two Artichokes on White: © MidoSemsem/ Shutterstock, Inc.

magnesium deficiency by itself is unusual.[38] Poor magnesium status also may occur with certain chronic illnesses, such as diabetes mellitus, renal disease, or cardiovascular disease, and is worsened by diarrhea and vomiting.[39]

In research studies, healthy people on magnesium-deficient diets have no symptoms for several weeks. Once bone reserves are depleted, loss of appetite, nausea, and weakness gradually develop. After more time, muscle cramps, irritability, and confusion occur. Low magnesium disrupts heart rhythm; if the deficiency becomes extreme, heart abnormalities can lead to death. Magnesium toxicity causes diarrhea, nausea, weakness, paralysis, and cardiac and respiratory failure.[40] In the absence of kidney disease, an abnormally high blood level of magnesium is uncommon. The UL for supplemental magnesium is 350 milligrams per day.

Key Concepts Magnesium participates in more than 300 reactions, including several in energy metabolism. It's required for cardiac and nerve function. Magnesium reserves are stored in bone. Whole grains and vegetables are good sources of magnesium. People with chronic diarrhea, poor diet, and heavy alcohol use are at risk of deficiency. Because magnesium ions help regulate heartbeat, heart rhythm irregularities occur if blood levels are too low.

Sulfur

Unlike the other minerals discussed in this chapter, sulfur does not function alone. In the body, sulfur is primarily a component of organic (carbon-containing) nutrients, such as the vitamins biotin and thiamin, as well as the amino acids methionine and cysteine. The sulfur in amino acids helps stabilize the three-dimensional shapes of proteins such as those in skin, hair, and nails. The liver's detoxification pathways require sulfur, and sulfate (sulfur combined with oxygen) helps maintain acid–base balance. Typical diets contain ample sulfur, and deficiency is unknown in humans.

Key Concepts Sulfur is a component of some amino acids and the vitamins biotin and thiamin. It helps proteins maintain their functional shapes. Sulfur is important in liver function and in maintaining acid–base balance. Human sulfur deficiency is unknown.

Trace Minerals

Despite the minute amounts in the body, trace minerals (microminerals) are crucial to many body functions. (See **FIGURE 8.17**.) Trace minerals serve as cofactors for enzymes, components of hormones, and participants in many chemical reactions. They are essential for growth and for normal functioning of the immune system. Deficiencies may cause delayed sexual maturation, poor growth, mediocre work performance, faulty immune function, tooth decay, and altered hormonal function.

Meats are the best food sources for some of these minerals—iron and zinc, for instance. Whole grains are also good sources of several minerals, including iron, copper, selenium, and manganese. Water is a major source of fluoride, a mineral that often occurs naturally in water or is added during municipal water treatment. Amounts in plant foods can differ dramatically from region to region, depending on the soil's mineral content. Even the maturity of a vegetable, fruit, or grain can influence its mineral content. A varied diet typically includes foods from many different locales and thus from a wide variety of soils.

Technological advances have triggered an explosion of exciting research because scientists can now track trace minerals throughout the body more effectively. Working together, nutritionists, biochemists, biologists, immunologists, geneticists, and epidemiologists are uncovering the mysteries behind many of these fascinating minerals and finding new links between trace minerals and a variety of diseases and genetic disorders.

Quick Bite

Do Onions Make You Cry?

The cabbage and onion families have sulfur-based compounds that are transformed into odiferous compounds when their tissues are broken. Cutting into a raw onion mixes the contents of its cells, bringing enzymes into contact with an odorless precursor substance apparently derived from the sulfur-containing amino acid cysteine. The volatile result, a powerful sulfur-containing irritant, causes most people's eyes to water, apparently by dissolving in fluids that surround the eye and forming sulfuric acid.

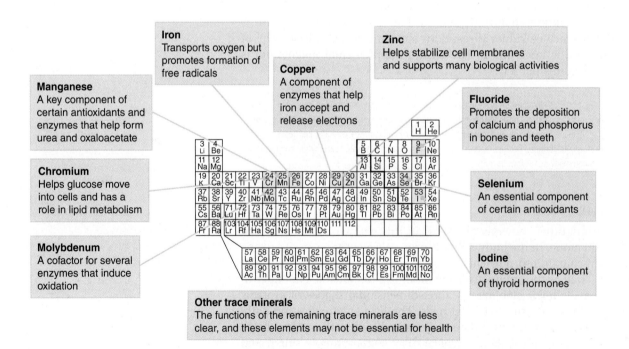

FIGURE 8.17 Trace minerals on the periodic table. Trace minerals are found in the body and required in the diet in small amounts, but they play important roles in the body.

Iron

Iron is among the most abundant minerals in the earth's crust. Yet iron deficiency is the most common nutrient deficiency in the world. Iron deficiency not only affects a large number of children and women in developing countries, but also is the only nutrient deficiency that is significantly prevalent in industrialized countries.[41] Iron has a special property that allows it to easily transfer electrons to and from other atoms. This ability makes iron essential for numerous reactions and allows it to easily bind and release oxygen. Iron's abilities also endow it with a dark side—the ability to promote formation of destructive free radicals.

Functions of Iron

Iron is well known for its role in transporting oxygen in the blood. Iron also is an essential component of hundreds of enzymes, many of which are involved in energy metabolism. In addition, iron plays a role in brain development and in the immune system. **FIGURE 8.18** shows the functions of iron.

Oxygen Transport

Iron is vital to oxygen transport and sits at the center of **heme**—the iron-containing portion of hemoglobin and **myoglobin**. (See **FIGURE 8.19**.) Hemoglobin carries oxygen in the blood; myoglobin resides in muscle and moves oxygen into muscle cells.

As blood passes through the lungs, hemoglobin loads up on oxygen and turns bright red. It transports oxygen through arteries to tissues throughout the body. Upon reaching its destination, hemoglobin flows through tiny capillaries, crossing capillary walls and delivering its oxygen cargo to target cells. Depleted of oxygen, hemoglobin turns a dark bluish-red and travels through veins back to the lungs for another load of oxygen.

Enzymes

Iron-containing enzymes play a vital role in reactions widespread in energy metabolism. Hundreds of enzymes contain iron or need iron as a cofactor. These enzymes drive reactions necessary for energy production, amino acid metabolism, and muscle function. Excess iron promotes the formation of highly reactive and destructive free radicals. Ironically, iron also is a cofactor of antioxidant enzymes that protect against free radical damage.

Immune Function

Optimal immune function requires iron. However, in areas of the world with rampant disease and iron deficiency, a dilemma arises. Iron nourishes certain bacteria, so iron supplementation can worsen an infection. In the absence of an infection, iron supplementation is appropriate for treating iron deficiency.

Brain Function

Iron is essential for optimal brain and nervous system development and function. Children with low iron status have impaired growth and intellectual development.[42] How does a lack of iron affect the brain? We know that iron is involved in producing the protective covering, or myelin sheath, that surrounds nerve cells. Iron also is involved in producing neurotransmitters, chemicals that carry messages between nerve cells.

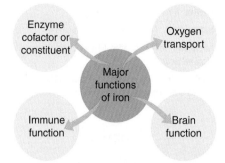

FIGURE 8.18 Major functions of iron. Well known for its role in transporting oxygen in the blood, iron also is essential for optimal immune function and nerve health. In addition, it is a cofactor in numerous reactions.

▶ **heme** A chemical complex with a central iron atom that forms the oxygen-binding part of hemoglobin and myoglobin.

▶ **myoglobin** The oxygen-transporting protein of muscle that resembles blood hemoglobin in function.

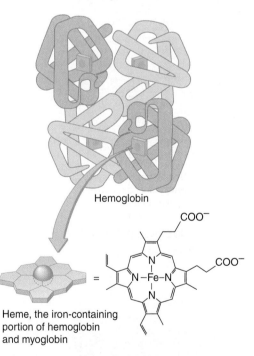

FIGURE 8.19 Heme in hemoglobin. Iron in the heme portion of hemoglobin and myoglobin binds and releases oxygen easily. Hemoglobin in red blood cells transports oxygen in the blood and gives blood its red color.

▶ **ferritin** A major storage form of iron.

▶ **hemosiderin** An insoluble form of storage iron.

▶ **heme iron** The iron found in the hemoglobin and myoglobin of animal foods.

▶ **nonheme iron** The iron in plants and animal foods that is not part of hemoglobin or myoglobin.

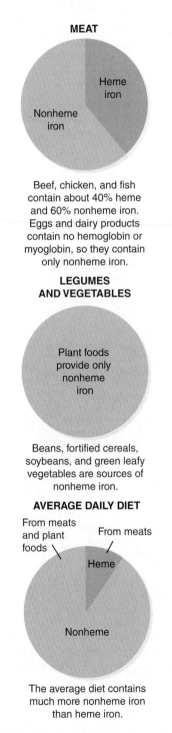

MEAT

Heme iron

Nonheme iron

Beef, chicken, and fish contain about 40% heme and 60% nonheme iron. Eggs and dairy products contain no hemoglobin or myoglobin, so they contain only nonheme iron.

LEGUMES AND VEGETABLES

Plant foods provide only nonheme iron

Beans, fortified cereals, soybeans, and green leafy vegetables are sources of nonheme iron.

AVERAGE DAILY DIET

From meats and plant foods

From meats

Heme

Nonheme

The average diet contains much more nonheme iron than heme iron.

FIGURE 8.20 Sources of heme and nonheme iron. Heme iron is found only in meats. Nonheme iron is found in both plant and animal foods.

Regulation of Iron in the Body

Total body iron averages about 4 grams in men and a little more than 2 grams in women.[43] Most of your body's iron is in hemoglobin, with the remainder in myoglobin and enzymes. If you're well nourished, you'll have good iron reserves stored as **ferritin** and **hemosiderin**.

But too much iron is toxic. Your body carefully performs a balancing act, adjusting iron absorption, transport, storage, and loss to optimize the amounts of actively functioning iron and iron reserves without exceeding safe levels.

Iron Absorption

Intestinal cells act as gatekeepers, absorbing needed iron but turning away excess (and potentially harmful) iron. The actual amount absorbed depends on the body's iron status and need, normal GI function, the amount and type of iron in the diet, and dietary factors that enhance or inhibit iron absorption. Once intestinal cells admit iron, they can use it immediately, release it to the blood, or store it for later. These cells have a major role in regulating the amount of iron in the body and help prevent toxic accumulations. During normal cell turnover, the GI tract sloughs intestinal cells. When excreted, these dead cells carry their stored iron out of the body.

Effect of Iron Status on Iron Absorption   Iron status is the primary factor in determining how much iron a person will absorb from food.[44] Depending on need, iron absorption can vary from less than 1 percent to greater than 50 percent. On average, adult men absorb about 6 percent of dietary iron, and nonpregnant women of childbearing age absorb about 13 percent. Women absorb a higher proportion to make up for iron losses from menstruation.

Normally, absorption is more efficient when circulating iron and iron reserves are low. Absorption is highest among iron-deficient people, and it slows as iron reserves become filled. An increase in red blood cell production—during pregnancy, for example, or after blood loss—increases the body's need for iron and can trigger a severalfold increase in iron uptake.

Effect of GI Function on Iron Absorption   To prepare iron for intestinal absorption, you need adequate stomach acid. Because stomach acid generally declines with aging, iron absorption tends to be less efficient in seniors. Overuse of antacids also can affect iron bioavailability.

Effect of the Amount and Form of Iron in Food   All other factors being equal, the less iron in your diet, the greater the proportion you absorb. This ability to conserve dietary iron no doubt helped people survive when iron-rich foods were scarce. But it has its limits—if iron intake is routinely too low, anemia will emerge over time.

Food contains two types of iron: **heme iron** and **nonheme iron**. Heme iron is a part of hemoglobin and myoglobin, so it is found only in animal tissue. Meat, fish, and poultry contain about 40 percent heme iron and 60 percent nonheme iron. In contrast, plant foods and iron-fortified foods contain only nonheme iron. (See **FIGURE 8.20**.) Eggs and dairy products contain small amounts of nonheme iron only. Vegan diets, by definition, contain no heme iron.

Heme iron is much more bioavailable than nonheme iron.[45] Therefore, meats, poultry, fish, and seafood have the most efficiently absorbed iron. Vegetarians need more iron than do people who eat foods with heme iron.

Dietary Factors That Enhance Iron Absorption   You can improve the bioavailability of nonheme iron with vitamin C. (See **TABLE 8.2.**) Eating fruits and vegetables—good sources of vitamin C—along with iron-containing foods enhances nonheme iron absorption. Eating heme iron foods (called the meat factor) along with nonheme iron foods also improves nonheme iron absorption.

Dietary Factors That Inhibit Iron Absorption   Whole grains contain phytate, which inhibits iron absorption. However, whole-grain foods are healthy in other respects, so don't avoid them. Instead, include vitamin C–rich fruits and vegetables, which counter the inhibitory effects of phytate.

Polyphenols, found in tea, coffee, other beverages, and many plants, limit nonheme iron absorption. Foods from soybeans, foods containing oxalates, and high-fiber foods in general also tend to inhibit nonheme iron absorption.

Calcium, zinc, and iron compete for absorption, and each can inhibit absorption of another mineral.[46] Many women take calcium supplements to reduce their risk of osteoporosis. To minimize interference with iron absorption, they should take their calcium supplements alone at bedtime rather than with meals.

Iron Transport and Storage

Transferrin is the carrier protein that ferries iron through the blood. It delivers iron from the intestines to the bone marrow for manufacture into hemoglobin, and it carries iron to all other body tissues as needed. (See **FIGURE 8.21.**)

The body stores surplus iron in two forms. Most iron is stored as ferritin, and smaller amounts are stored as hemosiderin. Although small amounts of ferritin circulate in blood, the liver, bone marrow, spleen, and skeletal muscle hold most iron reserves. Over time, a negative iron balance can deplete these reserves, and iron deficiency ensues.

Iron Turnover and Loss

The body is good at conserving iron, a trait probably acquired in ancient times when availability of high-iron foods was uncertain and irregular. The normal, routine destruction of old red blood cells releases iron, which the body recycles as it builds new red blood cells. A healthy adult man, for example, produces new red blood cells with about 95 percent recycled iron. Diet or iron stores must supply the remaining 5 percent. During periods of rapid growth and blood expansion, iron needs outstrip the supply of recycled and stored iron. Dietary iron makes up the difference. During infancy, for example, dietary iron supplies about 30 percent of iron for new red blood cells.

We lose small amounts of iron every day—a milligram or so in feces, sweat, and sloughed-off mucosal and skin cells. Women lose considerably more during menstruation. Pregnancy increases iron needs markedly to support growth of the fetus and expansion of the maternal blood supply. Blood loss with childbirth depletes iron; thus, women with repeated pregnancies close together are likely to have poor iron status and need extra iron.

Digestive disorders can increase blood and iron losses significantly. Any condition in which there is bleeding or accelerated destruction of intestinal cells—ulcer, cancer, inflammatory bowel disease, celiac disease, parasitic infection—can lead to iron-deficiency anemia.

TABLE 8.2
Factors That Affect Iron Absorption

Inhibitors	Enhancers
Fiber and phytate	Vitamin C (ascorbic acid)
Calcium and phosphorus (milk/dairy)	Factor in meat, poultry, fish, and eggs
Tannins, found in tea	Hydrochloric acid secreted in the stomach
Polyphenols	Citric, malic, and lactic acid
Oxalate	

▶ **polyphenols** Organic compounds that may produce bitterness in coffee and tea.

▶ **transferrin** A protein synthesized in the liver that transports iron in the blood to the red blood cells for use in heme synthesis.

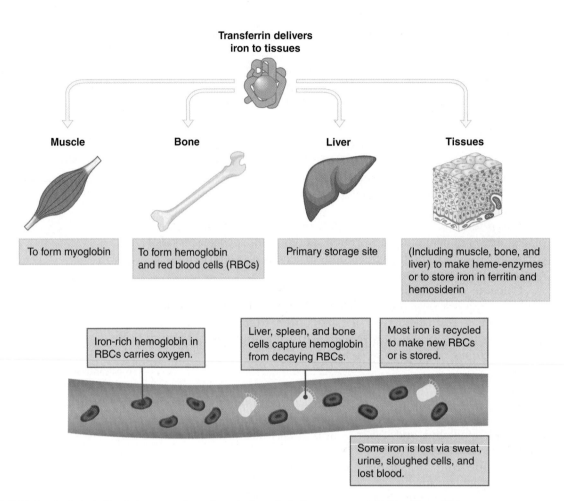

Transferrin delivers
iron to tissues

Muscle — To form myoglobin

Bone — To form hemoglobin and red blood cells (RBCs)

Liver — Primary storage site

Tissues — (Including muscle, bone, and liver) to make heme-enzymes or to store iron in ferritin and hemosiderin

Iron-rich hemoglobin in RBCs carries oxygen.

Liver, spleen, and bone cells capture hemoglobin from decaying RBCs.

Most iron is recycled to make new RBCs or is stored.

Some iron is lost via sweat, urine, sloughed cells, and lost blood.

FIGURE 8.21 Iron in the body. Transferrin transports iron to tissues for the synthesis of heme or storage in ferritin and hemosiderin.

Dietary Recommendations for Iron

The RDA for men and postmenopausal women is 8 milligrams per day. The RDA for women of childbearing age is 18 milligrams per day. Most men consume more than their RDA, but many women fall well short of recommended amounts.[47]

The iron needs of infants are a special concern. During the final weeks of pregnancy, babies ideally store enough iron in the liver, bone marrow, spleen, and hemoglobin-rich blood to see them through their first six months of life. However, if the mother's iron nutrition is poor or the baby is born early, the baby's iron stores are smaller and do not last. To help ensure that babies have adequate iron, pregnant women are urged to meet the RDA of 27 milligrams per day. Infant baby cereal and many infant formulas are fortified with iron.

Sources of Iron

In terms of both amount and bioavailability, beef is an excellent dietary source of iron. Other excellent sources include clams, oysters, and liver. Poultry, fish, pork, lamb, tofu, and legumes are also good sources. (See **FIGURE 8.22**.) Whole-grain and enriched-grain products contain less bioavailable iron than does meat, but are significant sources of iron because they make up a major part of our diets. Fortified cereals also make an important contribution to iron intake in the United States and Canada. Dairy products are low in iron.

Quick Bite

But It Worked in the Lab . . .

Carefully conducted clinical trials have shown that supplements reduce iron deficiency during pregnancy. However, public health programs that provide iron supplements in communities often are unsuccessful. Why? Programs in the "real world" have several limiting factors: inadequate supply of iron tablets, limited access to care, poor or nonexistent nutrition counseling, lack of knowledge, and the uncomfortable side effects experienced by some women. These are some reasons pregnant women don't take iron supplements even when programs to supply them are available.

THINK
About It

3

DV = 18 mg	Iron		
High: 20% DV or more	Whole-grain Total	1 cup	
	Rice Krispies cereals	1 ¼ cup	
	Lentils, cooked	1 cup	
	Spinach, cooked	1 cup	
	Semisweet chocolate	1 cup	
	Kidney beans, cooked	1 cup	
	Chickpeas, cooked	1 cup	
	Beets, canned	1 cup	
	Beef, flank, steak, cooked	3 oz	
	Raisins, seedless	1 cup	
Good: 10–19% DV	Turkey, roasted	1 cup	
	Peas, green, frozen, cooked	1 cup	
	Potato, baked, with skin	1 potato	
	Beef, ground (85% lean), cooked	3 oz	
	Collards, cooked	1 cup	

FIGURE 8.22 Food sources of iron. Iron is found in red meats, certain types of seafood, vegetables, and legumes, and is added to enriched grains and breakfast cereals.

Data from US Department of Agriculture, Agricultural Research Service, Nutrient Data Laboratory. USDA National Nutrient Database for Standard Reference, Release 28. Version Current: September 2015. Internet: http://www.ars.usda.gov/nea/bhnrc/ndl.

Cereal with milk and berries: © Aleksandrova Karina/ Shutterstock, Inc.; Pile of chickpeas: © homydesign/ Shutterstock, Inc.; flank steak: © Olena Kaminetska/ Shutterstock, Inc.; Fresh green peas: © ravl/ Shutterstock, Inc.

A varied diet (adequate in calories, rich in fruits and vegetables, and with small amounts of lean animal flesh) generally provides adequate iron. Vegetarians who consume no animal tissue can maximize iron bioavailability from other sources by consuming vitamin C–rich fruits and vegetables with every meal.

Iron Deficiency

Iron deficiency is the most common nutrient deficiency worldwide, especially in developing countries. Although less prevalent in the United States and Canada, it remains a public health concern. Infants and toddlers, adolescent girls, women of childbearing age, and pregnant women are particularly vulnerable.

Iron deficiency most commonly occurs in young children between 6 and 24 months old. Iron stores from fetal development have been depleted, and milk—a major source of energy in the young child's diet—is a poor source of iron. This is the age when cognitive and motor skills develop most rapidly, and inadequate iron during this critical time can cause irreversible developmental and intellectual deficits.

Progression of Iron Deficiency

Iron deficiency progresses through three stages. (See **TABLE 8.3**.) During the first stage of iron deficiency, the body depletes iron stores, but there are no physiological impairments. During the second stage, the body depletes its supply of iron in circulating transferrin, and heme production starts to slip. Enzymes that need an iron cofactor cannot function properly, and energy metabolism starts to suffer; an iron-deficient person may not be able to work at full capacity. The third and most severe stage is iron-deficiency anemia. (See **FIGURE 8.23**.)

During iron-deficiency anemia, a lack of iron inhibits production of normal red blood cells, while normal cell turnover continues to deplete

Quick **Bite**

Grandma's Cast-Iron Skillet Helped Her Avoid Iron Deficiency

Iron deficiency is the most common form of malnutrition in the United States. However, this is a relatively recent phenomenon. Americans used to cook using cast-iron pots and pans. A study showed that using these utensils to cook acidic foods such as spaghetti sauce and apple butter increases the iron content of such foods by 30- to 100-fold. Our preference for stainless steel, aluminum, and enamelware eliminates this fortification.

TABLE 8.3
Stages of Iron Deficiency

Stage	Functional Implications
Depletion of iron stores	None
Depletion of functional iron	Decreased physical performance
Iron-deficiency anemia	Cognitive impairment, poor growth, decreased performance, decreased exercise tolerance

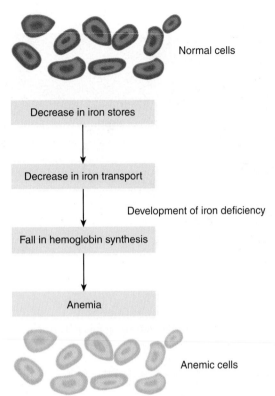

FIGURE 8.23 **Development of iron-deficiency anemia.** Iron deficiency can progress to iron-deficiency anemia, a severe form of iron deficiency that is accompanied by low hemoglobin levels.

Quick Bite

Bizarre Behavior or Nutritional Deficiency?

In all cultures, races, and geographic regions, certain people have strange cravings for non-food items. These cravings include ice (pagophagia), clay and dirt (geophagia), cornstarch (amylophagia), stone (lithophagia), paper, toilet tissue, soap, and foam. Pica, the compulsive consumption of nonfood items, often is associated with either iron or zinc deficiency, but it may also be the result of cultural beliefs or a response to family stresses. Whatever the cause, the behavior is not benign. It can injure teeth as well as cause constipation, intestinal obstruction or perforation, lead poisoning, pregnancy complications, poor growth in children, and mineral deficiencies.

▶ **hemochromatosis** A hereditary disorder in which excessive absorption of iron results in abnormal iron deposits in the liver and other tissues.

▶ **iron overload** Toxicity from excess iron.

the red blood cell population. Red blood cell production falters, producing red blood cells that are small and pale and lack sufficient hemoglobin (microcytic hypochromic anemia). Inadequate vitamin B_6 also can cause this type of anemia.

The symptoms of iron-deficiency anemia vary according to its severity and the speed of its development. They include fatigue, pale skin, breathlessness with exertion, poor tolerance to cold temperature, poor immune function, behavioral changes, cognitive impairment, and decreased work performance. In children, iron deficiency causes impaired growth, apathy, short attention span, irritability, and reduced ability to learn.[48]

Iron Toxicity

Iron pills can be hard on your digestive system. The UL for iron is based on the level that causes digestive distress. For adults, the UL for iron is 45 milligrams per day, although physicians may prescribe supplements with larger amounts for treating iron-deficiency anemia.

Iron Poisoning in Children

In the United States, accidental iron overdose is a leading cause of poisoning deaths in young children.[49] Parents who are cautious about keeping medications out of reach often do not realize that over-the-counter iron tablets and even iron-containing multivitamin/mineral supplements for children can be toxic. Just a few iron pills or a relatively moderate adult dose can be deadly for a small child. Symptoms of iron intoxication include nausea, vomiting, diarrhea, rapid heartbeat, dizziness, and confusion. Death can occur within hours of ingestion. If iron poisoning is suspected, the child must receive immediate emergency medical care.

Hereditary Hemochromatosis

In hereditary **hemochromatosis**, a genetic defect causes excessive iron absorption and chronic **iron overload**. Although it was once believed to be rare, scientists now know that mild forms are quite common and are estimated to affect 1 to 6 people per 100 in the United States.[50] Iron buildup over the years leads to severe organ damage, causing diabetes, heart disease, arthritis, liver cirrhosis, and liver cancer.

Men are more vulnerable to hemochromatosis than women, who lose iron through menstruation and pregnancy. Early diagnosis and treatment control the condition and prevent organ damage. Treatment includes minimizing iron intake, avoiding excess vitamin C, and periodically removing some blood. Iron chelation therapy has been used since the 1970s as a treatment for hemochromatosis. Another way to remove some excess iron is to donate blood. Chelation treatment for metal poisonings involves the use of certain drugs to bind and remove excess heavy metals from the body.

Key Concepts Iron is a key component of the oxygen transporters hemoglobin and myoglobin and of many enzymes involved in energy metabolism. The body carefully regulates iron absorption, based on its iron needs. Heme iron is absorbed more efficiently than nonheme iron. The best dietary sources of iron are organ meats and red meat. Plant foods contain only nonheme iron. Vitamin C–containing foods improve the bioavailability of nonheme iron. Iron deficiency develops gradually, and anemia is the most severe manifestation of deficiency. Iron poisoning, whether accidental or due to hemochromatosis, is potentially deadly.

Zinc

It's hard to believe that a nutrient so important to health could go unnoticed for so long. In fact, human zinc deficiency was not recognized until 1961.[51] A group of young men in Iran had a peculiar set of symptoms: severe growth retardation; poorly developed testicles (**hypogonadism**); anemia; and, among several, poor night vision. Their diet consisted mainly of wheat bread and was almost devoid of animal protein. They also ate clay (**geophagia**). Could their high-phytate, low-protein diet, along with geophagia, impair absorption of zinc and iron to such an extent? Six years later, a study in Egypt confirmed zinc's role; among a similar group of patients, zinc supplementation improved growth and genital development.[52]

▶ **hypogonadism** Decreased functional activity of the gonads (ovaries or testes) with retardation of growth and sexual development.

▶ **geophagia** Ingestion of clay or dirt.

▶ **galvanized** Describes iron or steel with a thin layer of zinc plated onto it to protect against corrosion.

Functions of Zinc

Your body contains a small amount of zinc—1.5 to 2.5 grams, or about the amount of zinc that's in the thin zinc layer on a **galvanized** nail. Yet zinc is found in every cell in the body.

The functions of zinc fall into three categories: catalytic, structural, and regulatory. Zinc is a cofactor for nearly 100 enzymes, representing all the major enzyme types. In its structural role, zinc helps fold proteins into functional shapes. As a regulator, zinc helps control many diverse functions, including gene expression, cell death, and nerve transmission.[53] (See **FIGURE 8.24**.)

Zinc and Enzymes

In many enzymes, zinc helps provide structural integrity or helps activate catalytic ability. For example, zinc performs a structural role in copper–zinc superoxide dismutase, an enzyme that speeds antioxidant reactions and helps protect cells from free radical damage. In the retina of the eye, the enzyme that activates vitamin A depends on zinc. Consequently, a lack of zinc can create a condition that resembles the night blindness caused by vitamin A deficiency.

Zinc and Gene Regulation

As a component of certain small proteins, zinc enables those proteins to fold into a special form that interacts with DNA. This interaction "turns on" a gene, beginning the steps to protein production and cell multiplication. Without zinc, that area of a gene won't function.[54]

In severe zinc deficiency, cells fail to replicate. This may explain zinc's importance for normal growth of children and sexual maturation of adolescents. Furthermore, certain tissues with high turnover rates, such as the cells lining the GI tract, skin cells, immune cells, and blood cells, are particularly vulnerable to a zinc deficiency. As a result, zinc-deficient people often have diarrhea, dermatitis, and depressed immunity.

Zinc and the Immune System

Zinc is vital to a vigorous immune response and is essential to the proper development and maintenance of the immune system. Without zinc, your body could not fight off invading viruses, bacteria, and fungi. Even mild deficiency may increase the risk of infection. (See the FYI feature "Zinc and the Common Cold.")

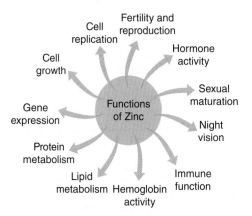

FIGURE 8.24 Functions of zinc in the body. Because zinc is involved in so many different functions, it is fortunate that overt zinc deficiency is rare.

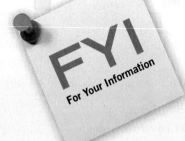

Zinc and the Common Cold

The common cold, one of our most common illnesses, affects U.S. adults 2 to 4 times per year and children 6 to 10 times per year.[a] Colds are even more frequent in young children in daycare settings and preschools. Because of missed work and decreased productivity, colds can be economically costly as well as a physical nuisance. A cure for the common cold would be of great benefit, and scientists have long pursued this goal.

Although scientists have suggested several hypotheses, the mechanism underlying a person's vulnerability to contracting a cold remains unclear. Zinc deficiency is known to impair immune function, but could all these people be zinc deficient? This is doubtful. Some speculate that zinc may reduce the severity and duration of cold symptoms by inhibiting viral replication. This is why products such as zinc lozenges and zinc syrups are under investigation.

Although overall zinc supplementation may be beneficial under certain circumstances, studies of zinc and colds have produced conflicting results. One study with positive results gained considerable attention from the press and, as a result, zinc lozenges are on nearly every pharmacy shelf in the United States. In this study, colds resolved in an average of four days for participants in the zinc group, as compared to seven days for the control group.[b] The same researchers then studied children who took zinc gluconate lozenges at the first sign of cold symptoms, but found no difference between those who took zinc and those who did not for all cold symptoms to resolve—a median of nine days.[c]

Research continues to provide conflicting results, with some studies finding a benefit of lozenges and others that zinc supplementation has no effect.[d,e] Review studies have also reported inconclusive findings.[f] More recently, a large systematic review of the scientific literature found benefits and concluded that "zinc (lozenges or syrup) is beneficial in reducing the duration and severity of the common cold in healthy people, when

taken within 24 hours of onset of symptoms. People taking zinc are also less likely to have persistence of their cold symptoms beyond seven days of treatment."[g]

High doses of zinc could have harmful effects beyond the mild side effects and cost of lozenges. People taking zinc lozenges (not syrup or tablet form) are more likely to experience adverse events, including bad taste and nausea.[h] Long-term use of high doses of zinc also could induce copper deficiency. In addition, loss of smell from the use of nasal zinc sprays prompted the FDA to issue a warning in 2009 instructing consumers to discontinue their use.[i]

Research to determine the effects of zinc for the treatment of the common cold is ongoing. Before a general recommendation can be made for using zinc in the treatment of the common cold, additional research is needed to determine the best formulation, dose, and treatment duration that provides a clinical benefit with minimal adverse effects.[j] Until there is more scientific agreement and standardized treatments, we should regard zinc as we would any other medical therapy and speak with a medical professional before routinely giving children (and ourselves) zinc lozenges every time a cold strikes.

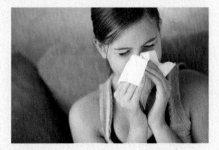

Zinc may reduce the severity and duration of cold symptoms, but research is ongoing.
© Grzegorz Placzek/Shutterstock.

a National Institute of Allergy and Infectious Diseases. Common colds: protect yourself and others. http://www3.niaid.nih.gov/healthscience/healthtopics/colds. Accessed June 16, 2014.

b Mossad SB, Macknin ML, Medendorp SV, Mason P. Zinc gluconate lozenges for treating the common cold: a randomized, double-blind placebo-controlled study. *Ann Intern Med.* 1996;125:81-88.

c Macknin ML, Piedmonte M, Calendine C, et al. Zinc gluconate lozenges for treating the common cold in children: a randomized controlled trial. *JAMA.* 1998;279:1962-1967.

d Prasad AS, Beck FW, Bao B, et al. Duration and severity of symptoms and levels of plasma interleukin-1 receptor antagonist, soluble tumor necrosis factor receptor, and adhesion molecules in patients with common cold treated with zinc acetate. *J Infect Dis.* 2008;197:795-802.

e Eby GA, Halcomb WW. Ineffectiveness of zinc gluconate nasal spray and zinc orotate lozenges in common-cold treatment: a double-blind, placebo-controlled clinical trial. *Altern Ther Health Med.* 2006;12:34-38.

f Caruso TJ, Prober CG, Gwaltney JM Jr. Treatment of naturally acquired common colds with zinc: a structured review. *Clin Infect Dis.* 2007;45:569-574.

g Singh M, Das RR. Zinc for the common cold. *Cochrane Database Syst Rev.* 2011;16(2):CD001364.

h Ibid.

i U.S. Department of Agriculture, U.S. Food and Drug Administration. Warnings on three Zicam intranasal zinc products. http://www.fda.gov/ForConsumers/ConsumerUpdates/ucm166931.htm. Accessed September 8, 2017.

j Singh M, Das RR. Op. cit.

Other Zinc Functions

Among zinc's many other functions, it interacts with hormones such as insulin and assists in linking oxygen to hemoglobin. Of special interest to nutritionists is zinc's role in the sense of taste. Zinc deficiency reduces taste perception, and poor appetite generally follows.

Regulation of Zinc in the Body

When dietary zinc is low, our bodies have no long-term storehouse of zinc to draw upon. We maintain zinc balance, even when confronted with varying needs and dietary conditions, by adjusting absorption and excretion.

Zinc Absorption

Much about absorption of dietary zinc is similar to that of iron. We absorb only about 10 to 35 percent of the zinc in our diets. The proportion that's absorbed depends on our zinc status, the zinc content of the meal, and the presence of competing minerals. People with zinc deficiency absorb zinc more efficiently than do people with optimal zinc status. Zinc absorption also increases during times of increased need, such as growth spurts, pregnancy, and lactation. As with iron, intestinal cells act as gatekeepers as they adjust their zinc absorption to maintain proper body levels.

Phytate from whole grains is the main dietary factor that inhibits zinc absorption.[55] For vegetarians whose diet consists of mainly phytate-rich unrefined grains and legumes, zinc requirements may exceed the RDAs.[56] Although calcium and iron supplements may interfere with the absorption of zinc, calcium and iron from food does not have the same effect.[57]

Zinc Transport, Distribution, and Excretion

Zinc circulates in the bloodstream bound to protein, traveling to the liver and tissues where it is most needed. Muscle and bone contain 90 percent of the body's zinc.

During digestion, the pancreas secretes a considerable amount of zinc in pancreatic juice. When needed, intestinal cells reabsorb most of this zinc. Otherwise, it is lost in feces, along with unabsorbed dietary zinc. Zinc is also lost from sloughed-off intestinal cells, skin, and hair; minor amounts are excreted in urine, sweat, and other fluids.

Dietary Recommendations for Zinc

The zinc RDA for men is 11 milligrams per day; for women it is 8 milligrams per day, increasing to 11 milligrams during pregnancy and to 12 milligrams while breastfeeding.[58] Most people in the United States and Canada consume more than the RDA, but a significant number do not.

Sources of Zinc

Zinc usually is abundant in foods that are good sources of protein, especially red meat and seafood such as oysters and clams. (See **FIGURE 8.25**.) For poultry, dark meat is a richer source than white meat. The zinc in animal foods is generally well absorbed. Conversely, whole grains have a relatively high amount of zinc, but it is poorly absorbed. Fruits and vegetables generally are poor zinc sources. Because diets that exclude meat are excluding the best zinc sources, adequate intake is a special concern for vegetarians.

Quick **Bite**

Hair Analysis Is a Misguided Measure

Although its use has been discredited, hair analysis is promoted with the claim that it can reveal mineral deficiencies. However, this measure lacks sensitivity and is unreliable. The color, diameter, and rate of growth of a person's hair; the season of the year; the geographic location; and the person's age and gender can affect the levels of minerals in hair. It is possible for hair concentration of an element (zinc, for example) to be high even though deficiency exists in the body. Hair dyes, perming agents, and certain shampoos also alter the mineral content of hair.

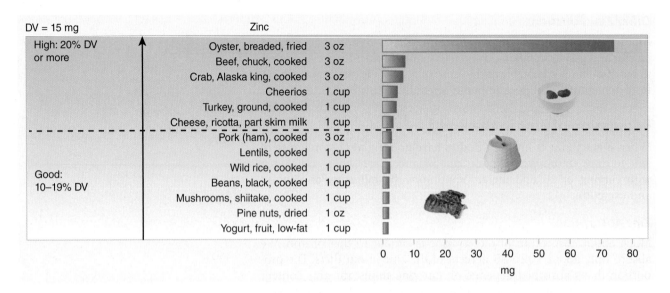

FIGURE 8.25 Food sources of zinc. Meat, organ meats, and seafood are the best sources of zinc. Data from U.S. Department of Agriculture, Agricultural Research Service, Nutrient Data Laboratory. USDA National Nutrient Database for Standard Reference, release 28. http://www.ars.usda.gov/Services/docs.htm?docid=8964. Accessed September 8, 2017.

Data from US Department of Agriculture, Agricultural Research Service, Nutrient Data Laboratory. USDA National Nutrient Database for Standard Reference, Release 28. Version Current: September 2015. Internet: http://www.ars.usda.gov/nea/bhnrc/ndl.

A grilled chuck roast: © MSPhotographic/ Shutterstock, Inc.; Fresh ricotta: © BrunoRosa/ Shutterstock, Inc.; Strawberry yogurt: © Watthano/ Shutterstock, Inc.; Japanese food, deep fried oyster: © jreika/ Shutterstock.com.

Zinc Deficiency

Zinc deficiency is uncommon in the United States and Canada. It usually occurs in people with illnesses that impair absorption. In other parts of the world, zinc deficiency is most prevalent in populations that subsist on cereals and little else. Zinc from cereal grains is poorly absorbed. Among these populations, infections with pneumonia and diarrhea are commonplace and cause significant zinc losses. A downward spiral results: Zinc deficiency lowers immunity, and infection causes zinc loss, more infection, and more zinc loss. In some regions, zinc supplementation programs have cut the incidence of childhood respiratory infections and diarrhea.

Symptoms of moderate to severe zinc deficiency include poor growth, delayed or abnormal sexual development, diarrhea, severe skin rash and hair loss, impaired immune response, and impaired taste acuity. During pregnancy, zinc deficiency may contribute to complications and low birth weight.[59]

Zinc Toxicity

Although toxicity from high dietary zinc intake is rare, chronic supplementation with too much zinc causes adverse effects. High doses of zinc may cause acute GI distress, nausea, vomiting, and cramping. The UL for zinc is set at 40 milligrams per day. Chronic high doses of zinc (100 to 150 milligrams per day) for prolonged periods can interfere with copper metabolism and cause low blood copper levels and impaired immunity.[60] Chronic high dosing of zinc relative to copper inhibits copper absorption and with time may induce a copper deficiency. Doctors use the interaction of zinc and copper to treat people with **Wilson's disease**, a genetic disorder of hyperabsorption and accumulation of copper. Zinc works by blocking copper absorption

▶ **Wilson's disease** Genetic disorder of increased copper absorption, which leads to toxic levels in the liver and heart.

and increasing its excretion, thus preventing its accumulation in the body.[61]

> **Key Concepts** Zinc is important for normal growth and development, immune function, and the function of many enzymes. Zinc balance is maintained by regulating intestinal absorption. The best food sources are good protein sources, especially red meats and seafood. Zinc deficiency occurs most often among populations that subsist on cereals and grains.

Selenium

The story of selenium is a recent one and becomes more complex as scientists continue to explore its roles. Historically, because animals grazing on selenium-rich soils suffered selenium poisoning, scientists focused on its toxicity. This changed in 1957, when researchers first demonstrated selenium's nutritional benefits in vitamin E–deficient animals. But not until 1979 did evidence emerge that selenium is essential for humans. Chinese scientists reported an association between low selenium status and **Keshan disease**, a heart disorder that strikes children in the Keshan province of China. The Chinese scientists demonstrated that selenium supplements could prevent the disease. Although selenium deficiency does not cause the disease, it predisposes a child to heart damage after a particular type of viral infection. When selenium intake is adequate, the virus apparently does not cause Keshan disease.

> ▶ **Keshan disease** Selenium-deficiency disease that impairs the structure and function of the heart.

Functions of Selenium

In your body, most selenium joins up with one of two amino acids, methionine or cysteine, for storage or for its role as an antioxidant. Selenium is a component of a well-known family of antioxidants, the glutathione peroxidases. Like vitamin E, these enzymes work to prevent oxidative damage. In fact, to some extent selenium and vitamin E "spare" each other in this protection. A generous intake of one reduces the requirement for the other.

Selenium-containing enzymes are also involved in thyroid metabolism, converting thyroid hormone to its most active form. A deficiency of selenium worsens the **hypothyroidism** caused by iodine deficiency. (See the discussion of iodine later in this chapter.)

> ▶ **hypothyroidism** The result of a lowered level of circulating thyroid hormone, with slowing of mental and physical functions.

Selenium is important to immune function. As the Keshan studies showed, the body needs selenium to fight infections. Animals with depleted selenium get sicker from viral infections, and low selenium levels are associated with faster progression of viral disease in humans. Selenium may have some anticancer benefits, but more research is needed to clarify the relationship.[62] Selenium is also under investigation for its role in heart disease, arthritis, and HIV.[63]

Absorption and Excretion of Selenium

Most selenium in food is bound to the amino acids methionine or cysteine, and in this form about 50 to 90 percent is bioavailable. Vitamins A, C, and E enhance selenium absorption, and phytate inhibits it. Excess selenium leaves the body mainly through feces and urine.

Dietary Recommendations and Sources of Selenium

For both men and women, the selenium RDA is 55 micrograms per day.[64] U.S. and Canadian diets generally provide these levels. Selenium

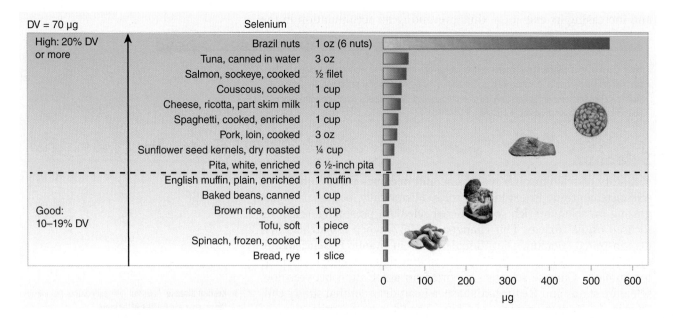

DV = 70 μg

Selenium

High: 20% DV or more	Brazil nuts	1 oz (6 nuts)
	Tuna, canned in water	3 oz
	Salmon, sockeye, cooked	½ filet
	Couscous, cooked	1 cup
	Cheese, ricotta, part skim milk	1 cup
	Spaghetti, cooked, enriched	1 cup
	Pork, loin, cooked	3 oz
	Sunflower seed kernels, dry roasted	¼ cup
	Pita, white, enriched	6 ½-inch pita
Good: 10–19% DV	English muffin, plain, enriched	1 muffin
	Baked beans, canned	1 cup
	Brown rice, cooked	1 cup
	Tofu, soft	1 piece
	Spinach, frozen, cooked	1 cup
	Bread, rye	1 slice

0 100 200 300 400 500 600

μg

FIGURE 8.26 Food sources of selenium. Selenium is found mainly in meats, organ meats, seafood, and grains.

Data from US Department of Agriculture, Agricultural Research Service, Nutrient Data Laboratory. USDA National Nutrient Database for Standard Reference, Release 28. Version Current: September 2015. Internet: http://www.ars.usda.gov/nea/bhnrc/ndl.

Brazil nuts: © Leonid Shcheglov/ Shutterstock, Inc.; Fresh raw organic broccoli: © poplasen/ iStock / Getty Images Plus; Grilled salmon: © amenic181/ Shutterstock, Inc.; Baked Beans: © Paul_Brighton/ Shutterstock, Inc.

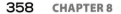

Quick Bite

On Your Next Moonlit Stroll, Think Selenium!

Selenium takes its name from the Greek word *Selénê* ("moon") because it has a pasty white color. In mythology, Selene is the Greek goddess of the moon. Ancient Greeks often blamed Selene and her brother Helios (god of the sun) for pestilent diseases and death.

▶ **cretinism** A congenital condition often caused by severe iodine deficiency during gestation; characterized by arrested physical and mental development.

is found in both plant- and animal-derived foods. Selenium levels are quite variable in plant foods and generally reflect the selenium content of the soil in which the plant was grown. Brazil nuts are particularly high in selenium. The soil in Venezuela, where most Brazil nuts are harvested, is rich in selenium. As a result, a single Brazil nut provides more than the RDA for selenium. The selenium content of animal-derived foods is much more consistent. Organ meats, fish, seafood, and meats are consistently good sources. (See **FIGURE 8.26**.)

Selenium Deficiency and Toxicity

Selenium deficiency is rare, although it can be seen where soil selenium concentrations are low. Chronic selenium deficiency interferes with immune function. Three conditions have been associated with selenium deficiency: Keshan disease, which occurs in selenium-deficient children and results in an enlarged heart and poor heart function; Kashin–Beck disease, which results in diseases of the joints and bones; and **cretinism**, which results in mental retardation.[65]

There are isolated reports of selenium toxicity. Outward signs are brittle hair and nails and a garliclike body odor. Excessive intake may be accidental or the result of overenthusiastic supplementation. Chronic selenium toxicity also exists in isolated regions of the world where soil levels are very high. The UL is set at 400 micrograms per day for adults.

Key Concepts Selenium functions in antioxidant systems and spares vitamin E. It is involved in thyroid metabolism and immune function. Good dietary sources are Brazil nuts, organ meats, and seafood. Selenium deficiency is associated with Keshan disease, a rare heart ailment. Marginal deficiency may compromise immune function and increase cancer risk.

Iodine

Iodine deficiency has existed for centuries. The ancient Chinese wrote about it, and European artists of the Middle Ages included iodine-deficient people in their paintings.[66] Iodine deficiency existed in the American Midwest, too, until supplementation and fortification programs were begun around the mid-1920s. Prior to that, deficiency was so common the region was nicknamed "the goiter belt." Iodine deficiency remains a significant nutritional problem in some parts of the world, and its eradication is an important goal of the World Health Organization, which it hopes to reach by encouraging universal salt iodization.[67]

Iodine is an essential component of thyroid hormones, which help regulate body temperature, basal metabolic rate, reproduction, and growth. Not surprisingly, most of the body's iodine is found in the thyroid gland. Selenium-dependent enzymes activate the major thyroid hormone, so a selenium deficiency can lead to inefficient use of iodine. In food, iodine is mostly in its ion form—iodide. Your intestines absorb nearly all dietary iodide. Raw vegetables in the cabbage family contain compounds known as **goitrogens**. These interfere with iodine absorption and can worsen deficiency. Cooking inactivates goitrogens. We excrete most excess iodine in urine, but also lose some in sweat, especially in hot, humid climates.

Dietary Recommendations and Sources of Iodine

The iodine RDA for men and women is 150 micrograms per day, an amount that replaces iodine losses and provides a generous margin of safety.[68] Because the ocean is the best iodine source, the best food sources are ocean products: fish, seafood, and seaweed. (See **FIGURE 8.27**.) Saltwater fish have higher concentrations of iodine than do freshwater

▶ **goitrogens** Compounds that interfere with iodine absorption and can induce goiter.

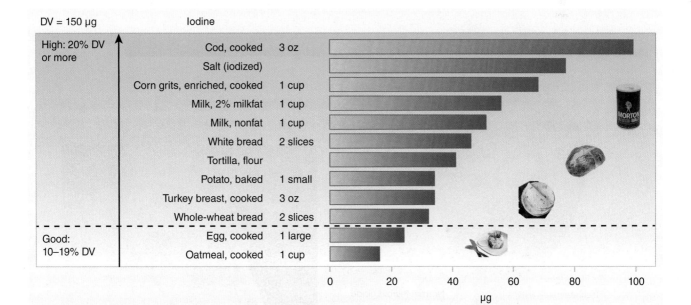

FIGURE 8.27 Food sources of iodine. Few foods are rich in iodine; it is found mainly in milk, seafood, and some grain products. Iodized salt is a primary source of iodine for many people.

Data from Pennington JAT. *Bowes and Church's Food Values of Portions Commonly Used.* 17th ed. Philadelphia, PA: Lippincott-Raven Publishers; 1998.

Baked cod served: © finaeva_i/ Shutterstock Inc.; Stack of homemade whole wheat flour tortilla on napkin: © Africa Studio/ Shutterstock, Inc.; Plain baked potato: © Joe Gough/ Shutterstock, Inc.; Iodized table salt by Morton Salt Company: © GIPhotoStock/ Getty Images, Inc.

fish. Natural iodine levels in plants reflect soil iodine levels, and foods grown near the ocean are considerably richer in iodine than foods grown far inland. Eons ago, the Midwestern United States and Canada were covered by glaciers rather than the ocean; therefore, these regions have iodine-poor soils and produce food with little iodine.

The dairy industry adds iodine to cattle feed and uses sanitizing solutions that contain iodine. This substantially increases the iodine in milk and dairy products, which are now major contributors of iodine to the American diet. For many people, iodized salt is their primary iodine source. In the United States, iodized salt contains an average of 76 micrograms of iodine per gram of salt. In addition to common iodized table salt, specialty sea salts are available that are usually not iodized. However, sea salts naturally contain trace amounts of iodine and other minerals because these salts are derived from evaporated salt water.

Iodine Deficiency

Iodine deficiency causes hypothyroidism, which is low levels of thyroid hormones. Its most apparent sign is **goiter**—an enlarged thyroid gland in the neck. (See **FIGURE 8.28**.)

Iodine deficiency inhibits thyroid hormone production. The body senses low levels of thyroid hormones and produces more and more **thyroid-stimulating hormone (TSH)**. The excessive TSH, in turn, stimulates the thyroid gland to grow, eventually causing a goiter. Other symptoms of hypothyroidism are intolerance to cold temperatures, decreased body temperature, weight gain, and sluggishness.

Severe iodine deficiency during pregnancy increases prenatal death and can result in birth defects, cretinism, and infant mortality.[69] Symptoms of cretinism are mental retardation, stunted growth, deafness, and muteness.

▶ **goiter** A chronic enlargement of the thyroid gland, visible as a swelling at the front of the neck; usually associated with iodine deficiency.

▶ **thyroid-stimulating hormone (TSH)** Hormone secreted from the pituitary gland at the base of the brain; regulates synthesis of thyroid hormones.

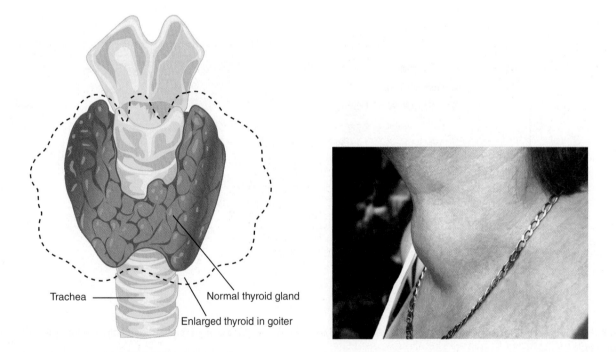

Trachea

Normal thyroid gland

Enlarged thyroid in goiter

FIGURE 8.28 Enlargement of the thyroid gland in goiter. Iodine deficiency results in goiter. Use of iodized salt dramatically reduces goiter rates. This finding led to the widespread fortification of table salt with iodine.

Photo of goiter: © Chris Pancewicz/Alamy.

Iodine deficiency has disappeared from the United States and Canada, but it still exists in the world's poor and isolated areas where the soils are low in iodine and little food from outside enters the local food supply. Deficiency may be worsened by diets low in selenium and high in goitrogenic vegetables.

Iodine Toxicity

Large amounts of iodine inhibit synthesis of thyroid hormone, surprisingly, and stimulate thyroid growth and goiter. In other words, both too much and too little iodine cause goiter. Overzealous supplementation is the most common cause of iodine toxicity. The UL for iodine is 1,100 micrograms per day.

> **Key Concepts** Iodine is an essential component of thyroid hormones. Iodine deficiency causes overstimulation of the thyroid gland and eventual goiter. Deficiency during pregnancy can cause cretinism in the offspring. Important food sources include ocean fish and seafood, dairy products, and iodized salt. Worldwide, iodine deficiency continues to exist in some regions. Iodizing salt is a powerful preventive measure.

Copper

During the 1960s, researchers learned that copper was essential when they uncovered **Menkes syndrome**, a rare genetic disease of copper deficiency. Dietary copper deficiency is not a significant public health concern, but excessive supplementation with other trace minerals can cause a secondary copper deficiency.

As a part of coenzymes, copper participates in dozens of reactions, among them energy release, skin pigment (melanin) production, and the production of the connective tissue proteins collagen and elastin. It plays a role in maintaining nerve health, immune function, and heart function. Copper is a component of the superoxide dismutases, enzymes involved in antioxidant reactions. Copper also is a component of **ceruloplasmin**, an enzyme required for iron transport. Without ceruloplasmin, iron accumulates in the liver, creating symptoms similar to hemochromatosis.

Copper Absorption and Storage

Copper absorption varies with dietary intake and can range from 20 to 50 percent. Most absorption takes place in the small intestine, though some occurs in the stomach. Some mineral supplements, most notably iron and zinc, can interfere with copper absorption. So can excessive use of antacids.

Albumin transports copper to the liver, where most is incorporated into ceruloplasmin. Little copper is stored. Unabsorbed copper, copper sloughed off in intestinal cells, and excess copper secreted in bile all leave the body via feces.

Dietary Recommendations and Sources of Copper

The copper RDA for both men and women is 900 micrograms per day.[70] It's not difficult to achieve because copper is widely distributed in foods. The richest food sources for copper include organ meats, shellfish, nuts and seeds, legumes, peanut butter, and chocolate. (See **FIGURE 8.29.**)

Quick **Bite**

Iodine or Iodide: What's in a Name?
Although the terms *iodine* and *iodide* often are used interchangeably, chemically they are not identical. Iodine (I_2) is a bluish-black solid that gives off a purple vapor, which gives the element its name. Iodine stems from the Greek word *iôdēdes*, meaning "violet-colored." Iodide (I^-) is the colorless negative ion of iodine. Iodine circulates in the body either bound to protein or as free iodide ions. Sodium iodide and potassium iodide are iodide salts commonly used in medicines.

▶ **Menkes syndrome** A genetic disorder that results in copper deficiency.

▶ **ceruloplasmin** A copper-dependent enzyme that enables iron to bind to transferrin. Also known as *ferroxidase I*.

Quick **Bite**

Egg Whites? Please Stand Up!
Although cooking food in a copper pot is inadvisable, copper mixing bowls can be a plus. Meringues made in ceramic or steel bowls tend to be snowy white and drier than those made in copper bowls. Making meringue in a copper bowl leads to a creamier, yellowish foam that is harder to overbeat into a lumpy liquid. The copper bowl contributes copper ions to conalbumin, a metal-binding protein, thus stabilizing the whipped egg whites.

▶ **albumin** A protein that circulates in the blood and helps transport many minerals and some drugs.

Quick **Bite**

A Penny for Your …
How do the amounts of zinc and copper in a U.S. penny compare with the amounts in your body? Today's penny is mostly zinc (2.4 grams), covered with some copper plating (62.5 milligrams). A penny's zinc is in the upper range of the body's zinc content, but the amount of copper falls short. It takes the copper in about 11/2 pennies to equal the amount of copper in your body.

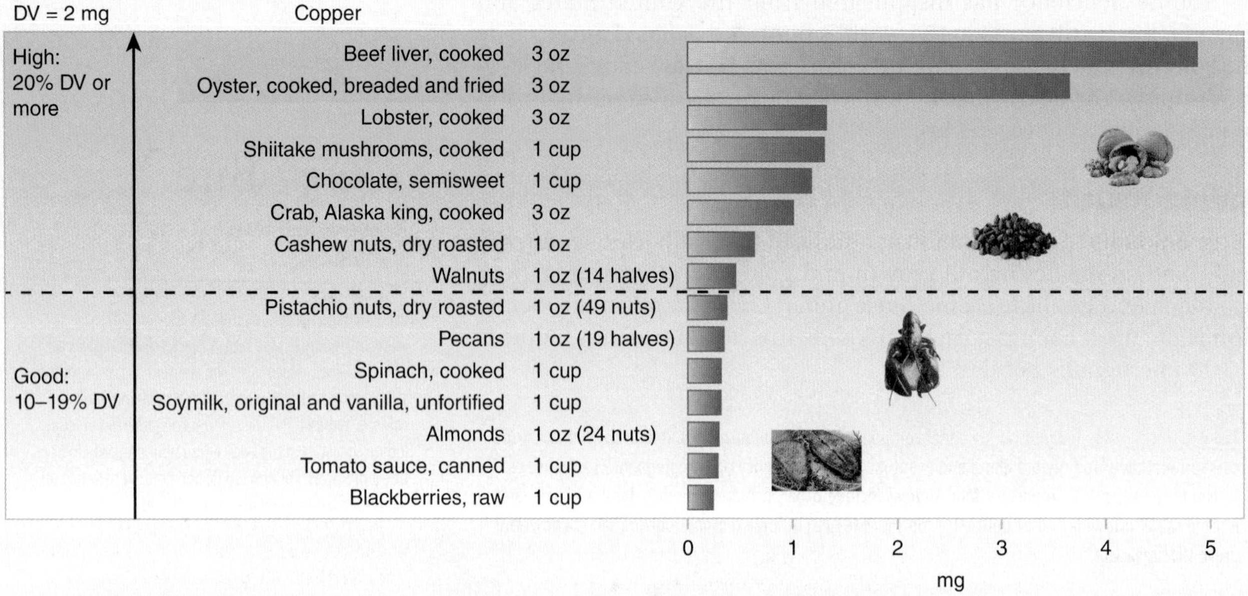

FIGURE 8.29 Food sources of copper. Copper is found in a limited variety of foods. The best sources are seafood, legumes, and nuts.

Data from US Department of Agriculture, Agricultural Research Service, Nutrient Data Laboratory. USDA National Nutrient Database for Standard Reference, Release 28. Version Current: September 2015. Internet: http://www.ars.usda.gov/nea/bhnrc/ndl.

Slices of liver cooked with rosemary and speck: © MauMar70/ Shutterstock, Inc.; Cooked lobster: © Alena Haurylik/ Shutterstock, Inc.; Chocolate Chips: © bonchan/ Shutterstock, Inc; walnut and a cracked walnut: © oriori/ Shutterstock, Inc.

Copper Deficiency

Copper deficiency is rare and occurs most often in infants born prematurely, who have low copper stores at birth and a very rapid growth rate. Cow's milk has little copper, so infants who are inappropriately fed cow's milk rather than human milk or formula could have low copper levels.

Copper deficiency reduces production of both red and white blood cells, causing anemia and poor immune function. Deficiency also causes bone abnormalities. Menkes syndrome is an extremely rare genetic copper absorption disorder that usually is fatal in infancy or early childhood.[71]

Copper Toxicity

Compared with other trace minerals, copper is relatively nontoxic. The UL for copper is 10 milligrams per day. However, in Wilson's disease, another rare genetic disorder, excessive copper accumulates in the liver, brain, kidneys, and eyes. Like copper deficiency, copper excess causes anemia. People with Wilson's disease now avoid serious liver and neurologic problems with therapies that bind and remove copper. Zinc supplements, which inhibit copper absorption, also are used in treating Wilson's disease.

> **Key Concepts** Copper is a component of ceruloplasmin, superoxide dismutase, and many other enzymes. Good food sources include organ meats, shellfish, nuts and seeds, legumes, peanut butter, and chocolate. Copper deficiency and toxicity are rare.

Manganese

The body contains only 10 to 20 milligrams of manganese, yet manganese is a cofactor in reactions of key importance. It's involved in energy metabolism and urea formation. Manganese-containing enzymes also are required for building cartilage. Like zinc and copper, manganese is a component of the antioxidant enzyme superoxide dismutase.

Absorption of manganese is very low, only 1 to 15 percent, probably a protection against toxicity. There is little storage, and any excess is excreted in bile and leaves via feces.

Dietary Recommendations and Sources of Manganese

Adequate Intake (AI) for manganese is 2.3 milligrams per day for men and 1.8 milligrams per day for women.[72] Tea, nuts, cereals, and some fruits are the best food sources of manganese. (See **FIGURE 8.30**.) Meat, dairy products, poultry, fish, and refined foods are poor sources.

Manganese Deficiency and Toxicity

Most people are not at risk of manganese deficiency. However, some illnesses, such as **Lou Gehrig's disease** and **multiple sclerosis**, may cause suboptimal manganese status. In animal studies, manganese deficiency impairs growth, impairs energy metabolism, and produces bone abnormalities.

Manganese toxicity is a greater threat than manganese deficiency. However, incidents of toxicity have been due not to food, but to air pollutants. Foundry workers exposed to airborne manganese dust experience severe manganese toxicity. Their symptoms include irritability, hallucinations, and severe lack of coordination. Lower doses of airborne manganese can impair memory and motor coordination. The UL for manganese is 11 milligrams per day.

▶ **Lou Gehrig's disease** A syndrome marked by muscular weakness and atrophy due to a degeneration of motor neurons of the spinal cord. Technically known as *amyotrophic lateral sclerosis (ALS)*.

▶ **multiple sclerosis** A progressive disease that destroys the myelin sheath surrounding nerve fibers of the brain and spinal cord.

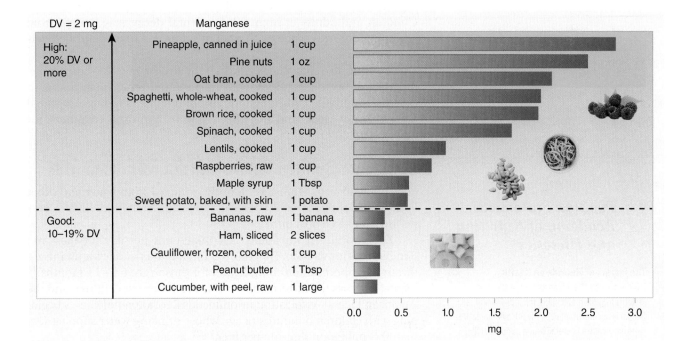

FIGURE 8.30 Food sources of manganese. Manganese is found mainly in plant foods such as grains, legumes, vegetables, and some fruits.

Data from US Department of Agriculture, Agricultural Research Service, Nutrient Data Laboratory. USDA National Nutrient Database for Standard Reference, Release 28. Version Current: September 2015. Internet: http://www.ars.usda.gov/nea/bhnrc/ndl.

> **Key Concepts** Manganese is a cofactor in several enzyme systems. Food sources for manganese are tea, coffee, cereals, and some fruits. Toxicity from airborne manganese is a greater threat than deficiency.

Fluoride

Fluoride is a form of the element fluorine. Large-scale studies undertaken during the 1940s convincingly demonstrated that fluoride has the ability to prevent dental caries. Since then, fluoride has been added to water supplies in many regions of the United States, and use of fluoridated toothpaste and mouthwash has become widespread.

Functions of Fluoride

Nearly 99 percent of the body's fluoride is in bones and teeth, where it promotes deposition of calcium and phosphate. During infancy and childhood, while new teeth are being formed, fluoride acts systemically. In other words, it arrives via the bloodstream to the site of new tooth formation. There it is incorporated into the tooth structure.

Every day there is a battle in your teeth between normal mineral loss and mineral deposition. When your mouth contains food, bacteria multiply and produce acids that eat away tooth enamel, especially beneath plaque. Fluoride inhibits bacterial activity and shifts the balance toward depositing minerals. This action in teeth helps counter normal mineral loss, a loss that acid-forming bacteria accelerate. Fluoride therefore inhibits tooth decay and loss of tooth enamel.

Children and adults at low risk for dental decay can stay cavity-free through frequent exposure to small amounts of fluoride by drinking fluoridated water and using a fluoride toothpaste twice daily. Children and adults at high risk for dental decay may benefit from additional fluoride, such as that found in professionally applied gels and varnishes.[73]

Fluoride also may play a role in bone health, and fluoride supplements have been used along with calcium and other medications to treat osteoporosis.[74] Although the risk of fracture is reduced, optimal dosage is not clear, and fluoride is not an approved treatment for osteoporosis.

Dietary Recommendations and Sources of Fluoride

Your body absorbs almost all fluoride extracted from water and other liquids, and about 50 to 80 percent of fluoride from food. Most excess fluoride is excreted in urine.

The fluoride AI for adults is 4 milligrams per day for men and 3 milligrams for women. The AI is 0.01 milligram per day for infants up through 5 months and 0.5 milligram for those ages 6 to 11 months.[75] Dental caries is the most common chronic disease in children, and the American Dental Association recommends fluoride supplements beginning with children 6 months of age whose drinking water supplies less than 0.3 milligram fluoride per liter.[76,77]

Water is the main source of fluoride. Water naturally may contain fluoride, or fluoride may be added to produce fluoridated water. Fluoride naturally present in drinking water varies from less than 0.1 milligram to more than 10 milligrams per liter. Where naturally occurring fluoride levels are low, many water companies add fluoride.

Position Statement: Academy of Nutrition and Dietetics

The Impact of Fluoride on Health

It is the position of the Academy of Nutrition and Dietetics to support optimal systemic and topical fluoride as an important public health measure to promote oral health and overall health throughout life.

Reprinted from *Journal of the Academy of Nutrition and Dietetics*, 112(9), Carole A. Palmer, Joyce Ann Gilbert, Position of the Academy of Nutrition and Dietetics: The Impact of Fluoride on Health, Page no. 129-147, 2012, with permission from Elsevier.

The U.S. Department of Health and Human Services recommends 0.7 milligram of fluoride per liter of water, based on an assessment of the benefits versus side effects by the Environmental Protection Agency and the U.S. Department of Health and Human Services.[78] The Environmental Protection Agency requires public drinking water systems to remove excess fluoride so that it does not exceed 4.0 milligrams per liter.[79] Community water fluoridation has been credited with reducing tooth decay by 50–60 percent in the United States since the 1940s. The Centers for Disease Control and Prevention named the fluoridation of drinking water one of the 10 great public health achievements of the twentieth century.[80]

Other fluoride sources have emerged since we first began fluoridating water supplies. Today's fluoride sources include fluoride supplements, mouthwash, toothpaste, and some beverages. Almost one-quarter of U.S. children younger than 12 years of age and 30 percent of 2 year olds use supplemental vitamins, fluoride, and iron in a given week.[81]

When Fluoride Balance Goes Awry

Low fluoride intake is associated with tooth decay. Adequate fluoride intake during infancy and childhood cuts the incidence of tooth decay by up to 30 to 60 percent. Prolonged excessive intake of fluoride causes **fluorosis**. (See **FIGURE 8.31**.) During tooth development, fluorosis damages teeth. In mild fluorosis, white specks form on the teeth. Severe fluorosis weakens teeth and produces permanent brownish stains. In adults, fluorosis is associated with hip fracture; weak, stiff joints; and chronic stomach inflammation. Fluorosis can occur in people living where water is naturally very high in fluoride, or in children who chronically swallow large amounts of fluoridated toothpaste. The UL for fluoride is 10 milligrams per day.

The Fluoridation Debate

Almost three-quarters of the U.S. population receive the benefit of optimally fluoridated public water.[82] In some communities, water fluoridation programs have been in place since the mid-1940s. Since the United States first began fluoridating water supplies, however, other fluoride sources have emerged, making it difficult to determine the current effectiveness of artificial fluoridation of the water supply.

Although the dramatic decline in dental caries since fluoridation was initiated is undeniable, the balance between the positive effects of just enough fluoride and the negative effects of too much fluoride has caused fluoridation to become hotly debated. Some groups are worried that the combination of fluoride sources may put children at increased risk for excessive fluoride intake and fluorosis. Opponents argue that fluoridation is outdated and involuntary: "If you administer fluoride by fluoridating the tap water in the community then you have no control of the dose an individual gets per day."[83] To retain the benefits yet avoid overconsumption, the American Dental Association supports the fluoridation of all water supplies and monitoring of other fluoride sources.[84,85]

THINK About It 4

The AI levels for infants and children have been reduced to account for increased fluoride in the food supply. Fluoride supplements are available only by prescription.

▶ **fluorosis** Mottled discoloration and pitting of tooth enamel caused by prolonged ingestion of excess fluoride that is characterized in children by discoloration and pitting of the teeth.

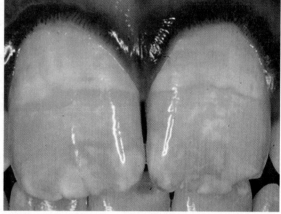

FIGURE 8.31 Tooth mottling in fluorosis. During tooth development, prolonged excessive fluoride intake can cause fluorosis, which discolors and damages teeth.
Centers for Disease Control.

Key Concepts Bones and teeth contain 99 percent of body fluoride. Fluoride supports mineralization of bones and teeth, and adequate intake reduces tooth decay. The main dietary source is water. The majority of municipal water supplies contain fluoride. Excess fluoride causes fluorosis with mottling of the teeth. Severe fluorosis causes weakened, brown-stained teeth.

Chromium

The best-understood role of chromium is in glucose metabolism. Chromium appears to enhance the ability of insulin to move glucose into cells. Other functions of chromium involve nucleic acid metabolism, growth, and immune function. The amount of chromium in the body is exceedingly tiny—only about 4 to 6 milligrams.

Dietary chromium is poorly absorbed, and levels decrease with age. Chromium absorption appears to increase with need and decrease as dietary intake rises. Absorption improves when chromium is combined with an organic acid, as in chromium picolinate supplements. Excess chromium is excreted in urine.

Dietary Recommendations and Sources of Chromium

The AI for adults 19 to 50 years of age is 35 micrograms per day for men and 25 micrograms per day for women; for older adults the daily AI decreases by 5 micrograms.[86] The chromium content of foods varies widely. Good sources include grape and orange juice, processed meats, whole grains, green beans, broccoli, and spices. Cooking acidic foods in stainless steel containers leaches some chromium into the food.

Chromium Deficiency and Toxicity

It is difficult to detect chromium deficiency in the general population. The only known cases of chromium toxicity are from airborne chromium compounds in industrial settings. To date, no UL has been set for chromium, but up to 200 micrograms of inorganic chromium appears to be a safe supplement dose.

The role of chromium supplements remains controversial. Supplementation with chromium has been shown to reduce risk factors for type 2 diabetes and cardiovascular disease and aid in mild weight loss in obese and overweight individuals.[87-89] The current body of evidence, however, does not support chromium supplementation as a tool for diabetes management.[90] Based on perceived but unfounded beneficial effects on body composition, chromium supplements are popular among many athletes, bodybuilders, and those seeking a weight loss aid. Results from systematic reviews have been inconsistent, and experts caution that there is little evidence that chromium supplementation is safe and effective in overweight or obese adults.[91,92] Hard evidence behind chromium's fat metabolism–enhancing properties is lacking, and supplement sales are driven by the industry marketing nonscientific evidence.[93]

Molybdenum

Molybdenum is essential to both plants and animals. In humans, molybdenum functions as a cofactor for several enzymes. Molybdenum is efficiently absorbed, and it's excreted rapidly in urine and bile. Dietary copper can inhibit molybdenum absorption, and vice versa. Doctors exploit the competition between copper and molybdenum by using a form of molybdenum to treat patients with Wilson's disease.

The RDA for molybdenum is 45 micrograms per day for adults.[94] Peas, beans, and some breakfast cereals are the richest food sources, and organ meats also are good sources.

Molybdenum deficiency does not occur in people who eat a normal diet. Deficiency symptoms of weakness, mental confusion, and night blindness have occurred in people on long-term intravenous feeding or people with a rare genetic disorder.

Although molybdenum is unlikely to cause toxicity in humans, a UL for molybdenum has been set at 2,000 micrograms per day.

> **Key Concepts** Chromium is involved in glucose metabolism and probably has other important roles as well. Molybdenum is required in several important enzyme systems. Deficiency or toxicity of chromium and molybdenum is very unlikely.

Other Trace Minerals and Ultratrace Minerals

Five of the minerals we have discussed—iodine, fluoride, manganese, molybdenum, and selenium—could be considered "ultratrace" minerals. They are found in the body in minuscule amounts, and for most of these we need less than 1 milligram daily. Although there is substantial research on these minerals, the functions of other trace and ultratrace minerals are less clear. Research and attention have focused on arsenic, boron, nickel, silicon, and vanadium. Although insufficient evidence exists to set an AI or RDA for these minerals, ULs have been established for boron, nickel, and vanadium.

Arsenic

Although arsenic has been an infamous poison for centuries, inorganic arsenic may actually be an essential ultratrace element. Although no studies have determined the nutritional importance of arsenic for humans, arsenic-deprived laboratory animals have poor growth and abnormal reproduction. Dairy products, as well as meat, poultry, fish, grains, and cereal products, contribute arsenic in the diet. Some water supplies contain considerable arsenic, and standards for safe arsenic levels are hotly debated. A UL has not yet been established.

Boron

Boron is essential for some animals and likely is essential for humans. Boron plays a role in promoting bone metabolism, brain health, and cancer prevention.[95] Americans generally seem to consume diets adequate in boron. Noncitrus fruits and leafy vegetables are good sources. Although coffee and milk are low in boron, Americans consume such large quantities of these beverages that they are among the top boron contributors to the American diet.

Chronic boron toxicity symptoms include poor appetite, nausea, weight loss, decreased sex drive, and low sperm count. The UL for boron is 20 milligrams per day.

Nickel

A few nickel-containing enzymes have been identified, and nickel can activate or inhibit a number of other enzymes. Although nickel is an essential trace element in animals, the specific function of nickel in

Quick **Bite**

Molybdenum Takes a Stand Against the Elements
Molybdenum is a silvery-gray metal that is not found free in nature. It has properties similar to those of tungsten and is used as an alloy to strengthen and protect metal from corrosion.

TABLE 8.4
Summary of Minerals

Mineral	Important Dietary Sources	Major Functions	Signs/Symptoms of Deficiency	Toxic Effects of Megadoses	Special Considerations
Macrominerals					
Sodium AI: Younger than age 51: 1,500 milligrams Ages 51–70: 1,300 milligrams Over age 70: 1,200 milligrams UL: 1,500 mg for those age 51 and older; African Americans; or those who have hypertension, diabetes, or chronic kidney disease	Salt Soy sauce Condiments Processed foods	Helps maintain normal fluid and acid–base balance	Muscle cramps and loss of appetite	High blood pressure	Getting enough sodium is not an issue for most people. Most people consume far too much sodium, which puts them at risk for high blood pressure.
Potassium AI: 4,700 milligrams	Meat Milk Fruits and vegetables Grains Legumes	Essential for fluid balance Involved in muscle contraction	Muscle weakness, paralysis, confusion; can cause death in severe cases	Toxicity from potassium from food is extremely rare. Potassium supplements should only be taken if prescribed by a healthcare provider due to the potential of large amounts of potassium slowing or even stopping the heart.	Moderate potassium deficiency may increase risk of high blood pressure.
Chloride AI: Younger than age 51: 2,300 milligrams Ages 51–70: 2,000 milligrams Over age 70: 1,800 milligrams UL: 3,600 milligrams	Table salt Processed foods Soy sauce Eggs Meat	One of the major extracellular anions in the body. Helps maintain fluid balance. As part of HCl, it is necessary for digestion.	Deficiency is very rare.	Excessive dietary chloride only occurs with consumption of large amounts of salt or potassium chloride. Toxic effects of such diets are attributed to the high sodium content of the diet as opposed to high chloride.	Deficiency can occur with extreme fluid loss that is associated with prolonged or repeated vomiting or diarrhea or extreme sweating for prolonged periods of time. When deficiency does occur, it results in alkalosis, a life-threatening condition where the blood becomes alkaline.
Calcium AI: Younger than age 51: 1,000 milligrams Age 51 and older: 1,200 milligrams UL: 2,500 mg	Milk and milk products Green leafy vegetables Soybeans Tofu processed with calcium carbonate	Essential for bone mineralization Involved in muscle contraction Needed for proper blood clotting	Bone loss in adults (osteoporosis) Improper growth in children	Toxicity is rare; however, calcium supplements may interfere with the absorption of other minerals, specifically iron, zinc, and magnesium.	The body keeps the calcium level in the blood constant. Even if calcium intake is very low, calcium will be pulled from the bones.
Phosphorus RDA: 700 milligrams UL: 4,000 milligrams	Meat Poultry Milk and milk products Soft drinks Processed foods	Involved in the mineralization of bones and teeth Essential for acid–base balance	Uncommon	Kidney stones	

Mineral	Sources	Function	Deficiency	Toxicity	Notes
Magnesium RDA: Women: 320 milligrams Men: 420 milligrams UL: 350 milligrams from nonfood sources	Nuts Legumes Green leafy vegetables Seafood	Involved in bone mineralization Essential for protein synthesis Needed for muscle contraction	Weakness, confusion, growth failure	Uncommon	
Sulfur No RDA	Protein foods	Helps proteins maintain their functional shapes Important in liver function and in maintaining acid–base balance	No known deficiency		
Microminerals					
Iron RDA: Women younger than age 51: 18 milligrams Women 51 and over: 8 milligrams Men: 8 milligrams UL: 45 milligrams	Meat Seafood Spinach Lentils Cereals fortified with iron	Transports oxygen in the blood Serves as a component of many enzymes	Anemia	Digestive problems. Accidental iron overdose is a leading cause of poisoning deaths in young children.	Cooking in an iron pan, especially acid foods such as spaghetti sauce, can increase the iron content of food dramatically.
Zinc RDA: Women: 8 milligrams Men: 11 milligrams UL: 40 milligrams	Meat Fish Shellfish Poultry Cereals fortified with zinc	Helps stabilize cell membranes Supports fertility and reproduction Involved in cell growth and replication	Uncommon	Uncommon from food sources. High doses of zinc through supplements can cause a decrease in immune function	Zinc lozenges are commonly used to decrease the duration of the common cold. There is conflicting evidence as to the effectiveness.
Selenium RDA: 55 micrograms UL: 400 micrograms	Meat Seafood Whole grains Vegetables				
Iodine RDA: 150 micrograms UL: 1,100 micrograms	Iodized salt Seafood Bread Eggs	Essential component of thyroid hormones	Low levels of thyroid hormones. Severe deficiency causes a goiter or enlargement of the thyroid gland—this is rare in North America.	Decreased thyroid activity	
Copper RDA: 900 micrograms UL: 10,000 micrograms	Shellfish Sunflower seeds Hazelnuts Mushrooms Beans Peanuts	Helps make hemoglobin Serves as a component of several enzymes	Uncommon	Uncommon	

(continues)

TABLE 8.4 *(continued)*
Summary of Minerals

Mineral	Important Dietary Sources	Major Functions	Signs/Symptoms of Deficiency	Toxic Effects of Megadoses	Special Considerations
Manganese AI: Women: 1.8 milligrams Men: 2.3 milligrams UL: 11 milligrams	Green leafy vegetables Whole grains Sweet potatoes	Involved in energy metabolism Serves as a component of several enzymes	Uncommon	Uncommon	Calcium can interfere with the absorption of manganese. If you take a calcium supplement, be sure to regularly include foods high in manganese in your diet.
Fluoride AI: Women: 3 milligrams Men: 4 milligrams UL: 10 milligrams	Water, if fluoridated or naturally containing fluorine Tea Seafood	Needed for proper bone and teeth formation Helps make teeth resistant to decay	Susceptibility to tooth decay	Discoloration of teeth (fluorosis), nausea, vomiting	
Chromium AI: Women under age 51: 25 milligrams Women 51 and over: 20 milligrams Men: 35 milligrams Men 51 and over: 30 milligrams	Whole grains Meats Vegetable oil	Helps glucose move into the cell Aids in lipid metabolism	Abnormal glucose metabolism	Only known toxicity is exposure to airborne chromium in industrial settings.	Chromium supplements are popular among athletes and body builders even though there is limited evidence of their effectiveness.
Molybdenum RDA: 45 micrograms UL: 2,000 micrograms	Grains Nuts Legumes	Serves as a component of several enzymes	Uncommon	Uncommon	

humans has not yet been identified. There is no known nickel deficiency in humans. Toxicity has occurred only in workers exposed to nickel dust or nickel carbonyl in industrial settings. The UL is 1 milligram per day.

Silicon

Experimental diets lacking silicon cause poor growth and skeletal abnormalities in baby chickens. Although there are no known deficiency symptoms in humans, silicon is believed to help strengthen collagen and elastin. Silicon plays a role in bone formation and growth. Silicon also may have a role in preventing atherosclerosis in the elderly. Chronic inhalation of silicon causes serious illness, but there's no evidence of dietary silicon toxicity. No UL has been set for silicon.

Vanadium

Scientists are not sure exactly what role vanadium plays in the body and have not observed deficiencies. Currently, vanadium supplements are available in amounts many times greater than that found in the diet. They are promoted to athletes and people trying to gain muscle mass. The UL for vanadium is 1.8 milligrams per day.

> **Key Concepts** Ultratrace minerals have very low estimated requirements. Although specific biochemical functions have not been defined for the minerals arsenic, boron, nickel, silicon, and vanadium, they are thought to be essential for humans.

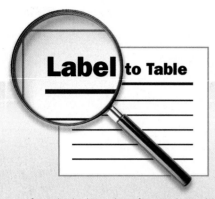

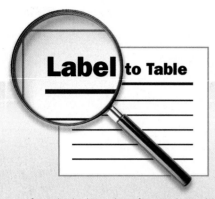

Label to Table

If you looked at a list of minerals, could you pick out the trace minerals? Let's see how well you do! Look at the accompanying Nutrition Facts label from a breakfast cereal and guess how many trace minerals are listed.

You should be able to spot three trace minerals on the label: iron, zinc, and copper. Looking at the "ingredients" and "vitamins and minerals" lists, you can see that the iron and zinc were added, but the copper appears to come naturally from the cereal. Why do you think these trace minerals are added to this cereal? Many people

(especially children) eat marginal amounts of iron and zinc. The best sources of these minerals are meats, liver, and shellfish. Most children don't eat much shellfish or liver, so adding the minerals to cereals, which they do eat, is an easy way to make sure they get 45 percent and 25 percent of the Daily Values for iron and zinc, respectively.

The last mineral you see listed is copper. There is 2 percent of the Daily Value for copper in one serving of this cereal. That's 0.04 milligram (2 percent of 2 mg).

Nutrition Facts

9 servings per container
Serving size   1 cup (30g)

Amount per serving	Cheerios	with 1/2 cup skim milk
Calories	**110**	**150**
	% DV**	% DV**
Total Fat	2g* 3%	2g* 3%
Saturated Fat	0g 0%	0.6g 3%
Trans Fat	0g	0g
Cholesterol	0g 0%	3g 1%
Sodium	280mg 12%	350mg 15%
Total Carbohydrate	22g 7%	28g 9%
Dietary Fiber	3g 11%	3g 11%
Total Sugars	1g	7g
Includes Added Sugars	1g 2%	1g 2%
Protein	3g	7g
Vitamin D	1mcg 10%	2.5mcg 25%
Calcium	40mg 4%	200mg 20%
Iron	8mg 45%	8mg 45%
Potassium	0mg 0%	300mg 9%
Vitamin A	150mcg 10%	225mcg 15%
Vitamin C	6mg 10%	6mg 10%
Thiamin	.4g 25%	.5g 30%
Riboflavin	.5mg 25%	.6mg 35%
Niacin	5mg 25%	5mg 25%
Vitamin B₆	.5mg 25%	.5mg 25%
Folic Acid	400mcg 50%	400mcg 50%
Vitamin B₁₂	1μg 25%	2μg 35%
Phosphorus	100mg 10%	250mg 25%
Zinc	4mg 25%	5mg 30%
Copper	.04mg 2%	.04mg 2%

* Amount in Cereal. A serving of cereal plus skim milk provides 2g total fat (0.5g saturated fat, 1g monosaturated fat). less than 5mg cholesterol, 350mg sodium, 300mg potassium, 28g total carbohydrate (7g sugars) and 7g protein.
** The % Daily Value (DV) tells you how much a nutrient in a serving of food contributes to a daily diet. 2,000 calories a day is used for general nutrition advice.

Learning Portfolio

Key Terms

	page
albumin	361
aldosterone	328
anions	325
antidiuretic hormone (ADH)	328
calmodulin	339
cations	325
ceruloplasmin	361
ciliary action	339
cretinism	358
electrolytes	325
ferritin	348
fibrin	339
fluorosis	365
galvanized	353
geophagia	353
goiter	360
goitrogens	359
heat capacity	326
heme	347
heme iron	348
hemochromatosis	352
hemosiderin	348
hydroxyapatite	338
hypertension	333
hypogonadism	353
hypothyroidism	357
insensible water loss	328
ions	325
iron overload	352
Keshan disease	357
Lou Gehrig's disease	363
major minerals	332
Menkes syndrome	361
mineralization	338
multiple sclerosis	363
myoglobin	347
nonheme iron	348
osmosis	326
osteoblasts	338
osteoclasts	338
oxalate (oxalic acid)	333
phytate (phytic acid)	333
plasma	325
polyphenols	349
salts	325
thyroid-stimulating hormone (TSH)	360
trace minerals	332
transferrin	349
Wilson's disease	356

Study Points

- Water is the most essential nutrient; we can live much longer without food than without water.

- Water is important for chemical reactions, temperature regulation, maintaining acid–base balance, and transporting nutrients and waste. Fluids in the body lubricate and cushion joints, cleanse the eyes, and moisten the food we eat.

- Water is lost through exhaled air, perspiration, feces, and urine. Insensible water loss is the continuous evaporation of water from the lungs and skin. Diuretics increase fluid excretion. When fluid loss exceeds intake, the resulting dehydration can seriously impair physical and mental performance.

- Minerals are inorganic elements and are categorized as major or trace depending on the amount in the body and the amount needed in the diet.

- The bioavailability of minerals may be affected by excess intake of single-mineral supplements; phytate, oxalate, and fiber in plant foods; and mineral status in the body.

- Sodium helps regulate water distribution and blood pressure. Most Americans eat too much dietary sodium, mainly from processed foods.

- Potassium is necessary for nerve and muscle function. Unprocessed foods, including fruits and vegetables, provide most dietary potassium. A diet high in potassium from fruits and vegetables may help to lower blood pressure.

- Chloride is a component of stomach acid. Chloride deficiency is most often associated with prolonged vomiting. Most Americans consume more chloride than recommended as part of salt (sodium chloride).

- Calcium, the most abundant mineral in the body, is found mainly in bones and teeth. It's required for blood clotting, nerve and muscle function, and cellular metabolism. Major dietary sources of calcium are dairy products and calcium-fortified foods.

- Phosphorus is a key component of ATP, DNA, RNA, phospholipids, and lipoproteins. Because phosphorus is widespread in foods, inadequate phosphorus intake is rare.

- Plant foods such as whole grains and vegetables are important sources of magnesium, which is a cofactor for hundreds of enzymes. Kidney disease, alcoholism, and overuse of diuretics may cause low magnesium levels.

Learning Portfolio (continued)

- Sulfur does not function alone as a nutrient, but as a component of certain amino acids and the vitamins biotin and thiamin.

- Hemoglobin and myoglobin contain iron, which transports oxygen. Iron is also an enzyme cofactor, important for immune function and brain function.

- Due to menstruation, women of childbearing age need more iron than men do. Meats are the best source of iron, but enriched and whole grains are also significant sources in the American diet.

- Iron deficiency is the most common nutritional deficiency worldwide. Anemia is the most severe stage of deficiency, occurring after iron stores are depleted. Iron toxicity can be acute or chronic. Accidental iron overdose is a leading cause of poisoning deaths of young children in the United States. Hemochromatosis is a disease of chronic excessive iron absorption.

- Zinc is a cofactor for numerous enzymes and is crucial for normal growth, sexual development, and immune function. It is found in protein-rich foods, particularly meats. Deficiency results in poor growth, impaired taste, and impaired immune response.

- Selenium is considered an antioxidant nutrient. It is also needed for thyroid function. Good sources of selenium are Brazil nuts, organ meats, and seafood. Deficiency of selenium in the Keshan region of China is associated with Keshan heart disease.

- Iodine is required for thyroid function. Iodine deficiency causes enlarged thyroid or goiter. Severe deficiency during pregnancy can cause cretinism in the baby. Much of the iodine in the American diet comes from iodized salt.

- Copper functions in many enzyme systems involved with antioxidant protection, iron utilization, and immune function. The richest food sources of copper include organ meats, shellfish, nuts and seeds, peanut butter, and chocolate. Copper deficiency is rare.

- Manganese functions in many enzyme systems. The best food sources include tea, coffee, nuts, cereals, and some fruits. Manganese deficiency and toxicity are uncommon; toxicity is from manganese air pollutants.

- Fluoride promotes mineralization of bones and teeth and protects teeth from decay. Water, which contains fluoride naturally or is fluoridated, is our main fluoride source. Excessive fluoride causes fluorosis, which mottles teeth.

- Chromium is involved in glucose metabolism. Some good sources of chromium are broccoli, grape juice, processed meats, and whole grains. Chromium toxicity is unlikely.

- Molybdenum functions as an enzyme cofactor. Good food sources are peas, beans, and some breakfast cereals. Molybdenum deficiency and toxicity are both rare.

- Ultratrace minerals are those required in extremely small amounts; the specific function of many of these nutrients is unknown. Some ultratrace minerals are arsenic, boron, nickel, silicon, and vanadium.

Study Questions

1. List the biological functions of water.
2. Which major minerals affect blood pressure?
3. What are the major functions of calcium, other than its relation to bone health?
4. Explain the differences between heme and non-heme iron. Which is absorbed better?
5. List the three stages of iron deficiency.
6. What are the main functions of selenium?
7. What is goiter?
8. How does fluoride prevent tooth decay? Other than water, what sources supply fluoride?
9. What is chromium's best-understood role in the body? Which foods are good sources of chromium?

Getting Personal

How Much Water Are You Drinking?

To better understand your fluid requirements and intake, keep a fluid journal for one day. Write down everything you drink and the quantity. (Although water from food contributes, too, this activity will at least give you a general guideline of how much you are drinking.) Assess your hydration status by the simple urine test described in this chapter.

Time	Water or Other Beverage	Amount
Example: 8 AM	Coffee	16 ounces

- Do you think you are well hydrated, based on your intake and output of fluids? Why or why not? (Keep in mind that physical activity and weather can affect output.)
- Jot down a list of foods you regularly eat that you think may be adding to your total water intake.
- What were the results of your urine test?
- How do the results of your urine test compare with your intake?

Try This

Osmosis Experiment

Purchase some celery and let it sit for a week or two until it becomes limp. When the celery looks limp and lifeless, fill your sink with cold water and soak the celery. When it has soaked for several hours, take the celery out and examine its appearance. Notice anything different? Because the crispness of celery is due to osmotic pressure, when you soaked the limp celery, it absorbed water into its cells and became crisp again.

A Simple Check on Your Zinc

A simple test can provide a rough signal of your zinc status. Buy some zinc sulfate at a health food store. Dissolve it in distilled water to make a 0.1 percent zinc sulfate solution. Refrain from eating, drinking, and smoking for at least an hour before the test. Then swish a teaspoon of the solution around your mouth for 10 seconds. If it tastes unpleasant or metallic, your level of zinc is probably adequate. However, if the solution tastes like water, you may be consuming less zinc than you need.

References

1. Institute of Medicine, Food and Nutrition Board. *Dietary Reference Intakes for Water, Potassium, Sodium, Chloride, and Sulfate*. Washington, DC: National Academies Press; 2004.
2. Popkin BM, D'Anci KE, Rosenberg IH. Water, hydration, and health. *Nutr Rev*. 2010;68(8):439-458.
3. Institute of Medicine, Food and Nutrition Board. Op. cit.
4. Ibid.
5. Popkin BM, D'Anci KE, Rosenberg IH. Op. cit.
6. Duff RL. *American Dietetic Association Complete Food and Nutrition Guide*. 4th ed. New York: Houghton Mifflin Harcourt; 2012.
7. Maughan RJ. Hydration, morbidity, and mortality in vulnerable populations. *Nutr Rev*. 2012;70(Suppl 2):S152-S155. doi: 10.1111/j.1753-4887.2012.00531.x
8. Armstrong LE. Challenges of linking chronic dehydration and fluid consumption to health outcomes. *Nutr Rev*. 2012;70(Suppl 2):S121-S127. doi: 10.1111/j.1753-4887.2012.00539.x
9. Stuempfle KJ. Exercise-associated hyponatremia during winter sports. *Phys Sportsmed*. 2010;38(1):101-106.
10. Institute of Medicine, Food and Nutrition Board. Op. cit.
11. Nevius CW. In hazing, dumb stunts can be fatal. *San Francisco Chronicle*. February 8, 2005. http://sfgate.com/cgi-bin/article.cgi?file=/c/a/2005/02/08/BAG61B7D341.DTL. Accessed September 9, 2017.
12. Medeiros DM, Wildman REC. *Advanced Human Nutrition*. 2nd ed. Burlington, MA: Jones & Bartlett Learning; 2012.
13. U.S. Department of Health and Human Services, U.S. Department of Agriculture. *2015–2020 Dietary Guidelines for Americans*. 8th ed. Washington, DC: U.S. Government Printing Office; 2015.
14. Institute of Medicine, Food and Nutrition Board. Op. cit.
15. U.S. Department of Health and Human Services, U.S. Department of Agriculture. Op. cit.
16. American Heart Association. The American Heart Association's diet and lifestyle recommendations. http://www.heart.org/HEARTORG/GettingHealthy/Diet-and-Lifestyle-Recommendations_UCM_305855_Article.jsp. Accessed September 9, 2017.
17. Institute of Medicine, Food and Nutrition Board. *Sodium Intake in Populations: Assessment of Evidence*. Washington, DC: National Academies Press; 2013.
18. Kretser A, Dunn C, DeVirgillis R, Levine D. Utility of a new food value analysis application to evaluate trade-offs when making food selection. *Nutr Today*. 2014;49(4):185-194.
19. Chen ST, Maruthur NM, Appel LJ. The effect of dietary patterns on estimated coronary heart disease risk: results from the Dietary Approaches to Stop Hypertension (DASH) trial. *Circulation*. 2010;3(5):484-489.
20. Institute of Medicine, Food and Nutrition Board. *Dietary Reference Intakes for Water, Potassium, Sodium, Chloride, and Sulfate*. Op. cit.
21. U.S. Department of Health and Human Services, U.S. Department of Agriculture. Op. cit.
22. Yang Q, Liu T, Kuklina EV, et al. Sodium and potassium intake and mortality among U.S. adults. Prospective data from the Third National Health and Nutrition Examination Survey. *Arch Intern Med*. 2011;171(13):1183-1191.
23. Institute of Medicine, Food and Nutrition Board. *Dietary Reference Intakes for Water, Potassium, Sodium, Chloride, and Sulfate*. Op. cit.
24. Ibid.
25. Howe TE, Shea B, Dawson LJ, et al. Exercise for preventing and treating osteoporosis in postmenopausal women. *Cochrane Database Syst Rev*. 2011;7:CD000333.
26. Institute of Medicine, Food and Nutrition Board. *Dietary Reference Intakes for Calcium and Vitamin D*. Washington, DC: National Academies Press; 2011.
27. Jung Yang Y, Martin BR, Boushey CJ. Development and evaluation of a brief calcium assessment tool for adolescents. *J Am Diet Assoc*. 2010;110:111-115.
28. National Institutes of Health, Office of Dietary Supplements. Calcium: fact sheet for health professionals. http://ods.od.nih.gov/factsheets/calcium. Accessed September 9, 2017.
29. Institute of Medicine, Food and Nutrition Board. *Dietary Reference Intakes for Calcium and Vitamin D*. Op. cit.
30. Ibid.
31. National Institutes of Health, Office of Dietary Supplements. Op. cit.
32. Institute of Medicine, Food, and Nutrition Board. *Dietary Reference Intakes for Calcium and Vitamin D*. Op. cit.
33. Institute of Medicine, Food and Nutrition Board. *Dietary Reference Intakes for Calcium, Phosphorus, Magnesium, Vitamin D, and Fluoride*. Washington, DC: National Academies Press; 1997.
34. Ibid.
35. Ibid.
36. Ibid.
37. Ibid.
38. Longo D, Fauci A, Kasper D, Hauser S, Jameson J, Loscalzo J. *Harrison's Principles of Internal Medicine*. 18th ed. New York: McGraw-Hill; 2011.
39. Gropper SS, Smith JL. *Advanced Nutrition and Human Metabolism*. 6th ed. Belmont, CA: Cengage Learning; 2012.

Learning Portfolio (continued)

40. Ibid.

41. World Health Organization. Micronutrient deficiencies: Iron deficiency anaemia. http://www.who.int/nutrition/topics/ida/en/. Accessed September 9, 2017.

42. Wessling-Resnick M. Iron. In Ross AC, Caballero B, Cousins RJ, et al. eds. *Modern Nutrition in Health and Disease.* 11th ed. Baltimore, MD: Lippincott Williams and Wilkins; 2014:176-188.

43. Institute of Medicine, Food and Nutrition Board. *Dietary Reference Intakes for Vitamin A, Vitamin K, Arsenic, Boron, Chromium, Copper, Iodine, Iron, Manganese, Molybdenum, Nickel, Silicon, Vanadium, and Zinc.* Washington, DC: National Academies Press; 2001.

44. Hurrell R, Egli I. Iron bioavailability and dietary reference values. *Am J Clin Nutr.* 2010;91(Suppl):1461S-1467S.

45. Ibid.

46. Gropper SS, Smith JL. Op. cit.

47. Institute of Medicine, Food and Nutrition Board. *Dietary Reference Intakes for Vitamin A, Vitamin K, Arsenic, Boron, Chromium, Copper, Iodine, Iron, Manganese, Molybdenum, Nickel, Silicon, Vanadium, and Zinc.* Op. cit.

48. Ibid.

49. Spanierman CS. Iron toxicity. Medscape. http://emedicine.medscape.com /article/815213-overview. Accessed September 9, 2017.

50. Centers for Disease Control and Prevention. Hemochromatosis (iron storage disease). https://www.cdc.gov/genomics/resources/diseases /hemochromatosis.htm. Accessed September 18, 2017.

51. Prasad AS, Helstead JA, Nadami M. Syndrome of iron deficiency anaemia, hepatosplenomegaly, hypogonadism, dwarfism, and geophagia. *Am J Med.* 1961;31:532-546.

52. Sandstead HH, Prasad AS, Schubert AR, et al. Human zinc deficiency endocrine manifestations and response to treatment. *Am J Clin Nutr.* 1967;20:422-442.

53. Institute of Medicine, Food and Nutrition Board. *Dietary Reference Intakes for Vitamin A, Vitamin K, Arsenic, Boron, Chromium, Copper, Iodine, Iron, Manganese, Molybdenum, Nickel, Silicon, Vanadium, and Zinc.* Op. cit.

54. King JC, Cousins RJ. Zinc. In Ross AC, Caballero B, Cousins RJ, et al. *Modern Nutrition in Health and Disease.* 11th ed. Baltimore, MD: Lippincott Williams and Wilkins; 2014:189-205.

55. Hambidge KM, Miller LV, Westcott JE, Sheng X, Krebs NF. Zinc bioavailability and homeostasis. *Am J Clin Nutr.* 2010;91(5):1478S-1483S.

56. Position of the Academy of Nutrition and Dietetics: vegetarian diets. *J Am Diet Assoc.* 2009;109(7):1266-1282.

57. Gropper SS, Smith JL. Op. cit.

58. Institute of Medicine Food, and Nutrition Board. *Dietary Reference Intakes for Vitamin A, Vitamin K, Arsenic, Boron, Chromium, Copper, Iodine, Iron, Manganese, Molybdenum, Nickel, Silicon, Vanadium, and Zinc.* Op. cit.

59. Johnson LE. Zinc. Merck Manual Professional Version. http://www.merck .com/mmpe/sec01/ch005/ch005j.html. Accessed September 9, 2017.

60. Ibid.

61. Johnson LE. Copper. Merck Manual Professional Version. http://www .merck.com/mmpe/sec01/ch005/ch005c.html. Accessed September 9, 2017.

62. Dennert G, Zwahlen M, Brinkman M, Vinceti M, Zeegers MP, Horneber M. Selenium for preventing cancer. *Cochrane Database Syst Rev.* 2011;5:CD005195.

63. National Institutes of Health, Office of Dietary Supplements. Selenium: dietary supplement fact sheet. http://ods.od.nih.gov/factsheets/selenium. Accessed September 9, 2017.

64. Institute of Medicine, Food and Nutrition Board. *Dietary Reference Intakes for Vitamin C, Vitamin E, Selenium, and Carotenoids.* Washington, DC: National Academies Press; 2000.

65. National Institutes of Health, Office of Dietary Supplements. Selenium: dietary supplement fact sheet. Op. cit.

66. Hetzel BS. *The Story of Iodine Deficiency: An International Challenge in Nutrition.* Oxford, UK: Oxford University Press; 1989.

67. World Health Organization. Micronutrient deficiencies: iodine deficiency disorders. http://www.who.int/nutrition/topics/idd/en/index.html. Accessed September 9, 2017.

68. Institute of Medicine, Food and Nutrition Board. *Dietary Reference Intakes for Vitamin A, Vitamin K, Arsenic, Boron, Chromium, Copper, Iodine, Iron, Manganese, Molybdenum, Nickel, Silicon, Vanadium, and Zinc.* Op. cit.

69. Johnson LE. Iodine. Merck Manual Professional Version. http://www .merck.com/mmpe/sec01/ch005/ch005e.html. Accessed September 9, 2017.

70. Institute of Medicine, Food and Nutrition Board. *Dietary Reference Intakes for Vitamin A, Vitamin K, Arsenic, Boron, Chromium, Copper, Iodine, Iron, Manganese, Molybdenum, Nickel, Silicon, Vanadium, and Zinc.* Op. cit.

71. Collins JF. Copper. In Ross AC, Caballero B, Cousins RJ, et al. *Modern Nutrition in Health and Disease.* 11th ed. Baltimore, MD: Lippincott Williams and Wilkins; 2014:206-216.

72. Institute of Medicine, Food and Nutrition Board. *Dietary Reference Intakes for Vitamin A, Vitamin K, Arsenic, Boron, Chromium, Copper, Iodine, Iron, Manganese, Molybdenum, Nickel, Silicon, Vanadium, and Zinc.* Op. cit.

73. American Dental Hygienists' Association. Fluoride facts. 2009. http:// www.adha.org/sites/default/files/7253_Fluoride_Facts.pdf. Accessed November 9, 2016.

74. Everett ET. Fluoride's effects on the formation of teeth and bones, and the influence of genetics. *J Dent Res.* 2011;90(5):552-560.

75. Institute of Medicine, Food and Nutrition Board. *Dietary Reference Intakes for Calcium, Phosphorus, Magnesium, Vitamin D, and Fluoride.* Op. cit.

76. Benjamin RM. Oral health. The silent epidemic. *Public Health Rep.* 2010;125(2):158-159.

77. American Dental Association. Oral health topics. Fluoride supplements. Facts about fluoride. http://www.ada.org/en/member-center/oral-health -topics/fluoride-supplements. Accessed September 9, 2017.

78. U.S. Department of Health and Human Services. HHS and EPA announce new scientific assessments and actions on fluoride: agencies working together to maintain benefits of preventing tooth decay while preventing excessive exposure. June 7, 2011. http://yosemite.epa.gov/opa /admpress.nsf/6427a6 b7538955c585257359003f0230/86964af577 c37ab285257811005a8417!OpenDocument&Start=1&Count=5&Ex pand=1. Accessed September 9, 2017.

79. Environmental Protection Agency. Basic information about fluoride in drinking water. http://water.epa.gov/drink/contaminants/basicinformation /fluoride.cfm. Accessed June 17, 2014.

80. U.S. Department of Health and Human Services. Op. cit.

81. Vernacchio L, Kelly JP, Kaufman DW, Mitchell AA. Vitamin, fluoride, and iron use among U.S. children younger than 12 years of age: results from the Slone Survey, 1998–2007. *J Am Diet Assoc.* 2011;111(2):285-289.

82. Position of the Academy of Nutrition and Dietetics: the impact of fluoride on health *J Acad Nutr Diet.* 2012;112:1443-1453.

83. George C. Battle renewed over value of fluoridation. *CMAJ.* 2011;183(10):1173.

84. American Dental Association. Fluoride in water. http://www.ada.org /fluoride.aspx. Accessed September 9, 2017.

85. Berg J, Gerweck C, Hujoel PP, et al. Evidence-based clinical recommendations regarding fluoride intake from reconstituted infant formula and enamel fluorosis. A report of the American Dental Association Council on Scientific Affairs. *J Am Dent Assoc.* 2011;142(1):79-87.

86. Institute of Medicine, Food and Nutrition Board. *Dietary Reference Intakes for Vitamin A, Vitamin K, Arsenic, Boron, Chromium, Copper, Iodine, Iron, Manganese, Molybdenum, Nickel, Silicon, Vanadium, and Zinc.* Op. cit.

87. Austin RP. Should I try chromium tablets? *Diabetes Forecast.* July 2011. http://www.diabetesforecast.org/2011/jul/should-i-try-chromium-tablets .html. Accessed September 9, 2017.

88. Sharma S, Agrawal RP, Choudhary M, Jain S, Goyal S, Agarwal V. Beneficial effect of chromium supplementation on glucose, HbA(1)C, and lipid variables in individuals with newly onset type-2 diabetes. *J Trace Elem Med Biol*. 2011;25(3):149-153.

89. Onakpoya I, Posadzki P, Ernst E. Chromium supplementation in overweight and obesity: a systematic review and meta-analysis of randomized clinical trials. *Obes Rev*. 2013;14(6):496-507. doi: 10.1111/obr.12026. Epub March 18, 2013.

90. Chehade JM, Sheikh-Ali M, Mooradian AD. The role of micronutrients in managing diabetes. *Diabetes Spectr*. 2009;22(4):214-218.

91. Tian H, Guo X, Wang X, He Z, Sun R, Ge S, Zhang Z. Chromium picolinate supplementation for overweight or obese adults. *Cochrane Database Syst Rev*. 2013;11:CD010063. doi: 10.1002/14651858.CD010063.pub2

92. Onakpoya I, Posadzki P, Ernst E. Op. cit.

93. Jeukendrup AE, Randell R. Fat burners: nutrition supplements that increase fat metabolism. *Obes Rev*. 2011;12(10):841-851.

94. Institute of Medicine, Food and Nutrition Board. *Dietary Reference Intakes for Vitamin A, Vitamin K, Arsenic, Boron, Chromium, Copper, Iodine, Iron, Manganese, Molybdenum, Nickel, Silicon, Vanadium, and Zinc*. Op. cit.

95. Eckhert CD. Trace minerals in modern nutrition in health and disease. In Ross AC, Caballero B, Cousins RJ, et al. *Modern Nutrition in Health and Disease*. 11th ed. Baltimore, MD: Lippincott Williams and Wilkins; 2014:245-257.

Spotlight on Metabolism and Energy Balance

Revised by Don Ross

THINK About It

1   You are driving on "the energy highway." You stop at the tollbooth. What kind of currency do you need to pay the toll?

2   When you think of "cell power," what comes to mind?

3   What do you think is meant by the saying "Fat burns in a flame of carbohydrate"?

4   When it comes to fasting, what's your body's first priority?

5   How often are you tempted by dessert after a big meal?

CHAPTER Menu

- Energy: Fuel for Work
- What Is Metabolism?
- Breakdown and Release of Energy
- Alcohol Metabolism
- Biosynthesis and Storage
- Special States

- Energy Balance: Finding Your Equilibrium
- Energy In
- Energy Out: Fuel Uses
- Body Composition: Understanding Fatness and Weight

LEARNING Objectives

1   Predict energy balance in the body.
2   Determine BMI and total energy expenditure using standard equations.
3   Differentiate between anabolic and catabolic reactions.
4   Describe the process of extracting ATP from carbohydrate, fat, and protein.
5   Discuss the role of insulin in energy storage and glucose regulation.
6   Explain how energy use differs in the states of psychological stress, diabetes, obesity, and exercise.

Your body is a wonderfully efficient factory. It accepts raw materials (food), burns some to generate power, uses some to produce finished goods, routes the rest to storage, and discards waste and byproducts. Constant turnover of your stored inventory keeps it fresh. Your body draws on these stored raw materials to produce compounds, and nutrient intake replenishes the supply.

Do you ever wonder how your biological factory responds to changing supply and demand? Under normal circumstances, the body hums along nicely with all processes in balance. When supply exceeds demand, your body stores the excess raw materials. When supply fails to meet demand, your body draws on these stored materials to meet its needs. Your biological factory never stops; even though a storage or energy-production process may dominate, all your factory operations are active at all times.

Collectively, we call these processes **metabolism**. (See **FIGURE SM.1**.) Whereas some metabolic reactions break down molecules to extract energy, others synthesize building blocks to produce new molecules. To carry out metabolic processes, thousands of chemical reactions occur every moment in cells throughout your body. The most active metabolic sites include your liver, muscle, and brain cells.

▶ **metabolism** All chemical reactions within organisms that enable them to maintain life. The two main categories of metabolism are catabolism and anabolism.

Energy: Fuel for Work

🍎 **Why Is This Important?** Energy in food is stored in the molecular bonds of carbohydrates, fats, and proteins. Our bodies extract this energy and convert it to a form that our cells can use.

To operate, machines need energy. Cars use gasoline for fuel, factory machinery uses electricity, and windmills rely on wind power. So what about you? All cells require energy to sustain life. Even during sleep your body uses energy for breathing, pumping blood, maintaining body temperature, delivering oxygen to tissues, removing waste products, synthesizing new tissue for growth, and repairing damaged or worn-out tissues. When awake, you need additional energy for physical movement (such as standing, walking, and talking) and for the digestion and absorption of foods.

▶ **chemical energy** Energy contained in the bonds between atoms of a molecule.

▶ **photosynthesis** The process by which green plants use light energy from the sun to produce carbohydrates from carbon dioxide and water.

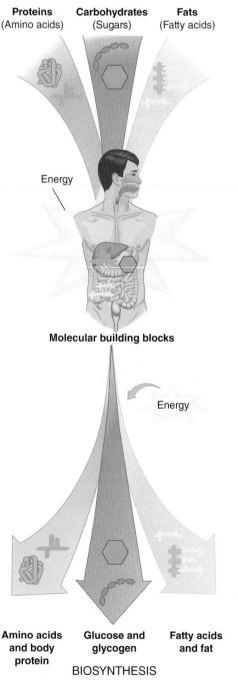

EXTRACTION OF ENERGY

Proteins   **Carbohydrates**   **Fats**
(Amino acids)   (Sugars)   (Fatty acids)

Energy

Molecular building blocks

Energy

Amino acids   **Glucose and**   **Fatty acids**
and body   **glycogen**   **and fat**
protein

BIOSYNTHESIS

FIGURE SM.1   Metabolism. Cells use metabolic reactions to extract energy from food and to form building blocks for biosynthesis.

Where does the energy come from to power your body's "machinery"? Our cells get their energy from **chemical energy** held in the molecular bonds of carbohydrates, fats, and proteins—the energy macronutrients—as well as alcohol.[1] The chemical energy in food and beverages originates as light energy from the sun. Green plants use light energy to make carbohydrate in a process called **photosynthesis**. In photosynthesis, carbon dioxide (CO_2) from the air combines with water (H_2O) from the earth to form a carbohydrate, usually glucose ($C_6H_{12}O_6$), and oxygen (O_2). Plants store glucose as starch and release oxygen into the atmosphere. Plants such as corn, peas, squash, turnips, potatoes, and rice store especially high amounts of starch in their edible parts. When our bodies extract energy from food and convert it to a form that our cells can use, we lose more than half of the total food energy as heat.[2]

Within any system (including the universe), the total amount of energy is constant. Although energy can change from one form to another and can move from one location to another, the system never gains nor loses energy. This principle, called the first law of thermodynamics, is known as conservation of energy.

Transferring Food Energy to Cellular Energy

Although burning food releases energy as heat, we cannot use heat to power the many cellular functions that maintain life. Rather than using combustion, we transfer energy from food to a form that our cells can use. This transfer is not completely efficient; we lose roughly half of the total food energy as heat as our bodies extract energy from food in three stages (see **FIGURE SM.2**)[3]:

- *Stage 1: Digestion, absorption, and transport:* Digestion breaks food down into small subunits—simple sugars, fatty acids, monoglycerides, glycerol, and amino acids—that the small intestine can absorb. The circulatory system then transports these nutrients to tissues throughout the body.
- *Stage 2: Breakdown of many small molecules to a few key metabolites:* Inside individual cells, chemical reactions convert simple sugars, fatty acids, glycerol, and amino acids into a few key **metabolites** (products of metabolic reactions). This process liberates a small amount of usable energy.
- *Stage 3: Transfer of energy to a form that cells can use:* The complete breakdown of metabolites to carbon dioxide and water liberates large amounts of energy. The reactions during this stage are responsible for converting more than 90 percent of the available food energy to a form of energy our bodies can use.

What Is Metabolism?

🍎 **Why Is This Important?** Metabolism is a general term for the chemical activity in our bodies. These activities enable us to eat, sleep, repair tissue, grow, think, and feel. They sustain life and are all that make us who we are.

Metabolism is a general term that encompasses all chemical changes occurring in living organisms. The term **metabolic pathway** describes a series of chemical reactions that either break down a large compound into smaller units (**catabolism**) or build more complex molecules from smaller ones (**anabolism**).[4] For example, when you eat bread or rice,

STAGES IN THE EXTRACTION OF ENERGY FROM FOOD

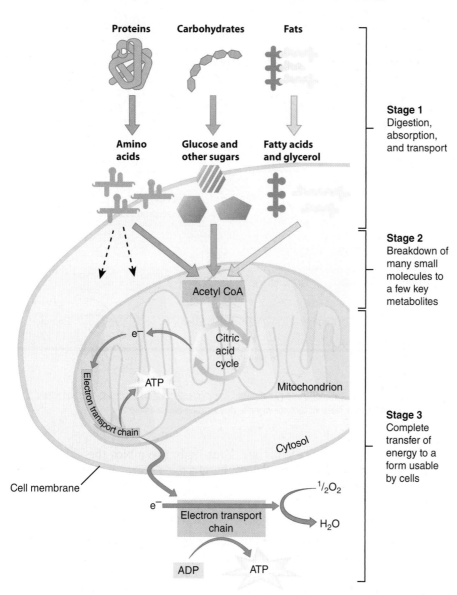

FIGURE SM.2 Energy extraction from food. In the first stage, the body breaks down food into amino acids, monosaccharides, and fatty acids. In the second stage, cells degrade these molecules to a few simple units, such as acetyl CoA, that are widespread in metabolism. In the third stage, the oxygen-dependent reactions of the citric acid cycle and electron transport chain liberate large amounts of energy in the form of ATP.

the GI tract breaks down the starch into glucose units. Cells can further catabolize these glucose units to release energy for activities such as muscle contractions. Conversely, anabolic reactions take available glucose molecules and assemble them into glycogen for storage. (See **FIGURE SM.3**.)

Metabolic pathways are never completely inactive. Their activity continually ebbs and flows in response to internal and external events. Imagine, for example, that your instructor keeps you late and you have only five minutes to get to your next class. As you hustle across campus, your body ramps up energy production to fuel the demand created by your rapidly contracting muscles. As you sit in your next class, your body continues to break down and extract glucose from

▶ **metabolites** Substances produced during metabolism.

▶ **metabolic pathway** A series of chemical reactions that either break down a large compound into smaller units (catabolism) or synthesize more complex molecules from smaller ones (anabolism).

▶ **catabolism [ca-TA-bol-iz-um]** Any metabolic process whereby cells break down complex substances into simpler, smaller ones.

▶ **anabolism [an-A-bol-iz-um]** Any metabolic process whereby cells build complex substances from simple, smaller units.

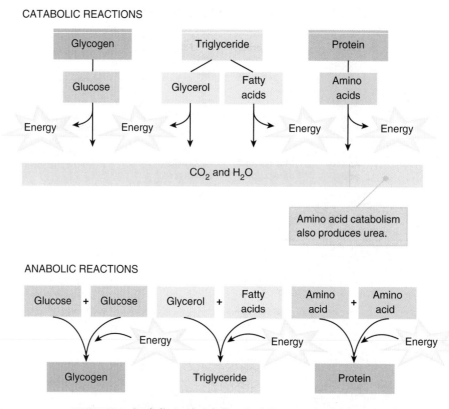

FIGURE SM.3 Catabolism and anabolism. Catabolic reactions break down molecules and release energy. Anabolic reactions consume energy as they assemble complex molecules.

the banana you recently ate. Your body assembles the glucose into branched chains to replenish the glycogen stores you depleted running across campus.

The Cell Is the Metabolic Processing Center

Cells are the work centers of metabolism. (See **FIGURE SM.4**.) Although our bodies are made up of different types of cells (e.g., liver cells, brain cells, kidney cells, muscle cells), most have a similar structure. The basic animal cell has two major parts—the cell **nucleus** and a membrane-enclosed space called the **cytoplasm**. As we zoom in for a closer look, we see that the semifluid **cytosol** fills the cytoplasm. Floating in the cytosol are many **organelles**, small units that perform specialized metabolic functions. A large number of these organelles—the capsule-like **mitochondria**—are power generators that contain many important energy-producing pathways.

To remember the major parts of a cell, think about a bowl of thick vegetable soup with a single meatball floating in it. For our example, think of the broth as having a runny, jelly-like consistency and the bowl as a thin, flexible structure with the consistency of a wet paper bag. The bowl surrounds and holds the mixture, similar to the way a cell membrane encloses a cell. The meatball represents the cell nucleus, and the remaining mixture is the cytoplasm. This cytoplasmic soup is made up of a thick, semiliquid fluid (cytosol) and vegetables (organelles). Among the vegetables, think of those kidney beans as mitochondria.

Enzymes speed up chemical reactions in metabolic pathways. Many enzymes are inactive unless they are combined with certain smaller

▶ **cells** The basic structural units of all living tissues. Cells have two major parts—the nucleus and the cytoplasm.

▶ **nucleus** The primary site of genetic information in the cell, enclosed in a double-layered membrane.

▶ **cytoplasm** The material of the cell, excluding the cell nucleus and cell membranes. The cytoplasm includes the semifluid cytosol, the organelles, and other particles.

▶ **cytosol** The semifluid inside the cell membrane, excluding organelles. The cytosol is the site of glycolysis and fatty acid synthesis.

▶ **organelles** Various membrane-bound structures that form part of the cytoplasm. Organelles perform specialized metabolic functions.

▶ **mitochondria (mitochondrion)** The sites of aerobic production of ATP, where most of the energy from carbohydrate, protein, and fat is captured. Called the "power plants" of the cell, the mitochondria are where the citric acid cycle and electron transport chain are located. A human cell contains about 2,000 mitochondria.

Organelles

Endoplasmic reticulum (ER)
- An extensive membrane system extending from the nuclear membrane.
- Rough ER: The outer membrane surface contains ribosomes.
- Smooth ER: Devoid of ribosomes, the site of lipid synthesis.

Golgi apparatus
- A system of stacked membrane-encased discs.
- The site of extensive modification, sorting, and packaging of compounds for transport.

Lysosome
- Vesicle containing enzymes that digest intracellular materials and recycle the components.

Mitochondrion
- Contains two highly specialized membranes, an outer membrane and a highly folded inner membrane. Membranes are separated by narrow intermembrane space. Inner membrane encloses space called mitochondrial matrix.
- Often called the power plant of the cell. Site where most of the energy from carbohydrate, protein, and fat is captured in ATP (adenosine triphosphate).
- About 2,000 mitochondria in a cell.

Ribosome
- Site of protein synthesis.

Nucleus
- Contains genetic information in the DNA of chromosomes.
- Site of RNA synthesis—RNA needed for protein synthesis.
- Enclosed in a double-layered membrane.

Cytoplasm
- Enclosed in the cell membrane and separated from the nucleus by the nuclear membrane.
- Filled with particles and organelles which are dispersed in a clear semiliquid fluid called cytosol.

Cytosol
- The semifluid inside the cell membrane.
- Site of glycolysis and fatty acid synthesis.

Cell Membrane
- A double-layered sheet, made up of lipid and protein, that encases the cell.
- Controls the passage of substances in and out of the cell.
- Contains receptors for hormones and other regulatory compounds.

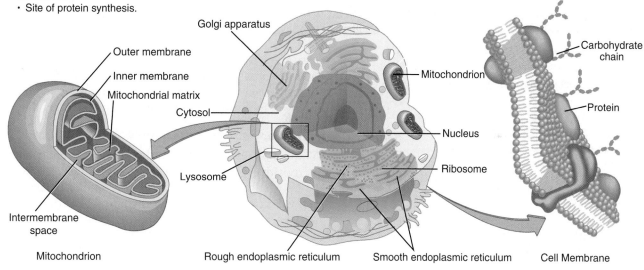

FIGURE SM.4 Cell structure. Liver cells, brain cells, kidney cells, muscle cells, and so forth all have a similar structure.

molecules called **cofactors**, which usually are derived from a vitamin or mineral. Vitamin-derived cofactors also are called **coenzymes**. All the B vitamins form coenzymes used in metabolic reactions.

▶ **cofactors** Compounds required for an enzyme to be active. Cofactors include coenzymes and metal ions such as iron, copper, and magnesium.

▶ **coenzymes** Organic compounds, often derived from B vitamins, that combine with inactive enzymes to form active enzymes.

Key Concepts Metabolism encompasses the many reactions that take place in cells to build tissue, produce energy, break down compounds, and do other cellular work. Anabolism refers to reactions that build compounds, such as protein or glycogen. Catabolism is the breakdown of compounds to yield energy. Mitochondria, the power plants within cells, contain many of the breakdown pathways that produce energy.

Who Are the Key Energy Players?

THINK
About It
1

Certain compounds have recurring roles in metabolic activities. Adenosine triphosphate (ATP) is the fundamental energy molecule used to power cellular functions, so it is known as the universal energy currency. Two other molecules, NADH

ATP: Adenosine triphosphate

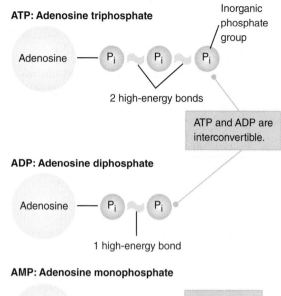

2 high-energy bonds

Inorganic phosphate group

ATP and ADP are interconvertible.

ADP: Adenosine diphosphate

Adenosine — P_i — P_i

1 high-energy bond

AMP: Adenosine monophosphate

Adenosine — P_i

No high-energy phosphate bonds

AMP is interconvertible with both ADP and ATP.

FIGURE SM.5 ATP and ADP. When extracting energy from nutrients, the formation of ATP from ADP + Pi captures energy. Breaking a phosphate bond in ATP to form ADP + Pi releases energy for biosynthesis and work.

▶ **adenosine triphosphate (ATP) [ah-DEN-oh-seen try-FOS-fate]** A high-energy compound composed of adenosine and three phosphate groups. ATP is the main direct fuel that cells use to synthesize molecules, contract muscles, transport substances, and perform other tasks. Breaking down ATP to adenosine diphosphate (ADP) releases energy, and forming ATP from ADP captures energy.

▶ **adenosine diphosphate (ADP) [ah-DEN-oh-seen di-FOS-fate]** A molecule composed of adenosine and two phosphate groups.

▶ **NAD⁺** Nicotinamide adenine dinucleotide (NAD$^+$), a coenzyme derived from the B vitamin niacin, becomes NADH as it accepts a pair of high-energy electrons for transport in cells.

▶ **FAD** Flavin adenine dinucleotide (FAD), a coenzyme derived from the B vitamin riboflavin, becomes FADH$_2$ as it accepts a pair of high-energy electrons for transport in cells.

and FADH$_2$, are important couriers that carry energy for the synthesis of ATP.

ATP: The Body's Energy Currency

To power its needs, your body must convert the energy in food to a readily usable form called **adenosine triphosphate (ATP)**. (See **FIGURE SM.5.**) ATP—the body's universal energy currency—kick-starts many energy-releasing processes, such as the breakdown of glucose and fatty acids, and powers energy-consuming processes, such as the building of glycogen from glucose. By breaking one of the high-energy bonds in an ATP molecule, cells can release usable energy as they convert high-energy ATP to lower-energy **adenosine diphosphate (ADP)**. That energy can then be used to make large molecules from smaller ones (anabolism).

Production of ATP is the fundamental goal of metabolism's energy-producing pathways. Just as the ancient Romans could claim that all roads lead to Rome, you can say that, with a few exceptions, your body's energy-producing pathways all lead to ATP production.

The body's pool of ATP is a small, immediately accessible energy reservoir rather than a long-term energy reserve. The typical lifetime of an ATP molecule is less than one minute, and ATP production increases or decreases in direct relation to energy needs. At rest, you use about 40 kilograms of ATP in 24 hours (an average rate of about 28 grams per minute). In contrast, if you are exercising strenuously, you can use as much as 500 grams per minute! On average, you turn over your body weight in ATP every day.[5]

NAD⁺ and FAD: The Body's Transport Shuttles

During the breakdown of the bonds in carbohydrate, fat, protein, and alcohol, protons (positively charged hydrogen atoms) and electrons are released. The body's transport shuttles, **NAD⁺** and **FAD**, accept pairs of high-energy electrons and transport them to ATP production sites. (See **FIGURE SM.6.**) When the empty shuttle molecules (NAD⁺

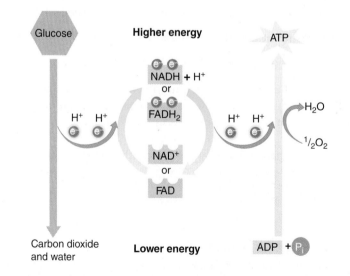

FIGURE SM.6 Energy transfer. As energy moves from glucose to ATP, molecules become high-energy or low-energy as they collect and transfer protons (positively charged hydrogen atoms) and high-energy electrons.

and FAD) pick up their high-energy electron cargo, they also pick up hydrogen and become NADH + H$^+$ and FADH$_2$. These shuttle molecules highlight the importance of B vitamins in metabolism. NAD$^+$ is derived from the B vitamin niacin, and FAD is derived from the B vitamin riboflavin.

> **Key Concepts** ATP is the energy currency of the body. Your body extracts energy from food to produce ATP. As energy-yielding compounds break down, the shuttle molecules NAD$^+$ and FAD transport high-energy electrons to ATP production sites.

Breakdown and Release of Energy

🍎 **Why Is This Important?** You can think of the food you eat as traveling on a journey along specific pathways within your body. As carbohydrate, fat, and protein are broken down into smaller and smaller parts, the ultimate destination is your mitochondria, where energy is extracted. Although carbohydrate, fat, and protein begin their journeys at unique entry points, all yield energy (ATP) and byproducts (carbon dioxide and water).

Bang! The starter's gun echoes in your ears as you leap out of the blocks. With legs pumping, you race to the finish 200 meters away. As you cross the finish line, you congratulate yourself on your best race yet.

Where did the energy come from to power your muscles at peak effort? Your stores of readily available ATP are used up within the first few seconds. To power the remainder of the race, **anaerobic** reactions (reactions that do not require oxygen) partially break down glucose. Needy cells gobble up glucose and rapidly pour out ATP. Although partial breakdown produces only a small amount of ATP per glucose molecule, it is extremely fast and powers maximal effort for short events.

Bang! The starter's gun signals the beginning of the marathon and you commence running at a moderate pace. For 26 miles, your feet pound the pavement over and over again. Rather than sprinting, you settle into a rhythm. The minutes and hours pass as you maintain your steady pace until reaching the finish.

Although anaerobic reactions can power a short, maximal burst of energy for a sprint, they cannot fuel a prolonged event. To sustain muscle contractions during endurance events, **aerobic** reactions (reactions that require oxygen) complete the breakdown of glucose. These aerobic pathways also extract energy from fat and a bit of protein. Compared with anaerobic energy production, aerobic metabolism produces much more energy but at a slower, more easily maintained rate. Anaerobic metabolism may be fast, but, for a single glucose molecule, complete aerobic breakdown produces more than 15 times as much ATP.

Although different pathways initiate the breakdown of carbohydrate, fat, and protein, complete breakdown of these nutrients eventually proceeds along two shared catabolic pathways—the citric acid cycle and the electron transport chain. The next section first describes the pathways that catabolize glucose. Then it discusses the breakdown of fat and protein.

Extracting Energy from Carbohydrate

Cells extract usable energy from carbohydrate via four main pathways: glycolysis, pyruvate to acetyl CoA, the citric acid cycle, and the electron transport chain. (See **FIGURE SM.7.**) Of these four pathways, the electron transport chain is the major ATP production site.

▶ **anaerobic [AN-ah-ROW-bic]** Referring to the absence of oxygen or the ability of a process to occur in the absence of oxygen. Glycolysis is an anaerobic pathway.

▶ **aerobic [air-ROW-bic]** Referring to the presence of or need for oxygen. The complete breakdown of glucose, fatty acids, and amino acids to carbon dioxide and water occurs only via aerobic metabolism. The citric acid cycle and electron transport chain are aerobic pathways.

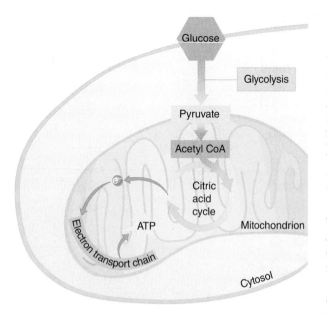

FIGURE SM.7 Obtaining energy from carbohydrate. The complete breakdown of glucose uses four major metabolic pathways: glycolysis, pyruvate to acetyl CoA, the citric acid cycle, and the electron transport chain. Glycolysis takes place in the cytosol of the cell. The remaining reactions take place in the mitochondria.

▶ **glycolysis [gligh-COLL-ih-sis]** The anaerobic pathway that breaks down a glucose molecule into two molecules of pyruvate and yields two molecules of ATP and two molecules of NADH. Glycolysis occurs in the cytosol of a cell.

▶ **pyruvate** The three-carbon compound that results from glycolysis. Cells also can make glucose from pyruvate, but this process requires energy and several enzymes not involved in glycolysis. Pyruvate also can be derived from glycerol and some amino acids.

▶ **acetyl CoA** A key intermediate product in the metabolic breakdown of carbohydrates, fatty acids, and amino acids. It consists of a two-carbon acetate group linked to coenzyme A, which is derived from pantothenic acid.

▶ **coenzyme A** A cofactor derived from the vitamin pantothenic acid.

▶ **lactate** A three-carbon compound that is produced when insufficient oxygen is present in cells to break down pyruvate to acetyl CoA. Often called *lactic acid*.

▶ **citric acid cycle** The metabolic pathway occurring in mitochondria in which the acetyl portion (CH_3COO-) of acetyl CoA is oxidized to yield two molecules of carbon dioxide and one molecule each of NADH, $FADH_2$, and GTP. Also known as the *Krebs cycle* and the *tricarboxylic acid cycle*.

▶ **oxaloacetate** A four-carbon intermediate compound in the citric acid cycle. Acetyl CoA combines with free oxaloacetate in the mitochondria, forming citric acid and beginning the cycle.

▶ **guanosine triphosphate (GTP)** A high-energy compound, similar to ATP but with three phosphate groups linked to guanosine.

Glycolysis

Glycolysis (glucose splitting), the first few steps in the "burning" of glucose, does not require oxygen. In the cytosol, this sequence of reactions splits one six-carbon glucose molecule into two three-carbon **pyruvate** molecules while producing a relatively small amount of energy. Just as a pump requires priming, glycolysis requires the input of two ATP to get started. Using several reactions, glycolysis then transfers high-energy electrons to NAD^+ shuttle molecules and produces four ATP. Finally, it forms two pyruvate molecules. (See **FIGURE SM.8.**)

What about the other simple sugars, fructose and galactose? In liver cells, glycolysis also breaks them down.[6] Although fructose and galactose enter glycolysis at intermediate points, the breakdown of each sugar yields the same results as the breakdown of glucose.

Once glycolysis is complete, the two pyruvate molecules easily pass from the cytosol to the interior of the mitochondria, the cell's power generators, for further processing.

Conversion of Pyruvate to Acetyl CoA

When a cell requires energy, and oxygen is readily available, an aerobic reaction in the mitochondria converts each pyruvate molecule to an **acetyl CoA** molecule and transfers a pair of high-energy electrons to an NAD^+ shuttle. (See **FIGURE SM.9.**) The shuttle carries the electrons to the electron transport chain. To form acetyl CoA, reactions remove one carbon from the three-carbon pyruvate and add **coenzyme A**, a molecule derived from the B vitamin pantothenic acid. After combining with oxygen, the carbon is released as part of carbon dioxide. Because glucose splits into two pyruvate molecules, two acetyl CoA molecules are produced from each molecule of glucose.

Although many metabolic pathways can proceed forward or backward, the formation of acetyl CoA from pyruvate is a one-way (irreversible) process. Acetyl CoA cannot exit through the mitochondrial membrane, so it is trapped inside the mitochondria, poised to enter the citric acid cycle.

In rapidly contracting muscles such as those that propelled you to the finish of your 200-meter sprint, oxygen is in short supply, and pyruvate cannot form acetyl CoA. Instead, pyruvate is rerouted to form lactate, another three-carbon compound. **Lactate** is an alternative fuel that muscle cells can use or that liver cells can convert to glucose. (See the FYI feature "Lactate Is Not a Metabolic Dead End.") When oxygen again becomes readily available, lactate converts back to pyruvate, which irreversibly forms acetyl CoA.

Citric Acid Cycle

A series of reactions called the **citric acid cycle** completes the breakdown of acetyl CoA. To begin the citric acid cycle, acetyl CoA combines with **oxaloacetate** to form citrate (citric acid) and release coenzyme A (CoA). Subsequent reactions release the two carbon atoms from acetyl CoA. These carbon atoms combine with oxygen to form carbon dioxide. Reactions of the citric acid cycle also produce one **guanosine triphosphate (GTP)**, which readily converts to ATP, and transfer pairs

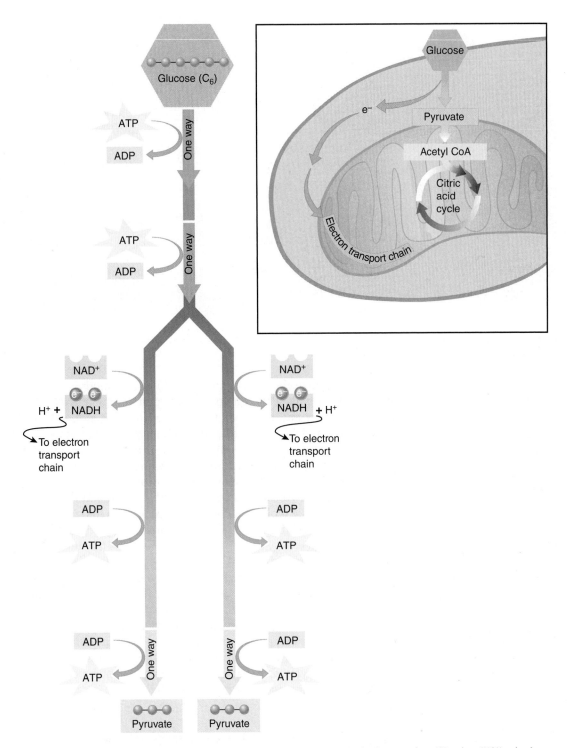

FIGURE SM.8 Glycolysis. The breakdown of one glucose molecule yields two pyruvate molecules, a net of two ATP and two NADH molecules. The two NADH molecules shuttle pairs of high-energy electrons to the electron transport chain for ATP production. Glycolytic reactions do not require oxygen, and some steps are irreversible.

of high-energy electrons to three molecules of NAD^+ and one molecule of FAD. The final reaction regenerates oxaloacetate. Because the breakdown of one glucose molecule produces two acetyl CoA molecules, the citric acid cycle will make two complete "turns"—one for each acetyl CoA.

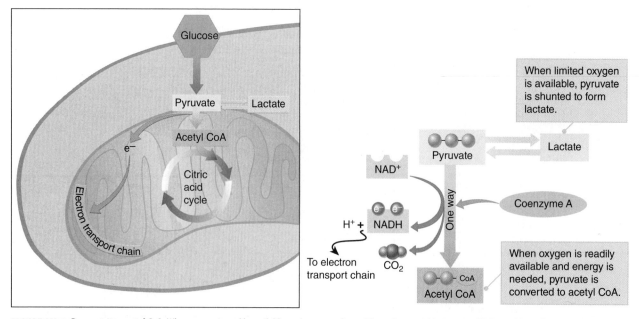

FIGURE SM.9 Pyruvate to acetyl CoA. When oxygen is readily available, each pyruvate formed from glucose yields one acetyl CoA, one CO_2, and one NADH. The NADH shuttles high-energy electrons to the electron transport chain for ATP production.

▶ **biosynthesis** Chemical reactions in which complex biomolecules, especially carbohydrates, lipids, and proteins, are formed from simple molecules.

▶ **electron transport chain** An organized series of protein carrier molecules located in mitochondrial membranes. As high-energy electrons delivered by NADH and FADH₂ traverse the electron transport chain to oxygen, it produces ATP and water.

▶ **mitochondrial membrane** The mitochondria are enclosed by a double shell separated by an intermembrane space. The outer membrane acts as a barrier and gatekeeper, selectively allowing some molecules to pass through while blocking others. The inner membrane is where the electron transport chain is located.

To help visualize the citric acid cycle, think of a merry-go-round at an amusement park. This is a special ride that completes only one revolution per rider and on which the ticket agent rides along. Acetyl CoA is the rider, and oxaloacetate is the ticket agent. Oxaloacetate welcomes acetyl CoA and, hand in hand, they climb aboard. Acetyl CoA's ticket (coenzyme A) is dropped into the recycling box. As the merry-go-round whirls by, two NAD⁺ shuttles swoop in and grab pairs of high-energy electrons as two carbons combine with oxygen and fly off the ride as carbon dioxide molecules. Who is jumping off in mid-cycle? It's GTP, a molecule similar to ATP. An FAD shuttle swoops in and grabs another pair of high-energy electrons. Nearing the end of the ride, a third NAD⁺ shuttle departs with a final pair of high-energy electrons. As the merry-go-round returns to the beginning, a new oxaloacetate beckons to the next acetyl CoA waiting in line. The cycle is ready to begin again. **FIGURE SM.10** shows an overview of the citric acid cycle.

The citric acid cycle also is an important source of building blocks for the **biosynthesis** of amino acids and fatty acids. Many of the cycle's intermediate molecules may be used for biosynthesis rather than the completion of the cycle. Oxaloacetate, for example, may be converted to glucose or to amino acids for protein synthesis.

Electron Transport Chain

The final step in glucose breakdown is a sequence of linked reactions that takes place in the **electron transport chain**, which is located in the inner **mitochondrial membrane**. Most ATP is produced here, and the outpouring of energy can fuel exercise for hours, such as during your marathon race. Because the mitochondrion is the site of both the citric acid cycle and the electron transport chain, it truly is the energy power plant of the cell.

When NAD⁺ accepts a pair of electrons, it becomes NADH. Similarly, FAD accepts electrons to become FADH₂. These shuttle molecules, NADH and FADH₂, deliver their cargo of high-energy electrons to the electron transport chain. As the electrons travel along the electron

THINK
About It

2

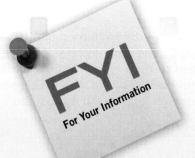

Lactate Is Not a Metabolic Dead End

Today's race is 200 meters, and you are in the lead. The crowd roars with excitement and your coach screams hoarsely as your feet slam over and over on the hard gray cinder track. Other runners are close behind, and you can feel them breathing and pounding at your heels. Air whistles in and out of your wheezing lungs as you doggedly push to stay ahead. Your muscles are screaming, but they carry you across the finish line. A winner!

As you slump in exhaustion, you wonder how your limp muscles carried you through to the end. Each leg seemed to weigh a thousand pounds. As your muscles tire, lactate levels rise and the pH in your muscle cells drops. Scientists, coaches, and athletes have long believed that lactate was a useless, even toxic, dead-end substance. Research proves otherwise. It is the overall acidification of the muscle tissue, rather than a buildup of lactate, that primarily causes muscle fatigue. Also, lactate is now recognized as a fuel in its own right. In addition to acting as a metabolic shunt, lactate is a useful fuel produced and consumed under all conditions of oxygen availability, while exercising or at rest.

Without the energy supplied by the lactic acid energy system, you would never have crossed the finish line. While your body anaerobically burned muscle glycogen, it produced large amounts of lactate. Where does this lactate come from, and how does your body handle it?

Cori Cycle

During vigorous exercise, your contracting muscle cells quickly extract small amounts of ATP from glucose. This simple pathway, called *glycolysis*, splits glucose into pyruvate molecules faster than the oxygen energy system can accept them for further processing. Cells divert excess pyruvate to lactate to help alleviate the backup.

Lactate accumulates rapidly in muscle cells, which receive a boost of energy by burning some lactate with oxygen—a strategy that yields more energy than glycolysis alone. In several types of exercise, lactate initially is released in the bloodstream, but after a given time, a shift occurs and active muscle starts to consume, rather than produce, lactate.[a] Most lactate easily diffuses through muscle cell membranes into the bloodstream. The liver picks up the circulating lactate and converts it back to pyruvate. Using energy-demanding reactions, the liver transforms pyruvate to glucose. Glucose enters the bloodstream and travels back to the skeletal muscle cells, where it reenters energy-producing pathways.

This recurring circular pathway is called the *Cori cycle* (see **FIGURE A**). When pyruvate is backed up in muscle cells, the Cori cycle buys time with a detour through the liver. When oxygen becomes readily available, the oxygen energy system becomes the main pathway.

Lactate Shuttle

The pathways of the Cori cycle are an important, but incomplete, part of the lactate picture. The use of the Cori cycle as a holding pattern led to the mistaken belief that lactate was simply a metabolic dead end. More recent studies described a more extensive role for this long-maligned substance.

Researchers now recognize lactate as an important means of distributing carbohydrate energy sources after a meal and during sustained physical exercise. Lactate's advantage is its ability to move rapidly between cells. It is a small molecule and, unlike glucose, does not need insulin to cross a cell membrane.

Under resting conditions of plentiful carbohydrate and oxygen, diverse tissues such as skeletal muscle, liver, and skin produce lactate.[b] In these conditions, the supply of raw materials, rather than limited oxygen, drives the formation of lactate.

According to the lactate shuttle hypothesis, lactate formed in muscle cells becomes an energy source at other sites, either adjacent or remote. Skeletal muscle, once thought simply to produce lactate, also directly uses lactate as fuel. At times, skeletal muscle actually removes more lactate than it produces. The heart muscle is fully aerobic, but it both produces and consumes lactate. Studies suggest that during exercise, lactate is the major fuel for the heart and the preferred fuel for certain muscle fibers.[c]

The next time you complain about sore, tired muscles, don't blame lactate. Instead, think about the daily usefulness of lactate and how this little-respected substance helped power you to the finish.

a   Cruz RS de O, de Aguiar RA, Turnes T, et al. Review article: intracellular shuttle: the lactate aerobic metabolism. *Sci World J.* 2012; 420984. *PMC* Web. December 18, 2014.

b   van Hall G. Lactate kinetics in human tissues at rest and during exercise. *Acta Physiol (Oxf).* 2010;199(4):499-508.

c   Brooks GA. Cell–cell and intracellular lactate shuttles. *J Physiol.* 2009;587:5591-5600.

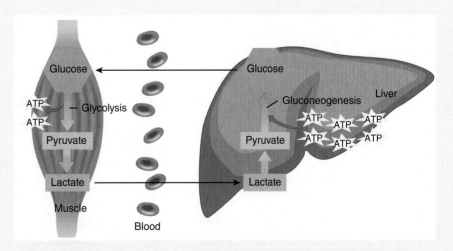

FIGURE A. The Cori cycle. The Cori cycle shifts some of the metabolic burden of contracting muscle to the liver. Lactate formed in contracting muscle travels to the liver, which uses it to form glucose. This glucose returns to the muscle to fuel further contractions.

Quick Bite

Cycling Down the Same Pathway

The citric acid cycle goes by many names. It may be called the **Krebs cycle** after Sir Hans Krebs, the first scientist to explain its workings, who was awarded the Nobel Prize in 1953 for his work. It also may be called the **tricarboxylic acid (TCA) cycle** because a tricarboxylic acid (citric acid) is formed in the first step. Most nutritionists use the term *citric acid cycle*.

▶ **Krebs cycle** See *citric acid cycle*.

▶ **tricarboxylic acid (TCA) cycle** See *citric acid cycle*.

transport chain, they give up energy to power the production of ATP. At the end of the chain, an oxygen "basket" accepts the energy-depleted electrons and combines with hydrogen to form water (H_2O). (See **FIGURE SM.11.**) Without oxygen, ATP production would stop, halting the supply of power for our body's essential functions. If our oxygen supply is not restored rapidly, we die.

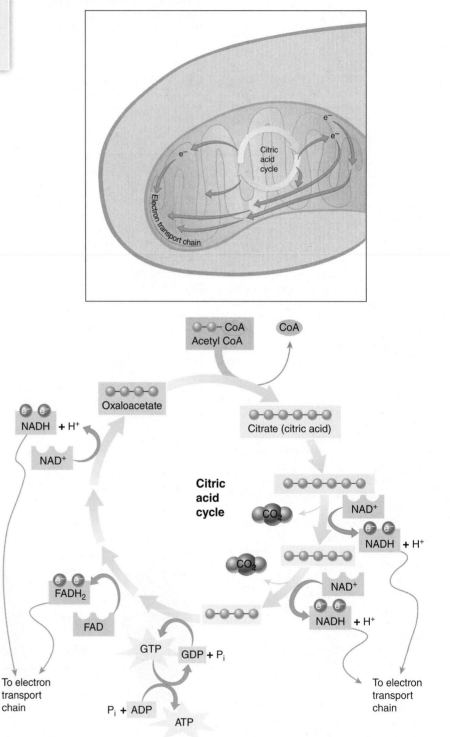

FIGURE SM.10 The citric acid cycle. This circular pathway accepts one acetyl CoA and yields two CO_2, three NADH, one $FADH_2$, and one GTP (readily converted to ATP). The electron shuttles NADH and $FADH_2$ carry high-energy electrons to the electron transport chain for ATP production.

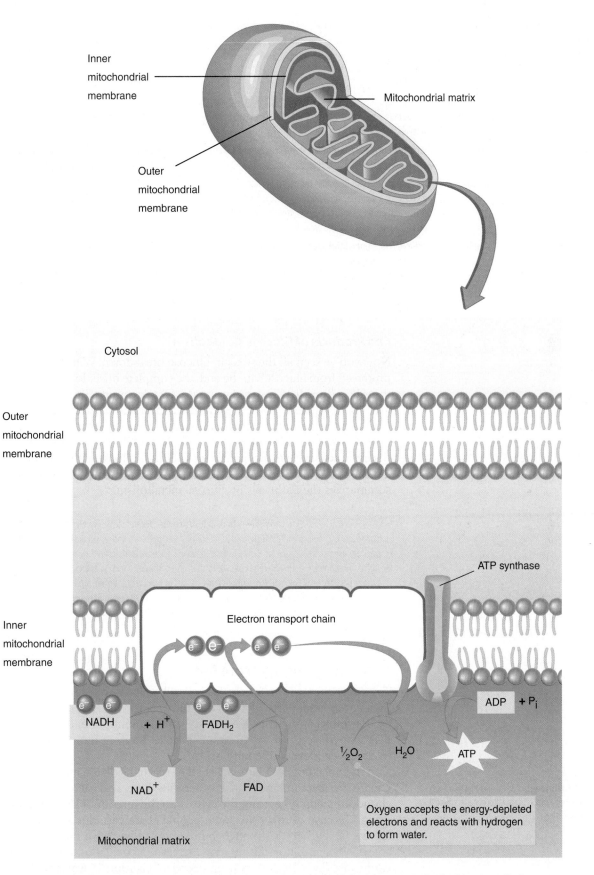

FIGURE SM.11 Electron transport chain. This pathway produces most of the ATP available from glucose. NADH shuttles deliver pairs of high-energy electrons to the beginning of the chain. The pairs of high-energy electrons carried by FADH₂ enter this pathway farther along and produce fewer ATP than electron pairs carried by NADH. Water is the final product of the electron transport chain.

TABLE SM.1
Summary of the Major Metabolic Pathways in Glucose

Phase	Location	Type	Summary	Starting Materials	End Products
Glycolysis	Cytosol	Anaerobic	A series of reactions that converts one glucose to two pyruvate molecules	Glucose, ATP	Pyruvate, ATP, NADH
Pyruvate to acetyl CoA	Mitochondria	Aerobic	Pyruvate from glycolysis combines with coenzyme A to form acetyl CoA while releasing carbon dioxide.	Pyruvate, coenzyme A	Acetyl CoA, carbon dioxide, NADH
Citric acid cycle	Mitochondria	Aerobic	This cycle of reactions degrades the acetyl portion of acetyl CoA and releases the coenzyme A portion. This cycle releases carbon dioxide and produces most of the energy-rich molecules, NADH and $FADH_2$, generated by the breakdown of glucose.	Acetyl CoA	Carbon dioxide, NADH, $FADH_2$, GTP
Electron transport chain	Mitochondria (membrane)	Aerobic	As the electrons from NADH and $FADH_2$ pass along this chain of transport proteins, they release energy to power the generation of ATP. Oxygen is the final electron acceptor and combines with hydrogen to form water.	NADH, $FADH_2$	ATP, water

End Products of Glucose Catabolism

Now you've seen all the steps in glucose breakdown. What has the cell produced from glucose? In the end, the complete breakdown of glucose to carbon dioxide (CO_2) and water (H_2O) takes about 30 steps and creates approximately 32 ATP.[7] Both the conversion of pyruvate to acetyl CoA and the citric acid cycle produce CO_2. The electron transport chain produces water. Although glycolysis makes small amounts of ATP and the citric acid cycle makes a little (as GTP), the electron transport chain generates the vast majority of this universal energy currency. **TABLE SM.1** summarizes the pathways of glucose metabolism.

> **Key Concepts** Extracting energy from glucose requires several steps. Glycolysis breaks the six-carbon glucose molecule into two pyruvate molecules. After glycolysis, the remaining breakdown pathways are used twice—once for each pyruvate molecule. Each pyruvate loses a carbon and combines with a coenzyme A to form an acetyl CoA, which then enters the citric acid cycle. Two carbons enter the cycle as part of acetyl CoA, and two carbons leave as part of two carbon dioxide molecules. Finally, the shuttle molecules NADH and $FADH_2$ carry high-energy electrons to the electron transport chain, where ATP and water are produced. When completely oxidized, each glucose molecule yields carbon dioxide, water, and ATP.

Extracting Energy from Fat

To extract energy from fat, the body first breaks down triglycerides into their component parts, glycerol and fatty acids. Glycerol, a small three-carbon molecule, carries a relatively small amount of energy, and the liver can convert it to pyruvate or glucose. Most of the energy stored in a triglyceride is in the fatty acids.

The breakdown of fatty acids takes place inside the mitochondria. **Carnitine** has the unique task of ferrying fatty acids across the mitochondrial membrane, from the cytosol to the interior of the mitochondrion. Because of this role, some people claim carnitine supplements act as "fat burners." Although numerous studies have mixed results, some indicate that carnitine may increase fat oxidation and improve cardiovascular efficiency during exercise. Caution is warranted. The C-carnitine form can cause muscular weakness.[8]

▶ **carnitine [CAR-nih-teen]** A compound that transports fatty acids from the cytosol into the mitochondria, where they undergo beta-oxidation.

Beta-Oxidation

Once inside a mitochondrion, a process called **beta-oxidation** disassembles the fatty acid chain. Like scissors, enzymes snip the chain into two-carbon "links." Reactions convert each link to acetyl CoA and transfer pairs of high-energy electrons to NAD$^+$ and FAD shuttles. (See **FIGURE SM.12**.) These shuttle molecules (now NADH and FADH$_2$) transport their high-energy cargo to the electron transport chain.

▶ **beta-oxidation** The breakdown of a fatty acid into numerous molecules of the two-carbon compound acetyl coenzyme A (acetyl CoA).

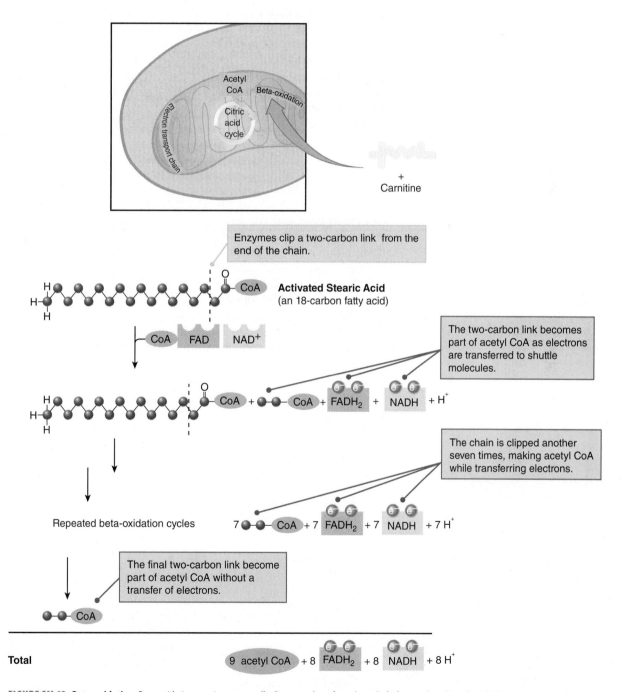

Enzymes clip a two-carbon link from the end of the chain.

Activated Stearic Acid (an 18-carbon fatty acid)

The two-carbon link becomes part of acetyl CoA as electrons are transferred to shuttle molecules.

The chain is clipped another seven times, making acetyl CoA while transferring electrons.

Repeated beta-oxidation cycles

$7 \bullet\!\!\bullet - CoA + 7$ FADH$_2$ $+ 7$ NADH $+ 7$ H$^+$

The final two-carbon link become part of acetyl CoA without a transfer of electrons.

Total

9 acetyl CoA $+ 8$ FADH$_2$ $+ 8$ NADH $+ 8$ H$^+$

FIGURE SM.12 Beta-oxidation. Beta-oxidation reactions repeatedly clip two carbons from the end of a fatty acid until it is degraded entirely to molecules of acetyl CoA.

Completing Fatty Acid Breakdown

Beta-oxidation of a fatty acid produces a flood of acetyl CoA. The citric acid cycle and electron transport chain complete the extraction of energy from fatty acids. Just as they processed acetyl CoA, NADH, and FADH$_2$ from glucose, these same pathways use acetyl CoA, NADH, and FADH$_2$ from fatty acids to produce ATP.

The end products of fatty acid breakdown are the same as those of glucose breakdown: carbon dioxide, water, and ATP. The exact amount of ATP depends on the length of the fatty acid chain. Because longer chains have more carbons than shorter chains, beta-oxidation of longer chains produces more acetyl CoA and thus more ATP. The complete breakdown of an 18-carbon fatty acid, for example, produces 120 ATP, whereas a 10-carbon fatty acid would produce only 66 ATP. A triglyceride, with its three fatty acids and glycerol, contains many more carbon atoms than a molecule of glucose, and thus produces substantially more ATP. In a single triglyceride with three 18-carbon fatty acids, completely breaking down the fatty acids produces 360 ATP—over 10 times the 32 ATP from glucose.

Fat Burns in a Flame of Carbohydrate

Acetyl CoA from beta-oxidation can enter the citric acid cycle only when fat and carbohydrate breakdown are synchronized. Without available oxaloacetate, acetyl CoA cannot start the citric acid cycle. Conditions such as starvation and very-low-carbohydrate diets can deplete oxalo-acetate, blocking acetyl CoA from entry. This reroutes the acetyl CoA to form a family of compounds called *ketone bodies*. (See the section "Making Ketone Bodies" later in this chapter.) Excess production of ketone bodies can occur with popular high-protein diets that are low in carbohydrate but high in fat.

For fatty acid oxidation to continue efficiently, reactions in the mitochondria help ensure a reliable supply of oxaloacetate. These reactions convert some pyruvate directly to oxaloacetate rather than to acetyl CoA. Because carbohydrate (glucose) is the original source of the pyruvate and, hence, this oxaloacetate, scientists coined the saying "Fat burns in a flame of carbohydrate."

THINK
About It
3

> **Key Concepts** Extracting energy from fat involves several steps. First, triglycerides are separated into glycerol and three fatty acids. Glycerol forms pyruvate and can be broken down to yield a small amount of energy. Beta-oxidation breaks down fatty acid chains to two-carbon links that form acetyl CoA, which enters the citric acid cycle. Beta-oxidation and the citric acid cycle transfer electrons to NAD$^+$ and FAD. As NADH and FADH$_2$, these shuttle molecules carry high-energy electrons to the electron transport chain, where ATP and water are made. The complete breakdown of a triglyceride yields water, carbon dioxide, and substantially more ATP than one glucose molecule.

Extracting Energy from Protein

Protein has vital structural and functional roles, so proteins and amino acids are not considered primary sources of energy. However, if energy production falters due to a lack of available carbohydrate and fat, protein comes to the rescue. During starvation, for example, energy needs take priority, so the body breaks down protein and extracts energy from the amino acid building blocks.

Our bodies can't use the nitrogen-containing portion of an amino acid in energy production, so a process called *deamination* strips down the amino acid to a "carbon skeleton" (see **FIGURE SM.13**)

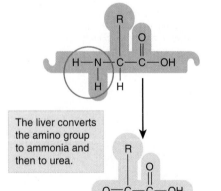

The liver converts the amino group to ammonia and then to urea.

The structure of the remaining carbon skeleton determines where it can enter the energy-producing pathways.

FIGURE SM.13 Deamination. A deamination reaction strips the amino group from an amino acid.

while producing a nitrogen byproduct that becomes urea. When you eat more protein than you need, your kidneys excrete urea in urine, and your liver uses carbon skeletons to produce energy, glucose, or fat. Much to the dismay of bodybuilders, when they attempt to build muscle by drinking pricey protein drinks, they can end up gaining fat instead!

Carbon Skeletons Enter Pathways at Different Points

Carbon skeletons—unlike glucose—can enter the breakdown pathways at several different points. Imagine arriving at an amusement park with five entrance gates. The ticket agent hands you a ticket that allows you to enter at your designated gate. Similarly, the structure of an amino acid's carbon skeleton determines which "entrance gate" it uses to enter the breakdown pathways. Some carbon skeletons directly enter the citric acid cycle, others enter at pyruvate, and still others at acetyl CoA. (See **FIGURE SM.14.**)

End Products of Amino Acid Catabolism

The complete breakdown of an amino acid yields urea, carbon dioxide, water, and ATP. The carbon skeleton's point of entry to the breakdown pathways determines the amount of ATP it produces. Whereas

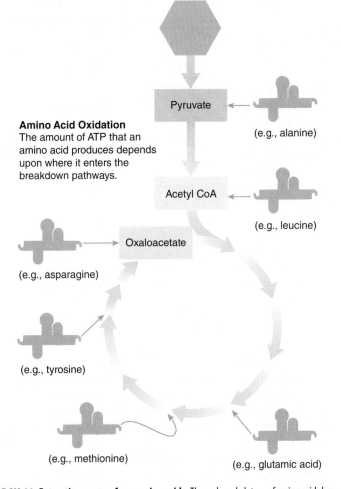

Amino Acid Oxidation
The amount of ATP that an amino acid produces depends upon where it enters the breakdown pathways.

Pyruvate

(e.g., alanine)

Acetyl CoA

(e.g., leucine)

Oxaloacetate

(e.g., asparagine)

(e.g., tyrosine)

(e.g., methionine)

(e.g., glutamic acid)

FIGURE SM.14 Extracting energy from amino acids. The carbon skeletons of amino acids have several different entrances to the breakdown pathways. Compared with glucose and fatty acids, amino acids yield much smaller amounts of energy (ATP).

Quick Bite

Sweet Origins
The word *gluconeogenesis* is derived from the Greek words *glyks*, meaning "sweet"; *neo*, meaning "new"; and *genesis*, meaning "origin" or "generation."

▶ **alcohol dehydrogenase (ADH)** The enzyme that catalyzes the oxidation of ethanol and other alcohols.

▶ **aldehyde dehydrogenase (ALDH)** The enzyme that catalyzes the conversion of acetaldehyde to acetate, which forms acetyl CoA.

▶ **fatty liver** Accumulation of fat in the liver, a sign of increased fatty acid synthesis.

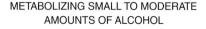

METABOLIZING SMALL TO MODERATE
AMOUNTS OF ALCOHOL

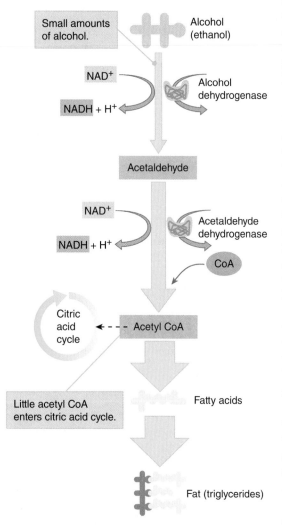

FIGURE SM.15 Metabolizing alcohol. The metabolism of alcohol inhibits the citric acid cycle and primarily forms fat.

the complete breakdown of alanine, for example, produces 12.5 ATP, methionine produces only 5 ATP. Compared with glucose and fatty acids, no amino acid produces much ATP.

Key Concepts To extract energy from amino acids, cells strip them down to carbon skeletons (deamination). The remaining nitrogen becomes urea, which is removed by the kidneys. The carbon skeleton structure determines where it enters the catabolic pathways. Some carbon skeletons become pyruvate, others become acetyl CoA, and still others become intermediate compounds of the citric acid cycle. Complete breakdown of amino acids yields water, carbon dioxide, urea, and ATP.

Alcohol Metabolism

🍎 **Why Is This Important?** Although alcohol can provide energy, the body primarily sees it as a substance to remove. One of the byproducts is toxic, and the liver works rapidly to convert it and avoid a buildup. Your liver is the major metabolic site for breaking down drugs and alcohol. Chronic excess alcohol consumption causes changes in the liver and can impact the body's response to certain medications.

Alcohol breakdown always takes priority over the breakdown of carbohydrates, proteins, and fats. To prevent alcohol from accumulating and destroying cells and organs, the body quickly metabolizes it and removes it from the blood. The liver is the primary site for alcohol metabolism and has special pathways to handle excess consumption.

Metabolizing Small Amounts of Alcohol

Alcohol dehydrogenase (ADH) is a zinc-containing enzyme that catalyzes the conversion of small to moderate amounts of alcohol to acetaldehyde, a toxic substance. To avoid a buildup of toxic acetaldehyde, another enzyme, **aldehyde dehydrogenase (ALDH)**, quickly and effectively converts it to acetate. (See **FIGURE SM.15**.) Chronic alcohol consumption increases the production of acetaldehyde and impairs the body's ability to metabolize it. Whereas normal circulating levels of acetaldehyde are low, levels usually are elevated in alcoholics.[9] Acetaldehyde can be more destructive than alcohol itself and can damage the mucous membranes lining the gut.

In certain people, usually of Asian heritage, a key enzyme that helps break down acetaldehyde is inactivated. In East Asia, this inactive version is found in 15 to 40 percent of the population. When people with the inactive enzyme consume alcohol, blood levels of acetaldehyde are 5- to 20-fold higher than levels in people with the normal active variant.[10]

Liver cells break down alcohol and use the products to synthesize fatty acids, which are assembled into fats. Fat accumulation in the liver can be seen after a single bout of heavy drinking, and fatty acid synthesis accelerates with chronic alcohol consumption. **Fatty liver** is the first stage of liver destruction in alcoholics.

Alcohol metabolism is higher in a fed nutritional state versus a fasting state. ADH levels are higher, and food also may increase blood flow to the liver. The sugar fructose increases alcohol metabolism by providing building blocks for key reactions and enhancing oxygen uptake. The effect of food increasing alcohol elimination was similar for meals of different compositions, with no difference among the effects of carbohydrate, fat, and protein on alcohol metabolism.[11]

Metabolizing Large Amounts of Alcohol

Large amounts of alcohol can overwhelm the alcohol dehydrogenase system, the usual metabolic path. As alcohol builds up, the body identifies it as a foreign substance and routes it into the primary overflow pathway, the **microsomal ethanol-oxidizing system (MEOS)**. (See **FIGURE SM.16.**) The liver ordinarily uses the MEOS bypass pathway to metabolize drugs and detoxify "foreign" substances. Chronic heavy drinking appears to activate MEOS enzymes, which may be responsible for transforming the pain reliever acetaminophen into chemicals that can damage the liver.

▶ **microsomal ethanol-oxidizing system (MEOS)** An energy-requiring enzyme system in the liver that normally metabolizes drugs and other foreign substances. When the blood alcohol level is high, alcohol dehydrogenase cannot metabolize it fast enough, and the excess alcohol is metabolized by MEOS.

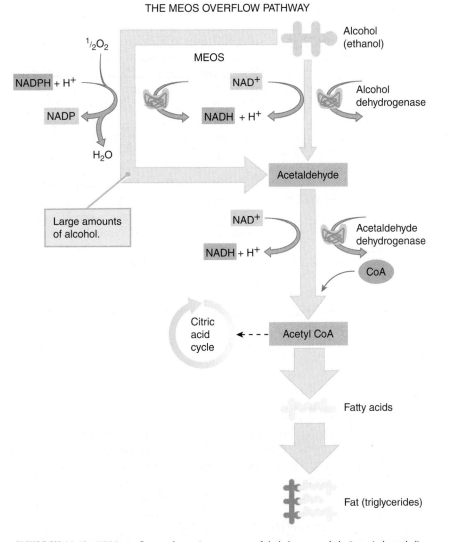

FIGURE SM.16 The MEOS overflow pathway. Large amounts of alcohol can overwhelm its typical metabolic route, so excess alcohol enters an overflow pathway called the microsomal ethanol-oxidizing system (MEOS).

To transform alcohol into acetaldehyde, the MEOS pathway uses different enzymes than the alcohol dehydrogenase system. When repeatedly exposed to large doses of alcohol, the MEOS pathway increases its capacity and processing speed. Whether alcoholics metabolize alcohol differently from nonalcoholics is unknown. Clearly, chronic ingestion of alcohol leads to changes in the liver, and the alcohol abuser acquires an increased tolerance to alcohol and to drugs such as sedatives, tranquilizers, and antibiotics.

Key Concepts The liver is the alcohol processing center. The primary metabolic enzymes are alcohol dehydrogenase and aldehyde dehydrogenase. When large amounts of alcohol are consumed, some alcohol is metabolized by the MEOS pathway.

Biosynthesis and Storage

Why Is This Important? Your body not only can break down food to extract energy, but also can assemble constituent parts to make carbohydrate (glucose), fat (fatty acids), and protein (from amino acids). Your body can make some types of amino acids from scratch, whereas others must be consumed directly from the diet.

Uh-oh! Surveying the results of those holiday dinners and treats, you cringe with regret. Your clothes no longer fit, and you hate the idea of stepping on the scale. Your biosynthetic pathways have been hard at work, building fat stores from your excess intake of energy.

You head for the gym. After sweating through many workouts, your body begins to firm. You drop fat and add muscle. Now any problem with clothes fitting is due to muscle gain, not fat gain. To build muscle protein, different biosynthetic pathways have been busy making amino acids and assembling proteins.

Perhaps you've heard of "carbo loading." This strategy uses high-carbohydrate meals to pack carbohydrate into your muscle glycogen stores before a competition. Biosynthetic pathways assemble glucose into glycogen chains for storage. When needed, your body also can make glucose from certain amino acids and other precursors.

Both the breakdown pathways and the biosynthetic pathways are active at all times. While some cells are breaking down carbohydrate, fat, and protein to extract energy, other cells are busy building glucose, fatty acids, and amino acids. When your body needs energy, the breakdown pathways prevail. When it has an excess of nutrients, the biosynthetic pathways dominate. The activities in these pathways ebb and flow so they proceed at just the right rate, not too fast and not too slowly. **FIGURE SM.17** illustrates the interconnections among the metabolic pathways.

Making Carbohydrate (Glucose)

Your body sets a high priority on maintaining an adequate amount of glucose circulating in the bloodstream. Blood glucose is the primary source of energy for your brain, central nervous system, and red blood cells. In fact, while you're at rest, your brain consumes about 60 percent of the energy consumed by your entire body.

Gluconeogenesis: Pathways to Glucose

When you are exercising intensely or when you aren't taking in enough carbohydrate, such as during a typical overnight fast, your body can make glucose by using a clever strategy called **gluconeogenesis**.

▶ **gluconeogenesis [gloo-ko-nee-oh-JEN-uh-sis]**
Synthesis of glucose within the body from noncarbohydrate precursors such as amino acids, lactic acid, and glycerol. Fatty acids cannot be converted to glucose.

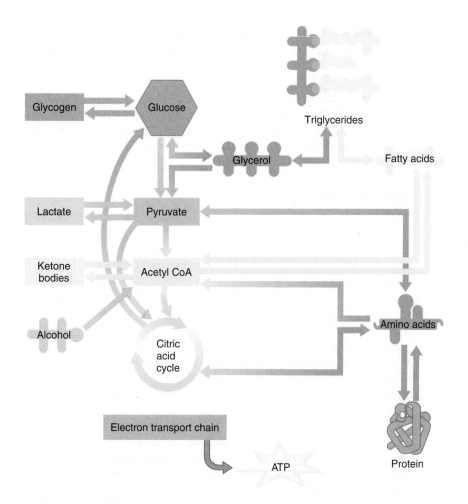

FIGURE SM.17 **Overview of metabolic pathways.** As if they were traveling a maze of city streets, molecules move through a network of breakdown and biosynthetic pathways. Not all pathways are available to a molecule. Just as traffic lights and one-way streets regulate traffic flow, cellular mechanisms control the flow of molecules in metabolic pathways. These mechanisms include hormones, irreversible reactions, and locations of reactions in the cell.

Gluconeogenesis is a pathway essential for the survival of humans that enables the body to maintain blood glucose levels after dietary sources of carbohydrate have been used up. Your liver is the major site of gluconeogenesis, accounting for about 90 percent of glucose production. Your kidneys make the rest.

Gluconeogenesis and glycolysis share many—but not all—reactions. During gluconeogenesis, reactions flow in the opposite direction as during glycolysis. Because some reactions of glycolysis flow only one way, gluconeogenesis must use energy-consuming detours to bypass them. Thus gluconeogenesis is *not* simply a reversal of glycolysis.

Your body can make glucose from pyruvate, lactate, and some noncarbohydrate sources—glycerol and most amino acids. Although gluconeogenesis can use the glycerol portion of fat, it cannot make glucose from fatty acids.

If the carbon skeleton of an amino acid can be made into glucose, the amino acid is called **glucogenic**. Glucogenic amino acids provide carbon skeletons that become pyruvate or they may directly enter the citric acid cycle at intermediate points other than forming acetyl CoA. If a carbon skeleton of an amino acid directly forms acetyl CoA (which

▶ **glucogenic** A term describing an amino acid whose carbon skeleton can be used in gluconeogenesis to form glucose.

▶ **ketogenic** A term describing an amino acid broken down to acetyl CoA (which can be converted into ketone bodies).

▶ **glycogenesis** The formation of glycogen from glucose.

▶ **lipogenesis [lye-poh-JEN-eh-sis]** Synthesis of fatty acids from acetyl CoA derived from the metabolism of fats, alcohol, and some amino acids.

your body can convert to ketone bodies but not glucose), the amino acid is called **ketogenic**. (See the "Ketogenesis" section.)

Storage: Glucose to Glycogen

By using a pathway called **glycogenesis**, our bodies store glucose as glycogen in the liver and muscles. Liver glycogen serves as a glucose reserve for the blood, and muscle glycogen supplies glucose to exercising muscle tissue. Glycogen stores are limited; fasting or strenuous exercise can deplete them rapidly.

Making Fat (Fatty Acids)

Your body can make long-chain fatty acids using a process called **lipogenesis**. To do this, your body assembles two-carbon acetyl CoA "links" into fatty acid chains. Where do these acetyl CoA building blocks come from? Ketogenic amino acids, alcohol, and fatty acids themselves supply acetyl CoA for lipogenesis.

Although you can think of fatty acid synthesis as reassembling the links broken apart by beta-oxidation, lipogenesis is not the reversal of beta-oxidation. These pathways use different reactions and take place in different locations—fatty acid synthesis occurs in the cytosol, whereas beta-oxidation operates inside the mitochondria. Your body assembles surplus fatty acids and glycerol to form triglycerides for storage as body fat.

Storage: From Dietary Energy to Stored Triglyceride

When you overeat, your body uses body fat as a long-term energy storage depot. When you eat an excess of fat, most extra dietary fatty acids head straight to your fat stores. If you eat more protein than your tissues can use, your body converts most of the excess protein to body fat. Interestingly, excess carbohydrate does not readily become fat. In research studies, massive overfeeding of carbohydrate in normal men caused only minimal amounts of fat synthesis. So are carbohydrate calories "free"? Unfortunately not. Although excess carbohydrate does not dramatically increase fat synthesis, it shifts your body's fuel preferences so it burns more carbohydrate and fewer fatty acids.[12] Thus, eating excess carbohydrate still can make you fat by allowing the fat you eat to go directly to storage rather than to make ATP. (See **TABLE SM.2**.)

TABLE SM.2
Summary of Energy Yield and Interconversions

Dietary Nutrient	Yields Energy?	Convertible to Glucose?	Convertible to Amino Acids and Body Proteins?	Convertible to Fat?
Carbohydrate (glucose, fructose, galactose)	Yes	Yes	Yes, can yield certain amino acids when amino groups are available	Insignificant
Fat (triglycerides)				
Fatty acids	Yes, large amounts	No	No	Yes
Glycerol	Yes, large amounts	Small amounts	Yes (see carbohydrate)	Insignificant
Protein (amino acids)	Yes, generally not much (see starvation in text)	Yes, if insufficient carbohydrate is available	Yes	Yes, from some amino acids
Alcohol (ethanol)	Yes	No	No	Yes

Key Concepts Your body can make glucose from pyruvate, lactate, glucogenic amino acids, and glycerol but not from fatty acids. The main storage form of glucose is glycogen. When your diet supplies an excess of energy, your body makes fatty acids and triglycerides. Excess dietary carbohydrate is not readily converted to fat but instead shifts the body's selection of fuel and encourages the accumulation of dietary fat in body fat stores.

Making Ketone Bodies

Ketone bodies (sometimes incorrectly called **ketones**) include three compounds, acetoacetate, beta-hydroxybutyrate, and acetone. Your body makes and uses small amounts of ketone bodies at all times. Although long considered to be just an emergency energy source or the result of an abnormal condition such as starvation or uncontrolled diabetes, ketone bodies are a normal, everyday fuel source for many tissues such as cardiac muscle, skeletal muscle, and the brain.[13]

Ketogenesis: Pathways to Ketone Bodies

During the breakdown of fatty acids, not all acetyl CoA enters the citric acid cycle. Your body converts some acetyl CoA to ketone bodies, a process called **ketogenesis**. (See **FIGURE SM.18**.) When a person has uncontrolled diabetes or is starving, ketone bodies help provide emergency energy to all body tissues, especially the brain and the rest of the central nervous system. Other than glucose, ketone bodies are your central nervous system's only effective fuel.[14]

To dispose of excess ketone bodies, your kidneys excrete them in urine and your lungs exhale them. If this removal process cannot keep up with the production process, ketone bodies accumulate in the blood—a condition called *ketosis*. There are two types of ketosis, normal ketosis that occurs with fasting and the medically dangerous hyperketonemia of diabetic **ketoacidosis**.[15] During even a brief overnight fast, the catabolism of fat and protein increases the production of ketone bodies. Hyperketonemia can occur in uncontrolled type 1 diabetes mellitus. In this situation, blood acidity rises quickly, leading to ketoacidosis, which can cause brain damage and eventually death if left untreated.[16] During a short fast, ketoacidosis rarely occurs.

Because "fat burns in a flame of carbohydrate," a very-high-fat, low-carbohydrate diet promotes ketosis. The lack of carbohydrate inhibits formation of oxaloacetate, slowing entry of acetyl CoA into the citric acid cycle and rerouting acetyl CoA toward the formation of ketone bodies. Given time, however, the body can adapt to a very-high-fat, low-carbohydrate diet and avoid ketosis. Eskimos, for example, sometimes live almost entirely on fat but do not develop ketosis.[17]

Key Concepts Three types of ketone bodies—acetoacetate, beta-hydroxybutyrate, and acetone—can be made from the precursor acetyl CoA. Ketone bodies are an important fuel source during starvation because they are able to be used in place of glucose by the brain. In uncontrolled type 1 diabetes mellitus, an accumulation of ketone bodies can acidify the blood, resulting in ketoacidosis.

Making Protein (Amino Acids)

Your body rebuilds proteins from a pool of amino acids in your cells. But how is that amino acid pool replenished? Your diet supplies some

▶ **ketone bodies** Molecules formed when insufficient carbohydrate is available to completely metabolize fat. Formation of ketone bodies is promoted by a low glucose level and high acetyl CoA level within cells. Acetone, acetoacetate, and beta-hydroxybutyrate are ketone bodies. Beta-hydroxybutyrate is sometimes improperly called a ketone.

▶ **ketones [KEE-tonez]** Organic compounds that contain a chemical group consisting of C=O (a carbon–oxygen double bond) bound to two hydrocarbons. Pyruvate and fructose are examples of ketones. Acetone and acetoacetate are both ketones and ketone bodies. Although beta-hydroxybutyrate is not a ketone, it is a ketone body.

▶ **ketogenesis** The process in which excess acetyl CoA from fatty acid oxidation is converted into ketone bodies.

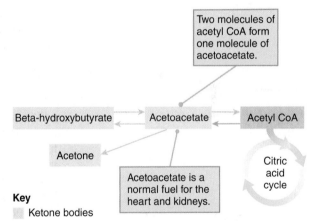

FIGURE SM.18 Ketogenesis (ketone body formation). For acetyl CoA from fatty acid oxidation to enter the citric acid cycle, fat and carbohydrate metabolism must be synchronized. When acetyl CoA cannot enter the citric acid cycle, it is shunted to form ketone bodies, a process called ketogenesis.

▶ **ketoacidosis** Acidification of the blood caused by a buildup of ketone bodies. It is primarily a consequence of uncontrolled type 1 diabetes mellitus and can be life threatening.

Quick Bite

Why Didn't My Cholesterol Levels Drop?

Your body can make cholesterol from acetyl CoA by way of ketones. In fact, all 27 carbons in synthesized cholesterol come from acetyl CoA. The rate of cholesterol formation is highly responsive to cholesterol levels in cells. If levels are low, the liver makes more. If levels are high, synthesis decreases. This is why dietary cholesterol in the absence of dietary fat often has little impact on blood cholesterol levels.

amino acids, the breakdown of body proteins supplies some, and your cells make some. During protein synthesis, your cells can make nonessential (dispensable) amino acids and retrieve essential (indispensable) amino acids from the bloodstream. Your cells cannot make essential amino acids, however. If a cell lacks an essential amino acid and your diet doesn't supply it, protein synthesis stops. The cell breaks down this incomplete protein into its constituent amino acids, which are returned to the bloodstream.

Biosynthesis: Making Amino Acids

To synthesize nonessential amino acids, your body uses many different pathways. Each pathway is short, involving just a few steps, and builds amino acids from carbon skeletons. Pyruvate and other compounds involved in glycolysis and the citric acid cycle supply the carbon skeletons.

Key Concepts Proteins are made from combinations of essential and nonessential amino acids. The body synthesizes nonessential amino acids from pyruvate, other compounds involved in glycolysis, and compounds from the citric acid cycle.

Special States

🍎 **Why Is This Important?** In times of feasting, your body stores excess energy as fat. In times of prolonged fasting or starvation, the body breaks down tissue and extracts energy. Understanding the details of these processes will help you appreciate how your body maintains homeostasis in times of stress.

Now you can put your new knowledge of metabolism to work by evaluating what happens when feasting or fasting. What do you think happens to your metabolism in each situation?

Feasting

You're stuffed. You just ate a huge holiday dinner: two servings of turkey with a big ladle of gravy and ample servings of dressing, mashed potatoes, caramelized sweet potatoes, green peas, and two bread rolls. To top it off, you ate a piece of pumpkin pie with whipped cream. You meant to stop there; you loudly proclaimed, "I'm so full—I can't eat another bite!" But, eventually your grandmother convinced you to taste her special pecan pie. Gosh, that was good! But now you are lying on the couch, uncomfortable and bloated, with your belt loosened. Your feasting may be finished for now, but your body's work has just begun.

Your meal led to a huge influx of carbohydrate, fat, and protein—a plentiful supply for your tissues and far more energy than you need for life as a couch potato. The influx of food signals your cells to "store, store, store!" Consequently, much of your holiday dinner will wind up stored as fat. The surplus carbohydrate first enters glycogen stores, filling their limited capacity. In the short term, excess carbohydrate adjusts your body's fuel preferences to maximize its use of carbohydrate and minimizes its use of fat, thereby promoting fat storage. Carbohydrate in excess of energy needs will be converted to fatty acids and stored in adipose tissue to provide an available source of fuel during fasting.[18]

What happens to the surplus fat and protein? Fat tissue is the perfect energy storage package for both. Although some ATP is produced from dietary fat, nearly all excess dietary fat becomes body fat. Excess protein, beyond what's needed to replenish the overall body pool of amino acids, also heads to fat storage. (See **FIGURE SM.19**.)

The Return to Normal

After this frenzied bout of storage, the amount of glucose and triglyceride circulating in the bloodstream drops to the fasting level roughly three to four hours after eating. The level of amino acids in the blood also returns to baseline.

Hours later, after a nap, and perhaps a game of touch football, a further decline in blood glucose levels triggers the signal "release the glucose!" and your body swings into action to counteract falling blood glucose levels. The body breaks down liver glycogen to glucose, which is released into the bloodstream. Synthesis and storage of glycogen and fatty acids slow. The body breaks down muscle glycogen to form glucose that muscles can use.

If low blood glucose levels persist for hours or days, most cells start shifting their fuel usage from glucose to fatty acids. Gluconeogenesis begins to ramp up and make glucose from circulating amino acids.[19] The body's metabolic pathways work in concert to maintain blood glucose levels and ensure a constant supply of glucose for the central nervous system and red blood cells[20]—until it is time to attack the leftovers!

> **Key Concepts** Feasting, or taking in too many calories, stimulates anabolic processes such as glycogen and fat synthesis. After a meal that contains dietary fat, carbohydrate, and protein, dietary fat will be deposited as fatty acids in adipose tissue. Dietary amino acids in excess of what is needed for protein synthesis and carbohydrate in excess of what is needed for glycogen synthesis and energy will also be converted to fatty acids and deposited in adipose tissue, leading to the accumulation of fat stores.

Fasting

Feasting on a holiday dinner floods your body with excess energy that is stored for future use. In contrast, fasting and starvation deprive you of energy, so your body must employ an opposing strategy—the mobilization of fuel. (See **FIGURE SM.20**.) Whether starvation occurs in a child during a famine, a young woman with anorexia nervosa, a patient with AIDS wasting syndrome, or a person intentionally fasting, the body responds in the same way. Some people deprive themselves of food for a particular purpose—to lose weight, to stage a political protest, to participate in a religious fast, or to "cleanse" their bodies.

Survival Priorities and Potential Energy Sources

Starvation confronts your body with several dilemmas. Where will it get energy to fuel survival needs? Which should it burn first—fat, protein, or carbohydrate? Can it conserve its energy reserves? Which tissues should it sacrifice to ensure survival?

THiNK About It 4

Your body's first priority is to preserve glucose-dependent tissue: red blood cells, brain cells, and the rest of the central nervous system. Your brain will not tolerate even a short interruption in the supply of adequate energy. Once your body depletes its carbohydrate reserves, it begins sacrificing readily available circulating amino acids to make glucose and ATP.

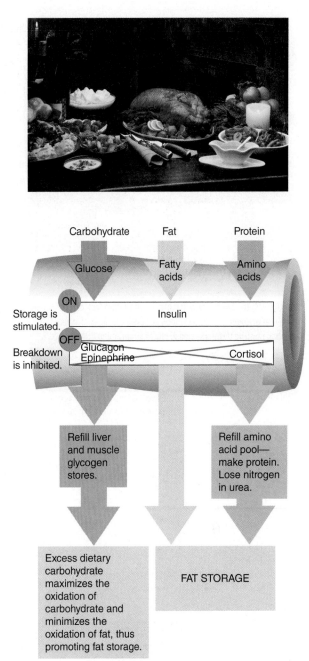

FIGURE SM.19 Feasting. Your body deals with a large influx of nutrients by increasing cellular uptake of glucose and promoting fat storage.

© Bob Montesclaros/Cole Group/Getty Images.

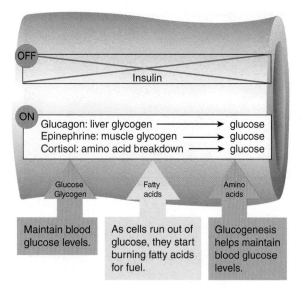

FIGURE SM.20 Short-term fasting. During a short fast, cells first break down liver glycogen to maintain blood glucose levels. They also burn fatty acids and ramp up the production of glucose from amino acids.

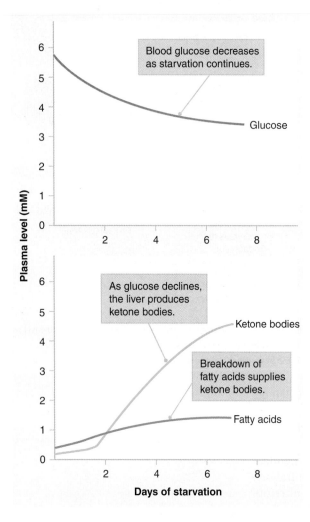

FIGURE SM.21 Shifting fuel selection during starvation. To fuel its needs as blood glucose levels decline, the body shifts from glucose to fatty acids and ketone bodies.

Your body's second priority is to maintain muscle mass. In the face of danger, we rely upon our ability to mount a "fight or flight" response. This survival mechanism requires a large muscle mass, allowing us to move quickly and effectively. Your body grudgingly uses muscle protein for energy and breaks it down rapidly only in the final stages of starvation.

Although your body stores most of its energy reserve in body fat, triglycerides are a poor source of glucose. Your body can make a small amount of glucose from the glycerol backbone, but it cannot make any glucose from fatty acids. As a consequence, your body's primary energy stores—fat—are incompatible with your body's paramount energy priority—glucose for your brain. To meet this metabolic challenge, your body's antistarvation strategies include a glucose-sparing mechanism. Your body shifts to fatty acids and ketone bodies for its primary fuel needs. In time, even your brain adapts as most, but not all, of its cells come to rely on ketone bodies for fuel.

The Prolonged Fast: In the Beginning

What happens during the fasting state? Let's take a metabolic look at Fasting Frank, a political activist determined to make a dramatic statement. Frank begins fasting at sundown, planning to drink nothing but water and to consume no other foods.

The first few hours are no different from your nightly fast between dinner and breakfast. As blood glucose drops to fasting baseline levels, the liver breaks down glycogen to glucose. Gluconeogenesis becomes highly active and begins churning out glucose from circulating amino acids. The liver pours glucose into the bloodstream to supply other organs and shifts to fatty acids for its own energy needs. Muscle cells also start burning fatty acids. After about 12 hours, the battle to maintain a constant supply of blood glucose exhausts nearly all carbohydrate stores.[21]

The First Few Days

During the next few days, fat and protein are the primary fuels. To preserve structural proteins, especially muscle mass, Frank's body first turns to easily metabolized amino acids. It uses some to produce ATP and others to make glucose. Glucogenic amino acids, especially alanine, furnish about 90 percent of the brain's glucose supply. Glycerol from triglyceride breakdown supplies the remaining 10 percent. After a couple of days, production of ketone bodies ramps up, augmenting the fuel supply. (See **FIGURE SM.21**.)

The Early Weeks

As starvation continues, Frank's body initiates several energy-conservation strategies. It ratchets down its energy use by lowering body temperature, pulse rate, blood pressure, and resting metabolism. Frank becomes lethargic, reducing the amount of energy expended in activity. He may begin to have detectable signs of mild vitamin deficiencies as his body depletes its small reserves of vitamin C and some B vitamins.

If Frank's body continued to rapidly break down protein, he would survive less than three weeks. To avoid such a quick demise, protein breakdown slows drastically and gluconeogenesis drops significantly.[22] To pick up the slack, Frank's body doubles the rate of fat breakdown to supply fatty acids for fuel and glycerol for glucose. Ketone bodies pour into the bloodstream and provide an important glucose-sparing energy source for the brain and red blood cells. After about 10 days of fasting, ketone bodies meet most of the nervous system's energy needs. Some brain cells, however, can use only glucose. To maintain a small, but essential, supply of blood glucose, protein breakdown crawls along, supplying small amounts of amino acids for gluconeogenesis.

Several Weeks of Fasting

During prolonged fasting, the main determinant of survival is the amount of body fat at the start of the fast. An average adult has about two months' worth of stored fat.[23] As the later stages of starvation exhaust the final fat stores, the body turns again to protein, its sole remaining fuel source. (See **FIGURE SM.22**.) You can see some of the effects of accelerated protein breakdown in starving children suffering from kwashiorkor. The loss of blood proteins leads to the swollen limbs and bulging stomachs that typify this type of protein-energy malnutrition (PEM).

Quick **Bite**

When Men Starve: A Starvation Study

During World War II, researchers at the University of Minnesota conducted a starvation study on 36 male volunteers, all conscientious objectors. Their typical food intake was cut in half, and they lost about 25 percent of their body weight. Researchers noted significant psychological changes as well. The subjects began obsessing about food, collecting recipes and cookbooks, and hoarding food-related objects. They became apathetic, chronically exhausted, and lost all interest in sex. Most were afraid to leave the experimental conditions for fear of losing control in the outside world.

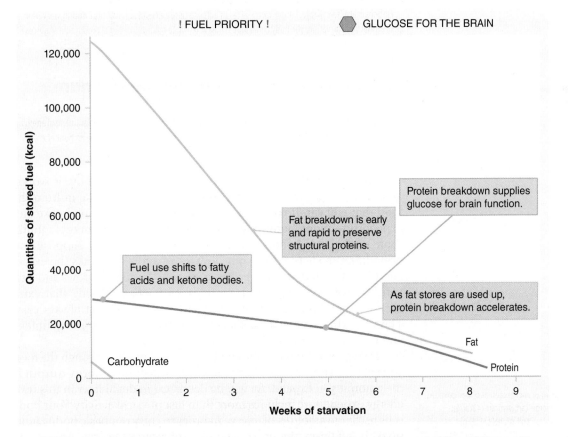

FIGURE SM.22 Starvation and fuel sources. During starvation, stored carbohydrate (glycogen) is exhausted quickly, and fat becomes the primary fuel. Burning fat without available carbohydrate produces ketone bodies, a byproduct that the body can use as fuel. Glucose produced from amino acids and the glycerol portion of fatty acids help fuel the brain. The body conserves protein and breaks it down rapidly only after most fat stores are depleted.

The End Is Near

In the final stage of protein depletion, the body deteriorates rapidly. You can see the severe muscle atrophy and emaciation in photos of Holocaust victims. Their bodies sacrificed muscle tissue in attempts to preserve brain tissue. Even organ tissues were not spared. The final stage of starvation attacks the liver and intestines, greatly depleting them. It moderately depletes the heart and kidneys and even mounts a small attack on the nervous system. Amazingly, starving people can cling to life until they lose about half their body proteins, after which death generally occurs.[24]

How long can a person survive total starvation? Several years ago, some Irish prisoners starved themselves to death—the average time was 60 days.[25] Most people survive total starvation for one to three months. Starvation survival factors include the following:

- *Starting percentage of body fat:* Ample fat tissue prolongs survival.
- *Age:* Middle-aged people survive longer than children and the elderly.
- *Gender:* Women fare better due to their higher proportion of body fat.
- *Energy expenditure levels:* Increased activity leads to an earlier death.

Key Concepts Fasting, or underconsumption of energy (calories), favors catabolic pathways. The body first obtains fuel from stored glycogen, then from stored fat and body proteins, such as muscle. Over time, the body adapts to using more and more ketone bodies as fuel because limited carbohydrate is available. Larger stores of fat in adipose tissue extend survival time during starvation. In prolonged starvation, the body catabolizes muscle tissue to continue minimal production of glucose from amino acids.

Energy Balance: Finding Your Equilibrium

🍎 **Why Is This Important?** Knowing your energy balance requires an understanding of energy intake—the amount of energy you consume from food—versus energy output—the amount of energy you expend for body functions and movement.

Your body is in the energy exchange business. Here's how it works: You balance the energy you expend with energy you take in from the food that you eat. If you do a fairly good job of equalizing intake and expenditure, your body does the rest—maintaining energy equilibrium, or "balance," and keeping your weight stable. But suppose you bring in more energy than your body can handle? It banks the excess energy as fat, and you gain weight. If your "account" grows too big, you become overweight and, perhaps, even obese. Losing that extra weight—withdrawing the fat from your account—is not always easy. Thus, weight management is a balancing act between energy intake and energy expenditure.

Energy intake is the amount of fuel you consume through the food you eat (i.e., carbohydrate, protein, fat, and alcohol). **Energy output** is the amount you expend. As will be described in detail later in this text, energy expenditure includes more than just physical activity. Your body cells use large amounts of energy in order to carry out basic bodily functions. In addition, the processing of food requires energy. An average adult consumes 1,800 to 3,000 kilocalories per day. In one year, that

▶ **energy intake** The caloric or energy content of food provided by the sources of dietary energy: carbohydrate (4 kcal/g), protein (4 kcal/g), fat (9 kcal/g), and alcohol (7 kcal/g).

▶ **energy output** The use of calories or energy for basic body functions, physical activity, and processing of consumed foods.

adds up to 657,000 to 1,095,000 kilocalories! Amazingly, despite such a huge intake of energy over time, most people maintain relatively stable body weights during most of their adult lives.

People who maintain a relatively constant weight are in **energy equilibrium**, such that, on average, the calories they consume are approximately equal to the calories they expend. Your body can be in energy equilibrium even if your energy intake is very high, as long as your expenditure also is high. Conversely, your body can be in energy equilibrium when you don't expend much energy, as long as your energy intake also is low.

When you consume more calories than you expend, you have a situation of **positive energy balance**. The surplus in calories will be stored as fat—the major energy reserve—and you will see the number on the bathroom scale go up. Now, positive energy balance is not always a bad thing. Pregnant women and growing children need a positive energy balance to increase energy stores. Strength and power athletes need to be in positive energy balance to increase lean body mass (e.g., muscle). But the positive energy balance that results from overeating and inactivity, a common occurrence in the United States and Canada, leads to unneeded weight gain.

When you consume fewer calories than you expend (or conversely, expend more calories than you consume), you are said to be in **negative energy balance**. To obtain the fuel it needs, your body uses its stores of glycogen and fat (and breaks down body protein, too, if the deficit is extreme), and body weight goes down. Thus, body weight change reflects overall **energy balance**. **FIGURE SM.23** shows three people with different ratios of energy intake to energy expenditure.

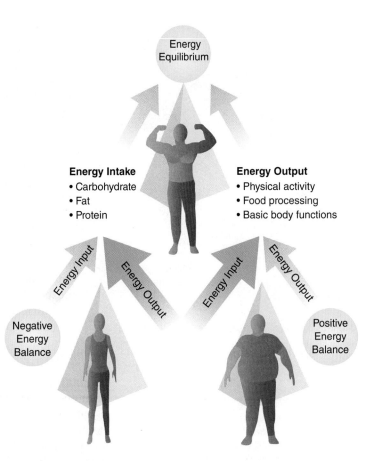

FIGURE SM.23 Energy balance. For most people, energy intake and output stay in balance, and weight remains stable. People in negative energy balance lose weight, and those in positive energy balance gain weight.

▶ **energy equilibrium** A balance of energy intake and output that results in little or no change in weight over time.

▶ **positive energy balance** Energy intake exceeds energy expenditure, resulting in an increase in body energy stores and weight gain.

▶ **negative energy balance** Energy intake is lower than energy expenditure, resulting in a depletion of body energy stores and weight loss.

▶ **energy balance** The balance in the body between amounts of energy consumed and expended.

> **Key Concepts** Energy balance is the relationship between energy intake and energy output. Energy intake is the number of calories consumed. Energy output is the number of calories expended, mainly for basic body functions, the processing of food, and physical activity.

Energy In

🍎 **Why Is This Important?** Both internal cues (such as hunger) and external cues (such as emotions) regulate your eating behavior. Knowing how these cues work can help you tap into them to help you eat more healthfully.

We know that energy intake is the number of calories consumed. But how does the body know how much energy it needs? A complex interaction between internal and external cues is believed to help the body regulate food intake and, thus, maintain energy equilibrium. Internal cues involve interactions and feedback mechanisms among neuropeptides, hormones,

Quick **Bite**

Early Energy-Balance Experiments

Erasistraus of Chios performed the first recorded experiment on energy balance in 280 BCE. Seeking to balance intake with output, he used a jar to fashion a kind of respiration apparatus. He then put two birds in the jar, weighing them and their excreta before and after feeding.

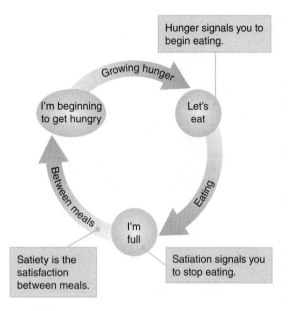

FIGURE SM.24 Hunger, satiation, and satiety. Hunger helps initiate eating. Satiation brings eating to a halt. Satiety is the state of nonhunger that determines the amount of time until eating begins again.

▶ **hunger** The internal, physiological drive to find and consume food. Unlike appetite, hunger is often experienced as a negative sensation, often manifesting as an uneasy or painful sensation; the recurrent and involuntary lack of access to food that may produce malnutrition over time.

▶ **satiation** Feeling of satisfaction and fullness that terminates a meal.

▶ **satiety** The effects of a food or meal that delay subsequent intake. Feeling of satisfaction and fullness following eating that quells the desire for food.

▶ **appetite** A psychological desire to eat that is related to the pleasant sensations often associated with food.

and other hormone-like compounds and organ systems. External cues are stimuli in the eating environment and include the sight, smell, and taste of food. Although these internal and external cues generally work together to ensure that we eat enough to survive, they can be readily overridden, such that we eat more than we need, resulting in positive energy balance and weight gain.

Hunger, Satiation, and Satiety

The internal cues that govern our energy intake are frequently classified as three distinct sensations, although there is some fundamental overlap in how we experience them. (See **FIGURE SM.24**.) The first, **hunger**, prompts eating ("I'm hungry"). Most of us recognize hunger as the empty or gnawing feeling in our stomachs, lightheadedness, and even headaches that signal the physiological need to eat. **Satiation**, the second internal cue, tells you when you've had enough to eat ("I'm full"). Finally, **satiety** represents the length of time that satiation lasts and generally tells you when you are ready to eat again ("I'm not ready to eat yet" or "I just ate an hour ago and I'm hungry already").

Appetite

External cues can stimulate **appetite**, which complicates the workings of hunger, satiation, and satiety. Appetite is the psychological desire to eat and is related to pleasant sensations associated with food. The eating environment often influences appetite. For example, exposure to a variety of tasty foods (such as at a buffet) can stimulate you to eat more than if you are served a limited number of foods. Hunger is the physiological need for food. In this sense, whereas appetite reflects our eating experiences, hunger is a basic drive. When you are truly hungry, any food will do, but your appetite can trigger your desire for a specific food or type of food, even though you may not be hungry. For example, after a big meal of steak, potato, salad, and bread, you probably wouldn't want a second helping of these foods. But you might be tempted by the dessert cart! That's appetite. Even when we are hungry, illness and medication can cause loss of appetite and a lack of interest in food.

THINK
About It

5

> **Key Concepts** Food intake is regulated by sensations of hunger, a physiological drive to eat; satiation, feelings of satisfaction that lead to ending a meal; and satiety, continued feelings of fullness that delay the start of the next meal. Appetite is the psychological urge to eat and often has no relation to hunger.

Control by Committee

What, then, stimulates hunger, satiation, satiety, and appetite? Internal responses in the digestive tract, central nervous system, and general circulation influence your eating behavior. Sites throughout the body monitor energy status and send reports to the brain, which can then stimulate feelings of hunger, satiety, and satiation. Externally, the eating environment—where we are eating, what we are eating, who we are eating with—can all influence what and how much we eat.

Gastrointestinal Sensations

As food fills your stomach and small intestine, they stretch and trigger signals to the brain. Your sense of fullness suppresses your urge to eat.

Just passing a reasonable amount of food through the mouth can satisfy hunger temporarily—even if the food never reaches the stomach. When researchers fed large amounts of food to a person with a hole in the esophagus, hunger decreased, even though the food never reached the stomach. As we taste, salivate, chew, and swallow, the brain probably measures the passage of food, much as a water meter measures the flow of water. After a certain amount of food passes through the mouth, hunger diminishes for 20 to 40 minutes.

Neurological and Hormonal Factors

More than 50 different chemicals are thought to be involved in the regulation of feeding. Determining the way these chemical factors work is an active research area that may lead to improved therapies for both the overweight and underweight.

Hormones, hormone-like factors, and some drugs (including appetite suppressants) influence eating behavior through their direct or indirect effects on the brain.[26] **Neuropeptide Y (NPY)** is a hormone-like factor in the brain and a powerful appetite stimulator that has been shown to cause people to hoard food.[27] Although a number of signals can affect NPY activity, opposing signals from the hormones **ghrelin** and **leptin** link NPY secretion to daily feeding patterns.[28]

Ghrelin, sometimes called the "hunger hormone," is produced in the stomach. Ghrelin levels rise prior to a meal and fall quickly after food is consumed. The rise in ghrelin levels appears to stimulate NPY, thus encouraging feeding. As you might expect, ghrelin levels increase in people who are undereating and decrease in those who are overeating.

Leptin, sometimes called the "satiety hormone," is produced in fat cells in direct proportion to the amount of fat stored and helps regulate fat storage.[29] Leptin levels are lower in thin people than in obese people. But unfortunately, many obese people have built up a resistance to the appetite-suppressing effects of leptin.[30] In normal weight people, a rise in leptin levels appears to inhibit NPY, thus suppressing appetite. A diet low in carbohydrates can lower leptin resistance, and a diet rich in whole grains or high in protein can suppress the "hunger hormone" ghrelin.[31]

Disruptions in the satiety signaling system can lead to consuming more calories, gaining weight, and storing fat. Stress-induced sleep loss, but not sleep loss per se, may result in decreased leptin levels, increased hunger, and a desire for "comfort foods."[32]

Key Concepts The interaction of internal factors, such as gastrointestinal sensations, hormonal responses, and neurological signals, helps regulate our feeding behavior. In obese people, these regulators can act inconsistently.

Diet Composition

The energy density (kilocalories per gram of food), balance of energy sources (carbohydrates, lipids, and protein), and the form (liquid versus solid) of your foods affect your energy intake. Overall, people tend to eat a fairly constant amount of food. If your diet includes a lot of energy-dense foods (typically high-fat, high-sugar, low-fiber foods), the way you eat likely will result in excess energy consumption, and in turn, weight gain.

Dietary protein and fiber may help control energy intake. Eating protein appears to increase satiety more than eating fat or carbohydrate.[33] Some types of fiber enhance satiation by slowing the rate at which the stomach empties, whereas others seem to enhance satiation

▶ **neuropeptide Y (NPY)** A neurotransmitter widely distributed throughout the brain and peripheral nervous tissue. NPY activity has been linked to eating behavior, depression, anxiety, and cardiovascular function.

▶ **ghrelin** A hormone produced by the stomach that stimulates feeding by increasing release of neuropeptide Y.

▶ **leptin** A hormone produced by adipose cells that signals the amount of body fat content and influences food intake.

by creating bulk.[34] Adding fiber to low-energy-dense foods may be an effective way to suppress appetite and control food intake.[35]

Simple carbohydrates and added sugars generally have low satiety value, and can be a significant source of calories. People eating low carbohydrate diets tend to have higher energy expenditures than people eating low fat diets. In general, liquid foods are less satiating than solid foods. One exception is soup, which despite its liquid form has relatively high satiety value.

Sensory Properties

The aroma of freshly baked bread or the warmth and chewiness of chocolate chip cookies right out of the oven can encourage us to eat more than our hunger dictates. Food's sensory properties—flavor, texture, color, temperature, and presentation—influence its appeal, and such external cues affect food intake.[36] (See **FIGURE SM.25**.) Taste often is the reason why people choose a particular food, and we are more likely to overconsume a food that tastes good.

Portion Size

Portion size plays a role in how much we eat, with larger portions generally leading to an increase in energy intake. Over the past two decades, portion sizes have increased for virtually all foods and beverages prepared for immediate consumption, including fast food, individually packaged food, and ready-to-eat prepared food. (See **TABLE SM.3**.)

Several studies have documented a "portion distortion" phenomenon. Rather than paying attention to internal feelings of satiation, we tend to respond to the visual stimulation of the amount of food on a plate or the serving size and consider that to be "normal." In a study of 110 undergraduate students, the group offered a larger plate of cookies consumed more than the group presented with a smaller plate of

Quick Bite

Supersize Me!

Morgan Spurlock wrote, directed, produced, and is the lead character in *Supersize Me*, a film that documents Spurlock's consumption of a 30-day, McDonald's-only diet. As part of the experiment, whenever offered the option to "supersize" his order, Spurlock always said "yes." Starting at 185 pounds, the 6-foot, 2-inch Spurlock packed on 25 pounds and weighed 210 pounds by the end of his experiment. His total cholesterol shot up from 165 to 230, his libido flagged, and he suffered headaches and depression.

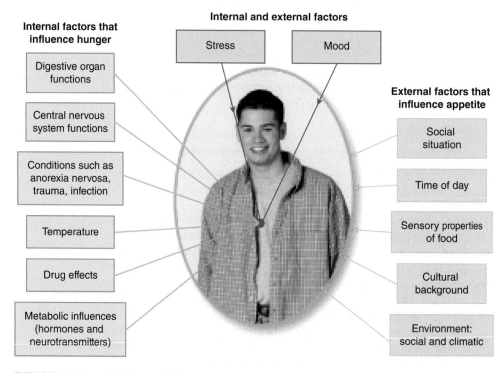

FIGURE SM.25 Internal and external influences on hunger and appetite.
© Photodisc.

TABLE SM.3

Comparison of Common Portion Sizes 20 Years Ago Versus Today

Food Item	20 Years Ago		Today	
	Portion	Calories	Portion	Calories
Bagel	3-inch diameter	140	6-inch diameter	350
Cheeseburger	1	330	1	590
Spaghetti with meatballs	1 cup spaghetti with sauce and 3 small meatballs	500	2 cups pasta with sauce and 3 large meatballs	1,025
Soda	6.5 oz	85	20 oz	250
Muffin	1.5 oz	210	4 oz	500

National Heart, Lung, and Blood Institute, National Institutes of Health, U.S. Department of Health and Human Services. Portion distortion. https://www.nhlbi.nih.gov/health/educational/wecan/eat-right/portion-distortion.htm. Accessed February 25, 2017.

cookies.[37] Another study looked at consumption of snack foods from different-sized containers. The results suggest that serving food in larger containers increases food intake.[38]

Children also are tempted by large portions. In a study of cereal consumption, children presented with a large bowl requested almost twice as much cereal as those presented with a smaller bowl.[39] In another study, children ate less when served smaller portions.[40] The ability of children to self-regulate energy intake at a meal is heavily influenced by portion size. A study of preschoolers found that the amount of food a child was served was highly predictive of the amount they consumed.[41]

Americans are living in a "super-size" culture in which portion sizes keep getting larger. Buffets, fast-food restaurants, and convenience stores offer "value meals" providing more food for less money. Consumers indicate that value for money is important when purchasing food and that large portion sizes offer more value for money than small portion sizes.[42] This dramatic increase in portion sizes eaten both at home and at restaurants may be a major contributing factor to excess energy intake and weight gain.

Environmental and Social Factors

We tend to eat more in cold weather and less in hot weather. Systems in the **hypothalamus** that regulate body temperature and food intake probably interact to link temperature and eating behavior. In cold temperatures, increased food intake helps us survive—increasing the metabolic rate, which helps generate heat, and increasing fat stores, which provide insulation to reduce heat loss.[43]

Plate size and shape, package sizes, lighting, color, convenience, and socializing are other factors that influence consumption.[44] Any change in our surroundings that inhibits our self-monitoring of consumption tends to increase the volume that we eat. Larger plates and bowls encourage larger servings. We tend to eat more in dimly lit situations than when the lights are brighter, perhaps because we are less inhibited and self-conscious.[45] Multitasking, such as watching television while eating, can draw attention away from the amount of food we're eating and increase consumption. We also tend to eat more when eating with others and less when eating alone.

Emotional Factors

Many people use food to cope with stress and negative emotions. Eating can provide a powerful distraction from loneliness, anger, boredom, anxiety, shame, sadness, and inadequacy. To combat low moods, low

▶ **hypothalamus [high-po-THAL-ah-mus]** A region of the brain involved in regulating hunger and satiety, respiration, body temperature, water balance, and other body functions.

energy levels, and low self-esteem, people often turn to the refrigerator. When we use food and eating to cope with our emotions, binge eating or other disturbed eating patterns can develop.

Key Concepts External factors such as portion size, aroma, weather, social circumstances, and emotions can enhance or suppress appetite. Our eating behaviors are determined by a complex interplay of physiological and psychological influences.

Energy Out: Fuel Uses

🍎 **Why Is This Important?** Understanding how your body expends energy will help you appreciate how you can make adjustments. Although intentional physical activity (exercise) is crucial, maintaining your body functions consumes the most energy. In addition to exercise, your body composition, and even your tendency to fidget, can impact your energy output significantly.

Our bodies use fuel (expend energy) for three primary purposes:

1. To maintain basic physiological functions such as breathing and blood circulation
2. To process the food we eat
3. To power physical activity

We also expend energy to support growth, stay warm in cold environments, metabolize drugs, and deal with physical trauma, fever, and psychological stress. The sum of all energy expended is the **total energy expenditure (TEE)**. **FIGURE SM.26** illustrates the major components of energy expenditure.

Major Components of Energy Expenditure

Energy Expenditure at Rest

We generally expend most of our energy on the basic body functions needed to sustain life at rest. This resting energy expenditure is the

▶ **total energy expenditure (TEE)** The total of the resting energy expenditure (REE), energy used in physical activity, and energy used in processing food (TEF); usually expressed in kilocalories per day.

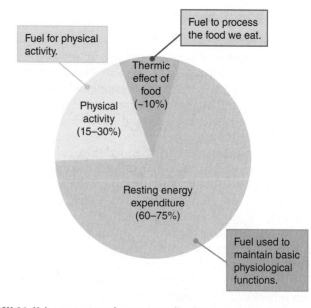

FIGURE SM.26 Major components of energy expenditure. You expend most of your energy to maintain basic body functions. Energy expended in physical activity can be significant and is the most variable component of total energy expenditure. The thermic effect of food is the energy needed to digest, absorb, transport, metabolize, and store ingested food.

energy needed to maintain heartbeat, respiration, nervous function, muscle tone, body temperature, and other bodily functions. Resting energy expenditure accounts for approximately 60 to 75 percent of total energy expenditure. The rate of energy expended at rest (kcal/hour) is called the **resting metabolic rate (RMR)**. Extrapolating the RMR over 24 hours (kcal/hr × 24) determines the **resting energy expenditure (REE)**.[46]

Energy expended by the vital organs (e.g., liver, brain, heart, kidneys, pancreas) and skeletal muscle makes up the greatest proportion of REE. Other tissues, such as fat, have lower metabolic activity and consume less energy. The vital organs and skeletal muscle, along with bones and fluids, make up most of what is known as the **lean body mass**—the total mass of the body that isn't fat. An exceptionally muscular person has more lean body mass and, thus, a higher RMR than an obese person of the same weight. Although differences in lean body mass explain most of the differences in RMR among people, extreme weight loss can depress RMR significantly.[47]

Lean body mass tends to decline as we age, and body fat tends to rise. Keeping physically active helps slow this age-related loss of lean tissue and discourages accumulation of fat so we maintain a higher RMR.

Women usually have lower RMRs than men. Women tend to be smaller, and pound for pound they generally have less lean body mass. A woman's RMR also varies during the menstrual cycle, fluctuating from a low point about one week before ovulation to a high point just before the onset of menstruation.[48]

Diet composition also can affect resting and total energy expenditures. Independent of the actual number of calories consumed, people eating a low-carbohydrate diet expend less energy that those eating a low-fat diet.[49] **FIGURE SM.27** shows the factors that affect RMR.

Key Concepts We use energy to fuel basic body functions, process the food we eat, and support physical activity. The energy used in these basic functions is called resting energy expenditure, or REE. Factors that affect resting energy expenditure include body composition, age, and gender.

Energy Expenditure in Physical Activity

Physical activity encompasses more than just exercise and participation in sports. It includes the activity you do at work, during leisure activities, and other everyday activities—even fidgeting. For most individuals, the energy expended in physical activity accounts for 15 to 30 percent of total daily energy expenditure (depending on whether you are mostly sedentary or very physically active).[50] For some elite athletes, training several hours each day, the energy expended in physical activity may be as high as 50 percent of total daily energy expenditure.

The energy cost of an activity depends on its type (i.e., walking, running, or typing, for example), duration, and intensity. **TABLE SM.4** shows the amounts of energy expended in specific activities. Body size affects energy cost, too—it takes more energy to move a bigger mass, so a large person expends more kilocalories per minute than a smaller person doing the same activity. Fitness level has an effect as well. A fit person exercises more efficiently, with lower energy costs. However, fit people also can exercise with greater intensity and duration, burning

▶ **resting metabolic rate (RMR)** A clinical measure of resting energy expenditure performed three to four hours after eating or performing significant physical activity.

▶ **resting energy expenditure (REE)** The minimum energy needed to maintain basic physiological functions (e.g., heartbeat, muscle function, respiration). The resting metabolic rate (RMR) extrapolated to 24 hours.

▶ **lean body mass** The portion of the body exclusive of stored fat, including muscle, bone, connective tissue, organs, and water.

Increase RMR

- Total body weight
- Large body surface area
- Hot and cold ambient temperature
- Fever
- Hyperthyroidism
- Stress
- Caffeine
- Smoking
- Increased lean body mass
- Rapid growth
- Pregnancy and lactation

- Genetics
- Some medications

- Aging
- Female gender
- Fasting/starvation
- Hypothyroidism
- Sleep
- Extreme weight loss

Decrease RMR

FIGURE SM.27 Factors that affect RMR. Inherited traits determine whether you have a generally high or low RMR. Many environmental and physiological factors may temporarily raise RMR, and other factors may temporarily lower it.

TABLE SM.4
Amount of Energy Expended in Specific Activities

Description	Kcal/hr/kg	Kcal/hr/lb	50 kg (110 lb)	Kcal/hr at Different Body Weights			
				57 kg (125 lb)	68 kg (150 lb)	80 kg (175 lb)	91 kg (200 lb)
Aerobics							
Light	3.0	1.36	150	170	205	239	273
Moderate	8.0	2.27	250	284	341	398	455
Heavy	8.0	3.64	400	455	545	636	727
Bicycling							
Leisurely (< 10 mph)	4.0	1.82	200	227	273	318	364
Light (10–11.9 mph)	6.0	2.73	300	341	409	477	545
Moderate (12–13.9 mph)	8.0	3.64	400	455	545	636	727
Fast (14–15.9 mph)	10.0	4.55	500	568	682	795	909
Racing (16–19 mph)	12.0	5.45	600	682	818	955	1,091
BMX or mountain	8.5	3.86	425	483	580	676	773
Daily Activities							
Sleeping	1.2	0.55	60	68	82	95	109
Studying, reading, writing	1.8	0.82	90	102	123	143	164
Cooking, food preparation	2.5	1.14	125	142	170	199	227
Home Activities							
House painting, outside	4.0	1.82	200	227	273	318	364
General gardening	5.0	2.27	250	284	341	398	455
Shoveling snow	6.0	2.73	300	341	409	477	545
Running							
Jogging	7.0	3.18	350	398	477	557	636
Running 5 mph	8.0	3.64	400	455	545	636	727
Running 6 mph	10.0	4.55	500	568	682	795	909
Running 7 mph	11.5	5.23	575	653	784	915	1,045
Running 8 mph	13.5	6.14	675	767	920	1,074	1,227
Running 9 mph	15.0	6.82	750	852	1,023	1,193	1,364
Running 10 mph	16.0	7.27	800	909	1,091	1,273	1,455
Sports							
Frisbee, ultimate	3.5	1.59	175	199	239	278	318
Hacky sack	4.0	1.82	200	227	273	318	364
Wind surfing	4.2	1.91	210	239	286	334	382
Golf	4.5	2.05	225	256	307	358	409
Skateboarding	5.0	2.27	250	284	341	398	455
Rollerblading	7.0	3.18	350	398	477	557	636
Soccer	7.0	3.18	350	398	477	557	636
Field hockey	8.0	3.64	400	455	545	636	727
Swimming, slow to moderate laps	8.0	3.64	400	455	545	636	727
Skiing downhill, moderate effort	6.0	2.73	300	341	409	477	545
Skiing cross country, moderate effort	8.0	3.64	400	455	545	636	727
Tennis, doubles	6.0	2.73	300	341	409	477	545
Tennis, singles	8.0	3.64	400	455	545	636	727

TABLE SM.4 (*continued*)
Amount of Energy Expended in Specific Activities

Description	Kcal/hr/kg	Kcal/hr/lb	50 kg (110 lb)	Kcal/hr at Different Body Weights			
				57 kg (125 lb)	68 kg (150 lb)	80 kg (175 lb)	91 kg (200 lb)
Strolling (< 2 mph), level	2.0	0.91	100	114	136	159	182
Moderate pace (~3 mph), level	3.5	1.59	175	199	239	278	318
Moderate pace (~3 mph), uphill	6.0	2.73	300	341	409	477	545
Brisk pace (~3.5 mph), level	4.0	1.82	200	227	273	318	364
Very brisk pace (~4.5 mph), level	4.5	2.05	225	256	307	358	409

Modified from Nieman DC. *Exercise Testing and Prescription*. 7th ed. New York: McGraw-Hill, 2010.

more kilocalories overall. **FIGURE SM.28** shows how energy expenditure is measured during exercise.

Mental activity—such as studying for an exam—uses little energy. But if you fidget when you study, you may expend a significant amount of energy. The acronym **NEAT** stands for **nonexercise activity thermogenesis**, which is the energy associated with activities other than purposeful exercise, such as fidgeting, maintenance of posture, occupational activities, and similar contributors to energy expenditure.[51] (See the FYI feature "What's Neat About NEAT?")

Energy Expenditure to Process Food

Our bodies expend energy to digest, absorb, and metabolize the nutrients we take in, and these processes generate heat. This energy output is collectively called the **thermic effect of food (TEF)**. TEF peaks about one hour after eating and normally dissipates within five hours. For a typical mixed diet, TEF accounts for about 10 percent of total energy expenditure and declines in older adults.[52] The daily TEF is determined primarily by the number of kilocalories an individual consumes—a higher intake of energy requires more energy for digestion, absorption, and metabolism. Research also suggests that TEF may be reduced in obese individuals, contributing to further weight gain.[53] It's possible to increase the TEF by altering the macronutrient composition of the diet, but not by much—only about 50 kilocalories or so daily.

> **Key Concepts** An individual's fitness level and weight and the type, duration, and intensity of activity affect the amount of energy expended in physical activity. The thermic effect of food is the energy needed to process the food we eat and is influenced by the amount and mix of nutrients in the diet.

Estimating Total Energy Expenditure

An adult's REE can be estimated using an abbreviated method. The 1.0 and 0.9 factors used in this method for kilocalories per kilogram reflect the differences in body composition between men and women. As previously described, men have proportionally more lean body mass and thus burn more kilocalories per kilogram of body weight. This abbreviated method dramatically underestimates children's REE, however, and somewhat overestimates the REE of elders.

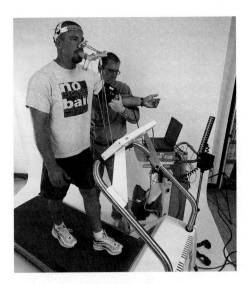

FIGURE SM.28 Measuring energy expended in physical activity. A technician can collect respiratory gases and indirectly calculate energy expenditure during exercise.

▶ **nonexercise activity thermogenesis (NEAT)** The output of energy associated with fidgeting, maintenance of posture, and other minimal physical exertions.

▶ **thermic effect of food (TEF)** The energy used to digest, absorb, and metabolize energy-yielding foodstuffs. It constitutes about 10 percent of total energy expenditure but is influenced by various factors.

Quick Bite

Brrr! Shivering Away Calories
Cold weather increases energy needs. Shivering alone can increase the RMR by 2.5 times. Although shivering bodies use both fat and carbohydrate, carbohydrates are the preferred fuel. In addition, people with less body fat shiver more in the cold.

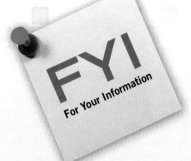

What's Neat About NEAT?

It seems Jan only has to look at food to gain weight. Yet her friend Schuling doesn't seem to gain weight no matter what she eats. Both have the same height and frame, eat about the same amount of calories, and have the same workout schedule. So what's missing? The answer is NEAT (nonexercise activity thermogenesis).

NEAT is the energy expenditure of all physical activities other than intentional exercise and participation in sports. "NEAT includes all those activities that render us vibrant, unique, and independent beings," says Mayo Clinic researcher James Levine, MD, PhD.[a] NEAT activities include fidgeting, daily living activities, posture maintenance, and occupational activities.

Among adults of similar size, total energy expenditures can vary widely, mainly due to differences in physical activity. Physical activity energy expenditure is divided into two categories—exercise and NEAT. Exercise is any exertion for the sake of developing and maintaining physical fitness. All other physical movement is NEAT. For most people who exercise, their exercise activity burns about 100 kilocalories per day.

NEAT includes occupational activity. Job-based activities account for the greatest differences in energy expenditures. For example, are you sitting at a desk all day or are you outside digging trenches? Active work easily can burn 1,000 kilocalories per day more than a sedentary job. After work you might burn 30 kilocalories watching TV or 600 kilocalories gardening in the yard. (See **TABLE A**.) Mostly due to differences in occupational activities, NEAT can vary by 2,000 kilocalories per day.[b]

Unfortunately, the American workforce has become sedentary, and this is an important

TABLE A
Occupational Nonexercise Activity Thermogenesis (NEAT)

Occupation Type	NEAT (kcal/day)
Chair-bound	300
Seated work (no option of moving)	700
Seated work (discretion and requirement to move)	1,000
Standing work (e.g., homemaker, cashier)	1,400
Strenuous work (e.g., farming)	2,300

*Data based on a basal metabolic rate of 1,600 kcal/day.

factor in the growing obesity epidemic. Due to technology and better mass transportation, people have become less active in their occupations and daily lives. Since 1950, sedentary jobs have increased 83 percent, and people with physically active jobs now make up less than 20 percent of our workforce.[c] Nearly half of Americans are not sufficiently active to receive health benefits, and about a quarter report doing no physical activity or exercise other than their regular job in the prior 30 days.[d] Increasing NEAT during work or leisure could be essential to maintaining a negative energy balance. NEAT can be applied by being upright, walking, and

redesigning workplace and leisure-time environments to encourage activity.

Increasing NEAT has significant health benefits. In patients with type 2 diabetes, NEAT may reduce obesity while improving insulin sensitivity and lipid profiles.[e] In general, NEAT not only reduces the occurrence of metabolic syndrome, but also lowers the long-term risk of cardiovascular disease and all-cause mortality.[f] Experts believe that to overcome the obesity epidemic and related health consequences, NEAT should become a part of current medical recommendations.

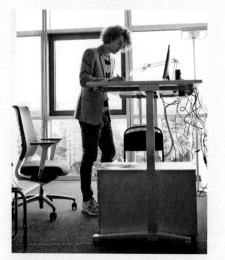

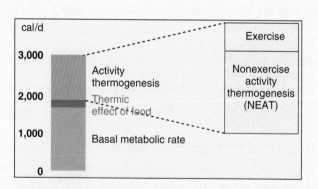

FYI SM.2A Energy expenditure. The three components of human daily energy expenditure are the basal metabolic rate (about 60 percent of daily energy expenditure), the thermic effect of food (i.e., the energy expended in response to a meal [about 10 percent of daily energy expenditure]), and activity thermogenesis (both exercise and nonexercise activity).

If we can get people out of their chairs, energy expenditures can be expected to increase by 350–750 kilocalories or more per day. But how can daily activity be tracked accurately? An application using accelerometers in smartphones was validated in the laboratory. Within six months of deployment, 28,000 people used it, and the results are being used to shape behavioral interventions.[g] Effective interventions can be simple, such as moving printers away from where computers are located, moving other commonly used items further away from your desk, and defining longer office walking pathways with floor tape. Each of these interventions has been validated in the laboratory.[h] To exploit NEAT in the fight against obesity, it's time to stand up and walk!

a   Young, Jr WF, ed. The "NEAT defect" in human obesity: the role of nonexercise activity thermogenesis. *Endocrinol Upd.* 2007;2(1):1-2. http://www.mayoclinic.org/documents/mc5810-0307-pdf/doc-20079082. Accessed September 11, 2017.

b   Villablanca PA, Alegria JR, Mookadam F, et al. Nonexercise activity thermogenesis in obesity management. *Mayo Clin Proc.* 2015;90(4):509-519.

c   American Heart Association. The price of inactivity. http://www.heart.org/HEARTORG/HealthyLiving/PhysicalActivity/FitnessBasics/The-Price-of-Inactivity_UCM_307974_Article.jsp#.WLSeOW_yuUk Accessed September 11, 2017.

d   Hamasaki H, Exaki O, Yanai H. Nonexercise activity thermogenesis is significantly lower in type 2 diabetic patients with mental disorders than in those without mental disorders. *Medicine.* 2016;95(2):e2517.

e   Ibid.

f   Villablanca PA, Alegria JR, Mookadam F, et al. Op. cit.

g   Manohar CU, McCrady SK, Fujiki Y, Pavlidis IT, Levine JA. Evaluation of the accuracy of a triaxial accelerometer embedded into a cell phone platform for measuring physical activity. *J Obes Weight Loss Ther.* 2012;1:106.

h   McCrady-Spitzer SK, Levine JA. Nonexercise activity thermogenesis: a way forward to treat the worldwide obesity epidemic. *Surg Obes Relat Dis.* 2012;8(5):501-506.

Abbreviated Method to Estimate REE for Adult Men
REE = weight (kg) $\times$ 1.0 kcal/kg $\times$ 24 hr/day
REE = weight (kg) $\times$ 1.0 $\times$ 24
For Adult Women
REE = weight (kg) $\times$ 0.9 kcal/kg $\times$ 24 hr/day
REE = weight (kg) $\times$ 0.9 $\times$ 24

The abbreviated method estimates only REE. To determine total energy expenditure (TEE), energy expended in physical activity and the thermic effect of food must be included. Energy expended in physical activity can be estimated as a percentage of REE based on a person's general activity level. (See **TABLE SM.5**.) Most adults in the United States and Canada have a light or moderate activity level. The

TABLE SM.5
Estimating Energy Expended in Physical Activity

Percentage of REE	Activity Level	Description
20–30	Sedentary	Mostly resting with little or no activity
30–45	Light	Occasional unplanned activity (e.g., going for a stroll)
45–65	Moderate	Daily planned activity (e.g., brisk walks)
65–90	Heavy	Daily workout routine requiring several hours of continuous exercise
90–120	Exceptional	Daily vigorous workouts for extended hours; training for competition

Data from Institute of Medicine, Food and Nutrition Board. *Dietary Reference Intakes for Energy, Carbohydrate, Fiber, Fat, Fatty Acids, Cholesterol, Protein, and Amino Acids (Macronutrients).* Washington, DC: National Academies Press; 2005.

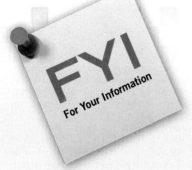

How Many Calories Do I Burn?

You can estimate the amount of energy you use each day by using some simple equations. Remember that there will be quite a lot of individual variation in actual energy output, so these calculated values are just estimates.

1. Convert your weight in pounds to weight in kilograms. For example, Carol is a 120-pound female. Her weight is 54.5 kilograms (54.5 = 120 ÷ 2.2).

$$\frac{}{\text{weight (lb)}} \div 2.2 = \frac{}{\text{weight (kg)}}$$

2. Estimate your personal REE.

   For adult women:

   $$\text{REE} = \frac{}{\text{weight (kg)}} \times 0.9 \times 24$$

   For adult men:

   $$\text{REE} = \frac{}{\text{weight (kg)}} \times 1.0 \times 24$$

For example, Carol has an estimated REE of 1,177 kilocalories (1,177 = 54.5 × 0.9 × 24).

3. Estimate your energy expended in physical activity (see Table SM.5).

$$\text{Energy}_{\text{physical activity}} = \frac{}{\text{from Table SM.5}} \times \text{REE}$$

For example, Carol has a light to moderate physical activity level. She expends about 530 kilocalories in physical activity (530 = 0.45 × 1,177).

4. Estimate your thermic effect of food (TEF).

$$\text{TEF} = 0.1 \times \left(\frac{}{\text{Energy}_{\text{physical activity}}} + \frac{}{\text{REE}} \right)$$

For our example, Carol's thermic effect of food is about 171 kilocalories (171 = 0.1 × [530 + 1,177]).

5. Estimate your personal total energy expenditure (TEE).

$$\text{TEE} = \frac{}{\text{REE}} + \frac{}{\text{Energy}_{\text{physical activity}}} + \frac{}{\text{TEF}}$$

For our example, Carol's total energy expenditure is about 1,878 kilocalories (1,177 + 530 + 171).

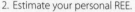

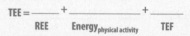

Quick Bite

The Fattest Mammals
Among mammals, humans carry the largest percentage of weight as body fat.

thermic effect of food can be estimated as roughly 6 to 10 percent of the sum of REE plus energy expended in physical activity. Summing the three estimated components—REE, physical activity, and TEF—delivers the estimated total energy expenditure. See the FYI feature "How Many Calories Do I Burn?" for an example of these estimates in action.

DRIs for Energy: Estimated Energy Requirements

Just as there are DRIs for nutrients, there are DRIs for energy, called estimated energy requirements (EERs). The EER is defined as the energy intake predicted to maintain energy balance in a healthy person of normal weight. The EER equations for adults (see **TABLE SM.6**) predict TEE from age, height, weight, gender, and physical activity level. Separate equations have been developed for infants, children, and teens, and adjustments are made for pregnancy and lactation.

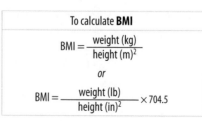

To calculate **BMI**
$$\text{BMI} = \frac{\text{weight (kg)}}{\text{height (m)}^2}$$
or
$$\text{BMI} = \frac{\text{weight (lb)}}{\text{height (in)}^2} \times 704.5$$

TABLE SM.6
Estimated Energy Requirements for Adults

Males		
EER = 662 − 9.53 × age [yr] + PA × (15.91 × weight [kg] + 539.6 × height [m])		
Physical activity =	1.0	Sedentary
	1.11	Low active
	1.25	Active
	1.48	Very active
Females		
EER = 354 − 6.91 × age [yr] + PA × (9.36 × weight [kg] + 726 × height [m])		
Physical activity =	1.0	Sedentary
	1.12	Low active
	1.27	Active
	1.45	Very active

Modified with permission from Institute of Medicine, Food and Nutrition Board. *Dietary Reference Intakes for Energy, Carbohydrate, Fiber, Fat, Fatty Acids, Cholesterol, Protein, and Amino Acids (Macronutrients)*. Copyright 2005 by the National Academy of Sciences, courtesy of the National Academies Press, Washington, DC.

Body Composition: Understanding Fatness and Weight

🍎 **Why Is This Important?** Understanding the distinction between body fat and body weight will give you insight into how nutritionists and other scientists determine an individual's energy expenditure and risk for certain diseases.

Stepping onto a scale provides quick and easy feedback about your body weight. Yet many people have a distorted notion of their weight—thinking they're too fat when they aren't or thinking their weight is just fine when it isn't. In terms of your health risks, body composition is more important than body weight.

Body composition is the relative amount of fat and lean body mass. Excess body fatness is linked with increased risk for heart disease, hypertension, cancer, diabetes, and other chronic diseases. Two people with the same high weight and height may have very different health risks. One may be obese and have many weight-related health risks. The other could be very fit and muscular, with no increased disease risk.

Assessing Body Weight

The **body mass index (BMI)** has become the accepted method for assessing body weight for height. This index, which is a ratio of weight to height squared, correlates reasonably well with body fatness and health risks. To determine your BMI, accurately measure your height without shoes and your weight with minimal clothing. Then plug these numbers into the provided equation. For adults, the *2015–2020 Dietary Guidelines for Americans* defines **underweight, normal weight, overweight,** and **obesity** as follows:

- *Underweight:* BMI < 18.5 kg/m²
- *Normal weight:* 18.5 kg/m² ≤ BMI < 25 kg/m²

▶ **body composition** The chemical or anatomical composition of the body. Commonly defined as the proportions of fat, muscle, bone, and other tissues in the body.

▶ **body mass index (BMI)** Body weight (in kilograms) divided by the square of height (in meters), expressed in units of kg/m².

▶ **underweight** BMI less than 18.5 kg/m².

▶ **normal weight** BMI at or above 18.5 kg/m² and less than 25 kg/m².

▶ **overweight** BMI at or above 25 kg/m² and less than 30 kg/m².

▶ **obesity** Excessive accumulation of body fat leading to a body weight in relation to height that is substantially greater than some accepted standard. A BMI at or above 30 kg/m².

- *Overweight:* $25 \text{ kg/m}^2 \leq \text{BMI} < 30 \text{ kg/m}^2$
- *Obese:* $\text{BMI} \geq 30 \text{ kg/m}^2$

TABLE SM.7 can help you determine whether your weight is a healthy weight according to the *Dietary Guidelines for Americans.*

As **FIGURE SM.29** shows, correlating BMI with mortality produces a *J*-shaped curve. Studies indicate that underweight (BMI less than 18.5 kg/m^2) is associated with increased mortality, as is obesity (BMI greater than or equal to 30 kg/m^2). Normal weight and overweight are not associated with excess overall mortality.[54,55]

Although your BMI can give you a general idea of your overall health risks, it still doesn't tell you enough about whether you are carrying muscle weight or excess fat and/or where that excess fat is (i.e., around your midsection or in your hips and thighs). A classic example is the heavy football player or bodybuilder with a large muscle mass who has a BMI greater than 30 kg/m^2 but is not overfat. For someone

Quick Bite

Is Tom Brady Too Fat?

Although BMI has become the standard reference for determining overweight and obesity, it has limitations at the extremes of body size and composition. Consider Tom Brady, quarterback for the New England Patriots. At 6 feet, 4 inches, and 225 pounds, Tom has a BMI of 27.4, which puts him in the category of "Overweight." This star athlete does not have too much body fat!

TABLE SM.7
Adult BMI Chart

BMI	19	20	21	22	23	24	25	26	27	28	29	30	31	32	33	34	35
Height								**Weight in Pounds**									
4'10"	91	96	100	105	110	115	119	124	129	134	138	143	148	153	158	162	167
4'11"	94	99	104	109	114	119	124	128	133	138	143	148	153	158	163	168	173
5'	97	102	107	112	118	123	128	133	138	143	148	153	158	163	158	174	179
5'1"	100	106	111	116	122	127	132	137	143	148	153	158	164	169	174	180	185
5'2"	104	109	115	120	126	131	136	142	147	153	158	164	169	175	180	186	191
5'3"	107	113	118	124	130	135	141	146	152	158	163	169	175	180	186	191	197
5'4"	110	116	122	128	134	140	145	151	157	163	169	174	180	186	192	197	204
5'5"	114	120	126	132	138	144	150	156	162	168	174	180	186	192	198	204	210
5'6"	118	124	130	136	142	148	155	161	167	173	179	186	192	198	204	210	216
5'7"	121	127	134	140	146	153	159	166	172	178	185	191	198	204	211	217	223
5'8"	125	131	138	144	151	158	164	171	177	184	190	197	203	210	216	223	230
5'9"	128	135	142	149	155	162	169	176	182	189	196	203	209	216	223	230	236
5'10"	132	139	146	153	160	167	174	181	188	195	202	209	216	222	229	236	243
5'11"	136	143	150	157	165	172	179	186	193	200	208	215	222	229	236	243	250
6'	140	147	154	162	169	177	184	191	199	206	213	221	228	235	242	250	258
6'1"	144	151	159	166	174	182	189	197	204	212	219	227	235	242	250	257	265
6'2"	148	155	163	171	179	186	194	202	210	218	225	233	241	249	256	264	272
6'3"	152	160	168	176	184	192	200	208	216	224	232	240	248	256	264	272	279
	Healthy Weight						**Overweight**					**Obese**					

Locate the height of interest in the leftmost column, and read across the row for that height to the weight of interest. Follow the column of the weight up to the top row that lists the BMI. A BMI of 19 to 24 is in the healthy range, a BMI of 25 to 29 is in the overweight range, and a BMI of 30 or above is in the obese range. Due to rounding, these ranges vary slightly from the NHLBI values.

A calculator for adult BMI is available at http://www.nhlbi.nih.gov/health/educational/lose_wt/BMI/bmicalc.htm. A child and adolescent BMI calculator is available at http://apps.nccd.cdc.gov/dnpabmi.

National Heart, Lung, and Blood Institute. National Institutes of Health. Body Mass Index Table. https://www.nhlbi.nih.gov/health/educational/lose_wt/BMI/bmi_tbl.htm. Accessed February 26. 2017. U.S. Department of Health and Human Services and U.S. Department of Agriculture. Table A6-1 Body Mass Index (BMI) and Corresponding Body Weight Categories for Children and Adults in *2015–2020 Dietary Guidelines for Americans*. 8th Edition. December 2015. Available at http://health.gov/dietaryguidelines/2015/guidelines/. Accessed February 26, 2017.

who has lost muscle mass, perhaps an older adult, BMI can underestimate health risks associated with excess body fat. BMI measurements should be interpreted cautiously when used for people who are petite, who have large body frames, or who are highly muscular.[56]

For children and teens, height and weight measurements can be compared to standard growth charts to see if the child is growing and gaining weight at the appropriate rate. For children and teens (2 to 20 years old), pediatric growth charts include age- and sex-specific percentile curves for BMI.[57] A BMI-for-age at or above the 95th percentile indicates overweight and the need for further evaluation and possible treatment. Further evaluation may also be indicated if the child's BMI-for-age is at or above the 85th percentile and is accompanied by other risk factors, such as high blood pressure, high blood cholesterol, diabetes, and family history of obesity-related disease. A BMI-for-age below the 5th percentile suggests the child is underweight.

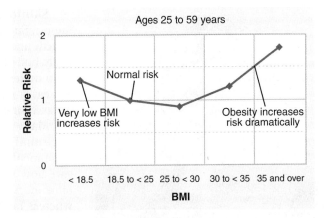

FIGURE SM.29 BMI and mortality. People with a high or very low BMI have a higher relative risk of mortality.
Modified from Flegal KM, Graubard BI, Williamson DF, Gail MH. Excess deaths associated with underweight, overweight, and obesity. *JAMA.* 2005;293:1861-1867.

> **Key Concepts** Body composition is a key element in determining energy expenditure and is an important factor in disease risk. Weight and height measures can be used to calculate BMI, which is correlated with body fatness and health risks. Elevated BMI in adults or children can increase health risks.

Assessing Body Fatness

Fat that is stored in adipose tissue that lies directly under the skin is referred to as *subcutaneous fat,* whereas fat that surrounds internal organs is called *visceral fat.* For healthy adult females, fat typically consists of 20 to 35 percent of total body weight; for adult men, the typical range is 8 to 24 percent. Risk of chronic disease appears to rise when body fat exceeds these levels.

Densitometry is the measure of body density (body mass divided by body volume). Because fat and lean tissues have different densities, if we know the person's volume and weight we can calculate the ratio of fat to lean body mass. The density of fat doesn't vary, but hydration status, age, gender, and ethnicity all influence the density of lean body mass. For example, bone loss in the elderly leads to a lower density of lean body mass.

Body fatness can be assessed by a number of methods. The current gold standard for measuring composition and determining body fatness is dual energy x-ray absorptiometry (DXA).[58] Originally developed for the measurement of bone mineral density (to test for osteoporosis), DXA is unique in that it measures the body's mineral content (bone), fat mass, and lean body mass (protein and water). Unfortunately, the equipment is expensive and not readily available, limiting its use to research settings. Another technique frequently used in research settings is **underwater weighing**, also called **hydrostatic weighing**. Because fat is less dense than muscle, a person with more body fat will have a lower underwater weight than a person with the same body weight but less fat. The newer **BodPod** uses the same principle of density, but it measures displacement of air to determine relative amounts of fat and fat-free mass. **FIGURE SM.30** illustrates underwater weighing, and **FIGURE SM.31** shows the BodPod.

▶ **underwater weighing** Determining body density by measuring the volume of water displaced when the body is fully submerged in a specialized water tank. Also called *hydrostatic weighing.*

▶ **hydrostatic weighing** See *underwater weighing.*

▶ **BodPod** A device used to measure the density of the body based on the volume of air displaced as a person sits in a sealed chamber of known volume.

▶ **skinfold measurements** A method to estimate body fat by measuring the thickness of a fold of skin and subcutaneous fat.

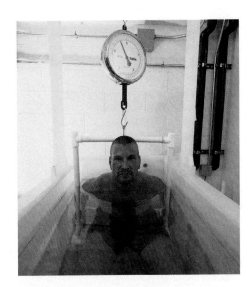

FIGURE SM.30 Underwater weighing. During underwater weighing, the subject must exhale completely, submerge without taking a breath, and remain motionless until the water is still and the scale is steady.

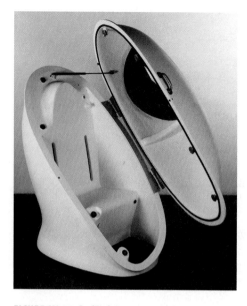

FIGURE SM.31 **BodPod.** By using air displacement, the BodPod provides an alternative to underwater weighing that is easier, cheaper, and of similar accuracy.
Courtesy of COSMED USA, Inc.

Skinfold measurements are a low-tech method for assessing body fatness. Special calipers are used to measure the thickness of fat deposits directly underneath the skin at several locations around the body. Done correctly, body composition estimates from skinfolds correlate well with those from underwater weighing, but an inexperienced or careless technician can easily make large errors. Skinfold measurements usually work better for assessing malnutrition than for identifying overweight and obesity.

Many health clubs and fitness centers use **bioelectrical impedance analysis (BIA)** to measure body fatness. A technician uses special equipment to pass a small electric current through the body and measure how well the body conducts electricity. Because lean tissue contains more water than fat tissue, it is a better conductor of electricity, whereas fat produces a greater impedance. Measurements are used to determine the amounts of lean and fat mass. Unfortunately, this method is readily affected by hydration status, with dehydration producing a falsely elevated impedance and overestimation of body fatness. Thus, the many factors that can impact hydration status (exercise, eating, drinking, medications, etc.) render this measure unreliable and inaccurate.

Body Fat Distribution

Measurements of body fatness tell you more about your health risks than your weight does, but they still don't tell the whole story. Where the fat is located—**body fat distribution**—can be an independent risk factor.[59] The "pear shape," or **gynoid obesity**, which is more common in women, has fat distributed predominantly around the hips and thighs. The "apple shape," or **android obesity**, typical of men, has extra fat distributed higher up, around the abdomen. You are at greater health risk with the apple pattern than with the pear pattern of fat distribution. In fact, excess abdominal fat may increase breast cancer risk for women.[60] **FIGURE SM.32** shows the gynoid and android distributions of body fat.

▶ **bioelectrical impedance analysis (BIA)** Technique to estimate amounts of total body water, lean tissue mass, and total body fat. It uses the resistance of tissue to the flow of an alternating electric current.

▶ **body fat distribution** The pattern of fat distribution on the body.

▶ **gynoid obesity** Excess storage of fat located primarily in the buttocks and thighs. Also called *gynecoid obesity*.

▶ **android obesity [AN-droyd]** Excess storage of fat located primarily in the abdominal area.

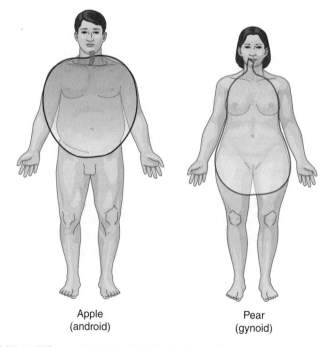

Apple
(android)

Pear
(gynoid)

FIGURE SM.32 **Differences in body fat distribution.** Men tend to carry excess fat around their abdomen (android obesity). Women tend to accumulate excess fat in their hips and thighs (gynoid obesity).

If your **waist circumference** increases, you are probably gaining abdominal fat. National Institutes of Health (NIH) clinical guidelines suggest that for people with a BMI of 25 kg/m² to 34.9 kg/m², a waist circumference greater than 40 inches (102 centimeters) in men or greater than 35 inches (88 centimeters) in women is a sign of increased health risk. When BMI is 35 kg/m² or higher, waist circumference measures do not accurately predict health risks. Combining measures of BMI and waist circumference is more predictive of cardiovascular disease risk than either measure alone.[61]

▶ **waist circumference** The waist measurement, as a marker of abdominal fat content, that can be used to indicate health risks.

Key Concepts Excess body fatness is associated with increased risk for chronic diseases, including heart disease and diabetes. Researchers use a number of different methods to assess body fatness. Skinfold measurements are better suited for assessing malnutrition than for detecting excess fat. Distribution of body fat is important in evaluating the risk of disease. Excess body fat around the abdomen (even with normal to slightly elevated BMI) is associated with higher disease risk than is excess fat around the hips and thighs. Waist circumference can be used to assess body fat distribution.

Learning Portfolio

Key Terms

Study Points

- Energy is necessary to do any kind of work. The body converts chemical energy from food sources—carbohydrates, proteins, and fats—into a form usable by cells.

- Anabolic reactions (anabolism) build compounds. These reactions require energy.

- Catabolic reactions (catabolism) break compounds into smaller units. These reactions produce energy.

- Adenosine triphosphate (ATP) is the energy currency of the body.

- NAD^+ and FAD accept pairs of high-energy electrons, becoming NADH and $FADH_2$ and shuttling the electrons to the electron transport chain to make ATP.

- Cells extract energy from carbohydrate via four main pathways: glycolysis, pyruvate to acetyl CoA, the citric acid cycle, and the electron transport chain.

- The citric acid cycle and electron transport chain require oxygen. Glycolysis does not.

- The electron transport chain produces more ATP than other catabolic pathways.

- To extract energy from fat, first triglycerides are separated into glycerol and fatty acids. Next, beta-oxidation breaks down the fatty acids to yield acetyl CoA and high-energy electrons that are shuttled to the electron transport chain. The acetyl CoA enters the citric acid cycle, which yields one GTP and more high-energy electrons. In the electron transport chain, the high-energy electrons give up energy to produce ATP.

- To extract energy from an amino acid, first the amino group is removed. Depending on the structure of the remaining carbon skeleton, it enters the catabolic pathways at pyruvate, acetyl CoA, or a citric acid cycle intermediate. The citric acid cycle and the electron transport chain complete the extraction of energy and production of ATP.

- The liver converts the nitrogen portion of amino acids to urea, which the kidneys excrete.

- Tissues differ in their preferred source of fuel. The brain, nervous system, and red blood cells rely primarily on glucose whereas other tissues use a mix of glucose, fatty acids, and ketone bodies as fuel sources.

- When carbohydrate is available, glucose can be stored as glycogen in liver and muscle tissue.

- Glucose can be produced from the noncarbohydrate precursors glycerol and some (glucogenic) amino acids, but not from fatty acids.

- Feasting, or overconsumption of energy, leads to glycogen and triglyceride storage.

- Fasting, or underconsumption of energy, leads to the mobilization of liver glycogen and stored triglycerides. Starvation, the state of prolonged fasting, leads to protein breakdown as well and can be fatal.

- Energy balance is the relationship between energy intake and energy output.

- Food intake is regulated by hunger, satiation, satiety, and appetite, which are influenced by complex factors. Hunger is the physiological need to eat. Satiation is the feeling of fullness that leads to termination of a meal. Satiety is the feeling of satisfaction and lack of hunger that determines the interval until the next meal. Appetite is a desire to eat that is influenced by external factors such as flavors and smells, environmental factors, and cultural factors.

- Gastrointestinal stimulation, circulating nutrients, neurotransmitters, and hormones signal the brain to regulate food intake.

- The major components of energy expenditure are resting energy expenditure, the thermic effect of food, and energy for physical activity.

- Estimated energy requirements (EERs) for adults predict total energy expenditure from age, height, weight, gender, and physical activity level.

- Body composition, age, gender, genetics, and hormonal activity affect the amount of energy used for resting metabolism.

- The energy cost of physical activity is affected by a person's size and the intensity and duration of the activity.

- Body composition, the relative amounts of fat and lean body mass, has a major influence on energy expenditure and risk of chronic disease.

- Body mass index—a ratio related to total body fatness and risk of chronic disease—is calculated with height and weight measurements.

Study Questions

1. What is the "universal energy currency"?

2. What four pathways are involved in extracting energy from carbohydrate? Which of these pathways are anaerobic, and which are aerobic?

3. What molecule does beta-oxidation form from the two-carbon links it "clips" off a fatty acid chain? What else does beta-oxidation produce that is important to producing ATP?

Learning Portfolio (continued)

4. What are ketone bodies, and when are they produced?

5. Name the three tissues where energy is stored. Which contains the largest store of energy?

6. Explain the concept of energy balance.

7. Define *hunger, satiation, satiety*, and *appetite*.

8. List and describe the three main components of energy expenditure.

9. Explain the three main factors that determine energy expenditure in activity.

10. What body mass index (BMI) values are associated with being underweight, overweight, and obese? Do these vary for men and women?

Try This

Comparing Fad Diets

The purpose of this exercise is to have you evaluate two fad diets in regard to their metabolic consequences. The two diets, Cabbage Soup and Super Protein, are described here. Once you've reviewed them, answer the following questions:

Will these diets result in weight loss? On the seventh day of each diet, which of the following metabolic pathways will be highly active?

- Glycogen breakdown
- Fat breakdown
- Gluconeogenesis
- Ketogenesis

Diet 1: The Cabbage Soup Diet

A person following the Cabbage Soup diet eats only a water-based soup made out of cabbage and a few other vegetables. Three to four meals per day of this restricted diet supply approximately 500 kilocalories per day. The diet is devoid of protein and fat and gets its calories from the small amount of carbohydrate in the vegetables. Think about what happens during starvation.

Diet 2: The Super Protein Diet

In the Super Protein diet, a person can eat an unlimited amount of protein-rich foods, such as meat, poultry, eggs, and seafood, but no added fats or carbohydrates are allowed. The average person can consume about 1,400 kilocalories if he or she eats three or four small meals each day. Think about what happens when little carbohydrate is available as a person metabolizes fat and protein.

Increasing Your Energy Output

Physical activity is the part of your energy output that varies the most. The purpose of this exercise is to increase your energy expenditure by committing to daily exercise for one week. Make each exercise session about 30 minutes long, and remember that the longer the duration, the harder the intensity, and the larger the muscle groups involved, the greater the energy expenditure. Choose an exercise you enjoy—such as walking, jogging, cycling, swimming, or rollerblading. Once your week is complete, ask yourself these questions: How did this week's daily exercise affect my energy balance? Have I gained or lost weight during the week? Did I compensate for the extra energy expenditure by increasing my calorie intake?

References

1. Gropper SS, Smith JL, Carr TP. *Advanced Nutrition and Human Metabolism*. 7th ed. Belmont, CA: Wadsworth; 2017.

2. Butte NF, Cabellero B. Energy needs: assessment and requirements. In: Ross AC, Caballero B, Cousins RJ, Tucker KL, Ziegler TR, eds. *Modern Nutrition in Health and Disease*. 11th ed. Philadelphia: Lippincott Williams & Wilkins; 2012:136-148.

3. Stipanuk MH, Caudill MA. *Biochemical and Physiological Aspects of Human Nutrition*. 3rd ed. Philadelphia: WB Saunders; 2012.

4. Nelson DL, Cox MM. *Principles of Biochemistry*. 6th ed. New York: WH Freeman; 2012.

5. Berg JM, Tymoczko JL, Gatto Jr GJ, Stryer L. *Biochemistry*. 8th ed. New York: WH Freeman; 2015.

6. Gropper SS, Smith JL, Carr TP. Op. cit.

7. Devlin TM. *Textbook of Biochemistry with Clinical Correlations*. 7th ed. Hoboken, NJ: John Wiley and Sons; 2011.

8. Kleiner S, Greenwood-Robinson M. *Power Eating*. Champaign, IL: Human Kinetics; 2014.

9. Cederbaum AI. Alcohol metabolism. *Clin Liver Dis*. 2012;16(4):667-685.

10. Ibid.

11. Ibid.

12. Gropper SS, Smith JL, Carr TP. Op. cit.

13. Devlin TM. Op. cit.

14. Ibid.

15. Ibid.

16. Oh S, Kalyani RR, Dobs A. Nutritional management of diabetes mellitus. In: Ross AC, Caballero B, Cousins RJ, Tucker KL, Ziegler TR, eds. *Modern Nutrition in Health and Disease*. 11th ed. Philadelphia: Lippincott Williams & Wilkins; 2012:1043-1066.

17. Hall JE. *Guyton and Hall Textbook of Medical Physiology*. 13th ed. Philadelphia: Elsevier Health Sciences; 2015.

18. Gropper SS, Smith JL, Carr TP. Op. cit.

19. Nelson DL, Cox MM. Op. cit.

20. Martini FH, Nath JL, Bartholomew EF. *Fundamentals of Anatomy and Physiology*. 10th ed. San Francisco: Benjamin Cummings; 2014.

21. Gropper SS, Smith JL, Carr TP. Op. cit.

22. Ibid.

23. Hoffer LJ. Metabolic consequences of starvation. In: Ross AC, Caballero B, Cousins RJ, Tucker KL, Ziegler TR, eds. *Modern Nutrition in Health and Disease*. 11th ed. Philadelphia: Lippincott Williams & Wilkins; 2012:660-677.

24. Ibid.

25. Barrett KE, Barmanv SM, Boitano S, Brooks H. *Ganong's Review of Medical Physiology*. 24th ed. New York: McGraw-Hill; 2012.

26. Kalafatakis K, Triantafyllou K. Contribution of neurotensin in the immune and neuroendocrine modulation of normal and abnormal enteric function. *Regul Pept*. 2011;170(1-3):7-17.

27. Bartness TJ, Keen-Rhinehart E, Dalley MJ, Teubner BJ. Neural and hormonal control of food hoarding. *Am J Physiol Regul Integr Comp Physiol*. 2011;301(3):R641-R655.

28. Karatas Z, Durmus Aydogdu S, Dinleyici EC, Colak O, Dogruel N. Breastmilk ghrelin, leptin, and fat levels changing foremilk to hindmilk: is that important for self-control of feeding? *Eur J Pediatr*. 2011;170(10):1273-1280.

29. Rosenbaum M, Leibel RL. Adaptive thermogenesis in humans. *Int J Obes*. 2010;34(Suppl):S47-S55.

30. Ozkan Y, Timurkan ES, Aydin S, et al. Acylated and deacylated ghrelin, preptin, leptin, and nesfatin-1 peptide changes related to the body mass index. *Int J Endocrinol*. 2013;2013:1-7.

31. Magee E, Nazario B. Your 'hunger hormones.' WebMD. http://www.webmd.com/diet/features/your-hunger-hormones#1. Accessed September 11, 2017.

32. Pejovic S, Vgontzas AN, Basta M, et al. Leptin and hunger levels in young healthy adults after one night of sleep loss. *J Sleep Res*. 2010;19(4):552-558.

33. Blatt AD, Roe LS, Rolls BJ. Increasing the protein content of meals and its effect on daily energy intake. *J Am Diet Assoc*. 2011;111(2):290-294.

34. Wanders AJ, Feskens EJ, Jonathan MC, et al. Pectin is not pectin: a randomized trial on the effect of different physicochemical properties of dietary fiber on appetite and energy intake. *Physiol Behav*. 2014;128:212-219.

35. Higgins JA. Resistant starch and energy balance: impact on weight loss and maintenance. *Crit Rev Food Sci Nutr*. 2014;54:1158-1166.

36. Spahn JM, Reeves RS, Keim KS, et al. State of the evidence regarding behavior change theories and strategies in nutrition counseling to facilitate health and food behavior change. *J Am Diet Assoc*. 2010;110(6):879-891.

37. Marchiori D, Papies EK. A brief mindfulness intervention reduces unhealthy eating when hungry, but not the portion size effect. *Appetite*. 2014;75:40-45.

38. Marchiori D, Corneille O, Klein O. Container size influences snack food intake independently of portion size. *Appetite*. 2012;58(3):814-817.

39. Wansink B, Van Ittersum K, Payne CR. Larger bowl size increases the amount of cereal children request, consume, and waste. *J Pediatr*. 2014;164(2):323-326.

40. Marchiori D, Waroquier L, Klein O. "Split them!" Smaller item sizes of cookies lead to a decrease in energy intake in children. *J Nutr Educ Behav*. 2012;44(3):251-255.

41. Johnson SL, Hughes SO, Li X, et al. Portion sizes for children are predicted by parental characteristics and the amounts parents serve themselves. *Am J Clin Nutr*. 2014;99(4):763-770.

42. Vermeer WM, Steenhuis IH, Seidell JC. Portion size: a qualitative study of consumers' attitudes toward point-of-purchase interventions aimed at portion size. *Health Educ Res*. 2010;25(1):109-120.

43. Hall JE. Op cit.

44. Wansink B. From mindless eating to mindlessly eating better. *Physiol Behav*. 2010;100(5):454-463.

45. Ibid.

46. Fink HH, Burgoon LA, Mikesky AE. *Practical Applications in Sports Nutrition*. 5th ed. Burlington, MA: Jones & Bartlett Learning; 2017.

47. Fothergill E, Guo J, Howard L, et al. Persistent metabolic adaptation 6 years after "The Biggest Loser" competition. *Obesity*. 2016;24:1612-1619. http://onlinelibrary.wiley.com/doi/10.1002/oby.21538/full. Accessed September 11, 2017.

48. Mahan LK, Raymond JL. *Krause's Food, Nutrition, and Diet Therapy*. 14th ed. Philadelphia: Saunders; 2016.

49. Ebbeling CB, Swain JF, Feldman HA, et al. Effects of dietary composition on energy expenditure during weight-loss maintenance. *JAMA*. 2012;307(24):2627-2634.

50. Kenny WL, Wilmore JH. *Physiology of Sports and Exercise with Web Study Guide*. 6th ed. Champaign, IL: Human Kinetics; 2015.

51. Villablanca PA, Alegria JR, Mookadam F, et al. Nonexercise activity thermogenesis in obesity management. *Mayo Clin Proc*. 2015;90(4):509-511.

52. Du S, Rajjo T, Santosa S, Jensen MD. The thermic effect of food is reduced in older adults. *Horm Metab Res*. 2014;46(5):365-369.

53. Piaggi P, Krakoff J, Bogardus C, Thearle MS. Lower "awake and fed thermogenesis" predicts future weight gain in subjects with abdominal adiposity. *Diabetes*. 2013;62(12):4043-4051.

54. Jørgensen TS, Osler M, Ängquist LH, et al. The U-shaped association of body mass index with mortality: influence of the traits height, intelligence, and education. *Obesity*. 2016;24(10):2240-2247.

55. Aune D, Sen A, Prasad M, et al. BMI and all cause mortality: systematic review and non-linear dose-response meta-analysis of 230 cohort studies with 3.74 million deaths among 30.3 million participants. *BMJ*. 2016;353:i2156.

56. National Heart, Lung, and Blood Institute, National Institutes of Health. Assessing your weight and health risk: body mass index (BMI). http://www.nhlbi.nih.gov/health/public/heart/obesity/lose_wt/risk.htm. Accessed September 11, 2017.

57. National Center for Health Statistics. CDC growth charts. https://www.cdc.gov/growthcharts/cdc_charts.htm. Accessed September 11, 2017.

58. Nana A, Slater GR, Hopkins WG, Burke LM. Effects of exercise sessions on DXA measurements of body composition in active people. *Med Sci Sports Exerc*. 2013;45(1):178-185.

59. Kishida K, Funahashi T, Matsuzawa Y. Visceral adiposity as a target for the management of the metabolic syndrome. *Ann Med*. 2012;44(3):233-241.

60. Yoshikawa K, Shimada M, Kurita N, et al. Visceral fat area is superior to body mass index as a predictive factor for risk with laparoscopy-assisted gastroectomy for gastric cancer. *Surg Endosc*. 2011;18(6):1-6.

61. Tybor DJ, Lichtenstein AH, Dallal GE, et al. Independent effects of age-related changes in waist circumference and BMI z scores in predicting cardiovascular disease risk factors in a prospective cohort of adolescent females. *Am J Clin Nutr*. 2011;93(2):392-401.

Chapter 9

Nutrition for Physical Performance

Revised by Don Ross

THINK About It

1   How much importance do you place on being physically active?

2   How often do you suffer muscle fatigue? What do you think causes it?

3   How often do you think about food choices when you're planning a physical activity?

4   What kind of protein do you emphasize in your diet?

LEARNING Objectives

1. Identify the components of and guidelines to physical fitness.
2. Distinguish among the different types of muscle fibers.
3. Apply nutrition concepts to a food plan for athletic performance.
4. Summarize the benefits of hydration and the dangers of dehydration.
5. Discuss nutrition supplements and ergogenic aids designed to enhance athletic performance.
6. Give examples of protein intake before, during, and after physical activity.

Today is the big 10,000-meter race. You've trained for months. Fans in the crowd shade their eyes as they watch you and your competitors walk onto the track. "Ready," shouts the starter. "Get set." You toe the starting line and adrenaline courses through your blood vessels, increasing your heart rate, diverting blood to your muscles, and mobilizing energy stores in your liver, muscles, and fat. "Go!" Within a fraction of a second, a torrent of calcium flows into your muscle cells, causing your muscles to contract and launch you away from the starting line.

How will you perform in this race? Will your breakfast help or hinder your performance? Will what you ate yesterday and the day before affect your stamina? Does it matter what you eat after you finish the race? Read on for the answers to these questions and to learn about the links between nutrition and physical performance.

Nutrition and Physical Performance

🍎 **Why Is This Important?** Even if you have difficulty meeting minimum recommendations for exercise, any level of physical activity is better than being sedentary. Get out and move! Incorporate activity into your regular routine. Exercises should promote strength, endurance, and flexibility. Optimal physical fitness also requires good nutrition practices.

THINK About It 1

Just how physically active do you need to be? (See **FIGURE 9.1**.) Both the National Institutes of Health (NIH) and Health Canada have found that small to moderate amounts of physical activity can produce substantial health benefits. Physically active people have a lower risk of developing many chronic diseases, such as coronary heart disease, diabetes, hypertension, osteoporosis, and obesity. Active people also experience an increased sense of well-being and are much better equipped to cope with stress. Health Canada recommends choosing a variety of activities from three types of exercise: endurance, flexibility, and strength. (See **FIGURE 9.2**.)

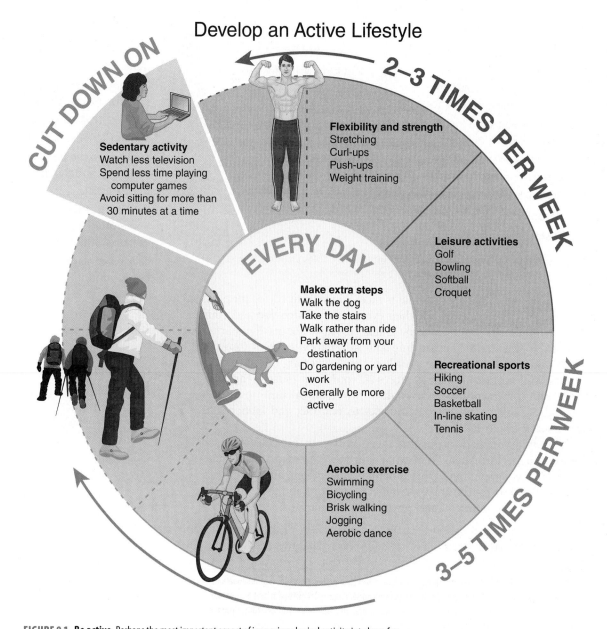

Develop an Active Lifestyle

CUT DOWN ON

Sedentary activity
Watch less television
Spend less time playing
computer games
Avoid sitting for more than
30 minutes at a time

2–3 TIMES PER WEEK

Flexibility and strength
Stretching
Curl-ups
Push-ups
Weight training

Leisure activities
Golf
Bowling
Softball
Croquet

Recreational sports
Hiking
Soccer
Basketball
In-line skating
Tennis

3–5 TIMES PER WEEK

Aerobic exercise
Swimming
Bicycling
Brisk walking
Jogging
Aerobic dance

EVERY DAY

Make extra steps
Walk the dog
Take the stairs
Walk rather than ride
Park away from your
destination
Do gardening or yard
work
Generally be more
active

FIGURE 9.1 Be active. Perhaps the most important aspect of increasing physical activity is to have fun.

"Exercise is Medicine" is a global collaboration focused on encouraging primary care physicians, nutritionists, and other healthcare providers to include exercise when designing treatment plans for patients. Launched by the American Medical Association and the American College of Sports Medicine (ACSM), Exercise is Medicine strives to make physical activity a "vital sign" that is routinely assessed at every patient interaction with a healthcare provider. The goals of this program include: (1) have healthcare providers assess every patient's level of physical activity at every clinic visit, (2) determine if the patient is meeting the U.S. National Physical Activity Guidelines, and (3) provide the patient with brief counseling to help him or her meet the guidelines and/or refer the patient to either healthcare or community-based resources for further physical activity counseling.[1]

The ACSM notes an important distinction between physical activity as it relates to health and exercise for physical fitness.[2] According

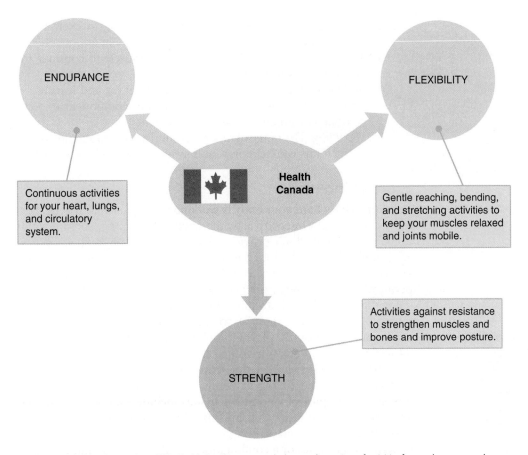

FIGURE 9.2 Variety is the spice of life. Health Canada recommends that you do a variety of activities from each group—endurance, flexibility, and strength—to receive the most health benefits.

Data from *Canada's Physical Activity Guide to Healthy Active Living.*

to the ACSM, the level of physical activity that may reduce the risk of various chronic diseases may not be enough—in quantity or quality— to improve physical fitness. The *Physical Activity Guidelines for Americans* state that adults need at least 150 minutes of moderate-intensity physical activity per week and should perform muscle-strengthening exercises on 2 or more days each week. Youth ages 6 to 17 years need at least 60 minutes of physical activity per day, including aerobic, muscle-strengthening, and bone-strengthening activities.[3] Unfortunately, physical inactivity is a fast-growing public health concern, and most U.S. adults fall short of meeting the activity recommendations. In 48 states, more than 75 percent of adults fail to meet the guidelines for aerobic and muscle-strengthening physical activity.[4]

What is physical fitness? The ACSM defines physical fitness as "the ability to perform moderate to vigorous levels of physical activity without undue fatigue and the capability of maintaining this level of activity throughout life."[5] In other words, fitness is more than being able to run a long distance or lift a lot of weight at the gym. Being fit is not defined only by what kind of activity you do, how long you do it, or at what level of intensity. Although these are important measures of fitness, they only address single areas. Overall fitness is made up of five main components:

1. *Cardiorespiratory fitness:* The ability of the body's circulatory and respiratory systems to supply fuel during sustained physical activity.

2. *Muscular strength:* The ability of the muscle to exert force during an activity.
3. *Muscular endurance:* The ability of the muscle to continue to perform without fatigue.
4. *Body composition:* The relative amounts of fat and lean body mass. Body composition is an important component to consider for health and weight management.
5. *Flexibility:* The range of motion around a joint. Good flexibility in the joints can help prevent injuries through all stages of life.

Exercise Intensity

Intensity is how hard your body is working during aerobic activity. For most people, light-intensity activities such as shopping, cooking, and doing the laundry don't provide health benefits. Why? Their bodies are not working hard enough to increase their heart rates. When you are working enough to raise your heart rate and break a sweat, you are performing a *moderate-intensity aerobic activity*. One way that you can tell is that you'll be able to talk, but not sing. Examples of moderate-intensity activities include brisk walking, doing water aerobics, riding a bike on level ground, playing doubles tennis, and pushing a lawn mower. Vigorous-intensity aerobic activity means that you are breathing hard and your heart rate has gone up quite a bit. At this level of activity, you will be able to say only a few words before pausing for a breath. Examples of vigorous activities include running, swimming laps, riding a bike fast or up hills, playing singles tennis, or playing basketball. To meet your activity goals for health, you can do moderate or vigorous activities or a combination of both. A rule of thumb is that 2 minutes of moderate-intensity activity is about the same as 1 minute of vigorous-intensity activity.

Muscle Strengthening Exercises

Muscle strengthening exercises (also called resistance training) should work all major muscle groups (legs, hips, back, abdomen, chest, shoulders, and arms). For maximal health benefits, these exercises should be done to the point where it's hard to do another repetition without assistance. A *repetition* is one complete movement, such as doing a sit-up or lifting a weight. A *set* is a minimum of 8–12 repetitions per activity. When exercising, try to do at least one set of muscle-strengthening activities; two to three sets are better. Strengthening activities include lifting weights, working with resistance bands, push-ups and sit-ups, digging and shoveling, and yoga.

Flexibility and Neuromotor Exercises

Flexibility exercises improve joint range of motion and are most effective after the muscles are warmed by at least five minutes of light- to moderate-intensity activities. Stretches should be to the point of feeling tightness or slight discomfort. Neuromotor exercises, such as yoga, improve balance, agility, coordination, and gait.

Some Is Better Than None

It's best to spread your activities throughout the week. You can even break sessions into smaller chunks of time during the day, as long as you're doing moderate or vigorous effort at least 10 minutes at a time.

TABLE 9.1
Physical Activity Guidelines for Americans

Age	Recommendations
6 to 17 years	Children and adolescents should do 60 minutes (1 hour) or more of physical activity daily. • *Aerobic:* Most of the 60 or more minutes a day should be either moderate-[a] or vigorous-intensity[b] aerobic physical activity, and should include vigorous-intensity physical activity at least 3 days a week. • *Muscle-strengthening* [c]: As part of their 60 or more minutes of daily physical activity, children and adolescents should include muscle-strengthening physical activity on at least 3 days of the week. • *Bone-strengthening* [d]: As part of their 60 or more minutes of daily physical activity, children and adolescents should include bone-strengthening physical activity on at least 3 days of the week. • It is important to encourage young people to participate in physical activities that are appropriate for their age, that are enjoyable, and that offer variety.
18 to 64 years	• All adults should avoid inactivity. Some physical activity is better than none, and adults who participate in any amount of physical activity gain some health benefits. • For substantial health benefits, adults should do at least 150 minutes (2 hours and 30 minutes) a week of moderate-intensity, or 75 minutes (1 hour and 15 minutes) a week of vigorous-intensity aerobic physical activity, or an equivalent combination of moderate- and vigorous-intensity aerobic activity. Aerobic activity should be performed in episodes of at least 10 minutes, and preferably, it should be spread throughout the week. • For additional and more extensive health benefits, adults should increase their aerobic physical activity to 300 minutes (5 hours) a week of moderate-intensity, or 150 minutes a week of vigorous-intensity aerobic physical activity, or an equivalent combination of moderate- and vigorous-intensity activity. Additional health benefits are gained by engaging in physical activity beyond this amount. • Adults should also include muscle-strengthening activities that involve all major muscle groups on 2 or more days a week.
65 years and older	• Older adults should follow the adult guidelines. When older adults cannot meet the adult guidelines, they should be as physically active as their abilities and conditions will allow. • Older adults should do exercises that maintain or improve balance if they are at risk of falling. • Older adults should determine their level of effort for physical activity relative to their level of fitness. • Older adults with chronic conditions should understand whether and how their conditions affect their ability to do regular physical activity safely.

[a] *Moderate-intensity physical activity:* Aerobic activity that increases a person's heart rate and breathing to some extent. On a scale relative to a person's capacity, moderate-intensity activity is usually a 5 or 6 on a 0 to 10 scale. Brisk walking, dancing, swimming, or bicycling on a level terrain are examples.

[b] *Vigorous-intensity physical activity:* Aerobic activity that greatly increases a person's heart rate and breathing. On a scale relative to a person's capacity, vigorous-intensity activity is usually a 7 or 8 on a 0 to 10 scale. Jogging, singles tennis, swimming continuous laps, or bicycling uphill are examples.

[c] *Muscle-strengthening activity:* Physical activity, including exercise that increases skeletal muscle strength, power, endurance, and mass. It includes strength training, resistance training, and muscular strength and endurance exercises.

[d] *Bone-strengthening activity:* Physical activity that produces an impact or tension force on bones, which promotes bone growth and strength. Running, jumping rope, and lifting weights are examples.

U.S. Department of Health and Human Services and U.S. Department of Agriculture. *2015–2020 Dietary Guidelines for Americans.* 8th Edition. December 2015. Available at http://health.gov/dietaryguidelines/2015/guidelines/ Accessed February 27, 2017.

TABLE 9.1 shows the recommended amounts of physical activity needed to promote good health.

Nutrition has taken its rightful place as a vital component of any program that seeks to enhance health, fitness, and athletic performance. In a joint position paper, the Academy of Nutrition and Dietetics, Dietitians of Canada, and the American College of Sports Medicine state that "physical activity, athletic performance, and recovery from exercise are enhanced by optimal nutrition."[6] But just what is "optimal nutrition"? Is it the same for a child who plays recreational softball and for a senior citizen who takes daily walks to reduce the risk of type 2 diabetes? What about the competitive athlete who strives to maximize athletic performance and uses nutrition to gain a competitive edge?

▶ **creatine phosphate** An energy-rich compound that supplies energy and a phosphate group for the formation of ATP. Also called *phosphocreatine*.

▶ **phosphocreatine** See *creatine phosphate*.

To understand the relationship between physical activity and nutrition, you first need to appreciate how we use energy during exercise.

Key Concepts Exercise provides numerous health benefits, including reduced risk of chronic disease. Physical fitness includes strength, endurance, and flexibility. For optimal physical performance, nutrition is an essential part of all athletic training programs.

Energy Systems, Muscles, and Physical Performance

🍎 **Why Is This Important?** Your body uses three distinct systems to generate energy. Although all are active, the primary system varies with the demand for energy—a quick burst, short duration, or long-term endurance. In addition, your body has two distinct types of muscle fibers, specialized for either short bursts of movement, such as sprinting, or endurance exercises, such as distance running.

Let's return to your race. As you leave the starting line, your body immediately ramps up energy production to meet the increased demand. Just as a rocket uses different fuel systems and stages to power its leap into space, your body uses three different energy systems to launch, accelerate, and maintain exercise intensity.

ATP–CP Energy System

As you launch yourself from the starting line, it takes less than a second for your contracting muscles to burn their entire reserve of adenosine triphosphate (ATP), the immediate energy source for cells. Luckily, your body has a small reservoir of **creatine phosphate** (also called **phosphocreatine**) that your muscles can convert quickly to ATP. (See **FIGURE 9.3**.) Muscle cells contain four to six times as much

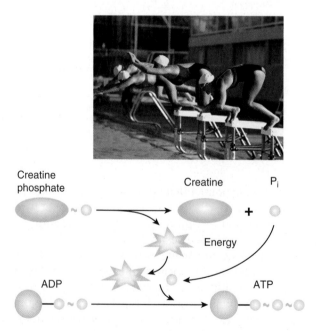

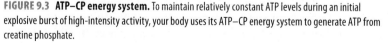

FIGURE 9.3 ATP–CP energy system. To maintain relatively constant ATP levels during an initial explosive burst of high-intensity activity, your body uses its ATP–CP energy system to generate ATP from creatine phosphate.

creatine phosphate as ATP.[7] Together, your available ATP and creatine phosphate, the **ATP–CP energy system**, can power an all-out effort for only about 10 seconds.[8] To continue the race, you must enlist carbohydrate stored as glycogen in your muscles and liver. Your cells rapidly disassemble glycogen to glucose, from which they can extract ATP.

Lactic Acid Energy System

During the acceleration stage (10–180 seconds), your body uses the simplest and speediest chemical pathways to produce ATP from glucose—the **lactic acid energy system**. (See **FIGURE 9.4**.) Please note that the term "lactic acid energy system" actually is a misnomer. Although "lactic acid" and "lactate" are used interchangeably, they are different chemically, and lactic acid is not produced in the body.

> **THINK**
> About It
> **2**

Like the ATP–CP energy system, these pathways are anaerobic—they do not require oxygen. The raw material, glucose, is much more plentiful than creatine phosphate, but its breakdown also produces a by-product—lactate (mistakenly called lactic acid). The rapid extraction of energy from ATP molecules produces ADP molecules and protons (hydrogen ions). During aerobic metabolism these protons are used by cells, but during anaerobic metabolism the protons accumulate and make the cells acidic. A rise in acidity impairs the breakdown of glucose and inhibits calcium binding. Without calcium, muscles cannot contract. For years, coaches and athletes have blamed "lactic acid" for muscle fatigue. But it's the change in pH due to excess protons that is the primary culprit.[9]

To continue running beyond the first few minutes, your body employs a sophisticated, oxygen-based system to process lactate and squeeze out much more ATP from glucose.

Oxygen Energy System

Beyond about two and a half minutes you enter the endurance stage, when cells use lengthy, complex chemical pathways in their mitochondria—small units within cells that function as power-generating plants—to convert food and oxygen to ATP. (See **FIGURE 9.5**.) These reactions are aerobic—they require abundant oxygen. In contracting muscle, blood vessels dilate and deliver a 20-fold increase in oxygen-rich blood to muscle cells,[10] a sufficient supply for mitochondria to produce ATP. In contrast to the two anaerobic systems (the ATP–CP system and lactic acid system), the **oxygen energy system** can produce a tremendous amount of ATP. Another advantage is that the oxygen energy system can extract energy from fat as well as from glucose. But, because the required oxygen must travel a long distance—from lungs to blood to muscle cells to mitochondria—the oxygen energy system produces ATP at a much slower rate than the anaerobic systems do.

Teamwork in Energy Production

The energy systems work together to fuel athletic performance. (See **FIGURE 9.6**.) The transitions between energy systems do not occur abruptly, nor does the body ever rely upon only one pathway exclusively for energy production. As the first two minutes of your race elapse, the oxygen energy system is supplying about half of your muscles' energy needs.

▶ **ATP–CP energy system** A simple and immediate anaerobic energy system that maintains ATP levels. Creatine phosphate is broken down, releasing energy and a phosphate group, which is used to form ATP.

▶ **lactic acid energy system** Anaerobic energy system; using glycolysis, the process rapidly produces energy (ATP) and lactate. Also called *anaerobic glycolysis*.

▶ **oxygen energy system** A complex energy system that requires oxygen. To release ATP, it completes the breakdown of carbohydrate and fatty acids via the citric acid cycle and electron transport chain.

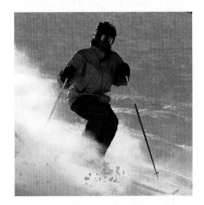

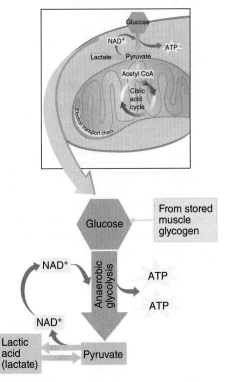

FIGURE 9.4 Lactic acid energy system. During short physical events requiring power and speed, the lactic acid energy system supplies much of the energy. Because the lactic acid system does not require oxygen, these events are anaerobic activities.

© Photodisc.

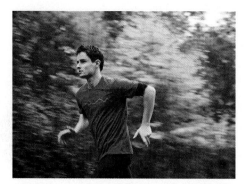

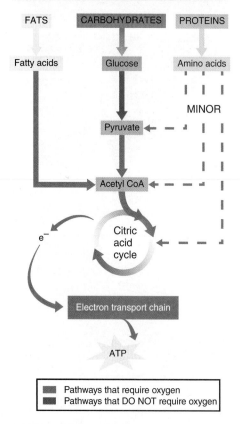

FIGURE 9.5 Oxygen energy system. During longer endurance events (aerobic events), the oxygen energy system supplies most of the energy. This energy system requires oxygen and primarily relies on carbohydrate and fat as fuels. Lightpoet/Shutterstock.

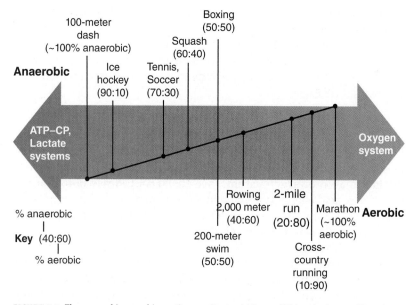

FIGURE 9.6 The anaerobic–aerobic continuum. Most activities use ATP from both anaerobic and aerobic energy systems. However, the 100-meter dash is considered completely anaerobic, and the marathon is considered completely aerobic.

(See **FIGURE 9.7**.) By the time you pass the 30-minute mark, this aerobic system is supplying 95 percent; and at two hours or more, the oxygen energy system is supplying 98 percent of your muscles' energy needs.[11]

As long as ATP production by the mitochondria meets energy needs, you are exercising aerobically; highly trained athletes can sustain such exercise for hours. If the exercise rate exceeds your body's ability to supply oxygen to your muscles, you are exercising anaerobically, rapidly depleting your creatine phosphate and glycogen reserves. Once these are exhausted, if the available oxygen cannot support the oxygen energy system, performance plummets.

Carbohydrate stores are limited. A 68-kilogram (150-pound) man with 10 to 20 percent body fat, for example, has carbohydrate stores of 1,800 to 2,000 kilocalories in muscle glycogen, liver glycogen, and blood glucose. Compare this with the energy he stores in fat. His fat tissue holds roughly 63,000 to 120,000 kilocalories.[12] Although the body can burn protein for energy, in well-fed people protein probably provides no more than 5 percent of energy expended in exercise.[13]

Glycogen Depletion

At the beginning of the race, your body rapidly uses muscle glycogen. But, as the race keeps going, the rate of glycogen use markedly slows. During the first one and a half hours, glycogen stores drop steadily to about one-third their starting levels. About three hours into the run, as glycogen stores become almost entirely depleted, you may "hit the wall." Your muscles become weak and heavy, your legs shake, and you become confused. Marathon runners commonly experience a sudden onset of exhaustive fatigue around the 18- to 20-mile mark. Drinking fluids that contain glucose can partially compensate for glycogen depletion and soften its effects. Dehydration can cause an even faster onset of fatigue, so drinking plenty of fluids is essential during endurance events.

As exercise intensity increases, glycogen depletion accelerates. Sprinting, for example, uses muscle glycogen 35 to 40 times faster

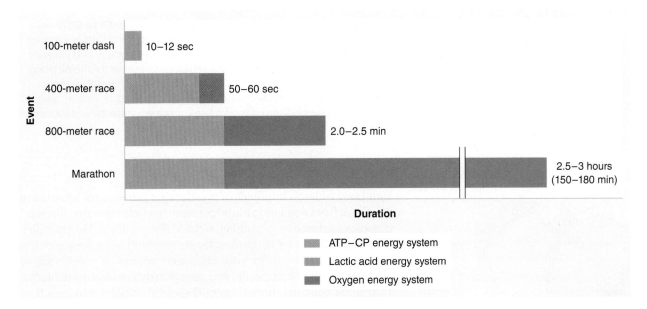

FIGURE 9.7 Sports events and energy systems. Short-term, explosive events rely upon the ATP–CP and lactic acid energy systems. For longer events, your body turns to the oxygen energy system. During endurance events, your body uses this system to burn fat as well as glucose.

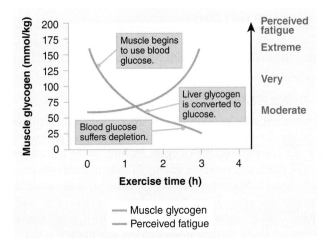
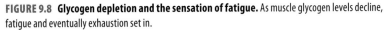

FIGURE 9.8 Glycogen depletion and the sensation of fatigue. As muscle glycogen levels decline, fatigue and eventually exhaustion set in.

than walking.[14] **FIGURE 9.8** illustrates how the sensation of fatigue relates to the depletion of muscle glycogen.

Endurance Training

Have you ever trained for a long run only to realize that what started off as a difficult distance gradually becomes a pretty easy run? Endurance training has effects on muscle capillaries that increase blood flow and produce marked improvement in endurance capacity.[15] Training enhances aerobic capacity by increasing the number of mitochondria and improving the body's ability to deliver oxygen to them. This decreases the reliance on anaerobic energy systems, extending the availability of glycogen reserves and delaying fatigue. Following weeks of endurance training, your long runs are much easier than before the start of your training cycle.

Quick **Bite**

Use It or Lose It!
After only two weeks of inactivity, the benefits of training begin to disappear. Muscular endurance—the ability of a muscle to avoid fatigue—declines, and activities of certain oxidative enzymes drop by as much as 40 percent. By the fourth week, muscle glycogen levels also may drop by 40 percent. Flexibility is quickly lost, and inactivity can substantially decondition the heart muscle and cardiovascular system.

Key Concepts Muscle cells use three different energy systems to produce ATP: the ATP–CP energy system, the lactic acid energy system, and the oxygen energy system. The ATP–CP and lactic acid energy systems rely on carbohydrate and do not require oxygen. The oxygen energy system requires oxygen and relies on carbohydrate and fat. During the early minutes of high-intensity exercise, the anaerobic systems are the predominant source of ATP. During lower-intensity endurance events, the third system supplies ATP, although at a much slower rate. Dehydration and depletion of glycogen stores are major factors in fatigue. Training increases the efficiency of oxygen delivery to muscle and increases the number of muscle mitochondria available for aerobic metabolism.

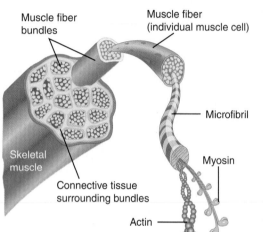

FIGURE 9.9 **Basic structure of skeletal muscle.** A muscle fiber is an individual muscle cell that usually extends the entire length of the muscle. Each muscle fiber contains hundreds to thousands of microfibrils. Each microfibril contains thousands of actin and myosin filaments, large protein molecules responsible for muscle contractions.

▶ **skeletal muscles** Muscles composed of bundles of parallel, striated muscle fibers under voluntary control. Also called *voluntary muscle* or *striated muscle*.

▶ **muscle fibers** Individual muscle cells.

▶ **slow-twitch (ST) fibers** Muscle fibers that develop tension more slowly and to a lesser extent than fast-twitch muscle fibers. ST fibers have high oxidative capacities and are slower to fatigue than fast-twitch fibers.

▶ **fast-twitch (FT) fibers** Muscle fibers that can develop high tension rapidly. These fibers can fatigue quickly but are well suited to explosive movements in sprinting, jumping, and weight lifting.

▶ **aerobic endurance** The ability of skeletal muscle to obtain a sufficient supply of oxygen from the heart and lungs to maintain muscular activity for a prolonged time.

Quick Bite

Pound for Pound?
Women's muscles have smaller muscle fiber cross-sections and less muscle mass than men. For a given amount of muscle, however, there is no difference in strength between men and women.

Muscles and Muscle Fibers

Your body contains hundreds of muscles that help control a myriad of functions, from regulating blood pressure to climbing stairs. **Skeletal muscles** are bundles of parallel, striated fibers attached to your skeleton. (See **FIGURE 9.9**.) These muscles are responsible for your physical movement and are under your conscious control. If you decide to bend your arm, for example, you consciously contract your biceps. Your body contains more than 600 skeletal muscles and uses 9 of them just to control your thumb!

Individual muscle cells are called **muscle fibers**; skeletal muscle has two primary types:

- **Slow-twitch (ST) fibers**
- **Fast-twitch (FT) fibers**

They derive their names from the difference in their speed of action. One type of fast-twitch fiber can contract 10 times faster than slow-twitch fibers.[16]

Slow-Twitch Fibers

To power their activity, slow-twitch fibers efficiently produce energy by breaking down carbohydrate and fat via aerobic pathways—metabolic reactions that require oxygen. As long as the aerobic pathways are active, ST fibers can produce energy to sustain their movement. With a sufficient supply of oxygen, ST fibers can maintain muscular activity for a prolonged time. This ability is known as **aerobic endurance**.

Because ST fibers have high aerobic endurance, your body predominantly relies on them during low-intensity endurance events, such as long-distance running, and during everyday activities such as walking.

Fast-Twitch Fibers

Compared with ST fibers, fast-twitch fibers have poor aerobic endurance. They are optimized to perform anaerobically (when the oxygen supply is limited). FT fibers can efficiently produce energy for their use via metabolic pathways that do not require oxygen. Bundles of FT fibers exert considerably more force than bundles of ST fibers; due to their limited endurance, however, FT fibers tire quickly.

The body recruits both ST and FT fibers during shorter, higher-intensity endurance events, such as the mile run or the 400-meter swim. During highly explosive events, such as the 100-meter dash and the 50-meter sprint swim, the body still recruits both types, but FT fibers contribute most of the muscle power.

Fiber Type and the Athlete

Genes determine the relative proportion of muscle fiber types in athletes. Although distance runners who have a high percentage of ST

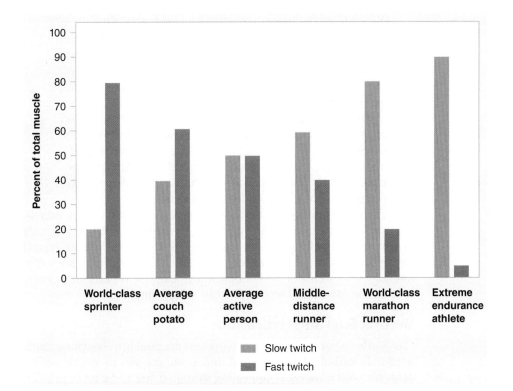

FIGURE 9.10 What's your mix of muscle fibers? If you are best at events requiring explosive movements, you may have a greater percentage of fast-twitch muscle fibers. If endurance events are your specialty, you may have more slow-twitch fibers.
Reproduced with permission. Copyright © 2000 *Scientific American*, a division of Nature America, Inc. All Rights reserved.

fibers are well suited for endurance events, they will not become elite sprinters. Conversely, sprinters who have predominantly FT fibers are better equipped for explosive events, but they will not become competitive marathon runners. (See **FIGURE 9.10**.)

> **Key Concepts** A muscle cell is called a muscle fiber. The two main types of skeletal muscle fibers are slow-twitch and fast-twitch fibers. Slow-twitch fibers generate fuel through aerobic pathways, whereas fast-twitch fibers produce energy using anaerobic pathways. Fast-twitch fibers can exert more force but have limited endurance.

Optimal Nutrition for Exercise Performance

🍎 **Why Is This Important?** Most physically active people do not need special nutrition workout strategies. The basic advice is to stay hydrated by sipping water during exercise and eat a snack before and after exercising. Your snacks should be a mix of carbohydrate and protein, and low in fat. If you are a competitive athlete, you can work with a specialized dietician to develop a personalized nutrition plan.

The one-minute video "We Are All Athletes" showcases U.S. Olympians, Paralympians, and recreational athletes of various backgrounds, including different genders, races and ethnicities, religions, sexual orientations, and abilities.[17] While promoting diversity, social inclusion, sportsmanship, and teamwork, it delivers the important message that each and every one of us is an athlete, albeit with different capabilities. Although there is no sharp dividing line between recreational athletes and competitive athletes, competitive athletes typically train at higher intensity levels and focus on specific events.

Quick Bite

Fast-Twitch Fish

A large percentage (40 to 60 percent) of a fish's body weight is muscle tissue. Although it spends much of its life slowly cruising, a fish must be able to execute occasional quick bursts of high speed to escape predators or catch a meal. Thus, fish muscle is composed of approximately 75 to 90 percent fast-twitch fibers, and fish flesh often is white. The slow-twitch fibers generally are concentrated just under the skin or near fins that are used during slow or high speeds. This arrangement is possible only because fish are buoyant. Land animals could not survive dragging around a large mass of muscle that they use only occasionally in extreme situations.

Most physically active people—from the college student who plays recreational basketball to the 50-year-old woman who enjoys walking during her lunch break—don't need special workout nutrition strategies. The American College of Sports Medicine says, "Adequate food and fluid should be consumed before, during, and after exercise to help maintain blood glucose concentration during exercise, maximize exercise performance, and improve recovery time. Athletes should be well hydrated before exercise and drink enough fluid during and after exercise to balance fluid losses."[18] In short, observe good nutrition practices and drink plenty of fluids. Special micronutrient supplementation also is unnecessary, unless addressing a deficiency.

THINK
About It

3

Although many people work out to lose or maintain weight, exercising burns fewer calories than you might think. For every mile you walk or run, for example, you burn about 100 kilocalories. Yet, the typical energy bar has about 250 kilocalories, and a 16-ounce fruit smoothie has 350–400 kilocalories. It's best not to exercise on an empty stomach, but be careful not to overdo your calorie intake.

Before: Fuel and Hydration

One to three hours before your workout, the goal is to consume easily digestible carbohydrates for fuel and some protein to supply amino acids for your muscles. Avoid eating saturated fats and a lot of protein. Either can slow digestion and cause your digestive system to compete with your muscles for oxygen and energy-delivering blood. If you only have time to grab a snack 5–10 minutes before working out, eat a piece of fruit (e.g., apple or banana) that is easily digestible.

Before Exercising

- Hydrate with water.
- Eat complex carbohydrates and some protein. Examples are:
    - Banana and nut butter; apple and nut butter
    - Oatmeal with low-fat milk and fruit
    - Yogurt and berries
    - Handful of nuts and raisins (one part nuts, two parts raisins)

During: Slowing Fluid and Energy Loss

During your workout, keep hydrated with small, frequent sips of water. For high-intensity workouts that last longer than an hour, eat small snacks every half hour. These snacks, such as raisins or a banana, should be rich in carbohydrates.

After: Time to Replenish (the Sooner, the Better)

After your workout (preferably within 20 minutes), you need to (1) restore your hydration and electrolytes, (2) replenish the glycogen your muscles used during exercise, and (3) provide a pool of amino acids as raw materials to rebuild and repair tired muscles.

After Exercising

- Rehydrate with water and some juice or a sports drink.
- Eat complex carbohydrates and some protein. Examples include:
    - Turkey on whole-grain with veggies
    - Yogurt with berries
    - Low-fat chocolate milk

Nutrition for the Competitive Athlete

Athletes, coaches, and scientists have long recognized that training and good nutrition go hand in hand when it comes to improving performance. Nutrition can profoundly influence the molecular and cellular processes that occur in muscle during exercise and recovery. Nutrition plans must be personalized to the individual athlete. A well-designed plan accounts for the specific competitive event, performance goals, practical challenges, food preferences, and personal responses to various strategies.

An athlete's skeletal muscle has a remarkable ability to respond quickly to mechanical loading and nutrient availability with metabolic adaptations, also known as **conditioning**. The well-conditioned athlete uses energy and other nutrients more efficiently than a poorly conditioned athlete.

Sports nutrition practice requires an integrated knowledge of several domains: clinical nutrition, exercise physiology, nutrition science, and evidence-based research. The Commission on Dietetic Registration (the credentialing agency for the Academy of Nutrition and Dietetics) has established a unique credential—the Board Certified Specialist in Sports Dietetics (CSSD)—for registered dietitians who specialize in sports nutrition. This is the premier sports nutrition credential in the United States and is available internationally, including in Canada.

The underlying foundations of a training diet are similar to the basic principles incorporated into the *Dietary Guidelines for Americans* and *Canada's Guidelines for Healthy Eating*. The primary differences are increased fluid needs to cover an athlete's sweat losses and increased energy needs to fuel physical activity. Let's take a closer look at the nutritional needs of athletes.

▶ **conditioning** The body's adaptations to exercise and activity. Endurance (aerobic) conditioning is the strengthening of the heart and lungs (cardiovascular system) through the rhythmic movement of large muscle groups. Strength conditioning is the strengthening of skeletal muscle through resistance training. To maintain or increase the level of conditioning, athletes must maintain or progressively increase their training level.

Quick Bite

The Weaker Sex?
Prior to the 1960s, women were banned from running any race longer than 800 meters, and they could not officially participate in marathon competitions until 1970. The race authorities mistakenly believed that women could harm themselves and were unsuitable for distance running. Imagine their amazement during the 1984 Olympic Games when Joan Benoit won the gold medal for the women's marathon with a time of 02:24:52—a time that would have won 11 of the previous 20 men's Olympic marathons!

Fluid Needs During Extensive Exercise

🍎 **Why Is This Important?** Proper hydration is key to dissipating heat and performing at your best. Because thirst lags fluid losses, active people must drink before becoming thirsty. Although water is the preferred beverage, sports drinks may help replace electrolytes lost during endurance exercise.

Exercise generates heat, and heavy exercise can increase heat production 15- to 20-fold. (See **FIGURE 9.11**.) The increase in body heat triggers sweating, and sweat cools your body as it evaporates on your skin. Why do some people sweat more than others? Sweat rate is affected by environmental temperature (extreme heat or extreme cold), humidity (higher humidity increases the rate of sweat production but reduces efficiency of evaporation), type of clothing, fitness level, and initial fluid balance. During exercise in hot weather, the risk of dehydration and heat injury increases dramatically. Normal sweat rates for athletes range from 0.5 to 2.0 liters per hour, depending on temperature, humidity, exercise intensity, and the personalized sweat response to exercise.[19] When possible, athletes should drink fluid at rates that most closely match their sweat rates.[20]

To prevent overheating, blood must flow to the skin, carrying core heat to the surface where evaporating sweat can dissipate heat. During exercise, the cooling demand for blood flow to the skin may compete with the cardiovascular demand for blood to deliver oxygen and nutrients to working muscles. Dehydration stresses

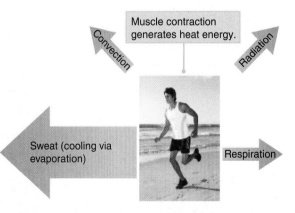

FIGURE 9.11 Dissipation of heat during exercise. During exercise, radiation, convection, and respiration are responsible for some heat loss, but evaporation of sweat dissipates more than 80 percent of the heat generated by increased physical activity.
© Yuri Arcurs/Shutterstock, Inc.

TABLE 9.2
Stages of Dehydration

	Percent Body Weight Change
Well hydrated	−1 to 1%
Minimal dehydration	−1 to −3%
Significant dehydration	−3 to −5%
Serious dehydration	Loss > −5%

Selectively and Effectively Using Hydration for Fitness. Reprinted with permission of the American College of Sports Medicine. 2011 American College of Sports Medicine.

▶ **perceived exertion** The subjective experience of how difficult an effort is.

both systems, making each less efficient. Without fluid replacement, a heavily sweating person can become dehydrated quickly; a water deficit of just 2 percent of body weight impairs exercise performance.[21]

One way to check your hydration status is to observe the color of your urine. A large amount of light-colored urine means you are well hydrated. The darker the color, the more you are dehydrated. Another method is to weigh yourself before and after exercise. Because any weight loss is likely from fluid loss, drinking enough to replenish those losses will maintain hydration. Because exercise inhibits the body's thirst signal, you need to begin drinking fluids before you feel thirsty to keep up with your losses. The stages of dehydration are shown in **TABLE 9.2**.

Signs of dehydration include:

- Elevated heart rate at a given exercise intensity
- Increased rate of **perceived exertion** during activity
- Decreased performance
- Lethargy
- Concentrated urine
- Infrequent urination
- Loss of appetite

Hydration

Active people must train themselves to consume adequate amounts of fluid before, during, and after exercise. Because each person has different water electrolyte losses based on factors such as body weight, genetic makeup, and metabolism, hydration strategies must be personalized.

The goal of hydrating before exercise is to start the physical activity with normal plasma electrolyte levels. Prior to strenuous exercise (optimally four hours prior), you should consume fluids by drinking beverages slowly. Beverages that contain sodium can help stimulate thirst and retain needed fluids.[22] Because even partial dehydration can compromise performance (see **TABLE 9.3**), athletes should maintain fluid balance by drinking fluids during the event.

The goal of drinking during exercise is to prevent excessive dehydration (> 2 percent body weight loss) and excessive changes in electrolyte balance.[23] A general recommendation for fluid and electrolyte replacement is difficult due to the differences in exercise tasks, weather

TABLE 9.3
Adverse Effects of Dehydration on Athletic Performance

Percent Body Weight Loss	Adverse Effects on Performance
1	The thirst threshold; leads to decrease in physical work capacity
2	Stronger thirst, vague discomfort, loss of appetite
3	Dry mouth, reduction in blood volume and urine output
4	Decrease of 20–30 percent in physical work capacity
5	Difficulty concentrating, headache, sleepiness
6	Severe impairment in ability to regulate body temperature during exercise; increased respiratory rate, leading to tingling and numbness of extremities
7	Collapse is likely if combined with heat and exercise

TABLE 9.4
American College of Sports Medicine Hydration Recommendations

Hydration Before Exercise

Check your hydration status before exercise because there is a wide variability in fluid needs for each person.
- Drink 16–20 fluid ounces of water or sports beverage at least four hours before exercise.
- Drink 8–12 fluid ounces of water 10–15 minutes before exercise.

Consuming a beverage with sodium (salt) and/or a small meal helps to stimulate thirst and retain fluids.

Hydration During Exercise

- Drink 3–8 fluid ounces of water every 15–20 minutes when exercising for less than 60 minutes.
- Drink 3–8 fluid ounces of a sports beverage (5–8 percent carbohydrate with electrolytes) every 15–20 minutes when exercising longer than 60 minutes.

Do not drink more than one quart/hour during exercise.

Hydration Guidelines After Exercise

Obtain your body weight and check your urine to estimate your fluid losses. The goal is to correct your losses within two hours after exercise.
- Drink 20–24 fluid ounces of water or sports beverage for every 1 pound lost.

Selectively and Effectively Using Hydration for Fitness. Reprinted with permission of the American College of Sports Medicine. 2011 American College of Sports Medicine.

conditions, fitness levels, and other factors. Active people should develop their own customized fluid-replacement programs that prevent excessive dehydration. Consumption of normal meals and beverages typically is sufficient to restore hydration status. For rapid recovery from excessive dehydration, the dehydrated person can drink approximately 1.5 liters of fluid for each kilogram of body weight lost.[24] See **TABLE 9.4** for a summary of the American College of Sports Medicine's position on the amount and type of fluid to consume before, during, and after activity.

Muscle Cramps

A muscle cramp is excruciatingly painful and often associated with dehydration. Although massage and stretching may provide immediate relief, the causes of cramps are not well understood. Likely related to overexertion, other contributing factors may include fluid loss, inadequate conditioning, and electrolyte imbalance. Lack of water, sodium, calcium, magnesium, and potassium, individually or together, may trigger a cramp during exercise. Before exercising, drink plenty of fluids and make certain that your diet is rich in these minerals.

Key Concepts Adequate intake of complex carbohydrates and protein, plus proper hydration, is important for optimal exercise performance. Exercise of any type increases fluid losses through sweat, and evaporation of sweat from the skin allows the body to cool itself. To avoid dehydration, fluid losses must be replaced. Athletes should drink plenty of fluid before, during, and after exercise. Fluid choices depend on the duration of activity and the preferences of the athlete. Optimal sports drinks provide energy and electrolytes in a solution that promotes rapid absorption.

Quick **Bite**

Alligator Water?
To enhance athletic performance, early research at the University of Florida developed a drink that combined water with electrolytes in a pleasant tasting solution. They named it Gatorade after the school's beloved alligator mascot.

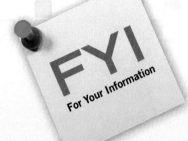

When Are Sports Drinks Recommended?

Water is now a designer beverage. On store shelves, you can find fortified water, fitness water, herbal water, electrolyzed water, and coconut water. Although some taste great, watch out for unsubstantiated claims and sugar content. Some sweetened waters have as much sugar as soda.

For rehydration, would you choose water, sports drinks, or other beverages? It depends on how long you are exercising. During activities that last fewer than 60 continuous minutes, water is your best sports drink. Drinking water can replace fluid lost in sweat and help offset the rise in core temperature. During exercise that lasts longer than 60 continuous minutes, electrolytes and glycogen stores become depleted. Consuming fluids that contain carbohydrate and sodium can delay fatigue, enhance taste, and promote fluid retention.

Optimal sports drinks provide energy (from glucose, glucose polymers, or sucrose) and electrolytes in a **palatable** (pleasant-tasting) solution that promotes rapid absorption, with less than 10 percent carbohydrate concentration. (See **TABLE A**.) The palatability of beverages containing electrolytes and 4 to 8 percent carbohydrate may increase the voluntary intake of fluid. Beverages such as fruit juices and soft drinks are concentrated sources of carbohydrates (more than 10 percent); the main carbohydrate is fructose, which is associated with slower stomach emptying (also called gastric emptying) and abdominal cramps. In addition, carbonated soft drinks may decrease the volume of fluid consumed and delay gastric emptying. Coconut water, on the other hand, contains no added sugars and is rich in potassium, vitamin C, antioxidants, and phytochemicals. Claims for coconut water beyond rehydration are not backed by scientific studies.

Athletes should avoid beverages that contain alcohol. Some athletes use alcohol for psychological benefits—calming nerves, improving self-confidence, and reducing anxiety, pain, and muscle tremor. This misguided effort fails to recognize alcohol's negative influence on physical performance. Alcohol slows reaction time, impairs coordination, and upsets balance. Its diuretic action contributes to dehydration and may impair regulation of body temperature.

For endurance events that last longer than four to five hours (or shorter events in high heat and humidity), athletes who do not replace electrolytes put themselves at risk for abnormally low levels of blood sodium. This life-threatening condition is associated with an excessive loss of electrolytes in sweat and with the excessive consumption of fluid, such as plain water, that does not replace electrolytes.

TABLE A Desirable Composition of Sports Beverages	
Characteristic	**Comment**
Fuel source	Contains carbohydrate: glucose, sucrose, and glucose polymers (maltodextrin). Goal intake is 60–70 g/hour (approximately 1 liter of a 6–8 percent carbohydrate drink).
Electrolytes	Contains sodium (70–165 mg per 240 mL) and potassium (30–75 mg per 240 mL) to replace sweat electrolyte loss when exercise is longer than 3–4 hours. Electrolytes also enhance palatability.
Rapid absorption	Contains 6–8 percent carbohydrate. Higher carbohydrate concentration slows gastric emptying and intestinal absorption.
Palatability	Flavored beverages enhance consumption. Electrolytes enhance flavor. Carbonation may decrease amount of fluid consumed.

Do you need a sports drink after mowing the grass? Although sports drinks have moved from the locker room to the mainstream, evidence does not support the use of commercial sports drinks for athletic events or other bouts of exertion lasting less than 60 minutes. Drink water after your burst of gardening. For people not engaged in athletics or heavy manual labor, sports drinks are not appropriate. At about 100 calories for 16 ounces, sports drinks contain significant calories (albeit less than other soft drinks) and have no redeeming nutritional qualities. For the nonathlete, these are little better than soft drinks.

▶ **palatable** Pleasant tasting.

Energy Intake and Exercise

🍎 **Why Is This Important?** Adequate energy intake is essential to optimal performance, and sports nutritionists tailor their recommendations to the large range of athlete body sizes and caloric expenditures.

Adequate energy intake is the first nutrition priority for athletes. Meeting energy needs is critical for athletic performance and for maintaining or increasing lean body mass. Appropriate energy intake supports optimal body function, determines the capacity for uptake of macronutrients and micronutrients, and assists in achieving the desired body composition. An athlete's energy requirements vary from day to day throughout the yearly training plan, relative to training intensity and duration. Other factors that increase energy needs include exposure to heat or cold, high altitude training, fear, stress, certain drugs or medications, and some physical injuries.

Sports nutritionists generally recommend eating small, frequent meals to maintain energy metabolism, improve nutrient intake, achieve desired body composition, support a training schedule, and reduce injuries.[25] During times of high physical activity, energy and macronutrient needs—especially carbohydrate and protein intake—must be met in order to maintain body weight, replenish glycogen stores, and provide adequate protein for building and repairing tissues.[26]

World-class athletes who train strenuously three to four hours each day can almost double their energy needs. The energy demand can be so high that some athletes have trouble consuming enough calories.[27] In contrast, athletes who compete in sports where they are judged by build and in sports with weight classifications often restrict energy intake to avoid weight gain. Energy intakes that are too low can lead to a loss of muscle mass, menstrual dysfunction, lower bone density, and increased risk of fatigue, injury, and illness.[28]

Because the *Dietary Guidelines* and *Dietary Reference Intakes* fail to cover the range of body sizes and activity levels of competitive athletes, these guidelines typically underestimate the energy requirements for this population. Experts in sports nutrition are using the concept of **energy availability (EA)**, which determines the energy intake needed for optimal health and fitness, rather than energy balance. EA is defined as dietary energy intake minus exercise energy expenditure adjusted to fat-free mass. It is the amount of energy available to the body to perform all functions after the energy cost of exercise is subtracted.[29]

To allow energy, carbohydrate, and protein recommendations to be scaled to the large range of athlete body sizes, sports nutritionist experts are providing guidelines based on grams of nutrient intake per kilogram of body mass. Sports nutrition guidelines also consider the importance of the timing of nutrient intake and nutritional support throughout the day and in relation to the specific sport rather than using general daily targets.

▶ **energy availability (EA)** The energy intake needed for optimal health and fitness, rather than energy balance. EA is the amount of energy available to the body to perform all functions after the energy cost of exercise is subtracted (thus EA = food energy intake − exercise energy expenditure).

Carbohydrate and Exercise

Carbohydrate has a number of key roles in adaptation to training and performance. Carbohydrate is a key fuel for the brain and central nervous system and supports muscular work over a broad range of intensities. As a fuel, carbohydrate yields more energy than fat per volume of oxygen, thus increasing gross exercise efficiency.[30] High carbohydrate availability enhances sustained or intermittent exercise, and depletion of carbohydrate stores is associated with fatigue. Because the stores of carbohydrate in the body are limited, they can be manipulated on a daily basis by adjusting intake or even by a single exercise session.[31] Sports nutrition strategies often target enhanced carbohydrate availability before, during, and in the recovery between events.

In addition to storing energy to power muscles, glycogen plays important roles in training adaptation. Specifically, starting a bout of endurance exercise when muscle glycogen stores are low results in an enhanced training response and adaptation (conditioning). In practice, an athlete may undertake a second training session in the hours immediately after the prior session has depleted glycogen stores.

Glycogen stores may be reduced, albeit to a lesser effect, by restricting carbohydrate intake. Increasingly, athletes are deliberately restricting carbohydrate within a training program ("train-low") combined with periodic dietary and training adjustments, although this practice also has the potential for misuse.[32] Individualized recommendations for daily intakes of carbohydrate must consider the athlete's training/competition program and when to target low- or high- carbohydrate intake. Although scheduled low-carbohydrate intake may enhance training adaptations, scheduled high-carbohydrate intakes may enhance performance during the competitive event. For a summary of generalized carbohydrate intake by athletes, see **TABLE 9.5**.

TABLE 9.5
General Guidelines for Carbohydrate Intake by Athletes

To provide high carbohydrate availability for training or competitive sessions, intake guidelines account for the athlete's body size (a proxy for muscle stores) and exercise session characteristics.

Daily Needs for Fuel and Recovery
The following targets are intended to provide high carbohydrate availability. These general recommendations should be fine-tuned with individual consideration of total energy needs, specific training needs, and feedback from training performance.

Exercise Intensity	Situation	Carbohydrate Targets	Comments on Type and Timing of Carbohydrate Intake
Light	Low-intensity or skill-based activities	3–5 g/kg of athlete's body weight (BW)/day	• Timing of intake of carbohydrate over the day may be manipulated to promote high carbohydrate availability for a specific session by consuming carbohydrate before or during the session, or in recovery from a previous session. • Otherwise, as long as total fuel needs are provided, the pattern of intake may simply be guided by convenience and individual choice. • Athletes should choose nutrient-rich carbohydrate sources to allow overall nutrient needs to be met.
Moderate	Moderate exercise program (e.g., ~1 hour/day)	5–7 g/kg/day	
High	Endurance program (e.g., 1–3 hours/day moderate- to high-intensity exercise)	6–10 g/kg/day	
Very high	Extreme commitment (e.g., > 4–5 hours/day moderate- to high-intensity exercise)	8–12 g/kg/day	

Acute Fueling Strategies
These guidelines promote high carbohydrate availability to promote optimal performance in competition or key training sessions.

Intake Goal	Situation	Carbohydrate Targets	Comments on Type and Timing of Carbohydrate Intake
General fueling up	Preparation for events < 90 min exercise	7–12 g/kg per 24 hours as for daily fuel needs	• Athletes may choose carbohydrate-rich sources that are low in fiber and easily consumed to ensure that fuel targets are met, and to meet goals for gut comfort or lighter "racing weight."
Carbohydrate loading	Preparation for events > 90 min of sustained/intermittent exercise	36–48 hours of 10–12 g/kg BW per 24 hours	
Speedy refueling	< 8 hours recovery between two fuel-demanding sessions	1–1.2 g/kg/hour for first 4 hours, then resume daily fuel needs	• Consuming small, regular snacks may be beneficial. • Carbohydrate-rich foods and drinks may help to ensure that fuel targets are met.
Pre-event fueling	Before exercise > 60 min	1–4 g/kg consumed 1–4 hours before exercise	• Timing, amount, and type of carbohydrate foods and drinks should be chosen to suit the practical needs of the event and individual preferences/experiences. • Choices high in fat/protein/fiber may need to be avoided to reduce risk of gastrointestinal issues during the event. • Low glycemic index choices may provide a more sustained source of fuel for situations where carbohydrate cannot be consumed during exercise.
During brief exercise	Exercise < 45 min	Not needed	

TABLE 9.5 *(continued)*
General Guidelines for Carbohydrate Intake by Athletes

Intake Goal	Situation	Carbohydrate Targets	Comments on Type and Timing of Carbohydrate Intake
Ensuring sustained high-intensity exercise	Exercise 45–75 min	Small amounts including mouth rinse	• A range of drinks and sports products can provide easily consumed carbohydrate. • The frequent contact of carbohydrate with the mouth and oral cavity can stimulate parts of the brain and central nervous system to enhance perceptions of well-being and increase self-chosen work outputs.
During endurance exercise, including "stop and start" sports	Exercise 1–2.5 hours	30–60 g/hour	• Carbohydrate intake provides a source of fuel for muscles to supplement glycogen stores. • Opportunities to consume foods and drinks vary according to the rules and nature of each sport. • A range of everyday dietary choices and specialized sports products ranging in form from liquid to solid may be useful. • The athlete should practice to find a refueling plan that suits their individual goals including hydration needs and gut comfort.
During ultra-endurance exercise	Exercise > 2.5–3 hours	Up to 90 g/hour	• As above. • Higher intakes of carbohydrate are associated with better performance. • Products providing multiple transportable carbohydrates (glucose/fructose mixtures) achieve high rates of oxidation of carbohydrate consumed during exercise.

Reprinted from *Journal of the Academy of Nutrition and Dietetics*, 116(3), D. Travis Thomas, Kelly Anne Erdman, Louise M. Burke, Position of the Academy of Nutrition and Dietetics, Dietitians of Canada, and the American College of Sports Medicine: Nutrition and Athletic Performance, Page no. 501–528, 2016, with permission from Elsevier.

Pre-exercise Carbohydrate Intake

By manipulating nutrition and exercise in the hours and days before an important competitive event, an athlete can begin the event with enough glycogen stores to meet the estimated fuel costs of the event. Carbohydrate-rich foods consumed one to four hours before an event can help increase body glycogen stores that have been depleted by an overnight fast. They also may provide a source of glucose to be released by the gut during exercise.

Events lasting longer than 90 minutes may benefit from higher glycogen stores, which can be achieved by a technique known as **carbohydrate loading** or **glycogen loading**. Just as you might top off the gas tank in a car before a long trip, athletes can fill their glycogen stores prior to training or competing by manipulating their carbohydrate intake and exercise regimen to maximize muscle glycogen stores. For prolonged exercise, sports nutritionists recommend pre-exercise carbohydrate intakes of 1 to 4 grams/kilogram body weight, with timing, amount, and food choices tailored to the individual.[33]

Even though "extra" glycogen prior to competition sounds like a perfect plan, there is a downside to carbohydrate loading. For each gram of glycogen stored in muscle tissue, the body also stores about 3 grams of water. Many athletes who carbohydrate-load complain about this weight gain and subsequent sluggishness. Some opt to train and compete without carbohydrate loading because, for them, the risk of physical discomfort outweighs the benefit of a greater carbohydrate store. If your competitive event or workout is expected to be shorter than 90 minutes, carbohydrate loading is unlikely to provide benefits.

▶ **carbohydrate loading** Changes in dietary carbohydrate intake and exercise regimen before competition to maximize glycogen stores in the muscles. It is appropriate for endurance events lasting 60 to 90 consecutive minutes or longer. Also known as *glycogen loading*.

▶ **glycogen loading** See *carbohydrate loading*.

In general, carbohydrate-rich foods with a low-fat, low-fiber, and low-to-moderate protein content are the preferred choice. These foods are less likely to cause gastrointestinal problems and promote gastric emptying. Athletes who suffer from pre-event jitters may prefer easily digested liquid meal supplements. When the energy and carbohydrate content of the athlete's diet is taken into account, neither glycemic load nor glycemic index of carbohydrate-rich meals affects the metabolic or performance outcomes of training.[34] Above all, the individual athlete should choose an eating strategy that suits their situation and past experience; this strategy can be fine-tuned with experimentation.

Carbohydrate Intake During Exercise

Consuming carbohydrate during exercise can enhance performance by replenishing expended energy, preventing hypoglycemia, and activating reward centers in the central nervous system.[35] These benefits depend on several factors, including type of exercise, the environment, the athlete's training and nutrition regimen, and the athlete's carbohydrate tolerance. Individualized amounts, timing, and types of carbohydrate are needed to achieve optimal effects.[36]

Postexercise Carbohydrate Intake

A key goal of postexercise carbohydrate consumption is restoration of glycogen stores. Proper refueling requires adequate carbohydrate intake and timing. Because the rate of glycogen resynthesis is only about 5 percent per hour, early carbohydrate intake after exercise (about 1–1.2 g carbohydrate/kg body mass/hour during the first four to six hours) can be most effective. As long as the athlete is consuming adequate energy, carbohydrate, and other nutrients, foods and fluids can be chosen according to personal preferences.

> **Key Concepts** Energy intake is the most important element of the athlete's diet, and the major source of energy should be carbohydrates. Foods rich in complex carbohydrates, which also can provide fiber, iron, and B vitamins, are best. A high-carbohydrate diet prior to competition helps to maximize glycogen stores and endurance. Carbohydrate loading is a process of adjusting carbohydrate intake and training intensity to maximize glycogen stores just before an event. Consuming carbohydrates soon after exercise enhances the rebuilding of glycogen stores. Individualized recommendations for daily intakes of carbohydrate must consider the athlete's training/competition program, personal preferences, and when to target low- or high-carbohydrate intake.

Dietary Fat and Exercise

🍎 **Why Is This Important?** In general, high-fat diets appear to reduce rather than enhance performance due to the accompanying reduction of carbohydrate availability and a reduced capacity to use carbohydrate as a fuel.

During exercise, carbohydrates and fats are the two main fuel sources. Endurance (aerobic) training increases the capacity of your oxygen energy system, enhancing your body's ability to use fat as a fuel. Exercise intensity also affects fuel use. During low- to moderate-intensity exercise, fatty acids are the major fuel source. During high-intensity exercise, the predominant energy source is glucose.

This does not mean that endurance athletes should consume diets high in fat. High-fat diets usually are lower in carbohydrate, thus limiting

Quick Bite

The First Sports Trainers

During the time of the ancient Olympic Games, sports trainers demanded that their athletes follow strict training regimens: 10 months of regulated diet, bathing, exercise, rest, and massage. Until 480 BCE, Olympic athletes consumed a mostly vegetarian diet of cheese, porridge, figs, wine, and meal cakes. After twice winning the Olympic long race, however, Dromeus of Stymphalus revolutionized the ancient training diet by advocating mammoth amounts of meat and exercise.

muscles' ability to replenish glycogen stores. High-fat diets often are high in calories, saturated fat, and cholesterol; your body also digests fat more slowly than carbohydrate.

Fat Intake and the Athlete

Intake of fat by athletes should be in accordance with public health guidelines and individualized for training level and body composition goals. In general, high-fat diets appear to reduce rather than enhance performance due to the accompanying reduction of carbohydrate availability and a reduced capacity to use carbohydrate as a fuel. Recall from the "Spotlight on Metabolism and Energy Balance" that "fat burns in a flame of carbohydrate."

Endurance training increases the availability of fatty acids as a fuel for muscles. Athletes may choose to restrict fat intake in an attempt to lose body weight or improve body composition. They should be discouraged from chronic dietary fat intakes below 20 percent of energy intake. Such restrictions likely will reduce the intake of fat-soluble vitamins and essential fatty acids, especially omega-3 fatty acids. However, fat intake may be restricted temporarily, such as during carbohydrate loading.

Protein and Exercise

🍎 **Why Is This Important?** Increases in strength and muscle mass are greatest with the immediate postexercise consumption of protein. High-quality dietary proteins, especially milk-based proteins, are most effective for the maintenance, repair, and synthesis of skeletal muscle proteins. Excessive protein intake can increase risk of dehydration and kidney problems.

All athletes, even those for whom building muscle is not the goal, benefit from well-timed protein intake. To maximize conditioning, there is now a good rationale to recommend daily protein intakes well above the Recommended Dietary Allowance (RDA). Although the adult RDA for protein of 0.8 gram of protein per kilogram of body weight per day is sufficient for sedentary people and those engaging in low-intensity exercise, it often is insufficient for athletes focused on conditioning and performance improvement. Thus, experts have moved beyond the DRIs to focus on the benefits of providing sufficient protein at optimal times to support tissues with rapid protein turnover and enhance conditioning. Dietary protein combined with exercise is both a stimulus and substrate for building body proteins, including proteins in muscle, tendons, and bone.

Protein Recommendations for Athletes

To support metabolic adaptation, repair, remodeling, and protein turnover, the recommended dietary protein intake ranges from 1.2 to 2.0 g carbohydrate/kg body mass/day.[37] During intensified training, even higher protein intake may be needed for short periods. In meeting daily protein intake goals, a meal plan should provide moderate amounts of high-quality protein across the day and following strenuous training sessions.

Athletes should not be solely categorized as strength or endurance athletes. Protein requirements fluctuate based on "trained" status (well-trained athletes require less), training (high-frequency and intense sessions or a new regimen stimulate protein needs), carbohydrate availability, and energy availability.[38] Consuming adequate energy, particularly from carbohydrate, is necessary to spare protein from oxidation so that it is available for synthesis. When an athlete is sidelined by an injury, elevating his or her protein intakes (as high as 2.0 g/kg/day) over the course of the day may help prevent loss of fat-free mass.[39]

Timing Protein Intake with Exercise

Increases in strength and muscle mass are greatest with the immediate postexercise consumption of protein. Whereas traditional protein intake guidelines focused on total protein intake over the day (g/kg), newer recommendations highlight that the conditioning can be maximized by ingesting these targets as 0.3 g/kg body weight after key exercise sessions and every three to five hours over multiple meals.[40] In response to a single bout of resistance exercise, the body has increased protein synthesis and enhanced sensitivity to dietary protein for a minimum of 24 hours. Aerobic and other types of exercise, such as intermittent sprints, produce similar results. Consuming protein before and during exercise appears to have a lesser effect on muscle protein synthesis.

Optimal Protein Sources for Athletes

High-quality dietary proteins, especially milk-based proteins, are effective for the maintenance, repair, and synthesis of skeletal muscle proteins. Dairy proteins appear to be superior to other tested proteins, largely due to leucine content and the way branched-chain amino acids in fluid-based dairy foods are digested.

THINK
About It
4

When considering protein supplements, the sports nutritionist should conduct a thorough assessment of the athlete's specific nutritional goals. Experts recommend using protein supplements conservatively while maintaining high diet quality overall.

Dangers of High Protein Intake

▶ **diuresis** The formation and secretion of urine.

Excessive protein intake from food or supplements enhances **diuresis** (loss of body water) as the body attempts to excrete excess nitrogen through the urine. This increases the risk for dehydration and may contribute to mineral losses. High-protein diets often are high in saturated and total fat and may contribute to obesity, osteoporosis, heart disease, and certain types of cancer.

High intakes of single-amino-acid supplements may impair absorption of other amino acids. Further, the amount of amino acids contained in supplements is very small compared with the amount in food. For example, one pill may contain 500 milligrams of an amino acid, but 1 ounce of meat, poultry, or fish provides more than 7,000 milligrams of essential and nonessential amino acids! And, milligram for milligram, the cost of supplements is higher.

Key Concepts Although fat is an important fuel for exercise, a high-fat diet is unnecessary and not recommended. Dietary protein both stimulates body protein synthesis and is a source of amino acids to build proteins. The protein requirements of athletes are higher than those of sedentary adults. Dairy proteins appear to be superior to other protein sources due to easier and quicker digestion. Amino acid supplements are neither recommended nor necessary.

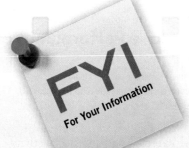

Nutrition Periodization: Tailoring Nutrition Intake to Exercise Goals

Athletes, competitive as well as recreational, adjust their training schedules based on desired performance outcomes. Athletes are not constantly "in season," and their training during a 12-month period can be described as consisting of three phases: (1) preparation, (2) competition, and (3) transition. This concept is referred to as exercise periodization.[a]

Let's take a look at each training phase more closely:

- *Preparation:* Also called the *macrocycle,* this phase leads up to the competition phase. Training is both general and specific, with goals to improve aerobic endurance, strength, and flexibility.
- *Competition:* Also called the *mesocycle,* the performance goals during this phase are to improve strength and speed.
- *Transition:* Also called the *microcycle,* this phase is the time spent between competition and the next preparation cycle. Also referred to as the "off-season" or "active recovery," workouts in this phase are generally less structured and are intended for the athlete to improve his or her weaknesses.

During exercise periodization, an athlete's nutrition needs will change. Adjusting macronutrient (carbohydrate, fat, and protein) intake to enhance the training cycle enables athletes to provide the best combination of fuel for their bodies all year long.[b] This process is referred to as *nutrition periodization,* and it goes hand-in-hand with exercise periodization:

- *Preparation:* This is the one phase where, if needed, athletes should focus on changing their weight, body fat percentage, and/or building muscle. This is a time when habits regarding diet can be changed and an in-depth evaluation of regular dietary habits can occur. Adjustments are made within the diet to work toward a desired competition weight and/or body composition.
- *Competition:* During this phase, a routine for eating during the competition season should be well established. The focus should not be on changing weight or experimenting with different food choices. Recovery after exercise is an important focus.
- *Transition:* This is a time to focus on calorie control and good nutrition. It is a time to experiment with and enjoy different types of foods.

Use **TABLES A**, **B**, and **C** as guidelines for successful nutrition periodization.[c]

a Seebohar B. *Nutrition Periodization for Endurance Athletes.* Boulder, CO: Bull Publishing; 2004. Reprinted with permission of Bull Publishing.
b Block O, Kravitz L. Tailoring nutrient intake to exercise goals. *IDEA Fitness J.* 2006;3:48-55.
c Seebohar B. Op. cit.

TABLE A
Daily Needs: No Weight Loss

Training Phase	Carbohydrate (g/kg)	Protein (g/kg)	Fat (g/kg)	Hydration (color of urine)
Preparation	5–12+	1.2–1.7	0.8–1.0	Lemonade
Prerace	7–13	1.4–2.0	0.8–2.0	Lemonade
Race	7–19	1.4–2.0	0.8–3.0	Diluted lemonade
Transition	5–6	1.2–1.4	0.8–1.0	Lemonade

Seebohar B. *Nutrition Periodization for Endurance Athletes.* Boulder, CO: Bull Publishing Co.; 2004. Reprinted with permission of Bull Publishing.

TABLE B
Daily Needs: Summary

Training Phase	Daily Calorie Difference	
	Low	High
Preparation	0	2,238
Prerace	+620	−1,007
Race	0	−2,322
Transition	−620	−5,101

Seebohar B. *Nutrition Periodization for Endurance Athletes.* Boulder, CO: Bull Publishing Co.; 2004. Reprinted with permission of Bull Publishing.

TABLE C
Example: 155-Pound Male

Training Phase	Carbohydrate g/kcal	Protein g/kcal	Fat g/kcal	Total Daily Kilocalories
Preparation	325–845+/1,408–3,380	85–120/340–480	56–70/504–630	2,252–4,490+
Prerace	493–916/1,972–3,664	99–141/396–564	56–141/504–1,269	2,872–5,497
Race	493–1,339/1,972–5,356	99–151/396–564	56–211/504–1,899	2,872–7,819
Transition	352–453/340–396	85–99/340–396	56–70/504–630	2,252–2,718

Seebohar B. *Nutrition Periodization for Endurance Athletes.* Boulder, CO: Bull Publishing Co.; 2004. Reprinted with permission of Bull Publishing.

Quick Bite

Vitamins, Minerals, and Exercise Performance

🍎 **Why Is This Important?** Exercise stresses many metabolic pathways that require micronutrients, but in general, single micronutrient supplements are appropriate only for correcting a clinically defined need, such as iron supplements for iron-deficiency anemia.

Many metabolic reactions that support exercise and physical activity require vitamins and minerals. They help extract energy from nutrients, transport oxygen, and repair tissues. The safest and most effective strategy regarding micronutrients is to consume a well-chosen diet containing nutrient-rich foods.

B Vitamins

Because B vitamins are essential for energy metabolism, wouldn't active people with high energy expenditures require more B vitamins? There is no need to run to the supplement counter. Although B vitamins are needed for chemical reactions that release energy, a diet with adequate calories and ample complex carbohydrates, fruits, and vegetables also supplies plenty of B vitamins. However, if overall diet quality is poor, with too few calories or mostly refined sugars in lieu of complex carbohydrates, B vitamin intake can be compromised.

Vegan athletes who do not include fortified foods, such as some soy products and ready-to-eat cereals, may have a problem with vitamin B_{12} intake. They should consult a medical advisor or registered dietitian to determine whether they need B_{12} supplements.

Calcium

Calcium is essential for normal muscle function and strong bones. Adequate calcium intake coupled with regular exercise slows the skeletal deterioration that occurs with age and can reduce the risk of osteoporosis.

Inadequate calcium may increase the risk of stress fractures in active people. This is of particular concern for women of reproductive age who exercise heavily and are not menstruating. Athletes should strive to meet the Adequate Intake (AI) for calcium from a variety of low-fat dairy products and other calcium-rich foods. This is especially true for teens, whose calcium needs (1,300 milligrams per day) are higher than those of adults (1,000 milligrams per day). In athletes with low energy intake or menstrual dysfunction, calcium intakes of 1,500 mg/day and vitamin D intakes of 1,500–2,000 IU/day are needed to optimize bone health.[41]

Iron

Iron is vital to oxygen delivery for aerobic energy production and may be the most critical mineral with implications for performance during endurance exercise. As an essential part of hemoglobin and myoglobin, iron helps deliver oxygen to active muscle cells. It also is a key component of several enzymes vital to the production of ATP by the oxygen energy system.

Because of menstrual losses and lower dietary iron intakes, active females have a greater risk of iron deficiency than active males. Iron requirements for all female athletes may be increased by up to 70 percent above the estimated average requirements.[42] In endurance athletes, the impact of running can cause mechanical trauma to capillaries in the feet and increase the breakdown of red blood cells. The increased breakdown contributes to low iron status. Some studies suggest that athletes involved in heavy training may need 30 to 70 percent more iron than nonathletes.[43] Endurance training also increases the volume of plasma in the blood without initially changing the amount of hemoglobin. This dilutes the hemoglobin, even though training typically maintains or increases the amount of total hemoglobin. This condition, called **sports anemia**, is a false anemia for most athletes and can be remedied with a few days of rest.

Although many elite athletes, especially females, have depleted iron stores (low serum ferritin), the incidence of iron-deficiency anemia in this population is similar to that of the nonathletic female population.[44] Anemia can seriously impair a person's capacity to perform activities, but there is disagreement about the impact of mild iron deficiency. Still, most authorities suggest iron supplementation for athletes who have a documented iron deficiency, even without anemia.[45] Because iron deficiency anemia can require three to six months to reverse, nutritional intervention should begin at the first sign of an impending deficiency. In iron-depleted female endurance athletes, iron supplementation appears to enhance their ability to expend energy, and they could train harder.[46] Iron supplements should not be taken immediately after strenuous exercise. Intense exercise may raise the level of an iron regulatory hormone (hepcidin) that impairs iron absorption.[47]

Vitamin D

In addition to supporting bone health, vitamin D also may support athletic performance. Athletes who live at latitudes above the 35th parallel or who primarily train indoors are at increased risk of low vitamin D levels. Other factors such as dark complexion, high body fat content, training only in the early morning or late evening when ultraviolet B (UVB) levels are low, and aggressive blocking of UVB exposure (with clothing, equipment, or sunscreen) increase the risk of inadequate vitamin D.[48] Dietary interventions alone are unreliable for resolving low vitamin D.[48] Vitamin D supplementation and/or responsible exposure to UVB may be required to maintain adequate vitamin D status. When vitamin D status is adequate, studies do not support use of vitamin D supplements to enhance athletic performance.

Other Trace Minerals

Strenuous exercise taxes the body's reserves of copper (essential for red blood cell synthesis) and zinc (vital to the work of many enzymes involved in energy production). During endurance events, increased fluid loss increases mineral losses—zinc in urine and relatively high amounts of both zinc and copper in sweat.

Although these losses may cause marginal deficiencies, supplementation is not necessarily recommended. High-dose supplements of iron, copper, or zinc can interfere with the normal absorption of these and other minerals, so an excess of one can cause a deficiency of the others. **TABLE 9.6** is an example of a training diet that would meet an athlete's needs for vitamins and minerals through food, which is preferable to taking supplements.

▶ **sports anemia** A lowered concentration of hemoglobin in the blood due to dilution. The increased plasma volume that dilutes the hemoglobin is a normal consequence of aerobic training.

TABLE 9.6
A Sample Training Diet

Athlete performs prolonged daily training.		
Body weight = 70 kilograms (154 pounds)		
Energy intake = 3,400 kilocalories		

Macronutrients

Carbohydrate	Protein	Fat
535 g	128 g	83 g
63 percent kcal	15 percent kcal	22 percent kcal
7.5 g/kg body weight[a]	1.8 g/kg body weight[b]	

Breakfast	Postexercise	
8 oz orange juice	1 bagel	
2 cups Cheerios cereal	2 oz string cheese	
8 oz 1% milk	16 oz apple juice	
1 large bran muffin	1 large baked potato with 2 tablespoons low-fat sour cream	

Lunch	Dinner	
2 slices whole wheat bread		
3 oz chicken breast		
2 oz turkey	2 whole wheat dinner rolls	
2 slices tomato	1 teaspoon margarine	
Lettuce leaf	1 cup cooked broccoli	
2 teaspoons mayonnaise	1 cup salad greens with 2 tablespoons Italian salad dressing	
1 medium apple	8 oz 1% milk	
12 oz cranberry juice	1 cup low-fat frozen yogurt	

Pre-exercise		
8 oz Gatorade		
1 cereal bar		

[a] Recommended carbohydrate intake goals for prolonged daily training

[b] Recommended protein intake goals up to 2 g/kg body weight for extreme training loads

Key Concepts Vitamins and minerals are important components of athletes' diets. B vitamins are necessary for normal energy metabolism. Adequate calcium intake can help protect against stress fractures and, coupled with exercise, delays the onset of osteoporosis. Iron is needed to carry oxygen. Vitamin D supports strong bones and athletic performance. Strenuous exercise can tax the body's reserves of both copper and zinc.

The Vegetarian Athlete

Athletes may choose a vegetarian diet for reasons ranging from ethnic, religious, and philosophical beliefs to health, food aversions, financial constraints, and attempts to disguise disordered eating. A vegetarian diet can be nutritionally adequate. Still, vegetarian athletes may have an increased risk of lower bone mineral density and stress fractures.

Vegetarian athletes may benefit from comprehensive dietary assessments and education to ensure nutritionally sound diets to support training and performance.

Nutrition Needs of Youth in Sport

Young athletes (younger than 19 years) should place a higher priority on nutritional needs for growth and development than on athletic performance.[49] Young athletes often consume insufficient calories. The consequences of chronic low energy intake include[50]:

- Short stature and delayed puberty
- Nutrient deficiencies and dehydration
- Menstrual irregularities
- Poor bone health
- Increased incidence of injuries
- Increased risk of developing eating disorders

Parents and youths must understand the energy and nutrient demands of growth and training, and many need help in planning meals and snacks to meet those needs. Many sport activities for this age group take place after school, and some schools serve lunch as early as 10:45 a.m. To provide energy for the activity and nutrients for recovery, young people should have meals and snacks before and after exercise. Easily portable snacks include fruit, pretzels, dry cereal, cereal bars, yogurt, sports drinks, sandwiches, and milk. Young athletes must drink adequate fluids during the day as well as at practice and competition. This is especially important because youths have a high tolerance for exercising in heat, which puts them at increased risk for heat exhaustion and heatstroke.

> **Key Concepts** Vegetarian athletes may have an increased risk of stress fractures and lower bone density. Nutrient intakes by young athletes must support both competition and continued growth.

Nutrition Supplements and Ergogenic Aids

🍎 **Why Is This Important?** Although supplements and ergogenic aids are highly popular, most are unnecessary for athletes who eat a variety of foods and meet their energy needs. Supplements are best used as adjuncts to a well-chosen nutrition plan.

The pressure to win contributes to the search for a competitive edge, and the use of dietary supplements in an attempt to enhance athletic performance is increasing. A study of young Canadian athletes found that 98 percent were taking at least one dietary supplement. Whereas athletes 11–17 years old focused on vitamin and mineral supplements, athletes 18–25 years old took **ergogenic aids** with the expectation of improved performance.[51] In a study of nearly 22,000 U.S. high school students, about 30 percent reported using energy drinks or shots.[52] Nutrition supplements and ergogenic aids include products and practices that:

- Provide calories (e.g., liquid supplements, energy bars)
- Provide vitamins and minerals (including multivitamin supplements)
- Contribute to performance during exercise and enhance recovery after exercise (e.g., sports drinks, carbohydrate supplements)

Quick **Bite**

Training: Young at Heart or Skeletal Old Age?

With endurance training, younger athletes largely achieve improvements as a result of increased cardiac output. Older athletes show greater improvement in the activities of the oxidative enzymes in their skeletal muscles.

Quick **Bite**

Climbing with Age

Aging does not seem to impair a healthy person's ability to perform activities at a high altitude. However, aging reduces our ability to sweat, and, as we age, our ability to regulate body temperature declines, thus reducing our ability to exercise safely in hot environments.

▶ **ergogenic aids** Substances that can enhance athletic performance.

▶ **creatine** An important nitrogenous compound found in meats and fish and synthesized in the body from amino acids (glycine, arginine, and methionine).

- Are believed to stimulate and maintain muscle growth (e.g., purified amino acids)
- Contain micronutrients, herbal, and/or cellular components that are promoted to enhance performance (e.g., caffeine, chromium, picolinate, **creatine**)
- Are used for nutritional, physiological, psychological, biomechanical, or pharmacological reasons (see **TABLE 9.7**)

Most nutritional supplements are unnecessary for athletes who eat a variety of foods and meet their energy needs. However, iron and calcium supplements may be recommended for female athletes if their diets are low in these nutrients. Liquid supplements and sports bars that contain carbohydrates, proteins, and fats can provide an easy way to increase energy intake. Sports drinks, gels, and recovery drinks also can contribute to needed fluids and carbohydrates before, during, and after exercise.

Dietary supplements marketed as performance enhancers are another matter. Herbals, glandulars, enzymes, hormones, and other compounds aimed at athletes carry many attractive claims. Although some products have been well researched, most lack rigorous clinical trials to evaluate efficacy, apply to only one gender (usually males), or are relevant to only one sport (e.g., weight lifting). Such products should be used only after careful evaluation for safety, efficacy, and potency.

Concerns About Supplements and Ergogenic Aids

Few athletes undertake professional assessment of their baseline nutritional habits. Furthermore, athletes' supplementation practices often are guided by family, friends, teammates, coaches, the Internet, and retailers, rather than sports nutrition professionals.

Safety concerns include the presence of overt and hidden ingredients that are toxic, the inappropriate consumption of large doses, and problematic combinations of products. Hidden ingredients also may not comply with anti-doping standards. A supplement manufacturer's claim of "100% pure," "pharmaceutical grade," "free of banned substances," or "Natural Product—NHPN/NPN" (in Canada) are unreliable and do not guarantee a supplement is free of banned substances.

Quick Bite

Placebo Power!

Athletes involved in a heavy weightlifting program volunteered to participate in a study in which they would take what they thought were anabolic steroids. The results were dramatic: during four weeks of treatment, these experienced weightlifters had a nearly 7.5-fold increase in the rate of their strength gain. However, they were taking a placebo—an inactive substance identical in appearance to the genuine drug. Because there was no pharmacological effect, gains were solely due to their belief in the treatment.

TABLE 9.7
Types of Ergogenic Aids

Type	Description	Examples
Nutritional	Any supplement, food product, or manipulation that enhances work capacity or athletic performance	Carbohydrate loading; amino acid and vitamin supplements
Physiological	Any practice or substance that enhances the functioning of the body's various systems (e.g., cardiovascular, muscular) and, thus, improves athletic performance	Any type of physical training (e.g., endurance, strength), blood doping via transfusions, warming up and/or stretching
Psychological	Any practice or treatment that changes mental state, and thereby enhances sport performance	Visualization, hypnosis, pep talks, relaxation techniques
Biomechanical	Any device, piece of equipment, or external product that can be used to improve athletic performance during practice or competition	Weight belts, knee wraps, oversize tennis rackets, body suits (swimming/track)
Pharmacological	Any substance or compound classified as a drug or hormonal agent that is used to improve output and/or sport performance	Hormones (e.g., growth hormones, anabolic steroids), caffeine

The ethical use of sports supplements is a personal choice and is controversial. It is the role of a sports dietitian to build rapport with the athlete and provide credible, evidence-based information regarding a supplement's appropriateness, efficacy, and dosage. After completing a thorough assessment of the athlete's nutritional status and dietary intakes, sports dietitians can assist the athlete in making a decision.

Few ergogenic aids have any benefits supported by sound evidence. Research methodologies on their efficacy often are limited by small sample size, enrollment of untrained subjects, and poor representation of athletic subpopulations (e.g., females, older athletes, athletes with disabilities). Studies often use unreliable or irrelevant performance tests, have poorly controlled confounding variables, and fail to include recommended nutrition practices or interactions with other supplements. Supplement use is best undertaken as an adjunct to a well-chosen nutrition plan. **TABLE 9.8** is a general guide that describes the ergogenic and physiological effects of potentially beneficial supplements and sports foods.

Quick **Bite**

The Burn to the Finish
The pain a runner feels when approaching the finish line and immediately after the event is called *acute muscle soreness*. The culprits include a buildup of metabolic by-products and tissue edema caused by fluid seeping from the bloodstream into surrounding tissues. The pain and soreness usually disappear within minutes or hours.

TABLE 9.8
Dietary Supplements and Sports Foods

Category	Examples	Use	Concerns
Sports food	Sports drinks Sports bars Sports confectionery Sports gels Electrolyte supplements Protein supplements Liquid meal supplements	Practical choice to meet sports nutritional goals, especially when access to food, opportunities to consume nutrients, or gastrointestinal concerns make it difficult to consume traditional food and beverages	Cost is greater than whole foods. May be used unnecessarily or in inappropriate protocols.
Medical supplements	Iron supplements Calcium supplements Vitamin D supplements Multivitamins/minerals Omega-3 fatty acids	Prevention or treatment of nutrient deficiency under the supervision of an appropriate medical/nutritional expert	May be self-prescribed unnecessarily without appropriate supervision or monitoring
Sports Performance Supplements	**Ergogenic Effects**	**Physiological Effects/Mechanism of Ergogenic Effect**	**Concerns**
Creatine	Improves performance of repeated bouts of high-intensity exercise with short recovery periods • Direct effect on competition performance • Enhanced capacity for training	Increases creatine and phosphocreatine concentrations May also have other effects such as enhancement of glycogen storage and direct effect on muscle protein synthesis	Associated with acute weight gain (0.6–1 kg), which may be problematic in weight-sensitive sports. May cause gastrointestinal discomfort. Some products may not contain appropriate amounts or forms of creatine.
Caffeine	Reduces perception of fatigue Allows exercise to be sustained at optimal intensity/output for longer	Adenosine antagonist with effects on many body targets including central nervous system Promotes Ca^{2+} release from sarcoplasmic reticulum	Causes side effects (e.g., tremor, anxiety, increased heart rate) when consumed in high doses. Toxic when consumed in very large doses. Rules of National Collegiate Athletic Association competition prohibit the intake of large doses that produce urinary caffeine levels exceeding 15 µg/mL. Some products do not disclose caffeine dose or may contain other stimulants.

(continues)

TABLE 9.8 (continued)
Dietary Supplements and Sports Foods

Sports Performance Supplements	Ergogenic Effects	Physiological Effects/Mechanism of Ergogenic Effect	Concerns
Sodium bicarbonate	Improves performance of events that would otherwise be limited by acid–base disturbances associated with high rates of anaerobic glycolysis • High-intensity events of 1–7 minutes • Repeated high-intensity sprints • Capacity for high-intensity "sprint" during endurance exercise	When taken as an acute dose pre-exercise, increases extracellular buffering capacity	May cause gastrointestinal side effects, which cause performance impairment rather than benefit
Beta-alanine	Improves performance of events that would otherwise be limited by acid–base disturbances associated with high rates of anaerobic glycolysis • Mostly targeted at high-intensity exercise lasting 60–240 seconds • May enhance training capacity	When taken in a chronic protocol, achieves increase in muscle carnosine (intracellular buffer)	Some products with rapid absorption may cause paresthesia (i.e., tingling sensation).
Nitrate	Improves exercise tolerance and economy Improves performance in endurance exercise, at least in nonelite athletes	Increases plasma nitrite concentrations to increase production of nitric oxide with various vascular and metabolic effects that reduce O_2 cost of exercise	Consumption in concentrated food sources (e.g., beetroot juice) may cause gut discomfort and discoloration of urine. Efficacy seems less clear cut in high-caliber athletes.

These supplements may perform as claimed, but this does not imply endorsement by this position stand. Athletes should be assisted to undertake a cost-to-benefit analysis before using any sports food and supplements with consideration of potential nutritional, physiological, and psychological benefits for their specific event weighed against potential disadvantages. Specific protocols of use should be tailored to the individual scenario, and specific products should be chosen with consideration of the risk of contamination with unsafe or illegal chemicals.

Reprinted from *Journal of the Academy of Nutrition and Dietetics*, 116(3), D. Travis Thomas, Kelly Anne Erdman, Louise M. Burke, Position of the Academy of Nutrition and Dietetics, Dietitians of Canada, and the American College of Sports Medicine: Nutrition and Athletic Performance, Page no. 501-528, 2016, with permission from Elsevier.

Weight and Body Composition

Why Is This Important? Athletes often seek to remodel their body composition by lowering weight and increasing lean body mass. Understanding safe methods of weight management is essential for optimal athletic performance and avoiding long-term, serious health consequences.

Pete, a bodybuilder, wants to bulk up by gaining 15 pounds of muscle, not fat. Sarah, on the other hand, wants to compete as a lightweight rower and needs to lose 7 pounds. Some athletes struggle to lose weight, but others find it nearly impossible to gain weight and muscle mass. Whether intentionally gaining or losing weight, weight change should be accomplished slowly—during the off-season or at the beginning of the season before competition starts.

Body composition and body weight are just two of many factors that affect exercise performance. Body composition can affect strength, agility, and appearance. Body weight can influence speed, endurance, and power. Because body fat adds weight without adding strength, many sports emphasize low body fat percentages. Yet, by themselves, body composition and body weight do not predict athletic performance accurately.

Weight Gain: Build Muscle, Lose Fat

Weight gain is influenced by genetics, stage of adolescent development, gender, body mass, diet, training program, prior resistance training, motivation, and use of supplements and **anabolic steroids**, among other factors. Complex interactions among these factors make it difficult to predict an athlete's ability to meet a weight goal. However, experience tells us the following:

- Untrained male athletes can gain approximately 3 to 4 pounds of lean body mass per month in the early stages of a rigorous resistance-training program.[53] Because of their smaller muscle mass and lean tissue, young women can achieve only 50 to 75 percent of the gains seen in male counterparts, but with the same relative strength.
- Approximately 20 percent of the increase in lean body mass occurs in the first year of resistance training, tapering to 1 to 3 percent in subsequent years. Scientists believe that the rate declines as muscle mass approaches the maximum potential amount determined by genetics.
- Some male athletes of high school age have difficulty gaining muscle mass. These athletes may be in the early stages of the adolescent growth spurt and may lack sufficient levels of the male hormones to stimulate muscle development.

Nutrition plays an important role in increasing lean body mass. Athletes must consume enough calories, along with adequate carbohydrate and protein, to gain the desired muscle mass.

> **Key Concepts** Athletes often seek to improve their power and strength by increasing muscle mass. Weight gain as muscle requires increased dietary calories, primarily as carbohydrate, combined with strength training.

▶ **anabolic steroids** Several compounds derived from testosterone or prepared synthetically. They promote body growth and masculinization and oppose the effects of estrogen.

Quick **Bite**

What's the Best "Fat-Burning" Exercise?

It's a common misconception that low-intensity exercise is superior for "fat burning." Aerobic activities do use a greater percentage of fat as fuel, but it is the total amount of energy (calories) expended during exercise that supports increased mobilization of fat in response to a caloric deficit. In terms of actual energy expenditure, higher-intensity exercise requires more calories for a given time period than exercise at a lower intensity. Thus, to lose body fat, the fuel (source of calories) is not as important as the amount of energy expended.

Weight Loss: The Panacea for Optimal Performance?

As the pressure to win increases, many coaches and athletes come to believe that weight loss and lower body fat composition will provide that competitive edge. Athletes strive for lower body weight and lower body fat for several reasons: (1) distance runners and cyclists benefit from a lower energy cost of movement and more efficient heat dissipation; (2) team athletes increase their speed and agility by being lean; (3) athletes in acrobatic sports (e.g., diving, gymnastics, dance) gain advantages in being able to move their bodies within a smaller space, and (4) some athletes, such as wrestlers, boxers, and body builders, must achieve a particular weight category or aesthetic to be competitive.[54] **FIGURE 9.12** illustrates the key factors in a successful weight-loss program.

As healthy young adults, men average 15 percent body fat and women average 25 percent.[55] Although these averages provide starting points, recommendations for individual athletes must account for genetic background, age, gender, sport, health, and weight history. Male athletes should not go below 5 to 7 percent body fat. For female athletes, at least 13 to 17 percent body fat is needed to maintain normal menstrual function, which in turn is important for maintaining bone health.

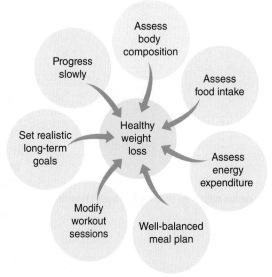

FIGURE 9.12 Keys to successful weight loss. Just as athletes focus on proper training techniques to avoid injury and improve performance, they should focus on proper weight-loss strategies to lose weight and maintain health.

Keeping accurate food and training records provides information on energy intake and expenditure. The best way for athletes to sustain a safe and sensible loss of body fat is to reduce calorie intake moderately and modify the training program. A combination of resistance training and aerobic activity is best for weight loss because it helps maintain or even increase lean body mass while simultaneously decreasing fat mass.

Beware of fad weight-loss methods such as ketogenic diets, high-protein diets, and semistarvation diets. These practices can compromise energy reserves, body composition, and psychological well-being, leading to decreased performance and increased health risks. Athletes often are alert to the latest supplements to hit the market. Many claim to accelerate the burning of body fat and augment weight loss. In reality, most "fat burners" are ineffective or associated with only very modest weight loss in obese subjects.

> **Key Concepts** Before embarking on a weight-loss program, athletes should carefully evaluate their goals and set a realistic plan for weight loss and maintenance. Safe weight-loss practices include modest changes in food intake accompanied by gradual increases in aerobic activity.

Weight Loss: Negative Consequences for the Competitive Athlete?

Although achieving a certain body composition has advantages, athletes may feel pressure to reach unrealistically low weights or percentage body fat, or they may attempt to reach their targets in an unrealistically short time. Such athletes may be susceptible to extreme and unhealthy weight-loss practices. Extreme methods of weight loss can be detrimental to both performance and health. When dieting goes awry, athletes risk serious medical problems.

Making Weight

▶ **pathogenic** Capable of causing disease.

Wrestlers, weightlifters, boxers, jockeys, rowers, and coxswains face competitive pressures to "make weight" to compete or to be certified in a lower weight classification. Such athletes often resort to the **pathogenic** weight-control behaviors summarized in **TABLE 9.9**. Repeated cycles of rapid weight loss and subsequent regain increase risk of disordered eating, fatigue, psychological distress (e.g., anger, anxiety, depression), dehydration, and sudden death.

Studies show that wrestlers, in attempts to gain a competitive advantage, will try to reduce weight a few days before or on the day of competition.[56] Athletes can achieve weight loss of up to 22 pounds (10 kilograms) of body water in one day by fasting, restricting fluids, using diuretics, sitting in a sauna, and exercising in a hot environment using rubber suits. A fluid loss of only 2 percent of initial body weight (3 pounds for a 150-pound individual) can decrease athletic performance by elevating heart rate and lowering **cardiac output**. Moderate to severe dehydration (more than 3 to 5 percent of body weight) can be dangerous because of increased core body temperature, electrolyte imbalances, and cardiac and kidney changes. These conditions may result in heat illness, including heat cramps, heat exhaustion, or heatstroke.

▶ **cardiac output** The amount of blood expelled by the heart.

Rapid weight loss can have serious health consequences. A tragic example occurred in 1998 and still serves as a cautionary warning. When trying to make weight, three previously healthy collegiate wrestlers died.[57] These athletes had not only dropped significant weight preseason—more than 20 pounds (9 kilograms)—but also lost between

TABLE 9.9
Pathogenic Weight-Loss Practices

Behavior	Consequence
Diet pills	Cardiovascular side effects and weight regained when discontinued
Fat-free diets	Deficiencies in fat-soluble nutrients, skin problems, impaired vision, impaired cognitive function
Self-starvation	Cardiovascular abnormalities, impaired growth, loss of lean body mass
Excessive exercise	Increased vulnerability to injury, overtraining, fatigue
Excessive sweating	Dehydration, impaired performance, impaired heat tolerance
Fluid restriction	Dehydration, impaired performance, impaired heat tolerance
Self-induced vomiting	Dehydration, impaired performance, electrolyte imbalance, inflammation or tears of the esophagus, GI bleeding, erosion of dental enamel, swollen glands
Diuretic abuse	Dehydration, impaired performance, electrolyte imbalance, impaired heat tolerance
Laxative abuse	Dehydration, impaired performance, cramps, nausea, rectal bleeding, dizziness, electrolyte imbalance, impaired GI functioning
Enemas	Dehydration, impaired performance, GI problems, fatigue, perforation or tearing of colon

3.5 and 9 pounds (1.6 and 4 kilograms) in the one to nine hours before their deaths. The wrestlers restricted food and fluid intake. To maximize sweat losses, they wore vapor-impermeable suits under cotton warm-up suits and exercised vigorously in hot environments. Dehydration and **hyperthermia** (elevated body temperature) led to their demise.

Today, the NCAA has better guidelines for monitoring weight-loss practices and weigh-in procedures. (See **FIGURE 9.13**.) These include educating coaches and athletic trainers about healthy weight-control strategies and limiting the amount of preseason and precompetition weight loss.[58] The NCAA weigh-in format requires athletes to have a season minimum weight established at the start of the year. This format attempts to prevent use of techniques and tools that have been used in the past for rapid dehydration resulting in rapid weight loss.[59]

Key Concepts Pathogenic weight-control practices increase risk of dehydration and compromise performance; they may have long-term serious consequences for athletes.

▶ **hyperthermia** A much higher than normal body temperature.

Quick Bite

Ouch! But I Felt Fine Yesterday …

After a bout of heavy exercise, a person may not feel muscle soreness for a day or two. We do not fully understand this painful phenomenon, which is called *delayed-onset muscle soreness*. Activities that lengthen muscles seem to be the primary cause. The muscles suffer damage with micro-tears in their structure. This leads to an inflammatory response, causing localized muscle pain, swelling, and tenderness.

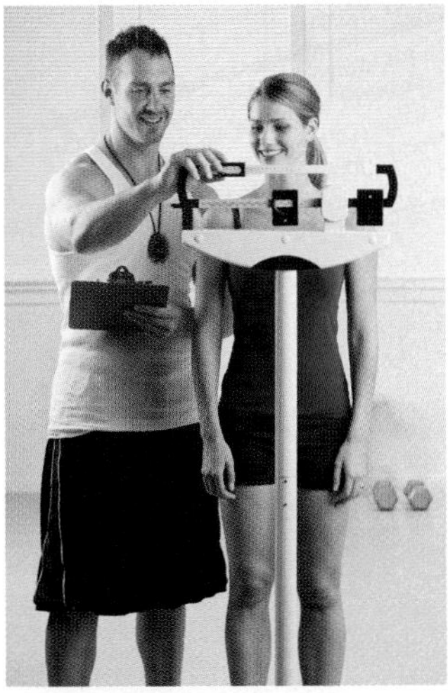

FIGURE 9.13 Weighing in. The NCAA discourages athletes from reducing their weight through intentional dehydration, a dangerous and potentially deadly practice.
© AVAVA/Shutterstock, Inc.

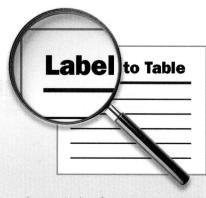

Label to Table

Sports drinks often are recommended instead of plain water for those who engage in vigorous physical activity. Their proponents claim that they quickly replenish the body's supply of nutrients, particularly electrolytes. Let's take a look at the Nutrition Facts panel from a popular sports drink, Gatorade.

First, look closely at the serving size—it's not the whole container. This is worth noting because many people might drink the whole container and assume they were getting 50 kilocalories. Not true! The whole container has 200 kilocalories (50 × 4 servings). It's always a good idea to look at the serving size when you are studying a nutrition label.

So, what makes this sports drink different from plain (and inexpensive) water? This one has added carbohydrate, sodium, and potassium. Replacing carbohydrate during long workouts prevents complete depletion of glycogen stores. Most sports drinks have between 5 and 8 percent simple sugar. Higher amounts would limit water absorption, and replacement of water is more critical than replacement of glucose.

Sodium and potassium are added to sports drinks to improve taste and help replace electrolytes that are lost during exercise. Gatorade contains 110 milligrams of sodium and 30 milligrams of potassium. For many athletes, and certainly for recreational exercisers, water really is the best fluid replacer. Although both sodium and potassium are lost in sweat, water is lost in greater quantities. Sports drinks have been shown to benefit only athletes who are strenuously exercising for longer than an hour. With prolonged exercise and sweat losses, large losses of electrolytes can make a person dizzy and weak, and may even lead to heat exhaustion or heatstroke.

The next time you head out for a bike ride, consider how long you'll be gone and how strenuous your ride will be, and then consider whether you'll need a sports drink. Also consider your personal taste—if a flavored sports drink will encourage you to replace fluids more than plain water will, that may be an important advantage. Just don't forget to read the label!

Nutrition Facts

4 servings per container

Serving size 8 fl oz (240mL)

Amount per serving

Calories 50

	% Daily Value*
Total Fat 0g	
Trans Fat 0g	
Sodium 110mg	0%
Total Carbohydrate 14g	5%
Dietary Fiber 0g	5%
Total Sugars 14g	0%
Includes 14g Added Sugars	28%
Protein 0g	
Vitamin D 0mcg	
Calcium 0mg	0%
Iron 0mg	0%
Potassium 30mg	0%
	1%

Not a significant source of Calories from Fat, Saturated Fat, Trans Fat, Cholesterol, Vitamin A, Vitamin C.

* The % Daily Value (DV) tells you how much a nutrient in a serving of food contributes to a daily diet. 2,000 calories a day is used for general nutrition advice.

Learning Portfolio

Key Terms

	page
aerobic endurance	438
anabolic steroids	459
ATP–CP energy system	435
carbohydrate loading	447
cardiac output	460
conditioning	441
creatine	456
creatine phosphate	434
diuresis	450
energy availability (EA)	445
ergogenic aids	455
fast-twitch (FT) fibers	438
glycogen loading	447
hyperthermia	461
lactic acid energy system	435
muscle fibers	438
oxygen energy system	435
palatable	444
pathogenic	460
perceived exertion	442
phosphocreatine	434
skeletal muscles	438
slow-twitch (ST) fibers	438
sports anemia	453

Study Points

- Exercise promotes health and reduces risk of chronic diseases.

- The ACSM defines physical fitness as "the ability to perform moderate to vigorous levels of physical activity without undue fatigue and the capability of maintaining this level of activity throughout life."

- There are two types of skeletal muscle fibers: slow-twitch (ST) and fast-twitch (FT). ST fibers have high aerobic endurance; FT fibers are optimized to perform anaerobically. Your body depends predominantly on ST fibers for low-intensity events and FT fibers for highly explosive events.

- The body uses three systems to produce energy for physical activity: (1) the ATP–CP energy system (anaerobic), (2) the lactic acid energy system (anaerobic), and (3) the oxygen energy system (aerobic).

- Anaerobic and aerobic metabolism work together to fuel all types of exercise. During the early minutes of high-intensity exercise, the ATP–CP energy system and the lactic acid energy system provide most of the energy. Endurance activities are fueled primarily by the metabolism of glucose and fatty acids in the oxygen energy system.

- Training improves use of fat as a fuel by enhancing oxygen delivery and increasing the number of mitochondria in muscle.

- Carbohydrate should be the major source of energy in the athlete's diet and should come from complex carbohydrates, which can provide fiber, iron, and B vitamins. Athletes need carbohydrate so muscle glycogen stores and blood glucose concentrations will be adequate for training and competitive events. Likewise, carbohydrate is necessary to replenish glycogen stores after intense exercise.

- Carbohydrate loading is a process of reducing activity while increasing carbohydrate intake to maximize glycogen stores.

- Fat is a major fuel source for exercise, but high fat intake is neither required nor recommended.

- Protein needs of athletes are higher than for sedentary individuals, but generally athletes who consume adequate amounts of energy get enough protein. High-quality dietary proteins, especially milk-based proteins, are effective for the maintenance, repair, and synthesis of skeletal muscle proteins.

- Micronutrients important to athletic performance include B vitamins, vitamin D, iron, zinc, and calcium.

- Water is the most essential nutrient and is easily lost from the body with heavy sweating. Replacing fluid with water or sports drinks is important to prevent dehydration. Optimal sports drinks provide energy and electrolytes in a palatable solution that is rapidly absorbed.

- Athletes who are still growing have even higher energy and nutrient needs to support both physical activity and normal growth.

- Many dietary supplements are promoted as ergogenic aids—substances that enhance performance. Few well-controlled studies on their efficacy and safety have been done, however.

- Many athletes strive to either gain or lose weight to improve performance. In both cases, realistic goals and gradual changes are necessary for long-term success. Gains in muscle mass require increased

Learning Portfolio (continued)

calorie intake and weight training. Successful weight loss requires modest reductions in energy intake and increases in aerobic activity.

■ Weight-control efforts that involve fasting, excessive sweating, purging, diuretics, or laxatives are detrimental to health.

Study Questions

1. List the three different energy systems that your body uses to generate energy during exercise. When is each active during exercise?

2. What are muscle fibers, and what are the two major types?

3. What are the general recommendations for the balance of carbohydrate, fat, and protein in a physically active person's diet?

4. What is carbohydrate loading?

5. How do protein recommendations for athletes vary from those for nonathletes?

6. Name three minerals that are of concern for athletes because they may not consume enough.

7. What is sports anemia, and why does it happen? How does it compare with other anemias?

8. Define the term *ergogenic aid*. Is there a clear, research-based answer as to whether ergogenic supplements work?

Try This

The Popularity of Ergogenic Aids

Take a trip to a health food store to see just how popular (and expensive!) ergogenic aids are. Try to locate each supplement listed in this chapter. Are they all available? What are their prices? Ask a salesperson what he or she knows about each of them. Do his or her answers match what you read in the text?

Commit to Get Fit

Do you meet the American College of Sports Medicine's (ACSM's) definition of fitness? Answer the questions below with a yes or no.

1. Do you exercise consistently three to five days per week?

2. When you exercise, does it include 20 to 60 minutes of continuous aerobic activity (20 minutes

for intense activity and 60 minutes for less intense activity)?

3. Does your type of exercise use large muscle groups? Can you maintain it? Is it rhythmical and aerobic?

4. Does part of your activity include strength training of a moderate intensity (a minimum of one set of 8 to 12 repetitions of 8 to 10 exercises) at least two days per week?

If you answer *no* to any of these questions, you are not following the ACSM's suggestions to develop and maintain cardiorespiratory and muscular fitness. Choose a question to which you answered *no* and set a specific goal to include that factor in your exercise routine.

References

1. American College of Sports Medicine. What is Exercise is Medicine. http://www.exerciseismedicine.org/support_page.php/about/. Accessed September 10, 2017.

2. Jonas S, Phillips E. *ACSM's Exercise Is Medicine: A Clinician's Guide to Exercise Prescription*. Philadelphia: Lippincott Williams & Wilkins; 2009.

3. U.S. Department of Health and Human Services. *Physical Activity Guidelines for Americans*. https://health.gov/paguidelines/guidelines/. Accessed September 10, 2017.

4. Centers for Disease Control and Prevention. *State Indicator Report on Physical Activity, 2014*. Atlanta, GA: U.S. Department of Health and Human Services; 2014.

5. Jonas S, Phillips E. Op. cit.

6. Thomas DT, Erdman KA, Burke LM. Position of the Academy of Nutrition and Dietetics, Dietitians of Canada, and the American College of Sports Medicine: nutrition and athletic performance. *J Acad Nutr Diet*. 2016;116(3):501-528.

7. Maughan R, Shirreffs S. Physiology of exercise. In: Rosenbloom C, ed. *Sports Nutrition: A Practice Manual for Professionals*. 5th ed. Chicago: Academy of Nutrition and Dietetics; 2012.

8. Thomas DT, Erdman KA, Burke LM. Op. cit.

9. McArdle WD, Katch FI, Katch VL. *Exercise Physiology: Nutrition, Energy, and Human Performance*. 8th ed. Philadelphia: Lippincott Williams & Williams; 2014.

10. Brown GC. Speed limits. *The Sciences*. 2000;40(5):32-37.

11. McArdle WD, Katch FI, Katch VL. Op. cit.

12. Ibid.

13. Thomas DT, Erdman KA, Burke LM. Op. cit.

14. Kenney WL, Wilmore JH, Costill D. *Physiology of Sport and Exercise*. 6th ed. Champaign, IL: Human Kinetics; 2015.

15. Jeukendrup A, Gleeson M. *Sport Nutrition: An Introduction to Energy Production and Performance*. 2nd ed. Champaign, IL: Human Kinetics; 2010.

16. Ibid.

17. U.S. Department of State. Sochi Olympics 2014: we are all athletes. [Video]. January 31, 2014. http://goo.gl/C4qpzR. Accessed September 10, 2017.

18. American Heart Association. Food as fuel before, during, and after workouts. http://www.heart.org/HEARTORG/HealthyLiving/PhysicalActivity/FitnessBasics/Food-as-Fuel---Before-During-and-After-Workouts

_UCM_436451_Article.jsp#.WLSuaW8rKUk. Accessed September 10, 2017.

19. Kreider RB, Wilborn DC, Taylor L, Campbell B. Exercise and sport nutrition review: research and recommendations. *J Int Soc Sports Nutr.* 2010;7:7.

20. Williams MH, Anderson DE, Rawson ES. *Nutrition for Health, Fitness, and Sport.* 10th ed. Boston: McGraw-Hill; 2012.

21. Thomas DT, Erdman KA, Burke LM. Op. cit.

22. American College of Sports Medicine, Sawka MN, Burke LM, et al. American College of Sports Medicine position stand. Exercise and fluid replacement. *Med Sci Sports Exerc.* 2007;39:377-390.

23. Ibid.

24. Ibid.

25. Mota J, Fidalgo F, Silva R, et al. Relationships between physical activity, obesity, and meal frequency in adolescents. *Ann Hum Biol.* 2008;35(1):1-10.

26. Thomas DT, Erdman KA, Burke LM. Op. cit.

27. Sundgot-Borgen J, Garthe I. Elite athletes in aesthetic and Olympic weight-class sports and the challenges of body weight and body composition. *J Sports Sci.* 2011;29(Suppl 1):S101-S114.

28. Thomas DT, Erdman KA, Burke LM. Op. cit.

29. Loucks AB. Energy balance and energy availability. In: Maughan RJ, ed. *Sports Nutrition, The Encyclopaedia of Sports Medicine, an IOC Medical Commission Publication.* West Sussex, UK: John Wiley & Sons; 2013:72-87.

30. Cole M, Coleman D, Hopker J, Wiles J. Improved gross efficiency during long duration submaximal cycling following a short-term high carbohydrate diet. *Int J Sports Med.* 2014;35(3):265-269.

31. Spriet LL. New insights into the interaction of carbohydrate and fat metabolism during exercise. *Sports Med.* 2014;44(Suppl 1):S87-S96.

32. Bartlett JD, Hawley JA, Morton JP. Carbohydrate availability and exercise training adaptation: too much of a good thing? *Eur J Sport Sci.* 2015;15(1):3-12.

33. Ormsbee MJ, Bach CW, Baur DA. Pre-exercise nutrition: the role of macronutrients, modified starches and supplements on metabolism and endurance performance. *Nutrients.* 2014;6(5):1782-1808.

34. Thomas DT, Erdman KA, Burke LM. Op. cit.

35. Cermak NM, van Loon LJ. The use of carbohydrates during exercise as an ergogenic aid. *Sports Med.* 2013;43(11):1139-1155.

36. Stellingwerff T, Cox GR. Systematic review: carbohydrate supplementation on exercise performance or capacity of varying durations. *Appl Physiol Nutr Metab.* 2014;39(9):998-1011.

37. Thomas DT, Erdman KA, Burke LM. Op cit.

38. Areta JL, Burke LM, Camera DM, et al. Reduced resting skeletal muscle protein synthesis is rescued by resistance exercise and protein ingestion following short-term energy deficit. *Am J Physiol Endocrinol Metab.* 2014;306(8):E989-E997.

39. Wall BT, Morton JP, van Loon LJ. Strategies to maintain skeletal muscle mass in the injured athlete: nutritional considerations and exercise mimetics. *Eur J Sport Sci.* 2015;15(1):53-62.

40. Phillips SM. A brief review of critical processes in exercise-induced muscular hypertrophy. *Sports Med.* 2014;44(Suppl 1):S71-S77.

41. Mountjoy M, Sundgot-Borgen J, Burke L, et al. The IOC consensus statement: beyond the female athlete triad—relative energy deficiency in sport (RED-S). *Br J Sports Med.* 2014;48(7):491-497.

42. DellaValle DM. Iron supplementation for female athletes: effects on iron status and performance outcomes. *Curr Sports Med Rep.* 2013;12(4):234-239.

43. Thomas DT, Erdman KA, Burke LM. Op. cit.

44. Ibid.

45. Rowland T. Iron deficiency in athletes: an update. *Am J Lifestyle Med.* 2012;6(4):319-327.

46. DellaValle DM, Haas JD. Iron supplementation improves energetic efficiency in iron-depleted female rowers. *Med Sci Sports Exerc.* 2014;46(6):1204-1215.

47. Peeling P, Sim M, Badenhorst CE, et al. Iron status and the acute post-exercise hepcidin response in athletes. *PloS ONE.* 2014;9(3):e93002.

48. Lagowska K, Kapczuk K, Friebe Z, Bajerska J. Effects of dietary intervention in young female athletes with menstrual disorders. *J Int Soc Sports Nutr.* 2014;11:21.

49. Armstrong N, McManus AM. The elite young athlete. *Med Sport Sci.* 2011;56:47-58.

50. Brown JE. *Nutrition Through the Life Cycle.* 4th ed. Belmont, CA: Wadsworth Cengage Learning; 2011.

51. Wiens K, Erdman KA, Stadnyk M, Parnell JA. Dietary supplement usage, motivation, and education in young Canadian athletes. *Int J Sport Nutr Exerc Metab.* March 25, 2014. [Epub ahead of print.]

52. Terry-McElrath YM, O'Malley PM, Johnston LD. Energy drinks, soft drinks, and substance use among United States secondary school students. *J Addict Med.* 2014;8(1):6.

53. Cormie P, McGuigan MR, Newton FU. Adaptations in athletic performance after ballistic power versus strength training. *Med Sci Sports Exerc.* 2010;42(8):1582-1598.

54. Thomas DT, Erdman KA, Burke LM. Op. cit.

55. McArdle WD, Katch FI, Katch VL. *Essentials of Exercise Physiology.* 5th ed. Philadelphia: Lippincott Williams & Wilkins; 2015.

56. Marttinen RH, Judelson DA, Wiersma LD, Coburn JW. Effects of self-selected mass loss on performance and mood in collegiate wrestlers. *J Strength Cond Res.* 2011;25(4):1010-1015.

57. Centers for Disease Control and Prevention. Rapid weight loss in wrestlers results in death. *MMWR.* 1998;47(6):105-108.

58. Kundrat S. Sport nutrition for coaches. *J Nutr Educ Behav.* 2010;42(6):430.

59. Center for Nutrition in Sport and Human Performance. Taking it to the mat: the wrestler's guide to optimal performance. http://www.sectiononewrestling.com/wrestlers_guide_optimal_performance.pdf. Accessed September 10, 2017.

Spotlight on Eating Disorders

Revised by Brian Cook

THINK About It

1   What's your view of the ideal female and male body?

2   When should you be concerned that you—or someone you know—is dieting obsessively?

3   What foods are you likely to binge on?

4   How often do you see magazine covers, social media posts, websites, or advertising that promote dieting or encourage a specific body type?

5   Do your dietary habits change when you are experiencing negative emotions such as stress, anxiety, or depression?

LEARNING Objectives

1 Describe the full range of the eating disorder continuum.

2 Identify common causes of eating disorders.

3 List risk factors, warning signs, and treatments of anorexia nervosa, bulimia nervosa, and binge-eating disorder.

4 Compare common risk factors for eating disorders in men with those in women.

5 Describe unique features of eating disorder in athletes.

6 Discuss each component of the female athlete triad.

A thin college freshman confides to her roommate that she's going to skip lunch because she feels chubby. After an enormous lunch, a secretary works her way through a bag of cookies and polishes off a box of chocolates. A swimming champion who obsesses over every calorie becomes concerned that she hasn't had a period in two months. Are these examples of disordered eating? Very likely. Eating disorder? Possibly.

The examples above illustrate that patterns of eating and self-evaluation of one's body may appear to fall outside of the realm of healthy or normal. They may be symptoms of an underlying eating disorder, or they may represent disordered eating. It is important to stress that eating disorders and disordered eating are not the same. **Eating disorders** are biologically based, serious psychiatric illnesses that result in severe detriment to mental and physical health, reduction in quality of life, and increased risk of mortality.[1,2] Currently, anorexia nervosa, bulimia nervosa, and binge-eating disorder are identified as eating disorders.

Disordered eating, in contrast, includes patterns of eating such as restrictive dieting, compulsive eating, and skipping meals. Many individuals will engage in disordered eating at some point in their lives, but not with the frequency or presence of other key psychological factors necessary to be diagnosed with an eating disorder. Although disordered eating is often a temporary or mild change in eating patterns, it can develop into an eating disorder as part of a continuum that includes all eating and weight-control behaviors.[3]

Although most of us take pleasure in eating, for people with an eating disorder, food is a source of continual fear, stress, and anxiety (see **FIGURE SED.1**). Individuals with eating disorders engage in behaviors such as fasting, bingeing, exercise, or vomiting in an attempt to relieve emotional distress.[4]

On particular occasions, most of us have eaten to the point of discomfort (Thanksgiving dinner comes to mind). And many of us have cut out desserts at one time or another, hoping to fit into a special outfit or to lose weight for an athletic event or job interview. But stuffing yourself at a holiday meal or going on an occasional diet does not constitute an eating disorder. According to the fifth edition of the *Diagnostic and Statistical Manual of Mental Disorders* (abbreviated *DSM-5*), defining characteristics of eating disorders include a fear of

▶ **eating disorders** Psychiatric disorders that include extreme emotional distress, disordered self-evaluation based primarily on faulty perceptions of one's body size or shape, and abnormal eating and compensatory behaviors performed in an attempt to alter body shape. Currently, the American Psychiatric Association recognizes three eating disorders: anorexia nervosa, bulimia nervosa, and binge-eating disorder. Several other unhealthy patterns of eating have been identified, but sufficient evidence does not yet exist to classify these as psychiatric disorders.

▶ **disordered eating** An abnormal change in eating pattern related to an illness, a stressful event, or a desire to improve one's health, appearance, or athletic performance. If it persists it can lead to an eating disorder.

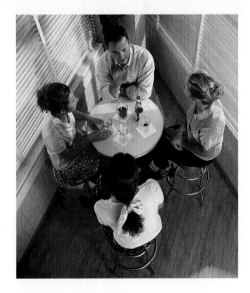

FIGURE SED.1 Can you spot the person with the eating disorder? Some people with eating disorders have normal body weights and are difficult to spot.
© Photodisc.

Body Dysmorphic Disorder

Some psychological conditions share key traits with eating disorders, even though the underlying obsession is with something other than food. For example, people with *body dysmorphic disorder* are preoccupied with an imagined or slight defect in appearance; they may worry that their skin is scarred, they are balding, or their nose is too big. They may engage in long rituals of grooming, repeatedly combing hair, applying makeup, or picking at their skin. They may have few friends, avoid dating, miss school or work, and feel self-conscious. The condition's severity varies. Whereas some people can manage it, for others it causes significant distress.

▶ **body image** A person's internal view of their own outer appearance.

A Matter of Degree

It's important to note that most high-school and college-age women (and men) engage in some behaviors that individuals with eating disorders also engage in, but this alone does not mean they have an eating disorder. What's more important is to recognize why they are engaging in such behaviors, how long they have been engaging in such behaviors, and how often these behaviors are occurring. The longer and more often someone shows unhealthy eating patterns and weight-control behaviors relating to body image dissatisfaction, the more likely he or she will move along the continuum towards an eating disorder.

becoming fat, an irrational evaluation of one's body and allowing that evaluation to influence self-concept, and/or bingeing on amounts of food that are more than what most people would eat during a similar period of time and under similar circumstances, experiencing a loss of control, and experiencing undue negative self-evaluation as a result of these types of eating-related behaviors.[5]

The Eating Disorder Continuum

🍎 **Why Is This Important?** The continuum of eating behaviors ranges from healthy eating, weight maintenance, and body acceptance, through varying levels of body dissatisfaction and behavioral attempts to change one's body, to serious psychiatric illnesses classified as eating disorders. It is important to distinguish disordered eating from actual eating disorders.

Labeling abnormal eating behaviors as an eating disorder may be as overstated as saying someone who sneezes has the flu. In fact, most people will face sociocultural pressures concerning weight and exhibit some type of disordered eating over the course of a lifetime.[6,7] Acknowledging where someone's behaviors fall on a continuum (see **FIGURE SED.2**) can help clarify when someone is at risk for severe health detriments related to dietary behaviors.

Body Image

How individuals internally perceive their outward appearance is called **body image**. It is basically a person's subjective evaluation of his or her own body, but it may not actually reflect the objective reality of body size and shape. Many of us are on the normal end of the continuum; that is, we are satisfied with our bodies. On the other hand, some people view their body image as negative. Sometimes this can be a motivating force for positive changes in lifestyle, as when an underweight person starts lifting weights to build muscle mass or when an overweight person starts eating smaller portions. But if a negative body

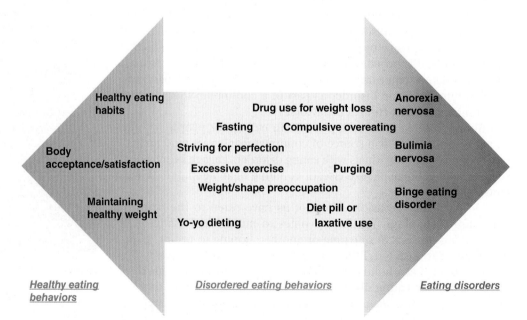

FIGURE SED.2 The eating disorder continuum.

image persists to **body dissatisfaction**, it may lead to depression, frustration, anger, or anxiety.

Societal trends that dictate our perceptions of the ideal body greatly influence how each of us sees and feels about our own body. The current emphasis on skinny female models dates back to the 1960s, when a British model named Twiggy, nicknamed for her stick-like appearance, ushered in an epidemic of unrealistic media portrayals of female bodies. Fashion magazine stories reported that she subsisted on water, lettuce, and a single daily serving of steak, and that she had learned to suppress her hunger pangs. Rather than condemn these clearly dangerous eating habits, the magazines held Twiggy up as a model of self-control for girls and young women (see **FIGURE SED.3**). It wasn't always so. Before Twiggy, style icons such as Marilyn Monroe were much more curvaceous and had BMIs much closer to average. Today young people are inundated with inaccurate and often dangerous advice about body image and related behaviors, especially on social media. This focus on culturally derived standards of beauty may inadvertently encourage some people to move away from the healthier end of the continuum and towards disordered eating or an eating disorder.

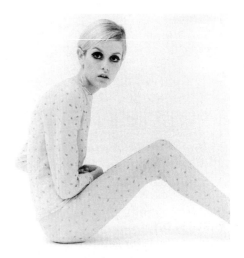

FIGURE SED.3 Eye of the beholder. In the 1960s, Twiggy became the new role model for young women who wanted to be thin and glamorous.

© Trinity Morror/Mirrorpix/Alamy Images.

Eating Disorders Defined

As discussed previously, healthy eating, appropriate amounts of exercise, and body acceptance represent one end of the continuum. Body image disturbance and disordered eating behaviors represent the middle part of the continuum. Most people will fall somewhere within this middle area. The pathological end of this continuum is defined by having an eating disorder. The *DSM-5* identifies three main variants of eating disorders.

Anorexia nervosa may be the easiest to identify because people with this disorder are considerably underweight for their age, height, and gender. Individuals with anorexia have a harmful level of body dissatisfaction. Even when they are dangerously underweight, people with anorexia typically see themselves as fat. Severely restricting food intake is another symptom of anorexia nervosa, but it is not the only way in which weight is controlled. People with anorexia may also engage in **purging** (self-induced vomiting) and excessive exercise.

Like people with anorexia, people with **bulimia nervosa** have a distorted perception of their body that results in distress and behaviors performed in an attempt to relieve this distress. Unlike individuals with anorexia, the distress in people with bulimia often leads to periods of loss of control in which they eat large amounts of food. After such **bingeing**, they often become disgusted with themselves and terrified of getting fat. People with bulimia then engage in behaviors intended to compensate for the massive amount of calories consumed during the binge. These behaviors are called compensatory behaviors and include purging, use of laxatives, excessive exercise, periods of fasting, and taking other actions to avoid gaining weight.

Finally, **binge-eating disorder**, formerly known as **compulsive overeating**, is the most common eating disorder. People with this disorder lose control while they are eating, consuming massive quantities of food in a short period of time. Binge eating occurs, on average, at least once a week for three months. Sufferers are typically obese; however, not all obese people binge eat. Similar to anorexia and bulimia,

▶ **body dissatisfaction** Body dissatisfaction is defined as a negative subjective evaluation of the weight and shape of one's own body.

▶ **anorexia nervosa [an-or-EX-ee-uh ner-VOH-sah]** An eating disorder marked by prolonged refusal to eat, self-starvation and excessive weight loss, distorted body image, and an intense and irrational fear of becoming fat.

▶ **purging** Emptying the gastrointestinal (GI) tract by self-induced vomiting and/or misuse of laxatives, diuretics, or enemas.

▶ **bulimia nervosa [bull-EEM-ee-uh ner-VOH-sah]** An eating disorder marked by binge eating followed by compensatory behaviors such as self-induced vomiting, use of laxatives or other drugs, excessive exercise, fasting, or other practices to avoid weight gain.

▶ **bingeing** Eating, in a discrete period of time (e.g., within a 2-hour period), an amount of food that is larger than most people would eat during a similar period of time and under similar circumstances, while simultaneously experiencing a loss of control or feeling that one cannot stop eating or control what or how much one is eating.

▶ **binge-eating disorder** An eating disorder marked by repeated episodes of binge eating and a feeling of loss of control. The diagnosis is based on a person's having an average of at least one binge-eating episode per week for three months. Also known as **compulsive overeating**.

▶ **compulsive overeating** An eating disorder marked by repeated episodes of binge eating and a feeling of loss of control. The diagnosis is based on a person's having an average of at least one binge-eating episode per week for three months.

episodes often are triggered by emotions such as frustration, anger, depression, and anxiety.[8]

Anorexia nervosa, bulimia nervosa, and binge-eating disorder may be experienced by the same person at different points of time. For example, a person may suffer from binge-eating disorder at one point in their lives, and anorexia or bulimia at another.[9] Studies also find that people with disordered eating behaviors during adolescence are at increased risk for dieting and disordered eating behaviors 10 years later.[10] **TABLE SED.1** shows the diagnostic criteria used to identify eating disorders.

TABLE SED.1
DSM-5 **Criteria for Eating Disorders**

Anorexia Nervosa

According to the DSM-5 criteria, to be diagnosed as having Anorexia Nervosa a person must display:
- Persistent restriction of energy intake leading to significantly low body weight (in context of what is minimally expected for age, sex, developmental trajectory, and physical health).
- Either an intense fear of gaining weight or of becoming fat, or persistent behaviour that interferes with weight gain (even though significantly low weight).
- Disturbance in the way one's body weight or shape is experienced, undue influence of body shape and weight on self-evaluation, or persistent lack of recognition of the seriousness of the current low body weight.

Subtypes:
Restricting type
Binge-eating/purging type

Bulimia Nervosa

According to the DSM-5 criteria, to be diagnosed as having Bulimia Nervosa a person must display:
- Recurrent episodes of binge eating. An episode of binge eating is characterised by both of the following:
  - Eating, in a discrete period of time (e.g. within any 2-hour period), an amount of food that is definitely larger than most people would eat during a similar period of time and under similar circumstances.
  - A sense of lack of control over eating during the episode (e.g. a feeling that one cannot stop eating or control what or how much one is eating).
- Recurrent inappropriate compensatory behaviour in order to prevent weight gain, such as self-induced vomiting, misuse of laxatives, diuretics, or other medications, fasting, or excessive exercise.
- The binge eating and inappropriate compensatory behaviours both occur, on average, at least once a week for three months.
- Self-evaluation is unduly influenced by body shape and weight.
- The disturbance does not occur exclusively during episodes of Anorexia Nervosa.

Binge-Eating Disorder

According to the DSM-5 criteria, to be diagnosed as having Binge Eating Disorder a person must display:
- Recurrent episodes of binge eating. An episode of binge eating is characterised by both of the following:
  - Eating, in a discrete period of time (e.g. within any 2-hour period), an amount of food that is definitely larger than most people would eat during a similar period of time and under similar circumstances.
  - A sense of lack of control over eating during the episode (e.g. a feeling that one cannot stop eating or control what or how much one is eating).
- The binge eating episodes are associated with three or more of the following:
  - eating much more rapidly than normal
  - eating until feeling uncomfortably full
  - eating large amounts of food when not feeling physically hungry
  - eating alone because of feeling embarrassed by how much one is eating
  - feeling disgusted with oneself, depressed or very guilty afterward
- Marked distress regarding binge eating is present
- Binge eating occurs, on average, at least once a week for three months
- Binge eating not associated with the recurrent use of inappropriate compensatory behaviours as in Bulimia Nervosa and does not occur exclusively during the course of Bulimia Nervosa, or Anorexia Nervosa methods to compensate for overeating, such as self-induced vomiting.

American Psychiatric Association. *Diagnostic and Statistical Manual of Mental Disorders*. 5th ed. (DSM-5). Washington, DC: American Psychiatric Publishing; 2013.

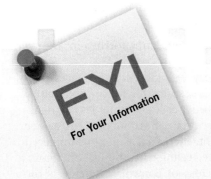

Night-Eating Syndrome: Not an Eating Disorder, but Sometimes a Concern

When a person grazes through the evening, finds him- or herself plotting midnight refrigerator raids, and wakes at night to eat, he or she might have *night-eating syndrome*. This syndrome is not an eating disorder, but some of its hallmarks are shared with people who suffer from binge-eating disorder. A person with night-eating syndrome:

- Eats more than half of daily calories during and after the evening meal
- Wakes up at least once a night to eat, especially high-carbohydrate snacks
- Feels tense, anxious, worried, or guilty while eating
- Lacks appetite for breakfast and postpones it for hours
- Persists in this behavior for at least three months

Night-eating syndrome is uncommon in the general population—about 1 to 2 percent of adults in the general population have this problem—but it affects up to a quarter of obese people. Although underlying causes are not fully understood, the disorder can result from a combination of biologic, genetic, and emotional factors. Several hormonal imbalances among night-eating syndrome sufferers have been noted, such as low levels of both melatonin (a sleep-inducing hormone) and leptin (an appetite-suppressing hormone). Cortisol—the so-called stress hormone that kicks in when we feel tense—appears higher at night in night eaters, perhaps arousing them to wake up and head for the kitchen. Stress, depression, and anxiety commonly affect mood among those with the condition.

The heavy preference for carbohydrates triggers the brain to produce immediate "feel-good" neurochemicals but a longer-term unsatisfied feeling because of blood sugar fluctuations. To reduce blood sugar fluctuations, a dietitian can help develop meal plans that emphasize protein over carbohydrate. Stress-reduction programs, including psychological therapy, can also be helpful.

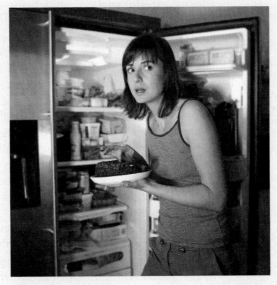

© Banana Stock/age fotostock.

Health Consequences of Eating Disorders

Eating disorders present a variety of serious physical and psychological health consequences throughout their duration. In fact, eating disorders have the highest mortality rate of any psychiatric illness. Up to half of the mortality rate of individuals with eating disorders can be attributed to cardiac and brain irregularities.[11] Other physical symptoms attributed to the poor nutrition that accompanies eating disorders include kidney dysfunction, electrolyte disturbances, dehydration, bone mineral and mass loss, and amenorrhea in women with anorexia nervosa.

Suicide, resulting from negative psychological consequences such as depression and irrational moods, is responsible for approximately half of the mortality rate in eating disorder cases.[12] Other less extreme, but still serious, psychological consequences are anxiety, obsessive thoughts concerning food and weight, increased isolation, impaired judgment, low self-esteem, guilt, shame, feelings of imperfection, diminished concentration, and feelings of loss of control.[13] Suicide is the most serious implication, yet self-injurious behaviors such as cutting, hitting, and scratching may also result from the psychological distress of eating disorders.[14]

Prevalence of Eating Disorders

Eating disorders, particularly bulimia nervosa, are secretive in nature.[15,16] For example, one of the best known prevalence studies on eating disorders found that only 43 percent of people with anorexia nervosa were recognized as having the disease by their primary care physicians; of those, 79 percent were referred for treatment. The secretiveness of eating disorders becomes more apparent when you consider that only 11 percent of people with bulimia were recognized by their primary care physicians; of those, only half (51 percent) were referred for treatment. In other words, most eating-disordered individuals do not receive adequate treatment.[17]

Anorexia is more prevalent in industrialized societies that have an abundance of food and a culture that equates beauty, particularly feminine beauty, with thinness. Nine out of 10 people with anorexia are female.[18] Studies show that the peak age of onset is between 15 and 19 years old.[19] Although anorexia was once predominantly reported in upper-class Caucasian adolescent females, physicians have reported cases of the disorder in young women from all social and ethnic backgrounds. In addition, anorexia has increased significantly among African American women.[20] A review of prevalence studies conducted throughout the world suggest prevalence rates of anorexia nervosa of between 1.2 percent and 4.2 percent in women and around 0.24 percent in men.[21] These percentages include reported cases as well as estimates of undiagnosed cases.

As noted, bulimia nervosa, particularly in its milder forms, often goes undetected. This is because people with bulimia are very secretive about their behaviors, typically limiting their binge-and-purge episodes to the middle of the night or times when they are assured of privacy. Also, unlike patients with anorexia or binge-eating disorder, whose body weights can hint at their underlying psychiatric disorder, the body weight of a patient with bulimia is usually average or only slightly above average. Several studies have found that as many as 40 percent of college-age women occasionally binge and purge—often enough to raise concern but too infrequently for an official diagnosis of bulimia.[22] A recent review of the literature concluded that the overall prevalence rate of bulimia nervosa (including undiagnosed cases) is approximately between 1.2 percent and 2.9 percent in women and approximately 0.5 percent in men.[23]

Prevalence estimates for binge-eating disorder are somewhat more difficult to estimate due to recent changes in how it is defined and diagnosed. Available data suggest that 3.5 percent of women and 2.0 percent of men in the United States have binge-eating disorder. Prevalence rates

Quick Bite

Estimates for Prevalence of Binge-Eating Disorder May Soon Rise

Prior to 2013, binge-eating disorder was included as part of a loose eating disorder diagnosis called Eating Disorder Not Otherwise Specified (EDNOS). A diagnosis of EDNOS was intended to describe cases of disordered eating in which abnormal behaviors were not yet frequent enough or causing the severe physical or psychological consequences necessary to meet the diagnostic criteria for anorexia or bulimia. Now that psychiatrists are starting to apply the updated criteria defined in *DSM-5*, experts estimate that the prevalence of binge-eating disorder in the United States will increase an additional 0.1 percent to 3.6 percent in women and 2.1 percent in men.

Vanucci A, Miller R, Pierpaoli C, Tanofsky-Kraff M. Overview of evidence on the biopsychosocial underpinnings of binge eating disorder. In Dancyger IF, Fornari VM, eds. *Evidence Based Treatments for Eating Disorders*. Hauppauge, NY; Nova Science; 2014:3-20.

in 13- to 18-year-old adolescents have been estimated as 2.3 percent for girls and 0.8 percent for boys.[24]

Key Concepts Eating disorders are unhealthy behavioral conditions that can have severe consequences on physical and psychological health. Eating disorders are alarmingly common in industrialized countries, particularly the United States. Eating disorders range from the self-starvation of anorexia nervosa to the compulsive overeating of binge-eating disorder.

No Simple Causes

🍎 **Why Is This Important?** The scientific understanding of causes of eating disorders has advanced considerably over the past few decades. Some risk factors are common to all eating disorders, whereas other risk factors are specific to anorexia, bulimia, or binge-eating disorder.

It's becoming clear that the causes of eating disorders are complex, multifaceted, and reflect a unique interaction of cultural, psychological, and biological factors.

The Cultural-Psychological Interaction

THINK
About It
1

Eating disorders can develop when people, especially women, feel social pressure to achieve an unrealistic standard of thinness. The pressure to achieve the "ideal" female form begins early, starting with girls' first Barbie doll, if not before.[25] Barbie and many other role-model dolls marketed to young girls often have grossly unnatural body dimensions (see **FIGURE SED.4**). Studies also suggest that television programing negatively affects the body image of young girls.[26]

How individuals feel about themselves can be a strong predictor of disordered eating patterns. Body dissatisfaction is a common problem among adolescent girls, and self-esteem is a relevant variable for helping to identify middle-adolescent girls who may be at risk for subsequent increases in body dissatisfaction.[27] Psychological factors are important as well. These encompass everything from peer relationships to relationships with parents. Studies have shown that adolescent girls who were teased about their weight by peers had a more negative image of their bodies and lower self-esteem, regardless of their actual weight.[28,29] Findings were similar for adolescent boys and for teens of varied racial and ethnic backgrounds. Studies also have linked more severe forms of emotional trauma to disordered eating. For example, trauma and the consequent distress have been linked to binge eating.[30]

Eating disorders also can be associated with dysfunctional family relationships. Some psychologists believe that people with anorexia and bulimia are trying to fulfill unrealistic parental expectations of perfection by succumbing to societal pressure to be very thin. Another strong predictor of dieting behavior is a woman's recollection of how much physical appearance was valued by her family members.[31] In addition, cross-sectional research suggests that friends are an important influence, especially among females. In this study, having friends who diet was positively associated with chronic dieting, unhealthy weight control behaviors, extreme weight control behaviors, and binge eating five years later among females, and with extreme weight control behaviors five years later among males.[32] **TABLE SED.2** summarizes the factors that increase risk of adolescent-onset eating disorders.

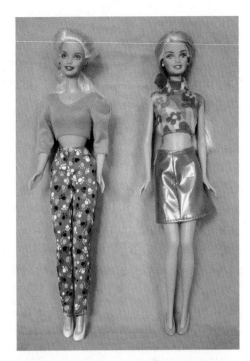

FIGURE SED.4 Thin is in. In 1998, Mattel overhauled Barbie's look for the millennium, giving her slimmer hips, a wider waist, and smaller breasts. Barbie's periodic overhauls are meant to fit the fashion of the times. Does the new Barbie (right) represent a realistic role model for today's young girls?

Quick Bite

Magazine Manipulations

When researchers studied fifth- through twelfth-grade girls in a working-class suburb in the northeastern United States, nearly 50 percent reported that they wanted to lose weight because of pictures in magazines. Frequent readers of fashion magazines were two to three times more likely to be influenced to diet or exercise to lose weight. Seventy percent of the girls reported that magazine pictures influenced their conception of the perfect body.

TABLE SED.2

Factors Increasing Risk for Adolescent-Onset Eating Disorders

Genetics
Body changes during puberty
Social pressures to be thin
Body image dissatisfaction
Restrictive diet
Impaired regulation of emotions
Depression
Low self-esteem

Worobey J. Barbie at 50: maligned but benign? *Eat Weight Disord.* 2009;14(4):e219-e224.

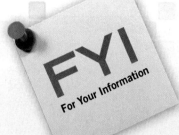

Exploring the Connection Between Negative Affect and Eating Disorders

The presence of body dissatisfaction, low self-esteem, anxiety, depression, obsessive-compulsive disorders, and emotional trauma in many individuals with eating disorders suggests that emotion (also called affect) plays a key contributing role as a potential cause of eating disorders. Collectively these emotional states share one thing in common—they are negative emotions. Psychologists refer to this as *negative affect*. Several models that theorize the causes of eating disorders have included negative affect as a major contributor. For example, the escape theory of binge eating hypothesizes that people binge because their self-perception causes feelings of negative affect.[a]

What causes eating disorders? Negative affect or negative emotions have often been cited as major contributors to the development of eating disorders. People with eating disorders, for example, often display heightened emotional sensitivity and reactivity to environmental triggers such as thoughts, beliefs, and attitudes about food and/or their own body. Such reactions to these environmental and personal stimuli then elevate a person's negative affect, which then prompts disordered eating in an attempt to relieve the negative emotional state.[b] This model is supported by several recent studies that suggest people with eating

disorders experience greater emotional swings around their eating-disordered behaviors than do people without eating disorders.[c]

a   Heatherton TF, Baumeister RF. Binge eating as escape from self-awareness. *Psychol Bull*. 1991;110:86-108.
b   Haynos AF, Fruzzetti AE. Anorexia nervosa as a disorder of emotion dysregulation: evidence and treatment implications. *Clin Psychol Sci Practice*. 2011;18:183-202.
c   Cook B, Wonderlich S, Lavender J. The role of negative affect in eating disorders and substance use disorders. In Brewerton T, Baker A, eds. *Eating Disorders, Addiction and Substance Use Disorders: Research, Clinical and Treatment Perspectives*. New York: Springer; 2014:363-378.

Biological Factors

Studies have linked abnormal levels of neurotransmitters, especially serotonin, in people with eating disorders.[33] Researchers, for example, have shown that bulimia patients experience spontaneous improvement in eating habits after taking antidepressants that increase brain levels of serotonin.[34] Many anti-obesity drugs also affect serotonin levels.[35]

Researchers have shown that eating disorders run in families with a history of **obsessive-compulsive disorder**, anxiety disorders, and depression.[36] Both depression and obsessive-compulsive behavior have been linked to atypical levels of serotonin and norepinephrine in the brain.[37] Finally, recent studies have found genetic evidence for anorexia nervosa[38] and binge-eating disorder,[39] and several other studies suggest bulimia nervosa runs in families.[40]

▶ **obsessive-compulsive disorder** A psychiatric disorder in which a person attempts to relieve anxiety by ritualistic behavior and continuous repetition of certain acts.

Key Concepts The precise causes of eating disorders remain obscure. Researchers have debated whether eating disorders are primarily psychological or genetic in origin. The current view is that eating disorders are a result of the complex interaction of cultural, psychological, and biological factors. In other words, eating disorders occur in biologically susceptible individuals exposed to particular types of environmental stimuli.

A Closer Look at Anorexia Nervosa

The term *anorexia nervosa*, which means "nervous loss of appetite," is misleading. People diagnosed with anorexia don't lose their appetites except in the final stages of the disorder. Instead, they are obsessed with food. Psychologists suggest that anorexia sufferers tend to be rigid, perfectionistic, all-or-nothing thinkers. Sufferers tend to lack a sense of independence and control. Parents may enable this illness by being overly protective or rigid or by holding a child to excessively high standards of achievement[41]; the child also may feel a significantly lower emotional connectedness, contributing to onset of an eating disorder.[42] Additional risk factors commonly associated with the onset of anorexia include extremely high levels of exercise, distorted body image, obsessive-compulsive disorders, and negative self-esteem.[43]

Warning Signs of Anorexia Nervosa

Parents and friends of people with anorexia often miss early signs of the disease. Avoidance of particular foods, unconventional food choices, or a rigorous exercise routine can easily be mistaken as a determination to lose a few pounds, rather than the warning signs of an underlying issue: an obsession with food and dieting. Many eating disorders start with a simple diet. Stress and a lack of appropriate coping mechanisms, dysfunctional family relationships, and drug abuse can cause dieting to get out of control.[44] Initially, someone with anorexia has a feeling of power. Sufferers enjoy a feeling of control as they learn to deny their hunger and limit their food intake. Early warning signs include obsessively counting calories; developing lists of "safe" foods and foods to avoid; cutting foods, even peas, into small pieces; and spending a great deal of time rearranging food on a plate. To suppress hunger, a person with anorexia may drink up to 30 cups of water or diet soda a day. Anorexia sufferers also may channel their obsessions with food into the preparation of elaborate meals for others without eating any of the food themselves.[45] **TABLE SED.3** shows the warning signs of anorexia.

THINK About It 2

As the disease progresses, anorexia sufferers become increasingly disillusioned, withdrawn, and hostile. Success always seems beyond their grasp. No matter how thin they are, they see themselves as overweight. (See **FIGURE SED.5.**) When they eat more than they think they should, they may induce vomiting or use **emetics**, **enemas**, **diuretics**, or **laxatives**. Or they might exercise relentlessly. Eventually, their efforts to avoid obesity take over their lives. They start to avoid social

▶ **emetics** Agents that induce vomiting.

▶ **enemas** Infusions of fluid into the rectum, usually for cleansing or other therapeutic purposes.

▶ **diuretics [dye-u-RET-iks]** Drugs or other substances that promote the formation and release of urine. Diuretics are given to reduce body fluid volume in treating such disorders as high blood pressure, congestive heart disease, and edema. Both alcohol and caffeine act as diuretics.

▶ **laxatives** Substances that promote evacuation of the bowel by increasing the bulk of the feces, lubricating the intestinal wall, or softening the stool.

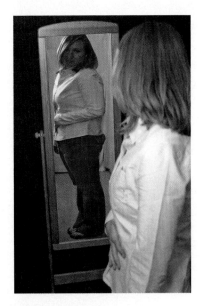

FIGURE SED.5. Distorted body image.

TABLE SED.3
Warning Signs of Anorexia

Anorexia nervosa is a disorder in which preoccupation with dieting and thinness leads to excessive weight loss. The person with anorexia may not acknowledge that weight loss and restricted eating are problems. Family and friends can help by recognizing the following warning signs:

- Loss of a significant amount of weight
- Continuing to diet (although thin)
- Pretending to eat or lying about eating
- Feeling fat, even after losing weight
- Fear of weight gain
- Cessation of menstrual periods for women
- Preoccupation with food, calories, nutrition, and/or cooking
- Strange or secretive food rituals
- Harshly critical of appearance
- Exercising compulsively
- Bingeing and purging

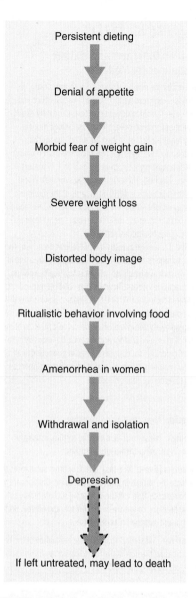

Persistent dieting

Denial of appetite

Morbid fear of weight gain

Severe weight loss

Distorted body image

Ritualistic behavior involving food

Amenorrhea in women

Withdrawal and isolation

Depression

If left untreated, may lead to death

FIGURE SED.6 The progression of anorexia.

situations that could expose their behaviors, and so withdraw more and more from friends and family. Groggy and irritable from food deprivation and sleep disturbances, people with advanced anorexia spend so little time on their schoolwork or jobs that their performance deteriorates. Yet when confronted with their obsessive dieting or deteriorating behavior, they will deny that anything is unusual.[46]

Treatment for Anorexia Nervosa

Just as there is no one cause for anorexia nervosa, there is no single way to treat it. Successful treatment of anorexia nervosa requires a collaborative approach by an interdisciplinary team of psychological, nutritional, and medical specialists.[47] With intensive therapy most patients can achieve normal weight; however, they may struggle all their lives with a moderate to severe preoccupation with food and body weight, poor social relationships, and depression. The longer someone suffers from anorexia nervosa before they receive treatment, the poorer the chances are for complete recovery; therefore, the earlier a patient begins treatment, the better the prognosis.

The course of anorexia varies. Typically, a patient recovers after a variety of treatments or enters a cyclical pattern of weight gain and relapse. Thirty to 50 percent of anorexia patients also have symptoms of bulimia, which can complicate diagnosis and treatment.[48] Tragically, in 6 to 18 percent of cases, the disease proves fatal (see **FIGURE SED.6**). Patients who have other emotional disorders, such as major depression or substance abuse, are the most likely to die from complications. Potentially fatal complications of anorexia include starvation and suicide.[49]

As with many psychiatric disorders, people with anorexia usually deny the danger of their situation. Family and friends often must intervene to get sufferers to treatment. The complex and multifaceted nature of anorexia requires a team of experienced healthcare professionals, including physicians, clinical dietitians, and psychotherapists. Some college counseling centers with a medical facility will treat college students or refer them to an eating disorders clinic.[50]

Restoring a patient's nutritional status is of prime importance. Otherwise, dehydration, starvation, and electrolyte imbalances can lead to serious health problems and even death (see **TABLE SED.4**). If a patient has lost more than 30 percent of body weight over a three-month period or weighs 70 percent or less of the standard weight considered healthy for height, hospitalization is essential. Restoration of body weight and return of menses are primary therapeutic goals.[51] Once the patient's physical condition has stabilized and physical symptoms of starvation have disappeared, psychotherapy can begin. Many therapists use a cognitive behavioral approach to help the patient challenge irrational beliefs and establish healthy attitudes and behaviors for gaining and maintaining weight.

To avoid detection, individuals with anorexia adopt behaviors to conceal their lack of weight gain. These include wearing concealing clothes or "bulking up" before weigh-ins by filling their pockets with coins or drinking large amounts of water or diet soda.[52] Psychologists use a variety of psychotherapeutic techniques to help the patient deal with underlying emotional issues such as depression. Treatment programs generally use a combination of behavioral therapy, individual psychotherapy, patient education, family education, and family therapy. Frequently, therapists find family conflicts at the heart of the eating

TABLE SED.4
Side Effects of Excessive Weight Loss in Anorexia Nervosa

Emaciation

- Loss of fat stores and muscle mass
- Reduced thyroid metabolism
- Cold intolerance
- Difficulty maintaining core body temperature

Hematological

- Leukopenia (abnormal decrease of white blood cells)
- Iron-deficiency anemia

Other

- Growth of lanugo (fine, baby-like hairs) over the trunk
- Osteopenia (mineral depletion in bone)
- Premature osteoporosis

Neuropsychiatric

- Abnormal taste sensation
- Depression
- Impaired thought process

Cardiac

- Loss of cardiac muscle, resulting in a smaller heart
- Abnormal heart rhythm
- Increased risk of sudden death

Gastrointestinal

- Delayed gastric emptying
- Bloating
- Constipation
- Abdominal pain

disorder. Ongoing therapy for the patient and family is key to successful recovery. As the patient's symptoms resolve, she or he must find new ways to relate to and communicate with family members. Family members must remain open and willing to change their behavior toward the person with the eating disorder.

Dietitians work closely with the psychotherapist to help patients develop a realistic view of food and to reshape their food selection and eating behaviors. Although no medication has been developed specifically to treat anorexia, some antidepressants have proved useful.

Most patients with anorexia nervosa require continued intervention after discharge from the hospital or treatment program. Support groups for people with eating disorders and their families can be an important link in the recovery process. Support groups also can be a useful technique for easing a resistant patient into treatment. With expert help and ongoing therapy, patients with anorexia can develop new mechanisms for coping with life's stresses, eventually replacing their disordered relationship with food with new, healthier interpersonal relationships.

Key Concepts The hallmark symptoms of anorexia nervosa are an obsession with thinness and self-imposed starvation. Sufferers manifest a body weight well below normal, a severely distorted body image, withdrawal from family and friends, and various physical and psychological changes related to starvation.

A Closer Look at Bulimia Nervosa

Gerald Russell, a British psychiatrist, first coined the term *bulimia nervosa* in 1979 to describe a syndrome of bingeing and purging in young women. The typical profile of an individual with bulimia is an unmarried Caucasian woman in her twenties or thirties with a normal or near-normal body weight. People with bulimia are more likely to be sexually active than are those with anorexia and often are involved in destructive relationships. However, almost anyone can be affected.

People with bulimia nervosa report suffering from depression and low self-esteem. Many were sexually abused as children. In general, food was a source of comfort, and eating gradually evolved into a tool for dealing with unpleasant events, from boredom to major life crises.

The relationships among dieting, severity of eating binges, and alcohol use have been studied in samples of college-age women. Researchers have found a relationship among drinking, dieting, and maladaptive coping patterns, such as using substances and/or denial as coping mechanisms.[53] It also has been shown that women who engage in binge eating or alcohol use act impulsively when distressed.[54]

Warning Signs of Bulimia Nervosa

A person with bulimia chronically binges and purges. The sufferer of bulimia feels out of control, has intense feelings of guilt or shame, and typically recognizes that the behavior is not normal. **TABLE SED.5** lists the warning signs of bulimia.

To meet the official *DSM-5* diagnostic criteria of bulimia nervosa, bingeing and purging occurs at least once per week for three or more months. Purging may be accompanied or replaced by fasting, excessive exercise, or other behaviors that compensate for the binge episode. Between binges, people with bulimia typically restrict their dietary intake to a limited number of low-calorie foods they consider "safe." This dietary control is an illusion, however. The average individual with bulimia is obsessed by thoughts of food and spends a great deal of time both planning the next binge and trying to resist the urge to binge.[55] **FIGURE SED.7** illustrates the binge-and-purge pattern of bulimia.

Just what triggers a binge is not clear. People with bulimia tend to be all-or-nothing thinkers. If they eat a single piece of food from their forbidden list, such as a cookie, they feel driven to consume the entire box. Some researchers believe that hunger caused by very restrictive

---

TABLE SED.5
Warning Signs of Bulimia

Bulimia nervosa involves frequent episodes of binge eating, almost always followed by purging and intense feelings of guilt or shame. The signs that a person may have bulimia include the following:

- Bingeing or eating uncontrollably
- Compensating for binges by strict dieting, fasting, vigorous exercise, vomiting, or abusing laxatives or diuretics in an attempt to lose weight
- Using the bathroom frequently after meals
- Preoccupation with body weight
- Depression or mood swings
- Irregular menstrual periods
- Dental problems, swollen cheeks or glands, heartburn, or bloating
- Personal or family problems with drugs or alcohol

dieting, combined with a buildup of everyday stresses, overwhelms the person's resolve and precipitates a binge.

During a binge, individuals with bulimia typically consume massive quantities of highly palatable "forbidden" foods such as pastry, ice cream, and candy. This gorging takes place over a relatively short time span—say, an hour or two. Binges may contain up to 10,000 kilocalories. Afterward, feeling physically ill from overindulgence, sufferers use a variety of purging techniques, such as self-induced vomiting or excessive quantities of laxatives, to rid themselves of the food. Or they may follow a binge with a period of very strict fasting and heightened exercise.

Purging leads to a variety of physical symptoms. Over time, gastric acid in vomit burns the lining of the pharynx, esophagus, and mouth; erodes tooth enamel; and can even result in loss of teeth. Repeated vomiting also can enlarge the salivary glands and erode the lining of the stomach and esophagus.

Excessive self-induced vomiting and diarrhea can upset the body's delicate biochemical balance through loss of electrolytes and body water. Among other dangers, changes in electrolyte balance can trigger an irregular heartbeat and precipitate a life-threatening medical crisis. Repeated use of emetics is toxic to the liver and kidneys, and abuse of laxatives can damage the lining of the large intestine. **TABLE SED.6** describes the side effects of bulimic purging.

Treatment for Bulimia Nervosa

It appears that bulimia may be more responsive to treatment than anorexia, perhaps because people with bulimia tend to recognize that their behavior is abnormal. Following treatment, more than half of patients report an improvement in their binge-eating and coping behaviors. About 30 percent of patients eventually become symptom-free. The rest, however, struggle with the disorder to some degree throughout their lives. To reduce the risk of relapse, therapists encourage patients to stay involved in support groups after completing formal therapy.

Cognitive behavior therapy is often used to help patients reshape their attitudes about food and identify situations that trigger bingeing. The therapist's goal is to help patients let go of their need to categorize foods as safe or dangerous, good or bad. Patients must learn techniques for dealing with stress and uncomfortable or painful memories and feelings. Depression, which typically accompanies this disorder, is often treated with antidepressants. Many patients with bulimia also require treatment for substance abuse. A patient is hospitalized when severely depressed or when purging is so frequent that physical damage has occurred or is imminent.

Medication can be an effective adjunct to psychotherapy. Serotonin-enhancing antidepressants have been used successfully to treat bulimia.

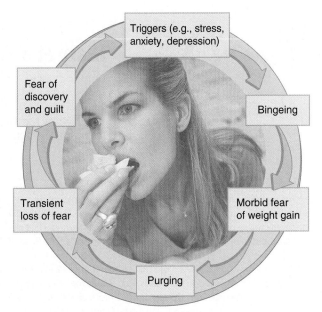

FIGURE SED.7 The binge-and-purge cycle of bulimia.
© Jack Star/PhotoLink/Photodisc/Getty Images.

TABLE SED.6
Side Effects of Purging in Bulimia Nervosa

Metabolic

- Electrolyte abnormalities
- Low blood magnesium

Gastrointestinal

- Inflammation of the salivary glands
- Pancreatic inflammation and enlargement
- Esophageal inflammation or ulcers
- Gastric erosion
- Dysfunctional bowel

Dental

- Erosion of dental enamel, particularly of front teeth, with corresponding decay

Neuropsychiatric

- Fatigue
- Weakness
- Impaired thought processes
- Seizures (related to large fluid shifts and electrolyte disturbances)
- Mild inflammation of peripheral nerves

Key Concepts Key symptoms of bulimia nervosa are binge-eating episodes at least once a week for three months, followed by behaviors that compensate for the binges, such as severe dieting, purging, or a combination of dieting and purging. The body weights of people with bulimia are typically close to or slightly above that considered healthy for their heights.

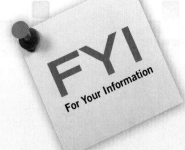

Diary of an Eating Disorder

Every time I leave one of my sessions I feel better. We talk about stuff; I feel, express, and even cry. Today was the third time since I left her office to come home and throw up. I think things are getting better despite the fact that my mind focuses 80 percent of the time on food during the 55 minutes. But it's like the kitchen is a refuge for my mind. I always know it will be there, waiting to embrace me when I get home.

Alone is how I hope to find it. I have been thinking of what I will sink my teeth into first. Usually I go for the fat-free chocolate cake, then to the frozen yogurt (which makes it all come up much smoother). I don't think this is normal, though I am not really concerned. I feel like a million-pound weight has been swept away by the effortless flush of the toilet. The hardest thing is to look in the mirror after I have thrown up. Sometimes I wipe my face before I look. Other times I leave the spit, bile, and food on my mouth and hands. I just stand there holding my hands up, with my shoulders slumped over. I produce this expression of absolute helplessness—then I laugh. I guess I am amazed by the act I've just committed. I can't explain why, I can't believe that it is really me doing this. Why would I do something like throw up? I really have no reason to torture myself. Bulimia was always them—I can't possibly be like that. I throw up, but I am not a bulimic. I sure as hell don't have an eating disorder.

I am totally for this whole counseling thing because I feel sad a lot and I want to feel better. But I can't leave there and not feel that I have to get this crap out. All this stuff that we talk about.

Today, Dr. Tant asked me when this all began. My first thought was, "Oh this throwing up thing? I can't remember." But I do recall one time when my ex-boyfriend Matt and I had gone to a really nice dinner. My recollection of the evening was that it was perfect. I remember thinking about how this food was really fattening, though, and how it would make me fat if I kept it down. I didn't know or have the willpower to just not eat it. Over and over I tortured and berated myself about the effects this dinner would have on my body. I couldn't bear it. This dinner was no longer one meal; it was going to ruin my body and make me fat. I couldn't stand that food being inside me another moment. Looking back I can't imagine how I could have thrown up right there on the side of the road. It was like I had no couth. I told Matt to pull over, and I just stuck my hand down my throat. Rationalizing the act while engaging in it, I then jumped back in the truck to carry on with the night. We never discussed my vile act other than Matt saying, "I can't believe you just did that."

"I know," I responded, "but it just was making me feel so sick. I mean, my stomach was really nauseous [sic]." Basically I don't know when I began this war with myself, but I know it caused me to fear myself. The rest is a blur—its beginning, its incentive. I heard Dr. Tant's question. I just didn't have the answer.

—Chelsea Browning Smith

Reproduced from Smith CB. *Diary of an Eating Disorder*. Dallas, TX: Taylor Publishing Company; 1998. Reprinted by permission of Taylor Trade Publishing, an imprint of Rowman & Littlefield Publishing Group.

A Closer Look at Binge-Eating Disorder

Overeating has been reported in the medical literature from the earliest records. However, the scientific understanding of when overeating becomes a diagnosable eating disorder (that is, *binge-eating disorder*) has only recently come into sharp focus, with its addition to the *DSM-5*. Accordingly, less is known about risk factors for this disorder compared with other eating disorders. What is known is that individuals with binge-eating disorder are usually overweight or obese and display more social problems during adolescence, show impulsive traits during youth, may be more likely to have dramatic or avoidant-type personality disorders, and may have difficulty regulating negative emotions. Additionally, adults with binge-eating disorder may experience weight-related teasing by close family members, social isolation, or some form of interpersonal violence.[56]

Warning Signs of Binge-Eating Disorder

Many binge eaters begin dieting in grade school and start bingeing during adolescence or in their early twenties. Typically, they try numerous weight-loss programs without long-term success. Binge eaters exhibit many of the same characteristics as individuals with bulimia. Previous research has found that approximately 20 percent have

TABLE SED.7
Warning Signs of Binge-Eating Disorder

Binge eaters, like bulimia sufferers, experience periods of uncontrolled eating that they usually keep secret. Binge eaters often are depressed and sometimes have other psychological problems. Signs that a person may have a binge-eating disorder include the following:

- Episodes of binge eating
- Eating when not physically hungry
- Frequent dieting
- Feeling unable to stop eating voluntarily
- Awareness that eating patterns are abnormal
- Weight fluctuations
- Depressed mood
- Attributing social and professional successes and failures to weight

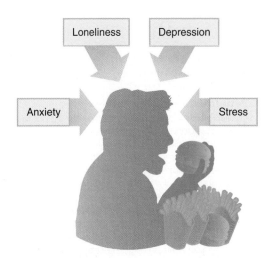

FIGURE SED.8 Emotions. Feelings of loneliness, depression, anxiety, or stress can trigger a binge-eating episode.

clinical depression.[57] Feelings of depression, loneliness, anxiety, or stress can precipitate a binge. Like other patients with eating disorders, those with binge-eating disorder may be all-or-nothing thinkers. They tend to categorize foods as safe or dangerous. Eating even a small serving of a forbidden food can trigger a binge.

THINK About It 3 Typical binge foods include sweets, pastries, ice cream, and high-fat snacks such as nuts and chips. However, if junk foods aren't handy, binge eaters might eat large quantities of starchy foods such as potatoes, bread, and pasta. **TABLE SED.7** lists the warning signs of binge-eating disorder, and **FIGURE SED.8** illustrates some factors that trigger binge eating.

During therapy sessions, many binge eaters report feeling helpless to influence the course of events or behaviors of others around them (see **FIGURE SED.9**).

Treatment for Binge-Eating Disorder

Compared to anorexia nervosa and bulimia nervosa, not as much is known about the course and prognosis of binge-eating disorder. People vulnerable to this disorder often suffer from weight-related health problems, including type 2 diabetes, hypertension, degenerative joint disease, heart disease, and even certain cancers.

Psychotherapy focused on changing the patient's thinking (cognition) and behaviors around bingeing has proven effective. Adding exercise to cognitive behavioral therapy for binge-eating disorder is associated with greater reductions in binge-eating frequency, as well as improvements in fitness and physical self-perceptions and greater weight loss compared to cognitive behavioral therapy without exercise.[58,59] Long-term support is key to keeping binge eaters from relapsing. Self-help groups such as Overeaters Anonymous are one source of support. These groups are organized according to the 12-step philosophy of Alcoholics Anonymous. In addition, many hospitals in large urban areas have support groups led by trained therapists.

Many patients with binge-eating disorder benefit from antidepressant medications. These drugs reduce the urge to binge, most likely by altering the brain's serotonin level. Various weight-management medications are now in development. These also can curb the urge to binge.

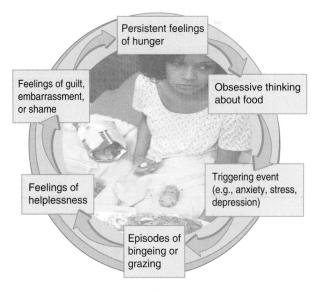

FIGURE SED.9 The vicious cycle of binge eating. Binge-eating disorder is the most common eating disorder.
© Jack Star/PhotoLink/Photodisc/Getty Images.

Quick **Bite**

When Plumpness Was Valued
In centuries past, extra pounds displayed one's wealth and prosperity. The wealthy could afford abundant food and didn't perform physical labor.

Quick Bite

Changing the Perception of Exercise to Help Combat an Eating Disorder

The value of exercise must be viewed carefully in the context of eating disorders. On the one hand, exercise may be used as a compensatory behavior, thereby exacerbating the progression and severity of an eating disorder. On the other hand, recent research has found that exercise can be used as a defense *against* eating disorders if patients are able to reverse their pathological attitudes and thoughts about exercise. Once a person relearns what healthy exercise is— by recognizing how the body feels after healthy amounts and types of exercise, and by understanding the need to properly support exercise with adequate nutrition—then exercise can help heal the damage done to the body by the eating disorder. A recent review of studies examining how to use exercise in the treatment of eating disorders has concluded that exercise may indeed be an efficacious add-on to standard eating disorders treatment.

Cook B, Wonderlich SA, Mitchell JE, Thompson R, Sherman R, McCallum K. Exercise in eating disorders treatment: systematic review and proposal of guidelines. *Med Sci Sport Exerc.* 2016;48(7):1408-1414.

Key Concepts Binge-eating disorder is the most common eating disorder seen in people of all ages and backgrounds. Like people with bulimia, those with binge-eating disorder consume significantly more food than is typically eaten in a given period of time. Unlike people with bulimia, those with binge-eating disorder do not purge or fast. Not all binge eaters are obese, although many obese people binge.

Eating Disorders: Specific Populations

Why Is This Important? Females suffer eating disorders at a much higher rate than males. Athletes of both genders can face distinct risks for developing eating disorders. Understanding the risks of eating disorders in men and in athletes of both genders is important to understanding the full picture of these serious psychiatric illnesses.

Males: An Overlooked Population

As many as a million boys and men in the United States struggle with eating disorders.[60] Yet males with eating disorders have been "ignored, neglected, or dismissed because of statistical infrequency of the disease, combined with the pervasive myth that eating disorders are a female disease," according to Arnold E. Andersen, former director of the Eating and Weight Disorders Clinic at Johns Hopkins University and scientific editor of the book *Males with Eating Disorders*.[61] Women who develop eating disorders may feel fat, but they typically are near average weight. In contrast, most men who develop these diseases are overweight. Many were seriously teased about their weight as children. Whereas women are concerned primarily with weight, men are concerned with shape and muscle definition. Indeed, men often develop disordered eating habits while trying to improve their athletic performance. More men than women diet to prevent medical consequences associated with being overweight.

Why do fewer males than females develop full-blown eating disorders? Some researchers suggest that there is a "dose-response" relationship between the amount of sociocultural pressure to be thin and the probability of developing an eating disorder. Note that articles and advertisements that promote dieting usually target young women rather than young men. When men are exposed to activities that require leanness, such as wrestling, swimming, and running, they exhibit a substantial increase in anorexic behavior. In fact, perceived pressure from social agents such as advertising, verbal messages, and social situations related to eating and dieting are strong predictors of eating disorders, indicating that cultural conditions, rather than gender, are the contributing factor for developing an eating disorder.[62]

THINK About It

4

Furthermore, the degree of thinness held up as desirable for women is 15 percent below a healthy body weight whereas the degree of thinness held up as desirable for men is well within the healthy limits of normal weight. Thus, women are more likely than men to alter their eating habits to achieve their desired appearance.

Like women, many men develop eating disorders during adolescence. But males can develop eating disorders during preadolescence and young adulthood as well. Doctors are so conditioned to viewing eating disorders as a female phenomenon that they often miss eating disorders in males. Likewise, the patient, his family, and friends may not recognize disordered eating patterns. Because our culture accepts overeating among men more readily than in women, binge eating in particular can go unrecognized in men. In addition, anorexia can elude diagnosis in men more often than in women because malnourished men don't experience definitive symptoms, such as a woman's loss of menstrual periods, that can alert professionals and others to the problem.

Athletes

Although participating in organized sports may benefit health, athletic competition complicates issues by contributing to psychological and physical stress. Add these pressures of competition to our cultural emphasis on thinness, and the risk of developing disordered eating increases for athletes. In a study of Division I NCAA athletes, over one-third of female athletes reported attitudes and symptoms that place them at risk for anorexia nervosa. Although most athletes with eating disorders are female, male athletes are also at risk—especially competitors in sports that tend to emphasize diet, appearance, size, and weight requirements, such as wrestling, bodybuilding, crew, and running.

Sports-related eating disorders are called **anorexia athletica**.[63] Athletes with anorexia athletica want to achieve an unrealistic body size that they consider desirable for competition, more so than their peers. In many cases, athletes with mild eating disorders are able to mask their illness as attention to fitness.

▶ **anorexia athletica** A generic term used to describe athletes with eating disorders.

Athletes who experience the following are at increased risk for eating disorders:

- Sports in which weight restrictions, muscularity, and general appearance are important, such as gymnastics, diving, bodybuilding, or wrestling
- Sports in which the individual, rather than a team, is the primary focus, such as gymnastics, running, figure skating, and diving
- Endurance sports such as track and field, running, and swimming
- A strong belief that reducing weight will improve performance
- Coaches who ignore the person and focus primarily on success and performance

Low self-esteem; family dysfunction (including parents who live through the success of their child in sport); families with eating disorders; chronic dieting; history of physical or sexual abuse; peer, family, and cultural pressures to be thin; and other traumatic life experiences are also risk factors.

Four risk factors are thought to particularly contribute to a female athlete's vulnerability to developing an eating disorder: social influences that emphasize thinness, performance anxiety, negative self-appraisal of athletic achievement, and identity based solely on participation in athletics.

The Female Athlete Triad

Although the majority of female athletes benefit from increased physical activity, there are those who go too far and risk developing a trio of medical problems (see **FIGURE SED.10**). Female athletes who fall prey to the "thin-at-any-cost" philosophy are at risk of developing a condition known as the **female athlete triad** (see **FIGURE SED.11**). This syndrome is characterized by problems with the interrelationship among energy availability, menstrual function, and bone mineral density, which can have clinical consequences including eating disorders, **amenorrhea**, and premature osteoporosis.[64]

Who is at the greatest risk of suffering from the female athlete triad? They tend to be female athletes who compete in endurance sports such as long-distance running, aesthetic sports such as gymnastics, antigravitational sports such as indoor rock climbing, and sports with weight classifications such as karate or wrestling.[65]

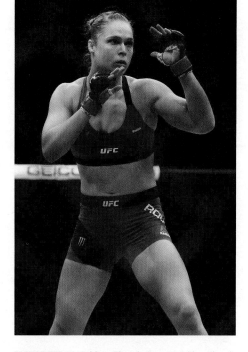

FIGURE SED.10 Athlete Rhonda Rousey. Athlete Rhonda Rousey has spoken about her experience overcoming an eating disorder, and the difficulty she has faced from being constantly in the public eye.

▶ **female athlete triad** A syndrome in young female athletes that involves disordered eating, amenorrhea, and lowered bone density.

▶ **amenorrhea [A-men-or-EE-a]** Absence or abnormal stoppage of menses in a female; commonly indicated by the absence of three to six consecutive menstrual cycles.

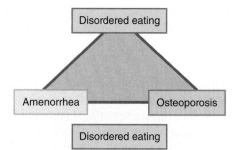

Disordered eating

The athlete develops one or more
harmful eating behaviors in an attempt
to lose weight. The result is an energy deficit.

Amenorrhea

An energy deficit leads to a reduction
in body fat. Once body fat falls below
about 20 percent, the athlete's body often
stops producing the hormones needed
to make estrogen, resulting in
menstrual cycle irregularities.

Osteoporosis

The lack of estrogen decreases calcium absorption
and retention. Dietary deficiency of calcium also is common.
Left untreated, this lack of calcium leads to bone loss,
stress fractures, and osteoporosis.

FIGURE SED.11 Female athlete triad. Disordered eating that results in excessive weight loss can lead to amenorrhea, which, in turn, can lead to osteoporosis.

Triad Factor 1: Disordered Eating

Restrictive eating behaviors practiced by girls and women in sports or physical activities that emphasize leanness are of special concern. When these athletes try to lose weight as a way to improve their athletic performance, they may be putting themselves at risk for disordered eating. Research suggests that female athletes are at greater risk for disordered eating than females not involved with an athletics program.[66]

Triad Factor 2: Amenorrhea

Once body fat falls below 20 percent, a woman's estrogen levels often drop significantly. As a result, women's bodies enter a menopause-like state years ahead of time. Their periods become irregular or cease altogether. Bone loss accelerates just as it would after natural menopause. Many female athletes who suffer from this triad have the decreased bone density of women in their fifties and sixties. Weakened bones are more likely to fracture during exercise or daily activities. Stress fractures can be a red flag for the female athlete triad. Because much of this bone loss is irreversible, women who suffer from the female athlete triad are at increased risk of developing osteoporosis.[67]

In the general population, 2 to 5 percent of women have amenorrhea. However, the prevalence is much higher in athletes.[68] Amenorrhea in athletic women is related to the combined effects of increased physical activity, weight loss, low body fat levels, and insufficient energy intake.

Triad Factor 3: Premature Osteoporosis

Health consequences of amenorrhea often include premature osteoporosis. Research shows that amenorrheic athletes experience rapid loss of bone mineral density in the spine, which can spread to other parts of the skeleton if amenorrhea continues for a long time.

Treatment involves replacing estrogen, which is low in amenorrheic females. Calcium supplementation is also recommended. Although bone mineralization may never return to normal in amenorrheic athletes, studies indicate that reducing the intensity of training, improving dietary intake, and increasing body weight can help restore menstruation and increase bone density.[69] To help combat this alarming trend, the American College of Sports Medicine and the National Collegiate Athletic Association (NCAA) have established an eating disorders awareness campaign aimed at coaches and trainers. The NCAA also has a three-part video series, *Nutrition and Eating Disorders*, to acquaint coaches and trainers with the causes and effects of eating disorders as well as the steps to take when they suspect an athlete has an eating disorder.

Screening, referral, and education are keys to preventing the female athlete triad. Prevention and treatment are most successful when they are interdisciplinary efforts provided by a team of medical, athletic, nutrition, and mental health experts. Proactive sports education includes reducing the emphasis on body weight, eliminating group weigh-ins, treating each athlete individually, and facilitating healthy weight management.

Key Concepts Like women, men typically develop eating disorders during adolescence and young adulthood, but they are more often overweight and striving for a particular body shape and muscularity. In addition, athletics can be a gateway to eating disorders in both men and women. Female athletes who develop restrictive eating habits are at risk for developing a severe syndrome known as the female athlete triad. Disordered eating, amenorrhea, and abnormally low bone density characterize this syndrome. If not corrected, the female athlete triad can hinder athletic performance and set the stage for lifelong health problems.

Combating Eating Disorders

Why Is This Important? Eating disorders should never be taken lightly or considered a phase that someone will outgrow. Accurate diagnosis and early treatment are imperative to improving the chances of recovery.

Eating disorders are extremely difficult to treat, although advances in neurochemistry and scientific understanding of the mind–body connection provide new avenues of treatment. Most experts agree that emphasis should be placed on preventing eating disorders through strong family support. See **TABLE SED.8**.

THINK About It 5

Preventing eating disorders depends on establishing appropriate mind–body–food relationships. Eating intuitively, an alternative approach to the diet mentality of our culture, suggests that we should trust ourselves and follow the body's signals. This approach might entail reframing our relationships to our body—for example, learning to distinguish physical from emotional feelings and gaining a sense of body wisdom. It's also a process of making peace with food and expunging constant "food worry" thoughts. One plan for learning to eat intuitively is presented in **TABLE SED.9**.

Although intuitive eating appears simple, it entails complex processes. For example, one basic principle of intuitive eating is the ability to respond to inner body cues. "Eat when you're hungry, and stop

TABLE SED.8
Combating Disordered Eating in Athletes

Deemphasize Body Weight

Do not view the athlete's weight as the primary contributor to, or detractor from, athletic performance. Research indicates that athletes can achieve appropriate weight and fitness when the focus is on physical conditioning and strength development, as well as the cognitive and emotional aspects of performance.

Eliminate Group Weigh-ins

Often viewed as a way to motivate the team, the practice of group weigh-ins can be destructive to people who are struggling with their body image and disordered eating. If there is a legitimate reason for weighing an athlete, explain the reason and weigh the athlete privately.

Treat Each Athlete Individually

Many athletes have an unrealistic perception of what an ideal body weight is, especially in sports for which leanness is considered important. Additionally, athletes may strive for weight and body composition that are realistic in only a few genetically endowed people. It is important to understand that genetic and biological processes, rather than one's willpower to control food intake, affect a person's weight.

Facilitate Healthy Weight Management

Be sensitive to issues related to weight control and dieting. Because many athletes have limited knowledge of sports nutrition, they resort to pathogenic weight-loss practices. Athletes can benefit from nutrition counseling by a sports nutritionist or a registered dietitian who has experience in working with athletes and disordered eating.

Thompson RA, Sherman RT. Reducing the risk of eating disorders in athletics. *Eating Disorders: Journal of Treatment and Prevention*. 1993;1:65-78. Reproduced by permission of Taylor & Francis Ltd, http://www.tandf.co.uk/journals.

TABLE SED.9
Intuitive Eating

1. Reject the Diet Mentality

Throw out the diet books and magazine articles that offer you false hope of losing weight quickly, easily, and permanently. Get angry at the lies that have led you to feel as if you were a failure every time a new diet stopped working and you gained back all of the weight. If you allow even one small hope to linger that a new and better diet might be lurking around the corner, it will prevent you from being free to rediscover intuitive eating.

2. Honor Your Hunger

Keep your body biologically fed with adequate energy and carbohydrates. Otherwise you can trigger a primal drive to overeat. Once you reach the moment of excessive hunger, all intentions of moderate, conscious eating are fleeting and irrelevant. Learning to honor this first biological signal sets the stage for rebuilding trust with yourself and food.

3. Make Peace with Food

Call a truce, stop the food fight! Give yourself unconditional permission to eat. If you tell yourself that you can't or shouldn't have a particular food, it can lead to intense feelings of deprivation that build into uncontrollable cravings and, often, bingeing. When you finally "give in" to your forbidden food, eating will be experienced with such intensity that it usually results in overeating and overwhelming guilt.

4. Challenge the Food Police

Scream a loud "NO" to thoughts in your head that declare you're "good" for eating minimal calories or "bad" because you ate a piece of chocolate cake. The Food Police monitor the unreasonable rules that dieting has created. The police station is housed deep in your psyche, and its loudspeaker shouts negative barbs, hopeless phrases, and guilt-provoking indictments. Chasing the Food Police away is a critical step in returning to intuitive eating.

5. Respect Your Fullness

Listen for the body signals that tell you that you are no longer hungry. Observe the signs that show that you're comfortably full. Pause in the middle of a meal or food and ask yourself how the food tastes, and what is your current fullness level?

6. Discover the Satisfaction Factor

The Japanese have the wisdom to promote pleasure as one of their goals of healthy living. In our fury to be thin and healthy, we often overlook one of the most basic gifts of existence—the pleasure and satisfaction that can be found in the eating experience. When you eat what you really want, in an environment that is inviting and conducive, the pleasure you derive will be a powerful force in helping you feel satisfied and content. By providing this experience for yourself, you will find that it takes much less food to decide you've had "enough."

TABLE SED.9 (*continued*)
Intuitive Eating

7. Honor Your Feelings Without Using Food

Find ways to comfort, nurture, distract, and resolve your issues without using food. Anxiety, loneliness, boredom, and anger are emotions we all experience throughout life. Each has its own trigger, and each has its own appeasement. Food won't fix any of these feelings. It may comfort for the short term, distract from the pain, or even numb you into a food hangover. But food won't solve the problem. If anything, eating for an emotional hunger will only make you feel worse in the long run. You'll ultimately have to deal with the source of the emotion as well as the discomfort of overeating.

8. Respect Your Body

Accept your genetic blueprint. Just as a person with a shoe size of 8 would not expect to realistically squeeze into a size 6, it is equally as futile (and uncomfortable) to have the same expectation with body size. But mostly, respect your body, so you can feel better about who you are. It's hard to reject the diet mentality if you are unrealistic and overly critical about your body shape.

9. Exercise: Feel the Difference

Forget militant exercise. Just get active and feel the difference. Shift your focus to how it feels to move your body, rather than the calorie-burning effect of exercise. If you focus on how you feel from working out, such as energized, it can make the difference between rolling out of bed for a brisk morning walk or hitting the snooze alarm. If when you wake up, your only goal is to lose weight, it's usually not a motivating factor in that moment of time.

10. Honor Your Health: Gentle Nutrition

Make food choices that honor your health and taste buds while making you feel well. Remember that you don't have to eat a perfect diet to be healthy. You will not suddenly get a nutrient deficiency or gain weight from one snack, one meal, or one day of eating. It's what you eat consistently over time that matters; progress, not perfection, is what counts.

Courtesy of Evelyn Tribole and Elyse Resch. http://www.intuitiveeating.com.

when you're full" may sound like a no-brainer, but it requires developing sensitivity to your body's signals.

The National Institutes of Health (NIH) believes that healthcare professionals should lead the eating disorder prevention effort by learning to promote self-esteem in their patients and teaching patients that people can be healthy at every size. Ideally, this approach would have a ripple effect: Patients would transmit these beliefs to others. A variety of public information campaigns aimed at parents and people who work with children and adolescents have evolved over the past decade to help promote eating disorder awareness. (See **TABLE SED.10**.) One of the most prominent examples is the Body Size Acceptance campaign coordinated through the University of California, Berkeley, under the direction of Joanne Ikeda.

Quick **Bite**

Scary Statistics
About 5 million Americans have anorexia nervosa, bulimia, or binge-eating disorders. Researchers estimate that 15 percent of young women have disordered eating attitudes and behaviors. Every year an estimated 1,000 people die from anorexia nervosa.

TABLE SED.10
Preventing Eating Disorders

To join the effort to prevent eating disorders, follow these tips:
- Celebrate the diversity of human body shapes and sizes.
- Present accurate information about nutrition, weight management, and health.
- Discourage restrictive eating practices, including skipping meals.
- Encourage people to eat in response to hunger, not emotions.
- Reinforce messages about good eating and activity patterns at school and at home.
- Carefully phrase comments about a person's weight, body, or fitness level.
- Teach children and young people how to constructively express negative emotions.
- Encourage parents, teachers, coaches, and other professionals who work with children to do likewise.
- Encourage people of all ages to focus on personal qualities rather than the physical appearance of themselves and others.
- Find and promote images of fit people of all sizes and shapes.

Learning Portfolio

Key Terms

Study Points

- An eating disorder is a complex emotional illness, the primary symptom of which is significantly altered eating habits. Eating disorders occur in susceptible people exposed to particular types of environmental stimuli.

- Although eating disorders existed even in ancient times, they have become alarmingly common in industrialized countries.

- Eating disorders involve highly restrictive eating patterns (seen in anorexia nervosa), a combination of compulsive overeating and purging (seen in bulimia nervosa), or unrestricted binge eating.

- Anorexia nervosa is an obsession with thinness manifested in self-imposed starvation.

- Key symptoms of bulimia nervosa are binge-eating episodes occurring at least once a week for three months, followed by severe dieting, purging, or a combination of dieting and purging.

- Binge-eating disorder is the most common eating disorder.

- Like those with bulimia, people with binge-eating disorder consume more food than is typically eaten in a given period of time.

- From 1 to 5 percent of people with eating disorders are male.

- Many competitive athletes, both male and female, have disordered eating behaviors.

- Eating disorders are common in people who participate in body-conscious activities such as dance, wrestling, gymnastics, and bodybuilding.

- Disordered eating, amenorrhea, and abnormally low bone density characterize the female athlete triad.

- The best treatment for eating disorders is prevention. Once an eating disorder has become entrenched, intensive and prolonged treatment is typically required. Many people require lifelong support to maintain healthful eating and lifestyle habits.

Study Questions

1. List the diagnostic criteria for anorexia nervosa, bulimia nervosa, and binge-eating disorder.

2. What are the warning signs of anorexia nervosa?

3. What is the usual treatment for people with anorexia nervosa, and what do most experts say about their recovery?

4. What is the typical profile of a person with bulimia nervosa?

5. Describe an eating binge and all the behaviors that constitute purging.

6. When boys and men develop eating disorders, are they typically near average weight or overweight?

7. What are the factors of the female athlete triad?

Try This

Is There Any Help Out There?

How much help is available in your community for people with eating disorders? Scan the Web for eating disorder clinics, programs, and centers. Call them to inquire about their services. Do they have a psychologist, medical doctor, dietitian, nurse, and/or social worker on staff? Is it an inpatient or outpatient program? What is their philosophy of therapy? What is their success rate? What are their payment plans?

Getting Personal

Why Are You Eating?

Use this worksheet to evaluate why you are eating, your emotional response to eating, and how this may relate to your body satisfaction. Using the table below, list all of the foods and drinks that you consume as you consume them. Next, honestly consider how you felt before and after eating. Were you anxious, depressed, happy, excited, numb, or experiencing any other emotion? Finally, list any compensatory behaviors you have performed in between snacks and meals.

- Was there one reason for eating that appeared more often than any other; if so, what was that reason?

- Are health and nutrition concerns ever a reason for your eating? If not, how can you make eating for health and nutrition concerns a priority?
- Looking at your emotions and the behaviors that follow, what changes can you make to become a more mindful, healthy eater who is comfortable with and accepting of your body?
- If you aren't sure if what you're feeling is healthy, you should have it checked out. For example, you can visit the campus health clinic or go to www.nationaleatingdisorders.org to get more information, take additional screening quizzes, or find information about referrals for help in your area.

Time	How Satisfied with Your Body Are You?	Food or Drink Amount	How Did I Feel Before Eating?	How Did I Feel After Eating?	Did I Engage in Any Compensatory Behaviors After Eating?

References

1. Klump KL, Bulik CM, Kaye WH, Treasure J. Academy for Eating Disorders position paper: eating disorders are serious mental illnesses. *Int J Eat Disord*. 2009;42:97-103.
2. Engel SC, Adair CE, Las Hayas C, Abraham S. Health-related quality of life and eating disorders: a review and update. *Int J Eat Disord*. 2009;42:179-187.
3. Fairburn CG, Bohn, K. Eating disorders NOS (EDNOS): an example of troublesome "not otherwise specified" (NOS) category in DSM-IV. *Behav Res Ther*. 2005;43:691-701.
4. American Psychiatric Association. *Diagnostic and Statistical Manual of Mental Disorders*. 5th ed. Washington, DC: American Psychiatric Publishing; 2013.
5. Position of the American Dietetic Association: nutrition intervention in the treatment of eating disorders. *J Am Diet Assoc*. 2011;111:1236-1241.
6. Tylka TL. The relationship between body dissatisfaction and eating disorder symptomatology: an analysis of moderating variables. *J Counsel Psychol*. 2004;51(2):178-191.
7. Tylka TL, Subich LM. Exploring young women's perceptions of the effectiveness and safety of maladaptive weight control techniques. *J Couns Dev*. 2002;80(1):101-111.
8. Academy of Nutrition and Dietetic. *Manual of Clinical Dietetics*. 6th ed. Chicago: American Dietetic Association; 2000.
9. Siegel M, Brisman J, Weinshel M. *Surviving an Eating Disorder, Strategies for Family and Friends*. 3rd ed. New York: Collins Living; 2009.
10. Neumark-Sztainer D, Wall M, Larson N, Eisenberg M, Loth K. Dieting and disordered eating behaviors from adolescence to young adulthood: findings from a 10-year longitudinal study. *J Am Diet Assoc*. 2011;111(7): 1004-1011.
11. Sobel SV. Eating disorders. *Contin Med Ed Resource*. 2004;118:69-114.
12. Ibid.
13. Ibid.

Learning Portfolio (continued)

14. Paul T, Schroeter K, Dahme B, Nutzinger DO. Self-injurious behavior in women with eating disorders. *Am J Psychiatry*. 2002;157:886-895.

15. Fairburn CG, Cooper PJ. Self-induced vomiting and bulimia nervosa: an undetected problem. *Br Med J*. 1982;284:1153-1155.

16. Hoek HW. The distribution of eating disorders. In KD Brownell, CG Fairburn, eds. *Eating Disorders and Obesity: A Comprehensive Handbook*. New York: Guilford; 1995:207-211.

17. Hoek HW, van Hoeken D. Review of the prevalence and incidence of eating disorders. *Int J Eat Disord*. 2003;34:383-396.

18. Stice E, Yokum S, Zaid D, Dagher A. Dopamine-based reward circuitry responsivity, genetics, and overeating. *Curr Top Behav Neurosci*. 2011;6:81-93.

19. American Medical Association. JAMA patient page; anorexia nervosa. *JAMA*. 2006;295(22):2684.

20. Urquhart CS, Mihalynuk TV. Disordered eating in women: implications for the obesity pandemic. *Can J Diet Pract Res*. 2011;72(1):50.

21. Smink FR, van Hoeken D, Hoek HW. Epidemiology of eating disorders: incidence, prevalence, and mortality rates. *Curr Psychiatr Rep*. 2012;14(4):406-414.

22. Keel PK, Dorer DJ, Eddy KT, et al. Predictors of mortality in eating disorders. *Arch Gen Psych*. 2003;60:179-183.

23. Smink FR, van Hoeken D, Hoek HW. Op. cit.

24. Ibid.

25. Dittmar H, Halliwell E, Ive S. Does Barbie make girls want to be thin? The effect of experimental exposure to images of dolls on the body image of 5- to 8-year-old girls. *Dev Psychol*. 2006;42(2):283-292.

26. Cho JH, Han SN, Kim JH, Lee HM. Body image distortion in fifth and sixth grade students may lead to stress, depression, and undesirable dieting behavior. *Nutr Res Pract*. 2012;6(2):175-181.

27. Wojtowicz AE, von Ranson KM. Weighing in on risk factors for body dissatisfaction: a one-year prospective study of middle-adolescent girls. *Body Image*. 2012;9(1):20-30.

28. Yoo JJ, Jonson KK. Effects of appearance-related testing on ethnically diverse adolescent girls. *Adolescence*. 2007;42(166):353–380.

29. Heijens T, Janssens W, Streukens S. The effect of history of teasing on body dissatisfaction and intention to eat healthy in overweight and obese subjects. *Eur J Public Health*. 2012;22(1):121-126.

30. Krukowski RA, West S, Perez P, et al. Overweight children, weight-based teasing, and academic performance. *Int J Pediatr Obes*. 2009;4(4):274-280.

31. Harrington EF, Crowther JH, Shipherd JC. Trauma, binge eating, and the "strong Black woman." *J Consult Clin Psychol*. 2010;78(4):469-479.

32. Tagay S, Schlegl S, Senf W. Traumatic events, posttraumatic stress symptomatology and somatoform symptoms in eating disorder patients. *Eur Eat Disord Rev*. 2010;18(2):124-132.

33. Eisenberg ME, Neumark-Sztainer D. Friends' dieting and disordered eating behaviors among adolescents five years later: findings from Project EAT. *J Adolesc Health*. 2010;47(1):67-73.

34. Portela de Santana ML, da Costa Ribeiro H Jr, Mora Giral M, Raich RM. Epidemiology and risk factors of eating disorder in adolescence: a review. *Nutr Hosp*. 2012;27(2):391-401.

35. Lock J, Fitzpatrick KK. Anorexia nervosa. *Clin Evid* [Online]. 2009;2009:1011.

36. Redman LM, Ravussin E. Lorcaserin for the treatment of obesity. *Drugs Today (Barc)*. 2010;46(12):901-910.

37. Ahren-Moonga J, Silverwood R, AF Klinteberg B, Koupil I. Association of higher parental and grandparental education and higher school grades with risk of hospitalization for eating disorders in females. The Uppsala Birth Cohort Multigenerational Study. *Am J Epidemiol*. 2009;170(5):566-575.

38. Federici A, Kaplan AS. Overview of the biopsychosocial risk factors underlying anorexia nervosa. In Dancyger IF, Fornari VM, eds. *Evidence Based Treatments for Eating Disorders*. Hauppauge, NY; Nova Science; 2014:3-20.

39. Kirkpatrick SL, Goldberg LR, Yazdani N, et al. Cytoplasmic FMR1-interacting protein 2 is a major genetic factor underlying binge eating. *Biol Psychiatr*. 2017 May 1;81(9):757-769. doi: 10.1016/j.biopsych.2016.10.021. Epub 2016 Oct 25.

40. Brewerton T, Cook B, Wonderlich S, Berg K. Overview of evidence on the underpinnings of bulimia nervosa. In Dancyger IF, Fornari VM, eds. *Evidence-Based Treatments for Eating Disorders*. Hauppauge, NY; Nova Science Publishers; 2014:21-56.

41. Stice E, Marti CN, Shaw H, Jaconis M. An 8-year longitudinal study of the natural history of threshold, subthreshold, and partial eating disorders from a community sample of adolescents. *J Abnorm Psychol*. 2009;118(3):587-597.

42. Wood NA, Petrie TA. Body dissatisfaction, ethnic identity, and disordered eating among African American women. *J Couns Psychol*. 2010;57(2):141-153.

43. Ma JL. Eating disorders, parent–child conflicts, and family therapy in Shenzhen, China. *Qual Health Res*. 2008;18(6):803-810.

44. Huemer J, Haidvogl M, Mattejat F, et al. Perception of autonomy and connectedness prior to the onset of anorexia nervosa and bulimia nervosa. *Z Kinder Jugendpsychiatr Psychother*. 2012;40(1):61-68.

45. Position of the American Dietetic Association: Nutrition intervention in the treatment of anorexia nervosa, bulimia nervosa, and other eating disorders. *J Am Diet Assoc*. 2006;109:2073-2082.

46. Byrd-Bredbenner C, Moe G, Beshgetoor D, Bernign J. *Wardlaw's Perspectives in Nutrition*. 8th ed. New York: McGraw-Hill; 2009.

47. Smith M, Segal J. Anorexia nervosa: signs, symptoms, causes, and treatment. https://www.helpguide.org/articles/eating-disorders/anorexia-nervosa.htm. Accessed September 15, 2017.

48. Position of the American Dietetic Association: nutrition intervention in the treatment of anorexia nervosa, bulimia nervosa, and other eating disorders. Op. cit.

49. Ibid.

50. Monteleone P, Di Genio M, Monteleone AM, Di Filippo C, Maj M. Investigation of factors associated to crossover from anorexia nervosa restricting type (ANR) and anorexia nervosa binge-purging type (ANBP) to bulimia nervosa and comparison of bulimia nervosa patients with or without previous ANR or ANBP. *Compr Psychiatry*. 2011;52(1):56-62.

51. Mehler PS, Winkelman AB, Anderson DM, Gaudiani JL. Nutritional rehabilitation: practical guidelines for refeeding the anorectic patient. *J Nutr Metab*. 2010:2010. http://www.hindawi.com/journals/jnume/2010/625782/. Accessed September 15, 2017.

52. Forcano L, Alvarez E, Santamaria JJ, et al. Suicide attempts in anorexia nervosa subtypes. *Compr Psychiatry*. 2011;52(4):352-358.

53. Lock J, Fitzpatrick KK. Op. cit.

54. Gentile MG, Manna GM, Pastorelli P, Oitolini A. Resumption of menses after 32 years in anorexia nervosa. *Eat Weight Disord*. 2011;16(3):e223-e225.

55. Strong KA, Parks SL, Anderson E, Winett R, Davy BM. Weight gain prevention: identifying theory-based targets for health behavior change in young adults. *J Am Diet Assoc*. 2008;108(10):1708-1715.

56. Vannucci A, Miller R, Pierpaoli C, Tanofsky-Kraff M. Overview of the evidence on the biopsychosocial underpinnings of binge eating disorder (BED). In Dancyger IF, Fornari VM, eds. *Evidence Based Treatments for Eating Disorders*. Hauppauge, NY: Nova Science; 2014:57-88.

57. Grilo CM, White MA, Masheb RM. DSM-IV psychiatric disorder comorbidity and its correlates in binge eating disorder. *Int J Eat Disord*. 2009;42:228–34.

58. Pendleton VR, Goodrick GK, Poston WSC, et al. Exercise augments the effects of cognitive-behavioral therapy in the treatment of binge eating. *Int J Eat Disord*. 2002;31(2):172-184.

59. Vancampfort D, Probst M, Adriaens A, et al. Changes in physical activity, physical fitness, self-perception and quality of life following a 6-month physical activity counseling and cognitive behavioral therapy program in outpatients with binge eating disorder. *Psychiatry Res*. 219(2):361-366.

60. Allen KL, Fursland A, Watson H, Byrne SM. Eating disorder diagnosis in general practice settings: comparison with structured clinical interview and self-report questionnaires. *J Ment Health*. 2011;20(3):270-280.

61. Neumark-Sztainer D, Wall M, Haines J, Story M, Eisenberg ME. Why does dieting predict weight gain in adolescents? Findings from Project EAT-II: a 5-year longitudinal study. *J Am Diet Assoc*. 2007;107(3):448-455.

62. Fenske JN, Schwenk TL. Obsessive-compulsive disorder: diagnosis and management. *Am Fam Physician*. 2009;80(3):239-245.

63. Hudson JI, Hiripi E, Pope HG, Kessler RC. The prevalence and correlates of eating disorders in the National Comorbidity Survey Replication. *Biol Psychiatry*. 2007;61:348-358.

64. Resch M. Eating disorders in sports—sport in eating disorders. *Orv Hetil*. 2007;148(40):1899-1902.

65. Schaal K, Tafflet M, Nassif H, et al. Psychological balance in high-level athletes: gender-based differences and sport-specific patterns. *PLoS One*. 2011;6(5):e19007.

66. Nattiv A, Loucks AB, Manore MM, Sanborn CF, Sundgot-Borgen J, Warren MP. American College of Sports Medicine position stand: the female athlete triad. *Med Sci Sports Exerc*. 2007;39(10):1867-1882.

67. Zach KN, Smith Machin A, Hoch AZ. Advances in management of the female athlete triad and eating disorders. *Clin Sports Med*. 2011;30(3):551-573.

68. Nattiv A, Loucks AB, Manore MM, et al. Op. cit.

69. Hoch AZ, Pajewski NM, Moraski L, et al. Prevalence of the female athlete triad in high school athletes and sedentary students. *Clin J Sport Med*. 2009;19(5):421-428.

Chapter 10

Diet and Health

Revised by Don Ross

THINK About It

1   Is there a history of heart disease in your family?

2   Do you know your blood pressure?

3   How often do you worry about your personal risk of cancer?

CHAPTER Menu

- Nutrition and Chronic Disease
- Genetics and Disease
- Cardiovascular Disease
- Hypertension
- Cancer
- Diabetes Mellitus
- Metabolic Syndrome
- Osteoporosis

LEARNING Objectives

1 Describe how nutrition and other lifestyle factors influence the risk of developing chronic diseases.

2 Define and describe cardiovascular disease and its risk factors, including dietary and lifestyle factors for reducing the risk of atherosclerosis.

3 Identify risk factors for diabetes and explain dietary and lifestyle factors for reducing diabetes.

4 Describe osteoporosis, its risk factors, and dietary and lifestyle factors for reducing osteoporosis risk.

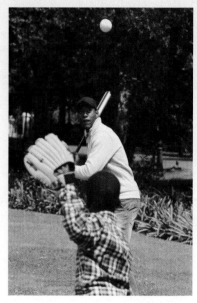

© Stockbyte/Thinkstock.

W hy did Joel Smith have a heart attack at age 48? Not his age. Few men suffer heart attacks before age 50. What about his cholesterol? Possibly. Joel inherited the tendency to have high levels of both low-density lipoprotein (LDL) cholesterol and homocysteine, an amino acid that is a risk factor for heart disease. Could his diet have been a contributing factor? Joel was a meat and potatoes guy. Over his lifetime, Joel enjoyed plenty of hearty meals with lots of meat, gravy, pie, and ice cream. He never developed the habit or pleasure of eating many fruits or vegetables.

Back in high school, Joel was a star athlete. Yet despite his enjoyment of sports, his current physical activity was limited to an occasional weekend basketball game. In fact, just prior to his heart attack, Joel was playing a spirited game of basketball with his kids. Sometime before his heart attack, Joel developed a respiratory infection from bacteria thought to contribute to arterial damage and atherosclerosis.

All these factors may have contributed to Joel's heart attack. It is difficult to separate out the relative importance of each factor, but, taken collectively, they culminated in a potentially fatal event. With some changes in his lifestyle, could Joel have avoided his early heart attack? Possibly. Some changes in his lifestyle, eating more fruits and vegetables, and limiting intake of fat may have helped, as would shooting hoops on a more regular basis or taking a brisk, 60-minute walk each day. You cannot change the inherited tendency to develop a disease, but many of us can reduce our risk by modifying our lifestyle.

Nutrition and Chronic Disease

🍎 **Why Is This Important?** Studying nutrition will give you insight into the prevention or reversal of many diseases. Furthermore, nutrition informatics can help you see trends across populations and show you which people will benefit most from nutrition interventions.

What does it mean to be healthy? The World Health Organization (WHO) defines health as "a state of complete physical, mental, and social well-being and not merely the absence of disease or infirmity."[1] Although most of us focus on the last part of that definition, "the absence of disease or infirmity," the first part is equally important. As you have learned, nutrition is an important part of physical, mental, and social well-being. It also is important for preventing disease.

Disease can be defined as "an impairment of the normal state of a living animal or one of its parts" and can arise from environmental factors or specific infectious agents, such as bacteria or viruses.[2] Diseases can be acute (short-lived illnesses that arise and resolve quickly) or chronic (diseases with a slow onset and long duration). Although nutrition can affect our susceptibility to acute diseases—and contaminated food is certainly a source of acute disease—our food choices are more likely to affect our risk for developing chronic diseases such as heart disease, diabetes, or cancer. In its report, *Diet, Nutrition, and the Prevention of Chronic Diseases*, the WHO states that "the diets people eat, in all their cultural variety, define to a large extent people's health, growth, and development."[3] Other lifestyle factors, such as tobacco use and exercise, in addition to genetic factors, also determine who gets sick and who remains healthy.

Nutrition Informatics

▶ **nutrition informatics** "The effective retrieval, organization, storage, and optimum use of information, data, and knowledge for food and nutrition related problem solving and decision-making. Informatics is supported by the use of information standards, processes, and technology." (Academy of Nutrition and Dietetics)

Nutrition informatics is the intersection of information, nutrition, and technology. With the U.S. healthcare system moving from a largely paper-based system to electronic records, dietitians have new tools and opportunities for chronic disease management through evidence-based decision support, quality management, outcomes reporting, and other strategies. As valued members and decision makers of the healthcare team, dietitians practice in a wide variety of settings from private practice to corporate wellness to the hospital clinic. Each setting has unique information needs, but all require skills in finding, evaluating, and sharing accurate food and nutrition information.

Nutrition informatics represents the next evolution in the practice of dietetics, and the Academy of Nutrition and Dietetics has established a collaboration with the Health Information Management Systems Society (HIMSS).[4] The academy has long been at the forefront of the exploration of biomedical informatics as it relates to nutrition, and HIMSS is a global organization focused on better health through information technology. The collaboration will support nutrition informatics competencies for Registered Dietitians/Dietetic Technicians, Registered (RDs/DTRs) and the nutrition community.

Healthy People 2020

Healthy People 2020, from the U.S. Department of Health and Human Services, is a comprehensive set of disease prevention and health promotion objectives for the nation.[5] Healthy People 2020's vision is to establish a society in which all people live long, healthy lives. The initiative includes four overarching goals, detailed in **FIGURE 10.1**. Because many diseases are impacted by diet, several goals of Health People 2020 can be reached in part by encouraging changes to the nation's eating habits. You will find these goals referred to throughout this chapter.

Health Disparities

▶ **health disparities** Differences in health outcomes and their determinants between segments of the population, as defined by social, demographic, environmental, and geographic attributes.

A key challenge to improving the diets of all Americans is overcoming the disparities in health associated with race/ethnicity, gender, income, education, disability status, and geography. **Health disparities** exist in

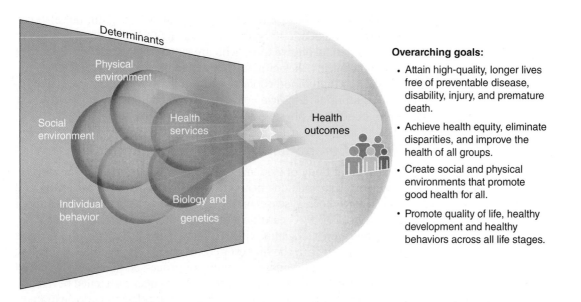

FIGURE 10.1 Healthy People 2020. Healthy People 2020 is a comprehensive set of disease prevention and health promotion objectives for the United States to achieve by the year 2020. This graphic framework illustrates the fundamental degree of overlap among the social determinants of health and emphasizes their collective impact and influence on health outcomes and conditions. For more on Healthy People 2020, visit www.healthypeople.gov.

Reproduced from U.S. Department of Health and Human Services. Office of Disease Prevention and Health Promotion. Healthy People 2020. Washington, DC. Available at http://healthypeople.gov/2020/about/GenHealthAbout.aspx. Accessed February 12, 2016.

people's access to doctors and health care, recreational opportunities, and healthful foods. For a tangible example of one way health disparities and nutrition intersect, think of a person on a tight income without a car whose closest food source is a convenience store with very limited fruits and vegetables. That person is likely to eat less healthfully than someone with more disposable income who lives close to a supermarket. The *CDC Heath Disparities and Inequalities Report* documents health disparities and provides a framework for comprehensive, community-driven approaches to reducing health disparities in the United States.[6,7]

Why are health and health outcomes so different among various groups? Beyond genetic susceptibility and traditional environmental factors are barriers to access found in our healthcare system. Consider for a moment the impact of cultural differences on nutritional advice from your healthcare provider. Does your provider speak your language and respect your culture and beliefs? When the answer is yes, trust is built between you and your provider. You are more likely to work hard to adjust your dietary habits according to your provider's advice. When the answer is no, suspicion and mistrust often result, and it is less likely that you follow your provider's recommendations carefully.

Obesity, Physical Inactivity, and Chronic Disease

Once considered merely an aesthetic issue, obesity is now widely recognized as a major public health problem. It is a risk factor for the major chronic diseases of public health significance in the United States and Canada: coronary heart disease, cancer, diabetes, hypertension, and metabolic syndrome. Good health habits and proper weight management are key components of a healthy lifestyle that avoids or at least delays the onset of these diseases. Often, weight loss—or, at a minimum, no further weight gain—can improve health outcomes dramatically.

A sedentary lifestyle not only promotes weight gain, but also is a significant independent risk factor for chronic disease. Physically active people generally outlive those who are inactive, and inactivity is almost as significant a risk factor for heart disease as high blood pressure, smoking, or high blood cholesterol. For all individuals, some activity is better than none. Physical activity is safe for almost everyone, and the health benefits of physical activity far outweigh the risks.

Dietary Components and Cardiometabolic Disease

A substantial body of evidence links diet with *cardiometabolic disease*, a category that includes heart disease (including atherosclerosis and hypertensive heart disease), stroke, and type 2 diabetes.[8] In a study of more than 700,000 cardiometabolic deaths, researchers found that nearly half were associated with 10 dietary factors. Excess sodium intake was associated with the highest percentage of deaths, followed by low intake of nuts and seeds, high intake of processed meats, low seafood omega-3 fats, low vegetables, low fruits, high sugar-sweetened beverages, low whole grains, low polyunsaturated fats (replacing carbohydrate or saturated fats), and high unprocessed red meats.[9]

Cardiometabolic mortality associated with each dietary factor was modestly higher in men than in women, primarily because of generally unhealthier dietary habits in men. Also, the top five dietary factors impacting men differed from those impacting women. (See **TABLE 10.1**.) Other observed health disparities included higher diet-related mortality for African Americans and Hispanics compared with whites, and for adults with low education versus high education.

Researchers also observed a few optimistic trends. Over a 10-year period, there was a decline in diet-related deaths associated with sugar-sweetened beverages, insufficient polyunsaturated fats, and low intake of nuts and seeds. Improvements were not uniform, however, and were small for less-educated people.

Public health strategies can help reduce health disparities. The Food and Drug Administration (FDA) recently announced voluntary sodium reduction targets for the food industry,[10] and several cities have imposed tax increases on sugar-sweetened beverages.[11] Federal government food programs for low-income people could be modified to encourage the purchase of fruits and vegetables as well as nuts and seeds, while discouraging sugar-sweetened beverages, processed meats, and high-sodium foods.

TABLE 10.1
Top Five Dietary Factors Associated with Cardiometabolic Deaths

Men			Women		
Rank	Factor	Intake	Rank	Factor	Intake
1	High processed meats	> 0 g/day	1	High sodium	> 2,000 mg/day
2	High sodium	> 2,000 mg/day	2	Low nuts and seeds	< 20.2 g/day
3	High sugar-sweetened beverages	> 0 g/day	3	Low vegetables	< 400 g/day
4	Low nuts and seeds	< 20.2 g/day	4	Low fruits	< 300 g/day
5	Low seafood omega-3 fats	< 250 mg/day	5	Low seafood omega-3 fats	< 250 mg/day

Data from Micha R, Peñalvo JL, Cudhea F, et al. Association between dietary factors and mortality from heart disease, stroke, and type 2 diabetes in the United States. *JAMA.* 2017;317(9):912-924.

Genetics and Disease

🍎 **Why Is This Important?** Nutritionists are combining genetic data with behavioral data, such as personal dietary practices, to find new connections to health and disease. Understanding the basics of genetics will help you appreciate the latest research findings.

In the last several years, knowledge has exploded regarding the relationship between our genetic makeup and disease. We now recognize that nearly all diseases have some genetic component. Most human illnesses occur because of the interaction of many genetic, environmental, nutritional, and lifestyle factors. (See **FIGURE 10.2**.) As the number one killer in the United States, cardiovascular disease is a good example of how genetic influences affect the development of disease.[12] A family history of heart disease indicates genetic vulnerability and is an important risk factor for developing the disease. Although some cancers, for example, breast cancer, have a genetic basis and affect many members of a given family, most cancers seem to be caused by a variety of factors.

THINK About It 1

Understanding how our **genes** influence our risk for disease has been a major goal of the **Human Genome Project**, an international effort spearheaded by the U.S. National Institutes of Health (NIH). The Human Genome Project is providing scientists with clues to the genetic variations that are responsible for common illnesses. Understanding the genetics of diseases will allow researchers to develop more effective medications and may lead to routine gene-based treatments.[13]

▶ **genes** Sections of DNA that contain hereditary information. Most genes contain information for making proteins.

▶ **Human Genome Project** An effort coordinated by the Department of Energy and the National Institutes of Health to map the genes in human DNA.

Quick **Bite**

Biological Blueprint
Nearly all 100 trillion cells in the human body contain a copy of the entire human genome, the complete set of genetic instructions necessary to build a human being.

Chronic diseases	High-fat diet	Excessive alcohol intake	Low complex carbohydrate/fiber	Low vitamin and/or mineral intake	High sugar intake	High intake of salty or pickled foods	Genetics	Age	Sedentary lifestyle	Smoking and tobacco use	Stress	Environmental contaminants
Cancers	X	X	X	X		X	X	X	X	X		X
Hypertension	X	X		X		in salt sensitive people	X	X	X	X	X	
Diabetes (type 2)	X		X				X	X	X			
Osteoporosis		X		X			X	X	X	X		
Atherosclerosis	X		X	X			X	X	X	X	X	
Obesity	X	X	X		X		X		X			
Stroke	X	X					X	X	X	X	X	
Diverticulosis	X		X	X			X	X				
Dental and oral diseases				X	X		X		X			

Dietary risk factors / Non-dietary risk factors

FIGURE 10.2 Risk factors for chronic diseases. Diet, lifestyle choices, and genetics interact to shape a person's risk profile.

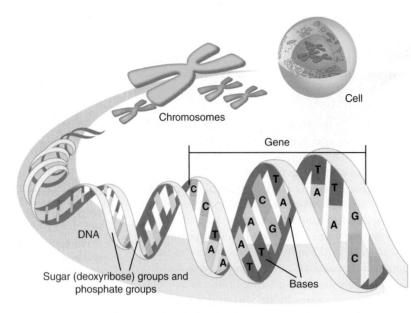

FIGURE 10.3 Structure of DNA. All the instructions needed to direct cellular activities are contained within the chemical DNA (deoxyribonucleic acid). The DNA sequence is the particular side-by-side arrangement of bases along the DNA strand (e.g., ATTCCGGA). This order spells out the exact instructions required to build proteins and create a unique person.

Courtesy of the Office of Biological and Environmental Research of the U.S. Department of Energy Office of Science. http://science.energy.gov/ber. Accessed February 12, 2016.

▶ **nucleotides** Subunits of DNA or RNA consisting of a nitrogenous base (adenine, guanine, thymine, or cytosine in DNA; adenine, guanine, uracil, or cytosine in RNA), a phosphate molecule, and a sugar molecule (deoxyribose in DNA and ribose in RNA). Thousands of nucleotides are linked to form a DNA or RNA molecule.

▶ **base pair** Two nitrogenous bases (adenine and thymine or guanine and cytosine), held together by weak bonds, that form a "rung" of the "DNA ladder." The bonds between base pairs hold the DNA molecule together in the shape of a double helix.

▶ **complementary sequence** Nucleic acid–base sequence that can form a double-stranded structure with another DNA fragment by following base-pairing rules (A pairs with T, and C pairs with G). The complementary sequence to GTAC, for example, is CATG.

▶ **genetic code** The instructions in a gene that tell the cell how to make a specific protein. A, T, G, and C are the "letters" of the DNA code; they stand for the chemicals adenine, thymine, guanine, and cytosine, respectively, which make up the nucleotide bases of DNA. Each gene's code combines the four chemicals in various ways to spell out three-letter "words" that specify which amino acid is needed at every step in making a protein.

▶ **mutation** A permanent structural alteration in DNA. In most cases, DNA changes either have no effect or cause harm. Occasionally, a mutation can improve an organism's chance of surviving and passing the beneficial change on to its descendants. Certain mutations can lead to cancer or other diseases.

The Workings of DNA and Genes

Our genetic instructions are carried by deoxyribonucleic acid (DNA), a molecule that can be visualized as an immensely long, corkscrew-shaped ladder—a double helix. (See **FIGURE 10.3**.) DNA is made of subunits called **nucleotides**. Each nucleotide contains one sugar molecule (deoxyribose—a five-carbon sugar), one phosphate molecule, and one base. The sugar and phosphate molecules make up the "side rails" of a DNA molecule, and the bases form the "rungs"; that is, the base in each nucleotide of one side rail joins with a base in a nucleotide on the opposite side rail. DNA has only four bases—adenine (A), thymine (T), guanine (G), and cytosine (C)—and each base is picky about its partner. To form a **base pair**, A always joins with T, and G always joins with C. Thus, the sequence of bases on one side of the ladder (for example, AGCGT) determines the **complementary sequence** on the other side (TCGCA). Using this "genetic alphabet," an enormous number of messages can be written.

Genes are sequences of DNA that carry the **genetic code** for making functional molecules, especially proteins. The genetic code combines the four "letters" of the genetic alphabet in various ways to spell out three-letter "words" that specify which amino acid is needed at each step in making a protein. Errors in the code can be harmless, or they can lead to serious disease. For example, people with sickle cell anemia have a mistake (called a **mutation**) in their genetic code for the amino acids making up the protein beta-globin. Beta-globin is part of the oxygen-carrying protein hemoglobin found in red blood cells. This mutated section of the genetic code in sickle cell anemia patients contains the sequence GTG (the code for valine) instead of GAG (the code for glutamate), so their cells manufacture beta-globin proteins with the wrong amino acid. Hemoglobin containing this faulty protein cannot carry a full load of oxygen and causes red blood cells to form a sickle shape.

Diet influences **gene expression**—the making of proteins. Components in the diet can enhance or inhibit gene expression, thereby increasing or decreasing protein synthesis. For example, folate status interacts with a genetic mutation that impacts the production of an enzyme that helps convert homocysteine to methionine. People with this particular DNA mutation have reduced enzyme activity and, as a result, higher homocysteine levels. When their folate status is low, their risk for heart disease is significantly elevated.[14] Scientists also are studying how folate status and this genetic mutation can influence cancer risk.

Nutritional genomics, or nutrigenomics, focuses on the influences of food components on gene expression and protection of the genome. Nutrigenomics integrates health, diet, and genetics, and it forms the foundation of *personalized nutrition*—the concept of adapting food intake to individual needs. If nutrigenomics can identify genetic predictors of diet-related disease risk, personalized nutrition practices may delay or avoid certain diseases. However, nutrigenomics and personalized medicine also have been the subject of much hyperbole. Unfortunately, current evidence does not yet demonstrate that personalized nutritional advice leads to improved health outcomes compared with following current dietary guidelines.[15]

Progress is being made. Big data analysis is rapidly advancing our understanding of the links between our DNA and disease risk. The study of nutrigenomics is increasing our understanding of how nutrition affects normal body functioning and the development or prevention of diet-related diseases. As we learn more about the genetic causes of disease and the lifestyle factors that influence them, we will be able to better screen individuals for disease susceptibility, and then target appropriate lifestyle interventions to reduce their risk.[16]

Key Concepts Diseases can be acute or chronic. Nutrition and other lifestyle factors such as obesity and physical inactivity strongly influence the risk of developing chronic diseases. Our genetic makeup also influences disease risk. Genes are segments of DNA that contain the code for making proteins. Gene expression can be modified by diet. Understanding how our genes can affect the course of a disease can influence future population screening and produce targeted interventions to reduce disease risk.

Cardiovascular Disease

🍎 **Why Is This Important?** Cardiovascular disease is the leading cause of death for Americans, with many links to poor diet. Dietary habits you can implement now to reduce your lifetime risk of heart disease include eating less fat while increasing intake of fruits, vegetables, whole grains, omega-3 fatty acids, and fiber.

Cardiovascular disease (CVD) is the leading cause of death in the United States and Canada, claiming one life every 40 seconds. More people die from CVD than from all forms of cancer combined. But not all the news is bad: Lifestyle changes and medical advances have led to significant progress in the fight against CVD.[17]

CVD is significantly related to what some people call the American way of life. Too many Americans eat a high-fat diet, are overweight and sedentary, smoke cigarettes, manage stress ineffectively, do not manage

▶ **gene expression** The process by which proteins are made from the instructions encoded in DNA.

Quick Bite

Adaptation Gone Awry
Sickle cell anemia is a hereditary blood disorder characterized by red blood cells that are a *C* or sickle shape. This disorder is a result of the human body adapting to resist malaria, a disease that attacks red blood cells, and is found primarily in people with sub-Saharan ancestry.

▶ **cardiovascular disease (CVD)** Any abnormal condition characterized by dysfunction of the heart and blood vessels. CVD includes atherosclerosis (especially coronary heart disease, which can lead to heart attacks), cerebrovascular disease (e.g., stroke), and hypertension (high blood pressure).

Quick Bite

Who Am I?
Our entire collection of genes, the human genome, contains about 25,000 genes. These genes consist of building blocks called base pairs. The human genome contains about 3 billion base pairs. Your mother supplied half of your genes and your father supplied the other half to create your unique combination. Unless you are an identical twin, no other person has your exact combination of genes.

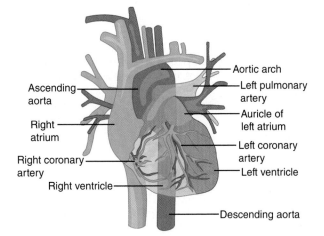

FIGURE 10.4 The heart and major arteries. Oxygenated blood is pumped through the arteries (red), and oxygen-depleted blood is returned to the heart via the veins (blue).

▶ **coronary heart disease (CHD)** A type of heart disease caused by narrowing of the coronary arteries that feed the heart, which needs a constant supply of oxygen and nutrients carried by the blood in the coronary arteries. When the coronary arteries become narrowed or clogged by fat and cholesterol deposits and cannot supply enough blood to the heart, CHD results.

▶ **atherosclerosis** A type of "hardening of the arteries" in which cholesterol and other substances in the blood build up in the walls of arteries. As the process continues, the arteries to the heart may narrow, cutting down the flow of oxygen-rich blood and nutrients to the heart.

▶ **plaque** A buildup of substances that circulate in the blood (e.g., calcium, fat, cholesterol, cellular waste, fibrin) on a blood vessel wall, making it vulnerable to blockage from blood clots.

▶ **endothelial cells** Thin, flattened cells that line internal body cavities in a single layer.

▶ **endothelium** See *endothelial cells*.

▶ **platelets** Tiny disk-shaped components of blood that are essential for blood clotting.

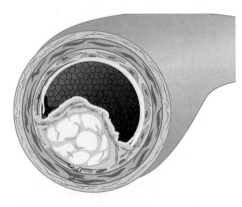

FIGURE 10.5 Development of atherosclerosis. Atherosclerotic plaque is formed by a buildup of fatty material in the wall of an artery. An artery narrowed by plaque is vulnerable to blockage by a blood clot, causing a heart attack or stroke.

their high blood pressure or high blood cholesterol levels, and do not know the signs of CVD. Of course, not all the risk factors for CVD are controllable—some people inherit a tendency toward persistent high blood pressure. But many factors can be changed, treated, or modified, so you have the power to significantly reduce your risk.

The Cardiovascular System and Cardiovascular Disease

The cardiovascular system consists of the heart and blood vessels (veins, arteries, and capillaries). (See **FIGURE 10.4**.) Together, they pump and circulate blood throughout the body. A person weighing 150 pounds has about 5 quarts of blood, which circulate about once every minute.

What Is Atherosclerosis?

When we talk about diet and heart disease, we are usually referring to **coronary heart disease (CHD)**. CHD is caused by **atherosclerosis**, a slow, progressive hardening and narrowing of the arteries by deposits of fat, cholesterol, and other substances. (See **FIGURE 10.5**.) When serious, atherosclerosis can result in angina pectoris (chest pain) or myocardial infarction (heart attack). Atherosclerosis of the cerebral arteries leading to the brain can cause a stroke.

Atherosclerosis is one type of arteriosclerosis, which literally means "hardening of the arteries." As deposits, called **plaque**, accumulate along the artery walls, the arteries lose their elasticity and their ability to expand and contract, thereby restricting blood flow. Once narrowed in this way, an artery is vulnerable to plaque rupture and blockage by blood clots.

Plaque buildup begins when excess lipid particles collect beneath the cells that line an artery, called **endothelial cells** or the **endothelium**. High cholesterol, high blood pressure, smoking, and diabetes can all damage the endothelium and initiate atherosclerosis. Certain viral and bacterial infections also can damage blood vessels, and a large number of infectious agents have been linked with an increased risk of vascular disease.[18] Infections can contribute to atherosclerosis by direct infection of vascular cells and indirect effects at other sites.[19]

Platelets, components of one of the body's protective mechanisms, collect at the damaged area and form a cap of cells, thereby isolating the plaque within the artery wall. The narrowed artery is vulnerable to blockage by clots that can form if the cap breaks and the fatty core of the plaque combines again with platelets and other clot-producing factors in the blood. If the heart, brain, or other organs are deprived of blood and the vital oxygen that blood carries, the effects of atherosclerosis can be deadly.

Cholesterol and Atherosclerosis

In the early 1960s, researchers identified high blood cholesterol, or **hypercholesterolemia**, along with smoking and high blood pressure, as a principal risk factor for coronary heart disease. They understood that a high-fat, high-cholesterol diet tends to raise blood cholesterol, and high blood cholesterol levels promote atherosclerosis. Atherosclerosis leads to artery disease and often causes heart attacks or strokes.

Total cholesterol levels do not tell the entire story. The levels of LDL and high-density lipoprotein (HDL) cholesterol predict a person's risk for developing atherosclerosis more accurately than the individual's total cholesterol levels. High LDL cholesterol is a greater risk than high total cholesterol, with some kinds of LDL being more dangerous than others. For example, high levels of **lipoprotein a [Lp(a)]**, a low-density lipoprotein, seem especially harmful. High levels of Lp(a) prevent the normal breakup of blood clots that cause heart attack or stroke. High levels of triglycerides and other blood lipids also increase the risk of cardiovascular disease, as do low HDL cholesterol levels.

Deaths from coronary heart disease have fallen dramatically over the past two decades. That drop seems to be correlated with a drop in total cholesterol levels (see **FIGURE 10.6**) and reductions in smoking. These gains, however, are threatened to be offset by substantial increases in obesity and diabetes mellitus.

To lower blood cholesterol, experts recommend lifestyle changes that include eating a healthful diet, managing weight, not smoking, engaging in physical activity, and when necessary, taking cholesterol-lowering drugs.[20] Although CHD can result from the interplay of genetic and environmental factors, modifiable lifestyle factors play a large role in the risk of disease. Multidimensional treatment of cholesterol and other heart disease risk factors that includes both lifestyle modifications and pharmacotherapy is likely the most beneficial way to prevent the vast majority of CHD events.

Inflammation and Atherosclerosis

The idea that chronic infection can lead to unsuspected disease is not new. Bacterial infection, for example, is known to cause stomach ulcers. Infection caused by bacteria or viruses is suspected to be a factor in heart disease as well. Infections are associated with atherosclerotic plaque, and a number of infectious agents have been linked with an increased risk of vascular disease. Current thinking, although still debated, is that an "infectious burden" of chronic infections from multiple agents, rather than the effects of a single organism, may contribute to atherosclerosis.[21]

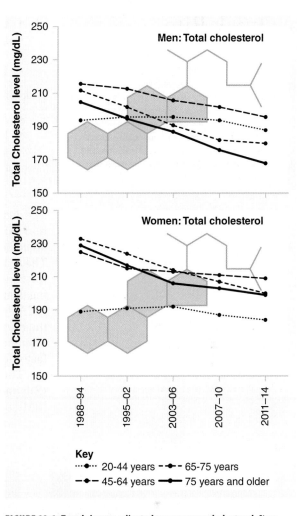

FIGURE 10.6 Trends in age-adjusted mean serum cholesterol. Since the 1960s, mean serum cholesterol levels have steadily declined, along with a decline in death rates from coronary heart disease.

Reproduced from National Center for Health Statistics. *Health, United States, 2015: With Special Feature on Racial and Ethnic Health Disparities.* Hyattsville, MD. 2016. http://www.cdc.gov/nchs/data/hus/hus15.pdf#055. Accessed April 30, 2016 [Note: See page 207].

Key Concepts Cardiovascular disease is the leading cause of death in the United States and Canada. CVD is significantly related to unhealthy aspects of the North American lifestyle, such as smoking, overeating, lack of exercise, high cholesterol levels, and uncontrolled blood pressure. An infection caused by bacteria or viruses can also lead to heart disease.

Risk Factors for Atherosclerosis

Risk factors are conditions or behaviors that increase your likelihood of developing a disease. When you have more than one risk factor for atherosclerosis, your chance of having a heart attack or stroke greatly multiplies. Fortunately, most heart disease risk factors are largely within your control. Risk factors for atherosclerosis that are under your control include:

- High blood pressure
- High blood cholesterol

Quick **Bite**

Who Discovered Atherosclerosis?
Leonardo da Vinci offered the first detailed analysis of diseased blood vessels and was also the first to attribute this pathology to diet.

▸ **hypercholesterolemia** The presence of greater than normal amounts of cholesterol in the blood.

▸ **lipoprotein a [Lp(a)]** A substance that consists of an LDL "bad cholesterol" part plus a protein (apoprotein a), whose exact function is currently unknown.

▸ **risk factors** Anything that increases a person's chance of developing a disease, including substances, agents, genetic alterations, traits, habits, or conditions.

Quick Bite

How Do Cholesterol-Lowering Medications Work?
One class of cholesterol-lowering medications, the bile acid sequestrants, works by combining bile acid and cholesterol in the small intestine to form compounds that the body cannot absorb. Because this cholesterol is then lost in feces, cholesterol must be taken from the blood to make more bile, thus lowering the blood cholesterol level. Another popular type of medication, the statins, interferes with cholesterol synthesis in the liver.

- Cigarette smoking
- Diabetes
- Overweight
- Physical inactivity

Risk factors beyond your control include:

- Age (45 or older for men; 55 or older for women)
- Family history of early heart disease (having a mother or sister who has been diagnosed with heart disease before age 65, or a father or brother diagnosed before age 55)

Dietary and Lifestyle Factors for Reducing Atherosclerosis Risk

The diet and lifestyle recommendations of the American Heart Association (AHA) are part of a comprehensive plan to reduce the incidence of atherosclerosis and are appropriate for anyone over the age of 2 years. The AHA has proposed "The 2020 Impact Goal: By 2020, to improve the cardiovascular health of all Americans by 20 percent while reducing deaths from cardiovascular diseases and stroke by 20 percent." The AHA defines "ideal cardiovascular health" as the absence of disease and the presence of seven key health factors and behaviors called "Life's Simple 7."[22] Unfortunately, U.S. adults have the poorest score on the factor for an overall healthy diet (Healthy Diet Score). (See **FIGURE 10.7**.)

The seven goals are: (1) consuming an overall healthy diet, (2) aiming for a healthy body weight (defined as a body mass index [BMI] of 18.5 to 24.9 kg/m^2), (3) aiming for a desirable lipid profile as

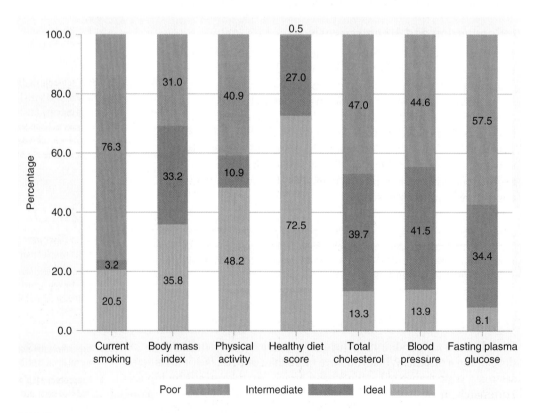

FIGURE 10.7 Life's Simple 7. Among the seven goals for cardiovascular health set by the American Heart Association, U.S. adults 20 years or older have the worst results for eating a healthy diet.
Reprinted with permission *Circulation*. 2014;129:e28-e292, © 2014 American Heart Association, Inc.

TABLE 10.2
Adult Blood Cholesterol and Triglyceride Levels

Total Cholesterol		LDL Cholesterol	
Desirable	< 200	Optimal	< 100
Borderline high	200–239	Near or above optimal	100–129
High	≥ 240	Borderline high	130–159
		High	160–189
		Very high	≥ 190
Triglycerides		**HDL Cholesterol**	
Normal	< 150	Low	< 40
Borderline high	150–199	High	≥ 60
High	200–499		
Very high	≥ 500		

Note: All units are mg/dL.

Data from National Cholesterol Education Program. *Third Report of the Expert Panel on Detection, Evaluation, and Treatment of High Blood Cholesterol in Adults (Adult Treatment Panel III), Final Report.* Washington, DC: U.S. Department of Health and Human Services, 2003. NIH publication 02-5215.

defined by the National Cholesterol Education Program (NCEP) of the National Heart, Lung, and Blood Institute (NHLBI) (see **TABLE 10.2**), (4) aiming for a normal blood pressure, (5) aiming for a normal blood glucose level, (6) being physically active, and (7) avoiding use of and exposure to tobacco products. Specific AHA recommendations, along with other diet and lifestyle factors related to cardiovascular disease risk reduction, are summarized in the following subsections.

Balance Calorie Intake and Physical Activity to Achieve or Maintain a Healthy Body Weight

Obesity is an independent risk factor for cardiovascular disease, and weight gain during the teen years and in adulthood is associated with increased risk of heart disease.[23] In an effort to avoid weight gain, calorie intake needs to match calorie output. Awareness of the calorie content of foods and beverages and control of portion sizes are major steps toward calorie control.

Physical activity helps reduce cardiovascular disease. Current recommendations suggest engaging in a minimum of 30 minutes of moderate-intensity activity on most days of the week; more activity would reduce heart disease risk further.

Consume a Diet Rich in Fruits and Vegetables

Fruits and vegetables are rich in nutrients and fiber and low in calories. Eating more fruits and vegetables helps meet nutrient intake requirements without overindulging in foods high in calories. In addition, diets that emphasize fruits and vegetables have consistently been shown to lower cardiovascular disease risk factors. A variety of vegetables and fruits, with an emphasis on whole, unprocessed sources, is recommended.

Brightly colored vegetables and fruits are not only nutrient-rich, but also good sources of phytochemicals, including antioxidants. In the blood, oxygen free radicals can attack and oxidize low-density lipoproteins; as these oxidized LDLs are deposited in blood vessel walls, the process of building up plaque begins. Despite the lack of significant randomized clinical trial data supporting antioxidant supplement use, Americans spend more than $20 billion annually on supplements for the antioxidant vitamins A, C, and E.[24] By comparison, higher fruit and vegetable intake, especially leafy green vegetables, has been shown to lower the risk of heart disease, and eating more fruits and vegetables is highly recommended. Because fruits and vegetables contain so many vitamins, minerals, and phytochemicals that could be working alone or in combination, diets rich in a variety of fruits and vegetables—sources of antioxidant vitamins and other antioxidant compounds—continue to constitute a cornerstone of dietary recommendations.

Choose Whole-Grain, High-Fiber Foods

Diets that emphasize whole grains and other foods rich in fiber have been linked to improved overall diet quality and reduced cardiovascular disease risk.[25] Certain types of fiber can bind to bile acids in the gastrointestinal tract. These bile acids are excreted in the feces rather than recycled and reused. Additional bile acids must then be made from cholesterol, lowering the total amount in the body. In the large intestine, intestinal bacteria partially digest fiber and then produce short-chain fatty acids, some of which may reduce cholesterol synthesis. The American Heart Association and the *2015–2020 Dietary Guidelines for Americans* recommend that at least half of grain intake come from whole grains. The Adequate Intake (AI) level for fiber (14 grams per 1,000 kilocalories) is based on the amount of fiber that has been shown to reduce CVD risk.[26] Despite FDA approval of health claims for fiber supplements, whether these supplements can provide protection against CVD similar to that of whole grain foods remains controversial.[27]

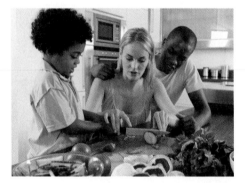

© Jupiterimages/Thinkstock.

Consume Fish, Especially Oily Fish, at Least Twice a Week

In the 1970s, a study of the Inuits (Greenland Eskimos) focused attention on the beneficial effects of EPA and DHA, the omega-3 fatty acids in fish fats.[28] Researchers were puzzled: This group of people had a high intake of fat, saturated fat, and cholesterol from marine mammals and fish, yet they showed little evidence of atherosclerosis. The Inuits were compared with the Danes, among whom atherosclerosis was common and whose diet was similarly high in fat, but from meats and dairy products. It became clear that the high EPA and DHA content of fish in the Inuit diet protects against heart disease by discouraging blood cells from clotting and from sticking to artery walls, and by reducing inflammation. Studies of other groups have since shown similar results. The Japanese, for example, with their generous fish intake, have low rates of atherosclerosis. Many other studies point in the same direction; some show that as few as two or three servings of fish weekly can be protective.

Fish is a good source of omega-3 fatty acids, which decrease risk of abnormal heartbeats that can lead to sudden deaths. Omega-3 fatty acids also decrease triglyceride levels, slow the rate of atherosclerosis, and slightly lower blood pressure.[29] Although consumption of foods rich in omega-3 fatty acids reduces CVD risk, the potential benefits from consuming omega-3 fatty acid supplements is less clear. A large review of data from 20 trials that included more than 60,000 people and more than 6,000 major cardiovascular events questioned the use

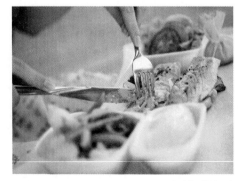

© iStockphoto/Thinkstock.

of fish oil supplements for the prevention of CVD.[30] All in all, there are certainly enough positive results to encourage further study and recommend regular consumption of cold-water fish (e.g., salmon, cod) for EPA and DHA as well as plant foods with alpha-linolenic acid.[31]

Controversy: Limiting Your Intake of Saturated and Trans Fat and Cholesterol

A major, but controversial, study questions the link between saturated fat and heart disease. The analysis included 27 clinical trials and 49 observational studies, totaling more than 600,000 participants. It concluded that "current evidence does not clearly support cardiovascular guidelines that encourage high consumption of polyunsaturated fatty acids and low consumption of total saturated fats."[32] The findings on omega-3 fatty acids and trans fats were mixed.

On the other hand, an extensive review and new guidelines released by the American College of Cardiology and the American Heart Association found strong evidence linking saturated fat and heart disease.[33] Still, modifying fat composition is less important than BMI, aging, and gender. In cross-sectional studies, differences in saturated fat intake account for only about 5 percent of the variance in blood cholesterol levels. The bottom line? Rather than focusing on a single dietary component, dietitians recommend that you "consume a heart-healthy diet that emphasizes vegetables, fruits, and whole grains; includes low-fat dairy products, poultry, fish, legumes, nontropical vegetable oils, and nuts; and limits intake of sweets, sugar-sweetened beverages, and red meats."[34]

Although saturated fat can raise total and "bad" LDL cholesterol, it also *raises* "good" HDL cholesterol. By comparison, trans fats raise total and "bad" LDL cholesterol, and *lower* "good" HDL cholesterol. The American Heart Association recommends limiting saturated fat intake to less than 5–6 percent of total calories, and trans fat intake to less than 1 percent.[35] (The *2015-2020 Dietary Guidelines* recommends keeping trans fat intake "as low as possible.")

Research shows that consuming monounsaturated fats, such as olive oil, lowers total and LDL cholesterol without lowering HDL.[36] This positive effect of olive oil may partially explain why Greeks, Turks, Italians, and others around the Mediterranean who eat a traditional diet higher in fat still have low rates of heart disease. The multi-center PREDIMED study identified the following average daily consumptions:

- *Dairy products:* 5.8 ounces for men, 7 ounces for women
- *Fruit:* 5 ounces for men, 4.4 ounces for women
- *Vegetables:* 4.4 ounces for men, 5 ounces for women
- *Cereals/grains:* 4.6 ounces for men, 4.4 ounces for women
- *Meat:* 2.7 ounces for men and women
- *Fish:* 0.7 ounce for men, 0.9 ounce for women
- *Legumes:* 0.35 ounce for men and women[37,38]

The overall diet pattern seems to model AHA recommendations. An average of 0.7 to 0.9 ounce of fish daily, for example, is about two 3-ounce servings per week (as is recommended by the AHA). Specific amounts were not identified for red wine, olive oil, or nuts, which also are important components of a Mediterranean diet. Moderate consumption of alcohol may account for about one-fourth or more of the positive health benefit.[39,40] Consistently favorable results from both epidemiological and intervention studies have made the Mediterranean diet popular.

Quick **Bite**

Hardy Hearts
By the end of a normal life span, the human heart has pumped more than 3 billion times. Despite this heavy use, heart failures are usually caused by heart attacks or problems with blood vessels and valves; heart muscle itself rarely wears out.

What about cholesterol intake? Some evidence links higher cholesterol intake to elevated blood cholesterol levels, and cholesterol is not essential in the diet. However, the AHA guidelines found insufficient evidence to determine whether lowering dietary cholesterol reduces LDL cholesterol in the blood.[41]

Minimize Your Intake of Beverages and Foods That Contain Added Sugars

Added sugar intake in the United States has risen dramatically in the last 20 years. Reducing consumption of added sugars helps to improve the nutrient quality of the diet and also reduces calorie intake. Paying attention to sources of added sugars will help individuals achieve weight goals.

Choose and Prepare Foods with Little or No Salt

Hypertension is a major risk factor for cardiovascular disease, and generally, blood pressure rises as salt intake rises. Further discussion of salt, sodium, other minerals, and blood pressure follows in the section "Hypertension" later in this chapter. The AHA suggests that reducing sodium intake to 2,300 milligrams (about 1 teaspoon of salt) per day or less is an achievable goal.

If You Consume Alcohol, Do So in Moderation

Moderate alcohol consumption is associated with a substantial decrease in heart disease risk.[42] However, alcohol can be addictive, and high intake can have adverse effects on the body. So, the *2015–2020 Dietary Guidelines* recommend limiting alcohol intake to no more than one drink per day for women and two drinks per day for men, and only by adults of legal drinking age.[43]

The positive effects of alcohol on heart disease risk provide at least a partial explanation for the "French paradox," the fact that the French eat rich cheeses and fatty meats, yet still have low rates of heart disease. They also have relatively high intakes of fruits, vegetables, and red wine—all rich sources of antioxidant phytochemicals. The active compound of the French paradox was recently identified to be a compound called resveratrol. In addition to its heart-protective effects, resveratrol also may have anticancer, anti-inflammatory, and antiaging benefits.

When You Eat Food That Is Prepared Outside of the Home, Follow the AHA's Diet and Lifestyle Recommendations

More and more of our meals are either eaten away from home or brought home as takeout food. All too often, our choices away from home are high in fat, added sugars, and sodium and low in fiber, fruits, and vegetables. Also, portion sizes at restaurants are typically more than those recommended by MyPlate. Consumers need to make wise choices both at home and away from home. Splitting entrée portions with a companion, choosing steamed vegetables instead of a loaded baked potato, or substituting a salad with low-fat dressing for french fries will help individuals follow the AHA guidelines. For more tips on heart-healthy choices when dining out, see **TABLE 10.3**.

Other Dietary Factors

The B vitamins folate, B_6, and B_{12} are involved in pathways that convert one amino acid, homocysteine, to another amino acid, methionine. As noted earlier, high levels of homocysteine can contribute to heart disease by promoting atherosclerosis, excessive blood clotting, or

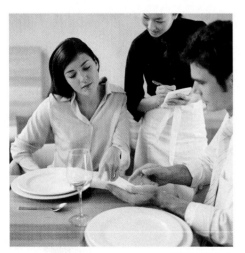

© Stockbyte/Thinkstock.

TABLE 10.3
Heart-Healthy Tips for Dining Out

Are you able to stick to your low-saturated-fat, low-cholesterol diet when eating out? If not, you will be able to if you follow these tips:

- Choose restaurants that have low-saturated-fat, low-cholesterol menu choices. Don't be afraid to make special requests—it's your right as a paying customer.
- Control serving sizes by asking for a side-dish or appetizer-size serving, sharing a dish with a companion, or taking some home.
- Ask that gravy, butter, rich sauces, and salad dressing be served on the side. That way, you can control the amount of saturated fat and cholesterol you eat.
- Ask to substitute a salad or baked potato for chips, fries, coleslaw, or other extras—or just ask that the extras be left off your plate.
- When ordering pizza, order vegetable toppings such as green peppers, onions, and mushrooms instead of meat or extra cheese. To make your pizza even lower in saturated fat and cholesterol, order it with half the cheese or no cheese.
- At fast food restaurants, go for salads, grilled (not fried or breaded) skinless chicken sandwiches, regular-sized hamburgers, or roast beef sandwiches. Go easy on the regular salad dressings and fatty sauces. Limit your consumption of jumbo or deluxe burgers, sandwiches, french fries, and other foods.

Reading the Menu

- Choose low-saturated-fat, low-cholesterol cooking methods. Look for terms such as the following: steamed, in its own juice (au jus), garden fresh, broiled, baked, roasted, poached, tomato juice, dry boiled (in wine or lemon juice), and lightly sautéed or lightly stir-fried.
- Be aware of dishes that are high in saturated fat and cholesterol. Watch out for terms such as the following: butter sauce, fried, crispy, creamed, in cream or cheese sauce, au gratin, au fromage, escalloped, Parmesan, hollandaise, béarnaise, marinated (in oil), stewed, basted, sautéed, stir-fried, casserole, hash, prime, pot pie, pastry crust.

Courtesy of National Heart Lung and Blood Institute.

blood vessel rigidity. Folate and vitamins B_6 and B_{12} can help reduce destructive levels of homocysteine. Scientists believe that consuming a diet rich in fruits, vegetables, and low-fat dairy products—such as the Dietary Approaches to Stop Hypertension (DASH) diet, which is also rich in these vitamins—helps lower blood homocysteine and therefore reduce risk of heart disease.[44]

Soy-based foods, such as soy milks, soy burgers, tofu, and tempeh, have become popular items in grocery stores. In October 1999, the U.S. Food and Drug Administration (FDA) approved labeling for foods containing soy protein as protective against coronary heart disease. Since then, many well-controlled studies on soy protein substantially added to our scientific knowledge base. The American Heart Association Nutrition Committee reevaluated the evidence on soy protein and found that the direct cardiovascular health benefit of soy protein is minimal at best.[45] In its assessment of 22 randomized trials, the AHA Nutrition Committee found that isolated soy protein with isoflavones (ISF) slightly lowered LDL cholesterol in hyperlipidemic people and had no effect on HDL cholesterol, triglycerides, lipoprotein a, or blood pressure.[46]

Other components in soybeans can provide favorable effects. Because many soy products have a high content of polyunsaturated fats, fiber, vitamins, and minerals, these foods are part of a heart-healthy diet.

Putting It All Together

Healthy People 2020 objectives target reducing deaths from heart disease and stroke as well as reducing the number of adults with high blood cholesterol levels. To accomplish these goals, dietitians recommend lowering total fat intake, maintaining a healthy body weight, and exercising on a regular basis. Eating fruits, vegetables, legumes, and grains that contain fiber helps lower cholesterol levels, too. These foods contain antioxidants and B vitamins, such as B_6 and folate, that also may reduce the risk of heart disease. Substituting fish or soy foods for high-fat meats and cheeses and choosing low-fat dairy products can be beneficial as well.

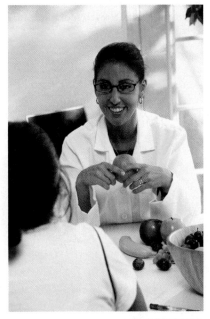

© LiquidLibrary/Thinkstock.

Key Concepts To reduce your risk of heart disease, get regular exercise, control your weight, and don't smoke. Dietary changes you can make to reduce your heart disease risk include eating less fat while increasing intake of fruits, vegetables, and whole grains. Look for sources of omega-3 fatty acids and fiber in your food choices.

Hypertension

🍎 **Why Is This Important?** High blood pressure is a risk factor for atherosclerosis, kidney disease, and stroke. Regulating dietary sodium and intake of other minerals is important to maintaining a healthy blood pressure.

Persistent high blood pressure (**hypertension**) often is called a "silent killer" because, although it usually has no specific symptoms or early warning signs and appears as no threat, it can kill you. You can be hypertensive for years without realizing it. During those years, untreated hypertension can cause damage to vital organs, particularly the heart, the brain, the kidneys, and the eyes. It increases the risk of heart attack, congestive heart failure, stroke, and kidney failure. Nearly half of American adults have hypertension. (Many don't even know they have it.)[47,48] The good news is that hypertension can be treated and controlled.

THINK
About It
2

What Is Blood Pressure?

Blood pressure is the force exerted by the blood on the walls of the blood vessels, especially the arteries. This force is created by the pumping action of the heart. Every time the heart contracts, or beats (systole), blood pressure increases. When the heart relaxes between beats (diastole), the pressure decreases. Blood pressure can fluctuate considerably, depending on various factors. When you are excited, afraid, or exercising, for example, your heart pumps more blood into your arteries and your blood pressure rises. Blood pressure rises and falls during the day. When it stays elevated over time, it's called hypertension.

Blood pressure is measured using a **sphygmomanometer** (blood pressure cuff) (see **FIGURE 10.8**) and is expressed as two numbers. The **systolic** pressure is the higher number and represents pressure during

▶ **hypertension** Condition in which resting blood pressure persistently exceeds 140 mm Hg systolic or 90 mm Hg diastolic.

▶ **blood pressure** The pressure of blood against the walls of a blood vessel or heart chamber. Unless there is reference to another location, such as the pulmonary artery or one of the heart chambers, this term refers to the pressure in the systemic arteries, as measured, for example, in the forearm.

▶ **sphygmomanometer [sfig-mo-ma-NOM-ehter]** An instrument for measuring blood pressure and especially arterial blood pressure.

▶ **systolic** Pertaining to a heart contraction. Systolic blood pressure is measured during a heart contraction, a time period known as systole.

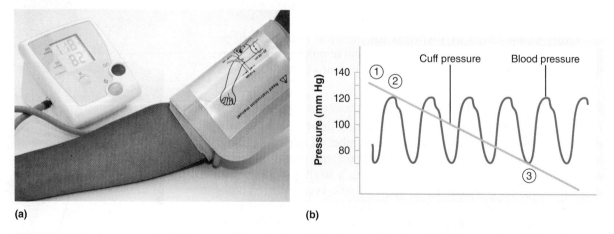

(a)   **(b)**

FIGURE 10.8 (a) A sphygmomanometer (blood pressure cuff) is used to determine blood pressure. **(b)** As shown, the blood pressure rises and falls with each contraction of the heart.
(a) © Paul Maguire/Shutterstock.

the heart's contraction. The **diastolic** pressure is the lower number, measured during the heart's resting phase. Normal blood pressure is defined as a systolic pressure less than 120 mm Hg (millimeters mercury) and a diastolic pressure less than 80 mm Hg.

What Is Hypertension?

Hypertension is a medical condition with chronic high blood pressure. (See **TABLE 10.4**.) Hypertension is classified as either primary (essential) hypertension or secondary hypertension. Most cases of hypertension (about 90 percent) are **essential hypertension**, which is defined by the lack of an obvious cause. Essential hypertension most likely has many contributing factors, including diet, obesity, alcohol abuse, lack of exercise, physical and emotional stress, and psychological and genetic factors. When hypertension results from another problem, such as a kidney defect, it is called **secondary hypertension**. In secondary hypertension, blood pressure usually returns to normal when the underlying defect is corrected.

Renin and Hypertension

The enzyme renin is associated with some cases of essential hypertension. This enzyme promotes the formation of angiotensin proteins, which cause the arteries to constrict. Some people with essential hypertension have higher than normal levels of renin in their blood. People with high renin levels have an increased incidence of heart attacks, strokes, and kidney failure.

Other people with essential hypertension have lower than normal levels of renin in their blood. Their hypertension may be caused primarily by increased blood volume. This condition could result either from decreased sodium excretion by the kidneys or from increased secretion of aldosterone, a hormone that causes the kidneys to retain sodium and water.

Stress and Hypertension

Stress can contribute to sustained high blood pressure. When stressors, either internal or external, activate the sympathetic nervous system, heart rate increases, arteries constrict, and the blood exerts greater force on the artery walls. Chronic stress has been implicated in heart disease.

▶ **diastolic** Pertaining to the time between heart contractions, a period known as diastole. Diastolic blood pressure is measured at the point of maximum cardiac relaxation.

▶ **essential hypertension** Hypertension for which no specific cause can be identified. Ninety to 95 percent of people with hypertension have essential hypertension.

▶ **secondary hypertension** Hypertension caused by an underlying condition such as a kidney disorder. Once the underlying condition is treated, the blood pressure usually returns to normal.

TABLE 10.4
Blood Pressure Classification for Adults

Blood Pressure Category	Systolic mm Hg (upper number)		Diastolic mm Hg (lower number)
Normal	less than 120	and	less than 80
Elevated	120–129	and	less than 80
High blood pressure (hypertension) stage 1	130–139	or	80–89
High blood pressure (hypertension) stage 2	140 or higher	or	90 or higher
Hypertensive crisis (consult your doctor immediately)	Higher than 180	and/or	Higher than 120

Reprinted with permission, www.heart.org, © 2017 American Heart Association, Inc.

Risk Factors for Hypertension

Even though the cause for most cases of hypertension is unknown, several factors clearly contribute to hypertension. As with heart disease risk, some hypertension risk factors are controllable and others are uncontrollable. Risk factors for hypertension under your control include the following:

- *Obesity:* People with a BMI of 30 kg/m² or higher are more likely to develop high blood pressure.
- *Eating too much salt:* High sodium intake increases blood pressure in some people.
- *Lack of physical activity:* A sedentary lifestyle is associated with overweight and increased blood pressure.
- *Drinking too much alcohol:* Heavy and regular use of alcohol increases blood pressure.

Risk factors for hypertension that are beyond your control include the following:

- *Race:* African Americans develop high blood pressure more often, at earlier ages, and with more severity than Caucasians do.[49]
- *Age:* Blood pressure risk rises with age; people with normal blood pressure at age 55 have a 90 percent lifetime risk of developing hypertension.[50]
- *Heredity:* Family history of hypertension is a strong predictive factor.

Dietary and Lifestyle Factors for Reducing Hypertension

The American Heart Association has guidelines for dietary approaches to prevent and treat hypertension in adults.[51] They direct you to do the following:

- *Maintain a healthy weight.* Strive for a body mass index (BMI) between 18.5 and 24.9.
- *Eat healthier.* Eat lots of fruit, veggies and low-fat dairy, and less saturated and total fat.
- *Reduce sodium.* Ideally, stay under 1,500 mg a day, but aim for at least a 1,000 mg per day reduction.
- *Get active.* Aim for at least 90 to 150 minutes of aerobic and/or dynamic resistance exercise per week and/or three sessions of isometric resistance exercises per week.
- *Limit alcohol.* Drink no more than 1-2 drinks a day. (One for most women, two for most men.)

Sodium

Excess sodium can hold excessive fluid in the body, at least temporarily. These excesses can be burdensome on the kidneys, heart, and blood vessels. The consensus among heart disease experts is that too much sodium, ingested routinely over the years, plays a role in the underlying causes of hypertension in genetically predisposed or "salt-sensitive" people. The more salt they eat, the higher their blood pressure.

Population studies appear to confirm this conclusion. Rates of hypertension are higher in countries with high sodium intakes. On the other hand, indigenous people, whose diets contain very little sodium, seldom have hypertension. If they continue to eat their traditional diet, their blood pressure does not rise with age. If they adopt a "modern" (higher-sodium) diet, however, their blood pressure tends to rise, and

Quick Bite

The Salt Wars

Salt was so precious historically that battles were fought over access to it. Of warring German tribes, the Roman historian Tacitus wrote, "These Chatti and Hermanduri! They fight bloody wars over who shall possess a salt stream." In Roman times, soldiers were paid a special allowance to buy salt. The allowance was called *salarium*, which gives us the word *salary*.

they are more likely to become hypertensive. In a multiethnic sample, for those born outside the United States, each 10 years of living in the United States has been associated with a higher prevalence of hypertension.[52]

Other Dietary Factors

Sodium is not the only dietary factor associated with hypertension. Excess weight tends to raise blood pressure; regular exercise and weight loss help to reduce blood pressure. Reducing consumption of alcohol also tends to reduce blood pressure and improves the effectiveness of antihypertensive medications. Eating a diet rich in calcium, magnesium, and potassium reduces blood pressure as well.[53] The mechanism by which these minerals act on hypertension in part reflects their interrelationship with sodium metabolism. Supplements of calcium, magnesium, and potassium do not have the same blood pressure–lowering effects as foods rich in these minerals.

The DASH Diet

The original **DASH (Dietary Approaches to Stop Hypertension)** study, a multicenter NHLBI-sponsored trial, tested the effects of different dietary patterns on blood pressure. After a control period, the 459 subjects in this study received one of three diets for an eight-week period[54]:

- *Control diet:* Macronutrient and fiber content equal to U.S. average; 4 servings of fruits and vegetables per day; 0.5 serving of dairy products per day; potassium, magnesium, and calcium levels close to the 25th percentile of U.S. consumption
- *Fruit and vegetable diet:* 8.5 servings of fruits and vegetables per day; potassium and magnesium levels at the 75th percentile of U.S. consumption; other nutrients similar to control diet
- *Combination diet:* 10 servings of fruits and vegetables per day; 2.7 servings of low-fat dairy products per day; less fat, saturated fat, and cholesterol than control diet; potassium, magnesium, and calcium levels at the 75th percentile of U.S. consumption

The sodium content of the diets averaged about 3,000 milligrams per day. The study excluded subjects who were taking antihypertensive medications, unless their physicians had given them permission to discontinue their medication for the course of the study.[55] **TABLE 10.5** shows sample meals from the three DASH diets used in the study.

Both the fruit and vegetable diet and the combination diet significantly lowered the systolic and diastolic blood pressure in all subjects and in subgroups analyzed by sex, ethnicity, and hypertensive/normotensive status. For hypertensive individuals, the DASH combination diet lowered blood pressure as much as antihypertensive drugs. Widespread adoption of the DASH eating plan could lead to a downward shift in the incidence and severity of the disease.

Results from a follow-up study, the DASH-Sodium trial, support both the DASH-style dietary changes and lower sodium intake. This study used different levels of daily sodium restriction (3,300 mg, 2,400 mg, and 1,500 mg) and two diet plans (a "typical" American diet and the DASH diet). Approximately 41 percent of the participants had hypertension. Reducing sodium intake lowered blood pressure for participants in both dietary treatment arms, but the DASH diet in combination with sodium restriction was more effective than the low-sodium control diet alone.[56]

Quick **Bite**

What Smells in Blood Pressure?

A family of complex cell receptors, some of which play a role in detecting odors in the nose, have been found to be involved in the kidneys' integration of signals from gut microbes and the regulation of blood pressure. Cell receptors in the kidneys are activated in response to short-chain fatty acids produced by bacteria in the gut during digestion of fats or fiber. These receptors appear to influence the release of hormones that help regulate blood pressure. This discovery identifies a previously unknown connection among the gut, kidney, and cardiovascular systems.

▶ **DASH (Dietary Approaches to Stop Hypertension)** An eating plan low in total fat, saturated fat, and cholesterol and rich in fruits, vegetables, and low-fat dairy products that has been shown to reduce elevated blood pressure.

TABLE 10.5
Sample Menus from the DASH Study

Meal	Control Diet	Fruit and Vegetable Diet	DASH Combination Diet
Breakfast	• Apple juice • Sugar-frosted flakes • White toast • Butter • Jelly • Whole milk	• Orange juice • Oat bran muffin • Raisins • Dried apricots • Butter	• Orange juice • Granola bar • Fat-free yogurt • 1% low-fat milk • Banana
Lunch	• Ham-and-chicken sandwich on white bread, with lettuce, pickles, mustard, and mayonnaise • Fruit cocktail	• Ham-and-Swiss cheese sandwich on whole-wheat bread • Banana	• Smoked turkey sandwich on whole-wheat bread with lettuce and mayonnaise • Fresh orange
Dinner	• Spiced cod • Scallion rice • Carrots • Butter • French rolls	• Spiced cod • Scallion rice • Lima beans • Butter • Dinner rolls • Melon balls	• Spiced cod • Scallion rice • Spinach • Margarine • Dinner rolls • Melon balls • 1% low-fat milk
Snack	• Graham crackers • Vanilla frosting • Tropical fruit punch	• Peanuts	• Peanuts • Dried apricots • Melon balls

Reprinted from *Journal of the American Dietetic Association*, 99(8), Karanja NM, Obarzanek E, Lin P-H, et al., Descriptive characteristics of the dietary patterns used in the Dietary Approaches to Stop Hypertension trial, Page no. S19-S27, 1999, with permission from Elsevier.

To help keep blood pressure at healthy levels, the DASH eating plan is rich in potassium. A potassium-rich diet can help to reduce elevated or high blood pressure, but be sure to get your potassium from food sources, not from supplements. Many fruits and vegetables, some milk products, and fish are rich sources of potassium. Because of the additional fruits and vegetables and therefore the antioxidant nutrients, phytochemicals, and fiber that people consume while following the DASH diet, the eating plan has the potential to extend beyond cardiovascular benefits.

The major landmark studies on the DASH diet used feeding trials with all food provided to the participants. A review of nine studies found that compliance is generally low when only counseling services were provided without food supplies. Given the health benefits of the DASH diet, studies for improving adherence are warranted.[57]

Putting It All Together

As previously described, hypertension can be controlled and even prevented by making modifications in diet and lifestyle. Blood pressure can be unhealthy even if it stays only slightly above the cutoff level of 120/80 mm Hg. The higher that blood pressure rises above normal, the greater the health risk. Recognition and control of high blood pressure are essential for avoiding damage to vital organs. Checking your blood pressure on a regular basis is the key to detecting this silent killer. Following diet and lifestyle recommendations, which includes the DASH eating plan, reducing dietary sodium, and regular physical activity, can be the key to prevention.

Key Concepts Hypertension is a risk factor for atherosclerosis, kidney disease, and stroke. Blood pressure tends to rise with age, and rates of hypertension are higher among African Americans. Sodium intake affects blood pressure, especially in those individuals who are salt sensitive. Low intake of potassium, calcium, and possibly magnesium also contribute to the development of hypertension. Eating a diet replete with fresh foods and avoiding processed foods not only will improve the balance of minerals in our diet, but also can reduce risk of disease.

Cancer

🍎 **Why Is This Important?** Diet is one of many factors that may influence cancer risk. Eating more fruits, vegetables, and whole grains; maintaining a healthy weight; and limiting alcohol consumption are three diet-related strategies you can take to reduce cancer risk.

THINK
About It
3

In the United States, **cancer** is the second leading cause of death (after heart disease).[58] In fact, one in every four deaths in this country can be attributed to cancer. Reducing both the number of new cancer cases and the death rates from cancer are key objectives of Healthy People 2020. Cancer comprises a group of more than 100 diseases that involve the uncontrolled division of the body's cells. Although it can develop in virtually any of the body's tissues, and each type of cancer has unique features, the basic processes that produce cancer are quite similar in all forms of the disease. To understand cancer, it is helpful to know what happens when normal cells become cancerous.

What Is Cancer?

The body consists of many types of cells. Normally, cells grow and divide to produce more cells only when the body needs them. This orderly process helps keep the body healthy. Sometimes, however, cells keep dividing when new cells are not needed. These extra cells form a mass of **tissue**, called a growth or **tumor**.

Tumors can be **benign** or **malignant**. Benign tumors are not cancer. They often can be removed and, in most cases, they do not regrow. Cells from benign tumors do not spread to other parts of the body. Most important, benign tumors rarely pose a threat to life. In contrast, malignant tumors are cancerous. Cells in these tumors are abnormal and divide without control or order. As a result, they can invade and damage nearby tissues and organs. Also, cancer cells can break away from a malignant tumor and enter the bloodstream or the lymphatic system. In this way, cancer can spread from the original site to form new tumors in other organs. The spread of cancer is called **metastasis**.

Most cancers are named for the organ or type of cell in which they originate. Cancer that begins in the colon is colon cancer, for example, and cancer that begins in skin cells known as **melanocytes** is called **melanoma**. **Leukemia** and **lymphoma** are cancers that arise in blood-forming cells. The abnormal blood cells circulate in the bloodstream and lymphatic system. They also may invade (infiltrate) body organs and form tumors.

Cancer develops in a multistage process that can take many years. There are typically three phases of development.

1. *Initiation* occurs when something alters a cell's genetic structure and prepares it to act abnormally during later stages.

▶ **cancer** A term for diseases in which abnormal cells divide without control. Cancer cells can invade nearby tissues and can spread through the bloodstream and lymphatic system to other parts of the body.

▶ **tissue** A group or layer of cells that are alike and that work together to perform a specific function.

▶ **tumor** An abnormal mass of tissue that results from excessive cell division. Tumors perform no useful body function. They can be benign (not cancerous) or malignant (cancerous).

▶ **benign** Not cancerous; does not invade nearby tissue or spread to other parts of the body.

▶ **malignant [ma-LIG-nant]** Cancerous; a growth with a tendency to invade and destroy nearby tissue and spread to other parts of the body.

▶ **metastasis [meh-TAS-ta-sis]** The spread of cancer from one part of the body to another. Tumors formed from cells that have spread are called "secondary tumors" and contain cells that are like those in the original (primary) tumor. The plural is *metastases*.

▶ **melanocytes [mel-AN-o-sites]** Cells in the skin that produce and contain the pigment called melanin.

▶ **melanoma** A form of skin cancer that arises in melanocytes, the cells that produce pigment. Melanoma usually begins in a mole.

▶ **leukemia [loo-KEE-mee-a]** Cancer of blood-forming tissue.

▶ **lymphoma [lim-FO-ma]** Cancer that arises in cells of the lymphatic system.

2. *Promotion*, a reversible stage, occurs when a chemical or other factor encourages initiated cells to become active.
3. *Progression* occurs when promoted cells multiply and perhaps invade surrounding healthy tissue.

When cancer spreads (metastasizes), cancer cells are often found in nearby or regional **lymph nodes** (sometimes called lymph glands). If the cancer has reached these nodes, it means that cancer cells may have spread to other organs, such as the liver, bones, or brain. (See **FIGURE 10.9.**) When cancer spreads from its original location to another part of the body, the new tumor has the same kind of abnormal cells and the same name as the primary tumor. If lung cancer spreads to the brain, for example, the cancer cells in the brain are actually lung cancer cells. The disease is called metastatic lung cancer (not brain cancer).

Risk Factors for Cancer

The more we can learn about what causes cancer, the more likely we are to find ways to prevent it. Although doctors can seldom explain why one person gets cancer and another does not, they know that cancer is not caused by an injury, such as a bump or bruise. Also, although being infected with certain viruses can increase the risk of some types of cancer, cancer is not contagious; no one can "catch" cancer from another person.

▶ **lymph nodes [limf nodes]** Rounded masses of lymphatic tissue that are surrounded by a capsule of connective tissue. Lymph nodes filter lymph (lymphatic fluid), and they store lymphocytes (white blood cells). They are located along lymphatic vessels. Also called *lymph glands*.

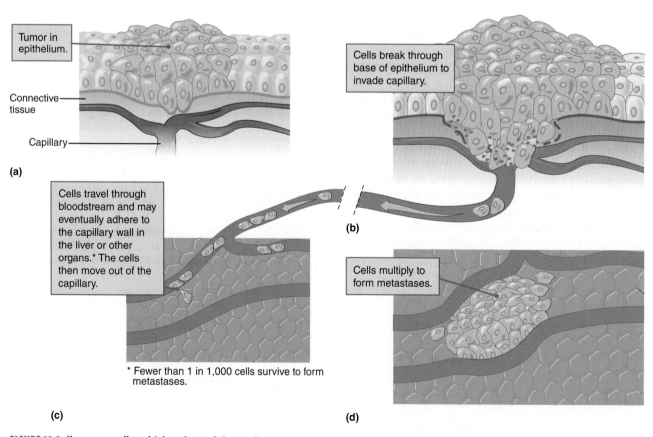

(a) Tumor in epithelium. / Connective tissue / Capillary

(b) Cells break through base of epithelium to invade capillary.

(c) Cells travel through bloodstream and may eventually adhere to the capillary wall in the liver or other organs.* The cells then move out of the capillary.

* Fewer than 1 in 1,000 cells survive to form metastases.

(d) Cells multiply to form metastases.

FIGURE 10.9 How cancer cells multiply and spread. Cancer cells can break away from a malignant tumor, enter the bloodstream or the lymphatic system, and travel to new sites to form new tumors in other organs.

Cancer usually develops over time. It results from a complex mix of factors related to lifestyle, heredity, and environment. Researchers have identified a number of factors that increase a person's chance of developing cancer. Many types of cancer are related to the use of tobacco, items that people eat and drink, exposure to ultraviolet (UV) radiation from the sun, and exposure to cancer-causing agents (**carcinogens**) in the environment and the workplace. Some people are more sensitive than others to factors that cause cancer.

▶ **carcinogens [kar-SIN-o-jins]** Any substances that cause cancer.

Nevertheless, some people who develop cancer have none of the known risk factors. And some people who do have risk factors do not develop the disease. Researchers have learned that cancer is caused by changes (called mutations or alterations) in genes that control normal cell growth and cell death. Most cancer-causing gene changes are generated by factors in a person's lifestyle or the environment. However, some alterations that lead to cancer are inherited; that is, they are passed from parent to child. Having such an inherited gene alteration increases the risk of cancer, but it does not mean that the person is certain to develop cancer.

The Diet–Cancer Link

Many studies have looked at the possibility that specific dietary components or nutrients increase or decrease cancer risk. Studies of cancer cells in the laboratory and of animal models have sometimes provided evidence that isolated compounds may be carcinogenic (cancer-causing) or, on the other hand, have anticancer activity.

But with few exceptions, studies of human populations have not shown definitively that any dietary component causes or protects against cancer. Still, some results from epidemiological studies that compare the diets of people with and without cancer have indicated intake of a particular dietary component differs significantly among these groups. **TABLE 10.6** summarizes dietary components and cancer risk.

Food choices interact with other lifestyle factors and also with genetics to affect cancer risk.[59] As the field of nutritional genomics evolves, it will enhance our ability to target dietary interventions for cancer prevention and treatment. Until that time, the general dietary guidelines from the American Cancer Society (ACS) can be used.

Dietary and Lifestyle Factors for Reducing Cancer Risk

In 2012, the American Cancer Society updated its *Nutrition and Physical Activity Guidelines for Cancer Prevention*.[60] These guidelines emphasize physical activity and weight control and also suggest how communities can provide opportunities for Americans to be physically active. Note that the four major recommendations for individual choices are similar to the guidelines for reducing the risk of heart disease.

Recommendations for community action connect directly to the recommendations for individual choices and include the integration of social, economic, and cultural factors that have the ability to influence an individual's choice regarding diet and physical activity. The ACS recommends that community organizations work to create social and physical environments that are supportive of healthy nutrition and physical activity so all people have the opportunity to make choices that can reduce their cancer risk.

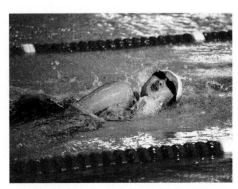
© Photos.com.

TABLE 10.6
Dietary Components and Cancer Risk

Scientists have studied many additives, nutrients, and other dietary components for possible associations with cancer risk. These include:

Alcohol

Although red wine has been suspected of reducing cancer risk, there is no scientific evidence for such an association. Also, alcohol is a known cause of cancer. Heavy or regular alcohol consumption increases the risk of developing cancers of the oral cavity (excluding the lips), pharynx (throat), larynx (voice box), esophagus, liver, breast, colon, and rectum. The risk of developing cancer increases with the amount of alcohol a person drinks.

Antioxidants

Antioxidants are chemicals that block the activity of other chemicals, known as free radicals, that may damage cells. Although laboratory and animal research has shown that antioxidants can help prevent the free radical damage associated with the development of cancer, research in humans has not demonstrated convincingly that taking antioxidant supplements can help reduce the risk of developing or dying from cancer. Some studies have even shown an increased risk of some cancers.

Artificial Sweeteners

Studies have been conducted on the safety of several artificial sweeteners, including saccharin, aspartame, acesulfame potassium, sucralose, neotame, and cyclamate. There is no clear evidence that the artificial sweeteners available commercially in the United States are associated with cancer risk in humans.

Calcium

Calcium is an essential dietary mineral that can be obtained from food and supplements. Research results overall support a relationship between higher intakes of calcium and reduced risks of colorectal cancer, but the results of studies have not always been consistent. Whether a relationship exists between higher calcium intakes and reduced risks of other cancers, such as breast and ovarian cancer, is unclear. Some research suggests that a high calcium intake may increase the risk of prostate cancer.

Charred Meat

Certain chemicals, called HCAs and PAHs, are formed when muscle meat, including beef, pork, fish, and poultry, is cooked using high-temperature methods. Exposure to high levels of HCAs and PAHs can cause cancer in animals; however, whether such exposure causes cancer in humans is unclear.

Cruciferous Vegetables

Cruciferous vegetables, such as bok choy, broccoli, Brussels sprouts, and kale, contain chemicals known as glucosinolates, which break down into several compounds that are being studied for possible anticancer effects. Some of these compounds have shown anticancer effects in cells and animals, but the results of studies with humans have been less clear.

Fluoride

Fluoride in water helps to prevent and can even reverse tooth decay. Many studies, in both humans and animals, have shown no association between fluoridated water and cancer risk.

Garlic

Some studies have suggested that garlic consumption may reduce the risk of developing several types of cancer, especially cancers of the gastrointestinal tract.

Tea

Tea contains polyphenol compounds, particularly catechins, which are antioxidants. Results of epidemiological studies examining the association between tea consumption and cancer risk have been inconclusive. Few clinical trials of tea consumption and cancer prevention have been conducted, and their results have also been inconclusive.

Vitamin D

Vitamin D helps the body use calcium and phosphorus to make strong bones and teeth. It is obtained primarily through exposure of the skin to sunlight, but it can also be obtained from some foods and dietary supplements. Epidemiological studies in humans have suggested that higher intakes of vitamin D or higher levels of vitamin D in the blood may be associated with a reduced risk of colorectal cancer, but the results of randomized studies have been inconclusive.

National Cancer Institute. Diet. (n.d.). Retrieved September 05, 2017, from https://www.cancer.gov/about-cancer/causes-prevention/risk/diet.

Recommendations for Individual Lifestyle Choices

1. Maintain a healthful weight throughout life.
   - Balance caloric intake with physical activity.
   - Avoid excessive weight gain throughout the life cycle.
   - Achieve and maintain a healthy weight if currently overweight or obese.

2. Adopt a physically active lifestyle.
   - *Adults:* Engage in at least 30 minutes of moderate to vigorous physical activity, above usual activities, on five or more days of the week. Forty-five to 60 minutes of intentional physical activity is preferable.
   - *Children and adolescents:* Engage in at least 60 minutes per day of moderate to vigorous physical activity at least five days per week.
3. Eat a healthy diet, with an emphasis on plant sources.
   - Choose foods and beverages in amounts that help achieve and maintain a healthy weight.
   - Eat five or more servings of vegetables and fruits each day.
   - Choose whole grains in preference to processed (refined) grains and sugars.
   - Limit consumption of processed meats and red meats.
4. If you drink alcoholic beverages, limit consumption.
   - People who drink alcohol should limit their intake: not more than two drinks per day for men and one drink a day for women.

Fat

High-fat diets have been associated with an increase in the risk of cancers of the colon and rectum, prostate, and endometrium. The association between high-fat diets and breast cancer appears to be much weaker. Several studies have evaluated the role of dietary fat on breast cancer risk, but the evidence has been inconclusive. Currently, the American Cancer Society considers the dietary fat recommendations for the general population for heart disease prevention appropriate for the population of cancer survivors due to shared risk factors between cancer and heart disease.[61]

High intake of red meat (e.g., beef, pork, lamb) and processed meat (e.g., bacon, sausage, hot dogs, lunch meat) is associated with some types of colorectal cancer; long-term consumption of poultry and fish is associated with reduced risk.[62,63]

Vegetables and Fruits

Evidence that vegetable and fruit consumption reduces cancer risk has led to attempts to isolate specific nutrients and to administer these in pharmacological doses to high-risk populations. Most have failed to prevent cancer and, in some cases, have produced adverse effects.

It remains unclear which components of vegetables and fruits are most protective against cancer. Vegetables and fruits are complex foods, with each containing more than 100 potentially beneficial substances, including vitamins, minerals, and fiber. Specific phytochemicals, such as carotenoids, flavonoids, terpenes, sterols, indoles, and phenols, show benefit against certain cancers in experimental studies. In addition to having antioxidant effects, nutrients and other phytochemicals might inhibit multiplication of cancer cells, alter enzymes, inhibit the conversion of chemicals into toxins, and alter hormone metabolism. Until more is known about specific food components, however, the best advice is to eat five or more servings of a variety of vegetables and fruits.

Despite strong encouragement from numerous health agencies to eat at least five servings of vegetables and fruits each day, intake of these foods remains below recommended levels among both adults and children. Many states are attempting to increase fruit and vegetable

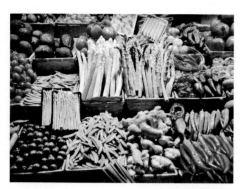

© Adisa/Shutterstock.

consumption with improved access and policies that make it easier to get fruits and vegetables in communities, schools, and child care. California and Oregon are above the national average on access to a healthier food retailer, density of farmers markets, and acceptance of nutrition assistance programs. These and other factors explain why adults in California and Oregon eat more vegetables than adults in other states. They also are among the highest in fruit consumption.[64] On the national scene, Fruit & Veggies—More Matters is a public health campaign that encourages people to eat more fruits and vegetables. Recommended intake is based on individual calorie needs, ranging from 4 to 13 servings daily.[65]

Whole Grains and Legumes

Whole grains are higher in fiber, certain vitamins, and minerals than are processed (refined) flour products. The Black Women's Health Study, a prospective study of 59,000 African American women, suggests that a diet containing more whole grains, vegetables, fruit, and fish (the "prudent diet") is associated with lower risk of breast cancer when compared with a Western diet containing refined grains, processed meats, and sweets.[66] In another study, adherence to a Mediterranean diet and dietary patterns characterized by low intake of meat and starches and high intake of legumes was found to reduce the risk of breast cancer in Asian American women.[67]

Evidence for the association between fiber intake and cancer risk supports consumption of high-fiber foods.[68] Because the benefits that grain-based foods impart might derive from their other nutrients and phytochemicals, as well as from fiber, it is best to obtain fiber from whole grains—and vegetables and fruits—rather than from fiber supplements.

Beans and other legumes are excellent sources of many vitamins and minerals, protein, and fiber. Legumes and, in particular, soy are especially rich in nutrients and phytochemicals that can protect against prostate cancer[69] and possibly breast cancer[70] and can be a useful low-fat, high-protein alternative to meat.

Putting It All Together

Some cancer risk factors can be avoided. Others, such as inherited factors, are unavoidable, but it is helpful to be aware of them. People can help protect themselves by avoiding known risk factors whenever possible. They can also talk with their doctors about regular checkups and the value of cancer screening tests. (See **FIGURE 10.10.**) Reducing both the number of new cancer cases and the death rates from cancer are key objectives of Healthy People 2020.

To reduce your cancer risk, eat a moderately low-fat diet and increase your consumption of fruits, vegetables, and whole grains. Maintain a healthy weight, exercise regularly, don't smoke, and don't use alcohol excessively. If these recommendations are beginning to sound like a broken record, you're right—the same lifestyle changes that reduce the risk of atherosclerosis and hypertension can reduce the risk of cancer.

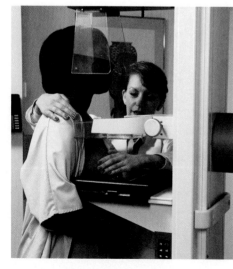

FIGURE 10.10 Cancer screening tests. Mammograms can detect breast cancer at an early stage and improve chances for successful treatment.
© Keith Brofsky/Photodisc/Getty Images.

Key Concepts Cancer develops when something alters cellular DNA so cells divide and multiply uncontrollably. Both genetic factors and environmental factors, including diet, influence cancer risk. Strategies for reducing cancer risk include eating more fruits, vegetables, and whole grains; increasing physical activity; maintaining a healthy weight; and limiting alcohol consumption.

Diabetes Mellitus

🍎 **Why Is This Important?** Diet and lifestyle play important roles in managing diabetes, especially the most common form—type 2 diabetes. The risk of developing type 2 diabetes increases progressively as body fat increases, especially around the midsection. Healthy eating, modest weight loss, and increases in physical activity can reduce type 2 diabetes risk substantially.

Almost everyone knows someone who has diabetes. An estimated 30.3 million people in the United States—9.4 percent of the population—have diabetes mellitus.[71] Although an estimated 23.1 million have been diagnosed, unfortunately 7.2 million people do not realize that they have this serious, lifelong condition.[72] If present trends continue, 1 in 3 American adults will have diabetes in 2050.[73] **FIGURE 10.11** shows the prevalence of obesity and diagnosed diabetes among U.S. adults.

What Is Diabetes?

Diabetes is a disorder of carbohydrate metabolism—the way our bodies use digested carbohydrates for growth and energy. Carbohydrates in food are digested and absorbed and end up as glucose in the blood. Glucose is a major source of fuel for the body. After digestion, glucose passes into the bloodstream and into cells, where it is used for growth and energy. For glucose to enter into most types of cells, insulin must be present. Insulin is a hormone produced by the pancreas.

When we eat carbohydrates, the pancreas should automatically produce the right amount of insulin to move glucose from blood into our cells. In people with diabetes, however, the pancreas either produces little or no insulin or the cells do not respond appropriately to the insulin that is produced. As a result, glucose builds up in the blood, causing **hyperglycemia**—an abnormally high blood glucose level that is the hallmark of diabetes mellitus.

Even though glucose in the blood is overabundant, it is unable to enter starving cells to fuel their needs. For this reason, diabetes often is called a disease of "starvation in the midst of plenty." In an ironic twist of fate, these starving cells signal the liver to make more glucose, worsening the hyperglycemia. The kidneys are taxed beyond their capacities to reabsorb glucose, and the excess spills into the urine, where it can be detected by urine glucose tests. Thus, even though the blood contains large amounts of glucose, the body loses access to its main source of fuel.

Unable to use glucose, cells turn to other energy sources—fat and protein. But these options can lead to other problems. Excessive use of fat as an energy source, without available glucose in the cell, causes ketosis and acidosis, dangerously high acidity levels in the blood. Breaking down muscle proteins to fuel the cells causes muscle wasting and weakness. Alterations in fat and protein metabolism often accompany hyperglycemia.[74]

Over time, abnormally high blood glucose levels increase the risk of high blood pressure, heart disease, and kidney disease. Excess glucose in the blood reacts with and damages body proteins and tissues, especially in the eyes, kidneys, nerves, and blood vessels. Complications of diabetes can contribute to degenerative conditions such as peripheral vascular disease (disease of blood vessels that supply the feet and legs), deterioration of the eye and eventual blindness, kidney disease, and progressive nerve damage. Diabetes is responsible for more than

Quick **Bite**

Smartphones Advance Artificial Pancreas

In an artificial pancreas, a computer calculates each insulin dose based on glucose levels and delivers insulin automatically through an insulin pump with minimal human input. Although significant progress has been made, laptops severely limit mobility. In tests, smartphone technology replaced laptops and had proper communication 98 percent of the time—far exceeding the 80 percent target. Participants stayed in real world settings, such as hotels, and ate whatever they wanted.

▶ **hyperglycemia [HIGH-per-gly-SEE-me-uh]** Abnormally high concentration of glucose in the blood.

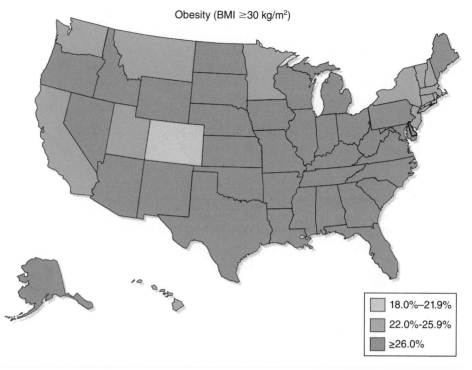

Obesity (BMI ≥30 kg/m²)

18.0%–21.9%

22.0%-25.9%

≥26.0%

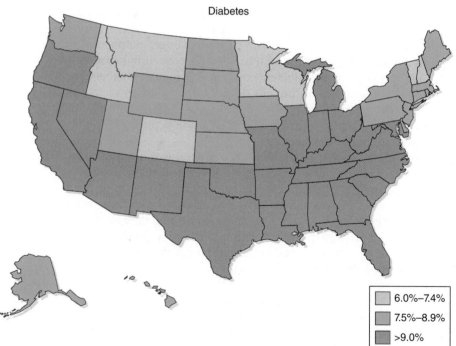

Diabetes

6.0%–7.4%

7.5%–8.9%

>9.0%

FIGURE 10.11 Prevalence of obesity and diagnosed diabetes among U.S. adults, 2015.

CDC's Division of Diabetes Translation. Maps of Diagnosed Diabetes and Obesity in 1994, 2000, and 2015. (2017, April). Retrieved September 5, 2017, from https://www.cdc.gov/diabetes/statistics/slides/maps_diabetesobesity94.pdf.

60 percent of all nontraumatic amputations of the lower extremities and 44 percent of all new cases of kidney failure in adults.[75] Diabetes is also the leading cause of blindness in adults.[76] Diabetics are 40 times more likely to develop glaucoma than nondiabetics.[77] Sixty-seven percent of people with diabetes have high blood pressure, and nearly all have one

or more lipid abnormalities.[78] People with diabetes are two to four times more likely to develop heart disease or have a stroke than people without diabetes.[79] In the United States and Canada, diabetes is one of the leading contributors to death and disability.

Diagnosis of Diabetes Mellitus

A diagnosis of diabetes mellitus is usually made by measuring plasma glucose concentration either after an overnight fast, as part of an oral glucose tolerance test (OGTT) (see **FIGURE 10.12**), or any time of the day if a patient presents with symptoms of diabetes. The classic symptoms of diabetes mellitus are polyuria (excessive urination), polydipsia (excessive thirst), and unexplained weight loss, sometimes with polyphagia (excessive eating). The diagnostic criteria for diabetes mellitus are shown in **TABLE 10.7**. Three major types of diabetes exist:

1. *Type 1 diabetes:* **Type 1 diabetes** usually is diagnosed in children and young adults and was previously known as insulin-dependent diabetes mellitus (IDDM) or juvenile diabetes. In type 1 diabetes, the body fails to produce insulin, the hormone that "unlocks" cells, allowing glucose to enter and fuel them. Roughly 5 to 10 percent of Americans who are diagnosed with diabetes have type 1 diabetes.[80]
2. *Type 2 diabetes:* In **type 2 diabetes**, either the body does not produce enough insulin or cells ignore the insulin. Type 2 diabetes was previously known as non-insulin-dependent diabetes mellitus (NIDDM) or adult-onset diabetes. Approximately 90 to 95 percent of all Americans with diabetes mellitus have type 2 diabetes.[81]
3. *Gestational diabetes:* **Gestational diabetes** occurs in a pregnant woman who has never had diabetes, but who develops hyperglycemia during pregnancy. In the United States, gestational diabetes affects 7 to 18 percent of pregnancies, and the number of cases is thought to be growing.[82]

Pre-diabetes (impaired glucose tolerance or impaired fasting glucose) is a condition in which a person's blood glucose levels are higher than normal but not high enough to warrant a diagnosis of type 2 diabetes. In 2012, an estimated 86 million American adults over the age of 20 had pre-diabetes, up from 79 million in 2010.[83]

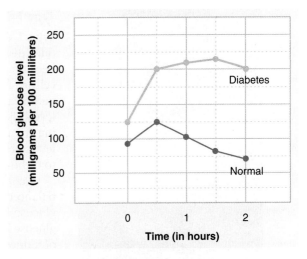

FIGURE 10.12 Glucose tolerance test. A glucose tolerance test measures the level of glucose in the blood following consumption of a standard dose of glucose. Glucose tolerance tests are used to diagnose diabetes.

▶ **type 1 diabetes** Diabetes that occurs when the body's immune system attacks beta cells in the pancreas, causing them to lose their ability to make insulin.

▶ **type 2 diabetes** Diabetes that occurs when target cells (e.g., fat and muscle cells) lose the ability to respond normally to insulin.

▶ **gestational diabetes** A condition that results in high blood glucose levels during pregnancy.

▶ **pre-diabetes** Blood glucose levels higher than normal but not high enough to warrant a diagnosis of diabetes.

TABLE 10.7
Diagnostic Criteria for Diabetes Mellitus

Blood Test Levels for Diagnosis of Diabetes and Pre-diabetes

	A1c (percent)	Fasting Plasma Glucose (mg/dL)	Oral Glucose Tolerance Test (mg/dL)
Diabetes	6.5 or above	126 or above	200 or above
Pre-diabetes	5.7 to 6.4	100 to 125	140 to 199
Normal	Below 5.7	99 or below	139 or below

National Institutes of Health. National Insititute of Diabetes and Digestive and Kidney Diseases. The A1C Test & Diabetes. https://www.niddk.nih.gov/health-information/diabetes/overview/tests-diagnosis/a1c-test. Accessed March 1, 2017; and Adapted from American Diabetes Association. Classification and diagnosis of diabetes. *Diabetes Care*. 2016;39(1):S14–S20, tables 2.1, 2.3.

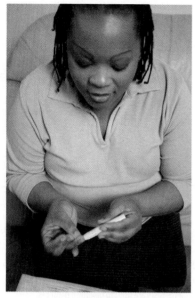

© Custom Medical Stock Photo/Alamy Images.

▶ **insulin resistance** State in which enough insulin is produced but cells do not respond to the action of insulin. Also called *insulin insensitivity*.

Type 1 Diabetes Mellitus

Type 1 diabetes usually occurs in people younger than 30 years and often develops suddenly. People with type 1 diabetes lack insulin, usually because an autoimmune response has destroyed the insulin-producing cells of the pancreas. Symptoms include excessive thirst, frequent urination, rapid weight loss, and blurred vision.[84] When blood glucose levels rise, glucose spills into the urine, taking water with it and causing frequent urination and increased thirst. Although blood glucose levels are high, the lack of insulin prevents glucose from entering cells to be burned for energy. The result is weight loss and feelings of hunger.

People with type 1 diabetes require lifelong, daily insulin injections balanced with a healthful diet and regular exercise to maintain blood glucose levels in the normal range. Initiating good control of blood glucose levels early reduces kidney damage and reduces long-term risk of kidney disease by 50 percent.[85] Because exercise lowers blood glucose levels, individuals must consider the timing of exercise in addition to food intake and insulin injections to avoid lowering blood glucose levels excessively.

Type 2 Diabetes Mellitus

In type 2 diabetes, glucose has trouble entering body cells because either the pancreas cannot produce enough insulin or cells in the body become resistant to the action of insulin. Although obesity contributes to **insulin resistance** in many people with type 2 diabetes, genetic factors also play a role. Type 2 diabetes usually develops in overweight individuals age 45 or older. However, with the rising prevalence of obesity, type 2 diabetes is occurring more frequently in adolescents.

The result is the same as for type 1 diabetes—glucose builds up in the blood, and the body cannot use its main source of fuel efficiently. Type 2 diabetes often is part of a metabolic syndrome that includes obesity, elevated blood pressure, and high levels of blood triglycerides. (See the "Metabolic Syndrome" section later in this chapter.)

In contrast to the sudden onset of type 1 diabetes, the symptoms of type 2 diabetes develop gradually, and some people may not show symptoms for many years. Symptoms of type 2 diabetes eventually include fatigue or nausea, frequent urination, unusual thirst, weight loss, blurred vision, frequent infections, and slow healing of wounds or sores.

Pre-diabetes

Before people develop type 2 diabetes, they usually have pre-diabetes—impaired glucose tolerance that results in a blood glucose level that is higher than normal yet not high enough to be diagnosed as diabetes. Some long-term damage to the body, especially to the heart and circulatory system, may already be occurring during the pre-diabetes stage.

People who have pre-diabetes are at increased risk for developing both type 2 diabetes and heart disease. Unless they take steps toward prevention, such as dietary changes, moderate weight loss, and regular exercise, many will develop type 2 diabetes within 10 years.

Gestational Diabetes Mellitus

During pregnancy—usually around the 24th week—some women develop gestational diabetes. These women may never have had diabetes before, but they developed impaired glucose tolerance during pregnancy. To check for gestational diabetes, many health practitioners routinely recommend a glucose test between 24 and 28 weeks of pregnancy.

Although the cause of gestational diabetes remains unknown, researchers have uncovered certain clues. The placenta produces hormones that help the baby develop. Unfortunately, these hormones also block the action of the mother's insulin in her body. This insulin resistance makes it difficult for the mother's body to use insulin and can triple the amount of insulin needed to get sufficient glucose into her cells. Gestational diabetes occurs more often in African Americans, Native Americans, and Hispanic Americans and is more common among obese women and women with a family history of diabetes.

In women with gestational diabetes, blood glucose levels usually decrease after pregnancy. Once a woman has had gestational diabetes, however, her chances are 2 in 3 that it will return in future pregnancies. In a few women, pregnancy reveals preexisting type 1 or type 2 diabetes that requires ongoing treatment after pregnancy. Women who have had gestational diabetes have a three- to seven-fold higher risk of developing type 2 diabetes within 5 to 10 years.[86] Both forms of diabetes involve insulin resistance.

Low Blood Glucose Levels: Hypoglycemia

Excess insulin results in low blood sugar, or **hypoglycemia**. Too much glucose enters cells, lowering blood glucose levels too far. When blood glucose levels drop too low, nervousness, irritability, hunger, headache, shakiness, rapid heartbeat, and weakness can develop. A further drop in blood glucose levels can cause coma and death.

A person with diabetes can develop hypoglycemia in response to an overdose of insulin or vigorous exercise. In nondiabetic individuals, two types of hypoglycemia occur—reactive hypoglycemia (related to the insulin drop after eating) and fasting hypoglycemia (which may be related to nondiabetic disease, medicines, or alcohol, especially binging). **Reactive hypoglycemia** occurs about one hour after eating carbohydrate-rich food. The body overreacts and produces too much insulin in response to the food. Individuals can prevent reactive hypoglycemia by eating frequent, smaller meals to smooth out blood glucose responses to food.

▶ **hypoglycemia [HIGH-po-gly-SEE-mee-uh]** Abnormally low concentration of glucose in the blood; any blood glucose value below 40 to 50 mg/dL of blood.

▶ **reactive hypoglycemia** A type of hypoglycemia that occurs about one hour after eating carbohydrate-rich food. The body overreacts and produces too much insulin in response to food, rapidly decreasing blood glucose.

> **Key Concepts** Approximately 29.1 million people in the United States have diabetes mellitus, a leading cause of death and disability. Unfortunately, 8.1 million of these people are unaware that they have the disease. If current trends continue, 1 in 3 Americans will have diabetes in 2050. Three major types of diabetes have been identified: type 1, type 2, and gestational diabetes. Type 1, the most severe form, requires a daily regimen of insulin, careful diet control, and physical activity. In type 2 diabetes, the treatment focuses on diet and weight loss. Gestational diabetes occurs during pregnancy and usually goes away after delivery.

Risk Factors for Diabetes

Some people are at higher risk than others for developing diabetes. **TABLE 10.8** lists the risk factors for type 1 and type 2 diabetes. Anyone with a family history of diabetes has an increased risk. In most cases of type 1 diabetes, people must inherit risk factors from both parents, and whites have the highest rate of this disease.[87,88] Yet genes do not tell the complete story. When one identical twin has type 1 diabetes, for example, the other twin gets the disease, at most, only half the time.[89] Possible environmental triggers include exposure to certain viruses or other infectious agents that activate the immune system. Type 1 diabetes develops more often in winter than summer and is more common in countries with cold climates (Sweden, Finland).

TABLE 10.8
Risk Factors for Type 1 and Type 2 Diabetes Mellitus

Risk Factors for Type 1 Diabetes

- First-degree relative (parent, sibling) with type 1 diabetes

Risk Factors for Type 2 Diabetes

- Age ≥ 45 years
- Overweight (BMI ≥ 25 kg/m²)
- First-degree relative with diabetes
- Sedentary lifestyle
- Ethnicity: African American, Latino, Native American, Asian American, Pacific Islander
- Previously identified pre-diabetes
- History of gestational diabetes or delivery of a baby weighing more than 9 pounds
- Hypertension (≥ 140/90 mm Hg)
- HDL cholesterol level < 35 mg/dL and/or triglyceride level > 250 mg/dL
- Polycystic ovary syndrome
- History of vascular disease

Reproduced from American Diabetes Association. Position statement: prevention of type 1 diabetes. *Diabetes Care*. 2004;27 (suppl 1):S133; and American Diabetes Association. Position statement: prevention or delay of type 2 diabetes. *Diabetes Care*. 2004;27 (suppl 1):S47–S54. Copyright © 2004 American Diabetes Association. Reprinted with permission from American Diabetes Association.

Early diet also can play a role. For example, type 1 diabetes is less common in people who were breastfed and began eating solid food at older ages.[90]

A family history of type 2 diabetes is one of the strongest risk factors for getting the disease.[91] As with gestational diabetes, the ethnic groups at highest risk of type 2 diabetes are Native Americans, Hispanic Americans, and African Americans. An increased risk of type 2 diabetes seems to occur more frequently in people who follow a "Western" lifestyle characterized by too much fat, too few fruits and vegetables, too little fiber, and not enough exercise.[92]

The risk of developing type 2 diabetes increases progressively as body fat increases, especially around the midsection. The dramatic surge in obesity rates in the United States is a major reason that the incidence of type 2 diabetes not only has increased dramatically in adults, but also has become a sizable and growing problem among U.S. children and adolescents.[93] Compared with a normal-weight person, an obese person has a significantly increased risk of developing type 2 diabetes.[94] Unfortunately, as more children and adolescents become overweight, type 2 diabetes is becoming more common in young people. Contrary to popular opinion, high sugar or high carbohydrate intake does not by itself cause diabetes, as long as it does not contribute to excess energy intake and obesity.

Do other dietary factors make a difference? Dietary fat is of interest to researchers due to its influence on glucose metabolism by altering cell function, enzyme activity, insulin signaling, and gene expression. A recent study found that people with the highest intakes of saturated and animal fat had about double the risk of type 2 diabetes than people with the lowest intakes.[95] Numerous studies have shown a protective effect of increased consumption of nonstarch polysaccharides (fiber). Conversely, drinking more sugar-sweetened beverages[96,97] or diet beverages[98] has been associated with an increased risk of type 2 diabetes.

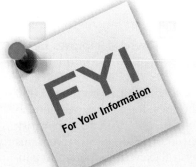

Nutrition, Health, and Wellness Coaching

Obesity, physical inactivity, and other unhealthy lifestyle conditions continue to be major health issues in this country and worldwide. In concert with this we have witnessed an incredible growth in health and wellness careers over the last few years. The expansion of various careers in nutrition and wellness has increased exponentially. You cannot pick up a magazine or newspaper, or visit a social media site without some discussion of nutrition or wellness.

Making lifestyle changes is difficult. Usually people need assistance. Many people will tell you that they have the knowledge of what to do to set their health goals, such as eating more vegetables and fruits and getting more exercise, but for various reasons they don't incorporate these recommendations into their daily lives. Life has become too busy or stressful, or they just don't know how to fit the needed changes into their current lifestyles. Consumers need to be supplied with accurate, doable information. People are always looking for a quick fix. That is why most have been unsuccessful in achieving their goals in the past.

One of the new occupations that can help the consumer achieve change goals is personal coaching. If coaching works for sports teams, if it can get them motivated to do their best and to be successful, then why can't it work for individuals? Individual plans, mutual goal setting, and positive motivation are all important components of making successful lifestyle changes. The main pillars of coaching are motivational interviewing, positive psychology, and mindfulness. All three of these components are necessary to help people change successfully. What works for one person may not work for another person. People achieve success by different means. Coaches help the individual choose the correct change process by using input from the client. Personal coaching appears to be meeting these needs of individuals and leading this trend of individualization, motivation, education, and positive support.

People have a tendency to be more successful at making lifestyle changes when they have continuous, positive support and they are allowed to actively participate in setting the goals they would like to achieve for themselves. This is one of the ways coaches differ from the traditional healthcare provider. In many cases the traditional healthcare provider *tells* the client what to do and how to achieve it. The coach gives the client equal authority in the relationship. The client actively participates in choosing what goal he or she would like to accomplish and how he or she is willing to change so the goal can be achieved. The coach is the listener, enabler, and positive motivator.

Coaches can play a valuable part in helping people change their lifestyle habits. It can be a rewarding career. Currently, however, there is no single professional organization overseeing the credentials of all coaches. Any individual or organization can offer a certificate in coaching. What does this mean to consumers? Some coaches may not be trained with the three pillars of coaching. Because there are no standard educational requirements, some coaches have no formal education in nutrition, health, or wellness and do not know or understand evidence-based science. What some teach may actually be harmful to certain people. So, whether you are looking to improve your health with a coach or you think you have what it takes to motivate and educate others and are interested in becoming a certified coach, look over training programs carefully. In other words, buyer beware!

For more information on coaching, visit the International Coach Federation (ICF) website at http://coachfederation.org.

Additional Resources

a Clark MM, Bradley KL, Jenkins SM, et al. The effectiveness of wellness coaching for improving quality of life. *Mayo Clin Proc.* 2014;89(11):1537-1544.

b Mettler EM, Preston HR, Jenkins SM, et al. Motivational improvements for health behavior from wellness coaching. *Am J Health Behav.* 2014;38(1):83-91.

c WebMD. Wellness coaching: the latest trend in fitness. http://www.webmd.com/balance/features/wellness-coaching-the-latest-trend-in-fitness. Accessed September 16, 2017.

d Brogen J. Are you ready for wellness coaching? *Boston Globe.* January 2, 2012. http://www.boston.com/lifestyle/health/articles/2012/01/02/are_you_ready_for_wellness_coaching/?page=2. Accessed September 16, 2017.

e National Consortium for Credentialing of Health and Wellness Coaches. Vision & mission. http://ichwc.org/mission-vision/. Accessed September 16, 2017.

f International Coach Federation. Code of ethics. http://coachfederation.org/about/ethics.aspx?ItemNumber=854&RDtoken=55851&userID=. Accessed September 16, 2017.

g Mayo Clinic. Wellness coaching: expert explains how it improves overall quality of life. *Science-Daily.* August 7, 2014. http://www.science-daily.com/releases/2014/08/140807104700.htm. Accessed September 16, 2017.

h International Coach Federation. Forbes columnist forecasts coaching as a top personal branding trend for 2015. http://coachfederation.org/newsdetail.cfm?ItemNumber=3776. Accessed September 16, 2017.

i Aruda W. The hottest personal branding trends that will impact your success in 2015. *Forbes.* http://www.forbes.com/sites/williamarruda/2014/12/02/the-hottest-personal-branding-trends-that-will-impact-your-success-in-2015-part-1/. Accessed September 16, 2017.

Dietary and Lifestyle Factors for Reducing Diabetes Risk

Obesity is the single largest modifiable risk factor in the development of type 2 diabetes. Therefore, the best measures for preventing prediabetes and obesity-related type 2 diabetes are a healthful diet and regular exercise. Reducing excess body fat improves glucose tolerance and reduces related risk factors for heart disease. Regular exercise improves carbohydrate and lipid metabolism and increases insulin sensitivity

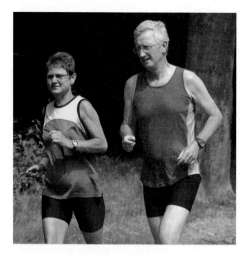

FIGURE 10.13 Exercise and diabetes. Regular physical activity improves glucose tolerance and helps reduce the risk of developing type 2 diabetes later in life.
© M.G. Mooij/Shutterstock, Inc.

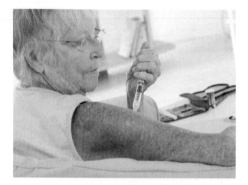

FIGURE 10.14 Insulin injections. In type 1 diabetes and some cases of type 2 diabetes, people need daily insulin injections to normalize blood glucose levels.
© CHASSENET/age fotostock.

(see **FIGURE 10.13**). As previously mentioned, exercise improves blood flow to the extremities, bringing blood pressure down to normal levels and reducing the risk of heart disease.

The Diabetes Prevention Program, a study of more than 3,000 people, 45 percent of whom were minorities, found that people who received intensive lifestyle intervention were able to reduce their risk of developing type 2 diabetes by 58 percent. The lifestyle interventions included walking or other moderate physical exercise for about 30 minutes per day and weight reduction of 5 to 7 percent.[99]

Online social media can support diabetes prevention. Use of an online social network program based on the Diabetes Prevention Program (Prevent) has been validated against the Centers for Disease Control and Prevention outcome standards for weight loss and blood glucose control. Online delivery platforms such as Prevent offer an effective and scalable solution for preventing diabetes.[100]

Management of Diabetes

Before the discovery of insulin in 1921, everyone with type 1 diabetes died within a few years after diagnosis. Although insulin therapy is not a cure, its discovery represented the first major breakthrough in diabetes treatment.

Today, healthy eating, physical activity, and insulin delivery by injection (see **FIGURE 10.14**) or an insulin pump are the basic therapies for type 1 diabetes. The amount of insulin must be balanced with food intake and daily activities. Blood glucose concentrations must be closely monitored.

Healthy eating, physical activity, and blood glucose testing are the basic management tools for type 2 diabetes, and weight loss often restores normal glucose metabolism. Weight loss can decrease insulin resistance and improve blood glucose levels. Exercise increases the sensitivity of body cells to insulin, so the body needs less insulin to get glucose into cells. "Small Steps, Big Rewards: Prevent Type 2 Diabetes" is a diabetes prevention campaign created by the National Diabetes Education Program based on the Diabetes Prevention Program.[101] Aimed at helping people lose a modest amount of weight, get 30 minutes of exercise five days a week, and make healthier food choices, the program enables people at risk to delay or prevent the onset of type 2 diabetes.

If diet and exercise fail to maintain blood glucose levels in the normal range, people with type 2 diabetes need medications to either increase insulin production or improve glucose uptake by cells. In some cases, insulin injections are needed to normalize blood glucose levels.

Nutrition

Although people with diabetes have the same nutritional needs as anyone else, good diabetes control requires that they monitor their food intake carefully. People with diabetes must take extra care to balance food intake with insulin and oral medications (if they take them), and exercise to help manage their blood glucose levels.

By eating well-balanced meals in the correct amounts, people can keep their blood glucose levels as close to normal (nondiabetes level) as possible. The American Diabetes Association offers My Health Advisor, an online resource that helps with diabetes management and includes a database of foods, recipes, and nutrient information.[102]

Specific meal plans should be based on an individual's usual food intake. People with type 1 diabetes should eat at about the same time each day and should try to be consistent regarding the types of food they choose. Keeping calorie and carbohydrate intake consistent helps to prevent blood glucose levels from becoming too high or too low. Although new rapid-acting insulin is providing greater freedom and flexibility, effects can vary among people. People with type 2 diabetes should consume a diet that is well balanced, low in fat, and promotes a healthy body weight. Dietary carbohydrates should come from fruits, vegetables, and whole grains. Having diabetes once meant a lifetime of meals that lacked one of the most pleasant aspects of taste: sweetness. Although in the past dietary treatment of diabetes eliminated simple sugars from the diet, current recommendations allow individuals with diabetes to include moderate amounts of simple sugars in their diet as long as sugar intake does not contribute to excess energy intake and obesity.

Putting It All Together

Researchers continue to search for the cause or causes of diabetes and ways to prevent and cure it. Some genetic markers for type 1 diabetes have been identified, and it is now possible to screen relatives of people with type 1 diabetes to see whether they are at increased risk. In the future, it may be possible to administer insulin through inhalers, a pill, or a patch.

For now, the challenge is to slow the rate at which diabetes incidence is increasing. Healthy People 2020 objectives include a reduction in incidence of diabetes along with the economic burden it presents. Results from the Diabetes Prevention Program show that relatively modest changes in weight and exercise can be enough to reduce the incidence of diabetes. We turn, once again, to advice encouraging healthful eating (consumption of more fruits, vegetables, and fiber), regular physical activity, and lifelong weight management.

Key Concepts Family history is a risk factor for both type 1 and type 2 diabetes. For type 2 diabetes, additional risk factors include increasing age, overweight, sedentary lifestyle, and ethnicity. Risk reduction can be achieved through healthy eating, modest weight loss, and increases in physical activity.

Metabolic Syndrome

Thirty-four percent of adults in the United States meet the criteria for **metabolic syndrome**, a group of symptoms that occur together and promote the development of coronary artery disease, stroke, and type 2 diabetes. The prevalence will continue to grow because of the widespread tendency toward a sedentary lifestyle, according to the Centers for Disease Control and Prevention.[103] Metabolic syndrome is usually indicated by a cluster of at least three of the following signs[104]:

▶ **metabolic syndrome** A cluster of at least three of the following risk factors for heart disease: hypertriglyceridemia (high blood triglycerides), low HDL cholesterol, hyperglycemia (high blood glucose), hypertension (high blood pressure), and excess abdominal fat.

- *Abdominal obesity:* For most men, a 40-inch waist or greater; for women, a waist of 35 inches or greater
- *High fasting blood glucose:* At least 100 mg/dL
- *High serum triglycerides:* At least 150 mg/dL
- *Low HDL cholesterol:* Less than 40 mg/dL for men; less than 50 mg/dL for women
- *Elevated blood pressure:* 130 mm Hg or above, systolic; or 85 mm Hg or above, diastolic

Taken individually, these risk factors might not look particularly serious. When you put them together, however, the problems rise substantially. Individuals with metabolic syndrome are at increased risk for both cardiovascular disease and type 2 diabetes.[105,106] More studies are needed to understand the relationship between the risk factors embodied in metabolic syndrome, but researchers have identified people with metabolic syndrome as having the greatest risk of death from heart attack.

Although some scientists think that metabolic syndrome is genetically based, it is unlikely that metabolic syndrome results from a single cause. The primary underlying diabetic and cardiac risk factors appear to be insulin resistance and abdominal obesity. For many people, poor diet and lack of physical activity combined with a genetic predisposition lead to the development of the syndrome. The high prevalence of metabolic syndrome underscores an urgent need to develop comprehensive efforts directed at controlling the obesity epidemic and improving physical activity levels.

People with metabolic syndrome should work with their medical team to do the following:

- Monitor blood glucose, lipoproteins, and blood pressure.
- Achieve and maintain a healthy body weight and increase physical activity—both are time-tested methods of improving insulin sensitivity, blood pressure, and lipoprotein levels.
- Treat diabetes and hyperlipidemia according to established guidelines.
- Choose drug therapy for hypertension with care—different medications have different effects on insulin sensitivity.

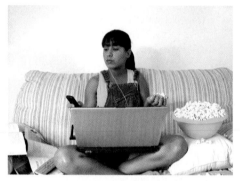

© Hemera/Thinkstock.

Key Concepts Metabolic syndrome, associated with an increased risk of death from heart attack, is a cluster including at least three of the following signs: abdominal fat, elevated blood glucose, elevated triglycerides and low HDL cholesterol, and elevated blood pressure. A poor diet and sedentary lifestyle combined with a genetic predisposition are thought to be the underlying causes.

Osteoporosis

🍎 **Why Is This Important?** Maximizing peak bone mass early in life can go a long way toward preventing or at least delaying osteoporosis. Adequate calcium and vitamin D intake throughout life, along with regular exercise, helps prevent osteoporosis.

Osteoporosis is a major public health problem, and in the United States more than 40 million people either already have osteoporosis or are at high risk because of low bone mass.[107] Although 80 percent of those with osteoporosis are women, up to one in four men over age 50 will break a bone due to osteoporosis.[108] However, women are most at risk for bone fractures related to osteoporosis. During their lifetimes, one in three women will suffer an osteoporotic fracture, and the risk increases with age.[109] Although we often associate osteoporosis with being elderly, the stage for its emergence is actually set much earlier in life, much like other chronic diseases. Fortunately, diet and lifestyle changes can help to delay the onset of osteoporosis and prevent related fractures.

What Is Osteoporosis?

Osteoporosis means "porous bone." It's a good description because bone mass or density declines and bone quality deteriorates, leaving the bones fragile and vulnerable to fracture. The hip, spine, and wrist bones are especially vulnerable. Often called a "silent disease," osteoporosis develops over several years without outward symptoms. Eventually bone loss makes bones so weak that they break with a mild strain, bump, or fall. In fact, in some cases, the break may occur first and cause the fall!

Bone strength depends on two main features: bone density and bone quality. Bone density is determined by peak bone mass and amount of bone loss. Bone quality refers to architecture, turnover, damage accumulation (e.g., microfractures), and mineralization. Currently, no accurate measure of overall bone strength exists. Bone mineral density (BMD) is frequently used as a proxy measure and accounts for approximately 70 percent of bone strength. Low bone mineral density is an important predictor of future bone fractures. Other predictors include a history of falls, low physical function such as slow gait speed and decreased leg muscle strength, impaired cognition, impaired vision, and the presence of environmental hazards (e.g., throw rugs). Some risks for fracture, such as age, low BMI, and low levels of physical activity, probably increase the rate of fractures through decreased bone density, increased propensity to fall, and inability to absorb impact.

Risk Factors for Osteoporosis

A common misperception is that osteoporosis always results from excessive bone loss. Bone loss commonly occurs as men and women age; however, a person who does not reach optimal (i.e., peak) bone mass during childhood and adolescence can develop osteoporosis without the occurrence of accelerated bone loss. Hence, suboptimal bone growth in childhood and adolescence is as important as bone loss in the development of osteoporosis. **TABLE 10.9** lists the risk factors for osteoporosis.

Bone mass typically peaks sometime around age 30. Starting in midlife, bone breakdown exceeds bone formation, and the progressive loss of bone begins. If you got enough calcium and vitamin D earlier in life so you maximized bone mass, then when bone loss begins you are likely to be a long way from low bone density and fractures.

Because declining estrogen levels accelerate bone loss, postmenopausal women have the highest risk of developing osteoporosis. By age 65, some women have lost half their skeletal mass, and they may show deformities of the upper spine, known as a "dowager's hump" (see **FIGURES 10.15** and **10.16**). Women who reach menopause with low bone mass have a greatly increased risk of fractures.

Many medical disorders, such as genetic disorders, endocrine disorders, congestive heart failure, kidney disease, and alcoholism, as well as administration of certain drugs such as steroids, also can lead to osteoporosis and increased fracture risk.

Dietary and Lifestyle Factors for Reducing Osteoporosis Risk

The main factor in reducing risk of osteoporosis and related fractures is maximum peak bone mass. Dietary components such as calcium and vitamin D help to achieve and maintain bone mass. Engaging in physical activity, especially weight-bearing exercise, helps to increase peak bone mass early in life and helps to maintain muscle strength and coordination that will reduce risk for falls later in life.

TABLE 10.9
Risk Factors for Osteoporosis
• Advanced age
• Female
• Thin and/or small frame
• Family history of osteoporosis
• Early menopause, whether natural or surgically induced
• Low testosterone levels in men
• Abnormal absence of menstrual periods (amenorrhea)
• Anorexia nervosa or bulimia nervosa
• Medical conditions such as thyroid disease, rheumatoid arthritis, and problems that block intestinal absorption of calcium
• Use of certain medications, such as corticosteroids and anticonvulsants
• Insufficient dietary calcium
• Lack of weight-bearing exercise
• Cigarette smoking
• Excessive use of alcohol or caffeine
• Insufficient vitamin D

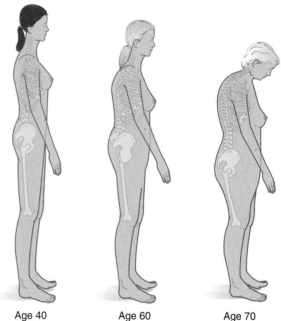

Age 40   Age 60   Age 70

FIGURE 10.15 Progression of dowager's hump.

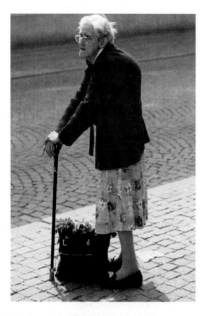

FIGURE 10.16 Dowager's hump. In people with osteoporosis, the bones in the upper spine develop small compression fractures. These bones heal into wedge shapes, and the upper spine assumes a deformed, curved shape known as a "dowager's hump."

© Bengt-Goran Carlsson/age fotostock.

Quick Bite

Lost in Space

Knowing that stress on bones maintains their strength, what would you guess happens in the gravity-free environment of outer space? Experience with prolonged space travel has made it clear that extensive bone and mineral loss are one health hazard of living without gravity's constant pull. Interestingly, changes in non-weight-bearing bones were not seen in studies of space travelers. As humans spend longer periods in space, scientists will be challenged to discover how to preserve bone strength without the constant stimulation of gravity on weight-bearing bones.

Calcium

Calcium is important for attaining peak bone mass and for preventing and treating osteoporosis. Adequate calcium intake throughout life helps prevent osteoporosis, and good calcium intake during childhood and adolescence helps maximize peak bone mass. Even in adulthood, adequate calcium slows bone loss, and it reduces fracture rates in postmenopausal women.

Calcium is clearly an important nutrient in bone health, but it's not the only one. Normal mineralization and maintenance of bone also require vitamins D, A, and K; the minerals phosphorus, fluoride, and magnesium; and protein.

Vitamin D

You need vitamin D for calcium absorption and bone maintenance. Because aging limits the ability to manufacture active vitamin D, older people should use vitamin D–fortified foods such as milk or consider taking vitamin D supplements. Phytate and oxalate, caffeine, and smoking can reduce calcium absorption or increase excretion rates. In Canada, Health Canada recommends that, in addition to following Canada's Food Guide, everyone over the age of 50 should take a daily vitamin D supplement of 400 IU.

Vitamin D deficiency, which occurs more often in postmenopausal women and older Americans,[110] has been associated with a greater risk of hip fractures. Because bone loss increases the risk of fractures, moderate doses of vitamin D supplementation (800 IU/day) can reduce bone turnover and increase bone density.[111] Because high doses of vitamin D can be highly toxic, it is important to be cautious with vitamin D supplements.

Vitamin A

Although vitamin A is essential for normal bone formation, some studies suggest an association between excessive vitamin A intake and weaker bones.[112] Researchers have also noticed that worldwide, the highest incidence of osteoporosis occurs in northern Europe, a population with a high intake of vitamin A.[113] However, this region has lower levels of sun exposure, which leads to decreased biosynthesis of vitamin D, which may be at least partially responsible for these findings.

Evidence does not indicate an association between beta-carotene intake and increased risk of osteoporosis. Instead, current evidence points to a possible association with vitamin A as retinol only. Because studies yield conflicting results, additional research is needed to clarify the association between high levels of vitamin A intake and osteoporosis.

Exercise

Regular weight-bearing and strength-training exercises enhance bone remodeling and strength. Exercise helps maximize bone mass when you're young and will slow bone loss during your later years. In addition to getting enough calcium and vitamin D to promote bone health and slow the development of osteoporosis, fitness experts make the following suggestions:

- Exercise should include weight-bearing and resistance training at least two days per week and should put stress on bones.
- For continued improvement, exercise intensity should increase progressively.

- There is a maximum achievable bone density. As this point is approached, greater efforts are needed to achieve smaller gains.
- Discontinuing an exercise program reverses the benefits.
- Don't smoke, and drink alcoholic beverages only in moderation.

Putting It All Together

Osteoporosis is a debilitating degenerative disease that contributes to poor quality of life in older adults. Although bone loss with age is a major contributor to osteoporosis, maximizing peak bone mass early in life can go a long way toward preventing or at least delaying osteoporosis. Reducing the proportion of adults with osteoporosis is one of the Healthy People 2020 objectives.

To improve your bone health, the U.S. Surgeon General suggests the following: Eat foods rich in calcium and vitamin D, be physically active every day, maintain a healthy body weight throughout your life, protect yourself from falls, avoid smoking, limit alcohol intake, and discuss increased risks with your doctor.[114] Postmenopausal women with low bone density might be advised to consider strength training to prevent or reduce bone loss.

Key Concepts Osteoporosis is the progressive loss of bone mass, resulting in fragile bones that break easily. Osteoporosis primarily affects postmenopausal women who have lower estrogen levels and accelerated rates of bone loss. Adequate calcium intake early in life helps maximize peak bone mass and reduces the risk of osteoporosis. Adequate amounts of vitamin D and regular exercise also are important for bone health.

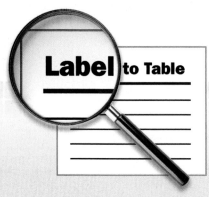

Label to Table

Sodium is found naturally in many foods, but processed foods account for most of the salt and sodium Americans consume. Processed foods with high amounts of salt include regular canned vegetables and soups, frozen dinners, lunch meats, instant and ready-to-eat cereals, and salty chips and other snacks. You can use food labels to choose products lower in sodium.

Compare Labels
Which of these two items is lower in sodium? To tell, check the Percent Daily Value.

The frozen peas are lower in sodium, with just 5 percent of the DV per 1/2 cup serving. The canned peas have three times more sodium than the frozen peas: 16 percent of the DV in one serving. Sodium is found in many foods that might surprise you, such as baking soda, soy sauce, and monosodium glutamate (MSG). Sodium is even found in some antacids—the range is wide. Before trying salt substitutes, check with your doctor, especially if you have high blood pressure. Many salt substitutes contain potassium chloride and can be harmful for individuals who have certain medical conditions or who take diuretic medications.

Nutrition Facts

3 servings per container
Serving size	1/2 cup

Amount per serving
Calories 60

	% Daily Value*
Total Fat 0g	**0%**
Saturated Fat 0g	**0%**
Trans Fat 0g	
Cholesterol 0mg	**0%**
Sodium 380mg	**16%**
Total Carbohydrate 12g	**4%**
Dietary Fiber 3g	**14%**
Total Sugars 4g	
Includes 4g Added Sugars	**8%**
Protein 4g	
Vitamin D 0mcg	0%
Calcium 20mg	2%
Iron 1.4mg	8%
Potassium 124mg	4%

* The % Daily Value (DV) tells you how much a nutrient in a serving of food contributes to a daily diet. 2,000 calories a day is used for general nutrition advice.

Nutrition Facts

3 servings per container
Serving size	1/2 cup

Amount per serving
Calories 60

	% Daily Value*
Total Fat 0g	**0%**
Saturated Fat 0g	**0%**
Trans Fat 0g	
Cholesterol 0mg	**0%**
Sodium 125mg	**5%**
Total Carbohydrate 11g	**4%**
Dietary Fiber 6g	**22%**
Total Sugars 5g	
Includes 5g Added Sugars	**10%**
Protein 5g	
Vitamin D 0mcg	0%
Calcium 300mg	30%
Iron 1.1mg	6%
Potassium 87mg	2%

* The % Daily Value (DV) tells you how much a nutrient in a serving of food contributes to a daily diet. 2,000 calories a day is used for general nutrition advice.

Learning Portfolio

Key Terms

Study Points

- Cardiometabolic disease includes heart disease, stroke, and type 2 diabetes. More than half of cardiometabolic-related deaths are associated with 10 dietary factors.

- Genetics plays a part in nearly all human diseases.

- Much of the prevalence of cardiovascular disease and cancer can be attributed to smoking, consumption of a high-fat diet, and a sedentary lifestyle.

- LDL and HDL cholesterol levels predict heart disease risks more accurately than do total cholesterol levels. Infection and the inflammatory process play a role in heart disease, and C-reactive protein might offer a new assessment of CVD risk.

- Ways to reduce risk for CVD include stopping smoking, exercising daily, managing weight, controlling blood pressure, and eating a healthful diet. Antioxidants, regular fish intake, and moderate alcohol consumption also can help protect against heart disease.

- Because hypertension usually has no specific symptoms or early warning signs, it is often called a silent killer.

- Added weight places greater demands on the cardiovascular system, so people who are overweight are at higher risk for hypertension. Rates of hypertension are higher in countries with high sodium intakes.

- The three phases in the development of cancer are initiation, promotion, and progression.

- Evidence shows that generous intake of vegetables and fruits reduces risk of cancer.

- An estimated 25.8 million people in the United States—8.3 percent of the population—have diabetes mellitus, and one-third of these are unaware of their condition.

- The three major types of diabetes are type 1, type 2, and gestational diabetes.

- The dramatic surge in obesity rates in the United States is a major reason why the incidence of type 2 diabetes has tripled since 1970.

Learning Portfolio (continued)

- Dietary recommendations for people with diabetes emphasize consuming diets rich in complex carbohydrates (including fiber) and low in fat.

- Often called a silent disease, osteoporosis develops over several years without outward symptoms or diagnosis. Osteoporosis affects more than 25 million Americans, making it a major public health problem.

- To promote bone health and slow the development of osteoporosis, fitness experts suggest that exercise should be weight-bearing and should put stress on bones. Examples include walking and running.

Study Questions

1. In what ways do diet and exercise affect your health?

2. What is the major goal of the Human Genome Project?

3. What are the diet-related guidelines for reducing heart disease risk?

4. How do high levels of homocysteine contribute to heart disease?

5. What are the risk factors for hypertension?

6. How can people with hypertension lower their blood pressure?

7. What is the difference between cancer initiation and cancer promotion?

8. What are the major types of diabetes? Describe the differences among them.

9. What is metabolic syndrome?

10. Which vitamin and mineral are most important for maximizing bone mass and reducing risk of osteoporosis?

Try This

Learn CPR!

The cardiopulmonary resuscitation (CPR) courses given by the American Red Cross, the American Heart Association, your local fire department, and other groups can help you save a life someday. Anyone can take these courses and become qualified to perform CPR. Investigate CPR courses in your community, and sign up to take one.

Getting Personal

What's Your Family History?

Look into your family medical history. Is there cardiovascular disease in your family, as indicated by premature deaths from heart attack, stroke, or congestive heart failure? Are there any cases of cancer in your family, and has anyone died of cancer? How about diabetes, hypertension, or osteoporosis? Interview your parents and other relatives and develop a history of chronic disease in your family. These diseases might be risk factors for you. Keep that point in mind as you consider whether you need to make lifestyle changes to stay healthy and avoid chronic disease.

References

1. World Health Organization. Constitution of WHO: principles. http://www.who.int/about/mission/en/. Accessed September 16, 2017.

2. MedlinePlus. Medical dictionary: disease. http://c.merriam-webster.com/medlineplus/disease. Accessed September 16, 2017.

3. World Health Organization. *Diet, Nutrition, and the Prevention of Chronic Diseases: A Report of a Joint WHO/FAO Expert Consultation.* Geneva, Switzerland: Author; 2003. WHO Technical Report Series 916. http://www.who.int/nutrition/topics/4_dietnutrition_prevention/en/. Accessed September 16, 2017.

4. Health Information Management Systems Society. Our partnership: the Academy of Nutrition & Dietetics & HIMSS. http://www.himss.org/ResourceLibrary/ContentReg.aspx?ItemNumber=17147. Accessed September 16, 2017.

5. U.S. Department of Health and Human Services. The vision, mission, and goals of Healthy People 2020. http://www.healthypeople.gov/sites/default/files/HP2020Framework.pdf. Accessed September 16, 2017.

6. Centers for Disease Control and Prevention. CDC health disparities and inequalities report—United States, 2013. *MMWR.* 2013;62 (Suppl 3)

7. Centers for Disease Control and Prevention. CDC strategies for reducing health disparities—selected CDC-sponsored interventions, United States, 2014. *MMWR.* 2014;63(Suppl 1).

8. Mueller NT, Appel LJ. Attributing death to diet: precision counts. *JAMA.* 2017;317(9):908-909.

9. Micha R, Peñalvo JL, Cudhea F, et al. Association between dietary factors and mortality from heart disease, stroke, and type 2 diabetes in the United States. *JAMA.* 2017;317(9):912-924.

10. U.S. Food and Drug Administration. Draft guidance for industry: voluntary sodium reduction goals: target mean and upper bound concentrations for sodium in commercially processed, packaged, and prepared foods. 2016. http://www.fda.gov/Food/GuidanceRegulation/GuidanceDocuments-RegulatoryInformation/ucm494732.htm. Accessed September 16, 2017.

11. Belluz J. In a devastating blow to the beverage industry, 4 cities passed soda taxes. November 9, 2016. http://www.vox.com/2016/11/9/13571902/soda-taxe s-vote-san-francisco-oakland-boulder-albany. Accessed September 16, 2017.

12. Centers for Disease Control and Prevention. Deaths and mortality. https://www.cdc.gov/nchs/fastats/deaths.htm. Accessed September 16, 2017.

13. U.S. Department of Energy, Genomic Science Program. Home page. http://genomicscience.energy.gov/index.shtml. Accessed September 16, 2017.

14. Singh PR, Lele SS, Mukheerjee MS. Gene polymorphisms and low dietary intake of micronutrients in coronary artery disease. *J Nutrigenet Nutrigenomics*. 2011;4(4):203-209.

15. Ferguson JF, Allayee H, Gerszten RE, et al. Nutrigenomics, the microbiome, and gene-environment interactions: new directions in cardiovascular disease research, prevention, and treatment: a scientific statement from the American Heart Association. *Circ Cardiovasc Genet*. 2016;9:291-313.

16. Sales NMR, Pelegrini PB, Goersch MC. Nutrigenomics: definitions and advances of this new science. *J Nutr Metab*. 2014:202759. doi: 10.1155/2014/202759. Epub March 25, 2014. http://www.ncbi.nlm .nih.gov/pmc/articles/PMC3984860/. Accessed September 16, 2017.

17. American Heart Association, American Stroke Association. Heart disease and stroke statistics 2017 at-a-glance. https://www.heart.org/idc /groups/ahamah-public/@wcm/@sop/@smd/documents/downloadable /ucm_491265.pdf. Accessed September 16, 2017.

18. Tufano A, Di Capua M, Coppola A, et al. The infectious burden in atherothrombosis. *Semin Thromb Hemost*. 2012;38(5):515-523.

19. Ibid.

20. National Institutes of Health. Cholesterol management. https://nccih.nih .gov/health/cholesterol.htm. Accessed September 16, 2017.

21. Tufano A, Di Capua M, Coppola A, et al. Op. cit.

22. American Heart Association. The 2020 impact goal. http://www.heart .org/idc/groups/heart-public/@wcm/@swa/documents/downloadable /ucm_425189.pdf. Accessed September 16, 2017.

23. Raj M. Obesity and cardiovascular risk in children and adolescents. *Indian J Endocrinol Metab*. 2012;16(1):13-19.

24. Pashkow FJ. Oxidative stress and inflammation in heart disease: do antioxidants have a role in treatment and/or prevention? *Int J Inflam*. 2011; Article ID 514623. http://dx.doi.org/10.4061/2011/514623. Accessed September 16, 2017.

25. Ye EQ, Chacko SA, Chou EL, Kugizaki M, Liu S. Greater whole-grain intake is associated with lower risk of type 2 diabetes, cardiovascular disease, and weight gain. *J Nutr*. 2012;142(7):1304-1313.

26. Institute of Medicine, Food and Nutrition Board. *Dietary Reference Intakes for Energy, Carbohydrate, Fiber, Fat, Fatty Acids, Cholesterol, Protein, and Amino Acids*. Washington, DC: National Academies Press; 2005.

27. Eilat-Adar S, Sinai T, Yosefy C, Henkin Y. Review: nutritional recommendations for cardiovascular disease prevention. *Nutrients*. 2013;5(9):3646-3683. http://www.ncbi.nlm.nih.gov/pmc/articles/PMC3798927/pdf /nutrients-05-03646.pdf. Accessed September 16, 2017.

28. Bang HO, Dyerberg J. The composition of food consumed by Greenlandic Eskimos. *Acta Med Scand*. 1973;200:69-73.

29. American Heart Association. Fish and omega-3 fatty acids. http://www .heart.org/HEARTORG/GettingHealthy/NutritionCenter/Healthy DietGoals/Fish-and-Omega-3-Fatty-Acids_UCM_303248_Article.jsp. Accessed September 16, 2017.

30. Kotwal S, Jun M, Sullivan D, et al. Omega 3 fatty acids and cardiovascular outcomes: systematic review and meta-analysis. *Circulation*. 2012;5: 808-818. http://circoutcomes.ahajournals.org/content/5/6/808.full .pdf+html. Accessed September 16, 2017.

31. American Heart Association. Fish and omega-3 fatty acids. Op. cit.

32. Chowdhury R, Warnakula S, Kunutsor S, et al. Association of dietary, circulating, and supplement fatty acids with coronary risk: a systematic review and meta-analysis. *Ann Intern Med*. 2014;160(6):398-406.

33. Eckel RH, Jakicic JM, Ard JD, et al. 2013 AHA/ACC guideline on lifestyle management to reduce cardiovascular risk. *Circulation*. 2014;129:S76-S99.

34. Tufts University. Does new study mean "butter is back"? Tufts University Health and Nutrition Letter. June 2014. http://www.nutritionletter .tufts.edu/issues/10_6/current-articles/Does-New-Study-Mean-Butter -Is-Back_1467-1.html?ET=tuftshealthletter:e1955:1459886a:&st=email &s=p_update052714&t=tl1. Accessed September 16, 2017.

35. Eckel RH, Jakicic JM, Ard JD, et al. Op. cit.

36. Baum SJ, Kris-Etherton PM, Lichtenstein AH, et al. Fatty acids in cardiovascular health and disease: a comprehensive update. *J Clin Lipidol*. 2012;6(3):216-234.

37. Ros E, Martinez-Gonzales MA, Estruch R, et al. Mediterranean diet and cardiovascular health: teaching of the PREDIMED study. *Adv Nutr*. 2014;5(3):330S-336S.

38. Fryxell DA. Forget pizza. TuftsNow. April 14, 2014. http://now.tufts.edu /articles/forget-pizza. Accessed September 16, 2017.

39. Arriola L, Martinez-Camblor P, Larranaga N, et al. Alcohol intake and the risk of coronary heart disease in the Spanish EPIC study. *Heart*. 2010; 96(2):124-130.

40. Phend C. Mediterranean diet still being refined. *Medpage Today*. April 23, 2013. http://www.medpagetoday.com/MeetingCoverage/EuroPRevent /38621. Accessed September 16, 2017.

41. Eckel RH, Jakicic JM, Ard JD, et al. Op. cit.

42. Arriola L, Martinez-Camblor P, Larranaga N, et al. Op. cit.

43. U.S. Department of Health and Human Services, U.S. Department of Agriculture. *2015–2020 Dietary Guidelines for Americans*. 8th ed. December 2015. http://health.gov/dietaryguidelines/2015/guidelines/. Accessed September 16, 2017.

44. Clarke R, Halsey J, Bennett D, Lewinston S. Homocysteine and vascular disease: review of published results of the homocysteine-lowering trials. *J Inherit Metab Dis*. 2011;34(1):83-91.

45. Sacks FM, Lichtenstein A, Van Horn L, et al. Soy protein, isoflavones, and cardiovascular health: an American Heart Association science advisory for professionals from the nutrition committee. *Circulation*. 2006;113:1034-1044.

46. Xiao CW. Health effects of soy protein and isoflavones in humans. *J Nutr*. 2008;138(6):1244S-1249S.

47. American Heart Association. The Facts About High Blood Pressure. Nov 17, 2017. http://www.heart.org/HEARTORG/Conditions/HighBlood Pressure/GettheFactsAboutHighBloodPressure/The-Facts-About-High -Blood-Pressure_UCM_002050_Article.jsp#.WhB4CFWnGUk Accessed Nov 18, 2017.

48. American College of Cardiology. New ACC/AHA High Blood Pressure Guidelines Lower Definition of Hypertension. ACC News Story. Nov 13, 2017. http://www.acc.org/latest-in-cardiology/articles/2017/11/08/11/47 /mon-5pm-bp-guideline-aha-2017 Accessed Nov 18, 2017.

49. American Heart Association. High blood pressure and African Americans. http://www.heart.org/HEARTORG/Conditions/HighBloodPressure /UnderstandYourRiskforHighBloodPressure/High-Blood-Pressure-and -African-Americans_UCM_301832_Article.jsp. Accessed September 16, 2017.

50. National Heart, Lung, and Blood Institute. Your guide to lowering your blood pressure with DASH—What is high blood pressure? https://www .nhlbi.nih.gov/health/resources/heart/hbp-dash-what-blood-pressure -html. Accessed September 16, 2017.

51. American Heart Association. Five Simple Steps to Control Your Blood Pressure. Nov 13, 2017. http://www.heart.org/HEARTORG/Conditions /HighBloodPressure/GettheFactsAboutHighBloodPressure/Five -Simple-Steps-to-Control-Your-Blood-Pressure_UCM_301806_Article .jsp#.WhB9alWnGUk Accessed Nov 18, 2017.

52. Yi S, Elfassy T, Gupta L, Myers C, and Kerker B. Nativity, language spoken at home, length of time in the United States, and race/ethnicity: associations with self-reported hypertension. November 4, 2013. http://ajh.oxfordjournals.org/content/27/2/237.short. Accessed September 16, 2017.

53. National Heart, Lung, and Blood Institute. In brief: your guide to lowering your blood pressure with DASH. NIH pub. no. 06-5834. http://www .nhlbi.nih.gov/files/docs/public/heart/dash_brief.pdf. Accessed September 16, 2017.

Learning Portfolio (continued)

54. Harsha DW, Lin PW, Obarzanek E, et al. Dietary approaches to stop hypertension: a summary of study results. *J Am Diet Assoc*. 1999;99 (8 Suppl):S35-S39.

55. Vogt TM, Appel LJ, Obarzanek E, et al. Dietary approaches to stop hypertension: rationale, design, and methods. *J Am Diet Assoc*. 1999;99(8 Suppl):S12-S18.

56. Sacks FM, Svetkey LP, Vollmer WM, et al. Effects on blood pressure of reduced dietary sodium and the Dietary Approaches to Stop Hypertension (DASH) diet. DASH-Sodium Collaborative Research Group. *N Engl J Med*. 2001;344(1):3-10.

57. Kwan WM, Wong MC, Wang HH, et al. Compliance with the Dietary Approaches to Stop Hypertension (DASH) diet: a systemic review. *PloS One*. 2013;8(10);e78412. http://www.ncbi.nlm.nih.gov/pmc/articles /PMC3813594/#!po=3.57143. Accessed September 16, 2017.

58. National Center for Health Statistics. Leading causes of deaths. https:// www.cdc.gov/nchs/fastats/leading-causes-of-death.htm. Accessed September 16, 2017.

59. National Cancer Institute. Risk factors for cancer. https://www.cancer .gov/about-cancer/causes-prevention/risk. Accessed September 16, 2017.

60. Kushi LH, Doyle C, McCullough M, et al., American Cancer Society 2010 Nutrition and Physical Activity Guidelines Advisory Committee. American Cancer Society guidelines on nutrition and physical activity for cancer prevention: reducing the risk of cancer with healthy food choices and physical activity. *CA Cancer J Clin*. 2012;62:30-67.

61. Makarem N, Chandran U, Bandera EV, Parekh N. Dietary fat in breast cancer survival. *Annu Rev Nutr*. 2013;33:319-348.

62. Rohmann S, Linseisen J, Nothlings U, et al. Meat and fish consumption and risk of pancreatic cancer: results from the European Prospective Investigation into Cancer and Nutrition. *Int J Cancer*. 2013;132(3):617-624.

63. Xu X, Yu E, Gao X, et al. Red and processed meat intake and risk of colorectal adenomas: a meta-analysis of observational studies. *Int J Cancer*. 2013;132(2):437-438.

64. Centers for Disease Control and Prevention. State indicator report on fruits and vegetables 2013. http://www.cdc.gov/nutrition/downloads /State-Indicator-Report-Fruits-Vegetables-2013.pdf. Accessed September 16, 2017.

65. Fruit and Veggies—More Matters. Home page. http://www.fruitsandveg giesmorematters.org. Accessed September 16, 2017.

66. Agurs-Collins T, Rosenberg L, Makambi K, et al. Dietary patterns and breast cancer risk in women participating in the Black Women's Health Study. *Am J Clin Nutr*. 2009;90(3):621-628.

67. Wu AH, Yu MC, Tseng C-C, et al. Dietary patterns and breast cancer risk in Asian American women. *Am J Clin Nutr*. 2009;89(4):1145-1154.

68. Bradbury KE, Appleby PN, Key TJ. Fruit, vegetable, and fiber intake in relation to cancer risk: findings from the European Prospective Investigation into Cancer and Nutrition (EPIC). *Am J Clin Nutr*. 2014;100(Suppl 1):394S-398S. http://ajcn.nutrition.org/content/100 /Supplement_1/394S.short. Accessed September 16, 2017.

69. Kushi LH, Doyle C, McCullough M, et al. Op. cit.

70. Khan MK, Ansari IA, Khan MS, Arif JM. Dietary phytochemicals as potent chemotherapeutic agents against breast cancer: inhibition of NF-kB pathway via molecular interactions in rel homology domain of its precursor protein p105. *Pharmacogn Mag*. 2013;9(33):51-57.

71. Centers for Diseases Control and Prevention, National Center for Chronic Disease Prevention and Health Promotion. National diabetes statistics report, 2017. https://www.cdc.gov/diabetes/pdfs/data/statistics/national -diabetes-statistics-report.pdf. Accessed November 6, 2017.

72. Ibid.

73. Boyle JP, Thompson TJ, Gregg EW, Barker LE, Williamson DF. Projection of the year 2050 burden of diabetes in the U.S. adult population: dynamic modeling of incidence, mortality, and prediabetes prevalence. *Popul Health Metr*. 2010;8:29.

74. Gropper SS, Smith JL, Carr TP. *Advanced Nutrition and Human Metabolism*. 7th ed. Belmont, CA: Wadsworth; 2017.

75. Centers for Disease Control and Prevention, National Center for Chronic Disease Prevention and Health Promotion. Op. cit.

76. Ibid.

77. American Diabetes Association. Complications. http://www.diabetes .org/living-with-diabetes/complications/. Accessed September 16, 2017.

78. Ibid.

79. National Stroke Association. Diabetes and Stroke. 2013. 1-12. http:// www.stroke.org/sites/default/files/resources/DiabetesBrochure.pdf Accessed November 6, 2017.

80. American Diabetes Association. Diagnosis and classification of diabetes mellitus. *Diabetes Care*. 2014;37(S1):S81-S90.

81. Ibid.

82. University of California San Francisco, Center for Vulnerable Populations. The prevalence of gestational diabetes is growing. February 2013. http://cvp.ucsf.edu/docs/gdm_factsheet_format.pdf. Accessed September 16, 2017.

83. Centers for Disease Control and Prevention, National Center for Chronic Disease Prevention and Health Promotion. Op. cit.

84. Ibid.

85. National Institute of Diabetes and Digestive and Kidney Diseases. The Diabetes Control and Complications Trial/Epidemiology of Diabetes Interventions and Complications Study: thirty years of research that has improved the lives of people with type 1 diabetes. In: *NIDDK Recent Advances & Emerging Opportunities*. March 2014:33. http://www.niddk .nih.gov/about-niddk/strategic-plans-reports/Documents/Feb%20Doc%20 2014/2014NIDDK_RecentAdvances_508c.pdf. Accessed September 16, 2017.

86. Centers for Disease Control and Prevention, National Center for Chronic Disease Prevention and Health Promotion. Op. cit.

87. American Diabetes Association. Genetics of diabetes. http://www .diabetes.org/diabetes-basics/genetics-of-diabetes.html. Accessed September 16, 2017.

88. Curry A. Exploring why gestational diabetes leads to type 2. *Diabetes Forecast*. January 2015. http://www.diabetesforecast.org/2015/jan-feb /exploring-gestational-diabetes-leads-type-2.html. Accessed September 16, 2017.

89. Ibid.

90. Frederiksen B, Kroehl M, Lamb MM, et al. Infant exposures and development of type 1 diabetes mellitus: the Diabetes Autoimmunity Study in the Young (DAISY). *JAMA Pediatr*. 2013;167(9):808-815.

91. American Diabetes Association. Genetics of diabetes. Op cit.

92. Ibid.

93. Centers for Disease Control and Prevention. Childhood obesity facts. http://www.cdc.gov/healthyyouth/obesity/facts.htm. Accessed September 16, 2017.

94. Hunger M, Schunk M, Meisinger C, Peters A, Holle R. Estimation of the relationship between body mass index and EQ-5D health utilities in individuals with type 2 diabetes: evidence from the population-based KORA studies. *J Diabetes Complications*. 2012;26(5):413-418.

95. Guasch-Ferré M, Becerra-Tomás N, Ruiz-Canela M, et al. Total and subtypes of dietary fat intake and risk of type 2 diabetes mellitus in the Prevención con Dieta Mediterránea (PREDIMED) study. *Am J Clin Nutr*. 2017;105:723-735.

96. Malik VS, Hu FB. Sweeteners and risk of obesity and type 2 diabetes: the role of sugar-sweetened beverages. *Curr Diabetes Rep*. 2012;12(2):195-203.

97. Lana A, Rodriquez-Artalejo F, Lopez-Garcia E. Consumption of sugar-sweetened beverages is positively related to insulin resistance and higher plasma leptin concentration in men and nonoverweight women. *J Nutr*. 2014;144(7):1099-1105. doi: 10.3945/jn.114.195230

98. Imamura F, O'Connor L, Ye Z, et al. Consumption of sugar sweetened beverages, artificially sweetened beverages, and fruit juice and incidence of type 2 diabetes: systematic review, meta-analysis, and estimation of population attributable fraction. 2015;351:h3576. http://www.bmj.com/content/351/bmj.h3576.full. Accessed September 16, 2017.

99. National Diabetes Information Clearinghouse. Diabetes prevention program. http://diabetes.niddk.nih.gov/dm/pubs/preventionprogram/#results. Accessed September 16, 2017.

100. Sepah SC, Jiang L, Peters AL. Translating the diabetes prevention program into an online social network: validation against CDC standards. *Diabetes Educ.* 2014;40(4):435-443.

101. National Diabetes Education Program. Small Steps, Big Rewards: prevent type 2 diabetes campaign. https://www.niddk.nih.gov/health-information/health-communication-programs/ndep/partnership-community-outreach/campaigns/small-steps-big-rewards/Pages/smallstepsbigrewards.aspx. Accessed September 16, 2017.

102. American Diabetes Association. My health advisor. http://www.diabetes.org/are-you-at-risk/my-health-advisor/. Accessed September 16, 2017.

103. Bankoski A, Harris TB, McClain JJ, et al. Sedentary activity associated with metabolic syndrome independent of physical activity. *Diabetes Care.* 2011;34(2):497-503. doi: 10.2337/dc10-0987. http://www.ncbi.nlm.nih.gov/pubmed/21270206. Accessed September 16, 2017.

104. Ibid.

105. Novo S, Peritore A, Guameri FP, et al. Metabolic syndrome (MetS) predicts cardio and cerebrovascular events in a twenty year follow-up. A prospective study. *Atherosclerosis.* 2012;223(2):468-472.

106. Ogbera AO. Relationship between serum testosterone levels and features of the metabolic syndrome defining criteria in patients with type 2 diabetes mellitus. *West Afr J Med.* 2011;30(4):277-281.

107. National Institutes of Health, Osteoporosis, and Related Bone Diseases National Resource Center. Osteoporosis overview. June 2015. http://www.niams.nih.gov/Health_Info/Bone/Osteoporosis/overview.asp. Accessed September 16, 2017.

108. National Osteoporosis Foundation. The man's guide to osteoporosis. 2011. https://cdn.nof.org/wp-content/uploads/2016/02/Mans-Guide-to-Osteoporosis-1.pdf. Accessed September 16, 2017.

109. Osteoporosis Canada. Osteoporosis facts & statistics. http://www.osteoporosis.ca/osteoporosis-and-you/osteoporosis-facts-and-statistics/. Accessed September 16, 2017.

110. National Institutes of Health Office of Dietary Supplements. Vitamin D: fact sheet for health professionals. https://ods.od.nih.gov/factsheets/VitaminD-HealthProfessional/#h6. Accessed September 16, 2017.

111. Cândido FG, Bressan J. Review: vitamin D: link between osteoporosis, obesity, and diabetes? *Int J Mol Sci.* 2014;15:6569-6591.

112. Mata-Granados JM, Cuenca-Acevedo JR, Luque de Castro MD. Vitamin D insufficiency together with high serum levels of vitamin A increases the risk for osteoporosis in postmenopausal women. *Arch Osteoporos.* 2013;8(1-2):124.

113. Lippuner K. Epidemiology and burden of osteoporosis in Switzerland. *Ther Umsch.* 2012;69(3):137-144.

114. National Institutes of Health, Osteoporosis and Related Bone Diseases National Resource Center. The Surgeon General's report on bone health and osteoporosis: what it means to you. December 2015. NIH pub. no. 15-7827. http://www.niams.nih.gov/Health_Info/Bone/SGR/surgeon_generals_report.asp. Accessed September 16, 2017.

Spotlight on Obesity and Weight Management

Revised by Don Ross

THINK About It

1   Do you think the problem of obesity is evidence of a genetic predisposition or simply the influence of lifestyle and more related to environment?

2   How might your friends and social network influence the development of overweight and obesity?

3   Why do you think that being overweight or obese as a child increases the likelihood of being an overweight adult?

4   What actions do you think people can take to help decrease the rising rate of obesity?

LEARNING Objectives

1 Describe the biological, lifestyle, and behavioral factors that contribute to the development of obesity.

2 Describe the factors involved in the development of overweight in childhood.

3 Identify the causes of the obesity epidemic in children.

4 Discuss approaches or solutions for the growing obesity epidemic.

5 Determine the corresponding disease risks associated with body fat distribution.

6 Recommend weight management strategies to overcome the risks of overweight, underweight, and obesity.

Amanda, a college senior, is late for her usual Thursday night date with her boyfriend Dan at the Campus Pizza Palace. She is annoyed because her weight has made it hard to be on her feet for long hours during her job at the campus bookstore. Dan, who is training to be an emergency medical technician, shares the news that his professor has said it will be difficult for him to land an ambulance job unless he loses weight and gets in shape.

Both are worried as they discuss their issues. Amanda suggests that maybe they should eat a healthier diet. Her action plan is to make an appointment at the campus health clinic on Monday. Nevertheless, they order their usual: a large pizza with pepperoni and a pitcher of beer.

Amanda makes her appointment at the health clinic and gets her test results back a couple of days later. The news is much more startling than she expected. The report shows she has an elevated blood pressure of 145/80 mm Hg, a body mass index (BMI) of 30, and a diagnosis of pre-diabetes and hypertension. The clinic recommends she make an appointment with the campus physician and registered dietitian as soon as possible. Amanda is obese. And she knows it. The campus dietitian suggests that Amanda is not just dealing with a metabolism problem, an exercise problem, or an eating problem.

Obesity is a behavioral problem that is shaped by the social environment. Susceptibility to obesity is also idiosyncratic, meaning that it differs among individuals. Some people are strongly influenced by the people they hang around with, whereas others can change their behaviors independently of other people. In this spotlight, we examine some possible causes of this serious epidemic and suggest how people can tailor strategies to meet their own idiosyncratic needs.

The Obesity Epidemic

🍎 **Why Is This Important?** Obesity is a global problem with far-reaching impacts on everyone. No matter your personal weight, obesity-related diseases are driving up healthcare costs and insurance rates. Preoccupation with weight consumes our attention, and the multi-billion-dollar weight loss industry consumes our dollars.

Amanda's problem is not unique. Obesity has become a major global epidemic and a burden to society and healthcare systems.[1] (See **FIGURE SO.1**.) Worldwide, 1.5 billion people are obese,[2] and obesity has emerged as the most important contributor to ill health, displacing undernutrition and infectious diseases. Obesity not only is prevalent in North America and Europe,[3] but also is on the rise in Southeast Asia, especially in China, India, and Japan. One-half of the children in Beijing are obese, and the rate of obesity in India is growing so fast that it threatens to slow India's economic growth.[4] In North Africa and the Middle East, overweight and obesity are common, with Kuwait having the highest rates—79 percent of adults are overweight and nearly 43 percent are obese.[5]

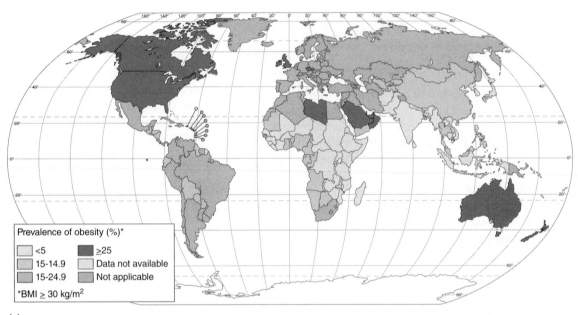

Prevalence of obesity (%)*

<5   ≥25
15-14.9   Data not available
15-24.9   Not applicable

*BMI ≥ 30 kg/m²

(a)

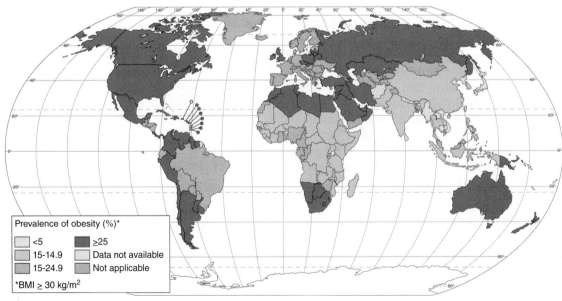

Prevalence of obesity (%)*

<5   ≥25
15-14.9   Data not available
15-24.9   Not applicable

*BMI ≥ 30 kg/m²

(b)

FIGURE SO.1   (a) Age-standardized prevalence of obesity in men aged 18 years and over (BMI ≥30 kg/m²), 2014, **(b)** Age-standardized prevalence of obesity in women aged 18 years and over (BMI ≥30 kg/m²), 2014.

World Health Organization, Global Status Report on noncommunicable diseases 2014. http://www.who.int/nmh/publications/ncd-status-report-2014/en/ Images from page 80. Data are on page 208.

In the United States, the prevalence of overweight and obesity has increased dramatically over the past three decades, jumping from 47 percent of the adult population to about 70 percent![6] What has caused this alarming increase? There are no simple answers. This spotlight discusses some possible answers and suggested solutions. Being overweight is a stepping stone to becoming obese. Obesity is not only a threat to health and physical appearance, but also a huge burden on society's wallets, leading to higher healthcare costs and reduced work productivity.

Perhaps most disconcerting is the prevalence of overweight and obesity among U.S. youth. Obesity starts young, and the prevalence increases with age: obesity rates are about 9 percent for ages 2–5 years, 17.5 percent for ages 6–11 years, and 20.5 percent for ages 12–19 years.[7] Childhood obesity is blamed on the overconsumption of energy-dense, sugar-laden, high-fat foods that are easily accessible, convenient, widely available, and inexpensive. (See **FIGURE SO.2**.) This overconsumption in combination with an increasingly sedentary lifestyle and decreased exercise and physical activity paves a path toward obesity. However, there is a glimmer of good news. The prevalence of obesity among children ages 2 to 5 years has decreased significantly, from 12.5 percent in 2006 to 8.9 percent in 2014.[8]

As the prevalence of overweight and obesity has increased, so has society's emphasis on thinness, as well as efforts at **weight management**. Every year, the diet industry rakes in more than $65 billion from weight-loss programs, diet books, pills, videos, and supplements.[9] The industry is experiencing relatively flat growth, however, as consumers strive to "eat clean" and shun highly processed foods, artificial ingredients, and preservatives in favor of fresh produce. Contrary to popular belief, diet and fitness apps for the smartphone are not the primary reason for lower enrollments at the large commercial weight-loss centers.

Quick **Bite**

BMI Distribution
If all countries had the BMI distribution of the United States, 58 million tons of human biomass would be added to the global population—equivalent to an extra 935 million people of average body mass—and energy requirements would be equivalent to that of 473 million adults.

▶ **weight management** The adoption of healthful and sustainable eating and exercise behaviors that reduce disease risk and improve well-being.

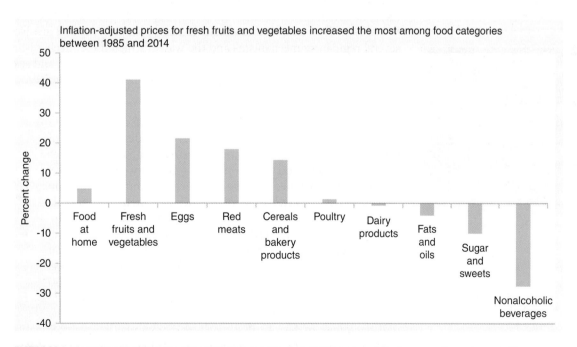

FIGURE SO.2 Changing cost of food. Over the past 30 years, real prices for fresh fruits and vegetables have grown the most compared to an inflation-adjusted Consumer Price Index. Meanwhile, prices for fats and oils, sugar and sweets, and nonalcoholic beverages have had a relative decline. A main ingredient in many nonalcoholic beverages is corn sweeteners.

Reproduced from USDA Economic Research Service. Growth in Inflation-Adjusted Food Prices Varies by Food Category. July 06, 2015. https://www.ers.usda.gov/amber-waves/2015/july/growth-in-inflation-adjusted-food-prices-varies-by-food-category/. Accessed March 4, 2017.

Nearly half of Americans worry about their weight. Among those who consider themselves to be overweight, about two-thirds are preoccupied with their weight.[10] Children and adolescents also are concerned about weight. In studies of grade-school girls from various socioeconomic backgrounds, 68 percent reported that they have attempted to lose weight because they very often worried about being fat.[11] Attempts to lose weight can be very costly and offer virtually no long-term assurance of keeping the weight off. About one-third of the lost weight typically is regained within the first year. By the fifth year, half the people return to their previous baseline weight. Among overweight and obese adults, a mere one in six report maintaining weight loss of at least 10 percent for at least 1 year, at any point in their lives.[12]

Key Concepts Worldwide, the number of overweight or obese people has increased markedly in recent years. The rising rates among children are especially disturbing. At the same time, more people are engaging in weight-control efforts, and they are starting to do so at younger ages.

Factors in the Development of Obesity

🍎 **Why Is This Important?** Underlying obesity are complex interactions among biological, social, environmental, lifestyle, and behavioral factors. Understanding these factors will give you insight into how they can influence weight status—either positively or negatively.

At its simplest, obesity results from a chronic positive energy balance—energy intake regularly exceeds energy expenditure, and weight is gained. But, although the cause of weight gain is simple, the factors that contribute to the energy imbalance are highly complex. As we learn more about the factors that regulate eating behaviors and energy metabolism, scientists are beginning to unravel the specific mechanisms at work and, from there, to determine what might go wrong in people who are obese. (See **FIGURE SO.3.**) The reality is that obesity is a complex disorder that involves several regulatory mechanisms and the way in which these mechanisms interact and respond to biological factors, such as heredity, age, and sex; social and environmental factors; and behavior and lifestyle choices.

Biological Factors

Genetics researchers have long recognized hereditary patterns of obesity. For example, when a parent is obese, an only child has double the likelihood of becoming obese. In two-child households, having an obese sibling is an even stronger association than parental obesity.[13] One might question, then, whether this is truly evidence of a genetic predisposition or simply the influence of family lifestyle and, thus, more related to environment. The answer is probably both. Studies using twins confirm that gene–environment interactions do influence energy balance. Researchers estimate that genes alone generally account for 50 to 90 percent of variations in the amount of stored body fat.[14]

Advances in genomics technologies are rapidly leading to new understandings of the roles that genetic variations play in obesity. Scientific advances, such as the identification of particular genes associated with regulating adipogenesis and adipocyte development in humans, suggest that genes have an effect on obesity.[15] Various studies have identified a number of genes associated with human body weight.[16] Although some of these genes have functional roles that explain their effect on human

THINK
About It

1

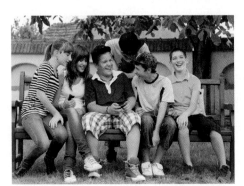

© prudkov/Shutterstock.

obesity, the majority do not have clearly defined roles linking them to how they might affect body weight.[17] Advances in genotyping technologies have raised great hope and expectations that, in the future, genetic testing will pave the way for personalized medicine and that complex traits such as obesity could be prevented even before birth.[18]

Gut Microbiota and Obesity

Our bodies are teeming with trillions of microorganisms. In fact, our bacterial partners outnumber our body cells by 10 to 1. From an ecological point of view, humans are superorganisms with a communal collective of human and microbial cells working as one. Gut microbes coevolved with the human host and affect digestion, production of vitamins B and K, energy metabolism, and immune function. For example, human gut microbes contribute 36 percent of the small molecules found in human blood.[19] In essence, our gut microbes function as a virtual, but vital, organ.

Our microbial partners may influence how many calories we are able to absorb from the food we eat, and various experiments suggest that gut microbes powerfully affect both obesity and the development of type 2 diabetes.[20] However, other experiments suggest that obesity and our diets can influence the composition of our gut microbial species; in other words, our gut microbiota may be a reflection of obesity (or leanness), as well as a cause of it.[21]

How to best manage our gut microbes to prevent obesity is hotly debated. Probiotics are well advertised, and manufacturers tout the virtues of "good bacteria." However, probiotic trials have failed to show a consistent preventive effect, and their use as a medical therapy has not been approved in the United States or Europe.[22]

Fat Cell Development

The number and size of fat cells in the body help determine how easily a person gains or loses fat. People with **hypercellular obesity**, an above-average number of fat cells, might have been born with them or might have developed them at certain critical times in their lives because of overeating. In **hypertrophic obesity**, fat cells are larger than normal. Fat cells continue to expand as they fill with more fat; when their capacity is reached, the body generates more cells. (See **FIGURE SO.4**.) Once body fat reaches three to five times the normal amount, fat tissue is likely to have both bigger fat cells and more of them, a condition called **hyperplastic obesity (hyperplasia)**.

Even with weight loss, the number of fat cells does not decline (though presumably some could be removed by liposuction). Fat cells do become smaller, but beyond a certain point they resist further shrinking, and the body strives to refill them with fat, making it difficult to maintain weight loss.

Sex and Age

The prevalence of obesity among men and women in the United States is similar, at about 36 percent.[23] Despite the similarities in obesity statistics, men and women seem to set different weight standards for themselves. Beginning in grade school, boys are less likely than girls to consider themselves overweight; in fact, males of all ages accept some degree of overweight. Boys typically are more concerned about

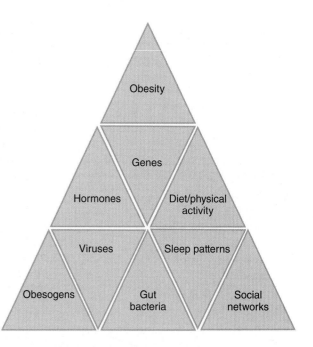

FIGURE SO.3 What influences obesity? Innovative views into individual and environmental interactions that contribute to obesity.

Quick Bite

Your Microbiota and You

Gut microbiota is the microbe population living in your intestines. It is composed of tens of trillions of microbes, can weigh up to 2 kilograms (4.4 pounds), and includes at least 1,000 different species with more than 3 million genes (150 times more than the number of human genes).

▶ **hypercellular obesity** Obesity due to an above-average number of fat cells.

▶ **hypertrophic obesity** Obesity due to an increase in the size of fat cells.

▶ **hyperplastic obesity (hyperplasia)** Obesity due to an increase in both the size and number of fat cells.

Quick Bite

Can You Pick Your Partners?

Liping Zhao, a professor of microbiology at Shanghai Jiao Tong University, adopted a dietary regimen involving Chinese yam, bitter melon, and whole grains. The yam and melon are fermented prebiotic foods believed to affect bacteria in the digestive system. After two years, he lost 20 kilograms (44 pounds); had lower blood pressure, heart rate, and cholesterol; and had an increase in a particular gut microbial species with anti-inflammatory properties. The changes persuaded him to focus his research on gut microbiota.

Quick Bite

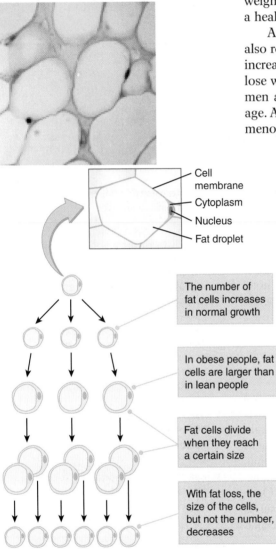

Cell membrane
Cytoplasm
Nucleus
Fat droplet

The number of fat cells increases in normal growth

In obese people, fat cells are larger than in lean people

Fat cells divide when they reach a certain size

With fat loss, the size of the cells, but not the number, decreases

FIGURE SO.4 The formation of fat cells. As body fat accumulates, fat cells enlarge and divide. Fat loss reduces the size of fat cells, but not their number.
© Donna Beer Stolz, Ph.D., Center for Biologic Imaging, University of Pittsburgh Medical School.

becoming taller and more muscular. As adolescents and young adults, most of us begin to worry about body weight and appearance.

By early adulthood, about the same percentage of men want to lose or gain weight, whereas significantly more women want to lose weight. As adults, males tend to see themselves as overweight at higher weights, whereas females describe themselves as overweight even when they are closer to a healthy body weight. (See **FIGURE SO.5**.) Adult women feel thin only when they weigh less than 90 percent of desirable body weight, whereas men rate themselves as thin even when they are above a healthy body weight.[24]

As we get older, we become more concerned with our weight as it also relates to health. Still, social acceptance of higher body weights is increasing, and the percentage of overweight or obese adults trying to lose weight has declined somewhat over the past two decades.[25] Both men and women gain the most weight between 25 and 34 years of age. After that, adults generally gain weight more slowly except during menopause, when many women will gain additional weight. Weight maintenance or slow gain often continues through adulthood until we reach old age, when frailty, disability, illness, and unintentional weight loss predict morbidity and mortality.

Race and Ethnicity

In the United States, the prevalence of obesity and attitudes about weight differ among racial and ethnic groups. African American and Hispanic women are more likely to be overweight compared to Caucasian women.[26] (See **FIGURE SO.6**.). Rates of overweight are similar for African American, Hispanic, and Caucasian men. Because of cultural factors, African Americans, Hispanic Americans, Native Americans, and Pacific Islanders typically value thinness less than Caucasian Americans do.[27,28]

Social and Environmental Factors

Socioeconomic Status

Americans are more likely to become obese if they have low socioeconomic status. Just as in some racial and ethnic groups, overweight and obesity are more socially acceptable in some lower socioeconomic settings. Compared to those with low socioeconomic status, people with higher socioeconomic status have better nutrition- and health-related psychosocial factors, such as more nutrition knowledge, aptitude for making better food choices, and more awareness of nutrition-related health risks.[29]

Lower socioeconomic status and food insecurity are associated with being overweight or obese.[30] The relationship between obesity and food insecurity might be related to the low cost of energy-dense foods and reinforced by the satisfying taste of sugar and fat. Periods of overeating when food is available, including binge-like patterns of eating or changes in eating habits that promote a metabolic-adaptive response, can account for overweight and obesity among adults from food-insecure households.[31]

Education is another factor associated with body weight. For both men and women, obesity prevalence was lowest among those with a college education; overall, prevalence was highest among those who did not graduate from high school.[32] See **FIGURE SO.7** for more on obesity and suggestions to reduce the problem.

Environment

Where you live also may affect your weight. Rural women tend to be heavier than women living in metropolitan areas.[33] Within the U.S., the prevalence of adult obesity in 2016 ranged from about 22 percent in Colorado to nearly 38 percent in West Virginia. A total of 47 states had a prevalence of obesity greater than or equal to 25 percent, and 25 of those states had a prevalence of obesity greater than or equal to 30 percent.[34] All states continued to have high obesity rates, and no state met the public health target of 15 percent. In fact, none were below 20 percent. (See the FYI feature "U.S. Obesity Trends: 1985 to 2015" for more information.)

Where you shop also may affect your weight. Obesity rates have been linked to the type of supermarket that people use, although proximity might be less important than food cost.[35] The prevalence of obesity is markedly lower, just 9 percent, among those who shop at higher-priced supermarkets, compared to 27 percent at lower-cost stores.[36] Over the past 40 years the actual cost of food has fallen. In the 1930s, Americans spent almost a quarter of their disposable income on food. Today, it's less than 10 percent.[37]

In addition, dietary behaviors are, in large part, the consequence of automatic responses to a particular situation with food, many of which lead to increased caloric consumption and poor dietary choices.[38] Individuals are subject to inherent cognitive limitations and mostly lack the capacity to consistently recognize, ignore, or resist contextual cues that encourage eating.

Take, for example, going to the movies. For many, a night at the movies also means sharing popcorn, candy, and soda. People often cannot resist this learned indulgence and are encouraged by the environment to

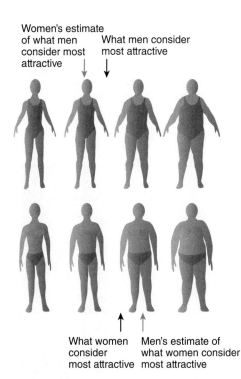

FIGURE S0.5 What men and women consider attractive. Compared with men, women perceive slimmer shapes to be more attractive.

Data from Bully P, Elosua P. Changes in body dissatisfaction relative to gender and age: the modulating character of BMI. *Span J Psychol.* 2011;14(1):313-322.

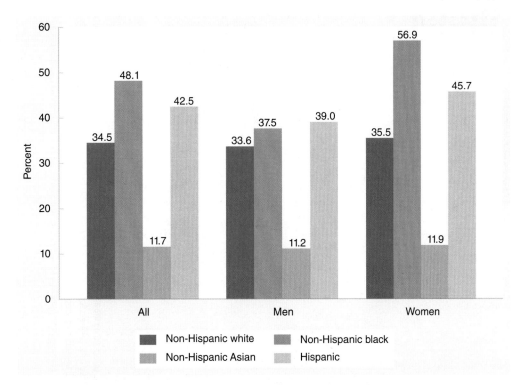

FIGURE S0.6 Rising obesity rates. Data from the Centers for Disease Control and Prevention show that the prevalence of obesity differs among men and women as well as among different racial and ethnic groups.

Ogden CL, Carroll MD, Fryar CD, Flegal KM. Prevalence of obesity among adults and youth: United States, 2011–2014. NCHS data brief, no 219. Hyattsville, MD: National Center for Health Statistics. 2015.

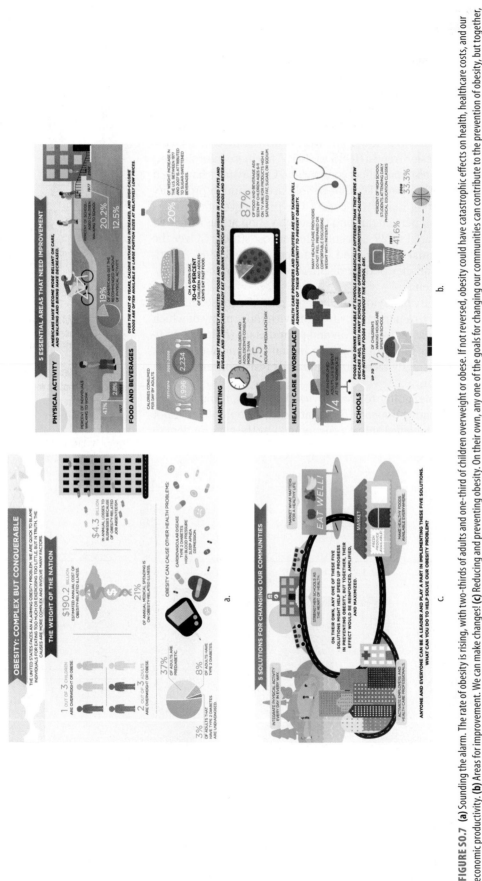

FIGURE SO.7 **(a)** Sounding the alarm. The rate of obesity is rising, with two-thirds of adults and one-third of children overweight or obese. If not reversed, obesity could have catastrophic effects on health, healthcare costs, and our economic productivity. **(b)** Areas for improvement. We can make changes! **(c)** Reducing and preventing obesity. On their own, any one of the goals for changing our communities can contribute to the prevention of obesity, but together, their effects will be reinforced, amplified, and maximized.

Reproduced with permission from Committee on Accelerating Progress in Obesity Prevention; Food and Nutrition Board; Institute of Medicine. Courtesy of the National Academies Press, Washington, DC, 2012.

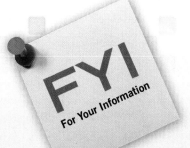

U.S. Obesity Trends: 1985 to 2015

During the past 20 years, there has been a dramatic increase in obesity in the United States, and rates remain high. The maps in **FIGURES A, B**, and **C** illustrate this trend by showing the increased prevalence of obesity across all of the states. Adult obesity rates now exceed 35 percent in five states, 30 percent in 25 states, and 25 percent in 46 states. West Virginia has the highest adult obesity rate at 37.7 percent and Colorado has the lowest at 22.3 percent. The adult obesity rate decreased in Kansas between 2015 and 2016, increased in Colorado, Minnesota, Washington, and West Virginia, and remained stable in the rest of the states. This supports trends that have shown overall leveling off of obesity rates in recent years. (see **TABLE A**).

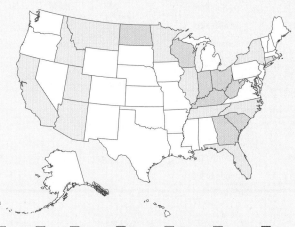

FIGURE A Percentage of obesity (BMI ≥ or equal to 30) in U.S. adults, 1985.
Reproduced from Centers for Disease Control and Prevention. Overweight and obesity. Obesity prevalence maps: Prevalence of self-reported obesity among U.S. adults by state and territory, BRFSS, 2013. http://www.cdc.gov/obesity/downloads/obesity_trends_2010.pdf. Accessed February 11, 2015.

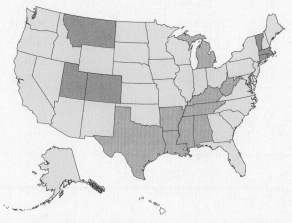

FIGURE B Percentage of obesity (BMI ≥ 30) in U.S. adults, 2004.
Reproduced from Centers for Disease Control and Prevention. Overweight and obesity. Adult obesity statistics. Obesity prevalence in 2011 varies across states and regions. http://www.cdc.gov/obesity/downloads/obesity_trends_2010.pdf. Accessed February 11, 2015.

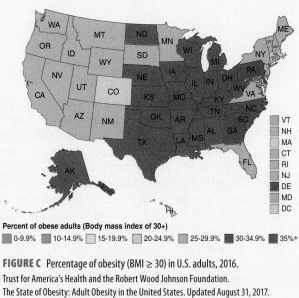

FIGURE C Percentage of obesity (BMI ≥ 30) in U.S. adults, 2016.
Trust for America's Health and the Robert Wood Johnson Foundation.
The State of Obesity: Adult Obesity in the United States. Updated August 31, 2017.
http://stateofobesity.org/adult-obesity/.

TABLE A
2016 State/Territory Obesity Rates

Rank	State	Adult Obesity Rate 2016	Rank	State	Adult Obesity Rate 2016
1	West Virginia	37.7%	26	Maryland	29.9%
2	Mississippi	37.3%	28	South Dakota	29.6%
3	Alabama	35.7%	29	Arizona	29.0%
3	Arkansas	35.7%	29	Virginia	29.0%
5	Louisiana	35.5%	31	Oregon	28.7%
6	Tennessee	34.8%	32	Washington	28.6%
7	Kentucky	34.2%	33	New Mexico	28.3%
8	Texas	33.7%	34	Minnesota	27.8%
9	Oklahoma	32.8%	35	Wyoming	27.7%
10	Michigan	32.5%	36	Florida	27.4%
10	Indiana	32.5%	36	New Jersey	27.4%
12	South Carolina	32.3%	36	Idaho	27.4%
13	Nebraska	32.0%	39	Vermont	27.1%
13	Iowa	32.0%	40	New Hampshire	26.6%
15	North Dakota	31.9%	40	Rhode Island	26.6%
16	North Carolina	31.8%	42	Connecticut	26.0%
17	Missouri	31.7%	43	Nevada	25.8%
18	Illinois	31.6%	44	New York	25.5%
19	Ohio	31.5%	44	Montana	25.5%
20	Georgia	31.4%	46	Utah	25.4%
20	Alaska	31.4%	47	California	25.0%
22	Kansas	31.2%	48	Hawaii	23.8%
23	Wisconsin	30.7%	49	Massachusetts	23.6%
23	Delaware	30.7%	50	District of Columbia	22.6%
25	Pennsylvania	30.3%	51	Colorado	22.3%
26	Maine	29.9%			

Trust for America's Health and the Robert Wood Johnson Foundation. The State of Obesity: Adult Obesity in the United States. Updated September 1, 2016. http://stateofobesity.org/adult-obesity/.

eat a particular food. Another example is eating potato chips or peanuts that have been set out during a friendly card game or conversation with others. Individuals often consume snacks not because they are hungry, but because they are prompted by the social environment that encourages them to eat. Grocery stores and restaurants have discovered the profits in suggestive selling, a sales technique where the customer is encouraged to make an additional purchase by taking advantage of a two-for-one sale or special discount. Grocery stores often use placement of items (candy bars at the checkout counter, or higher-priced snack foods at children's eye level on the shelves) to encourage impulse buying.

Our immediate surroundings influence our behaviors, and researchers have begun to link aspects of the **built environment** with obesity. The built environment can be defined as "human-formed, developed, or structured areas, including buildings, roads, parks, and transportation

▶ **built environment** Any human-formed, developed, or structured areas, including the urban environment that consists of buildings, roads, fixtures, parks, and all other human developments that form its physical character.

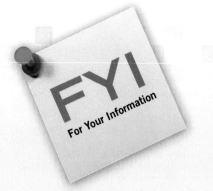

Does Our Environment Make Us Fat?

Colors affect our moods. Crowding can increase stress. Environmental psychologists have long known that elements of the built environment can influence our behaviors and physiology. An environment that promotes good health also is likely to promote well-being and security. In industrialized countries, our clean water, sewers, housing, and other material comforts have led to undeniable health benefits, but also to physical inactivity, poor eating choices, and related disease.[a]

Does the environment also contribute to the rise in the rate of obesity? The answer is yes. Both the social and built environments in which we live, work, and play influence both sides of the energy balance equation. An obesogenic environment promotes overconsumption of calories and discourages physical activity and caloric expenditure.

At the same time, our choices about the types and amounts of food we eat and which physical activities we prefer can be limited. In some neighborhoods, restaurants and stores offer mostly high-fat, high-salt foods. Often, the neighborhood offers few options for walking or parks for play and other activities. When the built environment lacks readily available healthful foods and restricts options for physical activity, it supports the development of obesity.

The social-ecological model illustrates the forces that shape our eating and activity choices.[b] (See **FIGURE A**.)

- *Individual factors* include personal genetics, physical characteristics, knowledge, beliefs, and attitudes.
- *Environmental settings* provide the context where we regularly make decisions and include schools, workplaces, recreational facilities, and food retail establishments.
- *Sectors of influence*, such as government, healthcare systems, agriculture, industry, and media, strongly affect the accessibility of healthful food.

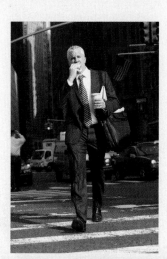

© Jupiterimages/Photos.com/Thinkstock.

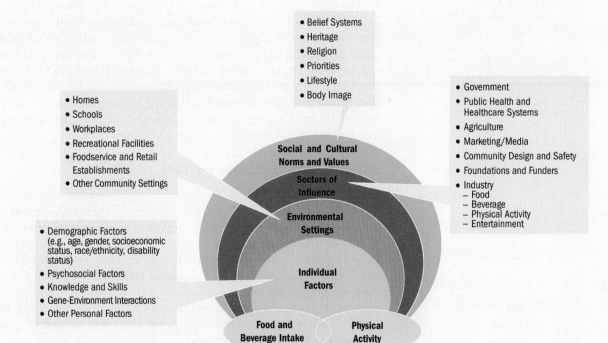

FIGURE A   A social-ecological framework for nutrition and physical activity decisions. Layers of influence and various factors intersect to shape a person's food and physical activity choices and ultimately health outcomes.

Modified from: (1) Centers for Disease Control and Prevention. Division of Nutrition, Physical Activity, and Obesity. *State Nutrition, Physical Activity and Obesity (NPAO) Program: Technical Assistance Manual*. January 2008, page 36. Accessed April 21, 2010. http://www.cdc.gov/obesity/ downloads/TA_Manual_1_31_08.pdf. (2) Institute of Medicine. *Preventing Childhood Obesity: Health in the Balance*, Washington (DC): The National Academies Press; 2005, page 85. (3) Story M, Kaphingst KM, Robinson-O'Brien R, Glanz K. Creating healthy food and eating environments: Policy and environmental approaches. *Annu Rev Public Health* 2008;29:253-272.

- *Social and cultural norms* are based on societal values and include religious dietary laws, personal expectations, expectations of friends and family members, lifestyles, and beliefs.
- *Cultural norms* shape choices for what, when, and how food and beverages are consumed. Cultural norms influence expectations for acceptable body weights and how much physical activity is a normal part of life.

Understanding the interactions among social-ecological factors can form the foundation for system-wide interventions to improve diet quality and increase physical activity. Nutritionists and public health experts expect this approach to have great potential in promoting a societal shift toward coping with the growing epidemic of obesity.

a Frank L, Kavage S, Devlin A. *Health and the built environment: a review.* June 2012. https://tennessee.gov/assets/entities/health/attachments/CMA_Health_Built_Environment_Review_2012.pdf. Accessed March 13, 2017.
b U.S. Department of Health and Human Services, U.S. Department of Agriculture. *2015–2020 Dietary Guidelines for Americans.* 8th ed. December 2015. http://health.gov/dietaryguidelines/2015/guidelines/. Accessed September 20, 2017.

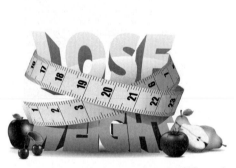
© graphit/Shutterstock.

systems."[39] These environments in which we live and work can either encourage or hinder physical activity and healthful eating.

People who live in and work in neighborhoods with sidewalks and safe streets are more physically active. But when neighborhoods have low "walkability," BMIs tend to be higher. Socioeconomic factors are at work, too—lower-income neighborhoods have fewer recreational facilities and healthful eating options. Fast food restaurants and convenience stores are more prevalent in low-income neighborhoods, a characteristic that is associated with higher obesity rates.[40] The number of supermarkets triples in wealthier neighborhoods.[41]

Many adults spend half (or more) of their day in sedentary activities, which often includes long hours at a computer or desk. Creating work environments that support and facilitate physical activity can have a large impact on health and body weight. Companies are beginning to feel the financial burden of obesity as well in terms of decreased worker productivity, number of lost workdays, and higher health insurance premiums. Many companies are now employing strategies such as the use of health and wellness coordinators or lifestyle coaches, gym facilities, organized fitness classes, running groups and walking tracks, and financial incentives for workers to make measureable improvements in their health such as weight loss or quitting tobacco use. Improvements in cafeteria and vending machine choices also are priorities for companies looking to reduce obesity in the workplace.

Lifestyle and Behavior Factors

How Often Do You Eat Out?

The average American eats out nearly four times a week, a choice that has been found to offer less nutritious food than food prepared at home.[42] According to a study that evaluated 28,433 regular menu items and 1,833 children's menu items at 245 restaurants around the country, 96 percent of U.S. chain restaurant entrées fell outside the range of the U.S. Department of Agriculture's recommendations for fat, saturated fat, and sodium per meal.[43] Putting the nutritional value of restaurant meals aside, let's look at how portion sizes at restaurants can contribute to overeating and ultimately to the obesity epidemic.

We have long recognized that many restaurants serve portions of foods that greatly exceed recommended sizes. Increased portion sizes can be a magnet to people who view large portions as appropriate and as providing more value for the money spent.[44] Super-sized portions affect not only adults, but also children. An evaluation of portion sizes of select key foods (soft/fruit drinks, salty snacks, desserts, french fries, burgers, pizzas, Mexican fast foods, and hot dogs) found that these foods represent more than one-third

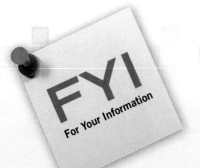

Is Food Addiction Real?

Palatable foods, which are typically associated with high energy content, lead to overeating, and it is almost a foregone conclusion that this is also an important contributor to the current obesity epidemic. How many of us are addicted to particular foods?[a] The tendency to indulge in unhealthy

eating and overconsumption of palatable food appears to be a crucial determinant in the rising prevalence of obesity.[b] This tendency to consume food in quantities that exceed energy requirements has been linked to an addiction-like process.[c] The existence of food addiction has not been conclusively proven, but as seen in drug addiction, evidence points to alterations in the brain–reward circuitry that are induced by overconsumption of palatable foods.[d]

There is evidence that bingeing on sugar-dense, palatable foods increases extracellular dopamine in part of the forebrain called the striatum, suggesting addictive potential.[e] Moreover, elevated blood glucose levels cause tryptophan to be absorbed and converted into the mood-elevating chemical serotonin.[f] Are there biological and psychological similarities between food addiction and drug dependence? What about loss of control? In some individuals, palatable foods even have

palliative properties and can be viewed as a form of self-medication.[g] In food environments where highly palatable foods are generally low in price and easy to obtain, and where increased portion size is routine, addictive-like behaviors seem to be encouraged.[h]

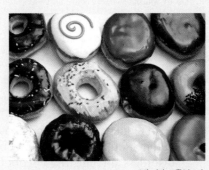

© iStockphoto/Thinkstock.

a Berthoud HR, Zheng H. Modulation of taste responsiveness and food preference by obesity and weight loss. *Physiol Behav*. 2012;107(4):527-532.

b Pandit R, Mercer JG, Overdium J, et al. Dietary factors affect food reward and motivation to eat. *Obes Facts*. 2012;5(2):221-242.

c Ibid.

d Ibid.

e Fortuna JL. The obesity epidemic and food addiction: clinical similarities to drug dependence. *J Psychoactive Drugs*. 2012;44(1):56-63.

f Ibid.

g Ibid.

h Allen PJ, Batra G, Geiger BM. Rationale and consequences of reclassifying obesity as an addictive disorder: neurobiology, food environment, and social policy perspectives. *Physiol Behav*. 2012;107(1):126-137.

of children's energy intake, and that the portion sizes increased significantly over the 30-year period studied, with increases in pizza size particularly pronounced in the last decade.[45]

Our Social Networks

Social factors also influence the development of obesity. (See **TABLE 50.1**.) Abundant high-calorie, highly palatable foods; pervasive advertising promoting their consumption; and the social enjoyment of eating all create pressures to overeat. At the same time, our culture tells us that we should be thin, and we might feel unhealthy pressures to diet.

Three interrelated social processes appear to explain the role of social networks in the development of overweight and obesity, namely *social contagion* (whereby the network in which people are embedded influences their weight over time), *social capital* (whereby sense of belonging and social support influence weight and weight-influencing behaviors), and *social selection* (whereby a person's network might develop according to his or her weight).[46]

THINK
About It

2

Our social networks shape the development of overweight and obesity, and obesity appears to spread through social ties (social contagion).[47] The impact of peer weight is larger among females and adolescents with high body mass index (social capital).[48] There is consistent evidence that school friends are significantly similar in terms of their body mass index, and friends with the highest body mass index appear to be most similar (social selection).

TABLE SO.1
Sociocultural Influences on Obesity

Social Contexts	
Culture	People in developed societies have more body fat than those in developing societies.
History	Fatness is increasing in the United States, but idealized weights are decreasing.
Social Characteristics	
Age and lifestyle	Fatness increases during adulthood and declines in older adults.
Gender	Obesity is more prevalent in women than in men.
Race and ethnicity	Obesity is more prevalent in African American, Hispanic, Native American, and Pacific Islander women.
Socioeconomic Status	
Income	Obesity is more prevalent in lower-income women.
Education	Less-educated women have a higher incidence of obesity.
Occupational prestige	Obesity is more prevalent in women in less prestigious jobs.
Employment	Adults who are unemployed have a higher incidence of obesity.
Household	Older adults who live with others have a higher incidence of composition obesity.
Marriage	Married men have a higher incidence of obesity.
Residence	Rural women have a higher incidence of obesity.
Region	People residing in the South have a higher incidence of obesity.

Modified from Dalton S. Body weight terminology, definitions, and measurements. In: Dalton S, ed. *Overweight and Weight Management: The Health Professional's Guide to Understanding and Practice.* Gaithersburg, MD: Aspen; 1997:314.

Frequency of fast food consumption also has been found to cluster within groups of boys, as have body image concerns, dieting, and eating disorders among girls.[49] School friends can be critical in shaping young people's eating behaviors and body weight. This suggests the potential that social networks are likely to have a powerful influence on health promotion interventions in schools.[50]

Lack of Physical Activity

Lack of exercise is a major contributing factor to weight gain and obesity. Still, one-third of adults never engage in any type of leisure-time physical activity.[51] (See **FIGURE SO.8**.) Inactivity is more common among women, older adults, less-affluent adults, and black and Hispanic adults. Children also exercise less. In both children and adults, research links excessive television viewing and computer use to overweight and obesity.[52] For all ages, obesity itself can lead to physical inactivity, although the strength of this relationship is unclear.

Psychological Factors

Some people adopt eating as a strategy for dealing with the stresses and challenges of life (others use drugs, alcohol, smoking, shopping, or gambling). Also, there's a pleasure in eating that alleviates boredom. Some people use eating as a pick-me-up when fatigued, and some use eating to distract themselves from difficult problems or as a means of punishing themselves or others for real or imagined transgressions.

Emotional Eating

Emotional eaters have a dysfunctional relationship with food, as illustrated by **restrained eaters** and **binge eaters**. Restrained eaters try to reduce their calorie intake by fasting or avoiding food for as long as possible. They skip meals, delay eating, or severely restrict the types of food they eat. Then, like a dam that bursts, they overeat when environmental or

▶ **restrained eaters** Individuals who routinely avoid food as long as possible, and then gorge on food.

▶ **binge eaters** Individuals who routinely consume a very large amount of food in a brief period of time (e.g., two hours) and lose control over how much and what is eaten.

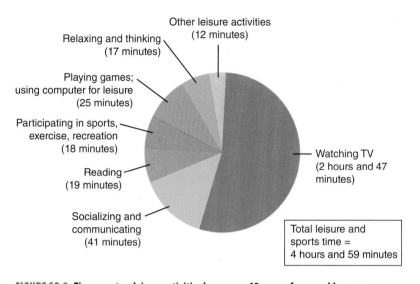

Leisure time on an average day

Other leisure activities
(12 minutes)

Relaxing and thinking
(17 minutes)

Playing games;
using computer for leisure
(25 minutes)

Participating in sports,
exercise, recreation
(18 minutes)

Reading
(19 minutes)

Socializing and
communicating
(41 minutes)

Watching TV
(2 hours and 47
minutes)

Total leisure and
sports time =
4 hours and 59 minutes

FIGURE S0.8 **Time spent on leisure activities by persons 15 years of age or older on an average day.**

Reproduced from U.S. Bureau of Labor Statistics. American Time Use Survey. https://www.bls.gov/tus/charts/chart9.pdf. Accessed March 3, 2017.

emotional stress triggers a complete release of inhibitions toward eating. Although not all obese binge eaters follow this pattern, the "fast, then binge" behavior is common in obese people who chronically attempt to lose weight.[53] This pattern also occurs in women of normal weight who perceive themselves as fat. These restrained eating patterns appear to be passed on from mother to daughter.[54] In adolescents, dieting predicts binge eating, decreased physical activity, and decreased breakfast consumption, and is also associated with increased BMI.[55] Therefore, in part, dieting during adolescence can lead to weight gain.

People with a healthy lifestyle have more effective ways to meet their personal needs. They communicate assertively and manage interpersonal conflict effectively, so they don't shrink from problems or overreact. The person with a healthy lifestyle is better suited to create and maintain relationships with others and often has a solid network of friends and loved ones. Food is used appropriately—to fuel life's activities and gain personal satisfaction, not to manage stress.

> **Key Concepts** Obesity tends to run in families. Sex, age, and social and environmental factors are related to weight. Lifestyle choices and behavioral factors also affect weight. Overly restrained eating can result in episodes of overeating and weight gain. Binge eating is common among people in weight-loss programs.

Childhood Overweight

🍎 **Why Is This Important?** Overweight and obesity in children is increasing rapidly, and overweight children are more likely to have social and academic difficulties. "Weight shaming" and bullying based on appearance can be devastating to young children. Obese children are more likely to become obese adults, and some overweight children already are dealing with obesity-related diseases such as type 2 diabetes.

In the United States, overweight and obesity are not only concerns for the adult population; childhood obesity also is increasing at an alarming rate. Approximately one-third of children ages 2 to 19 years are overweight (BMI from the 85th to 94th percentile) or obese (BMI greater than the

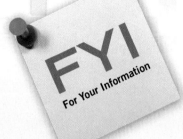

Childhood and Teenage Obesity: "The First Generation That Does Not Outlive Its Parents"

The most recent data on childhood obesity are frightening. Obesity affects 17 percent of all children and adolescents (ages 2–19 years) in the United States, triple the rate from just about one generation ago.[a] To meet the objective of promoting high-quality and longer lives free of preventable disease, disability, injury, and premature death, the Healthy People 2020 agenda calls for a 10 percent reduction in the percentage of children and adolescents considered obese in the United States.[b]

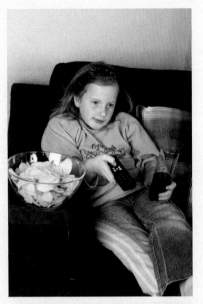

© Ivonne Wierink/Shutterstock.

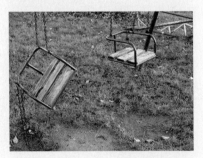

© Peter Gudella/Shutterstock.

Compared to their normal-weight counterparts, obese children and adolescents have increased risk of developing cardiovascular disease (CVD), metabolic syndrome, and type 2 diabetes, among others.[c] (See **TABLE A**.) These disorders can start as early as childhood, and such early onset increases the risk of premature death. Being obese as a child also increases the likelihood of being obese as an adult, and obesity in adulthood also leads to obesity-related complications. In addition to the burden of physical health problems, overweight/obese children and adolescents also are likely to be plagued with emotional challenges from teasing and harassment. Weight-based

bullying can lead to low self-esteem, poor body image, social isolation, eating disorders, poor academic performance, and even suicidal thoughts and attempts.

What's Causing the Epidemic?

The causes of childhood obesity are numerous and far-reaching but can be narrowed down to a few main contributors:

- *Meals consumed away from home:* What used to be a weekly treat—"eating out"—has become an almost daily occurrence in the United States. Of all the money spent on food, the percentage spent on food consumed away from home has risen from about 26 percent in 1970 to more than 43 percent in recent years. Meals and snacks based on food prepared away from home contained more calories per eating occasion than those based on at-home food. Away-from-home food was also higher in nutrients that Americans overconsume (such as fat and saturated fat) and lower in nutrients that Americans underconsume (calcium, fiber, and iron). Although progress is being made to improve the quality of Americans' diets, the rising popularity of eating out presents a challenge for Americans.[d]
- *Physical inactivity:* Only 29 percent of high school students met the *Physical Activity Guidelines for Americans*. Boys were more than twice as likely as girls to meet the *Guidelines* (38 percent versus 19 percent).[e] Children and adolescents spend approximately 7.5 hours per day using entertainment media that promote a sedentary lifestyle.[f]
- *Screen time:* For many of us, it takes a real effort to get ourselves away from overusing our screens—this includes television screens, computer monitors, and even the handheld devices we use for checking email, listening to music, watching television, and playing video games. According to researchers, 41 percent of high school students spend three or more hours per day playing video or computer games or using any computer device (including smartphones) outside of schoolwork.

About 25 percent watch three or more hours of television every day.[g] The more hours spent watching television or on electronic devices, the more likely children are to be both heavier and less physically active.[h] Even children under 5 years old who look at screens for more than three hours a day are fatter, have greater insulin resistance, and have an increased risk of type 2 diabetes.[i]

To make matters worse, it is not just the decrease in physical activity associated with screen use but that television advertising drives sales of junk food and that people tend to snack while watching television or using other screens.[j] In addition, media advertising for unhealthy foods contributes to obesity by influencing children's food preferences, requests, and diet.[k]

- *Lack of sleep:* Chronic partial sleep deprivation due to voluntary reasons (e.g., social activities, TV viewing) or involuntary reasons (e.g., work, caregiving, sleep disorders) contributes directly to weight gain by decreasing leptin (satiety hormone) and increasing ghrelin (hunger hormone).[l]
- *Food deserts:* Many rural, unsafe, lower-income, and minority neighborhoods have inadequate access to stores and supermarkets that offer healthy, reasonably priced food items such as fruits and vegetables. Adding to the food problem is the reality that in some neighborhoods, children do not have a safe place to play outside. Many children do not have parks, community centers, or sidewalks in their neighborhood.
- *Social networks and norms:* Close friends and associates of obese people are at higher risk of becoming obese themselves. For example, a study that tracked the same people over 32 years showed that a person's chance of becoming obese increased by 57 percent if he or she had friends who became obese in a given interval.[m] Social proximity (i.e., frequency and intensity of interactions between two parties) plays a stronger role than geographical distance in the spread of behaviors or norms associated with obesity. Three intertwined processes have been identified:

1. *social contagion* (the network in which people are embedded influences their weight over time. Components include:
    a. Mirroring weight-influencing behaviors of others
    b. Aspiring to the body size of others in one's social network
    c. Changing behavior in response to body sizes in a particular setting (e.g., desire to eat can be influenced by the body weight of others in the immediate setting)
2. *social capital* (the network provides a sense of belonging and social support for weight-influencing behaviors).
    a. Shared values within the network may promote healthy or unhealthy eating habits and other behaviors, such as physical activity.
    b. Social support provides structure, encouragement and purpose in relation to dietary habits and physical activity.
3. *social selection* (the network develops among people of similar BMI).
    a. For example, obese undergraduate students in the USA were more likely to prefer heavier partners than their non-obese peers (network of pairs).[n]

What Can Be Done?

The approach or solution to the childhood obesity epidemic in this country is not a simple one. This generation has been referred to as "the first generation not expected to outlive their parents."[o] The severity of the problem has increased over the past 30 years. Historically, the focus to reduce childhood overweight and obesity has concentrated mainly on school-age children, with only slight consideration to children under age 5. Today, preschool settings have been made a priority for obesity prevention.[p,q]

During their first years of life, children develop the eating patterns that can influence health and well-being throughout their life cycle. Childhood obesity predisposes individuals to become obese adults and increases the risks for obesity-related diseases and conditions. (See **TABLE A**.) Healthcare agencies should encourage pediatricians and other healthcare providers to emphasize to parents and caregivers the risks to their children's health, especially when they notice a trend toward unhealthy weight status.

The World Health Organization (WHO) has proposed that governments tax sugary drinks to increase prices by 20 percent and thus reduce consumption by about 20 percent. The WHO says there is increasingly clear evidence that taxes and subsidies influence purchasing behavior, and this could be used to curb consumption of sugar-sweetened beverages in

TABLE A
Health Problems That May Result from Childhood Obesity

Cardiovascular disease	Orthopedic complications
Metabolic syndrome	Infertility
Type 2 diabetes	Polycystic ovarian syndrome
Asthma	Social discrimination and other psychiatric problems
Obstructive sleep apnea	Cancer
Nonalcoholic fatty liver disease	

the fight against obesity, especially childhood obesity.[r] At the national level, some U.S. cities have imposed taxes on sugary drinks.

The complexity of childhood obesity requires states, communities, and parents to work together toward "helping children make the healthy choice the easy choice." (See **FIGURE A**.) The following are recommendations for reducing obesity in children and adolescents:

States and communities:

- Assess the retail food environment to determine the availability and accessibility of healthier foods.
- Develop incentive programs for supermarkets and farmer's markets to establish and maintain their businesses in low-income areas and to sell healthier foods.
- Increase the number of programs that provide local fruits and vegetables and increase the number of salad bars in schools.

- Implement regulations/licensing requirements for child-care providers to decrease the availability of less healthy foodstuffs and sugary beverages and to limit screen time in support of daily physical activities.
- Encourage schools to partake in programs such as the U.S. Department of Agriculture's Healthier U.S. School Challenge (HUSSC), increase free drinking water while limiting the sale of sugary beverages, support breastfeeding programs in schools and workplaces, and promote safe neighborhoods that encourage physical activity by improving access to parks and playgrounds.

Parents:

- *Limit screen time:* The American Academy of Pediatrics recommends: (a) For children younger than 18 months, avoid use of screen media other than video-chatting; (b) for children ages 2 to 5 years, limit screen use to 1 hour per day of high-quality programs; and (c) for children age 6 or older, place consistent limits on the time spent using media and the types of media, and make sure media does not take the place of adequate sleep, physical activity, and other behaviors essential to health.[s]
- Monitor the foods provided in school and child-care settings to ensure that healthier foods and beverages are provided and that physical activity is part of the curriculum.
- In the home, provide plenty of fruits and vegetables, limit foods high in fat and sugar (including sugary beverages), and promote physical activities.

a Ogden CL, Carroll MD, Fryar CD, Flegal KM. Prevalence of obesity among adults and youth: United States, 2011–2014. NCHS data brief, no 219. Hyattsville, MD: National Center for Health Statistics; 2015. https://www.cdc.gov/nchs/data/databriefs/db219.pdf. Accessed September 20, 2017.

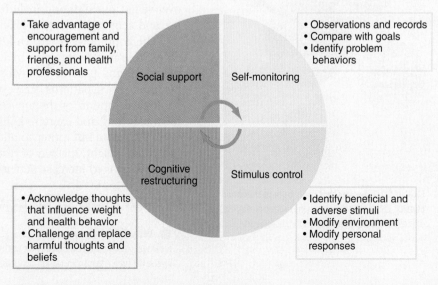

- Take advantage of encouragement and support from family, friends, and health professionals

Social support

- Observations and records
- Compare with goals
- Identify problem behaviors

Self-monitoring

- Acknowledge thoughts that influence weight and health behavior
- Challenge and replace harmful thoughts and beliefs

Cognitive restructuring

Stimulus control

- Identify beneficial and adverse stimuli
- Modify environment
- Modify personal responses

FIGURE A Behavior modification techniques to reduce obesity.

b HealthyPeople.gov. About Healthy People. http://www.healthypeople.gov/2020/about/default.aspx. Accessed September 20, 2017.

c Kelsey MM, Zaepfel A, Bjornstad P, Nadeau KJ. Age-related consequences of childhood obesity. *Gerontology.* 2014;60(3):222-228.

d U.S. Department of Agriculture, Economic Research Center. Food-away-from-home. https://www.ers.usda.gov/topics/food-choices-health/food-consumption-demand/food-away-from-home.aspx#nutrition. Accessed September 20, 2017.

e U.S. Department of Health and Human Services, Subcommittee of the President's Council on Fitness, Sports, & Nutrition. *Physical Activity Guidelines for Americans Midcourse Report: Strategies to Increase Physical Activity Among Youth.* Washington, DC: U.S. Department of Health and Human Services; 2012.

f Kaiser Family Foundation. Generation M2: media in the lives of 8- to 18-year-olds. January 2010. https://kaiserfamilyfoundation.files.wordpress.com/2013/01/8010.pdf. Accessed September 20, 2017.

g Kann L, McManus T, Harris WA, et al. Youth risk behavior surveillance—United States, 2015. *MMWR Surveill Summ.* 2016;65(6):40-41, 157.

h Boulos R, Vikre EK, Oppenheimer S, Chang H, Kanarek RB. ObesiTV: how television is influencing the obesity epidemic. *Physiol Behav.* 2012;107:146-153.

i Nightingale CM, Rudnicka AR, Donin AS, et al. Screen time is associated with adiposity and insulin resistance in children. *Arch Dis Child.* Epub March 13, 2017. doi: 10.1136/archdischild-2016-312016

j Smith M. *Screen Time Driving Youth Obesity Epidemic* [presentation]. School of Medicine, University of Pennsylvania, June 27, 2011.

k Hingle M, Kunkel D. Childhood obesity and the media. *Pediatr Clin North Am.* 2012;59(3):677-692.

l Miller AL, Lumeng JC, LeBourgeois, MK. Sleep patterns and obesity in childhood. *Curr Opin Endocrinol Diabetes Obes.* 2015;22(1):41-47.

m Christakis NA, Fowler JH. The spread of obesity in a large social network over 32 years. *N Engl J Med.* 2007;357:370-379.

n Powell K, Wilcox J, Clonan A, et al. The role of social networks in the development of overweight and obesity among adults: a scoping review. *BMC Public Health.* 2015;15:996.

o Bost EM. Testimony of Eric M. Bost, Under Secretary, Food, Nutrition, and Consumer Services, Before the House Committee on Government Reform Subcommittee on Human Rights and Wellness. U.S. Department of Agriculture. September 2004. http://www.gpo.gov/fdsys/pkg/CHRG-108hhrg98212/html/CHRG-108hhrg98212.htm. Accessed September 20, 2017.

p Birch LL, Parker L, Burns A. *Early Childhood Obesity Prevention Policies.* Washington, DC: National Academies Press; 2011.

q Centers for Disease Control and Prevention. Overweight and obesity: early care and education (ECE). https://www.cdc.gov/obesity/strategies/childcareece.html. Accessed September 20, 2017.

r World Health Organization. Fiscal policies for diet and the prevention of noncommunicable diseases. *WHO.* 2016;1-36.

s American Academy of Pediatrics. American Academy of Pediatrics announces new recommendations for children's media use. October 21, 2016. https://www.aap.org/en-us/about-the-aap/aap-press-room/pages/american-academy-of-pediatrics-announces-new-recommendations-for-childrens-media-use.aspx. Accessed September 20, 2017.

Quick Bite

Obesity and Car Seat Safety

A nationwide study found that 285,305 children age 6 or younger would have a difficult time fitting into most child safety seats because of their overweight status. More than half of these children are age 3 and weigh more than 40 pounds. The researchers found only four car seats on the market that could both accommodate these children and keep them safe.

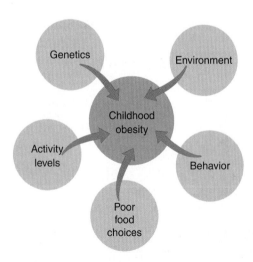

FIGURE S0.9 Factors that contribute to childhood obesity. Childhood obesity is on the rise and predisposes children to health problems when they become adults.

95th percentile).[56] An overweight child is likely to reach maturity earlier than a child of normal weight, but perhaps at the expense of height. Some overweight children already deal with the cardiovascular consequences of obesity, such as lipid abnormalities and hypertension, and many overweight children develop type 2 diabetes prior to their teen years. This public health problem is so drastic that many experts are saying this might be the first generation of people with shorter life expectancies than their parents. (See the FYI feature "Childhood and Teenage Obesity: 'The First Generation That Does Not Outlive Its Parents.'")

Overweight children are more likely to have social and academic difficulties[57] and experience the psychological trauma associated with obesity in our culture. In addition, obese children are more likely to become obese adults, and obesity in adulthood is likely to be more severe. Factors involved in the development of overweight in childhood include genetics, environment, behavior, and activity levels. (See **FIGURE S0.9**.)

THINK About It 3

The good news is that childhood obesity is preventable and treatable. Programs designed to treat childhood obesity are generally multifactorial and provide behavior modification to help children adopt healthier eating patterns, suggestions to increase physical activity, psychological support or therapy, and family counseling including family meal planning and exercise guidance. In some early stages the goal is not weight loss but rather to allow the child's height to catch up with his or her weight. Instead of restricting caloric intake or food choices, the strategy is to increase activity and improve food choices.

Health Risks of Overweight and Obesity

🍎 **Why Is This Important?** Overweight and obesity increase the risk of several diseases, and the longer obesity persists, the greater the risk. Within a few years, the rising rate of obesity is expected to reverse the current trend of increasing life spans.

TABLE S0.2
What Are the Risks of Being Overweight?

Hypertension	Overweight people are more likely to have high blood pressure, a major risk factor for heart disease and stroke, than are people who are not overweight.
Heart disease and stroke	Hypertension and very high blood levels of cholesterol and triglycerides (blood fats) can lead to heart disease and often are linked to being overweight. Being overweight also contributes to angina (chest pain caused by decreased oxygen to the heart) and sudden death from heart disease or stroke without any signs or symptoms.
Diabetes	Overweight people are twice as likely to develop type 2 diabetes as are people who are not overweight. Type 2 diabetes is a major cause of early death, heart disease, kidney disease, stroke, and blindness.
Cancer	Several types of cancer are associated with being overweight. In women, these include cancer of the uterus, gallbladder, cervix, ovary, breast, and colon. Overweight men are at greater risk for developing cancer of the colon, rectum, and prostate. For some types of cancer, such as colon or breast, it is not clear whether the increased risk is the result of the extra weight or a high-fat and high-calorie diet.
Sleep apnea	Sleep apnea is a serious condition that is closely associated with being overweight. Sleep apnea can cause a person to stop breathing for short periods during sleep and to snore heavily. Sleep apnea can cause daytime sleepiness and even heart failure. The risk for sleep apnea increases with higher body weights. Weight loss usually improves sleep apnea.
Osteoarthritis	Extra weight appears to increase the risk of osteoarthritis by placing extra pressure on weight-bearing joints and wearing away the cartilage (tissue that cushions the joints) that normally protects them. Weight loss can decrease stress on the knees, hips, and lower back and can improve the symptoms of osteoarthritis.
Gout	Gout is a joint disease caused by high levels of uric acid in the blood. Uric acid sometimes forms into solid stone or crystal masses that become deposited in the joints. Gout is more common in overweight people, and the risk of developing the disorder increases with higher body weights. Note: Over the short term, some weight-loss diets can lead to an attack of gout in people who have high levels of uric acid or who have had gout before. People who have a history of gout should check with their doctors or other health professionals before trying to lose weight.
Gallbladder disease	Gallbladder disease and gallstones are more common if you are overweight. Your risk of disease increases as your weight increases. It is not clear how being overweight causes gallbladder disease. Weight loss itself, particularly rapid weight loss or loss of a large amount of weight, can actually increase your chances of developing gallstones. Modest, slow weight loss of about 1 pound a week is less likely to cause gallstones.

Data from Weight Control Information Network. Do you know some of the health risks of being overweight? NIH Publication No. 07-4098; updated December 2012.

Overweight and obesity are major public health challenges. Obese people are at higher risk for heart disease, the leading cause of death in the United States and Canada, and for stroke, diabetes, hypertension, abnormal blood lipids, metabolic syndrome, some forms of cancer, **sleep apnea**, gallbladder and joint diseases, and psychosocial problems.[58] The longer obesity persists, the higher the risks. **TABLE S0.2** lists the effects that excess weight could have on your health. Scientists speculate that rising rates of obesity will soon reverse the increases in life expectancy that occurred throughout the twentieth century as a result of improved living conditions, advances in public health, and medical interventions.[59] The costs of obesity-related diseases are staggering. In the United States, the estimated annual healthcare costs of obesity-related illness are $190 billion.[60]

The blood lipid levels that typically accompany obesity—high serum triglycerides, low high-density lipoprotein (HDL), and a high low-density lipoprotein (LDL)/HDL ratio—increase the risk for atherosclerosis.[61] A person who is only mildly to moderately obese has an elevated risk of coronary heart disease. However, even modest weight loss (about 10 percent of body weight) reduces risk.

Type 2 diabetes, the most common form of diabetes in the United States and Canada, is three times more likely to develop in people who are obese, especially if they have abdominal obesity ("apple"-shaped body). Obesity increases insulin resistance and compromises the ability

▶ **sleep apnea** Periods of absence of breathing during sleep.

of body cells to take up glucose. Diabetes, in turn, is a risk factor for heart disease, kidney disease, and vascular problems. Again, even modest levels of weight reduction can improve glucose tolerance.

Overweight and obesity increase the risk of hypertension, probably because of increased resistance in the peripheral blood vessels, changes in the way the kidneys handle sodium, and other changes in kidney function. Weight loss lowers blood pressure in overweight people with hypertension.

Metabolic syndrome has become increasingly common and is linked to the rising incidence of obesity.[62] Metabolic syndrome is characterized by the combination of three or more metabolic risk factors that include elevated triglycerides, low levels of HDL ("good") cholesterol, elevated blood pressure, insulin resistance, and abdominal obesity. Although the exact reason is unknown, obesity also appears to increase the risk of certain types of cancer.

Being overweight or obese raises the risk for colon, breast, endometrial, and gallbladder cancers. The same food pattern that contributes to obesity (a diet high in calories and fat, plus low in fiber, fruits, and vegetables) also can be a cancer risk. Similarly, inactivity not only encourages obesity, but also increases cancer risk. Sedentary women, for example, have a higher risk of breast cancer compared to physically active women.[63]

Obese people are also more likely to have obstructive sleep apnea, a condition in which the airway collapses during sleep and breathing briefly stops. As the body struggles for air, blood pressure spikes upward. Typically, the individual wakes up, gasps for air, begins breathing again, and then falls asleep until the airway collapses again, and the cycle repeats. This pattern not only interrupts and prevents a good night's sleep, but also increases the risk of heart attack and stroke. Modest weight loss can alleviate sleep apnea, improve sleep quality, and reduce daytime drowsiness.[64]

Weight Cycling

Weight cycling (or yo-yo dieting) is a pattern of losing and regaining weight, over and over again. In national surveys, approximately 10 to 40 percent of adult women have a history of weight cycling.[65] The pattern of weight cycling often results when a person has success with rapid weight loss but regains the weight. This up-and-down pattern of weight changes over time has negative effects on health risks, body composition, body fat distribution, and energy expenditure. In addition, weight cycling has been associated with increased risk for metabolic syndrome, coronary heart disease, all-cause mortality, and reduced quality of life, even if BMI is at a healthy range. Obese individuals with large fluctuations in body weight have greater taste preference for fat and are prone to future weight gain.[66]

▶ **weight cycling** Repeated periods of gaining and losing weight. Also called *yo-yo dieting*.

Key Concepts Obesity is a risk factor for many chronic diseases, including heart disease, cancer, hypertension, and diabetes. In many cases, a modest amount of weight loss (about 10 percent) can improve symptoms and disease management.

Obesity Is a Preventable National Crisis

🍎 **Why Is This Important?** Obesity is not an inevitable condition. To reverse the obesity epidemic, Americans can employ several strategies, including dietary interventions, physical activity, environmental cue modifications, and, in certain cases, pharmaceuticals or even surgery.

THINK
About It
4

Although more than two-thirds of the U.S. population are over-weight or obese, much can be done to turn this epidemic around. Dietary interventions, physical activity, behavior and environmental modifications, and surgical and pharmacological treatments are the most widely accepted methods for weight loss and management.

Dietary interventions aimed at obesity prevention and treatment should focus on the development of healthy food choices and behaviors. The bottom line is that if you want to lose weight, you must take in fewer calories than you expend; however, a low-calorie diet is not necessarily a healthy diet. Following a healthy food plan such as MyPlate serves as a guide to including all food groups in a calorie-controlled diet. Commercial weight reduction programs should offer individualized nutrition, physical activity, and behavioral components and recommend slow and steady weight loss and maintenance.

Physical activity is a necessary component of any weight management program and essential for a healthy lifestyle. All adults should aim to be physically active on most, if not all, days of the week. Weight loss also is aided by reducing the amount of time each day spent in sedentary activities such as screen time in front of computers, televisions, and video games each day. In addition to the numerous benefits of the exercise itself, regular physical activity makes it easier to maintain a healthier weight.

Behavioral and environmental modification techniques can successfully help with weight loss and management. Identification of internal or environmental cues that trigger poor food choices or overeating should first be identified. Appropriate strategies to deal with challenging situations and encourage behavior changes that lead to lifelong weight management begin with appropriate and realistic goal setting. Goals should be both short term and long term and be specific, attainable, and forgiving to increase their effectiveness. Altering environmental cues so they prompt healthy behaviors and elicit positive self-worth is a valuable part of successful weight reduction.

Pharmaceutical treatment and surgery gained much media attention when the weight loss drugs Belviq (lorcaserin hydrochloride) and Qsymia (phentermine and topiramate extended-release) received approval by the U.S. Food and Drug Administration. These drugs, which must be obtained from a physician, are intended to help individuals eat less by activating hunger receptors in the brain. Surgical procedures are another option that can successfully treat morbidly or extremely obese adults. Common surgical procedures for weight management include bypassing some of the stomach or small intestine or gastric banding to reduce the amount of contents that can be held in the stomach.

Weight Management

🍎 **Why Is This Important?** For people facing overweight or obesity, a key first step is to stop weight gain. A modest weight loss of roughly 10 percent of initial body weight is enough to produce health benefits. A lifestyle focused on eating moderate amounts of healthful foods, getting plenty of exercise, thinking positively, and learning to cope with stress will help encourage continued success.

Each person has a unique set of interrelated factors that lead to weight gain. Approaches to weight management are just as complex, and, to be effective, they must be tailored to the individual. As you continue reading, keep in mind that weight management does not necessarily

Can Medicines Lead to Obesity?

After taking a steroid for asthma called prednisone for several months, 20-year-old Martha became painfully aware of a substantial weight gain. She immediately blamed her additional 20 pounds on increased snacking between meals, so she began exercising more. But her effort to exercise more wasn't working and she decided to curb her appetite. But this didn't work either. She felt depressed because she gained an additional 20 pounds and realized her BMI was now over 30: She was considered obese.

But, maybe it wasn't just the increased snacking that made Martha pack on the pounds. Obesogenic drugs also can cause weight gain. Although no one knows precisely how many prescription drugs promote weight gain, doctors suggest that there might be 40 or more of these common offenders. They can be found among drugs used to treat inflammation, diabetes, depression, psychosis, and other conditions. The effects of drugs are idiosyncratic; that is, they have different effects on different people. If you think your weight gain might be caused by a drug you are taking, work with your doctor—and your body—to find the drug that works best for you.

Martha's doctor thought her weight gain might be caused by the prednisone, an obesogenic drug, and substituted an inhaled steroid, which seemed to work. In the next few months, Martha lost most of the weight she had gained and felt that her normal optimism and positive attitude were back.

imply weight loss; rather, it is the adoption of healthful and sustainable eating and exercise behaviors indicated for reduced disease risk and improved feelings of energy and well-being.

The Perception of Weight

Over the course of the last few decades, the number of diet and exercise articles in the popular press has exploded, and diet books have become bestsellers. Dieting has become an institution, with its own magazines, television shows, camps and resorts, and weight-loss gurus. (See **FIGURE SO.10**.)

However, despite obesity's link to health risks, a backlash against dieting has emerged. The antidiet advocates' rallying cry is "Diets don't work!" While acknowledging that severe obesity is dangerous, they argue for size acceptance and challenge the notion that mild obesity is unhealthful. In fact, an analysis of 97 studies found that although obesity is associated with higher mortality, people who are overweight (BMI 25 to 30 kg/m^2) actually had a lower risk of mortality than people of normal weight.[67] Experts caution that relying on measures of weight alone is insufficient and does not account for substantial differences in nutritional status, disability, and disease that impact mortality risk. Still, when overweight or low obesity (BMI 30 to 35 kg/m^2) accompanies older age or chronic diseases, such as heart disease, there can be a protective effect. In this "obesity paradox," small excess amounts of adipose tissue may provide needed energy reserves during acute catabolic illnesses and may provide a cushion against some types of traumatic injuries.[68]

Health professionals now treat obesity as a complex disorder with multiple contributing factors. (See **FIGURE SO.11**.) They emphasize overall health and fitness rather than a number on the bathroom scale. Dietary recommendations emphasize moderation and a balanced diet that is low in fat and high in healthful foods such as fruits, vegetables, and whole grains. Behavior change is still an important part of weight management, but change is seen as an ongoing process that requires

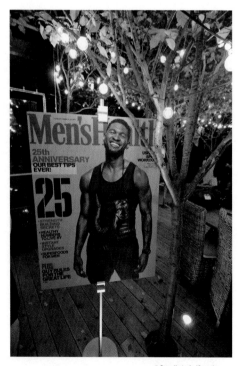

© Dave Kotinsky/Getty Images.

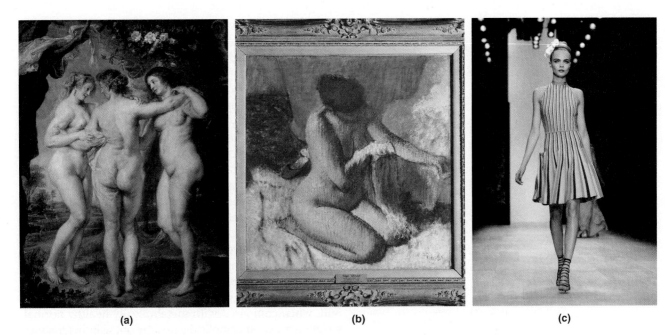

FIGURE S0.10 Society's changing standards of beauty. Over time, society has increasingly valued thinness. **(a)** Ruben's *The Three Graces*, 1639. **(b)** Degas's *After the Bath*, 1896. **(c)** Cara Delavigne, 2012.

(a) © Peter BarrittAlamy Images; (b) © The London Art Archive/Alamy Images; (c) © Featureflash Photo Agency/Shutterstock.

new skills for maintaining a healthy lifestyle over the long run. For weight maintenance, physical activity is part of a comprehensive weight-management program that should be individualized. The typical goal is to gradually accumulate 200 to 300 minutes or more of physical activity per week, depending on intensity.[69]

There are limitations as to what each of us can look like or what we can weigh. Although we shouldn't abandon efforts to achieve good health, we should balance our desire to lose weight with self-acceptance. If we engage in futile attempts to achieve an "ideal" body shape and weight, we may undermine our self-esteem and be harmed emotionally or even physically.

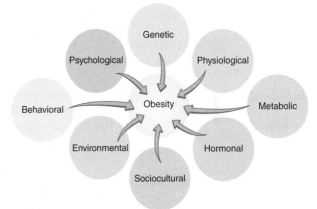

FIGURE S0.11 Multiple factors contribute to obesity. Obesity is a complex disorder that is not easy to treat.

Key Concepts Many factors contribute to the complex disorder of obesity. Currently, experts suggest that the best way to manage weight is to improve health by establishing healthful eating and exercise patterns and accepting the limitations of heredity.

What Goals Should I Set?

What are reasonable goals for weight management? Nutritionists recommend targeting the following behavior changes to manage body weight:

- Prevent and/or reduce overweight and obesity through improved eating and physical behavior.
- Control total calorie intake to manage body weight.
- Increase physical activity and reduce time spent in sedentary behaviors.
- Maintain appropriate calorie balance during each stage of life.

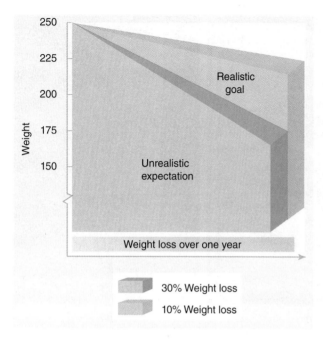

FIGURE SO.12 Expectations and reasonable weight goals. People who establish moderate rather than aggressive goals are more likely to succeed in their weight-loss program.

▶ **metabolically healthy obesity** A condition of reduced risk for obesity-related metabolic diseases.

If you are overweight, it doesn't take major weight loss to improve health; a modest weight loss of roughly 10 percent of initial body weight (e.g., a 20-pound weight loss if you weigh 200 pounds) is enough to produce health benefits and perhaps to encourage continued success. A key initial goal is to prevent or stop weight gain. An estimated 100 kilocalories per day change in energy balance (produced by any combination of decreases in energy intake and increases in energy expenditure) could theoretically prevent weight gain in 90 percent of the U.S. adult population.[70] Goals must be realistic and attainable. (See **FIGURE SO.12**.)

If you are metabolically fit, you don't have elevated metabolic or biochemical risk factors associated with obesity—such as high cholesterol (especially low HDL cholesterol), high levels of triglycerides, elevated blood glucose levels, insulin resistance, high blood pressure, and elevated fatty acids synthesis. Obese people who are metabolically fit are described as having **metabolically healthy obesity**. Still, when compared with metabolically healthy normal-weight persons, metabolically healthy obese individuals are at increased risk for all-cause mortality and cardiovascular events over the long term (10 years).[71] Often, you can reduce metabolic risk factors or even bring them within normal ranges through modest weight loss (5 to 10 percent of initial body weight) achieved by a low-fat, reduced-calorie diet and an increase in physical activity.

Don't focus on a particular weight as your goal. Instead, focus on living a lifestyle that includes eating moderate amounts of healthful foods, getting plenty of exercise, thinking positively, and learning to cope with stress. Learn to use your body's hunger and satiation signals to regulate eating and then let the pounds fall where they may. Most people who follow this advice will approach a healthy BMI range. Some will still weigh more than societal standards call for—but their weight will be right for them. By letting a healthy lifestyle determine your weight, you can avoid developing unhealthy patterns of eating and a negative body image.

Adopting a Healthy Weight-Management Lifestyle

Most weight problems are lifestyle problems. Even though more and more young people are developing weight problems, most arrive at early adulthood with the advantage of having a "normal" body weight—neither too fat nor too thin. In fact, many young adults get away with terrible eating and exercise habits and don't develop a weight problem. But as the rapid growth of adolescence slows and family and career obligations increase, maintaining a healthy weight becomes a greater challenge. If you develop a lifestyle for successful weight management during early adulthood, healthy behavior patterns have a better chance of taking a firm hold.

Permanent weight management is not something you start and stop. You need to adopt healthy behaviors that you can maintain throughout your life. People who have long-term success share common behavioral strategies that include eating a low-calorie, low-fat diet and performing high levels of regular physical activity. They also generally eat breakfast every day, weigh themselves at least once per week, watch less than

10 hours of TV per week, and exercise an average of 1 hour per day.[72] To maintain your weight over the long term, focus on healthy behaviors and develop coping strategies to deal with the stresses and challenges in your life. **FIGURE S0.13** shows the necessary components of an effective weight-management program.

> **Key Concepts** Healthy weight management means focusing on metabolic fitness—healthy levels of blood lipids, blood glucose, and blood pressure—rather than on achieving a specific weight. Permanent healthy behaviors are necessary for a long-term weight-management lifestyle.

Diet and Eating Habits

In contrast to "dieting," which involves some form of food restriction, "diet" refers to your daily food choices. Everyone has a diet, but not everyone is dieting. You need to develop a balanced diet of moderate caloric intake that includes foods you enjoy and that enables you to maintain a healthy body composition.

Total Calories

If you want to lose weight, you must take in fewer calories than you expend. Over the long term, you are more likely to control your weight successfully by cutting 200 to 300 kilocalories per day rather than drastically restricting your diet to only 1,000 to 1,200 kilocalories per day. Simply eliminating one can of regular soda from your daily routine would reduce your energy intake by about 150 kilocalories. Eating a half-serving of fries instead of a whole serving would save another 100 kilocalories. You don't need to make major diet changes; just make small, sustainable changes and focus on the balance of food groups suggested by MyPlate. The MyPlate website has interactive tools (www .choosemyplate.gov/tools.html) that can help you evaluate your intake and find small changes you can make.

Overconsumption of total calories is closely tied to portion sizes. Most of us significantly underestimate the amount of food we eat. Limiting portion sizes to those recommended in MyPlate is critical for weight management. You'll probably find it easier to monitor and manage your total food intake if you concentrate on portion sizes rather than counting calories.

Crash Diets Don't Work

Don't go on a "crash diet" that contains only minimal calories. You need to consume enough food to meet your need for essential nutrients. Once you lose weight, you probably won't maintain it unless you continue some degree of calorie restriction, so it is important that you adopt a level of food intake that you can live with. A highly restricted diet just won't work long term.

Balancing Energy Sources: Fat

Because fat is the most concentrated source of calories, limiting fat in the diet can help you limit your total calories. If you reduce your consumption of meats and processed foods and add whole grains, fresh fruits, and vegetables to your diet, you will reduce fat and total calorie consumption while increasing dietary fiber. But watch out for processed foods labeled "fat-free" or "reduced-fat"; they can be high in calories and added sugars despite their lower fat content.

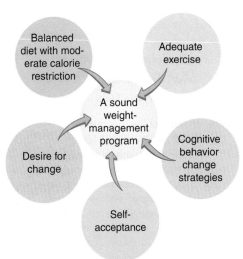

FIGURE S0.13 Components of a sound weight-management program. Recognizing the need for change, establishing reasonable goals, adopting goal-directed activities and self-monitoring, and rewarding goal attainment can help successfully implement the components of a sound weight-management program.

Quick **Bite**

Double-Checking Your Dietary Recall

When researchers checked the validity of food diaries and self-reports, they found that obese people underreport their energy intake by 20 to 50 percent and lean people underreport by 10 to 30 percent. Energy expenditure in the obese subjects was normal relative to their body size.

Position Statement: Academy of Nutrition and Dietetics

Interventions for the Treatment of Overweight and Obesity in Adults

It is the position of the Academy of Nutrition and Dietetics that successful treatment of overweight and obesity in adults requires adoption and maintenance of lifestyle behaviors contributing to both dietary intake and physical activity. These behaviors are influenced by many factors; therefore, interventions incorporating more than one level of the socioecological model and addressing several key factors in each level may be more successful than interventions targeting any one level and factor alone.

Reprinted from *Journal of the Academy of Nutrition and Dietetics*, 116(1), Hollie A. Raynor, Catherine M. Champagne, Position of the Academy of Nutrition and Dietetics: Interventions for the Treatment of Overweight and Obesity in Adults, Page no. 129-147, 2016, with permission from Elsevier.

Quick Bite

The Fletcherism Fad: Chew Until You …

At the turn of the twentieth century, a retired businessman named Horace Fletcher started a dietary craze known as "Fletcherism." Calling the mouth "Nature's Food Filter," he believed that the sense of taste and the urge to swallow are perfect guides to nutrition. Although he recommended chewing food at least 50 times before swallowing, preferably until tasteless, he far exceeded this by once chewing a piece of onion 722 times. His philosophy did lead to some weight loss; people adhering to Fletcherism cut back on energy intake due to the additional mechanical effort of chewing.

Balancing Energy Sources: Carbohydrates

In addition to balancing energy intake with energy output, balancing food sources of energy is important for successful weight management. Eating foods rich in complex carbohydrates and fiber, such as vegetables, legumes, and whole grains, can help you achieve and maintain a healthy body weight. Fiber-rich foods help provide a feeling of satiation, or fullness, that can keep you from overeating. Carbohydrates should make up about 45 to 65 percent of your total daily calories. Avoid foods with added sugars and foods rich in simple carbohydrates, such as potatoes and bread made with refined flour.

Diets high in added sugars tend to reduce satiation and encourage overeating. Also, high-sugar foods usually provide few nutrients to accompany their high caloric content. You should consume high-sugar foods sparingly, so choose fresh fruits and whole grains instead of candy, soft drinks, and sugary cereals. A good guide for choosing cereals is looking at the food label to pick ones with little added sugar and a moderate amount of fiber (at least 3 grams per serving).

Balancing Energy Sources: Protein

Most authorities recommend diets high in complex carbohydrates and moderate in protein consumption. (See the FYI feature "Learning Weight Management from Some of the 'Biggest' Weight Experts: Sumo Wrestlers.") Although protein promotes a sense of fullness, animal foods high in protein often are high in saturated fat. Vegetarian sources of protein (such as tofu, soymilk, beans, and lentils) and plant-based fats are healthier choices. Including some protein in each meal is a good idea, but stick to the recommended intake: 10 to 35 percent of total daily calories.

Eating Habits

Equally important to weight management is eating regularly. If you skip meals, you are apt to feel excessively hungry and deprived, and you will be more likely to snack or binge on high-calorie, high-fat, or sugary foods. A person who eats on a regular schedule is more likely to reduce total energy intake and improve lipid levels than a person who eats irregularly.[73] Also, a regular meal pattern usually includes breakfast—a benefit when trying to manage weight. Research shows that morning intake is much more satiating than late-night eating and will help reduce overall energy intake.[74] In a study of healthy, lean women, skipping breakfast lowered insulin sensitivity, raised LDL and total cholesterol, and led to higher energy intake.[75]

If you follow a regular pattern of eating and set up some "decision rules" that govern your food choices, you will be able to handle the many details that go into a healthful diet. Decision rules governing breakfast, for example, might be:

- Most of the time, choose a low-sugar, high-fiber cereal with nonfat milk or oatmeal with nonfat milk and fruit.
- Once in a while, have an egg that's prepared without added fat (e.g., hard boiled, scrambled) and a piece of whole-wheat toast.
- Sometimes have whole-grain pancakes and waffles topped with fruit.
- Occasionally have a donut or bagel with full-fat cream cheese.

When you proclaim some foods "off limits," you are setting up a rule to be broken. Instead, adopt the principle of "everything in moderation."

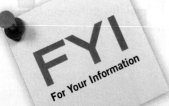

Learning Weight Management from Some of the "Biggest" Weight Experts: Sumo Wrestlers

Is it possible to work out three to five hours a day, seven days a week, eat a relatively low-fat diet, and still gain weight? Yes! This is the how Sumo wrestlers train, a life that allows them to pack on the pounds. The world's biggest people are experts at putting on fat, which means that the lessons they've learned can help teach us how to keep the weight off. If you do not want to gain weight, follow these tips. The wrestlers, of course, will be doing just the opposite[a]:

- *Make your workouts slow and steady, not fast and frantic.* Sustained moderate workouts lasting 30 to 60 minutes are more helpful at burning calories than exerting yourself in a brief, intense burst of exercise. Sumo wrestlers train to win at a sport whose rules are simple: A wrestler loses when he is forced out of the wrestling ring or if anything other than his feet touch the mat. The average sumo wrestler stands about 6 feet tall and weighs 336 pounds. Sumo wrestler training is focused on being powerful enough to push over something the size of a refrigerator. Going for a 3-mile run or riding a bicycle for 60 minutes is not a priority for sumo wrestler workouts.

- *Don't skip breakfast.* Try not to go longer than four to five hours without eating. Your body will adapt to the threat of starvation and decrease your metabolism so you can survive on fewer calories. Most sumo wrestlers eat only twice a day.
- *Eat small meals and snacks throughout the day.* Split up your daily calories among breakfast, lunch, dinner, and a couple of snacks. You're less likely to put on weight eating small meals and never overeating, rather than letting yourself get too hungry and then eating too much. Sumo wrestlers eat about one-half of their overall daily food calories at one meal. For a person the

size of a sumo wrestler, that can be over 3,000 calories every day just for lunch!
- *Choose a well-balanced diet with a lot of variety.* Remember that balance, variety, and moderation are cornerstones of good nutrition. Sumo wrestlers eat a relatively low-fat diet but tend to have a diet heavy in complex carbohydrates, protein, and vegetables, with little fruit.

a Anderson J, Christensen N, Hoffman E, et al. *Eat Right! Healthy Eating in College and Beyond.* San Francisco: Pearson Benjamin Cummings; 2007:67-79.

Troublesome foods might be placed off limits temporarily until you regain control. If you can learn to eat in moderation, you can achieve a healthful diet and manage your weight successfully; no foods need to be entirely off limits, though some should be eaten prudently. Making the healthier choice more often than not is the essence of moderation.

> **Key Concepts**   Although a highly restricted diet won't work long term, balancing energy sources and controlling portion sizes can help reduce overall energy consumption. Reducing fat intake is a major step toward lowering calorie intake. Fiber-rich foods and protein can provide a feeling of fullness that can help prevent overeating.

Physical Activity

Regular physical activity is a vital component of weight management and promotes fitness and good health. At the same time, it discourages overeating by reducing stress, produces positive feelings that reinforce self-worth and a sense of accomplishment, and often includes pleasant socialization.

Look for ways to incorporate more physical activity into your daily life. (See **FIGURE SO.14**.) To prevent weight gain and maximize health benefits, adults should aim for 60 minutes of moderate-intensity physical activity each day, but this doesn't have to be done all at once. Just walking more is beneficial. In many studies it has been shown that people who walk more tend to be thinner than those who do not walk as

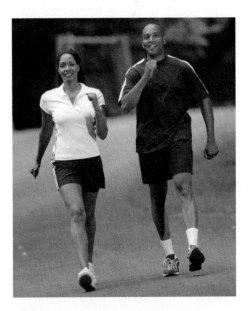

FIGURE SO.14 Weight management through lifetime habits. To achieve long-term weight management, healthy habits must become part of one's daily routine.
© Comstock Images/Alamy Images.

much. So, walk the dog for an extra half hour daily, for example. Use a stairway instead of an elevator. Walk briskly instead of using transportation. Take up an active hobby like bicycling, or if you live near the mountains, try hiking or skiing.

Increasing your activity level by just a small amount can help you maintain your current weight or lose a moderate amount of weight. "Going for the burn" and "no pain, no gain" were the mottoes of the aerobics movement during the 1970s and 1980s, but such intense activity is neither necessary nor desirable. Instead, regular exercise of moderate intensity—any activity that expends 4 to 7 kilocalories per minute (240 to 420 kilocalories per hour)—provides substantial health benefits.

Once you have increased your everyday activity level, consider beginning a formal exercise program that includes cardiorespiratory endurance exercise, resistance training, and stretching exercises. Regular, moderate cardiorespiratory endurance exercise, sustained for 45 minutes to 1 hour, can help trim body fat permanently. Strength training helps increase fat-free mass, which results in more calorie burning even outside of exercise periods.

One thing is clear: Regular exercise, maintained throughout life, makes weight management easier. The sooner you establish good habits, the better. You will succeed in maintaining your weight if you make exercise an integral part of the lifestyle you enjoy now and will enjoy in the future.

> **Key Concepts** Successful weight management involves regular physical activity as well as healthful food choices. Small increases in activity have significant health benefits and help weight loss and maintenance. To prevent weight gain and maximize health benefits, you should include at least 60 minutes of moderate physical activity in your daily routine.

Thinking and Emotions

What goes on in your head is another factor in a healthy lifestyle and successful weight management. The way you think about yourself and your world influences, and is influenced by, how you feel and how you act. Certain kinds of thinking produce negative emotions, which can undermine a healthy lifestyle.

When we compare ourselves to an internally held picture of an "ideal self," we are more likely to have low self-esteem and feel negative emotions. The ideal self we envision is often the result of having adopted perfectionistic goals and beliefs about how we and others "should" be. You might know someone who believes, "If I don't do things perfectly, I'm a failure" or "It's terrible if I'm not thin." When we accept these irrational beliefs, we may actually cause ourselves stress and emotional conflict. The remedy is to challenge such beliefs and replace them with more realistic ones.

The beliefs and attitudes you hold give rise to self-talk, an internal dialogue you carry on with yourself about events that happen to and around you. When you talk yourself through the steps of a job and then praise yourself when it's successfully completed, you are engaging in **positive self-talk**. When you make self-deprecating remarks or angry and guilt-producing comments and when you blame yourself unnecessarily, you are engaging in **negative self-talk**. Negative self-talk can undermine efforts at self-control and lead to feelings of anxiety and depression.

Your beliefs and attitudes influence how you interpret what happens to you and what you can expect in the future, as well as how you feel

▶ **positive self-talk** Constructive mental or verbal statements made to one's self to change a belief or behavior.

▶ **negative self-talk** Mental or verbal statements made to one's self that reinforce negative or destructive self-perceptions.

and react. Realistic beliefs and goals combined with positive self-talk and problem-solving efforts support a healthy lifestyle.

Stress Management

Stress management can be an important part of weight management, and you can use the **ABC model of behavior** (see **FIGURE SO.15**) to help cope with daily stresses and their impacts on eating behavior.

The ABC model helps you manage events that trigger behaviors and factors that reinforce them. Antecedents, the *A* part of the model, are the events that precede the behavior and trigger it. Overeating is one possible behavior, the *B* part of the model. The consequences, or *C*, follow and reinforce the *B*. The *C* may be desirable, such as relief from stress, or undesirable, such as guilt or weight gain. The consequences may be immediate or, like weight gain, occur in the future; consequences that occur immediately have the greatest influence.

Identifying the cues (*A*) that trigger overeating is the first step to changing or avoiding these triggers. You might remove problem foods from the house or avoid the grocery store's candy aisle. You can sometimes manipulate antecedents to trigger positive behaviors (e.g., putting exercise clothes by the door to prompt exercise).

You can change the behavior of overeating (*B*) by using positive self-talk to encourage a new behavior and by avoiding excuses and rationalizations to eat something inappropriate.

Positive consequences (*C*) help to reinforce new behaviors. You could sign a contract with a friend that rewards you for deciding not to overeat. Rewards such as time for physical activity not only reinforce behavior, but also develop fitness. **TABLE SO.3** summarizes cognitive-behavioral tools for changing habits and behavior patterns.

Balancing Acceptance and Change

It's not enough to change your behavior to manage obesity. Self-acceptance is equally necessary. (See **TABLE SO.4**.) Accepting yourself as

▶ **ABC model of behavior** A behavioral model that includes the external and internal events that precede and follow the behavior. The "A" stands for antecedents, the events that precede the behavior ("B"), which is followed by consequences ("C") that positively or negatively reinforce the behavior.

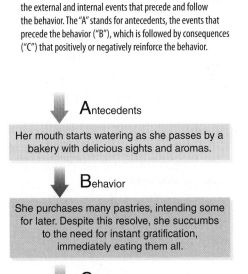

Antecedents

Her mouth starts watering as she passes by a bakery with delicious sights and aromas.

Behavior

She purchases many pastries, intending some for later. Despite this resolve, she succumbs to the need for instant gratification, immediately eating them all.

Consequences

She regrets her behavior and feels guilty. Overeating may leave her feeling ill and nauseated.

FIGURE SO.15 **The ABC model of eating behavior.** Conquering overeating often requires a psychological strategy for changing ingrained habits and other behaviors.

TABLE SO.3
Cognitive-Behavioral Tools for Changing Behavior

Self-monitoring	Prospectively recording information about behavior to identify the antecedents (what precedes and elicits a particular action), the behaviors of interest (usually eating behavior), and the consequences (the thoughts, feelings, and reactions that accompany the behavior of interest).
Environmental management	Avoiding or changing cues that trigger undesirable behavior (e.g., not driving by the doughnut shop, putting the cookie jar out of sight), or instituting new cues to elicit new behaviors (e.g., putting your walking shoes by the door as a reminder to exercise); also called *stimulus control*.
Alternate behaviors	Learning new ways of responding to old cues or circumstances that can't be changed or avoided (e.g., taking a walk when you get upset instead of getting something to eat).
Reward	Giving yourself, or arranging to be given, rewards for engaging in desired behaviors. Do not use food as a reward.
Negative reinforcement	Arranging to give up something desirable (e.g., money) or to endure something undesirable (e.g., wash your friend's car) for engaging in unwanted behaviors.
Social support	Getting others to participate in or otherwise provide emotional and physical support of your weight-management efforts.
Cognitive coping	Reducing negative self-talk, increasing positive self-talk, and challenging beliefs that undermine your resolve and contribute to negative emotions; setting reasonable goals and avoiding "thinking traps."
Managing emotions	Using reframing, disengagement, imagery, and self-soothing to reduce or manage negative emotions.
Relapse prevention and recovery	Identifying high-risk situations that pose a hazard for relapsing, and learning to recover from small indiscretions before they become major relapses.

Modified from Nash JD. *Maximize Your Body Potential.* 3rd ed. Palo Alto, CA: Bull Publishing Company; 2003. Used with permission from Bull Publishing Company.

TABLE SO.4

Basic Tenets of Size Acceptance

Human beings come in a variety of sizes and shapes. We celebrate this diversity as a positive characteristic of the human race.
There is no ideal body size, shape, or weight that every individual should strive to achieve.
Every body is a good body, whatever its size or shape.
Self-esteem and body image are strongly linked. Helping people feel good about their bodies and about who they are can help motivate and maintain healthy behaviors.
Appearance stereotyping is inherently unfair to the individual because it is based on superficial factors that the individual has little or no control over.
We respect the bodies of others even though they might be quite different from our own. Each person is responsible for taking care of his or her own body.
Good health is not defined by body size; it is a state of physical, mental, and social well-being. People of all sizes and shapes can reduce their risk of poor health by adopting a healthy lifestyle.

Data from Basic Tenets of Health at Every Size, developed by dietitians and nutritionists who are advocates of size acceptance; their efforts coordinated by Joanne P. Ikeda, MA, RD, Nutrition Education Specialist, Department of Nutritional Sciences, University of California, Berkeley.

you are will help your self-esteem and improve your general satisfaction with life. It is destructive to be overly concerned with the importance of body weight and shape or to have unattainable goals of idealized physical appearance. But don't confuse self-acceptance with complacency or a do-nothing attitude that ignores health risks.

If you must diet, do so in combination with exercise, and avoid very-low-calorie diets. Don't try to lose more than 1/2 to 1 pound per week. Realize that most low-calorie diets cause a rapid loss of body water at first. When this phase passes, weight loss declines. As a result, dieters often are misled into believing that their efforts are not working. They then give up, not realizing that smaller losses later in the diet actually are better than the initial big losses. In fact, the later loss is mostly fat loss, whereas the initial loss was primarily fluid loss.

> **Key Concepts**　Identifying cues that precede overeating can help a person make behavior changes. Long-term weight management should include self-acceptance and enhanced self-esteem. Goals of idealized body size and shape should be replaced with goals that promote good health and a lifetime of fitness.

Weight-Management Approaches

Do certain weight-loss diets have adverse health consequences? Is it unhealthy to lose weight quickly? Will the weight stay off? What motivates people to lose weight and to maintain weight? What are the barriers to losing weight and/or to maintaining weight?

All effective weight loss programs change the energy equation to achieve negative energy balance—generally by reducing energy input by restricting both overall intake and intake of calories, and by increasing energy output by adding physical activity. For any weight loss program to work, compliance is key. If you don't stick with the program, you won't lose weight. A program that best fits with your personal needs and motivations likely will be the most successful program for you.

A wide range of weight-management approaches is available to the consumer. It's important to investigate your options thoroughly to find the approach best suited to your personal needs.

Self-Help Books and Fad Diets

Some people respond well to simple information provided in an easy-to-understand format. By referring to good, well-researched self-help manuals and books, they work to improve their eating and lifestyle behaviors. Although such positive changes are desirable, few people achieve lasting weight loss.

Should you decide on the do-it-yourself route, develop specific goals for your diet, exercise, and maintenance plans. (See the FYI feature "Behaviors That Will Help You Manage Your Weight.") Keep tabs on your habits and become more involved in activities other than eating, especially fitness activities. Long-term success depends on maintaining the lifestyle changes that helped you lose the weight in the first place.

Fad diets promise easily-attainable weight loss and often are promoted with celebrity endorsements and exaggerated claims. In today's highly competitive marketplace, supporters claim that their diet is the "one true answer" to lose weight. Although these diets and associated products can generate substantial revenue for their promoters, they often require restrictive dietary behaviors that are unsustainable.

The proliferation of diet books and fad diets is nothing short of phenomenal, and each promotes their method as the ultimate "solution." (See **FIGURE S0.16**.) When sorting through the dozens of dubious weight-loss diet strategies that reach the market every year, be alert to the following warning flags:

- *Unbalanced diet patterns:* The recommended pattern should not stray too far from that of MyPlate.
- *Claims of a "scientific breakthrough" or promises of "quick and easy" weight loss:* There is no quick fix when it comes to weight management.
- *Irrational food instructions:* Food restrictions (e.g., no fruits), illogical overemphasis of some foods (e.g., five grapefruits daily) or supplements, and irrational food patterns (e.g., don't eat meat

There is always a new fad to try

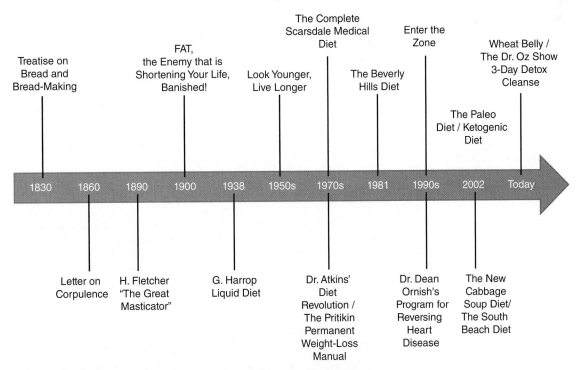

FIGURE S0.16 Fad diets. Over the last 200 years a variety of fad diets have captured the public imagination.

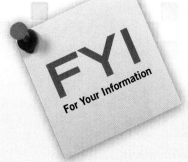

Behaviors That Will Help You Manage Your Weight

The following behaviors have been shown to be helpful in managing your weight.[a]

Set the Right Goals
Setting the right goals is an important first step. Most people trying to lose weight focus just on weight loss; however, you'll be more successful if you focus on dietary and exercise changes that lead to long-term weight change. Successful weight managers select no more than two or three goals at a time.

Effective goals are (1) specific, (2) attainable, and (3) forgiving. "Exercise more" is a commendable ideal, but it's not specific. "Walk 5 miles every day" is specific and measurable, but is it attainable if you're just starting out? "Walk 30 minutes every day" is more attainable, but what happens if you're held up at work or there's a thunderstorm? "Walk 30 minutes, five days each week" is specific, attainable, and forgiving. In short, a great goal!

Nothing Succeeds Like Success
Select a series of short-term goals that get you closer and closer to the ultimate goal (e.g., consider reducing fat intake from 40 percent of calories to 35 percent and later to 30 percent). Nothing succeeds like success. This strategy employs two important behavioral principles: (1) consecutive goals that move you ahead in small steps are the best way to reach a distant point, and (2) consecutive rewards keep the overall effort invigorated.

Reward Success (But Not with Food)
You're more likely to keep working toward your goal if you are rewarded—especially when goals are difficult to reach. An effective reward is something that is desirable, timely, and contingent on meeting your goal. Your rewards may be tangible (e.g., a movie, payment toward buying a more costly item) or intangible (e.g., an afternoon off from studying, an hour of quiet time away from the daily demands of school). As you meet small goals, give yourself numerous small rewards; don't wait to meet your ultimate goal for a large reward. The long, difficult effort might lead you to give up.

Balance Your (Food) Checkbook
Keeping track of your behavior—observing and recording calorie intake, servings of fruits and vegetables, exercise frequency and duration, or any other wellness behavior—can help alter that behavior. Self-monitoring usually changes a behavior in the desired direction and can produce "real-time" records for you and your healthcare provider. For example, you can track your exercise progress. A record of increasing exercise encourages you to keep up the good work. If the record shows little or no progress, you know that a change of strategy is needed. Some people find that specific self-monitoring forms make it easier, whereas others prefer to use their own recording system.

Although you don't need to step on the scale every day, monitoring your weight regularly (once a week) can help you maintain your lower weight. Use a graph rather than a list or calendar notations so you have a picture of cumulative progress. Changes in your body's water content, rather than fat content, are responsible for most of the up and down fluctuations from day to day. A long-term downward trend reflects fat losses.

Avoid a Chain Reaction
Identify the social or environmental cues that seem to encourage undesirable eating, and then change those cues. For example, you may learn from reflection or self-monitoring that you're more likely to overeat while watching television, when treats are on display at the campus cafe, or when you're around a certain friend. You might then try to break the association between eating and the cue (don't eat while watching television), avoid or eliminate the cue (avoid sitting near the display counter), or change the circumstances surrounding the cue (plan to meet with your friend in nonfood settings).

In general, visible and accessible food items often are cues for unplanned eating.

Get the (Fullness) Message
Changing the way you go about eating can make it easier to eat less without feeling deprived. It takes 15 or more minutes for your brain to get the message you've been fed. Slowing the rate of eating can allow satiation (fullness) signals to begin by the end of the meal. Eating lots of vegetables also can make you feel fuller. Another trick is to use smaller plates so moderate portions do not appear meager. Changing your eating schedule, or setting one, can be helpful, especially if you tend to skip or delay meals and overeat later.

The Backsliding Phenomenon
You've just signed a contract with yourself to avoid high-fat desserts for one month when you're presented with an array of your favorite "to die for" desserts. You say to yourself, "just this once" and satisfy your craving. Most of us have experienced the "backsliding phenomenon" in which we have lost our resolve and slipped back into a former bad habit. When it happens, be prepared for it and move on with your resolve. You're most apt to backslide when you're tempted by something unexpected and your self-control is threatened. You can remove high-fat snacks from your home but not from other places you eat. Imagine tempting situations in your mind's eye and practice coping with them successfully. If you do slip, don't waste time with self-blame. Learn from the experience and get back on track.

a National Heart, Lung, and Blood Institute. Guide to behavior change. http://www.nhlbi.nih.gov/health/public/heart/obesity/lose_wt/behavior.htm. Accessed September 20, 2017.

and bread at the same meal) set the stage for feelings of deprivation and binge eating.

- *The promise of a cure for some disease along with weight loss:* That's not only a waste of money, but also potentially dangerous.

- *Lack of an exercise plan or suggestions for physical activity throughout the day:* Physical activity is a fundamental component of any reputable weight management plan.

The website WebMD reviews popular diet plans.[76] Each review includes promises made by the diet plan promoters, a description of how the plan works and the level of effort required, and an opinion by a reputable doctor. To find these reviews, type "Weight Loss & Diet Plans A-Z" into your Internet search engine. To access the relevant pages, you may need to sign up for a free WebMD account.

Meal Replacements

Some people turn to meal replacements—shakes and bars, for example— to help lose weight. Meal replacements are convenient, often contain added vitamins and minerals, and reduce the choices and temptations available at mealtime. They also are highly processed and not as healthful as fresh, more natural foods. When compared with traditional, reduced-calorie diet programs, people using meal replacements lost slightly more weight and were less likely to stop the program.[77] The challenge is to learn long-term eating strategies that will allow weight management without reliance on special products.

Self-Help Groups

Self-help groups, often led by laypeople, help many people cope with their weight. Such groups can share experiences, reduce the isolation and alienation felt by many obese people, and provide an understanding and accepting community.

Commercial Programs

Commercial weight-loss programs provide group or individual counseling and group support. Some sell prepackaged foods or nutritional supplements. Some companies employ dietitians, health educators, psychologists, or physicians to develop and guide the program at the corporate level. The Federal Trade Commission (FTC) encourages commercial programs to release the following information to potential clients:

- Staff training and education
- Risks of overweight and obesity
- Risks of their products or program
- Cost
- Program outcomes: success and failure rates

Be sure to obtain this information before you register for a weight-loss program, and think twice about any program that does not willingly provide it.

Currently, three programs dominate the weight loss services industry—Weight Watchers, Jenny Craig, and Nutrisystem. A systematic review of 39 randomized controlled trials found consistent evidence supporting the long-term efficacy of Weight Watchers and Jenny Craig; Nutrisystem needs additional long-term studies for the researchers to be confident in its effects.[78]

The review also examined five self-directed programs—Atkins, Slim-Fast, Biggest Loser Club, eDiets, and Lose It!—all of which currently offer support through the Internet. Although Atkins showed results similar to Weight Watchers, additional randomized controlled trials are needed to evaluate the others. The self-directed programs typically are the most affordable options. The review did not include Ornish or

Quick **Bite**

Dangerous Caloric Restriction
Very-low-calorie diets (such as Optifast) promise substantial short-term weight loss. However, enthusiasm is dampened by the greatly increased risk of gallstones and the lack of evidence for sustained long-term weight loss. Very-low-calorie diets (less than 800 kilocalories per day) should be undertaken only with medical supervision.

the Zone, because Ornish does not focus on weight loss and the Zone offers no behavioral/social support. For several commercial programs (e.g., South Beach, Ideal Protein), published studies did not met eligibility criteria for review.

Smartphone-Based Interventions

Many people carry their smartphones everywhere they go, and the phones are almost always on. This enables real-time, on-demand interaction and provides the opportunity for frequent, interactive, and tailored messaging (via text or emails). Smartphones also enable immediate access to social support. Because interactive apps can provide real-time feedback, and even video "face-to-face" interactions, smartphones can help with decisions to modify behavior. Although smartphone apps are believed to have great promise in weight management, this is a new area in weight management and is not yet known to be effective.[79]

Professional Private Counselors

Private counselors can be physicians, psychotherapists, nutritionists, or registered dietitians. They provide individualized weight management and the support and attention that some obese people may need. Some programs use the Internet rather than face-to-face counseling sessions and have seen positive results. The Internet has shown potential for use in many areas of health behavior, including increased self-motivation and weight loss. Although Internet-based weight loss programs are popular, none have scientific evidence for superior long-term weight loss compared to conventional approaches.

Carefully scrutinize the training and credentials of private counselors before committing to any program. Effective weight-loss counselors should do the following:

- Assess obesity risk.
- Ask about readiness to lose weight.
- Advise in designing a weight-control program.
- Assist in establishing appropriate intervention.
- Arrange for follow-up.

Food and Drug Administration–Approved Weight-Loss Medications

The pharmaceutical industry has long searched for a "magic bullet" to battle obesity, but a cure has failed to emerge. With the recognition that obesity involves multiple factors, the focus is shifting to drugs with multiple mechanisms and drugs to be used in conjunction with proper diet and exercise. When combined with changes to eating and physical activity, prescription drugs may help some people lose weight (usually 3 to 9 percent of their body weight, although some can lose 10 percent or more). Results vary by drug and by person. Most weight loss takes place in the first 6 months of starting the medicine. After that time, the patient may lose weight more slowly or begin to regain weight.[80]

One should never take a weight loss medicine only for cosmetic benefit, and should only take the medicine under a doctor's supervision. The chance that side effects may outweigh benefits is of great concern. In the past, some drugs for obesity treatment were linked to serious health problems. For example, sibutramine (sold as Meridia) was recalled because of concerns related to heart disease and stroke.

The FDA has approved several prescription medications for weight loss. Five of these drugs—orlistat (Xenical, Alli), lorcaserin (Belviq),

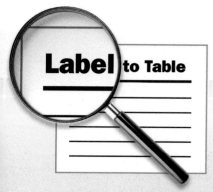

Label to Table

Do you believe that by choosing cookies or chips labeled "low-fat" or sticking with certain brand names associated with "diet foods" you are automatically making the right decisions? It may surprise you to know that many low-fat or fat-free products have nearly the same amount of calories as the full-fat versions! After reading this chapter, you now know that when it comes to weight loss, total calories are just as important as calories from fat. If you eat a fat-free food but eat so much of it that your calories are excessive, you will still gain weight. To illustrate this point, let's compare the nutrition labels from some leading cookie manufacturers. The lower-fat cookies (on the right) claim they are "better for you" and have "50% less fat" compared with regular cookies. Here are the labels:

Regular Cookie	Lower-Fat Cookie
Serving, 2 cookies (29 g)	Serving, 2 cookies (26 g)
Calories, 140	Calories, 110
Calories from fat, 50	Calories from fat, 25
Total fat, 6 g	Total fat, 3 g

True, there is a 50 percent reduction in fat content (6 grams versus 3 grams), which is an important part of the picture. However, take a look at the total calories. The lower fat cookies only have 30 fewer kilocalories than the regular cookies, which may be a surprise to those who think they are saving more.

There is another interesting piece of information on these labels—the serving size.

At first glance, you may think the serving sizes of the cookies are the same—two cookies. However, after further inspection you can see that the lower-fat cookies are slightly smaller. A 10 percent reduction in size/weight is certainly worth noting when you are trying to explain how a product can have fewer calories.

The next time you are in the cookie aisle debating whether you should settle a craving with a low-fat product or its full-fat version, be a smart consumer and read the label before you buy!

Regular cookie

Nutrition Facts
16 servings per container
Serving size 2 cookies (29g)

Amount per serving
Calories 140

	% Daily Value*
Total Fat 6g	9%
Saturated Fat 1.5g	8%
Trans Fat 0.5g	
Cholesterol 0mg	0%
Sodium 105mg	4%
Total Carbohydrate 21g	7%
Dietary Fiber less than 1g	3%
Total Sugars 8g	
Includes 8g Added Sugars	16%
Protein 2g	
Vitamin D 0mcg	0%
Calcium 0mg	0%
Iron 1mg	4%
Potassium 0mg	0%

* The % Daily Value (DV) tells you how much a nutrient in a serving of food contributes to a daily diet. 2,000 calories a day is used for general nutrition advice.

Lower fat cookie

Nutrition Facts
18 servings per container
Serving size 2 cookies (26g)

Amount per serving
Calories 110

	% Daily Value*
Total Fat 3g	5%
Saturated Fat 0.5g	3%
Polyunsaturated Fat 0g	
Monounsaturated Fat 1g	
Trans Fat 0g	
Cholesterol 0mg	0%
Sodium 130mg	5%
Total Carbohydrate 20g	7%
Dietary Fiber 0g	0%
Total Sugars 10g	
Includes 10g Added Sugars	20%
Protein 1g	
Vitamin D 0mcg	0%
Calcium 0mg	0%
Iron 1mg	4%
Potassium 0mg	0%

* The % Daily Value (DV) tells you how much a nutrient in a serving of food contributes to a daily diet. 2,000 calories a day is used for general nutrition advice.

Learning Portfolio

Key Terms

Study Points

- The prevalence of obesity and overweight is escalating worldwide, creating an epidemic responsible for numerous chronic diseases.

- The factors that cause obesity are not completely understood, but a complex interaction of hormonal and metabolic factors is believed to play a role, along with genetic, social, environmental, lifestyle, behavior, and psychological factors.

- In the United States, overweight and obesity are not only concerns for the adult population; childhood obesity is also increasing at an alarming rate.

- Compared to their normal-weight counterparts, obese children and adolescents are more likely to have risk factors associated with various chronic diseases.

- Eating meals away from home, physical inactivity, screen time, "competitive" foods, food deserts, and acceptance of obesity in social circles are all considered main contributors to childhood obesity.

- During the first years of life, children develop the eating patterns that can influence health and well-being throughout the life cycle.

- Obesity is a risk factor for many chronic diseases, including heart disease, cancer, hypertension, and diabetes. In many cases, a modest amount of weight loss can improve symptoms and disease management.

- Rather than focus on ideal body weight, many professionals now promote health and fitness goals.

- Physical activity improves fitness and helps achieve the negative energy balance needed for weight reduction.

- Abandoning unrealistic ideas of thinness and accepting body weight and shape are important elements in weight management.

- Long-term weight management includes a balanced diet of moderately restricted calorie intake, adequate exercise, cognitive-behavioral strategies for changing habits and behavior patterns, and attention to balancing self-acceptance and the desire for change.

- Surgical approaches to weight control should be considered only as a last resort for the morbidly obese.

- If the cause is not hereditary, being underweight can pose health problems.

- Gaining weight can be difficult for individuals who are underweight.

Study Questions

1. Obesity is seen as a complex disorder with multiple contributing factors. Give examples of each of the following factors: biological, social and environmental, lifestyle, and behavioral.

2. What is the difference between hyperplastic and hypertrophic obesity?

3. Think about the environment in which you live—your built environment, the human-formed, developed, or structured areas including roads, parks, sidewalks, and transportation system. Is your built environment conducive to a healthy lifestyle? Why or why not? Give examples of a built environment that would be different from where you currently live.

4. The causes of childhood obesity are numerous and far-reaching. List six main contributors to the childhood obesity epidemic.

5. List and identify the risks of being overweight.

6. Identify the negative consequences of weight cycling.

7. Discuss the four most widely accepted methods for weight loss and management.

8. Describe the concept of metabolically healthy obesity.

9. What are the four components of a sound approach to weight management?

10. Explain how the ABCs of behavior modification can assist with weight control.

Try This

"Watch" Your Screen Time

Monitor your screen time for a day. Keep track of the total amount of time you spend in any and all of the following activities: watching television; using a computer; playing video games; checking email; and using or playing games on handheld devices such as smartphones, iTouch devices, or iPads. In a 24-hour period, how many hours of screen time did you accrue? How does your use compare to the averages? If your screen time is too high, identify ways you can improve it.

Tracking Your Activity

Physical activity is a necessary component of a healthy lifestyle. All adults should aim to be physically active (30–60 minutes/day) on most, if not all, days of the week. Keep track of the amount of physical activity you get this week. Try to be more physically active in your everyday routine, such as walking short distances that you normally would drive and taking the stairs instead of the elevator. Do you notice a difference in your overall feeling of well-being on the days that you are physically active compared to the days that you are not?

References

1. Bahia L, Coutinho ES, Barufaldi LA, et al. The costs of overweight and obesity-related diseases in the Brazilian public health system: cross-sectional study. *BMC Public Health*. 2012;12(1):440.

2. McCrady-Spitzer SK, Levine JA. Keynote: nonexercise activity thermogenesis: a way forward to treat the worldwide obesity epidemic. *Surg Obes Rel Dis*. 2012;8:501-506.

3. Lien N, Henriksen HB, Nymoen LL, et al. Availability of data assessing the prevalence and trends of overweight and obesity among European adolescents. *Public Health Nutr*. 2010;13(10A):1680-1687.

4. McCrady-Spitzer SK, Levine JA. Op. cit.

5. Abdul Rahim HF, Sibai A, Hwalla N, et al. Non-communicable diseases in the Arab world. *Lancet*. 2014;383(9914):356-367.

6. National Center for Health Statistics. Health, United States, 2015: with special features on racial and ethnic health disparities. https://www.cdc.gov/nchs/data/hus/hus15.pdf#053. Accessed September 20, 2017.

7. Ibid.

8. Ibid.

9. MarketData Enterprises. *The U.S. Weight Loss & Diet Control Market*. 13th ed. April 2015.

10. Wilke J. Nearly half in U.S. remain worried about their weight. July 25, 2014. http://www.gallup.com/poll/174089/nearly-half-remain-worried-weight.aspx. Accessed September 20, 2017.

11. DeVault N, Kennedy T, Hermann J, et al. It's all about kids: preventing overweight in elementary school children in Tulsa, OK. *J Am Diet Assoc*. 2009;109(4):680-687.

12. Blomain ES, Dirhan DA, Valentino MA, et al. Mechanisms of weight regain following weight loss. *ISRN Obesity*. April 16, 2013. https://www.ncbi.nlm.nih.gov/pmc/articles/PMC3901982/pdf/ISRN.OBESITY2013-210524.pdf. Accessed September 20, 2017.

13. Pachucki MC, Lovenheim MF, Harding M. Within-family obesity associations: evaluation of parent, child, and sibling relationships. *Am J Prev Med*. 2014;47(4):382-391.

14. Llewellyn CH, Trzaskowski M, Plomin R, Wardle J. From modeling to measurement: developmental trends in genetic influence on adiposity in childhood. *Obesity*. 2014;22(7):1756-1761.

15. Yan H, Guo Y, Yang TL, et al. A family-based association study identified *CYP17* as a candidate gene for obesity susceptibility in Caucasians. *Genet Mol Res*. 2012;11(3):1967-1974.

16. Williams MJ, Almen MS, Fredriksson R, Schilth HB. What model organisms and interactomics can reveal about the genetics of human obesity. *Cell Mol Life Sci*. 2012;69(22):3819-3834.

17. Ibid.

18. Manco M, Dallapiccola B. Genetics of pediatric obesity. *Pediatrics*. 2012;130(1):123-133.

19. Hood L. Tackling the microbiome. *Science*. 2012;336(6086):1209.

20. Moreno-Indias I, Cardona F, Tinahones FJ, et al. Impact of the gut microbiota on the development of obesity and type 2 diabetes mellitus. *Frontiers Microbiol*. 2014;5(190):1-10.

21. Komaroff AL. The microbiome and risk for obesity and type 2 diabetes. *JAMA*. 2017;317(4):355-356.

22. Litonjua AA. Fat-soluble vitamins and atopic disease: what is the evidence? *Proc Nutr Soc*. 2012;71:67-74.

23. National Center for Health Statistics. Op. cit.

24. Acevedo P, Lopez-Ejeda N, Alferez-Garcia I, et al. Body mass index through self-reported data and body image perception in Spanish adults attending dietary consultation. *Nutrition*. 2014;30(6):679-684.

25. Snook KR, Hansen AR, Duke CH, et al. Change in percentages of adults with overweight or obesity trying to lose weight, 1988-2014. *JAMA*. 2017;317(9):971-973.

26. National Center for Health Statistics. Op. cit.

27. Vaughan CA, Sacco WP, Beckstead JW. Racial/ethnic differences in body mass index: the roles of beliefs about thinness and dietary restrictions. *Body Image*. 2008;5(3):291-298.

28. Gillen MM, Lefkowits ES. Gender and racial/ethnic differences in body image development among college students. *Body Image*. 2012;9(1):126-130.

29. Wang Y, Chen X. Between-group differences in nutrition- and health-related psychosocial factors among US adults and their associations with diet, exercise, and weight status. *J Acad Nutr Diet*. 2012;112(4):486-498.

30. Walker RE, Kawachi I. Use of concept mapping to explore the influence of food security on food buying practices. *J Acad Nutr Diet*. 2012;112(5):711-717.

31. Castillo DC, Ramsey NL, Yu SS, et al. Inconsistent access to food and cardiometabolic disease: the effect of food insecurity. *Curr Cardiovasc Risk Rep*. 2012;6(3):245-250.

32. Yu Y. Four decades of obesity trends among non-Hispanic whites and blacks in the United States: analyzing the influences of educational inequalities in obesity and population improvements in education. *PLoS One*. 2016;11(11):e0167193. doi:10.1371/journal.pone.0167193

33. Befort CA, Nazir N, Perri MG. Prevalence of obesity among adults from rural and urban areas of the United States: finding from NHANES (2005-2008). *J Rural Health*. 2012;28(4):392-397.

34. Trust for America's Health, the Robert Wood Johnson Foundation. The state of obesity: adult obesity in the United States. http://stateofobesity.org/adult-obesity/. Accessed September 20, 2017.

Learning Portfolio (continued)

35. Drewnowski A, Aggarwal A, Monsivais P, Moudon AV. Obesity and supermarket access: proximity or price? *Am J Public Health*. 2012;102(8):e74-e80.

36. Ibid.

37. Desilver D. Chart of the week: is food too cheap for our own good? Pew Research Center. May 23, 2014. http://www.pewresearch.org/fact-tank/2014/05/23/chart-of-the-week-is-food-too-cheap-for-our-own-good. Accessed September 20, 2017.

38. Cohen DA, Babey SH. Contextual influences on eating behaviors: heuristic processing and dietary choices. *Obes Rev*. 2012;13(9):766-779.

39. Durand CP, Andalib M, Dunton GF, et al. A systematic review of built environment factors related to physical activity and obesity risk: implications for smart growth urban planning. *Obes Rev*. 2011;12(5):e173-e182.

40. He M, Tucker P, Irwin JD, et al. Obesogenic neighbourhoods: the impact of neighbourhood restaurants and convenience stores on adolescents' food consumption behaviours. *Public Health Nutr*. 2012;15(12):2331-2339.

41. Safron M, Cislak A, Gasper T, Luszczynska A. Micro-environmental characteristics related to body weight, diet, and physical activity of children and adolescents: a systematic umbrella review. *Int J Environ Health Res*. 2011;27:1-25.

42. Todd JE. *Changes in Eating Patterns and Diet Quality Among Working-Age Adults, 2005-10*. ERR-161. Washington, DC: U.S. Department of Agriculture, Economic Research Service; January 2014.

43. Wu H, Sturm R. What's on the menu? A review of the energy and nutritional content of U.S. chain restaurant menus. *Public Health Nutr*. 2013;16(1):87-96.

44. Piernas C, Popkin BM. Food portion patterns and trends among U.S. children and the relationship to total eating occasion size, 1977–2006. *J Nutr*. 2011;141(6):1159-1164.

45. Ibid.

46. Powell K, Wilcox J, Clonan A. The role of social networks in the development of overweight and obesity among adults: a scoping review. *BMC Public Health*. 2015;15:996.

47. Zhang J, Tong L, Lamberson PJ, et al. Leveraging social influence to address overweight and obesity using agent-based models: the role of adolescent social networks. *Soc Sci Med*. 2015;125:203-213.

48. Ibid.

49. Fletcher A, Bonell C, Sorhaindo A. You are what your friends eat: systematic review of social network analysis of young people's eating behaviors and bodyweight. *J Epidemiol Community Health*. 2011;65(6):548-555.

50. Ibid.

51. Go AS, Mozaffarian D, Roger VL, et al. on behalf of the American Heart Association Statistics Committee and Stroke Statistics Subcommittee. Heart disease and stroke statistics—2013 update: a report from the American Heart Association. *Circulation*. 2013;127:e6-e245. http://circ.ahajournals.org/content/127/1/e6.full.pdf. Accessed September 20, 2017.

52. Gilbert-Diamond D, Li Z, Adachi-Mejia AM, McClure AC, Sargent JD. Association of a television in the bedroom with increased adiposity gain in a nationally representative sample of children and adolescents. *JAMA Pediatr*. 2014;168(5):427-434.

53. Mason TB, Robin JL. Profiles of binge eating: the interaction of depressive symptoms, eating styles and body mass index. *Eating Disord J Treat Prevent*. 2014;1:1-11.

54. Allen KL, Gibson LY, McLean NJ, Davis EA, Byrne SM. Maternal and family factors and child eating pathology: risk and protective relationships. *J Eating Disord*. 2014;2:11.

55. Lowe MR, Doshi SD, Katterman SN, Feig EH. Dieting and restrained eating as prospective predictors of weight gain. *Frontiers Psychol*. 2013;4:577.

56. Ogden CL, Carroll MD, Kit BK, Flegal KM. Prevalence of childhood and adult obesity in the United States, 2011-2012. *JAMA*. 2014;311(8):806-814.

57. Latzer Y, Stein D. A review of the psychological and familial perspectives of childhood obesity. *J Eating Disord*. 2013;1:7. Epub February 25, 2013. doi: 10.1186/2050-2974-1-7

58. National Heart, Lung, and Blood Institute. Risk factors. http://www.nhlbi.nih.gov/health/health-topics/topics/obe/risks.html. Accessed September 20, 2017.

59. Kitahara CM, Flint AJ, Berrington de Gonzalez A, et al. Association between class III obesity (BMI of 40-59 kg/m²) and mortality: a pooled analysis of 20 prospective studies. *PLOS Med*. 2014;11(7):e1001673.

60. Cawley J, Meyerhoefer C. The medical care costs of obesity: an instrumental variables approach. *J Health Econ*. 2012;31(1):219-230.

61. Kuller L. The great fat debate: reducing cholesterol. *J Am Diet Assoc*. 2011;111(5):663-664.

62. National Heart, Lung, and Blood Institute. What is metabolic syndrome? November 2011. http://www.nhlbi.nih.gov/health/health-topics/topics/ms/. Accessed March 3, 2017.

63. Land SR, Liu Q, Wickerham DL, Costantino JP, Gonz PA. Cigarette smoking, physical activity, and alcohol consumption as predictors of cancer incidence among women at high risk of breast cancer in the NSABP P-1 trial. *Cancer Epidemiol Biomarkers Prevent*. 2014;23(5):823-832.

64. Dobrosielski DA, Patil S, Schwartz AR, Bandeen-Roche K, Stewart KJ. Effects of exercise and weight loss in older adults with obstructive sleep apnea. *Med Sci Sports Exerc*. 2015;47(1):20-26.

65. Mason C, Foster-Schubert KE, Imayama I, et al. History of weight cycling does not impede future weight loss or metabolic improvements in postmenopausal women. *Metabolism*. 2013;62(1):127-136.

66. Ibid.

67. Flegal KM, Kit BK, Orpana H, Graubard BI. Association of all-cause mortality with overweight and obesity using standard body mass index categories: a systematic review and meta-analysis. *JAMA*. 2013;309:71-82.

68. Flegal KM, Kit BK, Orpana H, et al. Association of all-cause mortality with overweight and obesity using standard body mass index categories. *JAMA*. 2013;309(1):71-82. https://jamanetwork.com/journals/jama/fullarticle/1555137. Accessed November 6, 2017.

69. Raynor HA, Champagne CM. Position of the Academy of Nutrition and Dietetics: interventions for the treatment of overweight and obesity in adults. *J Acad Nutr Diet*. 2016;116(1):129-147.

70. Hill JO, Peters JC, Wyatt HR. Using the energy gap to address obesity: a commentary. *J Am Diet Assoc*. 2009;109(11):1848-1853.

71. Kramer CK, Zinman B, Retnakaran R. Are metabolically healthy overweight and obesity benign conditions? *Ann Intern Med*. 2013;159:758-769.

72. National Weight Control Registry. NWCR facts. http://www.nwcr.ws/Research/default.htm. Accessed September 20, 2017.

73. Kong A, Beresford SA, Alfano CM, et al. Self-monitoring and eating-related behaviors are associated with 12-month weight loss in postmenopausal overweight-to-obese women. *J Acad Nutr Diet*. 2012;112(9):1428-1435.

74. Kobayashi F, Ogata H, Omi N, et al. Effect of breakfast skipping on diurnal variation of energy metabolism and blood glucose. *Obes Res Clin Pract*. 2014;8(3):e201-e298.

75. Ibid.

76. WebMD. Weight loss and diet plans A-Z. http://www.webmd.com/diet/a-z/evaluate-latest-diets. Accessed September 20, 2017.

77. Soeliman FA, Azadbakht L. Weight loss maintenance: a review on dietary related strategies. *J Res Med Sci*. 2014;19(3):268-275.

78. Gudzune KA, Doshi RS, Mehta AK, et. al. Efficacy of commercial weight loss programs: an updated systematic review. *Ann Intern Med*. 2015;162(7):501-512.

79. Raynor HA, Champagne CM. Op. cit.

80. U.S. Department of Health and Human Services, National Institute of Diabetes and Digestive and Kidney Diseases. Prescription medications to treat

overweight and obesity. https://www.niddk.nih.gov/health-information/health-topics/weight-control/prescription-medications-treat-overweight-obesity/pages/facts.aspx. Accessed September 20, 2017.

81. Ibid.

82. Chang YY, Chiou WB. The liberating effect of weight loss supplements on dietary control: a field experiment. *Nutrition*. 2014;30(9):1007-1010.

83. Vaughan RA, Conn CA, Mermier CM. Effects of commercially available dietary supplements on resting energy expenditure: a brief report. *ISRN Nutr*. 2014 (2014), Article ID 650264.

84. U.S. Department of Health and Human Services, National Institute of Diabetes and Digestive and Kidney Diseases. Potential candidates for bariatric surgery. https://www.niddk.nih.gov/health-information/health-topics/weight-control/bariatric-surgery/Pages/potential-candidates.aspx. Accessed September 20, 2017.

85. U.S. Department of Health and Human Services, National Institute of Diabetes and Digestive and Kidney Diseases. Types of bariatric surgery. https://www.niddk.nih.gov/health-information/health-topics/weight-control/bariatric-surgery/Pages/types.aspx. Accessed September 20, 2017.

86. Inge TH, Courcoulas AP, Jenkins TM, et al. Weight loss and health status 3 years after bariatric surgery in adolescents. *New Engl J Med.* 2016;374(2):113-123.

87. Hoyuela C. Five-year outcomes of laparoscopic sleeve gastrectomy as a primary procedure for morbid obesity: a prospective study. *World J Gastrointest Surg* 2017 April 27;9(4):109-117. https://www.ncbi.nlm.nih.gov/pmc/articles/PMC5406732/pdf/WJGS-9-109.pdf. Accessed November 6, 2017.

88. U.S. Department of Health and Human Services, National Institute of Diabetes and Digestive and Kidney Diseases. Types of bariatric surgery. Op. cit.

89. Kreider RB, Serra M, Beavers KM, et al. A structured diet and exercise program promotes favorable changes in weight loss, body composition, and weight maintenance. *J Am Diet Assoc.* 2011;111(6):828-843.

Chapter 11

Life Cycle: Maternal and Infant Nutrition

Revised by Paul Insel

LEARNING Objectives

1 Discuss maternal physiological changes that occur during pregnancy, including the components of maternal weight gain and the corresponding nutritional needs.

2 Identify benefits of breastfeeding for both infant and mother.

3 Describe energy and nutrient needs during infancy.

4 Summarize the appropriate steps for introducing solid foods into an infant's diet.

5 Identify feeding problems during infancy and provide recommendations to overcome them.

I magine finding out you are pregnant. (If you are a guy, play along for a moment and imagine yourself as a woman, too!) Are your current eating habits sufficient to support the nutritional demands of pregnancy? If not, what changes should you make, and why? What about other aspects of your lifestyle that you may need to modify before pregnancy, such as smoking, alcohol use, or exercise? How would you feed a new baby? Breastfeeding imposes nutritional demands on the mother but provides many benefits for the infant. If you've never shopped for infant formula or baby food before, you may be surprised at the variety of choices and confused as to which is best. Imagining yourself in this scenario puts a spotlight on the many nutritional implications of pregnancy, breastfeeding, and infant feeding.

Nutrition Before Conception

🍎 **Why Is This Important?** Even before becoming pregnant, all women should ensure their folic acid intake meets recommended levels to reduce the risk of neural defects in the fetus. For both men and women, the use of alcohol, drugs, and tobacco should end well before conception, and women should continue to avoid their use throughout pregnancy to reduce the risk of poor fetal outcomes. Other healthy lifestyle behaviors—such as a nutritious diet, regular physical activity, and reducing caffeine—are also recommended before, during, and after pregnancy.

Once she becomes pregnant, a woman needs to focus on a healthful diet. But her nutritional status at the moment of conception also is important. Her vitamin status at conception, for example, can determine the difference between a healthy baby and one with a devastating birth defect. In addition, a woman's weight at conception can influence her pregnancy and delivery as well as the baby's health.

For these reasons, it's important for a woman to get health care and guidance before she gets pregnant. Many experts recommend extending prenatal care—the routine, professional health care that a woman receives during her pregnancy—to include the preconception period as well. (See **FIGURE 11.1**.) Although extending prenatal health care is a worthy goal, it is important to realize that about half the pregnancies in

---

📎 *Position Statement: Academy of Nutrition and Dietetics*

Nutrition and Lifestyle for a Healthy Pregnancy Outcome

It is the position of the Academy of Nutrition and Dietetics that women of childbearing age should adopt a lifestyle optimizing health and reduce the risk of birth defects, suboptimal fetal development, and chronic health problems in both mother and child. Components leading to healthy pregnancy outcomes include healthy prepregnancy weight, appropriate weight gain and physical activity during pregnancy, consumption of a variety of foods, appropriate vitamin and mineral supplementation, avoidance of alcohol and other harmful substances, and safe food handling. Pregnancy is a critical period during which maternal nutrition and lifestyle choices are major influences on mother and child health. Inadequate levels of key nutrients during crucial periods of fetal development may lead to reprogramming within fetal tissues, predisposing the infant to chronic conditions in later life. Improving the well-being of mothers, infants, and children is key to the health of the next generation.

Reprinted from *Journal of the Academy of Nutrition and Dietetics*, 114(7), Sandra B. Procter, Christina G. Campbell, Position of the Academy of Nutrition and Dietetics: Nutrition and Lifestyle for a Healthy Pregnancy Outcome, Page no. 1099-1103, 2014, with permission from Elsevier.

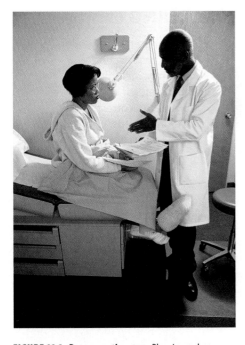

FIGURE 11.1 Preconception care. Planning and care before pregnancy are recommended for all prospective mothers.
© Photodisc.

the United States are unplanned. Hence, good nutrition for all women of childbearing age is an important public health objective.

Preconception care can be defined as a set of interventions that identify and modify biomedical, behavioral, and social risks to a woman's health or pregnancy outcome through prevention and management.[1] The overall goals are to (1) screen for risks; (2) promote health and education; and (3) identify, prevent, and manage risks. Nutrition is an important aspect of all three goals. Risk screening includes an evaluation of a prospective mother's vitamin status and weight as well as her health habits—including use of alcohol, tobacco, and other substances—and her overall medical condition. Health promotion and education means providing information to the would-be mother about steps she can take to maximize her chances of a trouble-free pregnancy, an uneventful delivery, and a healthy, full-term baby. Intervention can be as simple as recommending a folic acid supplement or as complex as treating an eating disorder or a substance abuse problem. Before conception, the goal is to resolve the nutrition and health issues that could harm a mother or her baby. **TABLE 11.1** lists 10 recommendations for preconception health developed by the Centers for Disease Control and Prevention.

Men's preconception health is also very important. Although some men are born with problems that affect fertility, lifestyle behaviors can also play a part. The CDC offers the following list of behaviors and conditions as potential risks to the health and number of sperm: type 1 diabetes; heavy alcohol use; use of some "street" drugs; smoking cigarettes; age; obesity; hazardous substances, including bug spray and metals such as lead; diseases such as mumps, serious conditions like kidney disease, or hormone problems; medicines (prescription, nonprescription, and herbal products); and radiation treatment and chemotherapy for cancer. All of these considerations should be discussed between the couple and their physicians.

Weight

Although everyone should be concerned about maintaining a healthful weight, a woman contemplating pregnancy needs to pay special attention to weight. Maternal obesity can complicate pregnancy and

TABLE 11.1
Recommendations for Preconception Health

Individual responsibility	Each woman, man, and couple should be encouraged to have a reproductive life plan.
Consumer awareness	Increase public awareness of appropriate preconception health behaviors.
Preventive visits	Provide risk assessment and health promotion counseling to all women of childbearing age during primary care visits.
Interventions for identified risks	Provide interventions to women following risk identification.
Interconception care	Use the time between pregnancies for intensive interventions.
Prepregnancy checkups	Offer prepregnancy visits as a component of maternity care.
Health insurance coverage	Increase coverage to ensure access for low-income women.
Public health programs	Integrate preconception health into existing public health programs.
Research	Increase the evidence base for methods to improve preconception health.
Monitoring	Use public health surveillance mechanisms to monitor the effectiveness of preconception care.

Modified from Centers for Disease Control and Prevention. Recommendations to improve preconception health and health care—United States. *MMWR.* 2006;55(RR-06):1-23. http://www.cdc.gov/mmwr/preview/mmwrhtml/rr5506a1.htm. Accessed May 13, 2017.

delivery and compromise a baby's health. Being too thin likewise carries its own risks.

Body mass index (BMI) is an indicator of a prospective mother's weight status. Lean women with a BMI less than 20 kg/m^2 have increased risks of **preterm delivery**.[2] Inadequate weight gain and poor nutrition—marked by a low white blood cell count and low iron levels—during the first stages of pregnancy are also associated with preterm birth,[3] as are inadequate intakes of protein and energy, calcium, zinc, omega-3 fatty acids, and multiple micronutrients.[4] At the other end of the spectrum, nearly two-thirds of U.S. women of childbearing age are overweight or obese, and one-fifth are obese at the start of pregnancy.[5] Overweight and obese women have increased risks of several problems, including preterm delivery and stillbirth.[6] In addition, obese women are at higher risk for the following[7]:

- High blood pressure
- Gestational diabetes—a form of diabetes associated with pregnancy that is often controlled through diet alone
- Preeclampsia—a condition marked by high blood pressure and protein in the urine
- Prolonged labor
- Unplanned cesarean section
- Difficulty initiating and continuing breastfeeding

Studies show that overweight and obesity during pregnancy are also linked to a variety of issues for the baby later in life, including higher BMI and waist circumference, increased subcutaneous adipose tissue, higher triglyceride levels, and reduced high-density lipoprotein (HDL) cholesterol.[8]

Of course, the time to lose or gain weight is well before a pregnancy begins. It is not a good idea for pregnant women, even obese pregnant women, to try to lose weight or follow a restrictive diet during pregnancy. Even a thin woman who finds it hard to put on weight under normal circumstances is unlikely to find it any easier when she's pregnant, especially if she experiences **morning sickness**.

Women with eating disorders have special pregnancy-related risks. Ideally, anorexia nervosa or bulimia nervosa is diagnosed and treated well before conception, to give the prospective mother's body plenty of time to recover and prepare for the demands of pregnancy, birth, and breastfeeding. A woman who begins her pregnancy with an active eating disorder may not gain enough weight—or may vomit too much—to sustain a growing fetus. Risks can include premature delivery, a **low-birth-weight infant**, and even fetal death.

Vitamins

A good diet goes a long way toward meeting the demands of pregnancy, but even a diet that includes all food groups can lack enough of specific nutrients. This is especially true for folic acid, a nutrient needed to prevent neural tube defects, which are birth defects that involve the spinal column.[9] A common neural tube defect is spina bifida, a birth defect in which part of the spinal cord protrudes through the spinal column, causing varying degrees of paralysis and lack of bowel and bladder control. (See **FIGURE 11.2**.)

The U.S. Preventive Services Task Force recommends that all women of childbearing age take a daily supplement of 400 to 800 micrograms

▶ **preterm delivery** A delivery that occurs before the thirty-seventh week of gestation.

▶ **morning sickness** A persistent or recurring nausea that often occurs in the morning during early pregnancy.

▶ **low-birth-weight infant** A newborn who weighs less than 2,500 grams (5.5 pounds) as a result of either premature birth or inadequate growth in utero.

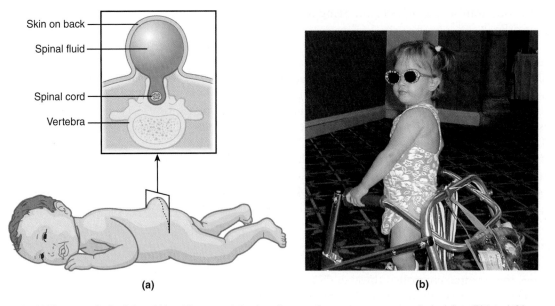

FIGURE 11.2 Spina bifida: a neural tube defect. (a) Low folate status during the early stages of pregnancy can cause neural tube defects. **(b)** Spina bifida causes varying degrees of limb paralysis. Some children will be able to walk using leg braces or crutches, whereas others will require a wheelchair.

(b) Courtesy of Spina Bifida Association of America.

TABLE 11.2
Folate in Grain Products

Foods	Folate (µg DFE)*
Ready-to-eat cereals (25% DV), 1 cup	170
Pasta, enriched, cooked, 1 cup	125–180
Rice, enriched, cooked, 1 cup	180
Tortilla, flour, enriched, 1 (10-inch diameter)	145
Bagel, enriched, 1 (3-inch diameter)	92
Bread, white, enriched, 1 slice	15–51

*DFE = Dietary Folate Equivalents

Data from U.S. Department of Agriculture, Agricultural Research Service. USDA National Nutrient Database for Standard Reference, Release 28. 2015. http://www.ars .usda.gov/ba/bhnrc/ndl. Accessed May 13, 2017.

of synthetic folic acid to reduce the risk of producing a fetal neural tube defect.[10] The CDC estimates that 50 to 70 percent of the birth defects spina bifida and anencephaly could be avoided if women consumed 400 micrograms of folic acid daily before and during pregnancy.[11]

This recommendation includes all women of childbearing age—not just pregnant women—because neural tube development occurs before the sixth week of fetal life. During this period, a woman may not know she is pregnant or may not have made appropriate dietary changes. This intake of folic acid is recommended in addition to folate (the natural form of the supplement) consumed from other foods. Folic acid is added to all enriched grain products and many ready-to-eat cereals. **TABLE 11.2** presents the folate content of selected grain products. The rate of neural tube defects has been declining in recent years, in part as a result of folic acid fortification.

Just as it is important to get enough folic acid, it is also crucial to avoid getting too much vitamin A (retinol) during pregnancy. Some vitamin A is good for you; too much can be teratogenic. A teratogen is a substance that causes birth defects—literally, the term means "monster-producing." The Institute of Medicine considered this link between excessive retinol intake and birth defects in setting the Tolerable Upper Intake Level (UL) of retinol for women of childbearing age. The UL is 3,000 micrograms (10,000 IU) of retinol from food and supplements for women older than age 18. For teens, the UL is 2,800 micrograms (9,300 IU).

Any woman who may become pregnant must avoid using drugs that contain vitamin A or vitamin A analogues; examples are the acne medications isotretinoin (Accutane) and tretinoin (Retin-A). Because these medications are potent teratogens, doctors prescribe such drugs to women of childbearing age only if tests show the woman is not pregnant and she practices two forms of birth control.

Pregnant women should eat fruits and vegetables rich in beta-carotene and other carotenoids. These foods pose no risk of birth defects and offer many health benefits.

Substance Use

Many women plan to give up cigarettes, alcohol, or other drugs if they get pregnant. But it is important to give up these substances well *before* becoming pregnant. This recommendation to plan ahead illustrates the importance of preconception guidance.[12] (See **FIGURE 11.3**.) A woman who uses tobacco, alcohol, or illicit drugs during pregnancy is more likely to have pregnancy-related complications and infant health problems.

> **Key Concepts** Ideally, the time to prepare nutritionally for pregnancy is well before conceiving. A woman who has adequate nutrient stores, particularly of folic acid, and is at a healthy weight can reduce the risk for maternal and fetal complications during pregnancy. In addition to healthful diet selections, avoiding tobacco, alcohol, and other drugs is important when contemplating pregnancy.

Physiology of Pregnancy

🍎 **Why Is This Important?** Pregnancy is an awe-inspiring interactive process of growth and development for both mother and fetus. An understanding of the stages of growth and development of the fetus, along with the physiological changes that occur in the mother during pregnancy, helps to explain the nutrient needs of a pregnant woman.

In both mother and fetus, pregnancy is a time of tremendous physiological change that demands healthful dietary and lifestyle choices. Energy and nutrient needs both increase, but the need for calories increases by a smaller percentage than the need for most vitamins and minerals. As a result, food choices during pregnancy must be nutrient dense.

What about tobacco and alcohol? Research clearly shows that both tobacco and alcohol inflict damaging effects on a developing fetus, and it's essential to abstain from both during pregnancy. Although research about the effects of caffeine is less conclusive, most healthcare professionals also recommend limiting caffeine intake during pregnancy.

Stages of Human Fetal Growth

How long does pregnancy last? Nine months, right? Well, it depends on when you start counting. When a healthcare provider gives an expectant mother a due date, it is typically calculated as 40 weeks from the start of her last menstrual period, roughly 10 to 14 days before the actual date of conception. This 40-week period is often considered as three **trimesters** of 13 or 14 weeks each; however, these time divisions do not coincide with specific stages in fetal development.

FIGURE 11.4 illustrates the early stages of pregnancy. Fertilization of the egg (ovum) sets off the **blastogenic stage**—a period of rapid cell division. As these cells divide, they begin to differentiate. The inner cells in this growing mass will form the fetus; the outer layer of cells will become the **placenta**. During this stage, which lasts about two weeks, the fertilized ovum implants itself in the wall of the mother's uterus.

The next period of pregnancy, the **embryonic stage**, extends from the end of the second week through the eighth week after conception. The placenta, a vital organ that serves as filter and conduit between mother and child, forms on the uterine wall during this stage. Attached to the placenta by the umbilical cord, the embryo now receives its nourishment from its mother; nearly everything the mother eats, drinks, or smokes is shared with the embryo.

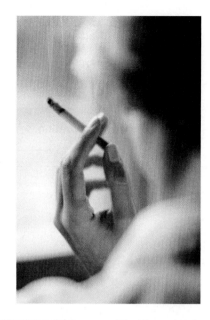

FIGURE 11.3 Substance use. Using tobacco, alcohol, or illicit drugs before and during pregnancy puts the baby at risk. If you use these substances, stop before becoming pregnant.
© Mel Curtis/Getty Images.

▶ **trimesters** Three equal time periods of pregnancy, each lasting approximately 13 to 14 weeks, that do not coincide with specific stages in fetal development.

▶ **blastogenic stage** The first stage of gestation, during which tissue proliferation by rapid cell division begins.

▶ **placenta** The organ formed in the mother's uterus during pregnancy that produces hormones to maintain the pregnancy, and across which the fetus receives oxygen and nutrients from the mother and empties its waste materials via the mother's circulatory system.

▶ **embryonic stage** The developmental stage between the time the egg implants in the uterine wall (about two weeks after fertilization) through the eighth week; the stage of major organ system differentiation and development of main external features.

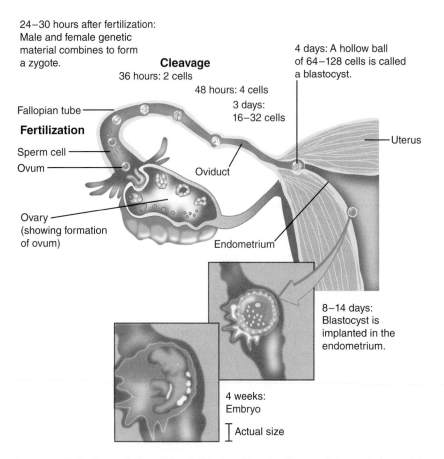

24–30 hours after fertilization:
Male and female genetic
material combines to form
a zygote.

Cleavage

36 hours: 2 cells

48 hours: 4 cells

3 days:
16–32 cells

4 days: A hollow ball
of 64–128 cells is called
a blastocyst.

Fallopian tube

Fertilization

Sperm cell

Ovum

Uterus

Oviduct

Ovary
(showing formation
of ovum)

Endometrium

8–14 days:
Blastocyst is
implanted in the
endometrium.

4 weeks:
Embryo

Actual size

FIGURE 11.4 Early stages of pregnancy. The fertilized egg divides rapidly, and cells begin to differentiate. The inner cells become the fetus, and the outer cells become the placenta.

▶ **organogenesis** The period when organ systems are developing in a growing fetus.

▶ **critical period of development** Time during which body structures are forming and environmental influences, such as drugs and infections, have the greatest impact on the developing embryo.

▶ **fetal stage** The period of rapid growth from the end of the embryonic stage, starting in the ninth week and lasting until birth.

The embryonic stage also is a period of **organogenesis**. By the time the embryo is eight weeks old, all its main internal organs have formed, along with the major external body structures. (See **FIGURE 11.5**.) Because embryonic nutrient deficiencies or excesses and intake of harmful substances during this time can result in congenital abnormalities (birth defects) or spontaneous abortion (miscarriage), this stage is a **critical period of development**.

The longest period of pregnancy is the **fetal stage**, the period from the end of the embryonic period (the ninth week) until the baby is born. During this time, the fetus is growing rapidly, with dramatic changes in body proportions. From the end of the third month of pregnancy until delivery at full term, fetal weight increases nearly 500-fold. The typical newborn is about 20 inches (50 cm) long and weighs approximately 7 pounds 7 ounces (3.4 kg).

Key Concepts From conception to full-term baby, the process of fetal development is typically described in three stages. The blastogenic stage involves rapid cell division of the fertilized ovum and its implantation in the uterine wall. During the embryonic stage, cells differentiate, and organ systems and body structures are formed. The fetal stage, the longest stage of pregnancy, is marked by growth in size and change in body proportions.

Maternal Physiological Changes and Nutrition

While the fertilized ovum is developing from a mass of dividing cells into an embryo, and then into a fetus, changes are occurring in the

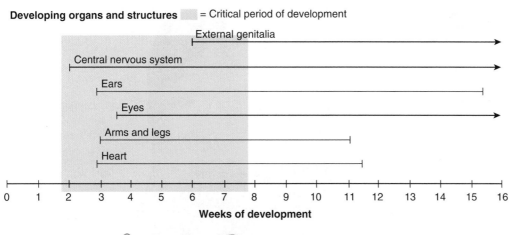

Developing organs and structures [ ] = Critical period of development

External genitalia

Central nervous system

Ears

Eyes

Arms and legs

Heart

0 1 2 3 4 5 6 7 8 9 10 11 12 13 14 15 16

Weeks of development

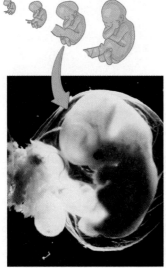

FIGURE 11.5 Embryonic development. During the embryonic stage—week 2 through week 8—all the major organ systems are forming. During this critical period of development, the embryo is highly vulnerable to nutrient deficiencies and toxicities as well as harmful substances, such as tobacco smoke.

Photo of baby in early development in uterus: © Claude Edelmann/Photo Researchers, Inc.

mother's body as well. (See **FIGURE 11.6.**) These changes occur as the result of various hormones, secreted mainly by the placenta.

Growth of Maternal Tissue

Maternal tissues, including breasts, uterus, and adipose stores, enlarge during pregnancy. Hormones promote growth and changes in the breast tissue to prepare for **lactation**. Fat stores increase to provide energy for late pregnancy and for lactation and are a major component of maternal weight gain.

Maternal Blood Volume

During the course of pregnancy, maternal blood volume expands by nearly 50 percent. Production of red blood cells also increases. Iron, folate, and vitamin B_{12} are all key nutrients in red blood cell production. Hemoglobin and hematocrit values during pregnancy are lower than when a woman is not pregnant, but this is more often the result

▶ **lactation** The process of synthesizing and secreting breast milk.

Quick Bite

Would It Be Healthier to Menstruate *Less* Often?

Women in industrialized countries, who start menstruating at an average age of 12.5 years, will generate 350 to 400 menstrual cycles in their lifetimes. In populations that do not use birth control, however, women spend the majority of their fertile years either pregnant or lactating, and therefore have fewer menstrual cycles. Menarche in these populations occurs later, at an average age of 16. In addition, because menstrual cycles do not occur during pregnancy and may not occur during lactation, women in natural-fertility populations experience only about 110 menstrual cycles in a lifetime, fewer than one-third as many cycles as women in industrialized countries. Women who produce fewer menstrual cycles are exposed to less estrogen and other steroid hormones. Researchers hypothesize that this can partly explain why nonindustrialized societies have lower cancer rates than do industrialized societies.

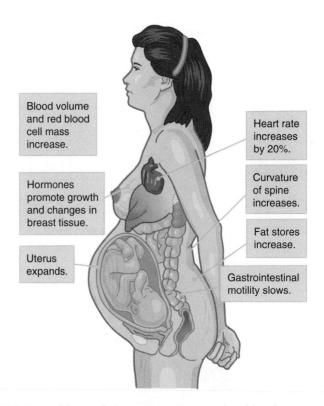

Blood volume and red blood cell mass increase.

Hormones promote growth and changes in breast tissue.

Uterus expands.

Heart rate increases by 20%.

Curvature of spine increases.

Fat stores increase.

Gastrointestinal motility slows.

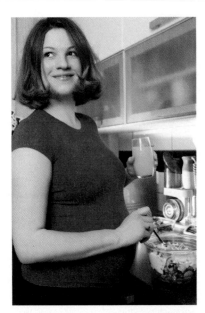

© Hemera/Thinkstock.

FIGURE 11.6 Maternal changes during pregnancy. Hormones released throughout pregnancy influence the growth of the baby and alter the way the mother's organs function.

of increased plasma volume diluting the blood cells than nutrient deficiency.

Gastrointestinal Changes

During pregnancy, gastrointestinal motility slows, and food moves more slowly through the intestinal tract. Because nutrients spend more time in the small intestine, their slower transit permits greater nutrient absorption. On the other hand, slower motility can contribute to nausea, heartburn, constipation, and hemorrhoids.

> **Key Concepts** The mother's body changes during pregnancy, responding to changing levels of hormones. Uterine, breast, and adipose tissues grow; blood volume expands; and gastrointestinal motility slows. All these changes have nutritional and dietary implications for pregnant women.

Maternal Weight Gain

How much weight should a woman gain during pregnancy? Doctors' recommendations have varied over the years from minimal weight gain to unlimited weight gain to recommendations based on prepregnancy BMI, as shown in **TABLE 11.3.** The most recent pregnancy weight gain guidelines from the Institute of Medicine and the National Research Council consider that a woman's health and that of her infant are affected by the woman's weight at the start of pregnancy as well as by how much she gains throughout the pregnancy.[13]

For underweight women with a BMI of less than 18.5 kg/m^2, the recommended weight gain is 28 to 40 pounds (12.5–18 kg). Normal-weight women with a starting BMI of 18.5 to 24.9 kg/m^2 should gain

TABLE 11.3
Guidelines for Weight Gain During Pregnancy

Prepregnancy BMI (kg/m²)	Weight Gain[a]	
	Pounds	Kilograms
Underweight (< 18.5)	28–40	12.5–18
Normal (18.5–24.9)	25–35	11.5–16
Overweight (25.0–29.9)	15–25	7.0–11.5
Obese (> 30.0)	11–20	5–9

[a] Young pregnant adolescents should strive for gains at the upper end of the recommended range. Short pregnant women (< 157 cm or 62 in.) should strive for gains at the lower end of the range.

Reprinted with permission from *Weight Gain During Pregnancy: Reexamining the Guidelines.* © 2009 by the National Academy of Sciences, Courtesy of the National Academies Press, Washington, DC.

25 to 35 pounds (11.5–16 kg). Women beginning pregnancy with an overweight BMI of 25.0 to 29.9 kg/m² are recommended to gain 15 to 25 pounds (7–11.5 kg). For the heaviest women—those with BMIs greater than 30.0 kg/m² at the start of pregnancy—a weight gain of 11 to 20 pounds (5–9 kg) is recommended. For women who are severely obese, some weight loss has been found to be reasonably safe when it results from healthy diet and lifestyle changes such as eating a balanced diet and regular moderate exercise.[14,15]

When maternal weight gain is within these limits, infants are more likely to be born normal weight and at term. These guidelines reflect the greater number of overweight and obese women currently in the United States and advise women to choose a healthy diet and exercise to achieve a normal BMI prior to getting pregnant. Although weight gain varies widely among women who give birth to healthy, full-term infants, pregnancy weight gain guidelines aim to lower risks associated with pregnancy weight change.[16]

Twin births account for 1 of every 34 live births in the United States. Of course, women who carry two or more fetuses need to gain more weight than women who carry just one. For normal-weight women, the recommended weight gain for carrying twins is 37 to 54 pounds (17–25 kg). Overweight women are recommended to gain 31 to 50 pounds (14–23 kg), and obese women should gain 25 to 42 pounds (11–19 kg).[17] There is currently not enough information to establish weight gain guidelines for underweight women with multiple fetuses. However, a higher weight gain is often recommended for women who were underweight prior to pregnancy.

The pattern of weight gain also is important to a healthy pregnancy outcome. During the first trimester, average weight gain is low, less than 5 pounds for most women. Over the second and third trimesters, the suggested weight gain for normal-weight women is a little less than 1 pound per week (0.4 kg per week), with more gain suggested for underweight women and those carrying twins and a lower gain for women who are overweight or obese.[18] Monitoring the amount and rate of weight gain is an important component of prenatal care.

The weight gained during pregnancy is divided between (1) the fetus and associated tissues and fluids and (2) maternal tissue growth. In a typical final weight gain of 27.5 pounds (12.5 kg), the fetus,

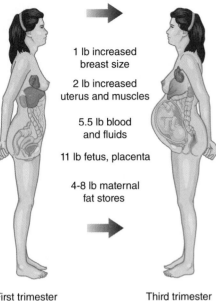

1 lb increased
breast size

2 lb increased
uterus and muscles

5.5 lb blood
and fluids

11 lb fetus, placenta

4-8 lb maternal
fat stores

First trimester   Third trimester

FIGURE 11.7 Components of maternal weight gain. During the first trimester, most women gain less than 5 pounds. Over the second and third trimesters, the suggested weight gain is a little less than 1 pound per week.

▶ **amniotic fluid** The fluid that surrounds the fetus; contained in the amniotic sac inside the uterus.

placenta, and **amniotic fluid** account for nearly 40 percent of that weight. Maternal tissues (i.e., adipose stores, breast and uterine growth, and expanded blood and extracellular fluid volumes) account for the remaining 60 percent. (See **FIGURE 11.7**.)

> **Key Concepts** Weight gained during pregnancy is a combination of increased weight in fetal and maternal tissues and fluids. Weight gain recommendations are based on BMI prior to pregnancy. Women of normal weight (BMI = 18.5–24.9 kg/m²) should gain 25 to 35 pounds over the course of pregnancy. Most of this weight gain occurs during the second and third trimesters.

Energy and Nutrition During Pregnancy

A pregnant woman requires added calories to grow and maintain not just her developing fetus, but also its support system: placenta, increased breast tissue, and fat stores. Growth and development of the fetus also require protein, vitamins, and minerals.

Energy

Resting energy expenditure (REE) increases during pregnancy because of the energy requirements of the fetus and placenta and the increased workload on the heart and lungs.[19] Energy also is needed to support weight gain, primarily in the second and third trimesters. Using median energy expenditure as a guide, pregnant women need approximately 340 extra kilocalories per day during the second trimester and an extra 450 kilocalories per day during the third trimester.[20] Because actual energy expenditure varies widely, weight gain during pregnancy is probably the best indicator of adequate calorie intake.[21]

THINK
About It

1

Nutrients to Support Pregnancy

Most healthy women who eat a well-balanced diet have no trouble meeting the majority of their nutrient requirements during pregnancy without vitamin and mineral supplements. However, despite even the best effort, many women have difficulty meeting increased recommendations during pregnancy for numerous nutrients, most often iron and folic acid. As a preventive measure, it is therefore recommended that all women planning to become pregnant take a multivitamin/mineral supplement containing folic acid.[22]

Essential nutrients can be divided into two broad categories: macronutrients (proteins, fats, and carbohydrates) and micronutrients (vitamins and minerals). **TABLE 11.4** shows the nutrient recommendations for pregnant women compared with nonpregnant women. The U.S. Department of Agriculture (USDA) Daily Food Plan for Moms is an interactive website that provides nutritional guidance to help pregnant and nursing mothers meet their individual nutritional requirements.[23]

Macronutrients

Macronutrients supply energy and provide the building blocks for protein synthesis. The recommended balance of energy sources does not change during pregnancy. A low-fat, moderate-protein, high-carbohydrate diet is still appropriate.

Protein Extra protein is needed during pregnancy for synthesizing new maternal, placental, and fetal tissues. A pregnant woman's Recommended Dietary Allowance (RDA) for protein is 1.1 grams per kilogram

TABLE 11.4

Nutritional Recommendations for Pregnancy

	Nonpregnant	Pregnant*	% Increase
Energy (kcal)	2,400	2,740/2,852	14–18
Protein (g)	46	71	54
Vitamin A (μg RAE)	700	770	10
Vitamin D (μg)	5	5	0
Vitamin E (mg)	15	15	0
Vitamin K (μg)	90	90	0
Thiamin (mg)	1.1	1.4	27
Riboflavin (mg)	1.1	1.4	27
Niacin (mg)	14	18	29
Vitamin B_6 (mg)	1.3	1.9	46
Folate (μg)	400	600	50
Vitamin B_{12} (μg)	2.4	2.6	8
Pantothenic acid (mg)	5	6	20
Biotin (μg)	30	30	0
Choline (mg)	425	450	6
Vitamin C (mg)	75	85	13
Calcium (mg)	1,000	1,000	0
Phosphorus (mg)	700	700	0
Magnesium (mg)	310	350	13
Iron (mg)	18	27	50
Zinc (mg)	8	11	38
Selenium (μg)	55	60	9
Iodine (μg)	150	220	47
Fluoride (mg)	3	3	0
Copper (μg)	900	1,000	11
Chromium (μg)	25	30	20
Manganese (mg)	1.8	2	11
Molybdenum (μg)	45	50	11
Sodium (mg)	1,500	1,500	0
Chloride (mg)	2,300	2,300	0
Potassium (mg)	4,700	4,700	0
Water (mL)	2,700	3,000	11

Needs for most nutrients increase during pregnancy. Generally, vitamin and mineral needs increase more than energy needs, which means that food choices should be nutrient dense. Values for energy are based on Estimated Energy Requirements (EERs) for a 19-year-old active woman. Values for protein, vitamins, minerals, and water are RDAs or AIs for ages 19 to 30.

*The first number for pregnancy represents the second trimester; the other number is for the third trimester.

per day (an additional 25 grams per day over nonpregnant needs). This amount of protein is easily supplied in typical American diets consumed by nonpregnant women. Thus, many women need not increase their protein intake to reach the levels recommended for pregnancy. Pregnant women who are vegetarians, including vegans, also should be able to meet their protein needs from food sources alone—as long as they select a variety of protein sources and consume enough total calories. (See the FYI feature "Vegetarianism and Pregnancy.")

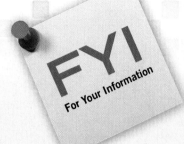

Vegetarianism and Pregnancy

Can pregnant women meet all their nutritional needs on a vegetarian diet? A fair question. Common vegetarian practices exclude meat, poultry, and fish to some degree (lacto-ovo-vegetarians eat milk and eggs, and vegans avoid all animal foods). These foods are important sources of iron, zinc, calcium, vitamin B$_{12}$, and other nutrients. Although vegetarian diets can provide reasonable quantities of trace elements, animal-derived foods frequently contribute larger amounts that the body absorbs more easily. To meet the demands of pregnancy, fortified foods as well as vitamin and mineral supplements may be in order.

Supplemental iron is generally recommended for all pregnant women. Supplemental vitamin B$_{12}$ (2.0 micrograms per day) is also recommended for vegan mothers. If the mother's sun exposure is limited, she also may need a daily supplement of 10 micrograms of vitamin D.[a] Vegetarians with low calcium intake (< 600 milligrams per day) should consume a supplement that provides at least 500 milligrams per day. Some vegan foods, such as fortified soy milks, may contain these important nutrients. It is a good idea to check the label to be sure.

The overall nutrient content of a vegetarian diet depends on both the energy content and the variety of the foods consumed. The sample meal plan in **TABLE A** provides an example of a vegan diet for pregnant women.

Institute of Medicine, Food and Nutrition Board. *Dietary Reference Intakes for Calcium and Vitamin D*. Washington, DC: National Academies Press; 2011.

TABLE A
Sample Meal Plan for a Vegan Pregnancy

Breakfast
1/2 cup oatmeal with maple syrup
1 slice whole wheat toast with
Fruit spread
1 cup fortified soy milk
1/2 cup calcium-fortified orange juice
Morning Snack
1/2 whole-wheat bagel with
Margarine
1 banana
Lunch
Veggie burger on whole-wheat bun with
Mustard
Ketchup
1 cup steamed collard greens
Medium apple
1 cup fortified soy milk
Afternoon Snack
3/4 cup ready-to-eat cereal with
1 cup blueberries
1 cup fortified soy milk
Dinner
3/4 cup tofu stir-fried with
1 cup vegetables
1 cup brown rice
1 medium orange
Evening Snack
Whole-grain crackers with
2 tablespoons peanut butter
4 oz apple juice

Fats   Dietary fats provide vital fuel for the mother and for the development of placental tissues. Needs for essential fatty acids during pregnancy are slightly higher than those of nonpregnant women.[24] The pregnant woman's body also stores fats to support breastfeeding after childbirth. Very-low-fat diets (in which less than 10 percent of daily calories comes from dietary fats) are not recommended for pregnancy. Such diets are unlikely to supply sufficient amounts of essential fatty acids, fat-soluble vitamins, or calories.

Carbohydrate   Carbohydrates provide the main source of extra calories during pregnancy. Food choices should emphasize complex carbohydrates such as whole-grain breads, and fortified cereals, rice, and pasta. In addition to supplying vitamins and minerals, these foods can increase fiber intake substantially. A fiber-rich diet is recommended during pregnancy to help prevent constipation and hemorrhoids. The Adequate Intake (AI) for fiber increases from 25 to 28 grams per day during pregnancy.

Key Concepts   Most healthy women with well-balanced diets meet the majority of their nutrient requirements during pregnancy. The actual increase in energy needs varies substantially among women. The adequacy of energy intake can be measured by the amount of weight gained. Weight loss is not advised during pregnancy, even for obese women. As long as energy intake is adequate and a variety of foods is eaten, protein intake should be more than adequate to support prenatal growth and development.

Micronutrients

A pregnant woman has an increased need for many vitamins and minerals that support fetal growth and development. In addition, her increased energy needs mean she requires greater amounts of nutrients such as the B vitamins thiamin, riboflavin, niacin, and pantothenic acid, which are essential for energy metabolism.

Needs for the other B vitamins (except biotin) also increase. Folate and vitamin B_{12} are used to synthesize DNA and red blood cells, and vitamin B_6 is crucial for metabolizing amino acids. Of these vitamins, folate needs increase most, from 400 to 600 micrograms per day during pregnancy. Vitamin C needs increase slightly during pregnancy, from 75 to 85 milligrams per day for women ages 19 to 50 years. For the fat-soluble vitamins, the RDA for vitamin A increases slightly during pregnancy, whereas recommended intake levels for vitamins D, E, and K are unchanged.

For most minerals, recommended intakes are higher during pregnancy—most dramatically for iron. The RDA for iron increases from 18 milligrams per day to 27 milligrams per day. Iron is necessary to make red blood cells and is important for normal growth and energy metabolism. Iron deficiency and its associated anemia is the most common nutrient deficiency in pregnancy. **TABLE 11.5** lists the characteristics of women who are at particularly high risk for iron deficiency.

Because getting 27 milligrams of iron in the daily diet is not easy, experts recommend iron supplementation for the general population of pregnant women.[25] A woman can maximize absorption of an iron supplement by eating it on an empty stomach (between meals or at bedtime) and washing it down with liquids other than milk, tea, or coffee, which inhibit absorption.

Key Concepts   Needs for vitamins and minerals increase during pregnancy, some more than others. Extra vitamins and minerals are needed to support growth and development as well as increased energy use. Recommended intake levels increase most dramatically for folate and iron.

TABLE 11.5
Factors Associated with Increased Risk for Iron Deficiency During Pregnancy

- Young age (e.g., 15 to 19 years)
- Multiple sequential pregnancies
- Twin or triplet pregnancy
- Diet low in meat
- Diet high in coffee and tea
- Low socioeconomic status
- Low level of education
- Black or Hispanic ethnicity
- Previous diagnosis of iron deficiency or iron-deficiency anemia

Food Choices for Pregnant Women

You may be surprised to learn that the recommended diet for a pregnant woman is not much different from that for adults in the general population. Variety is the key to a well-balanced diet. The extra calories needed for pregnancy are easy to obtain from an additional serving from each of the following food groups: grains, vegetables, fruits, and low-fat milk. Because the increased need for energy is proportionately less than the increased need for most nutrients, nutrient-dense foods are important. There is little room in the diet plan for high-calorie, high-fat, low-nutrient "extras."

Supplementation

Other than iron and folate, a pregnant woman can usually get all the nutrients she needs by making healthful choices, guided by the food intake patterns of MyPlate. Healthcare providers often evaluate the dietary intake of all prenatal patients and recommend dietary changes to improve nutrition where needed. However, to reduce preventable complications of nutrient deficiencies, pregnant women in the United States and Canada routinely receive prescriptions for prenatal vitamin/mineral supplements. The amount and balance of nutrients in prenatal formulations is appropriate for pregnancy. Because toxic levels can be reached quickly, especially for vitamins A and D, pregnant women should avoid high doses and multiple supplements. In addition, because most herbal preparations have not been evaluated for safety during pregnancy, they are not recommended.

Foods to Avoid

Alcohol is completely off-limits to pregnant women. And if a mother-to-be is experiencing problems with nausea and vomiting, she may want to abstain for a while from foods that aggravate these symptoms. Cultural traditions can dictate changes in diet during pregnancy, but these tend to reflect traditional beliefs and practices rather than health science.

The *2020 Dietary Guidelines for Americans* advised that women who are pregnant or breastfeeding consume 8 to 12 ounces of a variety of seafood types weekly; however, because of high mercury content, it advised limiting albacore tuna to 6 ounces per week and suggested avoiding tilefish, shark, swordfish, and king mackerel.[26] In addition, the Food and Drug Administration (FDA) and the Environmental Protection Agency (EPA) advise that women who may become pregnant, pregnant women, lactating mothers, and young children check local advisories about the safety of fish caught by family and friends in local lakes, rivers, and coastal areas.[27] (See **FIGURE 11.8**.)

The question of whether to reduce or eliminate caffeine intake during pregnancy continues to be debated. High caffeine intake has been linked to delayed conception, spontaneous miscarriage, and low birth weight.[28,29] However, caffeine intake during pregnancy does not appear to be associated with birth defects[30] or preterm birth.[31] The Academy of Nutrition and Dietetics recommends that pregnant women consume less than 300 milligrams of caffeine per day.[32] **TABLE 11.6** shows the caffeine content of common beverages and foods.

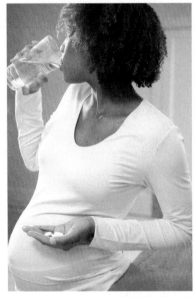

© Brand X Pictures/Thinkstock.

Key Concepts With the exception of iron and folate, a well-balanced, varied diet can often meet all of a pregnant woman's nutrient needs. Pregnant women should choose nutrient-dense and high-carbohydrate foods in the proportions found in MyPlate. Although vitamin/mineral supplementation is common during pregnancy, it probably is not needed other than for iron and folate. When supplements are used, they should be designed for pregnant women. Pregnant women should avoid alcohol and moderate their intake of caffeine.

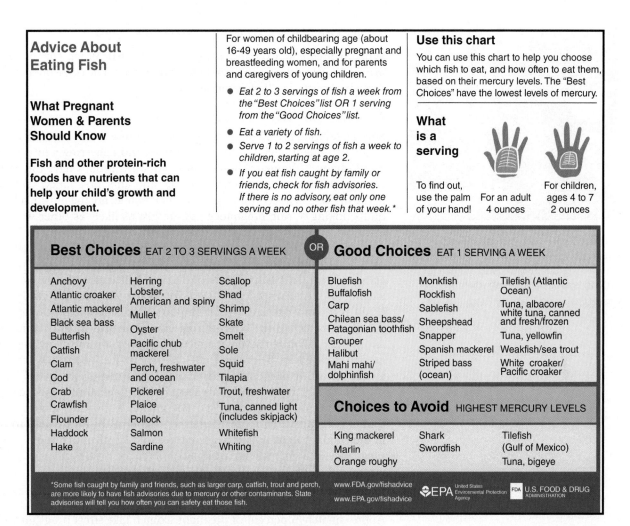

FIGURE 11.8 Choose healthy and safe fish options. Women who are pregnant or may become pregnant, breastfeeding mothers, and parents of young children should make informed choices and select fish that are healthy and safe to eat.

US Department of Health and Human Services U.S. Food and Drug Administration. Eating Fish: What Pregnant Women and Parents Should Know. http://www.fda.gov/Food/FoodborneIllnessContaminants/Metals/ucm393070.htm Page updated 1/18/17. Accessed January 24, 2017.

TABLE 11.6
Caffeine Content of Common Beverages and Foods

Food	Serving Size	Caffeine (mg)
Coffee, regular, brewed	8 fl. oz.	130
Coffee, Starbucks, brewed	8 fl. oz.	160
Espresso, regular	1 fl. oz.	40
Espresso, Starbucks	1 fl. oz.	75
Frappuccino beverage, Starbucks	9.5 fl. oz.	115
Tea, regular, brewed	8 fl. oz.	50
Tea, fruited, Snapple	8 fl. oz.	20
Tea, latte, Starbucks Tazo Chai	8 fl. oz.	50
Vault	12 fl. oz.	70
Mountain Dew	12 fl. oz.	55
Coca-Cola/Pepsi, regular, flavored, diet	12 fl. oz.	35–45
Sprite/7-Up	12 fl. oz.	0
Red Bull	8.3 fl. oz.	80
Ice cream, coffee	8 fl. oz.	50–80
Milk chocolate, Hershey's	1.55 oz.	10
Dark chocolate, Hershey's	1.45 oz.	20

Modified from Center for Science in the Public Interest. Caffeine content of food and drugs. http://www.cspinet.org/new/cafchart.htm. Accessed May 13, 2017.

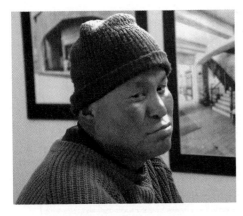

FIGURE 11.9 Fetal alcohol syndrome. The facial characteristics of a person with fetal alcohol syndrome include a short nose with a flattened bridge, eyelids with extra folds, and a thin upper lip with no groove below the nose.

© Richard Pipes, Albuquerque Journal/AP Photos.

Substance Use and Pregnancy Outcome

When a pregnant woman eats, she eats for two. When she smokes, drinks, or uses drugs, she does so for two as well. The consequences of these behaviors can be felt for generations.

Tobacco and Alcohol

Smoking during pregnancy increases the risks of miscarrying, delivering a stillborn infant, giving birth prematurely, and delivering a low-birth-weight baby.[33] Women in lower socioeconomic groups have the highest rates of cigarette use before, during, and after pregnancy. Women in the highest socioeconomic groups, meanwhile, are the most likely to quit smoking during pregnancy but are just as likely as other women to take up the habit again after giving birth.

All women of childbearing age should be aware of alcohol's effects on a developing fetus. Exposure to alcohol can lead to a range of physical, cognitive, and behavioral conditions collectively known as fetal alcohol spectrum disorders (FASD), of which fetal alcohol syndrome (FAS) is the most severe.[34] Most importantly, alcohol exposure affects the development of the brain during critical periods of differentiation and growth. Children severely afflicted by the syndrome show marked growth deficiencies before and after birth; physical anomalies such as a small head, certain characteristic facial deformities (see **FIGURE 11.9**), heart defects, and joint and limb irregularities; mental retardation; and central nervous system disorders. The greater a mother's alcohol use during pregnancy, the more severe the symptoms of FASD tend to be in the child. There is no known safe threshold for alcohol use in pregnancy. The only way to avoid alcohol-related risks to a fetus is to avoid all alcohol during pregnancy.

THINK
About It

2

Drugs

Approximately 5 percent of pregnant women take street drugs, including cocaine, ecstasy, heroin, or marijuana, or abuse prescription drug such as narcotics.[35]

Marijuana use increases the risk for premature delivery and low birth weight. In addition, maternal marijuana use can result in some of the same physical abnormalities seen in infants with FAS. Effects on the fetus vary depending on the mother's diet, frequency of marijuana use, and the use of other drugs. Marijuana also reduces fertility in both women and men.

Cocaine use increases risks of stroke, prematurity, fetal growth retardation, miscarriage, and certain birth defects. Some of these problems could stem from nutritional deficiencies in the mother both before and during pregnancy, as well as from concurrent tobacco and alcohol use, which is common among cocaine users. **FIGURE 11.10** illustrates the possible effects of drug, alcohol, or tobacco use on a pregnant woman.

> **Key Concepts** Smoking, alcohol, and illicit drug use during pregnancy can all have devastating effects on fetal development. Low birth weight, preterm delivery, and birth defects are some of the consequences. Fetal alcohol syndrome is a specific set of physical, mental, and behavioral defects caused by maternal alcohol consumption during pregnancy. A pregnant woman should avoid all these substances.

Special Situations During Pregnancy

Some women progress through pregnancy with no more than a mild period of morning sickness or problems with constipation or heartburn. However, even these conditions, as well as complications such as abnormal glucose tolerance or elevated blood pressure, can affect dietary choices and nutritional status. In addition, some women have unique nutritional needs during pregnancy.

Gastrointestinal Distress

Morning sickness, or nausea associated with pregnancy, is most common early in pregnancy as the mother's body adjusts to changes in hormone levels. Many pregnant women find they experience less morning sickness if they eat dry cereal, toast, or crackers about half an hour before getting out of bed (see **FIGURE 11.11**). Keeping some food in the stomach throughout the day helps, too. This means eating smaller, more frequent meals and drinking liquids between meals instead of with food. Avoiding food aromas that trigger nausea is another useful tactic.

Heartburn and constipation are the result of slowed gastrointestinal (GI) movement. Remaining upright for at least an hour after eating and having smaller, more frequent meals can prevent heartburn. Getting plenty of fiber and fluids in the diet and getting regular mild to moderate exercise can limit constipation. Of course, a pregnant woman should always consult her healthcare provider before using a prescription drug, over-the-counter medicine, herbal supplement, or home remedy for nausea, vomiting, heartburn, or constipation.

Food Cravings and Aversions

Many pregnant women experience specific food cravings and/or aversions, and we often laugh at stories about unusual combinations such as pickles and ice cream. These changes in food preferences can be linked to taste and metabolic changes, but they rarely are based on a nutrient deficiency or other physiological conditions. Most cravings and aversions do not affect the quality of the diet unless food choices become very narrow.

Some pregnant women crave nonfood items such as starch or clay. The term *pica* describes routine consumption of nonfood items such as dirt, clay, laundry starch, ice, or burnt matches. Although this behavior may seem outlandish, in many cases it is a culturally accepted practice that affects significant numbers of pregnant women worldwide.[36] Pica can be harmful if nonfood items crowd nutritious foods out of the diet. In addition, nonfood items can contain toxins, bacteria, and parasites; and in the case of laundry starch, a significant number of calories can be consumed without providing any vitamins or minerals.

Hypertension

Measurement of maternal blood pressure is a routine part of prenatal care. When not accompanied by other symptoms, increased blood pressure during pregnancy is usually temporary and carries little risk.

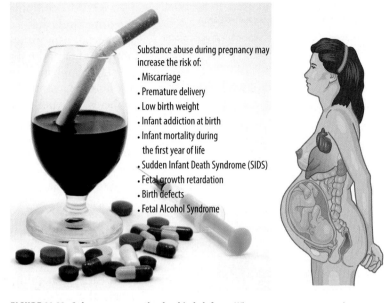

Substance abuse during pregnancy may increase the risk of:
- Miscarriage
- Premature delivery
- Low birth weight
- Infant addiction at birth
- Infant mortality during the first year of life
- Sudden Infant Death Syndrome (SIDS)
- Fetal growth retardation
- Birth defects
- Fetal Alcohol Syndrome

FIGURE 11.10 Substance use can lead to birth defects. When a pregnant woman smokes, drinks, or uses drugs, so does her growing baby. The consequences of these behaviors can be felt for generations.

Photo showing alcohol, tobacco, and prescription pills: ©iStockphoto/Thinkstock.

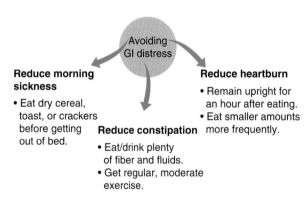

Avoiding GI distress

Reduce morning sickness
- Eat dry cereal, toast, or crackers before getting out of bed.

Reduce heartburn
- Remain upright for an hour after eating.
- Eat smaller amounts more frequently.

Reduce constipation
- Eat/drink plenty of fiber and fluids.
- Get regular, moderate exercise.

FIGURE 11.11 Strategies for avoiding GI distress. During pregnancy, most women experience GI distress as morning sickness, constipation, or heartburn.

▶ **preeclampsia** A condition of late pregnancy characterized by maternal hypertension, edema, and proteinuria.

▶ **eclampsia** The occurrence of seizures in a pregnant woman that are unrelated to brain conditions.

However, the combination of hypertension and proteinuria (protein in the urine) indicates a serious medical condition called **preeclampsia**. If preeclampsia progresses to **eclampsia**, it can threaten the lives of both mother and baby.

Preeclampsia is more common in first pregnancies, as well as in adolescents, women older than 35 years, and women with preexisting diabetes or hypertension. In mild cases, bed rest and close monitoring are the treatments of choice. Sodium restriction and drug therapy are not recommended. Ensuring adequate intake of zinc may help early detection of gestational hypertension. Early identification of preeclampsia through routine prenatal care is important for good maternal and fetal outcomes.

Diabetes

A woman with diabetes faces special challenges in pregnancy. She has an increased risk of developing preeclampsia and a greater-than-average chance of problems that affect the fetus, including fetal death. However, with early prenatal intervention and careful control of blood glucose levels, these risks can be reduced to the same level as in nondiabetic pregnancies.[37]

Pregnancy can require frequent adjustments of both diet and insulin to keep blood glucose in check. Insulin requirements often decrease during the first half of pregnancy but increase during the second half. Women who did not need insulin before they became pregnant and were able to control their blood glucose through diet alone may begin to need insulin during their pregnancy.

TABLE 11.7

Factors Associated with Risk for Gestational Diabetes

- Being older than 25 years
- Obesity, at any age
- Family history of diabetes mellitus
- Previous poor pregnancy outcome
- History of abnormal glucose tolerance
- Ethnicity associated with high incidence of diabetes

Gestational Diabetes

Gestational diabetes is a condition in which abnormal glucose tolerance exists only during pregnancy and resolves after delivery. The hormones of pregnancy tend to counteract insulin, and in about 4 percent of pregnancies, this results in a rise in blood glucose. **TABLE 11.7** lists factors associated with an increased risk of gestational diabetes. Gestational diabetes often can be controlled through diet, although some cases require insulin therapy.

HIV/AIDS

Women with the human immunodeficiency virus (HIV) can potentially pass the virus to their children during pregnancy, delivery, or breastfeeding. Medical treatments used routinely in the United States and other developed countries reduce the risk of transmission during pregnancy and delivery in the approximately 6,000 HIV-infected women who give birth each year.[38] More than 90 percent of all cases of childhood HIV infection are attributable to mother-to-child transmission of HIV, especially in countries where effective HIV/AIDS drugs are not available.[39] In developing countries where treatments are not available, women with HIV or acquired immune deficiency syndrome (AIDS) are likely to have multiple nutrition problems, including protein-energy malnutrition, vitamin and mineral deficiencies, and inadequate weight gain, all of which pose risks to the fetus.

Adolescence

Despite prevention efforts, about 229,715 infants were born to teenagers in 2015; the majority of these pregnancies were unintended.[40] Pregnant adolescents are nutritionally at risk. Their own needs for growth

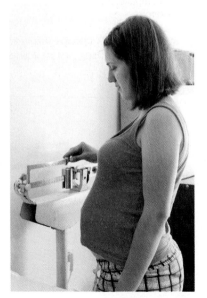

© Iakov Filimonov/Shutterstock, Inc.

LACTATION   601

and development are compromised by the extra demands posed by the growth and development of the fetus. Risks for preeclampsia, anemia, premature birth, low-birth-weight babies, infant mortality, and sexually transmitted diseases are all increased for pregnant adolescents under the age of 16.[41]

Even before becoming pregnant, many teenagers do not demonstrate healthful eating patterns. Their diets are likely to be inadequate in total calories, calcium, iron, zinc, riboflavin, folic acid, and vitamins A, D, and B_6. Poverty, smoking, and abuse of alcohol and other substances compound the negative effects of adolescent nutritional inadequacies.

Nutrition care for pregnant teens starts with determining daily energy needs. The Institute of Medicine recommends that pregnant adolescents be encouraged to strive for weight gains toward the upper end of the range recommended for adult mothers. (See Table 11.3.) The need for supplemental vitamins and minerals is also greater in this age group.

Key Concepts Numerous factors affect the dietary needs and choices of pregnant women. Routine prenatal care is important to identify unhealthful eating behaviors and potential complications such as preeclampsia and gestational diabetes. Pregnant women with diabetes or HIV/AIDS need special dietary intervention. Pregnant teens have especially high nutrient needs to support not only fetal growth, but also their own adolescent growth.

Lactation

🍎 **Why Is This Important?** Knowing about the physiology of lactation and the nutritional qualities of breast milk will help you understand the importance and significance of breastfeeding.

During pregnancy, physiological changes in breast tissue and fat stores prepare the woman's body for the demands of lactation. Preparation for lactation also involves education. Although breastfeeding is a natural function of a woman's body, knowledge about lactation can make breastfeeding a success for both mother and infant.

Breastfeeding Trends

Public health goals since the late 1970s have sought to increase the percentage of infants who are breastfed. The goal of Healthy People 2020 is to increase the proportion of newborns who are initially breastfed to almost 82 percent.[42] Efforts to promote breastfeeding have been successful; 74 percent of infants are now breastfed initially.[43] However, only 44 percent of infants are still being breastfed at 6 months of age.[44] What are the reasons for this trend? Lack of knowledge about the benefits of breastfeeding for both mother and baby surely plays a role. Societal attitudes regarding the acceptability of breastfeeding also are influential and vary across cultural and demographic groups. Some states have actually had to pass laws stating that breastfeeding in public is not indecent exposure. In addition, the decline in breastfeeding through the 1950s and 1960s affected the attitudes and knowledge base of today's grandmothers.

Parents should make decisions about feeding their infants based on accurate information: providing information about the mechanics of breastfeeding as well as the benefits for both mother and baby should therefore be an integral part of prenatal care.

Position Statement: Academy of Nutrition and Dietetics

Promoting and Supporting Breastfeeding
It is the position of the Academy of Nutrition and Dietetics that exclusive breastfeeding provides optimal nutrition and health protection for the first 6 months of life and that breastfeeding with complementary foods from 6 months until at least 12 months of age is the ideal feeding pattern for infants. Breastfeeding is an important public health strategy for improving infant and child morbidity and mortality, improving maternal morbidity, and helping to control health care costs.

Reprinted from *Journal of the American Dietetic Association*, 105(5), Position of the American Dietetic Association: Promoting and Supporting Breastfeeding, Page no. 810-818, 2005, with permission from Elsevier.

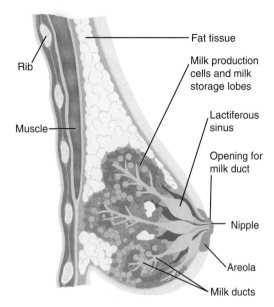

FIGURE 11.12 Anatomy of the breast. During pregnancy, breasts increase in size and undergo internal development. By the start of the third trimester, breasts are capable of producing milk.

▶ **colostrum** A precursor of breast milk; a thick, yellow fluid rich in immune factors and secreted during pregnancy and the first days after delivery.

▶ **prolactin** A pituitary hormone that stimulates the production of milk in breast tissue.

▶ **oxytocin** A pituitary hormone that stimulates the release of milk from the breast.

▶ **let-down reflex** The release of milk from the breast tissue in response to the stimulus of the hormone oxytocin. The major stimulus for oxytocin release is the infant suckling at the breast.

Quick Bite

Breastfeeding and Birth Control

Does breastfeeding prevent pregnancy? No. But under certain conditions, breastfeeding can dramatically reduce the chances of becoming pregnant. During the first six months after giving birth, a woman who has not yet had a period and fully breastfeeds her baby (no other liquids or solids) has less than a 2 percent chance of pregnancy. Still, it's important to use a reliable method of birth control while breastfeeding.

Physiology of Lactation

Although a significant number of women face social and physiological challenges, almost every woman who wants to breast-feed her newborn can do so. Only a small percentage of women are completely unable to lactate. The size and shape of the breast have no impact on the lactation process. **FIGURE 11.12** shows the anatomy of a normal breast.[45]

Changes During Adolescence and Pregnancy

Although mammary tissue is present in newborns, that tissue does not grow and develop until the onset of puberty. Throughout adolescence, the amount of breast tissue grows and the mammary glands and ducts develop. An adolescent who becomes pregnant shortly after her first period or a woman who has had only irregular periods prior to becoming pregnant may have underdeveloped mammary glands and insufficient breast tissue to support lactation. However, most teen mothers have no difficulty breastfeeding their babies.

During pregnancy, breast tissue changes so that milk production is possible. Not only does the breast change in size, but the structure of the glands and ducts also become more intricate, and secretory cells form. Mammary tissue is mature and capable of producing milk by the start of the third trimester.

After Delivery

Although birth triggers a rapid increase in a mother's milk production and secretion, full lactation does not begin as soon as the baby is born. An efficient way to establish lactation is to put the newborn to the breast as soon after delivery as possible. During the first two or three days after birth, a nursing infant receives **colostrum**, an immature milk that is quite high in protein and immunoglobulins (immunoprotective factors). If the newborn is fed regularly at the breast, lactation will be firmly established within two to three weeks after birth, and mature milk will be produced.

Hormonal Controls

Several hormones control the maturation of breast tissue and the production and release of breast milk (see **FIGURE 11.13**). During lactation, the pituitary gland produces two important hormones—**prolactin** and **oxytocin**. The infant suckling at the breast stimulates the release of prolactin from the mother's pituitary gland. In turn, prolactin stimulates the production of milk in the breast tissue. Giving water or infant formula to the baby reduces the time spent nursing at the breast, and milk production declines.

The second hormone, oxytocin, allows milk to be released from the mammary glands to the nipple and therefore to the hungry infant. It would be inconvenient and messy if milk were released from the breast as soon as it was produced! So, the infant suckling at the breast signals the pituitary gland to release oxytocin, which in turn stimulates the release of milk. This process, often called the **let-down reflex**, may be accompanied by a tingling or burning sensation in the breast that lets the mother know the infant is receiving milk. Let-down can be inhibited by anxiety, stress, and fatigue. It can be stimulated by thoughts of the baby or hearing the baby cry.

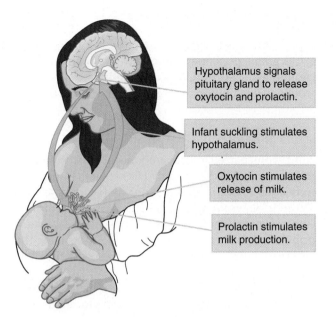

Hypothalamus signals pituitary gland to release oxytocin and prolactin.

Infant suckling stimulates hypothalamus.

Oxytocin stimulates release of milk.

Prolactin stimulates milk production.

FIGURE 11.13 Hormonal control of lactation. When an infant nurses, the infant's suckling stimulates the nipple, which sends nerve signals to the hypothalamus. In turn, the hypothalamus signals the pituitary gland to release hormones that stimulate milk production and release.

Key Concepts Increasing the proportion of infants who are breastfed is an important public health goal. Prenatal care should include information about the physiology of lactation and its benefits for mother and baby. Changes in breast tissue that allow lactation culminate at delivery. Breast milk composition changes in the two or three weeks following the infant's birth. The first milk, colostrum, is high in protein and immune factors. Key hormones that regulate milk production and release are prolactin and oxytocin.

Nutrition for Breastfeeding Women

To provide adequate nutrition for her baby while protecting her own nutritional status, a breastfeeding mother must choose a varied, healthful, nutrient-dense diet. Dietary inadequacies will lead to mobilization of stored maternal nutrients in an effort to produce nutritionally complete breast milk. For example, insufficient dietary calcium could hurt the mother's bone health, as her body frees up stored calcium in her bones for breast milk. A breastfeeding mother's needs for energy and most nutrients are higher or the same as for pregnancy.

Energy

The energy needed to support milk production is obtained in part by mobilization of fat stores, with the remaining kilocalories provided by the diet. On average, well-nourished breastfeeding women lose weight slowly, about 0.8 kilograms (approximately 1¾ pounds) per month, with weight stabilizing after about six months. Based on this rate of weight loss, a breastfeeding woman needs an extra intake of about 330 kilocalories per day during the first six months of lactation and about 400 extra kilocalories daily during the second six months.[46] However, this may be an overestimation of actual needs for many women, especially those who are sedentary. To ensure adequate milk production and avoid nutrient deficiencies, a nursing mother should consume at least 1,800 kilocalories per day.

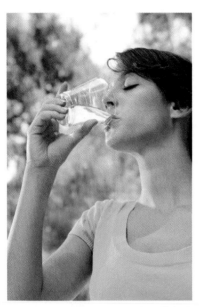

© iStockphoto/Thinkstock.

▶ **colic** Periodic inconsolable crying in an apparently healthy infant that appears to result from abdominal cramping and discomfort.

Protein

Adequate protein intake is very important while nursing. The RDA for protein is 1.3 grams per kilogram per day, or an additional 25 grams over the nonpregnant RDA. Unless calorie intake is very low, lack of dietary protein is uncommon among women in the United States and Canada.

Vitamins and Minerals

Breastfeeding women need greater amounts of most vitamins than they do during pregnancy. Exceptions include vitamins D and K, for which the recommended intake is the same during lactation and pregnancy, and niacin and folate, for which the RDA is lower during lactation than during pregnancy (although still higher than for women in the general population). When vitamin intake is inadequate, the vitamin content of breast milk can diminish, and that puts the infant at risk for deficiency.

For minerals, current RDA and AI values suggest increased needs during lactation (as compared with pregnancy) for all minerals except sodium, chloride, calcium, phosphorus, magnesium, fluoride, and molybdenum. Iron needs decrease below nonpregnant values because iron losses from menstruation often do not occur during the early months of exclusive breastfeeding. Maternal intake of minerals has less influence on levels in breast milk than is true for vitamins.

Water

Breastfeeding women require plenty of fluids. A nursing mother should drink about 2 liters (about 8 cups) of water per day and at least 1 cup of water each time she breastfeeds her baby. The AI for total water (beverages plus foods) is 3.8 liters per day. Coffee and other caffeinated beverages are acceptable if limited to 1 to 2 cups per day—and if they do not replace other fluids. Because caffeine passes into the breast milk, caffeine can make some breastfed infants wakeful and jittery.

Food Choices

Choosing a variety of foods from MyPlate for Pregnancy and Breastfeeding is the best way to meet the nutritional demands of lactation. Following the food intake patterns of MyPlate for Pregnancy and Breastfeeding, diets of 2,000 to 2,800 kilocalories per day can easily meet most nutrient needs.

Nursing mothers should eat plenty of vegetables, a source of many essential micronutrients. Although vegetables in the cabbage family, including broccoli, cauliflower, kale, and Brussels sprouts, have long been considered causes of **colic** symptoms in breastfed infants, their bad reputation may be unwarranted. Scientific evidence that these vegetables cause distress for infants remains weak. Removal of numerous foods from the diet should be done only under the supervision of a registered dietitian.

Supplementation

Some breastfeeding women need routine vitamin/mineral supplementation.[47] This group would include, for example, those women who do not follow dietary guidelines and vegan women, who avoid all animal products. Vitamin B_{12} is likely to be too low in the milk of nursing vegans, and they should take a B_{12} supplement.[48] For breastfeeding women who do not get regular sun exposure and do not drink milk or other fortified products, a vitamin D supplement can be warranted.[49] For most nursing mothers, though, dietary counseling to improve food choices is the preferred way to address nutrient imbalances.

> **Key Concepts** Energy and nutrient needs are usually even higher during lactation than during pregnancy. Intake recommendations suggest an additional 330 to 400 kilocalories and 25 extra grams of protein each day above nonpregnant needs. Low vitamin intake affects the nutritional quality of breast milk. Recommended intake levels for minerals are generally higher during lactation than during pregnancy. Fluids are also important for adequate milk production. Food choices during lactation should follow MyPlate for Pregnancy and Breastfeeding and emphasize nutrient-dense foods. With good choices and adequate calories, a lactating woman may not need vitamin and mineral supplements.

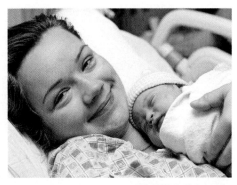

Practices to Avoid During Lactation

When a nursing mother smokes or uses alcohol or other drugs, these substances wind up in her breast milk. Women who smoke are encouraged to quit. However, breast milk remains the ideal food for their infants.[50] It is a myth that drinking alcohol enhances the letdown reflex, making it easier to nurse. Rather, alcohol inhibits the milk-ejection reflex so that the baby gets less milk, and milk more concentrated with alcohol. An occasional drink may not be harmful, but breastfeeding should be avoided for two hours after drinking alcohol.[51] Drugs also show up in breast milk and can be transferred to the infant. If a new mother cannot abstain from using illicit drugs, she should not breastfeed.

Benefits of Breastfeeding

THINK
About It

3

Breast milk is the optimal food for the health, growth, and development of infants. Both infants and mothers benefit from breastfeeding: breastfed infants have lower rates of childhood obesity and higher protection from infections and illnesses such as diarrhea; mothers have reduced risk of breast and ovarian cancers.[52] It is estimated that $13 billion in U.S. healthcare costs could be saved annually if 90 percent of babies were breastfed exclusively for six months.[53]

Benefits for Infants

Human milk provides optimal nutrition for babies, as you will see in the section "Energy and Nutrient Needs During Infancy." Breast milk provides more than nutrients, however, and the health-promoting factors in breast milk are difficult, if not impossible, to replicate in infant formula.

Breast milk has been shown to protect infants from infections and illnesses, including diarrhea, ear infections, pneumonia, and asthma,[54] leading to fewer healthcare visits, less prescription medication use, and fewer hospitalizations and resulting in decreased healthcare costs.[55] Breastfeeding also reduces an infant's risk of sudden infant death syndrome (SIDS).[56] In addition, a baby's risk of obesity declines with each month of breastfeeding.[57] Babies who are breastfed for at least six months are less likely to develop obesity, and breastfeeding for nine months reduces a baby's chance of being overweight by more than 30 percent.[58] Evidence suggests that these effects occur in a dose–response relationship, with the best outcomes for infants who are exclusively breastfed for at least six months.[59] Prolonged and exclusive breastfeeding also improves children's cognitive development.[60]

What makes human milk so important for infant health? Colostrum contains substantial amounts of antibodies, including immunoglobulin A (IgA), the first line of defense against most infectious agents.[61] Breastfeeding also appears to stimulate development of the infant's own immune system.[62]

Breastfeeding promotes a close bond between mother and infant that can be important to normal psychological development. It is important for mothers (and fathers) who bottle-feed to promote the same type of closeness while feeding.

As long as mother and baby are in relatively close proximity, breast milk is always ready when the baby is ready to eat. There's nothing to prepare, mix, or heat; and for a hungry infant who doesn't want to wait, that's an important advantage! Breast milk is always the perfect temperature and is sterile. In addition, links between breastfeeding and reduced risk of disorders such as type 1 diabetes, cardiovascular diseases, childhood obesity, and Crohn's disease have been suggested, although these links need further study. **TABLE 11.8** lists some possible protective benefits of human milk.

Benefits for Mother

Following childbirth, breastfeeding stimulates uterine contractions, which help the uterus return to its normal size. If the baby is put to the breast immediately after delivery, these same contractions (an effect of oxytocin)

TABLE 11.8
Potential Benefits of Breastfeeding for Infants and Mothers

Benefits for Infants

- Optimal nutrition for infant
- Strong bonding with mother
- Safe, fresh milk
- Enhanced immune system
- Reduced risk for acute otitis media, nonspecific gastroenteritis, severe lower respiratory tract infections, and asthma
- Protection against allergies and intolerances
- Promotion of correct development of jaw and teeth
- Association with higher intelligence quotient and school performance through adolescence
- Reduced risk for chronic disease such as obesity, types 1 and 2 diabetes, heart disease, hypertension, hypercholesterolemia, and childhood leukemia
- Reduced risk for sudden infant death syndrome
- Reduced risk for infant morbidity and mortality

Benefits for Mothers

- Strong bonding with infant
- Readily available and convenient
- Increased energy expenditure, which may lead to faster return to prepregnancy weight
- Faster shrinking of the uterus
- Reduced postpartum bleeding and delayed menstrual cycle
- Decreased risk for chronic diseases such as type 2 diabetes, and breast and ovarian cancer
- Improved bone density and decreased risk for hip fracture
- Decreased risk for postpartum depression
- Enhanced self-esteem in the maternal role
- Time saved from preparing and mixing formula
- Money saved from not buying formula and increased medical expenses

Reprinted from *Journal of the American Dietetic Association*, 109(11), Position of the American Dietetic Association: Promoting and Supporting Breastfeeding, Page no. 1926-1942, 2009, with permission from Elsevier.

also can help control blood loss. Although not an effective method of birth control, exclusive breastfeeding suppresses ovulation in many women. There is some evidence that breastfeeding will reduce a woman's risk of ovarian cancer, breast cancer, and osteoporosis, as well as postpartum depression.

Still, some women find breastfeeding difficult due to physiological and social challenges. Milk supply may be low or not able to circulate well. Some babies refuse to breastfeed. Nipples might get tender or infected. Sometimes employers and others can be unsupportive of breastfeeding in public places.

Contraindications to Breastfeeding

Nearly all women who want to breastfeed can do so successfully, and breastfeeding rates are steadily increasing. There are times, however, when breastfeeding is inappropriate because of infant or maternal disease or drug use.[63]

In the case of infectious or chronic diseases, individual situations should be discussed with the healthcare provider. For example, a woman with untreated tuberculosis should not breastfeed because the illness can be transmitted to her child. In the United States and Canada, where safe feeding alternatives exist, women infected with HIV are advised not to breastfeed because HIV can be transmitted to the baby through breast milk.

Some medications pass directly into human milk, and some prescribed medications preclude breastfeeding. If the mother is using an illegal drug such as cocaine, she should not breastfeed. Women taking prescription or over-the-counter medicines or herbal supplements should discuss the effects of these products on breast milk with their healthcare providers.[64]

> **Key Concepts** Health benefits and convenience are key advantages of breastfeeding. For the infant, breastfeeding has been linked to reduced incidence of many infectious diseases, as well as other conditions. For a mother, breastfeeding speeds recovery of normal uterine size and can reduce her disease risk. Although breastfeeding is the preferred method of infant feeding, there are times when breastfeeding is contraindicated. These situations should be identified and discussed as part of prenatal care.

Resources for Pregnant and Lactating Women and Their Children

Many agencies support research and education programs that promote the health of pregnant and breastfeeding women and their children. You may be familiar with the March of Dimes and its efforts to reduce birth defects and prematurity through optimal nutrition during pregnancy. La Leche League is a voluntary health and education organization that offers programs and educational materials to help breastfeeding mothers learn about the benefits and practice of breastfeeding.

The **Special Supplemental Nutrition Program for Women, Infants, and Children (WIC)** is a much-acclaimed program of the Food and Nutrition Service of the U.S. Department of Agriculture. WIC provides food assistance, nutrition education, and referrals to healthcare services for low-income pregnant, postpartum, and breastfeeding women, as well as for infants and children up to age 5.

Although WIC services include breastfeeding education and support, WIC participants are less likely to breastfeed their infants.[65] Continued promotion of breastfeeding by WIC and other public health programs can have both health and economic benefits, including improved household food security and reduced hunger.[66] Periodically,

▶ **Special Supplemental Nutrition Program for Women, Infants, and Children (WIC)** A USDA program that provides federal grants to states for supplemental foods, healthcare referrals, and nutrition education for low-income pregnant, breastfeeding, and nonbreastfeeding postpartum women, and to infants and children at nutritional risk.

Quick Bite

Breastfeeding to Control a Mother's Blood Pressure?
Oxytocin, the hormone produced while breastfeeding, can lower the blood pressure of nursing mothers. Research shows that breastfeeding mothers have lower blood pressures after nursing than do bottle-feeding mothers. When asked to discuss stressful events, nursing mothers show smaller increases in blood pressure than the bottle-feeders. Mothers often claim that they feel relaxed during breastfeeding, which can account for the difference in blood pressure.

WIC participants are required to bring their infants into the local WIC office. These visits give WIC staff an opportunity to evaluate the infant's growth and provide the caregiver with additional nutrition education.

🍎 **Why Is This Important?** The nutritional needs of infants are unique from those of older children and adults. For one, they grow faster than at any other time in their lives and thus have far greater energy needs, met largely by a high-fat diet. Infants have some dietary restrictions and special considerations, too. Proper nutrition sets infants on the path for healthy development.

Infancy

Infancy is the period of a child's life between birth and 1 year. Because of the rapid growth that occurs during this time, nutritional needs are higher per unit of body weight than at any other time in the life cycle. Despite the critical importance of nutrition at this stage, feeding an infant is a fairly simple process. Human milk provides all the nutrients an infant needs and is the model for infant formulas. By 4 to 6 months, the infant's physical development and physiological maturation signal readiness for the addition of "solid" foods to the diet.

Human infants need love as much as they need food. Without love and nurturing, a baby can fail to thrive even if she is offered all the right nutrients. If an infant is not nourished emotionally, nutrition recommendations and requirements become meaningless.

Infant Growth and Development

Birth weight is the best predictor of a child's health in the first year of life; however, it is important to correlate weight with length of development. The risk profile of an infant who has a low birth weight because of **prematurity** differs from that of a **full-term baby** with a low birth weight.

Immediately after birth, an infant loses about 6 percent of his body weight. This is normal and expected. By 10 to 14 days, the infant should return to his birth weight. Over the next 12 months, the infant's growth will be phenomenal.

By the age of 4 to 6 months, a healthy infant will have doubled his birth weight. By his first birthday, the infant will have tripled his birth weight and increased his length by about 50 percent. The infant's body proportions change, too, so that by age 1 he is looking less like a baby and more like a **toddler** (see **FIGURE 11.14**).

Length (a measurement used instead of height because infants can't stand) and **head circumference** are more sensitive measures than weight for assessing a baby's growth and nutritional status. Weight alone reflects just recent nutritional intake. Head circumference measures brain

▶ **infancy** The period between birth and 12 months of age.

Quick Bite

Flavored Breast Milk

When lactating mothers exercise vigorously, the amount of lactic acid in breast milk can increase. Some babies dislike the taste and tend to nurse less. Alcohol also can cause a taste that babies dislike. What flavors do babies like? When mothers consume vanilla, mint, or garlic, some babies nurse more.

▶ **prematurity** Birth before 37 weeks of gestation.

▶ **full-term baby** A baby delivered during the normal period of human gestation, between 38 and 41 weeks.

▶ **toddler** A child between 12 and 36 months of age.

▶ **head circumference** Measurement of the largest part of the infant's head (just above the eyebrows and ears); used to determine brain growth.

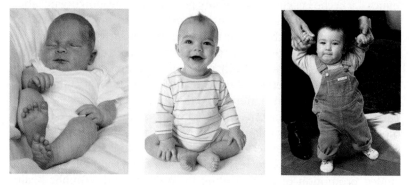

FIGURE 11.14 Different stages of infancy. (a) Newborn. **(b)** 4 to 6 months. **(c)** 12 months.
(a) © Johanna Goodyear/Shutterstock, Inc.; (b) © picturepartners/Shutterstock, Inc.; (c) © Gelpi/Shutterstock, Inc.

growth and development. Chronic malnutrition can limit this growth and is reflected in inadequate gains in head size. Regular measurements of head circumference, therefore, can verify desirable growth. Head circumference measurements are useful in infants and children up to age 2.

Growth Charts

During routine checkups throughout infancy (and during childhood and adolescence), healthcare practitioners measure weight, length or height, and head circumference and plot these values on **growth charts** (see **FIGURE 11.15**).

▶ **growth charts** Charts that plot the weight, length, and head circumference of infants and children as they grow.

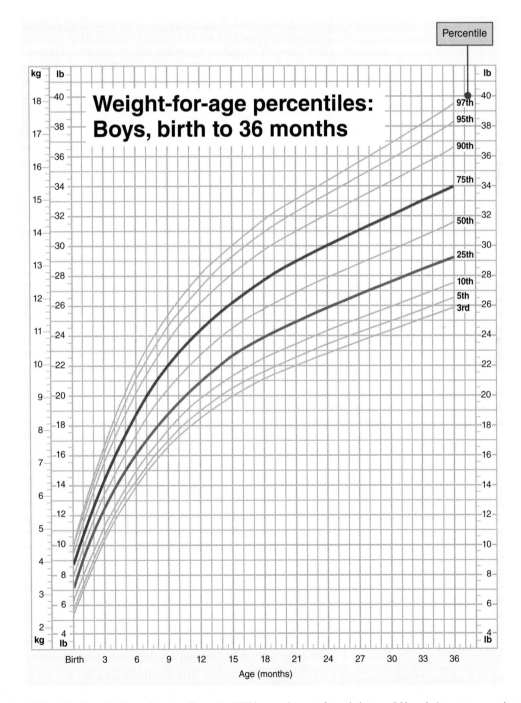

FIGURE 11.15 Growth chart. The Centers for Disease Control and Prevention (CDC) has complete sets of growth charts available on the Internet at www.cdc.gov/growthcharts.

Reproduced from the National Center for Health Statistics in collaboration with the National Center for Chronic Disease Prevention and Health Promotion (2000).

Charts for weight-for-age, length- (or height-) for-age, head circumference-for-age, weight-for-length, and BMI-for-age are available for boys and girls and for two age ranges: birth to 36 months and 2 to 20 years. Healthcare practitioners use growth charts to show the growth of an individual child over time. These charts also allow comparison of one child's growth to that of children in the general population.

> **Key Concepts** A typical infant doubles his or her birth weight by age 4 to 6 months and triples it by 12 months. Infant length increases about 50 percent during the first year. Healthcare practitioners use growth charts to follow and assess an infant's growth in weight, length, and head circumference.

Energy and Nutrient Needs During Infancy

How do you suppose scientists determine the nutrient needs of newborns and young infants? Studies with babies as subjects are rare—the logistical and ethical questions are daunting! So, how else can we know what babies need? It's simple; we just look at human milk—the food designed especially for babies. The composition of human milk is the gold standard by which infant nutrient needs are determined. Babies who are not breastfed are given infant formula. In the United States, most infant formulas have a base of modified cow's milk or soy protein. To ensure that formula meets all of an infant's nutrient needs, federal regulations require that the formula's composition comply with nutritional standards.

Energy

An infant's energy need is the amount of energy he or she requires for basal functions, such as respiration and metabolism, in addition to growth and activity. An infant's basal energy needs, relative to his or her size, are about twice those of an adult. The amount of energy an infant needs for activity varies throughout the first year of life, increasing as the child becomes more mobile (see **FIGURE 11.16**). In general, a newborn requires about 100 kilocalories per kilogram of body weight.[67] **TABLE 11.9** lists the specific equations for calculating infants' Estimated Energy Requirements (EER).

The appropriate balance of energy sources (carbohydrate, fat, and protein) for infants differs from that of adults (see **FIGURE 11.17**). The best diet for infants (as modeled by human milk) is high in fat and moderate in carbohydrate. Infants have high calorie needs but can consume only a small amount at any one time. An infant's stomach is quite small; a newborn can consume only about 1 to 2 ounces of liquid at a feeding. Because fat is the most concentrated source of calories, a high-fat diet supplies adequate calories in a smaller volume. A high-fat diet also is necessary for normal brain growth, which continues until about 18 to 24 months of age. **FIGURE 11.18** shows the primary functions of energy-yielding nutrients in infants, which are discussed in the next sections.

Protein

Infants need proportionately more protein than at any other time in the life cycle. In fact, protein needs (measured in grams per kilogram of body weight) during the first six months of life are nearly twice as high as an adult's needs. **TABLE 11.10** lists protein recommendations for infants. Both human milk and infant formula provide complete protein with all

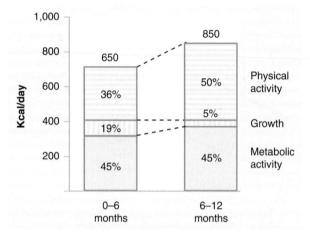

FIGURE 11.16 Allocation of energy expenditure. During the second six months, infants increase their energy expenditure for physical activity.

Modified from Foman SJ, Bell EF. Energy. In: Foman SJ, ed. *Nutrition of Normal Infants.* St. Louis: Mosby; 1993.

TABLE 11.9
Estimated Energy Requirement RDA During Infancy

Age (mo)	EER Equation
0–3	(89 × wt [kg] − 100) + 175 kcal/day
4–6	(89 × wt [kg] − 100) + 56 kcal/day
7–12	(89 × wt [kg] − 100) + 22 kcal/day

Reproduced from Institute of Medicine, Food and Nutrition Board. *Dietary Reference Intakes for Energy, Carbohydrate, Fiber, Fat, Fatty Acids, Cholesterol, Protein, and Amino Acids (Macronutrients).* © 2005 by the National Academy of Sciences, courtesy of the National Academies Press, Washington, DC.

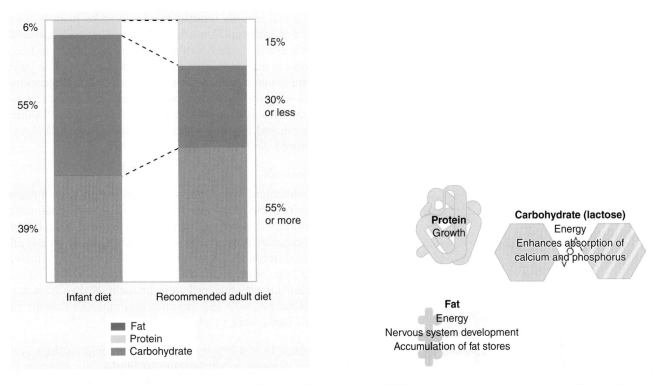

FIGURE 11.17 Percentages of energy-yielding nutrients in infant and adult diets. The best diets for infants are high in fat and moderate in carbohydrate. Infants need a high-fat diet for normal brain growth and to provide adequate calories in a smaller volume.

FIGURE 11.18 Primary functions of energy-yielding nutrients for infants. To support growth, protein needs (per kg body weight) are higher in infancy than in any other life stage.

the essential amino acids. The types of proteins found in human milk make it easier to digest and absorb than cow's milk.

Carbohydrate and Fat

Carbohydrates and triglycerides are the major energy sources for infants. This allows protein to be used primarily for growth and not as an energy source. Nearly all carbohydrate in human milk and in infant formulas made from cow's milk is lactose. Infants digest lactose easily and tolerate it well.

Triglycerides are the major energy source in human milk, providing about 50 to 55 percent of the calories. Fats in milk also enhance a baby's sense of fullness between feedings. Experts recommend that infants get at least 30 grams of fat per day.[68] Human milk is rich in essential fatty acids: the omega-6 fatty acid arachidonic acid and two long-chain omega-3 fatty acids, eicosapentaenoic acid and docosahexaenoic acid. These fatty acids have roles in neurological development. The Food and Nutrition Board has set an AI for newborns (0 to 6 months of age) of 4.4 grams per day of linoleic acid and 0.5 gram per day of alpha-linolenic acid. Infants also need cholesterol for brain development. Human milk is rich in cholesterol, containing about 20 to 30 milligrams per 100 milliliters.[69]

Water

Because water as a percentage of body weight is greater in babies than in adults, infants need more fluids. The AI for water during infancy is

TABLE 11.10
Protein AI or RDA for Infants

Age (mo)	g/kg	g/day[a]
0–6	1.52	9
7–12	1.2	11

[a] The value for grams per day is based on reference weights of infants.

Data from Institute of Medicine, Food and Nutrition Board. *Dietary Reference Intakes for Energy, Carbohydrate, Fiber, Fat, Fatty Acids, Cholesterol, Protein, and Amino Acids (Macronutrients).* © 2005 by the National Academy of Sciences, courtesy of the National Academies Press, Washington, DC.

▶ **neonate** An infant less than four weeks old.

0.7 liter per day in the first six months (assumed to be from human milk) and 0.8 liter per day from 7 months to 1 year of age. Human milk fulfills not only the nutrient needs of the **neonate**, but also the fluid requirements. Properly prepared formula accomplishes the same task. During the first four to six months, supplemental water is not necessary for healthy infants who are exclusively breastfed or who receive properly mixed formula. This is true even in hot, humid weather.[70] Once solid foods are introduced, a baby's water needs change, and additional water may be required.

Vitamins and Minerals

Human milk provides vitamins and minerals in the amounts that human babies need. Therefore, the micronutrient composition of human milk is the reference point for designing infant formula. As long as an infant receives adequate calories from breast milk or infant formula, nearly all vitamin and mineral needs also are being met. Human milk is lower in a few nutrients (e.g., iron, vitamin D) than is formula, but infants absorb these nutrients more efficiently from breast milk than from formula. This section focuses on a few vitamins and minerals that are of concern for infants (see **FIGURE 11.19**).

Vitamin D   Vitamin D is a key nutrient for absorbing calcium and mineralizing bone. Rickets is attributable to inadequate vitamin D intake and insufficient sunlight exposure in infants and children.[71] Recent evidence also suggests a role for vitamin D in maintaining innate immunity and preventing diseases such as cancer and diabetes.[72] Although human milk is low in vitamin D, infants absorb it well. Despite this, inadequate vitamin D levels are a concern for those infants who are exclusively breastfed, those not exposed to sunlight, and those with darkly pigmented skin who make less vitamin D from the same amount of sunlight exposure than do lighter-skinned infants. If a breastfed baby does not get adequate sunlight exposure and if the baby's mother is deficient in vitamin D, the infant's risk is especially high. In 2008 the American Academy of Pediatrics (AAP) increased its recommendation for daily vitamin D to 400 IU for all infants, children, and adolescents, beginning the first few days after birth.[73]

Vitamin K   Vitamin K is necessary for the production of prothrombin, a substance needed for blood to clot. Although intestinal bacteria synthesize vitamin K, the gut is sterile at birth. Because babies are born with minimal stores of vitamin K, it is recommended that a single dose of vitamin K be given at birth. Both human milk and infant formula provide adequate vitamin K, and as feeding begins, helpful bacteria begin to flourish in the infant's intestinal tract.

Vitamin B₁₂   Vitamin B_{12} is essential for cell division and normal folate metabolism. Mothers who include meat, fish, and dairy products in their diets produce milk that is adequate in vitamin B_{12}. This may not be true of strict vegetarians, whose diet—and therefore breast milk—can be deficient in vitamin B_{12}. Breastfed infants of vegan mothers may need a vitamin B_{12} supplement.

Iron   Iron is essential for growth and development, and iron-deficiency anemia is the most common nutritional deficiency in

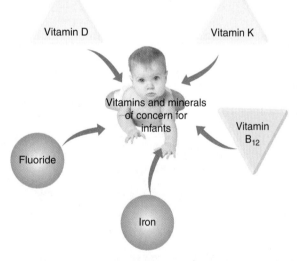

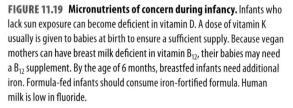

FIGURE 11.19 Micronutrients of concern during infancy. Infants who lack sun exposure can become deficient in vitamin D. A dose of vitamin K usually is given to babies at birth to ensure a sufficient supply. Because vegan mothers can have breast milk deficient in vitamin B_{12}, their babies may need a B_{12} supplement. By the age of 6 months, breastfed infants need additional iron. Formula-fed infants should consume iron-fortified formula. Human milk is low in fluoride.

the United States. Human milk is not a rich source of iron, but it does not need to be. Approximately 50 percent of the iron in breast milk is absorbed, compared with only 4 percent of the iron in infant formula. If the mother has consumed an iron-rich diet during pregnancy, the fetus builds up large enough iron stores during gestation to meet most of its iron needs for the first few months of life. These stores begin to diminish during the fourth month of life. By the age of 6 months, a breastfed infant needs an additional iron source. Iron-fortified infant cereals can meet this need. For formula-fed babies, iron supplementation is needed from birth. The AAP therefore recommends iron-fortified formula for all formula-fed babies.[74]

Fluoride   Human milk, although optimal in so many ways, is low in fluoride, a mineral important for dental health. Current research has led the American Dental Association and the AAP to recommend fluoride supplements for breastfed infants after the age of 6 months, depending on the fluoride content of the local water supply.[75] If the local water supply has adequate fluoride and the formula is mixed with tap water, formula-fed infants do not need fluoride supplements. If the water used to mix formula has inadequate fluoride, fluoride supplements are indicated. Fluoridation policies and the fluoride content of tap water vary among municipalities. Oversupplementation with fluoride in children has been associated with mild fluorosis in developing teeth; therefore, ingestion of higher than recommended levels is discouraged.[76]

> **Key Concepts** Energy and nutrient needs for infants are estimated based on the composition of human milk. Because of their rapid growth and development, infants have high energy and nutrient needs per kilogram of body weight. Caregivers must give special attention to vitamin D, iron, and fluoride to ensure that the infant obtains enough. If breast milk or formula (properly mixed) is meeting energy needs, the fluid needs of the infant also are being met.

Newborn Breastfeeding

The AAP has identified breastfeeding as the ideal method of feeding to achieve optimal growth and development[77] and recommends that breastfeeding begin as soon after birth as possible and continue at least through the first 12 months of life.[78] Feedings should occur at least every two to three hours, for a total of 8 to 12 feedings per day. Duration of feedings is guided by the infant's behavior and can last from 10 to 15 minutes per breast. Hospitals should provide every opportunity for breastfeeding to begin before the baby goes home. Nurses or **lactation consultants** should be available to offer professional breastfeeding support to new mothers. The AAP recommends that no supplements of formula or water be given to breastfed neonates unless medically indicated.

Alternative Feeding: Infant Formula

Women may decide not to breastfeed or to breastfeed only briefly. Their infants need infant formulas designed to provide adequate nutrition.

Standard Infant Formulas

Standard infant formulas have cow's milk as a base. In making infant formula, manufacturers first remove the milk fat and replace it with vegetable oils. Infant formula is fortified with all the essential vitamins and minerals according to guidelines established by the AAP and enforced

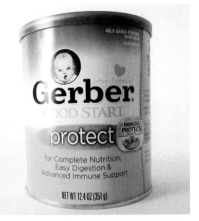

© Jones & Bartlett Learning. Photo by Amy Rathburn.

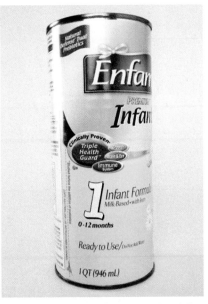

Jones & Bartlett Learning. Photo by Amy Rathburn.

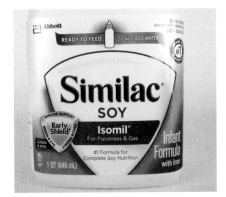

Jones & Bartlett Learning. Photo by Amy Rathburn.

▶ **lactation consultants** Health professionals trained to specialize in education about and promotion of breastfeeding; can be certified as an International Board Certified Lactation Consultant (IBCLC).

by the Food and Drug Administration. Infant formulas are available with or without added iron, but because of the decreased bioavailability of iron in infant formulas and the infant's high needs, the AAP recommends using only iron-fortified formulas.

Although formula manufacturers try to mimic the composition of human milk, formula remains an imperfect copy. Several brands of infant formula contain three fatty acids that are prevalent in human milk: arachidonic acid (ARA), eicosapentaenoic acid (EPA), and docosahexaenoic acid (DHA). Some studies show that supplemental ARA and EPA benefit infants' visual function and cognitive development; however, a large review of studies found that most randomized controlled trials have not shown a beneficial effect of long-chain polyunsaturated fatty acid supplementation of formula milk on the neurodevelopmental, visual, and physical outcomes of full-term newborns.[79] Human milk also contains more cholesterol than infant formulas.

Soy-Based Formulas

Formula-fed infants who develop vomiting, diarrhea, constipation, abdominal pain, or colic are frequently switched to soy-based formulas. In these formulas, soy is the source of protein. To compensate for the inferior digestibility of soy protein, soy formulas contain more protein than formulas based on cow's milk. Soy formulas are lactose-free and iron-fortified. Corn syrup and sucrose are the carbohydrate sources.

Other Types of Formula

Formulas can be classified according to three basic criteria: caloric density, carbohydrate source, and protein composition.[80] Special formulas are available for infants who are allergic to both cow's milk and soy protein, those who are premature, and those who have rare defects in metabolic pathways. These special formulas often have their protein content modified in either its digestibility or its amino acid composition. Antireflux formulas are designed to decrease vomiting and regurgitation. Many special formulas contain medium-chain triglycerides as the major fat source. This type of fat is very well digested and absorbed. These special formulas are expensive and often taste bad, but they are essential for many infants.

Formula Preparation

Formulas come in three forms: ready-to-feed, concentrate, and powdered. Although the ready-to-feed version is the most convenient, it is also the most expensive. As the name implies, the formula can be poured directly into a bottle and fed to the baby. Liquid concentrate formula is mixed with an equal amount of water before feeding. Powdered formula also is mixed with water and is the least expensive.

When using infant formulas, principles of food safety must be observed. Infants have immature immune systems and can develop infections from improperly prepared or stored formula. Prepared formula should be refrigerated immediately and kept in the refrigerator until needed. If formula is not used within 48 hours, it should be discarded. For at least the first few months, the AAP recommends sterilizing all equipment used for feeding.

Failure to follow instructions can result in an improperly mixed formula. Some caregivers on limited budgets may purposefully overdilute formula to make it last longer. This deprives the infant of necessary calories and protein and provides too much water. Other caregivers may overconcentrate the formula in the misguided belief that this may encourage faster growth. Overconcentrated formula provides too much protein and too little water and can cause problems with an infant's kidney function and hydration.

Breast Milk or Formula: How Much Is Enough?

It is fairly simple to use Dietary Reference Intake (DRI) values and breast milk or formula composition to estimate an infant's needs based on body weight. For example, a newborn who weighs 7 pounds, 11 ounces (3.5 kilograms) requires approximately 390 kilocalories and 5 grams of protein each day. This amount is provided by approximately 600 milliliters (approximately 20 fluid ounces) of breast milk or infant formula.

It's easy to keep track of how much formula an infant has consumed, but what about the breastfed baby? Although you can't see how much breast milk a nursing infant is consuming, there are other ways to tell that a baby is getting enough to eat. An adequately fed newborn will breastfeed daily 8 to 12 times, wet at least six diapers, and have at least three loose stools each day in the first week of life. The newborn will also regain his or her birth weight within the first two weeks. Normal growth, regular elimination patterns, and a satisfied demeanor are the best indicators that a baby is getting enough to eat.

Feeding Technique

Feeding should take place in a loving and affectionate environment. A breastfeeding mother holds her baby close, at a distance that encourages mother–baby eye contact. (See **FIGURE 11.20**.) During bottle-feeding, the caregiver should also hold the baby close and make eye contact. Propping the bottle against a pillow or other object so that the baby can feed alone should be avoided.

Babies swallow air while feeding, whether at the breast or with a bottle, and they need to be burped. Babies generally need to be burped after 15 minutes or 2 to 3 ounces of formula. Just as the infant sends signals of readiness for feeding, he also signals fullness. Fullness cues include fussiness, playfulness, sleep, or just turning away. Parents need to learn these cues and respond to them.

> **Key Concepts** Human milk provides all the necessary nutrients for growth and development and enhances the immune system of the maturing infant. Infants who are not breastfed receive infant formula, which should be fortified with iron. Careful preparation and storage of the formula ensures proper nutrient composition and food safety. Formula feedings should nourish the baby emotionally as well as nutritionally.

Introduction of Solid Foods into the Infant's Diet

Based on an infant's physiological needs (e.g., depletion of iron stores) and physical development (e.g., the ability to sit up), solid foods, also called **complementary foods**, are introduced. To say that we are introducing solid foods is a bit of a misnomer: We are really referring to pureed and liquefied cereals, fruits, vegetables, and meats that are added to the infant's diet of breast milk or infant formula. According to the AAP, solid foods should be introduced when infants are developmentally ready, around 4 to 6 months of age, to ensure that they get adequate nutrition.[81]

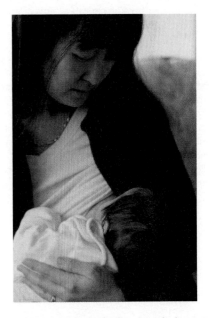

FIGURE 11.20 Breastfeeding. Breastfeeding nurtures an infant emotionally as well as physically. This intensely rewarding time helps to bond a mother and her child.

▶ **complementary foods** Any foods or liquids other than breast milk or infant formula fed to an infant.

Quick Bite

Ancient Baby Bottle
The earliest infant feeding vessel ever discovered is Egyptian and dates from 2000 BCE. Art found in the ruins of the palace of King Sardanapalus of Nineveh, who died in 888 BCE, depicts a mother holding a modern-looking baby bottle.

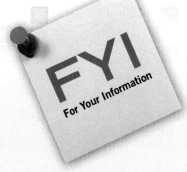

New Guidelines for Introducing Peanut Products

After almost two decades of warning parents to withhold peanut foods from infants to prevent life-threatening allergies, the National Institute of Allergy and Infectious Diseases (NIAID) recently released new guidelines in favor of feeding infants peanut foods in an attempt to prevent allergies. In a shift from earlier guidelines, the U.S. National Institutes of Health (NIH) is now recommending early introduction of peanut products into the diets of babies considered at high or moderate risk of developing peanut allergy.[a,b] The new guidelines are based largely on a randomized clinical trial, Leaning Early About Peanut allergy (LEAP),[c] which studied 600 infants and demonstrated that regular peanut consumption beginning in early infancy and continued to age 5 reduces the rate of peanut allergy in at-risk infants by about 80 percent.

The specific recommendations are[d]:

- Babies at "high risk" of peanut allergy because of severe eczema and/or egg allergy should have peanut-containing foods introduced as early as 4 to 6 months of age.
- Babies at "moderate risk" because of mild to moderate eczema should have peanut-containing foods introduced around six months.
- Babies at "low risk" because they lack eczema or any other food allergy should have peanut-containing foods freely introduced into their diets.

Ideally, parents will work with their pediatrician or allergy specialist, rather than going it alone. The topic should routinely be discussed at the four-month visit to the pediatrician, where parents and doctor together can set a plan for introducing peanut-containing foods. The doctor may first want to do an allergy test, to see if the baby is already sensitized to peanuts. To make sure these foods are introduced in a safe, age-appropriate manner, parents can mix smooth peanut butter with breast milk, formula, or warm water. Babies should first start some other solid foods before peanut products are added.

A follow-up study, the LEAP-ON study, examined whether infants who had consumed peanuts for more than four years were protected against allergy if they stopped eating peanuts.[e] LEAP-ON demonstrated that the immune system "remembers" the exposure, and a smaller number of peanut consumers were found to be allergic than those who avoided peanuts.

a National Institutes of Health. NIH-sponsored expert panel issues clinical guidelines to prevent peanut allergy. January 5, 2017. https://www.nih.gov/news-events/news-releases/nih-sponsored-expert-panel-issues-clinical-guidelines-prevent-peanut-allergy. Accessed September 17, 2017.

b Fleischer DM, Sicherer S, Greenhawt M, et al. Consensus communication on early peanut introduction and the prevention of peanut allergy in high-risk infants. *Pediatrics.* 2015;136(3). http://pediatrics.aappublications.org/content/136/3/600. Accessed September 17, 2017.

c Du Toit G, Roberts G, Sayre PH, et al. Randomized trial of peanut consumption in infants at risk for peanut allergy. *New Engl J Med.* 2015;372:803-813. http://www.nejm.org/doi/full/10.1056/NEJMoa1414850. Accessed September 17, 2017.

d National Institute of Allergy and Infectious Diseases. Guidelines for clinicians and patients for diagnosis and management of food allergy in the United States and 2017 addendum guidelines for the prevention of peanut allergy in the United States. https://www.niaid.nih.gov/diseases-conditions/guidelines-clinicians-and-patients-food-allergy. Accessed September 17, 2017.

e Du Toit G, Roberts G, Sayre PH, et al. Effect of avoidance on peanut allergy after early peanut consumption. *N Engl J Med.* 2016;374:1435-1443. http://www.nejm.org/doi/full/10.1056/NEJMoa1514209. Accessed September 17, 2017.

Physiological Indicators of Infant Readiness for Solid Foods

Before a baby reaches 6 months of age, solid food is not necessary for nutrition; in fact, early introduction of supplemental foods can be detrimental. By the age of 4 to 6 months, however, an infant is physiologically ready to expand his or her diet. For example, at this age a baby has increased levels of digestive enzymes so that foods other than human milk or formula can be digested with ease. In addition, the infant is better able to maintain adequate hydration by the age of 6 months. Before this age, adding cereals or other solid foods to the diet can negatively affect an infant's hydration. It is probably no coincidence that the iron stores acquired in the mother's womb become depleted at the same time the baby is physiologically ready to expand his or her diet. However, solid food is a supplement to, not a replacement for, human milk or formula at this time.

THINK About It 4

Developmental Readiness for Solid Foods

If you attempt to spoon-feed a very young infant, for example, at 3 weeks of age, the infant's tongue will push the spoon and food right back out. This **extrusion reflex** is a sign that the infant is not ready for solid

▶ **extrusion reflex** A young infant's response when a spoon is put in its mouth; the tongue is thrust forward, indicating that the baby is not ready for spoon feeding.

foods. By 4 to 6 months of age, the infant will no longer push the food out and is capable of transferring food from the front of the mouth to the back, an ability necessary for swallowing solid foods. Also, the infant can purposefully bring her hand to her mouth, an ability necessary for self-feeding. In addition, if the baby is able to control her head and neck while sitting with minimal support, she is ready to be fed solids.

Start Healthy Feeding Guidelines

The *Start Healthy Feeding Guidelines for Infants and Toddlers* are science-based, practical guidelines for feeding healthy babies for the first two years.[82] The *Start Healthy Feeding Guidelines* were designed to answer parents' and caregivers' questions, such as "When is my baby ready for complementary foods? What foods should I feed my baby? How do I feed these foods?"[83] The appropriate age for introduction of complementary foods balances physiological and developmental readiness with nutritional requirements for growth and development. **FIGURE 11.21** summarizes the *Start Healthy Feeding Guidelines*.

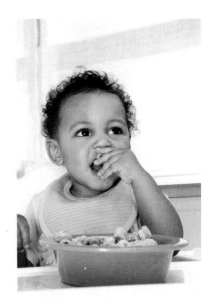

© James Woodson/Digital Vision/Thinkstock.

Signs of readiness for the introduction of infant cereals and thin, pureed foods include the ability to sit with support and the ability to take food from a spoon and move it forward and backward in the mouth with the tongue. As the infant's body control improves and he or she can sit independently, she will also develop the ability to pick up and hold objects in her hand. She will be able to take in thicker, pureed foods and soft, mashed foods without lumps.

Babies who can crawl also are likely to be ready to self-feed finger foods such as baby biscuits or crackers. Babies at this stage can hold small foods between the thumb and first finger and also hold a cup (preferably one with a cap and spout) independently. A baby is able to participate in the feeding process, and as his dexterity improves, he will be able to pick up small pieces of food. It is important that caregivers monitor the child's eating to make sure the youngster does not choke on food or on nonfood items.

At the end of the first year, when a baby is standing alone and beginning to walk, his diet can expand even further with bite-size pieces of table foods and a wider variety of textures. Self-feeding with his fingers is much easier, and he desires to self-feed with a spoon as well—a messy but developmentally appropriate thing to do. Most table foods are appropriate for the child at this stage.

There is no scientific evidence to support introduction of complementary foods in any particular order; cultural practices play a large role in determining which foods are introduced first. Introducing a source of iron, such as an iron-fortified infant cereal or pureed meats, is necessary because iron stores developed in pregnancy are declining. No matter what food is introduced first, new foods should be introduced one at a time, at intervals of about one week, to see how well the infant tolerates each food and to be on the lookout for allergic reactions. Throughout the first year, breast milk or infant formula still forms the major portion of the infant's diet. Ideally, however, the child will have been introduced to a variety of foods by his or her first birthday.

Parents and caregivers should take care that complementary foods are soft in texture to avoid the risk of choking. Delaying—until age 1—the introduction of common food allergens, particularly cow's milk, egg whites, and wheat, can prevent food allergies for many infants. In addition to its allergic potential, whole cow's milk provides too much protein and too little iron, is low in essential fatty acids, can impair kidney

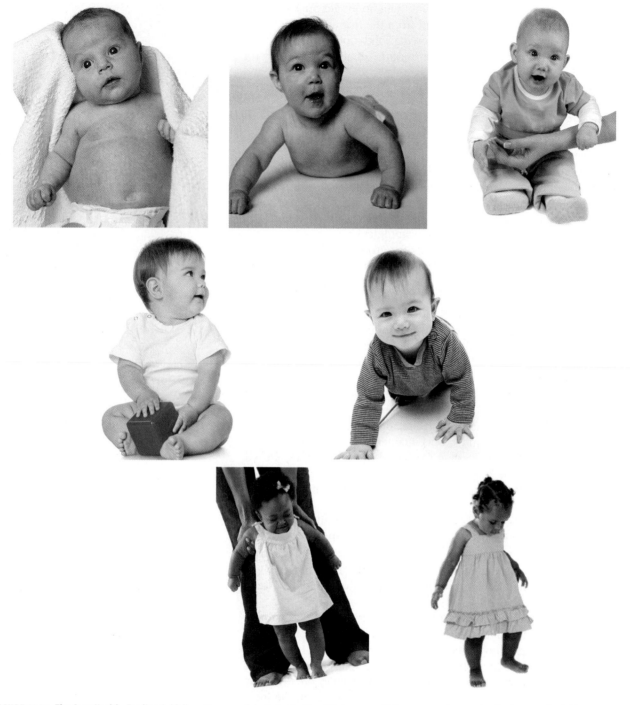

FIGURE 11.21 **The *Start Healthy Feeding Guidelines*.** Summary of physical and eating skills, hunger and fullness cues, and appropriate food textures for children 0 to 24 months of age.

Reprinted from *Journal of the American Dietetic Association*, 104(3), Butte N, Cobb K, Dwyer J, et al, The *Start Healthy Feeding Guidelines* for Infants and Toddlers, Page no. 442-454, 2004, with permission from Elsevier.

Newborn and Head Up: © Barbara Penoyar/Stockbyte/Getty Images; Supported Sitter: © Olga Sapegina/Shutterstock, Inc.; Independent Sitter, Crawler, Beginning to Walk: © iStockphoto/Thinkstock; Independent Toddler: © Hemera/Thinkstock.

function and lead to dehydration, and has been linked to development of type 1 diabetes.[84] In families with a history of allergies, introduction of eggs should be delayed until age 2, and fish and shellfish should not be introduced before age 3.

TABLE 11.11
Suggestions for Establishing a Healthy Feeding Relationship with a Child

Do	Why
Wash the baby's hands before feeding.	To clean any dirt or germs off the hands to keep the baby's food clean
Use a small spoon or let the baby use his or her fingers.	To help the baby learn proper eating habits
Place food on the tip of the spoon and put food in the middle of the baby's tongue.	To make it easy for the baby to swallow
Remove food from the jar before feeding. Do not feed the baby food from the jar.	To prevent the saliva from the baby's mouth from spoiling the remainder of the food in the jar
Give only one new food at a time, and wait at least 1 week before giving another new food.	To give the baby time to get used to each new flavor and texture, and to see if the baby is allergic to the new food

Reproduced from U.S. Department of Agriculture, Food and Nutrition Service. *A Guide for Use in the Child Nutrition Programs*. FNS-258. 2002. https://www.fns.usda.gov/tn/feeding-infants-guide-use-child-nutrition-programs. Accessed May 17, 2017.

Along with observing the infant's developmental readiness for complementary foods, parents and caregivers need to be alert to an infant's hunger and satiety cues. Hunger cues include crying and fussing, reaching for spoonfuls of food, opening mouth and leaning toward bowl or spoon, and also staring at you while you are eating. Conversely, if full, the infant may turn away from food, push the bowl or food away, clench her mouth shut, and spit out food. The suggestions in **TABLE 11.11** can help new parents establish a healthy feeding relationship with their child.

Various caregivers may be involved in a child's nutrition. In today's society, it is inappropriate to assume that the caregiver is solely the mother, father, grandparent, or even a relative of the child. Many children spend the majority of their feeding time in a child-care setting. Child-care staff can develop and implement strategies to overcome challenges and support healthy eating behaviors of children.[85]

> *Quick* **Bite**
>
> **Pumping Iron**
> The use of cow's milk for children younger than 1 year is a common cause of iron deficiency. Cow's milk is low in iron, and drinking it can cause intestinal bleeding in infants. Although the amount of iron in breast milk also is low, this iron is highly bioavailable. Breast milk also contains proteins that bind iron, thereby inhibiting the growth of diarrhea-causing bacteria that feed on iron. If formula is used, the AAP recommends that it be iron-fortified.

Key Concepts An infant's physiological needs and developmental readiness usually indicate the appropriate time to introduce solid foods. Semisolid and solid foods should be introduced slowly to check for infant food intolerances and allergic reactions. The caregiver should choose foods that meet the child's nutritional needs and suit his or her developmental capabilities.

Feeding Problems During Infancy

Colic

The term *colic* refers to continuous crying and distress in a healthy infant—apparently because of abdominal cramping and discomfort. Infants with colic usually cry for hours, despite efforts to comfort them. In some cases, a change in formula or a change in the breastfeeding mother's diet provides some relief. However, diet (of either mother or infant) is not considered a cause of colic.[86] Often, colic goes away on its own, usually by the age of 3 to 4 months, but the infant should be evaluated by a pediatrician to rule out a more serious cause of distress.

Early Childhood Caries

Decay in the primary teeth, known as early childhood caries and sometimes called "baby-bottle tooth decay" (see **FIGURE 11.22**), can result if baby teeth are bathed too long in milk, formula, or juice, which nourish decay-producing bacteria. Other factors, such as inadequate development of tooth enamel, can also contribute to tooth decay.[87] The problem

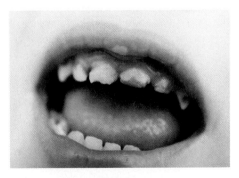

FIGURE 11.22 Early childhood caries. A baby routinely put to bed with a bottle can develop extensive tooth decay.
© RusN/ iStock/ Getty Images, Inc.

▶ **gastroesophageal reflux disease (GERD)** A backflow of stomach contents into the esophagus, accompanied by a burning pain because of the acidity of the gastric juices.

▶ **failure to thrive (FTT)** Abnormally low gains in length (height) and weight during infancy and childhood; can result from physical problems or poor feeding, but many affected children have no apparent disease or defect.

is often associated with routinely putting a baby to bed with a bottle so the baby's teeth are awash in formula or juice for much or all of the night. Children with early childhood caries are more susceptible to caries in the permanent teeth and lifelong dental problems.[88]

Iron-Deficiency Anemia: Milk Anemia

Human milk and cow's milk both are low in iron. As discussed earlier, this is usually not a problem: The iron in breast milk is well absorbed, and regular cow's milk is not recommended for babies younger than 1 year; however, iron deficiency may develop in older infants who do not eat enough iron-rich foods.

Gastroesophageal Reflux

Gastroesophageal reflux disease (GERD) is the regurgitation of the stomach contents into the esophagus after a feeding. This type of spitting up occurs in 3 percent of newborns, usually males, and typically disappears within 12 to 18 months. Concern is warranted if reflux makes a child difficult to feed or results in coughing, choking, or frequent vomiting. Adding cereal to bottle feedings is not recommended for a baby who has reflux.

Diarrhea

Stool patterns vary from infant to infant, as well as in the same infant over time. Healthy, thriving breastfed infants can have up to 12 stools per day—or only 1 per week. Formula-fed infants usually have one to seven bowel movements per day. Diarrhea—the frequent passage of loose, watery stools—can rapidly dehydrate an infant. Infants with diarrhea require increased fluids, and caregivers should consult the child's pediatrician for specific advice about how to meet this need.

Failure to Thrive

Full-term infants who experience poor growth in the absence of disease or physical defect suffer from **failure to thrive (FTT)** (see **FIGURE 11.23**). Although this can occur at any age, in infancy it usually occurs in the second half of the first year. Common causes include poverty and a resulting shortage of food, inappropriate foods in an infant's diet, improper formula preparation, or excessive consumption of fruit juice or fruit drinks. (See the FYI feature "Fruit Juices.") In addition, well-meaning parents may introduce low-fat or nonfat milk in an attempt to prevent obesity. Babies need a high-fat diet to support normal growth and brain development. As stated, regular cow's milk should not be introduced before age 1. Low-fat milks are inappropriate for children younger than 2 years.

Untreated, FTT can delay cognitive, motor, and language development. Studies indicate, however, that intensive intervention can correct FTT and allow resumption of a normal growth pattern. Such intervention includes nutrition education for caregivers, maintenance of food records by the caregiver, frequent weight checks of the infant, and perhaps social service intervention for the family.

Although there is nothing complex about the nutrient needs and food choices appropriate for babies, it is important for caregivers to receive some education about proper feeding. Some practices that we learn from friends, parents, and other family

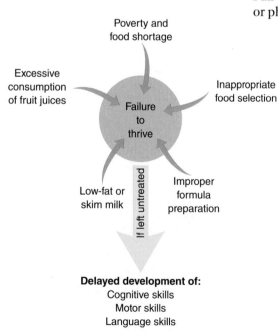

FIGURE 11.23 Failure to thrive. Failure to thrive can result from many different causes. If untreated, the effects are lifelong.

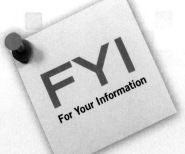

Fruit Juices

Fruit juices are popular beverages for children ages 6 months to 5 years. Apple, citrus, and other fruit juices, in addition to bananas and dried fruits, constitute a large amount of their total fruit intake, compared to youth ages 6 to 11 years.[a] An 8-oz glass of 100-percent fruit juice counts as one fruit serving. If juice is being used as a source of vitamin C, drinking just 3 to 6 fluid ounces per day meets vitamin C intake recommendations.

Juices do provide benefits to the diet. They are refreshing and sweet; accessible and affordable; more healthful than soft drinks; and provide energy, water, and selected minerals and vitamins. "Fruit drinks" on the other hand, can be nothing more than fruit-flavored beverages that are high in sugar and low in nutrients.

High fruit juice consumption among young children, however, may contribute to obesity and a failure to thrive. The link between excessive juice consumption and obesity has not been proven; however, studies suggest that it is more likely to be a factor in those children who are at risk for overweight and obesity.[b] Failure to thrive may result if fruit juices replace other food sources (particularly milk) or if sorbitol and fructose, found in higher amounts in apple and pear juice, cause diarrhea and malabsorption. If juice is substituted with fresh fruit, energy intake could be reduced and the adequacy of fiber intake improved. This would likely increase costs for schools, childcare providers, and families, but nutritional gains would be achieved.[c]

To keep intake of fruit juices to a healthy level, the American Academy of Pediatrics (AAP) recommends the following practices[d]:

- Wait until at least 6 months of age before introducing juice.
- Avoid giving infants juice in bottles or other containers that allow easy consumption throughout the day. Avoid giving juice at bedtime.
- Limit consumption of fruit juice to 4 to 6 fluid ounces per day for children 1 to 6 years old.
- Encourage caregivers to offer fruit rather than fruit juice to children.
- Determine the amount of juice being consumed when evaluating children with malnutrition (overnutrition and undernutrition) and in children with dental caries.
- Educate parents about the differences between fruit juice and fruit drinks.
- Fruit juice should be pasteurized (e.g., children should not drink fresh-pressed apple cider).
- Make sure that juice does not replace breast milk, formula, or cow's milk.

a Herrick KA, Rossen LM, Nielsen SJ, et al. Fruit consumption by youth in the United States. *Pediatrics*. 2015;136(4):664-671.
b Monsivais P, Rehm C. Potential nutritional and economic effects of replacing juice with fruit in the diets of children in the United States. *Arch Pediatr Adolesc Med*. 2012;166(5):459-464.
c Ibid.
d Kleinman RE, Greer FR, eds., *Pediatric Nutrition*. 7th ed. Elk Grove Village, IL: American Academy of Pediatrics; 2014:123.

members, or remember from our own childhood, are inappropriate for babies. Studies show that even people who receive nutrition education in the WIC program introduce solid foods much too early and feed infants sweetened tea, soft drinks, and other inappropriate foods.[89] Newborns don't come with instructions, but caregivers can always turn to a pediatrician or registered dietitian/registered dietitian nutritionist for answers to feeding questions.

Key Concepts Feeding-related problems of infancy include colic, baby-bottle tooth decay, iron-deficiency anemia, gastroesophageal reflux, diarrhea, and failure to thrive. Usually minor adjustments in food choices or feeding techniques solve these problems; however, caregivers may need the guidance of a pediatrician or registered dietitian/registered dietitian nutritionist.

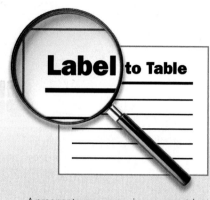

A pregnant woman requires more nutrients than usual. The RDA for both iron and folate increases by 50 percent during pregnancy. Iron, especially, is difficult to get in this quantity from the diet. Enriched grains and fortified foods, such as cereals, make it easier to obtain these essential nutrients. Let's take a look at the Nutrition Facts label from a popular breakfast cereal.

Take a look at how much folic acid a 1-cup serving of this breakfast cereal contains—50% Daily Value (DV = 400 micrograms). The DV for folate is the same as the RDA for nonpregnant women; for pregnancy, the RDA increases to 600 micrograms. If orange juice accompanies the cereal, another 15% DV (60 mg) is added for a 1-cup serving. So, these two foods provide a substantial amount of the folate that a pregnant woman would need.

Iron also is extremely important for pregnancy because of its role in growth and its importance as blood volume increases during pregnancy. One serving of this breakfast cereal provides almost half the DV of 18 milligrams (45 percent of 18 milligrams equals 8 milligrams). However, during pregnancy, the RDA for iron is 27 milligrams. So, one serving of this cereal provides nearly one-third of the iron needed each day—a good start. Having orange juice with the cereal will enhance iron absorption.

Nutrition Facts

9 servings per container
Serving size 1 cup (30g)

Amount per serving

	Cheerios	% DV**	with 1/2 cup skim milk	% DV**
Calories	110		150	
Total Fat	2g*	3%	2g*	3%
Saturated Fat	0g	0%	0.6g	3%
Trans Fat	0g		0g	
Cholesterol	0mg	0%	3g	1%
Sodium	280mg	12%	350mg	15%
Total Carbohydrate	22g	7%	28g	9%
Dietary Fiber	3g	11%	3g	11%
Total Sugars	1g		7g	
Includes Added Sugars	1g	2%	1g	2%
Protein	3g		7g	
Vitamin D	1mcg	10%	2.5mcg	25%
Calcium	40mg	4%	200mg	20%
Iron	8mg	45%	8mg	45%
Potassium	0mg	0%	300mg	45%
Vitamin A	150mcg	10%	225mcg	15%
Vitamin C	6mg	10%	6mg	10%
Thiamin	.4g	25%	.5g	30%
Riboflavin	.5mg	25%	.6mg	35%
Niacin	5mg	25%	5mg	25%
Vitamin B6	.5mg	25%	.5mg	25%
Folic Acid	400mcg	50%	400mcg	50%*
Vitamin B12	1µg	25%	2µg	35%
Phosphorus	100mg	10%	250mg	25%
Zinc	4mg	25%	5mg	30%
Copper	.04mg	2%	.04mg	2%

* Amount in Cereal. A serving of cereal plus skim milk provides 2g total fat (0.5g saturated fat, 1g monosaturated fat). less than 5mg cholesterol, 350mg sodium, 300mg potassium, 28g total carbohydrate (7g sugars) and 7g protein.
** The % Daily Value (DV) tells you how much a nutrient in a serving of food contributes to a daily diet. 2,000 calories a day is used for general nutrition advice.

Learning Portfolio

Key Terms

Study Points

- Nutritional status before pregnancy is an important part of having a healthy baby. Moreover, it is an integral part of all aspects of preconception care: risk assessment, health promotion, and intervention. Being either overweight or underweight prior to pregnancy increases the risk of complications.

- Folic acid supplementation before pregnancy has been shown to reduce the risk of neural tube defects such as spina bifida.

- Excessive intake of some vitamins (vitamin A, in particular) and use of tobacco, alcohol, and narcotic drugs increase the risk of poor pregnancy outcomes; women should discontinue these practices before they become pregnant.

- Gestation can be divided into three stages: blastogenic, embryonic, and fetal. In the blastogenic stage, the fertilized ovum begins rapid cell division and implants itself in the uterine wall. During the embryonic stage, organ systems and other body structures form. During the fetal stage, the longest period of gestation, from the ninth week to birth, the fetus grows in size and changes in proportions.

- Women who enter pregnancy at a normal BMI should gain 25 to 35 pounds during pregnancy. Underweight women should gain more weight, and overweight women less. Energy needs increase by 340 to 450 kilocalories per day for the second and third trimesters.

- By using MyPlate for Pregnancy and Breastfeeding to plan food intake, pregnant women who consume enough energy should be able to meet all their nutrient needs with the exception of iron and folate. They should get needed extra calories mainly from grains, fruits, and vegetables.

- Limiting caffeine intake during pregnancy is recommended. Smoking during pregnancy increases the risk of preterm delivery and low birth weight. Alcohol and drug use can interfere with normal fetal development and should be avoided during pregnancy.

- Gastrointestinal distress such as morning sickness, heartburn, and constipation are common during pregnancy and result from the action of various hormones on the GI tract.

- Although most food cravings or aversions present no problems, excessive consumption of nonfood items, known as pica, interferes with adequate nutrition.

- During pregnancy, hormones control the development of breast tissue in preparation for milk production. Colostrum, the first milk, which is rich in protein and antibodies, is produced soon after delivery. By two to three weeks after delivery, lactation is well established, and mature milk is being produced.

- The pituitary hormone prolactin stimulates milk production. Oxytocin, another pituitary hormone, stimulates milk release, which is known as the let-down reflex.

Learning Portfolio (continued)

- Unless they reduce their physical activity, breastfeeding women need 330 to 400 more kilocalories per day than they did when they were not pregnant. By obtaining adequate energy and using MyPlate for Pregnancy and Breastfeeding to balance choices, most lactating women can obtain all the nutrients they need from their diet.

- Cigarettes, alcohol, and illicit drugs should not be used while breastfeeding.

- Mothers benefit from breastfeeding through enhanced physiological recovery, convenience, and emotional bonding. Contraindications to breastfeeding include infection with HIV or active tuberculosis, and regular use of certain medications.

- Infants receive optimal nutrition from human milk. Breastfeeding can reduce the incidence of infectious diseases, allergies, and other problems during infancy.

- La Leche League, the March of Dimes, and the WIC program for low-income women are among the numerous resources for support and education of pregnant and breastfeeding women.

- Infancy is the fastest growth stage in the life cycle; infants double their birth weight in 4 to 6 months and triple it by 1 year of age. The nutritional status of infants is assessed primarily through measurements of growth.

- Infants' energy needs must be met through a high-fat diet, which provides the maximum calories in minimal volume. Infants' protein and fluid needs also are high.

- Human milk is low in vitamin D; breastfed babies need regular sun exposure or supplemental vitamin D. For breastfed infants, iron-fortified foods need to be introduced by 6 months of age. Formula-fed infants should be given iron-fortified formula.

- Infant formulas usually are based on either cow's milk or soy protein. Unmodified cow's milk is inappropriate for infants throughout the first year of life.

- The FDA regulates the vitamin and mineral composition of infant formulas to ensure adequate infant nutrition. Formula is available in ready-to-feed, liquid concentrate, and powdered forms.

- A nurturing environment is important to the feeding of infants, no matter what the milk source.

- Solid foods are introduced to the infant one at a time, usually beginning with iron-fortified infant cereal. Potential allergens, such as cow's milk, egg whites, and wheat, should be delayed until the baby is at least 12 months old. Developmental markers, such as head and body control and the absence of the extrusion reflex, show readiness for solid foods.

- Colic, although troublesome to infant and caregiver, is not caused by diet. Iron-deficiency anemia is common in infants who lack iron-rich foods. Infants are susceptible to dehydration, especially when diarrhea is prolonged. Failure to thrive describes an infant who is not growing well; intervention can be required to correct the feeding practices of caregivers.

Study Questions

1. Describe the three stages of fetal growth.
2. What physiological changes occur in a woman during pregnancy?
3. How do the recommended intake values for calories, protein, folate, and iron change for pregnancy?
4. What contributes to morning sickness, and how can a woman minimize its effects?
5. What are the benefits of breastfeeding for the infant? For the mother?
6. Is it okay for an infant to experience weight loss immediately after birth? If an infant does lose weight, does it mean he or she is at nutritional risk?
7. How much water does a breastfed or formula-fed infant need each day?
8. Is it necessary to give breastfed infants supplements of vitamins and/or minerals? If so, which ones?
9. Describe the process for introducing solid foods into an infant's diet.
10. List the feeding problems that can occur during infancy.

Try This

For Just One Week, Can You Eat Like You're Expecting?

The purpose of this exercise is to see if you can follow the nutrition guidelines for pregnancy for just one week. Keep in mind that pregnant women attempt to do this for

38 to 40 weeks! Your goal is to reduce or eliminate caffeine, alcohol, and over-the-counter medications. Make an effort to eat according to MyPlate each day, selecting the most nutrient-dense choices from each group. You should also take a basic multivitamin/mineral tablet (in place of a woman's prenatal supplement) daily. This will ensure that you consume the amounts of vitamins and minerals recommended for pregnancy.

Costs of Infant Formula

The purpose of this exercise is to find out how much it may cost to feed an infant. An average 3-month-old baby weighs about 13 pounds (6 kilograms) and would need about 650 kilocalories per day. Using standard infant formula, this baby would need about 32 ounces of formula each day. Now, go to a grocery store and find the infant formulas. If you were to purchase ready-to-feed formula, how much would it cost to feed this baby for one day? What if you were to use concentrated liquid formula? Powdered formula?

References

1. Farahi N, Zolotor A. Recommendations for preconception counseling and care. *Am Fam Physician.* 2013;88(8):499-506.
2. Salihu HM, Mbah AK, Alio AP, et al. Low pre-pregnancy body mass index and risk of medically indicated versus spontaneous preterm singleton birth. *Eur J Obstet Gynecol Reprod Biol.* 2009;144(2):119-123.
3. Hsu WY, Wu CH, Hsieh CT, et al. Low body weight gain, low white blood cell count and high serum ferritin as markers of poor nutrition and increased risk for preterm delivery. *Asia Pac J Clin Nutr.* 2013;22(1):90-99.
4. Ramakrishnan U, Imhoff-Kunsch B, Martorell R. Maternal nutrition interventions to improve maternal, newborn, and child health outcomes. *Nestle Nutrition Institute Workshop Series.* 2014;78:71-80.
5. Rasmussen KM, Yaktine AL, eds. *Weight Gain During Pregnancy: Reexamining the Guidelines.* Washington, DC: National Academies Press; 2009.
6. Ibid.
7. Ibid.
8. Kaar JL, Crume T, Brinton JT, et al. Maternal obesity, gestational weight gain, and offspring adiposity: the Exploring Perinatal Outcomes Among Children Study. *J Pediatr.* 2014;165(3):509-515.
9. Centers for Disease Control and Prevention. Folic acid. http://www.cdc.gov/ncbddd/folicacid/index.html. Accessed September 17, 2017.
10. U.S. Preventive Services Task Force. Folic acid to prevent neural tube defects: preventive medication. 2017. https://www.uspreventiveservicestaskforce.org/Page/Document/UpdateSummaryFinal/folic-acid-for-the-prevention-of-neural-tube-defects-preventive-medication. Accessed September 17, 2017.
11. Centers for Disease Control and Prevention. Folic acid. Op cit.
12. Lum KJ, Sundaram R, Buck Louis GM. Women's lifestyle behaviors while trying to become pregnant: evidence supporting preconception guidance. *Am J Obstet Gynecol.* 2011;205(3):203.e1-203.e7.
13. Rasmussen KM, Yaktine AL, eds. Op. cit.
14. Effects of interventions in pregnancy on maternal weight and obstetric outcomes: meta-analysis of randomised evidence. *BMJ.* 2012;344:e0288. doi: 10.1136/bmj.e2088
15. Blomberg M. Maternal and neonatal outcomes among obese women with weight gain below the new Institute of Medicine recommendations. 2011;117(5):1065-1070. doi: 10.1097/AOG.0b013e318214f1d1 http://journals.lww.com/greenjournal/Abstract/2011/05000/Maternal_and_Neonatal_Outcomes_Among_Obese_Women.7.aspx. Accessed September 17, 2017.
16. Ibid.
17. Ibid.
18. Ibid.
19. Institute of Medicine, Food and Nutrition Board. *Dietary Reference Intakes for Energy, Carbohydrate, Fiber, Fat, Fatty Acids, Cholesterol, Protein, and Amino Acids.* Washington, DC: National Academies Press; 2005. https://www.nap.edu/read/10490. Accessed May 13, 2017.
20. Ibid.
21. Procter S, Campbell C. Position of the Academy of Nutrition and Dietetics: nutrition and lifestyle for a healthy pregnancy outcome. *J Acad Nutr Diet.* 2014;114(7):1099-1103.
22. U.S. Preventive Services Task Force. Folic acid supplementation for the prevention of neural tube defects. U.S. Preventive Services Task Force Recommendation Statement. *JAMA.* 2017;317(2):183-189.
23. U.S. Department of Agriculture. Moms/moms-to-be. http://www.choosemyplate.gov/moms-pregnancy-breastfeeding. Accessed September 17, 2017.
24. Institute of Medicine, Food and Nutrition Board. Op. cit.
25. National Institutes of Health, Office of Dietary Supplements. Dietary supplement fact sheets. http://ods.od.nih.gov. Accessed September 17, 2017.
26. U.S. Department of Health and Human Services, U.S. Department of Agriculture. *2015–2020 Dietary Guidelines for Americans.* 8th ed. Washington, DC: U.S. Government Printing Office; December 2015.
27. U.S. Food and Drug Administration, Environmental Protection Agency. Eating fish: what pregnant women and parents should know. August 17, 2017. https://www.fda.gov/Food/FoodborneIllnessContaminants/Metals/ucm393070.htm. Accessed September 17, 2017.
28. Higdon JV, Frei B. Coffee and health: a review of recent human research. *Crit Rev Food Sci Nutr.* 2006;46:101-123.
29. Greenwood DC, Alwan N, Boylan S, et al. Caffeine intake during pregnancy, late miscarriage and stillbirth. *Eur J Epidemiol.* 2010;25(4):275-280.
30. Browne ML, Hoyt AT, Feldkamp ML, et al. Maternal caffeine intake and risk of selected birth defects in the National Birth Defects Prevention Study. *Birth Defects Res A Clin Mol Teratol.* 2011;91(2):93-101.
31. Maslova E, Bhattacharya S, Lin SW, Michels KB. Caffeine consumption during pregnancy and risk of preterm birth: a meta-analysis. *Am J Clin Nutr.* 2010;92(5):1120-1132.
32. Academy of Nutrition and Dietetics. Procter S, Campbell C. Op. cit.
33. Phelan S. Smoking cessation in pregnancy. *Obstet Gynecol Clin North Am.* 2014;4(2):255-266.
34. Ungerer M, Knezovich J, Ramsay M. In utero alcohol exposure, epigenetic changes, and their consequences. *Alcohol Res.* 2013;35(1):37-46.
35. March of Dimes. Street drugs and pregnancy. http://www.marchofdimes.org/pregnancy/street-drugs-and-pregnancy.aspx. Accessed September 17, 2017.
36. Young SL. Pica in pregnancy: new ideas about an old condition. *Ann Rev Nutr.* 2010;21:30:403-422.
37. Tande DL, Ralph JL, Johnson LK, et al. First trimester dietary intake, biochemical measures, and subsequent gestational hypertension among nulliparous women. *J Midwifery Women Health.* 2013;58(4):423-430.
38. American Pregnancy Association. HIV and AIDS in pregnancy. http://americanpregnancy.org/pregnancy-complications/hiv-aids-during-pregnancy/. Accessed September 17, 2017.
39. U.S. Department of Health and Human Services, National Institutes of Health, National Institute of Allergy and Infectious Diseases.

Learning Portfolio (continued)

Family planning. http://www.health.ri.gov/diseases/hivaids/about/stayinghealthy/. Accessed May 13, 2017.

40. Centers for Disease Control and Prevention. Reproductive health: teen pregnancy. http://www.cdc.gov/TeenPregnancy/index.htm. Accessed September 17, 2017.

41. Ibid.

42. U.S. Department of Health and Human Services. Healthy People 2020. Maternal, infant, and child health. https://www.healthypeople.gov/2020/topics-objectives/topic/maternal-infant-and-child-health. Accessed September 17, 2017.

43. Ibid.

44. Centers for Disease Control and Prevention. Breastfeeding report card—United States, 2016. https://www.cdc.gov/breastfeeding/pdf/2016breastfeedingreportcard.pdf. Accessed September 18, 2017.

45. Office of the Surgeon General, Centers for Disease Control and Prevention, Office on Women's Health. *The Surgeon General's Call to Action to Support Breastfeeding*. Rockville, MD: Office of the Surgeon General; 2011. https://www.ncbi.nlm.nih.gov/books/NBK52687/. Accessed September 18, 2017.

46. Institute of Medicine, Food and Nutrition Board. Op. cit.

47. Statement from Surgeon General Dr. Regina M. Benjamin on World Breastfeeding Week, August 1–7, 2011. Press release. August 1, 2011.

48. National Institutes of Health, Office of Dietary Supplements. Vitamin B12: dietary supplement fact sheet. http://ods.od.nih.gov/factsheets/VitaminB12-HealthProfessional. Accessed September 18, 2017.

49. U.S. Department of Agriculture. Health & nutrition programs for pregnant & breastfeeding women. https://www.nutrition.gov/subject/life-stages/women/pregnancy. Accessed October 3, 2017.

50. American Academy of Pediatrics policy statement. Breastfeeding and the use of human milk. *Pediatrics*. 2012;115(2):496-506. http://pediatrics.aappublications.org/content/early/2012/02/22/peds.2011-3552. Accessed September 23, 2017.

51. Ibid.

52. Academy of Nutrition and Dietetics. Position of the Academy of Nutrition and Dietetics: promoting and supporting breastfeeding. *J Acad Nutr Diet*. 2015;115:444-449.

53. Bartick M, Reinhold A. The burden of suboptimal breastfeeding in the United States: a pediatric cost analysis. *Pediatrics*. 2010;125(5):e1048-e1056.

54. SurgeonGeneral.gov. The surgeon general's call to action to support breastfeeding. Fact sheet. January 20, 2011. http://www.surgeongeneral.gov/topics/breastfeeding/factsheet.html. Accessed September 18, 2017.

55. National Conference of State Legislatures. Breastfeeding state laws. http://www.ncsl.org/default.aspx?tabid=14389. Accessed September 18, 2017.

56. Academy of Nutrition and Dietetics. Position of the Academy of Nutrition and Dietetics: promoting and supporting breastfeeding. Op. cit.

57. SurgeonGeneral.gov. Op. cit.

58. Centers for Disease Control and Prevention. CDC vital signs. Hospital support for breastfeeding. Preventing obesity begins in hospitals. http://www.cdc.gov/vitalsigns/BreastFeeding/?s_cid=vitalsigns_081. Accessed September 18, 2017.

59. Ibid.

60. Hogue MM, Ahmed NU, Khan FH, et al. Breastfeeding and cognitive development of children: assessment at one year of age. *Mymensingh Med J*. 2012;21(2):316-321.

61. American Academy of Pediatrics policy statement. Breastfeeding and the use of human milk. Op. cit.

62. Ibid.

63. Ballard O, Morrow AL. Human milk composition: nutrients and bioactive factors. *Pediatr Clin North Am*. 2013;60(1):49-74.

64. Hennet T, Weiss A, Borsig L. Decoding breast milk oligosaccharides. *Swiss Med Wkly*. 2014;144:w13927.

65. Hadberg IC. Barriers to breastfeeding in the WIC population. *MCN Am J Matern Child Nurs*. 2013;38(4):244-249.

66. Metallinos-Katsaras E, Gorman KS, Wilde P, Kallio J. A longitudinal study of WIC participation on household food insecurity. *Matern Child Health J.* 2011;15(5):627-633.

67. Institute of Medicine, Food and Nutrition Board. Op. cit.

68. Ibid.

69. Ibid.

70. Riordan J, Wambach K. *Breastfeeding and Human Lactation*. 4th ed. Burlington, MA: Jones & Bartlett Learning; 2010.

71. Institute of Medicine, Food and Nutrition Board. *Dietary Reference Intakes for Water, Potassium, Sodium, Chloride, and Sulfate*. Washington, DC: National Academies Press; 2005.

72. Ibid.

73. Ibid.

74. American Academy of Pediatrics policy statement. Breastfeeding and the use of human milk. Op. cit.

75. Vernacchio L, Kelly JP, Kaufman DW, Mitchell AA. Vitamin, fluoride, and iron use among US children younger than 12 years of age: results from the Slone survey, 1998–2007. *J Am Diet Assoc.* 2011;111:285-289.

76. National Treasury Employees Union. Why EPA's headquarters union of scientists opposes fluoridation. May 1, 1999. http://fluoridation.com/epa2.htm. Accessed September 18, 2017.

77. American Academy of Pediatrics policy statement. Breastfeeding and the use of human milk. Op. cit.

78. Ibid.

79. Simmer K, Patole SK, Rao SC. Long-chain polyunsaturated fatty acid supplementation in infants born at term. *Cochrane Database Syst Rev.* 2011, December 7;12.

80. Kleinman RE, Greer FR, eds. *Pediatric Nutrition*. 7th ed. Elk Grove Village, IL: American Academy of Pediatrics; 2013.

81. American Academy of Pediatrics. Ages and stages. Starting solid foods. http://www.healthychildren.org/english/ages-stages/baby/feeding-nutrition/pages/Switching-To-Solid-Foods.aspx. Accessed September 18, 2017.

82. Pac S, McMahon K, Ripple M, et al. Development of the *Start Healthy Feeding Guidelines* for infants and toddlers. *J Am Diet Assoc.* 2004;104:455-467.

83. Butte N, Cobb K, Dwyer J, et al. The *Start Healthy Feeding Guidelines* for infants and toddlers. *J Am Diet Assoc.* 2004;104:442-454.

84. Thorsdottir L, Thorisdottir AV. Whole cow's milk in early life. *Nestle Nutrition Workshop Series Pediatric Program.* 2011;67:29-40.

85. Academy of Nutrition and Dietetics. Position of the American Dietetic Association: benchmarks for nutrition in child care. *J Am Diet Assoc.* 2011;111:607-615.

86. U.S. Department of Agriculture, Food and Nutrition Service. Special Supplemental Nutrition Program for Women, Infants, and Children (WIC). Infant nutrition and feeding. http://www.nal.usda.gov/wicworks/Topics/FG/CompleteIFG.pdf. Accessed September 18, 2017.

87. Sheiham A, James WPT. A reappraisal of the quantitative relationship between sugar intake and dental caries: the need for new criteria for developing goals for sugar intake. *BMC Public Health.* 2014;14:863.

88. Ibid.

89. American Academy of Pediatric Dentistry. Policy on early childhood caries (ECC): unique challenges and treatment options. http://www.aapd.org/media/Policies_Guidelines/P_ECCUniqueChallenges.pdf. Accessed September 18, 2017.

Chapter 12

Life Cycle: From Childhood to Adulthood

Revised by Paul Insel

THINK About It

1 Were you a "picky" eater as a child? What about now?

2 What's your experience with acne and eating particular foods?

3 What behavior changes would you now consider making that would help you live longer?

4 Your grandfather lives by himself and relies on frozen foods for his nutritional needs. How do you feel about his diet?

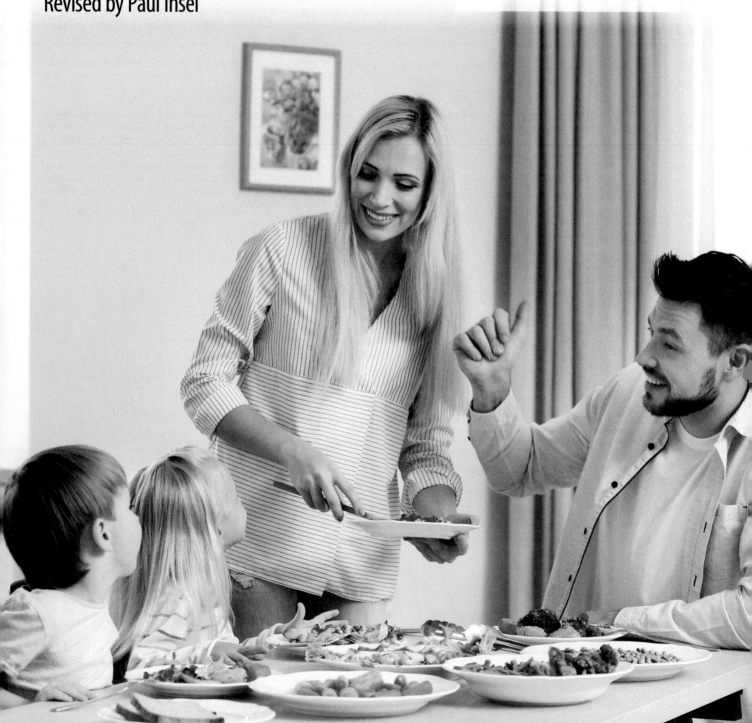

CHAPTER Menu

- Childhood
- Adolescence
- Staying Young While Growing Older

LEARNING Objectives

1 Discuss nutritional needs and concerns during childhood.

2 Discuss nutritional needs and concerns during adolescence.

3 Discuss age-related changes, nutritional needs, and concerns with aging.

4 Analyze nutrition-related issues and concerns associated with older adults.

5 Apply meal management strategies to older adults.

It's the year 2060. Who are you? Where do you live? What is your life like? How healthy are you? If projections made earlier in the century were accurate, you are part of the largest segment of the population—in 2060, between one-third and one-fourth of Americans are older than 65. Perhaps you have retired recently, or maybe you continue to work in your profession. Think about how technology has changed in your lifetime; new methods of communication have been developed that make email and the Internet seem old-fashioned, so late twentieth century!

Consider how much you have changed over the years. Throughout childhood and adolescence you were growing, sometimes quite rapidly! Whether you fueled that growth with burgers and fries, black beans and rice, chips and soft drinks, or yogurt and salads will have determined a lot about your health status in 2060. Did you continue the eating habits you had in college, and did these allow you to control your weight, blood cholesterol, and blood pressure? Or perhaps, in the year 2060, these conditions are no longer of concern. Advances in genetics may have allowed gene therapy to replace diet therapy and medications for chronic diseases.

This chapter looks at how continued growth in childhood and adolescence affects nutritional needs. In addition, we'll see how nutritional needs change as we age, and we'll consider feeding practices, meal planning, and obstacles to healthful eating for each age group.

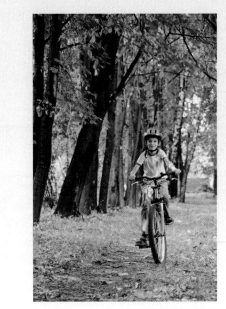

© Dmitry Naumov/Shutterstock, Inc.

Childhood

🍎 **Why Is This Important?** Challenges for caregivers during childhood include ensuring children get enough calcium and vitamin D and avoiding food wars while guiding children to choose foods that are healthful and nutritious. The serious problem of adult obesity can begin in childhood, so the importance of limiting sugar-sweetened beverages and other food behavior related to excessive weight gain should not be underestimated.

Childhood is the term that refers to the period of life spanning the years from age 1 through the beginning of **adolescence**. Growth in childhood, although continuous, occurs at a significantly slower rate than

▶ **childhood** The period of life from age 1 to the onset of puberty.

▶ **adolescence** The period between onset of puberty and adulthood.

in infancy. During the childhood years, a typical child will gain about 5 pounds and grow 2 to 3 inches each year. Children can be grouped based on their age and development: toddlers (ages 1–3), preschoolers (ages 4–5), and school-aged children (ages 6–10).

Energy and Nutrient Needs During Childhood

An average 1-year-old requires about 850 to 1,000 kilocalories per day.[1] This daily energy requirement gradually increases until it almost doubles by around age 10.

Energy and Protein

Estimated Energy Requirements (EERs) for children can be calculated based on sex, age, height, weight, and activity level. (See **TABLE 12.1**.) In contrast to the 175 kilocalories per day needed during early infancy, the added energy cost for growth during childhood is only 20 kilocalories per day.

Although total energy requirements increase, the kilocalories needed per kilogram of body weight slowly decrease as children move through childhood. The same is true for protein requirements. (See **TABLE 12.2**.)

Vitamins and Minerals

As long as a healthy child cooperates by eating a variety of healthful foods, a well-planned diet should provide most of the nutrients a child needs. One exception is iron. Children ages 4 to 8 years require

---

TABLE 12.1
Estimated Energy Requirement Equations for Children (Ages 3 Through 8)

Males

$EER = 88.5 - 61.9 \times age\ [y] + PA \times (26.7 \times weight\ [kg] + 903 \times height\ [m]) + 20\ kcal/day$
Physical activity (PA): Sedentary = 1.00; Low active = 1.13; Active = 1.26; Very active = 1.42

Females

$EER = 135.3 - 30.8 \times age\ [y] + PA \times (10.0 \times weight\ [kg] + 934 \times height\ [m]) + 20\ kcal/day$
Physical activity (PA): Sedentary = 1.00; Low active = 1.16; Active = 1.31; Very active = 1.56

Reproduced from Institute of Medicine, Food and Nutrition Board. *Dietary Reference Intakes for Energy, Carbohydrate, Fiber, Fat, Fatty Acids, Cholesterol, Protein, and Amino Acids (Macronutrients)*. Copyright © 2005 by the National Academy of Sciences, courtesy of the National Academies Press, Washington, DC.

TABLE 12.2
Protein RDAs for Childhood

Age (y)	Protein (g/kg)	Reference Weight[a] (kg)	Protein (g/day)
1–3	1.05	12	13
4–8	0.95	20	19
9–13	0.95	36	34

[a] Reference weights are based on median weights of children in that age group.

Reproduced from Institute of Medicine, Food and Nutrition Board. *Dietary Reference Intakes for Energy, Carbohydrate, Fiber, Fat, Fatty Acids, Cholesterol, Protein, and Amino Acids (Macronutrients)*. © 2005 by the National Academy of Sciences, courtesy of the National Academies Press, Washington, DC.

10 milligrams of iron per day but may not get that amount without careful meal planning.

Children should limit their consumption of sugar-sweetened beverages and calorie-dense snack foods, which are poor sources of iron. This allows room in the diet for high-iron food sources such as lean meats, legumes, fish, poultry, and iron-enriched breads and cereals. (See **TABLE 12.3**.) Iron deficiency not only affects growth, but also can impair the child's mood, attention span, focus, and ability to learn.[2,3]

Seventy percent of U.S. children do not get enough vitamin D. Among U.S. children ages 1 to 17, 7.6 million, or 9 percent, are vitamin D deficient, and another 50.8 million, or 61 percent, have insufficient levels of vitamin D.[4] A child's diet also may be low in calcium, potassium, and dietary fiber.[5] (See **FIGURE 12.1**.) U.S. children do not consistently meet the recommendations of MyPlate for the fruit, grain, and dairy groups, important sources of these nutrients.

Vitamin and Mineral Supplements

Many caregivers would rather simply give a child a multivitamin/mineral pill than plan and prepare the meals necessary to ensure an adequate diet. However, the balanced diet a child needs does not differ much from the diet an adult needs. In fact, MyPlate Kid's Place (see **FIGURE 12.2**) shows the same balance of food groups as is recommended for adults. Caregivers who understand this may be less tempted to rely on supplements and make the effort to achieve a balanced diet.

Some children should receive supplements. Among them are children whose diets are restricted for medical reasons, those with chronic diseases, those who are malnourished, and those with food allergies that require them to avoid multiple foods or food groups.[6] (For more

TABLE 12.3
Iron-Rich Foods and Snacks

Iron-Rich Foods

- Ground beef
- Poultry
- Fish
- Legumes
- Dark-green vegetables
- Protein
- Sloppy Joes
- Casseroles with meat

Iron-Rich Snacks

- Cream of wheat
- Cooked macaroni or pasta
- Enriched cereals, either dry or with milk
- Tortillas filled with refried beans
- Dried apricots
- Raisins (for older children)
- Bean dip
- Chili, mildly seasoned
- Peanut butter on enriched bread or graham crackers
- Enriched breads, cereals, rice, and pasta

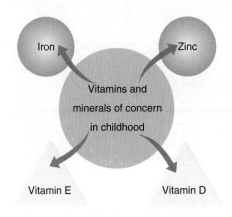

FIGURE 12.1 Micronutrients of concern in childhood.
Milk is low in iron, and small children also might have low intakes of magnesium, potassium, calcium, vitamins E and D, and zinc.

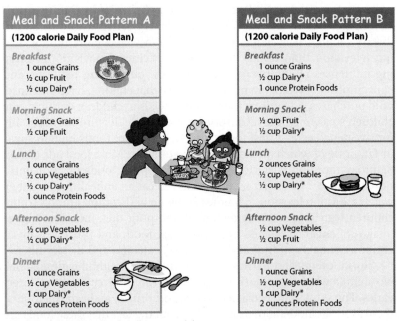

Meal and Snack Pattern A	Meal and Snack Pattern B
(1200 calorie Daily Food Plan)	**(1200 calorie Daily Food Plan)**
Breakfast 1 ounce Grains ½ cup Fruit ½ cup Dairy*	*Breakfast* 1 ounce Grains ½ cup Dairy* 1 ounce Protein Foods
Morning Snack 1 ounce Grains ½ cup Fruit	*Morning Snack* ½ cup Fruit ½ cup Dairy*
Lunch 1 ounce Grains ½ cup Vegetables ½ cup Dairy* 1 ounce Protein Foods	*Lunch* 2 ounces Grains ½ cup Vegetables ½ cup Dairy*
Afternoon Snack ½ cup Vegetables ½ cup Dairy*	*Afternoon Snack* ½ cup Vegetables ½ cup Fruit
Dinner 1 ounce Grains ½ cup Vegetables 1 cup Dairy* 2 ounces Protein Foods	*Dinner* 1 ounce Grains ½ cup Vegetables 1 cup Dairy* 2 ounces Protein Foods

*Offer your child fat-free or low-fat milk, yogurt, and cheese.

FIGURE 12.2 MyPlate Meal and Snack Patterns for a 1,200-calorie daily food plan for preschoolers. Sample patterns also are available for 1,000, 1,400, and 1,600 calories at ChooseMyPlate.com.

Reproduced from U.S. Department of Agriculture. Meal and Snack Patterns and Ideas. http://www .choosemyplate.gov/preschoolers/meal-and-snack-patterns-ideas.html. Accessed September 18, 2017.

Position Statement: Academy of Nutrition and Dietetics

Dietary Guidance for Healthy Children Ages 2 to 11 Years

It is the position of the Academy of Nutrition and Dietetics that children ages 2 to 11 years should achieve optimal physical and cognitive development, attain a healthy weight, enjoy food, and reduce the risk of chronic disease through appropriate eating habits and participation in regular physical activity.

Reprinted from *Journal of the Academy of Nutrition and Dietetics*, 114(8), Beth N. Ogata, Dayle Hayest, Position of the Academy of Nutrition and Dietetics: Nutrition Guidance for Healthy Children Ages 2 to 11 Years, Page no. 1257-1276, 2014, with permission from Elsevier.

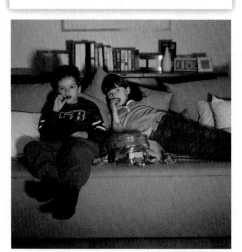

© BananaStock/age fotostock.

Position Statement: Academy of Nutrition and Dietetics

Benchmarks for Nutrition in Child Care

It is the position of the Academy of Nutrition and Dietetics that child-care programs should achieve recommended benchmarks for meeting children's nutrition needs in a safe, sanitary, and supportive environment that promotes optimal growth and development. Use of child care has become increasingly common and is now the norm for the majority of families in the United States.

Reprinted from *Journal of the American Dietetic Association*, 111(4), Sara E. Benjamin Neelon, Margaret E. Briley, Position of the American Dietetic Association: Benchmarks for Nutrition in Child Care, Page no. 607-615, 2011, with permission from Elsevier.

on food allergies, see the FYI feature "Food Hypersensitivities and Allergies.") Caregivers should be aware that vitamin and mineral supplements for children are dangerous in large doses. Like all medicines, vitamin and mineral preparations must be kept safely out of children's reach. Supplements containing iron in doses of more than 30 milligrams are especially dangerous to children. Accidental consumption of vitamin and mineral or iron supplements should be treated as a poisoning emergency.

Influences on Childhood Food Habits and Intake

Children develop food preferences at an early age. Toddlers start to exhibit unique feeding practices and styles. For some, this means that one food cannot touch another, or that foods cannot be green, or that all foods must be green. All these "preferences" are merely the toddler's way of exhibiting control over his or her environment while experimenting and exploring. Although this stage may seem to last an eternity to even the most patient caregiver, the food habits explored during this time are usually temporary. The wise caregiver allows this process to occur naturally, rather than wage food battles that the child ultimately wins. Nutrition professionals advocate feeding practices in which caregivers are responsible for positive structure, age-appropriate support, and healthful food and beverage choices. Within reason, children are responsible for whether and how much to eat. This division of responsibility promotes self-regulation of energy intake.[7]

THINK
About It

1

More and more children spend time in organized daycare settings. In these early years, child-care workers are playing an increasingly important role in the development of children's health and nutritional habits.[8]

As a child's environment expands, an increasing number of external factors influence the child's diet. Sedentary behavior in children, such as long periods of television watching, is associated with unhealthful dietary habits.[9] It is estimated that children spend more time watching television than doing most other activities. Television advertising influences children's food preferences, purchasing requests, and consumption.[10] Recognizing the influence that children have on household purchases, advertisers focus commercials at children during prime children's viewing hours. Cartoons, for example, feature countless ads for sweetened cereals, fast foods, candy, and other foods high in sugar or fat, none of which are necessary or desirable. Most food ads during Saturday morning television programming push foods of poor nutritional quality.[11] Children are more likely to eat an unhealthy diet if they watch a lot of television.[12] Studies show an association among young children watching morning television and poor diet, including higher intakes of sugar-sweetened beverages, fast food, and processed meat, and lower intakes of fruit and vegetables, calcium, and dietary fiber.[13]

Social events and parties often promote unhealthful eating habits. No matter what the occasion, the menu for children's parties rarely varies. The staples are pizza, ice cream, soft drinks, and candy. None of these foods in moderation is a problem, but the fact that these foods are offered at the majority of social gatherings is. Popular snacks and beverages also tend to be too high in sugar and fat. Serving more healthful but still child-friendly snacks, such as those in **TABLE 12.4**, breaks this tradition.

Who has the most important influence on the development of healthful eating habits? Parents![14] Parents not only are models for

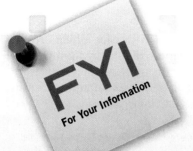

Food Hypersensitivities and Allergies

Proteins that trigger allergies are known as *allergens*. Food allergies, or food hypersensitivities, are allergic reactions to food proteins. Allergies are different from food intolerances (such as lactose intolerance), which involve digestive problems rather than an immune response. Allergies are less likely than intolerances to be transient, and they tend to have more serious consequences. The most common food allergens are found in milk, eggs, tree nuts, peanuts, soy, wheat, fish, and shellfish.

Food allergies occur when the immune system mounts a specific reaction to a food protein. About 25 percent of people in the general population believe they suffer from food allergies. According to Food Allergy Research and Education (FARE), 1 in 13 children in the United States has a food allergy, and about 30 percent of children with food allergies are allergic to more than one food.[a] In a true allergic reaction, the immune system responds to an allergen with a cascade of chemical reactions that can cause wheezing, difficulty breathing, and hives as well as a host of other symptoms. (See **TABLE A**.) Food allergy symptoms often affect more than one body system and may change in severity from one reaction to the next.

Anaphylaxis, the most severe allergic reaction, usually takes place within the first hour after eating the offending food. Shock and respiratory failure can rapidly ensue. Anaphylaxis can be fatal, so immediate emergency care is essential.

Allergy symptoms that occur immediately after a food is eaten make detective work easier. If symptoms are slow to evolve, a child may suffer chronic diarrhea and even experience failure to thrive before the problem is identified.

When identification of the food culprit isn't so obvious, an elimination diet can help. All suspected foods are eliminated from the diet and slowly reintroduced, one by one, on a specific schedule. Both intake and reactions are carefully recorded. Prolonged or improper use of such a diet can have severe nutritional consequences. A registered dietitian nutritionist can help with diet planning to ensure nutritional adequacy.

The double-blind, placebo-controlled food challenge is the gold standard of food allergy testing. Although definitive, it can be dangerous for people prone to anaphylactic reactions. In this test, increasing amounts of a suspected food are given to the child under the supervision of a physician, who looks for allergy symptoms and signs. This test must be done by trained personnel with emergency equipment handy.

The treatment for food allergy is avoidance of the offending allergen. Each child with a food allergy needs a nutrition assessment that pays attention to the specific nutrients missing from the diet because the child avoids the offending foods. For example, if a toddler is avoiding milk and milk products because of a cow's milk allergy, the nutrients most at risk would be protein, vitamin D, and calcium. As a child's diet includes more and more foods, careful label reading is the key to identifying allergen-containing foods. Organizations such as the Food Allergy and Anaphylaxis Network (FAAN) provide materials for deciphering food labels. FAAN also offers tips for successful traveling and dining with a child who has food allergies.

Some children naturally outgrow food allergies by the time they are 3 years old.[b] Allergies to milk, egg, wheat, and soy can resolve in childhood, but many children remain allergic after 5 years of age. However, allergies to peanuts, tree nuts, fish, and shellfish are generally not outgrown.

a Food Allergy Research & Education. Facts and statistics. https://www.foodallergy.org/facts-and-stats. Accessed September 18, 2017.
b Ibid.

TABLE A
Symptoms of Food Allergies
Gastrointestinal Tract
• Itching of the lips, mouth, and throat
• Swelling of the throat
• Abdominal cramping and distention
• Diarrhea
• Colic
• Gastrointestinal bleeding
• Protein-losing enteropathy
Skin
• Hives
• Swelling
• Eczema, contact dermatitis
Respiratory Tract
• Runny or stuffed-up nose, sneezing, and postnasal discharge
• Recurrent croup
• Chronic pneumonia
• Middle-ear infections
Systemic
• Anaphylaxis
• Heart rhythm irregularities
• Low blood pressure

TABLE 12.4
Healthy Snacks

- Cereal and milk
- Yogurt shake: plain yogurt, fresh fruit
- Popcorn sprinkled with Parmesan cheese
- Fresh vegetables and a yogurt dip
- Pretzels
- Peanut butter on celery
- Bananas with peanut butter
- Graham crackers and peanut butter
- Sliced apples with cheese
- Bagel and melted cheese
- Bran muffins
- Pumpkin, banana, or zucchini bread
- Mini pizza on English muffin
- Homemade pita pocket sandwiches
- Yogurt with fresh fruit or granola
- Vegetable soup
- Fresh fruit
- Colored peppers and hummus
- Cucumbers with plain yogurt
- Cheese and whole-grain crackers

children's eating behaviors, but also can make it easier for children to accept new foods. Parents can offer a variety of healthy food choices that help ensure that their children get all the nutrients they need from each food group. Eating healthy meals together as a family has also been found to reduce the risk of obesity in children.[15]

Key Concepts Children grow at a slower rate than they did as infants but still gain 2 to 3 inches and about 5 pounds per year. They should be able to obtain adequate energy and nutrients from their meals and snacks. Iron-deficiency anemia is the most common nutritional deficiency among U.S. children. Many children in the United States also do not get enough calcium and vitamin D. Sugar-sweetened beverages and high-calorie snacks fail to provide needed nutrients and contribute to obesity. Outside influences, such as television viewing, affect children's preferences for foods with low nutrient density. Parents are the most important influence on the food habits of their children.

Nutritional Concerns of Childhood

The major challenges to promoting healthful childhood nutrition are combating malnutrition and hunger, chronic disease, overweight, lead toxicity, food and behavior, and nutrition concerns regarding vegetarian practices.

Malnutrition and Hunger in Childhood

Of all issues facing children with respect to growth and nutrition, none is so devastating as hunger and malnutrition. Throughout the world, approximately 50 percent of the deaths of young children can be attributed to undernutrition.[16] Deficiencies in vitamin A, zinc, iron, and protein also result in illness, stunted growth, limited development, and, in the case of vitamin A, possibly permanent blindness. In the United States, in 2015, 3 million households failed at times to provide adequate, nutritious food for their children.[17]

By creating a safety net, federal programs help to protect young children from substantial reductions in food intake. The U.S. Department of Agriculture (USDA) has 15 nutrition assistance programs that address hunger, including the Supplemental Nutrition Assistance Program (SNAP)—formerly the Food Stamp Program—the National School Breakfast and Lunch Programs, and the Special Supplemental Nutrition Program for Women, Infants, and Children (WIC). (See **FIGURE 12.3**.) For many children, the meals provided through the National School Lunch, Breakfast, and Summer Food Service Programs are the major—and, in some cases, the only—sources of calories and other nutrients. Those who plan and serve meals have the challenge of balancing popular foods that children will eat with foods that provide good nutrition. To ensure that the nutritional needs of the more than 31 million children receiving meals through school lunch programs are met, the Child Nutrition Reauthorization Healthy Hunger-Free Kids Act of 2010 represents a national effort to provide children with healthier and more nutritious food choices.[18] The main objectives of the Healthy Hunger-Free Kids Act focus on improving nutrition and reducing childhood obesity, increasing access to school meal programs, and increasing monitoring and the integrity of school meal programs.[19]

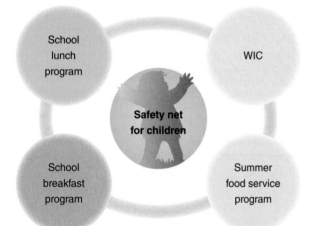

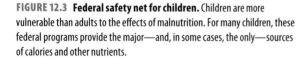

FIGURE 12.3 Federal safety net for children. Children are more vulnerable than adults to the effects of malnutrition. For many children, these federal programs provide the major—and, in some cases, the only—sources of calories and other nutrients.

Food and Behavior

The term **hyperactivity** describes an abnormal increase in activity that is maladaptive and inconsistent with developmental level. Although

▶ **hyperactivity** A maladaptive and abnormal increase in activity that is inconsistent with developmental levels. Includes frequent fidgeting, inappropriate running, excessive talking, and difficulty engaging in quiet activities.

hyperactivity has often been attributed to high sugar intake, most studies have failed to support a relationship between them.

Attention-deficit hyperactivity disorder (ADHD) is characterized by inattentive, hyperactive, and impulsive behavior that is unrestrained and frenetic. ADHD is estimated to affect 5 percent of children worldwide.[20] Genetic and environmental factors are both involved in the etiology of ADHD. Sugar and certain food additives, including preservatives and colorings, have all been thought to cause or exacerbate behavioral disorders. Many parents and caregivers often blame sugar for "hyper" behavior in children. However, this association has not been clearly demonstrated.[21] Although the cause remains controversial, studies do suggest that certain food colorings and additives enhance hyperactive behaviors in some children. Further research is needed.[22,23] For some children, ADHD can be triggered by various foods, and a diet that eliminates these foods has been shown to produce a favorable response in sensitive children.[24]

Caffeine products can make children jittery and interfere with their sleep. Because children have small body sizes, the effects of a caffeinated beverage are intensified. Many soft drinks are high in caffeine; examples include Mountain Dew (55 milligrams per 12-oz can), Surge (51 milligrams per 12-oz can), and Coca-Cola (37 milligrams per 12-oz can). Popular energy drinks can also be substantial sources of caffeine.

Childhood Overweight

In the United States, overweight in childhood is increasing at an alarming rate. Approximately 32 percent (nearly 1 in 3) of children ages 2 to 19 years are overweight (body mass index in the 85th to 94th percentile) or obese (body mass index at or above the 95th percentile).[25] An overweight child is likely to reach maturity earlier than a child of normal weight, but perhaps at the expense of height. Some overweight children already deal with the cardiovascular consequences of obesity, such as lipid abnormalities and hypertension, and many overweight children develop type 2 diabetes prior to the teen years. Finally, overweight children are likely to have social and academic problems[26] and experience the psychological trauma associated with obesity in our culture. Factors involved in the development of overweight in childhood include genetics, environment, behavior, and activity levels. (See **FIGURE 12.4**.)

Programs designed to treat childhood obesity generally provide behavior modification, exercise counseling, psychological support or therapy, family counseling, and family meal-planning advice. In some cases, the goal is not weight loss, but rather to allow the child's height to catch up with his or her weight. Instead of restricting caloric intake or food choices, the first strategy is usually to increase physical activity and improve food choices. To meet the challenge of childhood obesity and direct children toward healthy, active lifestyles, the White House Task Force on Childhood Obesity launched a comprehensive campaign, called Let's Move![27] Let's Move! aims to end childhood obesity within a generation with strategies that include providing parents with helpful information, creating environments that support healthy choices, providing healthier foods in schools, ensuring that every family has access to healthy and affordable foods, and helping children become more physically active.[28]

Nutrition and Chronic Disease in Childhood

When is it appropriate to adopt adult dietary guidelines for children? It is well documented that early signs of chronic disease can appear in

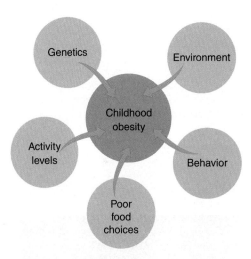

FIGURE 12.4 Factors that contribute to childhood obesity. Childhood obesity is on the rise and predisposes children to health problems when they become adults.

Quick Bite

Are Minority Children at High Risk for Cardiovascular Disease?

Early risk factors for cardiovascular disease are increasing in the United States. African American and Mexican American children are more likely to exhibit high blood pressure and high body mass index and to consume a higher percentage of calories from fat than are Caucasian children. The three ethnic groups have similar blood cholesterol levels, however, and Caucasian children are more likely to smoke.

Quick Bite

Television Tubbies

The number of obese children in the United States has doubled in the past 20 years, and one in five U.S. children is now overweight. Today's kids spend more time watching television and playing video games than engaging in physical activity. Advertisers know it. When programs for children are broadcast, 80 percent of commercials advertise food, most of it high in sugar and fat.

childhood. Evidence of early plaque development has been seen in the coronary arteries of adolescents and is associated with adult cardiovascular diseases. However, the low-fat, high-fiber diet advocated for adults can jeopardize a very young child's growth. Infants and toddlers younger than 2 years old need fat in their diets for growth, organ protection, and central nervous system development. Dietary restrictions at this age are not appropriate.

For children older than 2 years, however, efforts to lower sugar and saturated fat intake can reduce risks of chronic disease. Dietary choices in line with the *2015–2020 Dietary Guidelines for Americans* are recommended. But it's important that parents and caregivers not misinterpret the recommendations and restrict children's energy intake. During the preschool and school years, gradual changes can bring food choices in line with the *Dietary Guidelines for Americans.* Caregivers should offer children healthful choices and, as they grow, educate them about proper nutrition.

Because of the rising rates of childhood obesity and incidence of chronic diseases related to weight, the American Academy of Pediatrics (AAP) now recommends screening children who have a positive family history of abnormal blood lipids or premature cardiovascular disease for blood lipid abnormalities.[29] For those children with high levels of low-density lipoprotein (LDL) cholesterol, lifestyle interventions such as changes in diet and physical activity are recommended. In some circumstances, medication may be warranted.

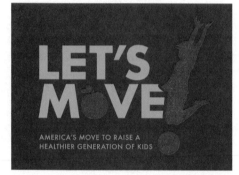

Courtesy of Let's Move!.

Lead Toxicity

Reducing elevated blood lead levels among children is one of the Healthy People 2020 objectives.[30] The Centers for Disease Control and Prevention (CDC) reports that the percentage of children with elevated levels (equal to or greater than 10 micrograms per deciliter) dropped significantly, from 7.61 percent in 1997 to 0.50 percent in 2015.[31] Lead toxicity can result in slow growth and iron-deficiency anemia and can damage the brain and central nervous system, leading to a host of learning disabilities and behavior problems. Increased blood lead levels are associated with reduced IQ, even at levels less than the CDC's reference value of 5 micrograms per deciliter.[32]

Lead is present in the plumbing of old homes, old paint, house dust in homes with cracked or peeling lead-based paint, and, in some areas, the soil. Children can ingest lead by drinking contaminated water, eating paint chips, or sucking their fingers after playing in or around lead-contaminated house dust or soil. Lead toxicity occurs more frequently in areas of poverty, where lead contamination is more common and where iron-deficiency anemia is present.

Low intake of iron, calcium, and zinc tend to result in increased lead absorption. Children with an adequate intake of these micronutrients show less incidence of lead toxicity. Therefore, many programs established to reduce the incidence of lead toxicity in children also promote good nutrition, with an emphasis on adequate iron, calcium, and zinc consumption.

Vegetarianism in Childhood

Well-planned lacto-vegetarian, lacto-ovo-vegetarian, and vegan diets can satisfy the nutrient needs of children.[33] Vegetarian children have lower intakes of total fat, saturated fat, and cholesterol, and higher intakes of fruits, vegetables, and fiber. Sources of calcium, iron, zinc, vitamin B_{12},

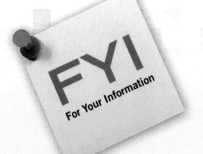

Farmers' Markets

Farmers' markets serve up a fresh harvest for those of us who don't have gardens. Direct from the grower, the produce of farmers' markets supports healthy lifestyles by offering unique varieties of fresh, nutritious food at the peak of flavor. By increasing children's access to fresh fruits and vegetables, these markets promote child health and reduce childhood obesity.

Patrons can redeem vouchers for the Women, Infants, and Children (WIC) and Senior Farmers' Market Nutrition Program (SFMNP) at participating markets, thus providing fresh fruits and vegetables to more than 2.3 million low-income families and more than 817,751 low-income seniors.[a] Many farmers' markets also accept electronic benefit transfer (EBT) cards that accompany the Supplemental Nutrition Assistance Program (formerly known as the Food Stamp Program). They also donate hundreds of thousands of pounds of unsold, fresh produce to food banks, shelters, and other social service agencies.

Farmers' markets support small family farms and preserve America's rural landscapes. They maintain opportunities for farmers, promote diversity, preserve agricultural land from overdevelopment, and keep farmers farming. Farmers' markets strengthen communities and stimulate local economies by creating jobs, reducing the distance food travels, and making local food affordable.

a U.S. Department of Agriculture, Food and Nutrition Service. Senior Farmers' Market Nutrition Program. http://www.fns.usda.gov/sfmnp/overview. Accessed September 18, 2017.

U.S. Department of Agriculture, Food and Nutrition Service. Senior Farmers' Market Nutrition Program. http://www.fns.usda.gov/sfmnp/overview. Accessed May 18, 2017.

and vitamin D need to be emphasized, especially for children following vegan diets. For a vegan child, legumes and nuts should be substituted for meats, and calcium- and vitamin B_{12}–fortified soy or almond milk can be substituted for cow's milk. Because of the risks associated with direct sunlight exposure, current AAP guidelines advocate decreasing sunlight exposure,[34] recommending daily intake of 400 IU of vitamin D per day for all infants beginning in the first few days of life. Children and adolescents who do not get regular sunlight exposure or drink at least 32 ounces of vitamin D–fortified milk each day should take supplemental vitamin D daily.[35]

> *Overweight in Children*
>
> The American Heart Association suggests that overweight children are more likely to be overweight adults. Successfully preventing or treating overweight in childhood may reduce the risk of adult overweight. This may help reduce the risk of heart disease and other diseases.
>
> Reproduced from American Heart Association, Inc.

Key Concepts Hunger and malnutrition affect a significant number of our nation's children. To combat the growing number of hungry children, programs such as WIC, SNAP, and the National School Breakfast and Lunch Programs are vital. Other concerns common to childhood include overweight, lead toxicity, and chronic disease prevention. Infants and toddlers should not be given low-fat, high-fiber diets; when children reach the age of 2, caregivers should begin to adjust children's diets to follow appropriate dietary guidelines. For vegetarian children, dietary sources of calcium, iron, zinc, vitamin D, and vitamin B_{12} require special attention.

Adolescence

🍎 **Why Is This Important?** Understanding common adolescent behaviors can give insight into some of the nutritional concerns specific to this life stage. For example, as teens replace milk with soft drinks, they reduce their calcium and vitamin D intake. Also, teens who spend a great deal of their free time online or texting instead of engaging in physical activity are at greater risk for obesity.

Adolescents seem to add inches overnight. Many caregivers complain that they cannot keep enough food in the house to satisfy an adolescent's appetite. Adolescence commonly is defined as the time between the onset of **puberty** and adulthood. This maturation process involves both physical growth and emotional maturation.

▶ **puberty** The period of life during which the secondary sex characteristics develop and the ability to reproduce is attained.

Physical Growth and Development

Hormones drive growth, which varies from child to child. In general, growth spurts begin between ages 10 and 12 for girls and between ages 12 and 14 for boys.[36] This spurt, or period of maximal growth, lasts about two years.

Height

The first phase of adolescent growth is linear. On average, boys grow 8 inches and girls grow 6 inches during puberty. This growth is uneven. The hands and feet enlarge first. The calves and forearms lengthen next, followed by expansion of the hips, chest, shoulders, and trunk. As a result, adolescents often appear awkward or clumsy. After the main growth spurt, growth continues for two to three years, but at a much slower rate.

▶ **menarche** First menstrual period.

For girls, peak growth occurs about one year before **menarche**, the onset of menstruation. A typical girl has achieved about 95 percent of her adult height by menarche and grows only 2 to 4 inches during the remainder of adolescence. Growth rates are closely related to sexual maturation, reflected in breast development (girls), change of voice (boys), development of sexual organs, and growth of pubic hair. When the growth plates at the ends of the long bones (**epiphyses**) close, skeletal growth is complete. This is a critical point in development. An adolescent who is malnourished and of small stature at the point of epiphyseal closure may not achieve his or her full potential height.

▶ **epiphyses** The heads of the long bones that are separated from the shaft of the bone until the bone stops growing.

Weight

The second growth phase of adolescence involves lateral growth. Here, the adolescent "fills out," or gains weight. External factors such as diet and exercise affect weight gain more than linear growth, so weight gain can vary widely among adolescents. However, a typical healthy girl will gain 35 pounds during adolescence; a typical boy will gain 45 pounds. In our weight-sensitive society, adolescents should be prepared for this normal, expected weight gain. Although the bulk of an adolescent's lateral growth occurs after the linear growth spurt, a significant portion of the two growth stages overlap. For girls, for example, peak weight gain usually occurs around the time of menarche.

Body Composition

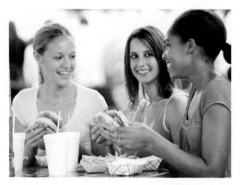

© iStockphoto/Thinkstock.

Before puberty, the body composition of boys and girls does not differ greatly. This changes dramatically during adolescence. Boys experience greater increases in lean body mass, resulting in more obvious muscle definition. Girls accumulate greater stores of body fat, specifically around the hips and buttocks, upper arms, breasts, and upper back.

Emotional Maturity: Developmental Tasks

Adolescence is a time not only of great physical growth, but also of tremendous emotional growth. This psychological development affects food choices, eating habits, and body image. Many teens become more interested in the healthful aspects of nutrition. Others experiment with unhealthful food choices, as an exercise in independence or in an attempt to achieve an idealized body.

Nutrient Needs of Adolescents

Although growth, not age, should be the ultimate indicator of nutrient needs, Daily Reference Intakes (DRIs) are established based on age.

TABLE 12.5
Estimated Energy Requirement Equations for Adolescence (Ages 9 Through 18)

Males

EER = 88.5 − 61.9 × age [y] + PA × (26.7 × weight [kg] + 903 × height [m]) + 25 kcal/day
Physical activity (PA): Sedentary = 1.00; Low active = 1.13; Active = 1.26; Very active = 1.42

Females

EER = 135.3 − 30.8 × age [y] + PA × (10.0 × weight [kg] + 934 × height [m]) + 25 kcal/day
Physical activity (PA): Sedentary = 1.00; Low active = 1.16; Active = 1.31; Very active = 1.56

Reproduced from Institute of Medicine, Food and Nutrition Board. *Dietary Reference Intakes for Energy, Carbohydrate, Fiber, Fat, Fatty Acids, Cholesterol, Protein, and Amino Acids (Macronutrients)*. © 2005 by the National Academy of Sciences, courtesy of the National Academies Press, Washington, DC.

Separate recommendations for males and females reflect the differences in growth rates and body composition during adolescence.

Energy and Protein

With the exception of pregnancy and lactation, energy needs are greater during adolescence than at any other time of life. Equations used to calculate Estimated Energy Requirements (EERs) are the same as for children, except for the added energy factor for growth, which is higher for adolescents. (See **TABLE 12.5**.) Recommended energy intakes are guidelines only; adjustments often are needed to meet individual requirements.

To support growth, an adolescent's protein needs per unit body weight are higher than an adult's, but less than a rapidly growing infant's. (See **TABLE 12.6**.) By age 14 to 18, the protein RDA has declined nearly to adult levels (as g/kg body weight), reflecting the end of linear growth for most teens. American teens rarely have a problem with adequate protein intake, but teen girls risk a lack of protein if they cut calories too drastically in attempts to control weight.

Vitamins and Minerals

Along with increased needs for energy and protein, adolescents have higher vitamin and mineral needs compared with people at most other life stages. Vitamin A, vitamin D, calcium, and iron all play an important role in the growth and development of adolescents. (See **FIGURE 12.5**.)

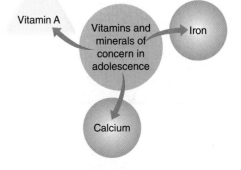

FIGURE 12.5 Micronutrients of concern in adolescence. Vitamin A is important for growth, and calcium and vitamin D are essential for building strong bones. Teen girls especially need adequate iron intake to replace iron lost during menstruation.

TABLE 12.6
Protein RDAs for Adolescence

Age (years)	Protein (g/kg)	Reference Weight[a] (kg)	Protein (g/day)
14–18, female	0.85	54	46
14–18, male	0.85	61	52

[a] Reference weights are based on median weights for that sex and age group.

Reproduced from Institute of Medicine, Food and Nutrition Board. *Dietary Reference Intakes for Energy, Carbohydrate, Fiber, Fat, Fatty Acids, Cholesterol, Protein, and Amino Acids (Macronutrients)*. © 2005 by the National Academy of Sciences, courtesy of the National Academies Press, Washington, DC.

Teens can improve their vitamin A intake by eating more fruits and vegetables. Adequate calcium and vitamin D are essential for bone formation, and maximal bone density can be hard to obtain if diets are deficient in these nutrients. Many teens, especially girls, actually reduce their calcium and vitamin D intake by replacing the milk in their diets with soft drinks. During puberty, adolescents gain 15 percent of their full adult height and accumulate half their ultimate adult bone mass. Adolescents who do not achieve sufficient bone density have a greater risk of developing osteoporosis later in life. The RDA for calcium for adolescents ages 9 to 18 years is 1,300 milligrams per day, and the RDA for vitamin D is 600 IU every day.[37] Fortified milk and dairy products are rich in these nutrients and convenient to eat; without these or other fortified products, meeting the recommended intake is difficult.

Adolescent boys need added iron to support growth of muscle and lean body mass. Teenage girls need added iron to replace what is lost in blood during menstruation. The recommended iron intake for boys ages 14 to 18 years is 11 milligrams per day; for teen girls, it is 15 milligrams per day. As long as they take in enough calories, both groups should be able to obtain this iron from nutrient-dense foods. During adolescence, however, food selection often is less than optimal. Careful meal planning is required to maximize teenagers' iron consumption.

Influences on Adolescent Food Intake

Teenagers want to choose and purchase their own food, and some may want to take over preparing it as well. Although parents can set an example of healthy eating patterns, their influence becomes weaker. In contrast, the influence of the food industry becomes stronger, as they market foods and beverages directly to teens. The message is enjoyment and pleasure, and advertised products may not be nutritionally adequate. Other factors that influence an adolescent's food selection and consumption are shown in **FIGURE 12.6**.

Vending machines are common in U.S. schools, placing schools in a unique position to influence the diet of their students.[38] (See FYI "School Vending Machines and the Teen Diet"). Consistent with the recommendation of the *2015–2020 Dietary Guidelines for Americans* to reduce the intake of calories from solid fats and added sugars, the American Academy of Pediatrics states that routine ingestion of sports drinks by children and adolescents should be avoided or restricted.[39] To reduce consumption of sugar-sweetened beverages (SSBs), the CDC is encouraging schools to improve access to free drinking water and to implement other strategies to reduce student consumption of SSBs through changes in school policies.[40] Also necessary is the involvement of families, media, and other institutions that interact with adolescents to discourage their consumption of SSBs and increase their awareness of the potential detrimental health effects of a poor diet.[41]

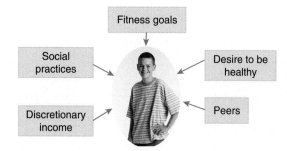

FIGURE 12.6 Factors that influence adolescent food choices.
Social, cultural, and psychological factors, especially peer pressure, strongly influence adolescent food choices.
© Patrick Foto/Shutterstock, Inc.

Key Concepts Apart from during pregnancy and lactation, humans need more calories and nutrients during adolescence than at any other stage of life. During this stage, boys grow about 8 inches, gain about 45 pounds, and increase their lean body mass. Girls grow about 6 inches, gain about 35 pounds, and increase their body fat. As at earlier ages, calcium, vitamin D, iron, and vitamin A are often lacking in adolescent diets. Factors that determine food selection and consumption include the desire to be healthy, fitness goals, amount of discretionary income, social practices, and peers.

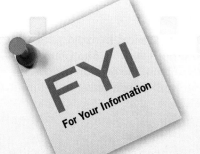

School Vending Machines and the Teen Diet

Teens perceive benefits to eating healthful foods, such as enhanced physical and mental performance, increased energy, and psychological well-being. However, while at school, teens are faced with more food choices than ever before. In addition to the standard school lunch or breakfast program outlined earlier, most middle schools and high schools have vending machines, snack carts, school stores, or even private vendors supplying foods for cafeteria meals. Vending and other food sales can be a major source of revenue for many schools, supporting athletic programs and other after-school activities. However, the food choices offered by vending machines can have a negative effect on teen diets.

The strongest risk factor for eating unhealthy snacks and beverages is simply the proximity of vending machines in schools.[a] More than half of middle and high schools in the United States offer sugary drinks and less healthy foods for their students to purchase.[b,c] Sugar-sweetened beverages (SSBs) are the largest source of added sugars, usually in the form of high fructose corn syrup, in the diets of children and adolescents in the United States. The increased caloric intake resulting from SSBs is a leading dietary contributor to the prevalence of obesity among adolescents.[d]

Health professionals and others have expressed concern about the presence of low-nutrient-density "competitive" foods (e.g., snacks and soft drinks sold side-by-side with school lunches), and many states have pursued legislation to either remove vending machines or change the products available during the school day. The Healthy Hunger-Free Kids Act of 2010 gives the USDA authority to establish national nutrition standards for all food and beverages sold and served in schools at any time during the school day.[e,f]

a Fox MK, Dodd AH, Wilson A, Gleason PM. Association between school food environment and practices and body mass index of US public school children. *J Am Diet Assoc.* 2009;109(2 Suppl):S108-S117.
b Centers for Disease Control and Prevention. Childhood obesity causes & consequences. http://www.cdc.gov/obesity/childhood/causes.html. Accessed September 18, 2017.
c Reedy J, Krebs-Smith SM. Dietary sources of energy, solid fats, and added sugars among children and adolescents in the United States. *J Am Diet Assoc.* 2010;110:1477-1484.
d Let's Move! Child Nutrition Reauthorization Healthy, Hunger-Free Kids Act of 2010, Healthy Hunger-Free Kids Act of 2010, Pub. L. No. 111-296, 124 Stat. 3183.
e Rovner AJ, Nansel TR, Wang J, Iannotti RJ. Food sold in school vending machines is associated with overall student dietary intake. *J Adolesc Health.* 2011;48(1):13-19.
f American Academy of Pediatrics Committee on Nutrition and the Council on Sports Medicine. Clinical report—sports drinks and energy drinks for children and adolescents: are they appropriate? *Pediatrics.* 2011;127:1182-1189.

Nutrition-Related Concerns for Adolescents

Adolescents are often preoccupied with weight, appearance, and eating habits. They need to know whether and how their eating practices can affect body image and development, fitness, acne, and obesity.

Fitness and Sports

For many adolescents, an interest in fitness becomes the catalyst for learning about nutrition and improving dietary habits. Some teens, unfortunately, become obsessed with their athletic performance, food intake, and body appearance and go to extremes that can jeopardize not only their current athletic performance, but also their long-term health.

Acne

THINK About It 2

Many teens blame certain foods for their **acne**. Myths surrounding acne and diet abound, but research has not found any correlation between acne and chocolate, greasy foods, soft drinks, nuts, or milk. Nevertheless, differences in acne incidence between Westernized and non-Westernized societies are striking, and researchers are investigating the connections between diets and acne.[42,43] Specifically, dietary components such as dairy products, high-glycemic-index foods, fat intake, and fatty acid composition have recently been investigated as contributors to acne.[44] Preliminary research suggests that a low-glycemic-load diet can be helpful, but further controlled testing is needed before specific recommendations can be made.[45]

▶ **acne** An inflammatory skin eruption that usually occurs in or near the sebaceous glands of the face, neck, shoulders, and upper back.

Effective treatments for acne include topical benzoyl peroxide, low-dose oral antibiotics, and two medications derived from vitamin A—Retin-A and Accutane. Although both of these medications are derivatives of vitamin A, there is no correlation between dietary vitamin A and acne.

Eating Disorders

Eating disorders frequently begin during adolescence. Adolescents often become preoccupied with their weight, appearance, and eating habits. Although eating disorders are still found more often in girls than in boys, the prevalence in males is increasing. Thus, eating disorders shouldn't be ignored or dismissed as only a "girl's problem."

Adolescent Obesity

As in childhood, obesity rates in adolescence are climbing. One contributing factor is a decline in physical activity by many teens.[46] Obese adolescents have an increased risk of developing high blood pressure, abnormal glucose tolerance and type 2 diabetes, breathing problems, joint pain, and heartburn.[47] They also suffer psychologically with poor self-esteem from teasing, being ostracized by peers, and longing to be slimmer. In addition, adolescent obesity sets the stage for adult obesity, with all its attendant health consequences.[48] Finally, overweight adolescents who spend on average 7.5 hours daily watching television or using other forms of entertainment media could be otherwise spending some of this time being physically active.[49] Nutrition education can positively influence the knowledge, attitudes, and eating behaviors of high school students, leading to a healthier lifestyle and reducing their risk of becoming overweight.[50] See **TABLE 12.7** for factors that put an adolescent at risk for obesity.

Tobacco, Alcohol, and Other Drugs

Developmentally, adolescence is a period of exploration in which many adolescents experiment with smoking, alcohol use, misuse of over-the-counter and prescription medications, and abuse of other illegal substances. Although survey results from 2014 show a continuing decline in alcohol use and binge drinking among teenagers, alcohol use remains widespread in this group.[51] Marijuana use, along with use of tobacco, illicit drugs, and the nonmedical use of prescription medications, continues to be high.[52] Nearly one-fourth of high school seniors graduate as users of tobacco products. An adolescent who smokes tobacco often has a lower energy intake and subsequently decreased nutrient intake. Although the use of cigarettes declined among middle and high school students between 2011 and 2014, there was no decline in overall tobacco use in this period, in part due to a rise in the use of electronic cigarettes. Between 2013 and 2014 alone, e-cigarette use more than tripled among middle and high school students, increasing from 4.5 percent to 13.4 percent. With 2 million American students now using e-cigarettes, 2014 marked the first year in which e-cigarette use surpassed the use of every other tobacco product, including conventional cigarettes.[53] Studies have not yet reported consistent results on the potential risks they carry.

Marijuana has the opposite effect on hunger. Many teens who smoke marijuana experience "the munchies," a desire to snack and munch—usually on snacks high in calories but with low nutrient density. Smoking marijuana carries the same risks as smoking tobacco.

TABLE 12.7
Risk Factors for Obesity in Adolescents

- Genetics
- Extent and duration of breastfeeding
- Early menarche
- Participation in high-risk behaviors such as smoking, alcohol use, and sexual experimentation
- Family and parental dynamics
- Food insecurity
- Socioeconomic status
- Lack of safe place for physical activity
- Inconsistent access to healthful food choices
- Low cognitive stimulation at home
- Parental food choices
- Parental food-related behaviors
- Lack of regular family meals
- Low level of physical activity—leisure time activities and activities of daily living, school physical activity programs
- Television, computer, and video games

Data from American Academy of Pediatrics. Prevention of pediatric overweight and obesity. *Pediatrics.* 2003;112(2):424-430.

Position Statement: Academy of Nutrition and Dietetics

Child and Adolescent Nutrition Assistance Programs

It is the position of the Academy of Nutrition and Dietetics that children and adolescents should have access to an adequate supply of healthful and safe foods that promote optimal physical, cognitive, and social growth and development. Nutrition assistance programs, such as food assistance and meal service programs and nutrition education initiatives, play a vital role in meeting this critical need.

Reprinted from *Journal of the American Dietetic Association*, 110(5), Jamie Stang, Position of the American Dietetic Association: Child and Adolescent Nutrition Assistance Programs, Page no.791-799, 2010, with permission from Elsevier.

In addition, marijuana sometimes is laced with other drugs, including LSD and amphetamines.

Almost all alcohol consumed by those younger than the age of 21 occurs during binge drinking—more than five drinks within two hours for men and four drinks within two hours for women. Through violence and accidental injury, adolescents who drink alcohol are at increased risk of harming themselves or others.[54] In addition, teens who drink are replacing needed nutrients with empty alcohol calories. Finally, alcohol can interfere with the absorption and metabolism of necessary nutrients. Growing adolescents cannot afford to have nutrients replaced or poorly absorbed during growth.

Other drugs, such as cocaine, pose further risks. In using illegal drugs, the adolescent becomes preoccupied with both the acquisition and use of the drug; these activities take priority over food intake or selection. Teens who use drugs are usually underweight and report poor appetites.

> **Key Concepts** Adolescence can be an uncomfortable time for the teen who is concerned with body image and weight, body changes, or athletic activities. Although many teens blame certain foods for their acne, research has not found a definite correlation between acne and diet. Adolescent obesity is on the rise, and eating disorders frequently begin during adolescence. Use of tobacco, alcohol, or recreational drugs can influence nutrient intake and interfere with good nutrition.

Staying Young While Growing Older

> 🍎 **Why Is This Important?** Knowing the changes in lifestyle typical of aging adults will reveal some of the accompanying nutritional concerns for this age group. For example, a sedentary lifestyle correlates to increasing overweight and obesity. Also, poor diet and lack of strengthening exercises in people over 50 years of age results in bone loss and a decrease in muscle tone, which can affect physical function, mobility, and balance.

Just when does old age begin? The answer is increasingly elusive, as more people remain healthy and active well into their 70s, 80s, and even 90s. Today, older adults represent the fastest-growing segment of the U.S. population; in 2015, the percentage of the older population (Americans age 65 years and older) had more than tripled since 1900, from 4.1 percent to 14.9 percent of the U.S. population.[55] (See **FIGURE 12.7**.) The baby boomers started turning 65 in 2011, and experts estimate that by 2060 approximately 98 million Americans will be older than 65 years. During the next few decades, the population age 85 or older is projected to double, from 6.5 million in 2015 to 14.6 million by 2040.[56]

Age-related changes in body composition, sensory abilities, organ systems, and immune function are normal. (See **FIGURE 12.8**.) We age at different rates, and many age-related declines will have little impact on our day-to-day lives. Other changes affect our nutrient needs and nutrient status (see **TABLE 12.8**), so it becomes especially important to eat nutrient-dense food.

As we get older, many of us fear loss of mental function even more than loss of physical function. Yet, as the years advance, most people maintain cognitive function with only subtle changes. Staying physically and mentally active is a key factor in maintaining function and independence. In most cases, slight changes involving sensory acuity,

Quick **Bite**

The Dangers of Teenage Smoking

The CDC estimates that more than 3 million adolescents smoke regularly. Each day, more than 3,200 young people try a cigarette for the first time, and more than 2,100 become regular smokers. The CDC predicts that if smoking continues at the current rate among U.S. youth, 5.6 million of today's Americans younger than 18 years of age will die prematurely from a smoking-related illness. Research shows that the earlier a person begins to smoke, the greater the damage.

Quick **Bite**

Longevity Champions

In the United States, women live an average of five years longer than men.

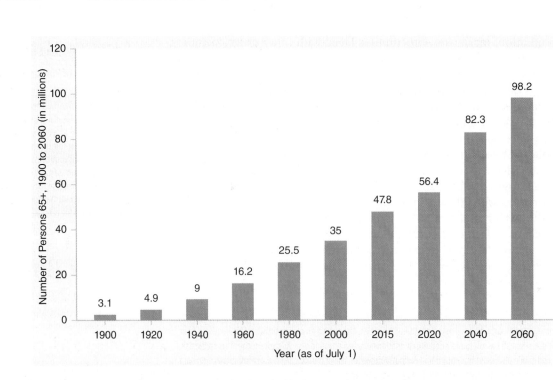

FIGURE 12.7 The aging U.S. population. The number of people older than age 65 is growing rapidly.
Reproduced from Administration on Aging. A Profile of Older Americans, 2016. https://www.acl.gov/aging-and-disability-in-america/data-and -research/profile-older-americans. Accessed May 20, 2017.

Saliva production
Digestive secretions
Lactase secretions
Gastrointestinal motility
Cardiac output
Blood volume
Kidney function   Blood pressure
Liver function
Immune function   Body weight
Vitamin absorption   Bone loss

FIGURE 12.8 Age-related physiological changes. As we age, most physiological changes emerge gradually.

secondary memory, and information-processing speed do not affect quality of life or lead to progressive or rapid declines in mental function. However, when depression or dementia is suspected, professional evaluation becomes necessary. Overmedication or drug interactions, rather than disease, could be responsible for the changes in behavior.

Although it is not possible to stop the aging process, we can control aspects of our lifestyle that contribute to a healthier old age. Many of

TABLE 12.8
Age-Related Changes and Nutrient Needs

Change in Body Composition or Physiologic Function	Impact on Nutrient Requirements
Decreased muscle mass	Decreased need for energy Increased need for high-quality protein
Decreased bone density	Increased need for calcium and vitamin D
Decreased immune function	Increased need for vitamin B_6, antioxidants, vitamin E, zinc, and high-quality protein
Increased gastric pH	Increased need for vitamin B_{12}, folic acid, calcium, iron, and zinc
Decreased skin capacity for cholecalciferol synthesis	Increased need for vitamin D
Decreased kidney ability to concentrate urine, constipation, and reduced thirst sensation	Increased fluid needs
Increased oxidative stress, cognitive impairment, cataracts, and age-related macular degeneration	Increased need for antioxidants such as beta-carotene, vitamin C, and vitamin E
Slowed gastric motility	Increased need for fiber

our choices—food, exercise, smoking, and alcohol—affect not only our risk for chronic disease, but also the rate at which we age. Nutrition is a key factor in promoting health and ability to function at advanced ages and plays a role in medical nutrition therapy for disease management.[57] Eating is not only a necessity of everyday life, but also an important pleasure and social component at every age.

Weight and Body Composition

Poor food choices and too many calories combined with a sedentary lifestyle have resulted in a growing number of overweight and obese older adults.[58] Older people who are overweight or who gain weight with age have an increased risk of chronic diseases such as heart disease, diabetes, metabolic syndrome, and cancer.[59] In addition, many older adults who have an increase in body fat and loss of muscle mass decline physically and are unable to function independently in their normal activities of daily living.

THINK About It 3   In contrast, people who enter their mature years on the lean side—and who remain lean as a result of a healthy, active lifestyle—increase their chances of enjoying a healthy old age. But thinness alone is not always a health advantage. Obviously, older adults who lose weight because of illness enjoy no health benefits from losing these pounds. Weight loss puts them at increased risk for further illness, including cardiovascular disease and osteoporosis—especially if the original illness also limits activity. And, of course, leanness caused by tobacco use or alcoholism increases a person's vulnerability to a decline in health.

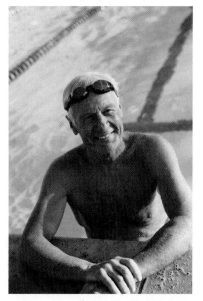

© Joaquin Palting/Photodisc/Getty Images.

Physical Activity

Lean body mass (muscle mass) and strength are commonly observed to decline with age. However, this decline might not be a simple physiological consequence of aging. Decreases in physical activity that accompany age contribute to loss of lean mass and muscle strength, a condition called sarcopenia.[60] Sarcopenia contributes to functional disability and loss of independence. Our posture begins deteriorating in our fifties—a result of bad habits, bone loss, and a decrease in muscle tone. Poor posture can affect lung and cardiovascular function, mobility, and balance. Diseases such as stroke, heart disease, arthritis, and diabetes become more common and can cause severe physical disability. These conditions, however, do not automatically preclude older adults from participating in physical activity with qualified supervision. In fact, they might instead provide additional justification for appropriate exercises for the older adult.[61] Medications and nutritional deficiencies can lead to impaired motor function; therefore, older adults should be evaluated by their physician prior to beginning a new exercise program.

Although physical activity cannot stop biological aging, regular exercise can help to minimize the physiological effects of a sedentary lifestyle and limit the progression of disabling conditions and chronic diseases.[62] The U.S. Department of Health and Human Services' 2008 *Physical Activity Guidelines for Americans* states that "regular physical activity is essential for healthy aging" and that all adults should avoid inactivity.[63] These recommendations for physical activity for older adults are included in the *2015–2020 Dietary Guidelines for Americans*. Canada also addresses this issue in its *Physical Activity Guide for Older Adults*.

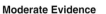

Moderate Evidence
Lower risk of hip fracture and increased bone density
Lower risk of lung and endometrial cancers
Weight maintenance after weight loss
Improved sleep quality

Moderate to Strong Evidence
Better functional health (for older adults)
Reduced abdominal obesity

Strong Evidence
Lower risk of early death
Lower risk of coronary heart disease, stroke,
high blood pressure,
    type 2 diabetes, metabolic syndrome, colon cancer,
    and breast cancer
Prevention of weight gain
Weight loss, particularly when combined with
reduced calorie intake
Improved cardiorespiratory and muscular fitness
Prevention of falls
Reduced depression
Better cognitive function (for older adults)

FIGURE 12.9 The health benefits associated with regular physical activity for adults and older adults. Physical activity helps adults maintain their health and independence as they age.

Modified from U.S. Department of Health and Human Services. 2008 *Physical Activity Guidelines for Americans*. ODPHP Publication No. U0036. Washington, DC: U.S. Department of Health and Human Services; 2008. http://www.health.gov /paguidelines/guidelines/chapter2.aspx. Accessed September 18, 2017.

▶ **urinary tract infection (UTI)** An infection of one or more of the structures in the urinary tract; usually caused by bacteria.

The benefits of an individualized exercise prescription designed to increase physical activity that includes aerobic activities, flexibility exercises, and progressive resistance strength training can be most profound for those who are aging. Increased self-confidence, better balance and mobility, fewer falls and fractures, enhanced mental acuity, and improved appetite and nutrient intake are but a few of the physical and psychological benefits of exercise during our older years. The bottom line is that all adults should avoid inactive lifestyles and regularly engage in various forms of physical activity.[64] (See **FIGURE 12.9** and **TABLE 12.9**.)

Immunity

Starting in one's 40s, the body's defense mechanisms begin to weaken, and the process continues over the next several decades into old age. The immune system loses some of its ability to fight viruses, bacteria, and other foreign bodies. Older adults are thus more vulnerable to upper respiratory tract infections such as influenza, pneumonia, **urinary tract infections (UTIs)**, pressure sores, and foodborne illnesses. Physical barriers to infectious agents, foreign bodies, and chemicals weaken as well. These barriers include the skin, the acid environment in the stomach, and the swallowing and coughing reflexes.

Inadequate consumption of protein and some antioxidant nutrients can compromise immunity and health in older adults. Because of poor appetite, difficulty chewing, financial constraints, concerns about fat intake, or lactose intolerance, older adults might reduce their intake of meat, dairy products, and fresh fruits and vegetables, making it difficult for them to get all the calories, protein, and other essential nutrients they need. (See **FIGURE 12.10**.) Poor dietary intake can lead to suppressed immunity, decreased muscle mass, slowed wound healing, and osteoporosis.

TABLE 12.9
2008 Physical Activity Guidelines for Americans: Key Guidelines for Adults and Older Adults

The following guidelines are the same for adults and older adults:
- All older adults should avoid inactivity. Some physical activity is better than none, and older adults who participate in any amount of physical activity gain some health benefits.
- For substantial health benefits, older adults should do at least 150 minutes (2 hours and 30 minutes) a week of moderate-intensity, or 75 minutes (1 hour and 15 minutes) a week of vigorous-intensity aerobic physical activity, or an equivalent combination of moderate- and vigorous-intensity aerobic activity. Aerobic activity should be performed in episodes of at least 10 minutes, and preferably, it should be spread throughout the week.
- For additional and more extensive health benefits, older adults should increase their aerobic physical activity to 300 minutes (5 hours) a week of moderate-intensity, or 150 minutes a week of vigorous-intensity aerobic physical activity, or an equivalent combination of moderate- and vigorous-intensity activity. Additional health benefits are gained by engaging in physical activity beyond this amount.
- Older adults should also do muscle-strengthening activities that are moderate or high intensity and involve all major muscle groups two or more days a week, as these activities provide additional health benefits.

The following guidelines are just for older adults:
- When older adults cannot do 150 minutes of moderate-intensity aerobic activity a week because of chronic conditions, they should be as physically active as their abilities and conditions allow.
- Older adults should do exercises that maintain or improve balance if they are at risk of falling.
- Older adults should determine their level of effort for physical activity relative to their level of fitness.
- Older adults with chronic conditions should understand whether and how their conditions affect their ability to do regular physical activity safely.

Reproduced from U.S. Department of Health and Human Services. 2008 *Physical Activity Guidelines for Americans*. Chapter 5: active older adults. http://www.health.gov/paguidelines/guidelines/chapter5.aspx. Accessed May 20, 2017.

Key Concepts Lifestyle choices, such as diet and exercise, affect how we age. Control of body weight can reduce our risk for many chronic diseases associated with aging. Adequate nutrient intake can protect our immune status. Regular physical activity not only helps us to maintain the ability to function in daily activities and enables our independence, but also reduces disease risk and overall well-being.

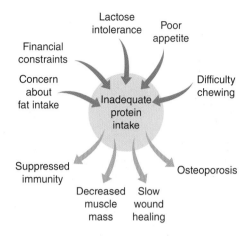

FIGURE 12.10 **Protein malnutrition in older adults.** A combination of several factors can lead to inadequate protein intake that compromises immunity and health.

▶ **taste threshold** The minimum amount of flavor that must be present for a taste to be detected.

Taste and Smell

In older adults, the **taste threshold**—the minimum amount of a flavor that must be present to detect the taste—is more than double that of college-aged adults. Sensitivity to sweet and salty tastes goes first, so older adults often increase their intake of foods high in sugar and sodium—increasing health problems that stem from overconsumption of these nutrients. Along with taste, our sense of smell diminishes with age, especially in the seventh decade of life (60 to 70 years old) and beyond. Medication use also can alter taste and flavor perception. The idea that older adults should be served bland foods is misguided. Intensifying flavors and aromas of food and varying temperature and textures are strategies older adults can use to compensate for the diminished taste and smell of foods. (See **FIGURE 12.11**.)

Gastrointestinal Changes

Saliva production tends to decrease as we age, especially in people who take medications for conditions such as congestive heart failure. Lack of saliva affects the preparation of food for digestion and contributes to gum disease—a breach in one of the immune system's first lines of defense against infection.

With age, digestive secretions decline. Most significant are reductions in the stomach secretions of hydrochloric acid and pepsin. These reductions can allow the development of atrophic gastritis—a chronic inflammation of the stomach lining that is common among older adults. Atrophic gastritis can interfere with normal absorption of vitamin B_{12}, leading to a deficiency of this vitamin.[65] Although reduced

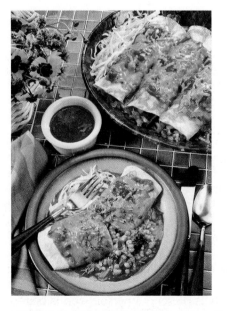

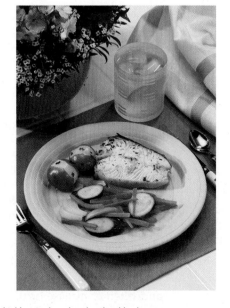

FIGURE 12.11 **Older adults need stronger flavors.** More highly spiced meals rather than bland ones can encourage an older adult to eat more.

(a, b) © Photodisc.

lactase production also is associated with aging, a complete intolerance to milk and dairy products is less common than older adults often suspect. Most people with reduced lactase production can include some milk, cheese, and yogurt in their diets.

Constipation, gas, and bloating are common complaints of old age. These problems are caused by a slowing of gastrointestinal motility with age, along with decreased physical activity, a diet low in fiber, and low fluid intake. Feelings of fullness can cause older adults to eat less. Reduced digestive secretions lower the amount of nutrients older adults absorb from the foods they do eat. Myths and misinformation about the gastrointestinal (GI) effects of various foods, even among the medical community, can steer a person away from nutrient-dense foods such as dairy products, legumes, broccoli, cauliflower, tomatoes, and citrus products. Although many older adults mistakenly blame these foods for causing problems with gas, others may be sensitive to lactose in dairy products or may have had an adverse reaction to members of the cabbage family or "acid"-containing foods. GI distress also can be caused by factors totally unrelated to the food itself—inappropriate food preparation, lack of adequate fluid, and physical inactivity. Regardless of the cause, once people have an adverse reaction, they may associate it with a recently consumed food and become reluctant to try it again.

Key Concepts   The perception of taste declines with age. To detect flavors, older adults often need food with stronger flavors and odors. This loss of taste can contribute to loss of appetite and poor food intake. Age-related changes in the GI tract reduce nutrient absorption. Decreased motility contributes to constipation.

Nutrient Needs of the Mature Adult

🍎 **Why Is This Important?**   Getting the right nutrition throughout the life span helps reduce risks of developing certain diseases later in life. Water, protein, vitamin D, vitamin B$_{12}$, calcium, and antioxidants are nutrients that are especially important with advancing age.

At any age, to live life to its fullest, you need good nutrition. A lifestyle that incorporates the *Dietary Guidelines for Americans* and MyPlate eating plan, together with regular physical activity, is essential to a long and productive life. **FIGURE 12.12** shows how MyPlate has been adapted to illustrate the nutritional concerns of older adults.

Energy

Mainly because of reduced physical activity and loss of lean body mass, our energy requirements decline as we age. In other words, a 60-year-old man will need to increase his physical activity and/or decrease his caloric intake to maintain his weight as he ages. Physical activity increases energy requirements while also helping to delay some of the loss in lean mass, thus allowing us to eat more without gaining weight and increasing the likelihood that our diets will be adequate in essential nutrients.

The EER equations are the same for older adults as for younger adults. Individual energy needs depend on activity, lean body mass, and whether disease or disability is present; a person who is bed- or chair-ridden, for example, usually requires fewer calories than a mobile person.

Quick Bite

Losing Water

At birth, 75 percent of the body is composed of water. By the time a person reaches old age, that number has dwindled to 50 percent as a result of changes in body composition.

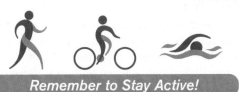

MyPlate for Older Adults

Fruits & Vegetables

Whole fruits and vegetables are rich in important nutrients and fiber. Choose fruits and vegetables with deeply colored flesh. Choose canned varieties that are packed in their own juices or low-sodium.

Healthy Oils

Liquid vegetable oils and soft margarines provide important fatty acids and some fat-soluble vitamins.

Herbs & Spices

Use a variety of herbs and spices to enhance flavor of foods and reduce the need to add salt.

Fluids

Drink plenty of fluids. Fluids can come from water, tea, coffee, soups, and fruits and vegetables.

Grains

Whole grain and fortified foods are good sources of fiber and B vitamins.

Dairy

Fat-free and low-fat milk, cheeses and yogurts provide protein, calcium and other important nutrients.

Protein

Protein rich foods provide many important nutrients. Choose a variety including nuts, beans, fish, lean meat and poultry.

Remember to Stay Active!

Tufts UNIVERSITY   JEAN MAYER USDA HUMAN NUTRITION RESEARCH CENTER ON AGING   HNRCA   **AARP** Foundation

FIGURE 12.12 MyPlate for older adults.

Protein

Protein needs (as grams per kilogram of body weight) can be somewhat harder for us to meet as our overall energy needs decrease and our tastes change. As our caloric needs decrease and our protein needs remain constant, an adequate diet must contain relatively more protein. For healthy older adults, the RDA for protein is 0.8 gram per kilogram of body weight, or on average 46 grams per day for women and 56 grams for men. However, some experts argue that the current RDA is not sufficient to meet protein needs and maximize muscle protein synthesis, and therefore recommend that older adults aim to include 25 to 30 grams of high-quality protein with each meal.[66] Eating enough protein can be challenging for older adults, so choosing foods with high-quality protein as recommended by MyPlate throughout the day is a helpful strategy. Chronically ill individuals might need more protein to maintain nitrogen balance. Trauma, stress, and infection also increase protein needs. However, there are risks associated with high protein intake, including dehydration, nitrogen overload, and adverse effects on the kidneys.

Carbohydrate

After infancy, carbohydrates should make up 45 to 65 percent of the calories in the diet. Because foods with primarily simple carbohydrates provide little nutrient value, the best choices are foods with complex carbohydrates.

Fiber, a complex carbohydrate, has many potential benefits, including preventing constipation and diverticulosis, helping to promote a healthy body weight, and reducing risk for diabetes. Older adults generally do not eat enough dietary fiber. Foods low in fiber tend to be nutritionally inferior and may take the place of more nutritious foods essential to the health and weight management goals of older adults. Because the AI for fiber is based on calorie intake (14 grams per 1,000 kcal per day), and energy needs decline with age, the AI for fiber is 30 grams per day for men older than age 50 and 21 grams per day for women in that age group. Fiber also can help to reduce blood cholesterol, making these recommendations especially important for those who are at risk for heart disease. Five or more servings of fruits and vegetables daily, accompanied by whole-grain breads or cereals high in bran, will supply this amount easily while also providing vitamins, minerals, and phytochemicals needed by older adults. To avoid abdominal discomfort, increase dietary fiber intake gradually. When increasing dietary fiber intake, it is essential to consume adequate fluids—ideally water—to avoid dehydration and constipation.

Fat

Excess dietary fat can lead to obesity, which in turn increases the risk for diabetes, heart disease, and some types of cancer. Younger people should limit their dietary cholesterol and fat, but severe restrictions in older adults may be counterproductive. Extreme fat phobia could contribute to nutritional deficiencies among older adults who are afraid to drink milk, eat red meat, or even eat poultry or fish. Too few animal products in the diet can contribute to a lack of dietary protein; deficiency of minerals such as calcium, iron, and zinc; and poor vitamin D and vitamin B_{12} intake.

Healthy people who are at low risk for heart disease should obtain 20 to 35 percent of their daily calories from fat, with no more than 8 to 10 percent of the calories from saturated fat. They should limit their cholesterol intake to 300 milligrams per day. People at increased risk for heart disease should limit saturated fat and cholesterol even more, according to their physicians' advice. Older adults in general should limit excess dietary fat to prevent eating too many calories, which could contribute to difficulty maintaining a healthy body weight.

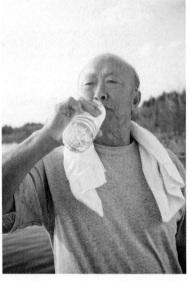

© Suprijono Suharjoto/123RF.

Water

Nutritionists often call water the forgotten nutrient. Water is essential to all body functions; if intake is inadequate, cellular metabolism becomes difficult, if not impossible. In older adults, a decreased thirst response and a reduction in kidney function can increase the risk of dehydration.[67] Diuretic medications, alcohol, and caffeine all increase fluid excretion and can contribute to dehydration. Fluid recommendations for older adults–from all foods and beverages–are the same as for younger adults: 3,700 milliliters (125 fluid ounces) per day for men, and 2,700 milliliters (91 fluid ounces) per day for women.[68]

Key Concepts Although caloric needs decline with loss of lean tissue and reduced physical activity, protein needs do not change for older adults. A high-carbohydrate, moderate-fat diet is still recommended. Water is important; because of their diminished thirst response, older adults may not drink enough.

Vitamins and Minerals

As we age, our micronutrient status changes, especially our needs for vitamin D, vitamin B_{12}, and calcium. (See **FIGURE 12.13**.) In many cases, our vitamin needs remain stable, while our energy needs decline. This often creates a challenge for older adults who become inactive with age, reducing their calorie needs. To maintain body weight or prevent gaining, this means that older adults must eat a more nutrient-dense diet to eat all the nutrients they need for good health without overeating calories. In other cases, age-related declines in absorption, use, or activation of nutrients lead to increased dietary vitamin and mineral needs. Therefore, it is especially important for older adults to eat nutrient-dense foods.

Vitamin D

Vitamin D promotes bone health; too little dietary vitamin D can lead to brittle and porous bones that are susceptible to fracture. Recently, vitamin D has been investigated for its role in the prevention and treatment of cancer, types 1 and 2 diabetes mellitus, hypertension, glucose metabolism, heart disease, arthritis, and multiple sclerosis.[69] Older adults often have low vitamin D status.[70] Not only are aging tissues less able to take up vitamin D from the blood, but also aging skin is less effective in synthesizing vitamin D when exposed to sunlight. In addition, many older adults spend more time indoors and have reduced exposure to sunlight. When they go outside, many avoid the sun and use sunscreens—a good strategy for skin cancer prevention, but one that reduces vitamin D synthesis. Older adults with lactose intolerance often avoid dairy products, reducing their vitamin D intake and further compromising vitamin D status. The RDA for vitamin D for adults ages 51 through 70 years is 600 IU per day. Younger adults also need 600 IU per day. For adults 70 years and older, the RDA is 800 IU per day.[71]

B Vitamins

The B vitamins deserve special consideration in adults and aging adults. Extensive research links inadequate folate, vitamin B_6, and vitamin B_{12} to elevated levels of plasma homocysteine, a protein breakdown product that may damage arterial walls, causing plaque to form. Homocysteine is associated with an increased risk for cardiovascular disease and mortality.[72] High homocysteine levels also have been found to be an independent risk factor for cognitive impairment and dementia.[73] Since the 1998 fortification of the food supply with folic acid, ready-to-eat cereals and grain products now play a significant role in the dietary folic acid intake of older adults.[74]

The prevalence of vitamin B_{12} deficiency increases with age. Six percent of adults age 60 years or older are vitamin B_{12} deficient, and close to 20 percent have marginal status.[75] Although most adults

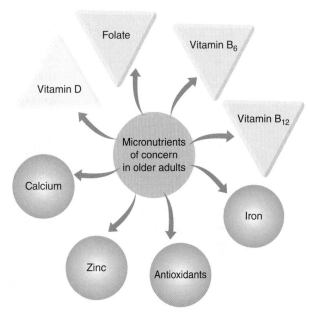

FIGURE 12.13 Micronutrients of particular concern for older adults. As we age, our energy needs decline, but our vitamin and mineral needs remain stable. This makes nutrient-dense foods especially important for older adults.

consume adequate amounts of dietary vitamin B_{12}, 10 to 30 percent of older adults lose their ability to absorb protein-bound vitamin B_{12} from foods. Folic acid intake in excess of recommended levels can mask a vitamin B_{12} deficiency and delay diagnosis.[76] Neurological symptoms such as changes in mental status require further investigation in older adults and should not simply be attributed to old age. An intake of 2.4 micrograms per day of vitamin B_{12} is recommended for all adults older than 51 years. Because it is easier to absorb synthetic B_{12} than food-bound B_{12}, scientists suggest that adults older than 50 years use fortified foods or B_{12}-containing supplements to meet their vitamin B_{12} requirements.

Antioxidants

Antioxidants such as those found in fruits and vegetables are important to reduce oxidative stress and degenerative diseases common in older adults. Cataracts and age-related macular degeneration (ARMD) are common conditions that affect the vision of older adults. Antioxidants can have a beneficial role in preventing, slowing the progression of, and treating cataracts and ARMD.[77] In addition, antioxidants protect against damage to the brain that can lead to Alzheimer's disease and other declines in cognition that are common in aging.[78]

> **Key Concepts** Vitamin D, folate, vitamin B_6, vitamin B_{12}, and antioxidants are key nutrients for older adults. Vitamin D status can decline as a result of reduced intake, synthesis, and activation. Poor folate, vitamin B_6, and vitamin B_{12} status might result in high homocysteine levels, a risk factor for heart disease. Excessive folic acid intake can mask a vitamin B_{12} deficiency. Vitamin B_{12} absorption declines with age; vitamin B_{12} is more easily absorbed from fortified foods and supplements, so these become important sources for older adults. Antioxidants help to lower the prevalence and progression of degenerative diseases such as ARMD and Alzheimer's.

Calcium

Maintaining adequate calcium intake reduces the rate of age-related bone loss and the incidence of fractures, especially of the hip.[79] For women ages 51 to 70 years, the RDA for calcium is 1,200 milligrams per day, 200 milligrams per day higher than the RDA for men of the same age. For both men and women older than the age of 70, the RDA for calcium is 1,200 milligrams per day.[80]

As we age we are less able to absorb calcium, partly because of a loss of vitamin D receptors in the gut. Stomach inflammation also reduces calcium absorption, as does an increase in the consumption of fiber—a practice that doctors recommend for its laxative effects. Because of real or perceived lactose intolerance, many older adults have a low intake of dairy foods and therefore of calcium.

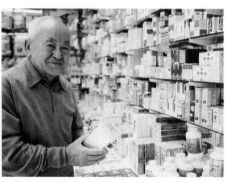

© Paul Edmondson/Corbis.

Zinc

Although clinical zinc deficiencies are uncommon, older adults frequently have marginal zinc intakes. Stress, especially in hospitalized older adults, appears to increase the risk of zinc deficiency and suppress immune function. Studies show that zinc supplementation hastens wound healing, but only in those who are zinc deficient. Because excess zinc can lead to a metallic taste, can interfere with immune function and the absorption of other minerals, and may work to lower high-density lipoprotein (HDL) cholesterol, people of all ages should avoid excessive and continuous zinc supplementation.

Iron

Iron remains an important nutrient throughout the life cycle. Following menopause, the RDA for women drops to the same level as for men, 8 milligrams per day. Iron deficiency is a concern for older adults who have limited intake of iron from the best sources—red meats, fish, and poultry. Reduced meat consumption may result from taste changes, economics, poor dentition, or a combination of factors.

To Supplement or Not to Supplement

Increased use of dietary supplements, including vitamins, minerals, and herbal and botanical products, is widespread.[81] Although food is "the best medicine," some older adults feel they need a supplement to meet their nutrient needs. Older adults take nutritional supplements for two main reasons: first, to delay age-related chronic diseases, and second, for the potential health-promoting effects of these nutrients.[82] Food is more than the sum of its known nutrients, however, and replacing food with supplements is a poor trade-off. In addition, some nutrients in large amounts can be toxic; they also can affect the absorption of other nutrients or interfere with the absorption and metabolism of prescription medications.

Excessive use of vitamin supplements by older adults might result in **hypervitaminosis**. The need for vitamin A decreases with age, increasing the chances that supplementation might lead to liver dysfunction, bone and joint pain, headaches, and other problems. Also, taking large amounts of vitamin C can increase the likelihood of kidney stones and gastric bleeding. Because we know that many older adults use vitamin supplements and that megadoses can have negative effects on health, it is important to inform older adults of the Tolerable Upper Intake Levels (ULs) for micronutrients. The UL represents a level of intake from a combination of food and dietary supplements that should not be exceeded on a routine basis. (See **TABLE 12.10**.)

▶ **hypervitaminosis** High levels of vitamins in the blood, usually a result of excess supplement intake.

> **Key Concepts** Important minerals for older adults are calcium, zinc, and iron. Calcium is important to reduce the risk for osteoporosis. Marginal zinc deficiency has been suspected in many older adults and might be the result of reduced intake of red meats. Iron needs decline for women as they go through menopause. Excessive supplementation with certain vitamins or minerals can lead to health problems.

Nutrition-Related Concerns of Mature Adults

🍎 **Why Is This Important?** Aging takes a toll on certain body functions, including metabolism, digestion, absorption, and elimination. Ensuring adequate intake of essential nutrients, taking part in regular physical activity, and avoiding negative drug–food interactions are key to staying healthy at this stage of life.

Many factors can interfere with intake or use of nutrients by older adults. Therefore, caretakers, healthcare practitioners, and seniors themselves must pay attention to nutritional status. To manage acute or chronic nutrition-related conditions, older adults may need to make specific dietary changes.

Drug–Drug and Drug–Nutrient Interactions

Drugs not only affect the way the body uses nutrients, but also can alter the activities of other drugs. In turn, foods and nutrients can enhance or interfere with the effects of drugs. (See **TABLE 12.11**.) Some drugs

TABLE 12.10
The UL Values for Vitamins and Minerals for Adults

Vitamin/Mineral	Daily UL
Vitamin A (as retinol)	3,000 µg/day
Vitamin C	2,000 mg/day
Vitamin D	4,000 IU/day
Vitamin E[a]	1,000 mg/day
Niacin[a]	35 mg/day
Vitamin B$_6$	100 mg/day
Folic acid	1,000 µg/day
Choline	3,500 mg/day
Boron	20 mg/day
Calcium	2,500 mg/day (19–50 years) 2,000 mg/day (51+ years)
Chloride	3,600 mg/day
Copper	10,000 µg/day
Fluoride	10 mg/day
Iodine	1,100 µg/day
Iron	45 mg/day
Magnesium	350 mg/day
Manganese	11 mg/day
Molybdenum	2,000 µg/day
Nickel	1 mg/day
Phosphorus	4,000 mg/day 3,000 mg/day (70+ years)
Selenium	400 µg/day
Sodium	2,300 mg/day
Vanadium	1.8 mg/day
Zinc	40 mg/day

[a] From fortified foods and supplements only.

interfere with appetite; others cause a dry mouth. Because many older adults take several medications or are on long-term drug therapy, they can find themselves at increased nutritional risk.

Herbal supplements and vitamins or minerals in high doses should be viewed as drugs, particularly when taken in conjunction with prescription or over-the-counter medications. Although herbal products almost certainly interact with other medicines, many interactions are not well documented. In addition to the health and safety issues, supplement therapies can be costly. It is critical that older adults tell their healthcare providers all the drugs and supplements that they take on a regular basis so that possible interactions can be identified and avoided.

Depression

Many studies report high levels of well-being among older adults, especially those who remain independent. Although depression is one of the most common psychological effects of aging, it is most common among institutionalized and low-income people.

TABLE 12.11
Examples of Food–Drug Interactions

Drug	Food That Interacts	Effect of the Food	What to Do
Analgesic			
Acetaminophen (Tylenol)	Alcohol	Increases risk for liver toxicity	Avoid alcohol.
Antibiotic			
Tetracyclines	Dairy products; iron supplements	Decreases drug absorption	Do not take with milk. Take 1 hr before or 2 hr after food or milk.
Amoxicillin, penicillin	Food	Decreases drug absorption	Take 1 hr before or 2 hr after meals.
Azithromycin (Zithromax), erythromycin	Food	Decreases drug absorption	Take 1 hr before or 2 hr after meals.
Nitrofurantoin (Macrobid)	Food	Decreases GI distress, slows drug absorption	Take with food or milk.
Anticoagulant			
Warfarin (Coumadin)	Foods rich in vitamin K	Decreases drug effectiveness	Limit foods high in vitamin K: liver, broccoli, spinach, kale, cauliflower, and Brussels sprouts.
Antifungal			
Griseofulvin (Fulvicin)	High-fat meal	Increases absorption	Take with high-fat meal.
Antihistamine			
Diphenhydramine (Benadryl), chlorpheniramine (Chlor-Trimeton)	Alcohol	Increases drowsiness	Avoid alcohol.
Antihypertensive			
Felodipine (Plendil), nifedipine	Grapefruit juice	Increases drug absorption	Consult physician or pharmacist before changing diet.
Anti-inflammatory			
Naproxen (Aleve)	Food or milk	Decreases GI irritation	Take with food or milk.
Ibuprofen (Advil, Motrin)	Alcohol	Increases risk for liver damage or stomach bleeding	Avoid alcohol.
Diuretic			
Spironolactone (Aldactone)	Food	Decreases GI irritation	Take with food.
Psychotherapeutic (MAO inhibitors)			
Tranylcypromine (Parnate)	Foods high in tyramine: aged cheeses, Chianti wine, pickled herring, brewer's yeast, fava beans	Risk for hypertensive crisis	Avoid foods high in tyramine.

Note: This table includes major food–drug and drug–nutrient interactions. This is only a sample of the medications and interactions in each of these common medication categories. Not all categories of medications are included in the table. Check with your doctor or pharmacist for specific information about your medications.

Reproduced from Bobroff LB, Lentz A, Turner RE. *Food/Drug and Drug/Nutrient Interactions: What You Should Know About Your Medications*. Gainesville, FL: University of Florida; 2009. Publication FCS 8092 in a series of the Department of Family, Youth and Community Sciences, Florida Cooperative Extension Service, Institute of Food and Agricultural Sciences. http://edis.ifas.ufl.edu/pdffiles/HE/HE77600.pdf. Accessed May 20, 2017. Reprinted by permission.

In older adults, life transitions and stressful events can become frequent companions that increase the likelihood and severity of depression. Among these stressors are the loss of loved ones, including spouse and friends; physical disability; perceived loss of physical attractiveness; inability to psychologically defend oneself from unpleasant events; inability to care for oneself, which forces one to depend upon caregivers and long-term care; social isolation; and, inevitably, the approach of death. In later life, depression often leads to malnutrition and can manifest itself as either anorexia (loss of appetite) or obesity.

Alcoholism is prevalent among socially isolated or depressed older adults. People who consume excessive amounts of alcohol often have diets low in essential nutrients.

▶ **anorexia of aging** Loss of appetite and wasting associated with old age.

Anorexia of Aging

Poor food intake that accompanies age can result from **anorexia of aging**. Reductions in appetite and food intake contribute to undernutrition in older adults.[83] Malnutrition, in turn, can contribute to numerous problems, including immune deficiencies, anemia, falls, and cognitive decline.

It can be difficult to pinpoint treatment strategies for anorexia in older adults. However, treating even one aspect of the problem can provide at least temporary improvement. Unfortunately, lifelong inappropriate food habits, social factors, living conditions, and fear of injury can interfere with a person's ability and desire to stay or become healthy.

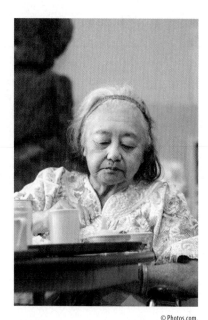

© Photos.com.

Key Concepts Among the problems older adults face are lack of appetite and the side effects and interactions of medications they use. Medicines have the potential to interact with food and nutrients in the diet, and a lack of knowledge of these possibilities increases the risk for harmful effects. Although many older adults have high levels of well-being, depression is common among institutionalized and low-income seniors.

Arthritis

Arthritis is a general term that describes more than 100 diseases that cause pain and swelling of joints and connective tissue. (See **FIGURE 12.14**.) Arthritis is a chronic, lifelong affliction that, at its worst, can make movement difficult or even impossible. Unfortunately, there is no proven cure for arthritis. At best, appropriate treatment programs reduce symptoms. In terms of nutrition, arthritis pain can impair appetite or make it hard to prepare meals, and some arthritis medications interfere with nutrient absorption. These factors underscore the importance of a nutrient-dense diet for arthritis sufferers.

Weight management is important in treating arthritis. Excess weight puts undue pressure on the hips and knees. Weight loss by people who are overweight or obese can reduce the risk of developing osteoarthritis, particularly of the knee.[84]

People who have rheumatoid arthritis can benefit from adding foods that are high in unsaturated fatty acids, particularly the omega-3 fatty acids in flaxseed and cold-water fish. There is some evidence that the right ratio of these fatty acids has beneficial effects on chronic inflammatory diseases such as rheumatoid arthritis, thus helping to reduce discomfort.[85] Other factors found to be protective against arthritis include dietary antioxidants; however, high coffee consumption, alcohol intake (especially among smokers), and obesity tend to increase risk of rheumatoid arthritis.[86]

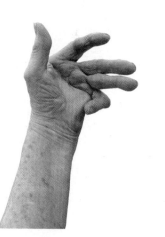

FIGURE 12.14 Arthritis. Degeneration of finger joints can cause a debilitating lack of function.

© Peterfactors/Dreamstime.com.

Bowel and Bladder Regulation

As a result of physiological and lifestyle changes, older adults are susceptible to problems with their bowels and bladder. Inadequate hydration not only affects the bladder, but also makes constipation more likely. Age-related decreases in intestinal motility and transit time, accompanied by poor food intake, can exacerbate the problem. In addition, lack of physical activity contributes to loss of muscle tone needed for regular elimination.

Chronic constipation is one of the most common health complaints among older adults. Excessive use of laxatives can cause nutritional deficiencies by decreasing transit time and preventing adequate absorption of nutrients. Decreased transit time also reduces water re-absorption by the GI tract and contributes to dehydration.

Increasing dietary fiber and fluid is one of the most effective treatments for bowel and bladder problems. Older adults should gradually switch to—and then maintain—a high-fiber diet. They also should be careful to maintain adequate fluid intake and exercise regularly. Supplementation with prebiotics, such as inulin, and probiotics, such as *Lactobacillus acidophilus*, can also improve their gastrointestinal health.[87]

Key Concepts Arthritis and changes in bowel and bladder habits are common problems in older adults. Weight management is an important component of arthritis treatment. Because of an increased risk of dehydration and constipation, older adults should be encouraged to follow a high-fiber diet and consume plenty of fluids.

Dental Health

The mouth is the gateway to the rest of the gastrointestinal system. Poor oral health can impair the ability to eat and obtain adequate nutrition. Missing teeth or poorly fitting dentures make some older adults self-conscious about eating, which leaves them unable to eat comfortably in public. Mouth pain and difficulty swallowing interfere with the process of eating, and tooth loss can alter choices and quality of food. Meats, fresh fruits, and fresh vegetables often are avoided. Oral infections affect the whole body and increase the risk of other chronic diseases, including heart disease.

Vision Problems

Poor vision and blindness interfere with the ability to buy and prepare food; people with visual impairments cannot read food labels, cookbooks, or the settings on stoves or microwave ovens. **Macular degeneration** is a common disease of the eye that gradually leads to loss of vision. It affects about 6 percent of people between the ages of 65 and 74 years, and about 20 percent of those ages 75 to 85 years. Research has found that people with a higher intake of green leafy vegetables are less likely to develop this sight-robbing disorder. Foods that contain the carotenoids lutein and zeaxanthin are widely investigated for their ability to reduce risk.[88] By preventing free radical damage, antioxidants in these foods may protect the eye and the blood vessels that supply it. The National Eye Institute's Age-Related Eye Disease Study (AREDS) found that taking a specific high-dose formulation of antioxidants and zinc (beta-carotene; vitamins A, C, and E; copper; and zinc) significantly reduces the risk of advanced age-related macular degeneration and its associated vision loss.[89] Preventing or slowing progression of the disease will save the vision of many people.

▶ **macular degeneration** Progressive deterioration of the macula, an area in the center of the retina, that eventually leads to loss of central vision.

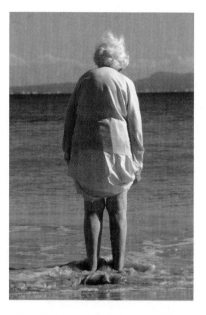

FIGURE 12.15 Osteoporosis. A hunched back (sometimes called a dowager's hump) caused by collapsed vertebrae is a visible symptom of osteoporosis.

© TravelStockCollection-Homer Sykes/Alamy Images.

▶ **Alzheimer's disease (AD)** A presenile dementia characterized by accumulation of plaques in certain regions of the brain and degeneration of a certain class of neurons.

Osteoporosis

Although osteoporosis affects older adults of both genders, it is most common in postmenopausal women. Osteoporosis is the deterioration of bone structure (see **FIGURE 12.15**) until, often without warning, the fragile bone breaks upon the slightest impact.

Nutritional factors, particularly early in life, are thought to play an important role in the development of osteoporosis. Whereas regular weight-bearing exercise helps prevent osteoporosis, inactivity increases osteoporosis risk. Long periods of inactivity, such as may be imposed by complete bed rest or illnesses that limit mobility, can promote the disease.

Although prevention is the best treatment for osteoporosis, many people enter later life with bad habits—poor nutrition and physical inactivity—that put them at risk. Adopting a diet that is rich in calcium and vitamin D and engaging in regular physical activity, particularly weight-bearing exercises, minimizes osteoporosis risks.

Alzheimer's Disease

Among its other ravages, **Alzheimer's disease (AD)** eventually destroys the ability to obtain, prepare, and consume an optimal diet. Although genetic factors can affect the risk for Alzheimer's disease, other risk factors include age, head trauma, and possibly exposure to environmental toxins. Although much more research is needed to determine their effects, antioxidants offer some protection from the disease.[90] Antioxidant supplements, however, have not been shown conclusively to be beneficial and can lead to undesirable side effects. Therefore, antioxidants from food should be encouraged for older adults to reduce risk of Alzheimer's disease.[91]

Most cases of Alzheimer's disease begin after age 70, but it can strike genetically predisposed people at a younger age. During the first stage of the disease, the afflicted person can have difficulty recalling names, frequently lose possessions, and easily become lost. Sensory sensitivity, such as loss of the sense of smell, is common, but because changes often occur gradually, they may not be readily noticed.

As the disease progresses, the person becomes unable to complete simple tasks that require learned motor movement, such as using a can opener. There is an increase in behavior problems and wandering that can affect the person's ability to maintain weight and nutritional status.

In late stages of the disease, about one-third of those with AD develop overactivity, which drains the nutritional reserve and increases calorie needs. At each stage the caregiver must carefully plan the person's diet to meet psychological and physical needs, paying particular attention to optimum nutrition without excess weight gain.

Overweight and Obesity

Maintaining a healthy body weight is critical at every life stage, the importance of which is underscored in older adults. Both underweight and overweight have significant consequences for the quality of life, health, and well-being of older adults. In addition to the health implications that accompany too much body weight, obesity in older adults can affect their ability to remain independent and accomplish their daily activities by interfering with normal physical functioning. Weight loss in this population is complicated by other health risks; however, additional weight gain is discouraged for overweight and obese older adults.[92] The presence of nutritional deficiencies in over-weight and obese older adults can be a consequence of the long-term consumption of a high-calorie, poor-nutrient diet and a physically inactive lifestyle.[93]

> **Key Concepts** Oral health, vision, and bone health all decline with aging. Tooth loss and oral pain can reduce food intake and nutrient quality. Loss of vision can make food shopping and preparation difficult. Osteoporosis, most common in postmenopausal women, can cause debilitating fractures. Alzheimer's disease eventually destroys the ability to obtain, prepare, and consume an optimal diet. Overweight and obesity are increasingly common and significantly affect the quality of life and health of older adults. Management of these conditions depends first on their identification by healthcare professionals.

Meal Management for Mature Adults

Many older adults are at nutritional risk because of economics, social isolation, physical restrictions, inability to shop for or prepare food, and medical conditions. Fortunately, there are a number of ways that older adults can remain independent and have access to an adequate diet.

Managing Independently

Independent and assisted-living programs allow people to live relatively carefree yet independent lives. Senior citizen apartment buildings and retirement villages offer a variety of services, including balanced meals. Programs such as **Meals on Wheels** and the **Older Americans Act Nutrition Program** (formerly known as the Elderly Nutrition Program) provide meals to home-bound people as well as those in congregate (group) settings. Most programs provide meals at least five times per week. The Older Americans Act Nutrition Program is supported primarily with federal funds; volunteer time, in-kind donations, and participant contributions make up the remainder. The **Supplemental Nutrition Assistance Program (SNAP)**, formerly the Food Stamp Program, is another option that provides low-income older adults with the means to purchase food. Unfortunately, because SNAP carries a "welfare" stigma, some older adults are reluctant to participate. In addition, many people who need some help buying food do not meet the eligibility requirements.

An evaluation of the Older Americans Act Nutrition Program showed that program participants had higher nutrient intake levels than nonparticipants and had a higher number of regular social contacts—another important factor in eating well.[94] Participation in food assistance programs can reduce the incidence of depression and overweight associated with food insecurity.[95]

Wise Eating for One or Two

Preparing meals that are healthful and tasty is a challenge for those living alone or in small households. As discussed earlier in this chapter, our nutrition needs—with the exception of calories—do not decrease as we age, but our ability to meet them does. Reliance on convenience foods, fast foods, and eating out can adversely affect the nutritional status of older adults. Men who live alone are especially likely to eat out or skip meals rather than prepare food for themselves. For both men and women, physical disability or illness can diminish the desire to prepare and eat meals.

▶ **Meals on Wheels** A voluntary, not-for-profit organization established to provide nutritious meals to homebound people (regardless of age) so they can maintain their independence and quality of life.

▶ **Older Americans Act Nutrition Program** A federally funded program (formerly known as the Elderly Nutrition Program) that provides older persons with nutritionally sound meals through home-delivered nutrition services, congregate nutrition services, and the nutrition services' incentive.

▶ **Supplemental Nutrition Assistance Program (SNAP)** A USDA program that helps single people and families with little or no income to buy food. Formerly known as the Food Stamp Program.

> ### Position Statement: Academy of Nutrition and Dietetics
>
> **Food and Nutrition for Older Adults: Promoting Health and Wellness**
>
> It is the position of the Academy of Nutrition and Dietetics that all Americans aged 60 years and older receive appropriate nutrition care; have access to coordinated, comprehensive food and nutrition services; and receive the benefits of ongoing research to identify the most effective food and nutrition programs, interventions, and therapies.
>
> Reprinted from *Journal of the Academy of Nutrition and Dietetics*, 112(8), Melissa Bernstein, Nancy Munoz, Position of the Academy of Nutrition and Dietetics: Food and Nutrition for Older Adults: Promoting Health and Wellness, Page no. 1255-1277, 2014, with permission from Elsevier.

Some simple changes in appliances and food-preparation techniques can help older adults overcome common obstacles to food preparation. Those who can't or won't cook can use microwaves, toaster ovens, and small appliances to prepare simple meals. A meal based on a lower-sodium, low-fat convenience entrée can meet nutritional needs if accompanied by vegetables, whole-grain bread, milk, and fruit.

THINK
About It
4

Finding Community Resources

An older person's need for community support typically changes from decade to decade. Sometimes, identifying community resources can be challenging, and financial considerations might further limit access to resources that can assist older adults in their own homes. Within local communities, area agencies on aging, social and rehabilitation services, cooperative extension services, churches, and extended-care facilities might have lists of resources and educational programs for older adults. **TABLE 12.12** lists important resources for older adults.

Key Concepts Older adults who obtain adequate food and nutrient intake while living independently can require assistance from time to time. This assistance might take the form of help with food shopping or preparation or identification of community resources that can stretch the food dollar. Numerous resources exist to assist older adults in maintaining a productive, high-quality life.

TABLE 12.12
Important Resources for Older Adults

The Eldercare Locator: www.eldercare.gov and (800) 677-1116 (toll free)
The National Association of Area Agencies on Aging and the National Association of State Units on Aging administer the Eldercare Locator, a public service of the Administration on Aging in the U.S. Department of Health and Human Services. The Eldercare Locator is a nationwide directory-assistance service that helps older persons and their families identify resources for aging Americans.

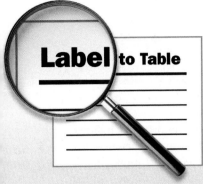

What is it about fruit snacks that makes them so attractive to kids? The sweet flavors, bright colors, different shapes, or logos of favorite movie or TV characters? Probably all of these. Parents may be attracted by claims for vitamins. So, are these nutritious snacks or little more than candy? Let's look at the label.

On the positive side, this is a fat-free snack and contains little sodium. However, most of the calories—56 of 80—come from sugar (14 g × 4 kcal/g), and the remainder from starch and protein. The ingredient list shows that the first three ingredients are sugars: high fructose corn syrup, sucrose, and fruit juice from concentrate.

The vitamins added to fruit snacks are the only redeeming feature of the product,

providing 25 percent of the DV for vitamins A, C, and E. But is there a better way to get these nutrients? One-half cup of orange juice provides two-thirds of the DV for vitamin C and significant amounts of thiamin, folate, and potassium as well. Just a handful of baby carrots provides more than 100 percent DV for vitamin A, along with some fiber. Vitamin E is widespread in the food supply—a small amount of salad dressing as a dip for the carrots would add vitamin E.

So, the fruit snacks are not as devoid of nutrients as candy, but are not as nutrient dense as fruits and vegetables. The fruit snacks may have some nutrient value, but they are high in sugar and, like all sugary snacks, should be limited.

Nutrition Facts

10 servings per container

Serving size   1 pouch (26g/0.9 oz)

Amount per serving

Calories 80

	% Daily Value*
Total Fat 0g	0%
Sodium 15mg	1%
Total Carbohydrate 19g	6%
Total Sugars 14g	
Includes 14g Added Sugars	28%
Protein 1g	
Vitamin D 0mcg	0%
Calcium 0mg	0%
Iron 0mg	0%
Potassium 2mg	0%
Vitamin A 375mcg	25%
Vitamin C 15mg	25%
Vitamin E 5mg	25%

Not a significant source of calories from fat, trans fat, cholesterol, dietary fiber, calcium, or iron.

* The % Daily Value (DV) tells you how much a nutrient in a serving of food contributes to a daily diet. 2,000 calories a day is used for general nutrition advice.

Learning Portfolio

Key Terms

Study Points

■ For children and adolescents, growth is the key determinant of nutrient needs. If diets are planned carefully, children do not need vitamin/mineral supplementation.

■ Federally funded nutrition and feeding programs reduce malnutrition and hunger among U.S. children.

■ Adoption of adult food plans to reduce risk of chronic disease should begin gradually after the age of 2.

■ The prevalence of obesity and eating disorders is rising among U.S. children and teens; treatment programs should address food choices and activity levels rather than impose strict calorie limits. Vegetarian diets for children need to be planned carefully to avoid nutrient deficiencies.

■ The total energy and nutrient needs of adolescents are high to support growth and maturation. Girls need more iron than boys do to compensate for losses after the onset of menstruation. Active teens need more calories and nutrients than sedentary teens; fluid intake is also a priority.

■ Nutrition and physical activity are two important, controllable components of a healthy life and healthful aging. Moreover, numerous physiological and psychological aspects of the aging process affect food intake and nutritional status.

■ Energy needs decline with age, reflecting loss of lean body mass and reduced physical activity.

The protein RDA and the recommended balance of carbohydrate and fat calories in the diet are similar for young and older adults. Fluid intake needs special attention because of the reduced thirst response that occurs with age.

■ Because of reduced intake, synthesis, and activation, vitamin D status declines with age; recommended intake levels are therefore raised. Vitamin B_{12} status might be compromised by inadequate absorption. Antioxidants can help in the protection against degenerative diseases.

■ Calcium and zinc intakes are likely to be marginal in the diets of older adults. Iron also remains important.

■ Dietary supplements, both vitamin/mineral and herbal/botanical, should be used with caution, preferably with professional advice.

■ Because many older adults take multiple medications, they are at risk for drug–nutrient, food–drug, and drug–drug interactions. Anorexia of aging is also a major public health problem.

■ Arthritis is a prevalent chronic health problem in this age group. Weight management is a key element of arthritis treatment.

■ Chronic constipation is a common complaint among older adults. Fluids, fiber, and regular exercise can reduce the likelihood of constipation.

■ Poor oral and visual health both can compromise the ability of older adults to consume a nutritionally adequate diet.

■ Osteoporosis is a major health problem that can be addressed through adequate calcium and vitamin D, regular weight-bearing exercise, and medication if needed.

■ Adults can maintain independence while aging but may require special assistance to obtain and prepare food. Community resources can help respond to the needs of older adults and those of their caretakers and family.

Study Questions

1. Which vitamins and minerals are most likely to be deficient in a child's diet?

2. Identify several chronic nutrition problems that can affect children. How can these problems be avoided?

3. What are typical nutritional concerns for adolescents?

4. What are some consequences of decreased immunity among older adults?

5. Compared with a younger adult, does a person older than 65 years need more, less, or about the same amount of protein?

6. Why are older adults at risk of vitamin D deficiency?

7. Discuss minerals that may need special attention in assessment of an older adult's nutrition status.

8. What problems might older adults encounter with dietary supplements?

9. What is the role of physical activity in osteoporosis prevention? What nutritional factors are important?

Try This

Eat Like a Kid

Children, especially toddlers, tend to be exploratory and take in the sensory nature of food—the textures, smells, and tastes. In fact, you were probably once this way. The purpose of this exercise is to eat a meal like a kid and gain an appreciation of food's textures and taste. Make some mashed potatoes, macaroni and cheese, buttered peas, or spaghetti (favorite "kid food") and eat it with your fingers. Explore your food and play with it. Try mixing foods. How does this experience make you feel?

Aging Simulation

The purpose of this exercise is to simulate what it can be like to age and experience age-related declines in health. Have you ever thought of how difficult it is to be an older person with health problems and do routine tasks? Invite a few friends over and do the following:

- Put gloves on to simulate the difficulty of losing sensitivity in your hands.

- Use cotton balls in your ears to decrease your hearing ability.

- Apply some petroleum jelly to a pair of glasses or sunglasses to give yourself poor vision.

Now try a simple activity. Make a salad, send a text message, or play a video. After completing the activity, switch disabilities with your friends so that everyone has experienced each of the limitations. What is it like to do these activities with your impairment?

Getting Personal

You have just graduated. Revisit your eating habits as a child, teenager, and college student, and assign the most appropriate descriptor to each item. Consider how your past nutritional behavior has helped determine your current health status.

0 = seldom or never true

1 = sometimes true

2 = frequently true

As a child,

1. I was a picky eater, rejecting the food usually offered.

2. I was not permitted to decide how much to eat.

3. I rarely drank milk.

4. I ate candy every day.

As an adolescent,

5. I let peer pressure influence my nutrition choices.

6. I ate in front of the TV.

7. I worried about my weight.

As a college student,

8. I didn't think about healthy food choices.

9. I resisted changing my eating habits.

10. I was influenced by food fads.

Add up your score. Scores over 12 should signal that your healthy nutrition behavior can be improved. Highlight the items you feel can be affected by behavior change.

References

1. Institute of Medicine, Food and Nutrition Board. *Dietary Reference Intakes for Energy, Carbohydrate, Fiber, Fat, Fatty Acids, Cholesterol, Protein, and Amino Acids.* Washington, DC: National Academies Press; 2005.

2. Kleinman RE, Greer FR, eds. *Pediatric Nutrition Handbook.* 7th ed. Elk Grove Village, IL: American Academy of Pediatrics; 2014.

3. Ogata B, Hayes D. Position of the Academy of Nutrition and Dietetics: nutrition guidance for healthy children ages 2 to 11 years. *J Acad Nutr Diet.* 2014;114:1257-1276.

4. Kumar J, Muntner P, Kaskel FJ, et al. Prevalence and associations of 25-hydroxyvitamin D deficiency in U.S. children: NHANES 2001–2004. *Pediatrics.* 2009;124(3):e362-e370.

5. Ogata B, Hayes D. Op. cit.

6. Kleinman RE, Greer FR. Op. cit.

7. Ogata B, Hayes D. Op. cit.

8. Neelon SE, Briley ME. Position of the American Dietetic Association: benchmarks for nutrition in child care. *J Am Diet Assoc.* 2011;111:607-615.

9. Pearson N, Biddle SJ. Sedentary behavior and dietary intake in children, adolescents, and adults: a systematic review. *Am J Prev Med.* 2011;41(2):178-188.

Learning Portfolio (continued)

10. Kelly B, Halford JCG, Boyland EJ, et al. Television food advertising to children: a global perspective. *Am J Pub Health*. 2011;100(9):1730-1736.

11. Batada A, Seitz M, Wootan M. Nine out of 10 food advertisements shown during Saturday morning children's television programming are for foods high in fat, sodium, or added sugars, or low in nutrients. *J Am Diet Assoc*. 2008;108(4):673-678.

12. Boyland EJ, Harrold JA, Kirkham TC, et al. Food commercials increase preference for energy-dense foods, particularly in children who watch more television. *Pediatrics*. 2011;128(1): e93-e100.

13. Miller SA, Taveras EM, Rifas-Shiman SL, Gillman MW. Association between television viewing and poor diet quality in young children. *Int J Pediatr Obes*. 2008;3(3):168-176.

14. U.S. Department of Agriculture, ChooseMyPlate.gov. 10 tips: be a healthy role model for children. https://www.choosemyplate.gov/10-tips-be-healthy-role-model-children. Accessed September 18, 2017.

15. Lehto R, Ray C, Roos E. Longitudinal associations between family characteristics and measures of childhood obesity. *Int J Public Health*. 2012;57(3):495-503.

16. World Food Programme. Nutrition. http://www1.wfp.org/nutrition. Accessed September 18, 2017.

17. Coleman-Jensen A, Rabbitt M, Gregory C, Singh A. Household food security in the United States in 2015. U.S. Department of Agriculture. https://www.ers.usda.gov/webdocs/publications/79761/err-215.pdf?v=42636. Accessed September 18, 2017.

18. American Heart Association, American Stroke Association. Facts: child nutrition reauthorization: a healthy recipe for school nutrition. http://www.heart.org/idc/groups/ahaecc-public/@wcm/@adv/documents/downloadable/ucm_463491.pdf. Accessed September 18, 2017.

19. Ibid.

20. American Psychiatric Association. *Diagnostic and Statistical Manual of Mental Disorders*. 5th ed. Arlington, VA: Author; 2013.

21. Kim Y, Chang H. Correlation between attention deficit hyperactivity disorder and sugar consumption, quality of diet, and dietary behavior in school children. *Nutr Res Pract*. 2011;5(3):236-245.

22. Stevens LJ, Kuczek T, Burgess JR, Hurt E, Arnold LE. Dietary sensitivities and ADHD symptoms: thirty-five years of research. *Clin Pediatr (Phila)*. 2011;50(4):279-293.

23. McCann D, Barrett A, Cooper A, et al. Food additives and hyperactive behaviour in 3-year-old and 8/9-year-old children in the community: a randomized, double-blinded, placebo-controlled trial. *Lancet*. 2007;370:1560-1567.

24. Pelsser LM, Frankena K, Toorman J, et al. Effects of a restricted elimination diet on the behaviour of children with attention-deficit hyperactivity disorder (INCA study): a randomised controlled trial. *Lancet*. 2011;377:494-503.

25. Ogden CL, Carroll MD, Curtin LR, Lamb MM, Flegal KM. Prevalence of high body mass index in US children and adolescents, 2007–2008. *JAMA*. 2010;303:242-249.

26. Let's Move! Health problems and childhood obesity. https://letsmove.obamawhitehouse.archives.gov/health-problems-and-childhood-obesity. Accessed September 18, 2017.

27. Let's Move! Home page. https://letsmove.obamawhitehouse.archives.gov. Accessed September 18, 2017.

28. Ibid.

29. National Heart, Lung, and Blood Institute. Expert panel on integrated guidelines for cardiovascular health and risk reduction in children and adolescents: summary report. http://www.nhlbi.nih.gov/files/docs/peds_guidelines_sum.pdf. Accessed September 18, 2017.

30. Office of Disease Prevention and Health Promotion. Healthy People 2020: environmental health. http://www.healthypeople.gov/2020/topicsobjectives2020/overview.aspx?topicid=12. Accessed September 18, 2017.

31. Centers for Disease Control and Prevention. Lead: CDC's national surveillance data (1997–2015). 2016. http://www.cdc.gov/nceh/lead/data/national.htm. Accessed September 18, 2017.

32. Centers for Disease Control and Prevention. Lead. http://www.cdc.gov/lead. Accessed September 18, 2017.

33. Melina V, Craig WJ, Levin S. Position of the Academy of Nutrition and Dietetics: vegetarian diets. *J Acad Nutr Diet*. 2016;116:1970-1980.

34. Wagner CL, Greer FR, Section on Breastfeeding and Committee on Nutrition. Prevention of rickets and vitamin D deficiency in infants, children, and adolescents. *Pediatrics*. 2008;122(5):1143-1152.

35. American Academy of Pediatrics. Vitamin D: on the double. http://www.healthychildren.org/English/healthy-living/nutrition/Pages/Vitamin-D-On-the-Double.aspx. Accessed September 18, 2017.

36. Kleinman RE, Greer FR. Op. cit.

37. Institute of Medicine. *Dietary Reference Intakes for Calcium and Vitamin D*. Washington, DC: National Academies Press; 2011.

38. Park S, Sappenfield WM, Huang Y, Sherry B, Bensyl DM. The impact of the availability of school vending machines on eating behavior during lunch: the Youth Physical Activity and Nutrition Survey. *J Am Diet Assoc*. 2010;110(10):1532-1536.

39. Minaker LM, Storey KE, Raine KD, et al. Associations between the perceived presence of vending machines and food and beverage logos in schools and adolescents' diet and weight status. *Public Health Nutr*. 2011;14(8):1350-1356.

40. Centers for Disease Control and Prevention. Trends in beverage consumption among high school students—United States, 2007–2015. *MMWR*. 2017;66(4):112-116.

41. Ibid.

42. Danby FW. Nutrition and acne. *Clin Dermatol*. 2010;28(6):598-604.

43. Spencer EH, Ferdowsian HR, Barnard ND. Diet and acne: a review of the evidence. *Int J Dermatol*. 2009;48:339-347.

44. Marcason W. Milk consumption and acne—is there a link? *J Am Diet Assoc*. 2010;110(1):152.

45. Berra B, Rizzo AM. Glycemic index, glycemic load: new evidence for a link with acne. *J Am Coll Nutr*. 2009;28(Suppl):450S-454S.

46. Nader PR, Bradley RH, Houts RM, et al. Moderate-to-vigorous physical activity from ages 9 to 15 years. *JAMA*. 2008;300:295-305.

47. Centers for Disease Control and Prevention. Childhood obesity causes & consequences. http://www.cdc.gov/obesity/childhood/causes.html. Accessed September 18, 2017.

48. Ibid.

49. Ibid.

50. Watson LC, Kwon J, Nichols D, Rew M. Evaluation of the nutrition knowledge, attitudes, and food consumption behaviors of high school students before and after completion of a nutrition course. *Fam Consumer Sci Res J*. 2009;37(4):523-534.

51. Dryden-Edwards R. *Teen drug abuse. What are some adolescent drug use statistics?* MedicineNet. http://www.medicinenet.com/teen_drug_abuse/page2.htm. Accessed September 18, 2017.

52. Ibid.

53. Centers for Disease Control and Prevention. E-cigarette use triples among middle and high school students in just one year. http://www.cdc.gov/media/releases/2015/p0416-e-cigarette-use.html. Accessed September 18, 2017.

54. Centers for Disease Control and Prevention. Alcohol and public health: fact sheets—binge drinking. http://www.cdc.gov/alcohol/quickstats/binge_drinking.htm. Accessed September 18, 2017.

55. U.S. Department of Health and Human Services, Administration for Community Living. Profile of older Americans: 2016 profile. https://www.acl.gov/aging-and-disability-in-america/data-and-research/profile-older-americans. Accessed September 18, 2017.

56. Ibid.

57. Position of the Academy of Nutrition and Dietetics: food and nutrition for older adults: promoting health and wellness. *J Acad Nutr Diet.* 2012;112:1255-1277.

58. Federal Interagency Forum on Aging Related Statistics. Older Americans 2016: key indicators of well-being. 2016. https://agingstats.gov. Accessed September 18, 2017.

59. Bernstein MA, Munoz NM, eds. *Nutrition for the Older Adult.* 2nd ed. Burlington, MA: Jones & Bartlett; 2016.

60. Sayer AA, Robinson SM, Patel HP, Shavlakadze T, Cooper C, Grounds MD. New horizons in the pathogenesis, diagnosis and management of sarcopenia. *Age Ageing.* 2013;42(2):145-150. doi: 10.1093/ageing/afs191

61. Bernstein MA, Munoz NM. Op. cit.

62. Salem GJ, Skinner JS, Chodzko-Zajko WJ, et al. Exercise and physical activity for older adults. *Med Sci Sports Exer.* 2009;41(7):1510-1530.

63. U.S. Department of Health and Human Services. Active older adults. In: *2008 Physical Activity Guidelines for Americans.* Rockville, MD: Author; 2008:1-61.

64. Chodzko-Zajki W, Proctor D, Fiatarone-Singh M, et al. American College of Sports Medicine position stand. Exercise and physical activity for older adults. *Med Sci Sport Exerc.* 2009;41(7):1510-1530.

65. Ravindran NC, Moskovitz DN, Kim YI. The aging gut. In: Chernoff R, ed. *Geriatric Nutrition: The Health Professional's Handbook.* 4th ed. Sudbury, MA: Jones & Bartlett; 2014:235-274.

66. Paddon-Jones D, Rasmussen BB. Dietary protein recommendations and the prevention of sarcopenia. *Curr Opin Clin Nutr Metab Care.* 2009;12(1):86-90.

67. Institute of Medicine, Food and Nutrition Board. *Dietary Reference Intakes for Water, Potassium, Sodium, Chloride, and Sulfate.* Washington, DC: National Academies Press; 2005.

68. Ibid.

69. National Institutes of Health, Office of Dietary Supplements. Vitamin D: fact sheet for health professionals. http://ods.od.nih.gov/factsheets/vitamind/. Accessed September 18, 2017.

70. Ibid.

71. Institute of Medicine. 2011. Op. cit.

72. Bernstein MA, Munoz NM. Op. cit.

73. Schalinske KL, Smazal AL. Homocysteine imbalance: a pathological metabolic marker. *Adv Nutr.* 2012;3(6):755-762. doi: 10.3945/an.112.002758

74. Position of the Academy of Nutrition and Dietetics: food and nutrition for older adults. Op. cit.

75. Allen LH. How common is vitamin B-12 deficiency? *Am J Clin Nutr.* 2009;89(2):693S-696S.

76. Position of the Academy of Nutrition and Dietetics: food and nutrition for older adults. Op. cit.

77. Academy of Nutrition and Dietetics. Food and nutrition for older adults (FNOA) promoting health and wellness (2011-2012). Evidence Analysis Library. http://www.andevidenceanalysislibrary.com/topic.cfm?cat=3987. Accessed September 18, 2017.

78. Devore E, Kang J, Stampfer M, Grodstein F. Total antioxidant capacity of diet in relation to cognitive function. *Am J Clin Nutr.* 2010;92:1157-1164.

79. Institute of Medicine. *2011.* Op. cit.

80. Ibid.

81. Nahin R, Pecha M, Welmerink D, et al. Concomitant use of prescription drugs and dietary supplements in ambulatory elderly people. *J Am Geriatr Soc.* 2009;57(7):1197-1205.

82. Buhr G, Bales CW. Nutritional supplements for older adults: review and recommendations—part II. *J Nutr Elder.* 2010;29(1):42-71.

83. Bernstein MA, Munoz NM. Op. cit.

84. National Institute of Arthritis and Musculoskeletal and Skin Diseases. Handout on health: osteoarthritis. May 2016. http://www.niams.nih.gov/Health_Info/Osteoarthritis. Accessed September 18, 2017.

85. Patterson E, Wall R, Fitzgerald GF, Ross RP, Stanton C. Health implications of high dietary omega-6 polyunsaturated fatty acids. *J Nutr Metab.* 2012;2012:539426.

86. Lahiri M, Morgan C, Symmons DP, Bruce IN. Modifiable risk factors for RA: prevention, better than a cure? *Rheumatology (Oxford).* 2012;51(3):499-512.

87. Sarubin Fragakis A, Thomson CA. *The Health Professional's Guide to Popular Dietary Supplements.* 3rd ed. Chicago: American Dietetic Association; 2006.

88. Position of the Academy of Nutrition and Dietetics: food and nutrition for older adults. Op. cit.

89. National Eye Institute. The AREDS formulation and age-related macular degeneration. Are these high levels of antioxidants and zinc right for you? https://nei.nih.gov/amd/summary. Accessed September 18, 2017.

90. Devore E, Kang J, Stampfer M, Grodstein F. Op. cit.

91. Position of the Academy of Nutrition and Dietetics: food and nutrition for older adults. Op. cit.

92. U.S. Department of Agriculture, U.S. Department of Health and Human Services. *2015–2020 Dietary Guidelines for Americans.* http://www.cnpp.usda.gov/2015-2020-dietary-guidelines-americans. Accessed September 18, 2017.

93. Position of the Academy of Nutrition and Dietetics: food and nutrition for older adults. Op. cit.

94. Position Paper of the American Dietetic Association: nutrition across the spectrum of aging. *J Am Diet Assoc.* 2005;105(4):616-633.

95. Kim K, Frongillo EA. Participation in food assistance programs modifies the relation of food insecurity with weight and depression in older adults. *J Nutr.* 2007;137:1005-1010.

Spotlight on World Nutrition: The Faces of Global Malnutrition

Revised by Tara LaRowe

THINK About It

1   Have you ever experienced hunger without being able to satisfy it within a day?

2   Have you seen evidence of hunger or malnutrition in your community?

3   How do you feel about the United States sending food to impoverished nations?

4   What can you do to help eliminate hunger in North America?

CHAPTER Menu

- Malnutrition in the United States
- Malnutrition in the Developing World

LEARNING Objectives

1. Define *food insecurity*.
2. List populations at risk for malnutrition.
3. Discuss domestic food programs that combat hunger.
4. Explain the causes of world hunger.
5. Describe the key features of protein-energy malnutrition.
6. Identify and discuss the major nutritional deficiencies worldwide.

E ach day on your way to class, you pass a soup kitchen. You look at the long line of men and women waiting to get their meals and wonder what brought them to this point. You wonder how many similar soup lines exist in your community and how many people need food assistance but can't get it. If **hunger** exists in our rich country, what about people living in poor countries?

Despite progress in reducing world hunger in the past two decades, between the years 2014 and 2016 there were still nearly 795 million people worldwide that did not have enough to eat. This figure includes 14.7 million people in developed countries,[1] although most of the world's hungry live in developing countries. (See **FIGURE SW.1**.)

▶ **hunger** The internal, physiological drive to find and consume food. Unlike appetite, hunger is often experienced as a negative sensation, often manifesting as an uneasy or painful sensation; the recurrent and involuntary lack of access to food that may produce malnutrition over time.

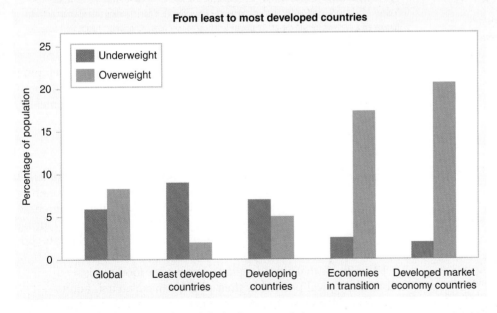

FIGURE SW.1 Global nutrition transition and obesity. As poor countries become more prosperous, they acquire some of the problems, including obesity, along with the benefits of becoming a more developed nation. In the developing world, a number of changes in diet, physical activity, health, and nutrition, collectively known as the "nutrition transition," lead to increased rates of obesity.
Courtesy of the Food and Agriculture Organization of the United Nations using data from WHO.

▶ **malnutrition** Failure to achieve nutrient requirements, which can impair physical and/or mental health. It may result from consuming too little food or from a shortage or imbalance of key nutrients.

▶ **food insecurity** (1) Limited or uncertain availability of nutritionally adequate and safe foods or (2) limited or uncertain ability to acquire acceptable foods in socially acceptable ways.

▶ **food security** Access to enough food for an active, healthy life, including (1) the ready availability of nutritionally adequate and safe foods and (2) an assured ability to acquire acceptable foods in socially acceptable ways.

Quick Bite

Food Recovery and Gleaning

Each year more than 40 percent of food in the United States goes uneaten. That is more than 20 pounds of food per person every month. Programs throughout the country are rescuing much of this wholesome food and distributing it to people in need. *Gleaning* is harvesting excess food from farms, orchards, and packing houses. Perishable items also are salvaged from wholesale and retail markets; fresh foods that are wholesome but will spoil before they can be sold are given to local food pantries and meal providers. Canned goods and other staples are collected from groceries, distributors, food processors, and individual homes. Even surplus food from restaurants, caterers, and other food services is collected by some charities for local food programs.

The majority of undernourished people live in Asia and the Asian Pacific region (over 500 million people); the region with the highest proportion of undernutrition is sub-Saharan Africa (23.2 percent of the population).[2] Worldwide, more than half the deaths of children younger than 5 years are caused directly or indirectly by **malnutrition**, which kills more than 3.1 million children per year.[3]

In this chapter, we look at hunger and malnutrition. By *hunger*, we don't mean that mildly empty feeling one gets before mealtime. We mean the inability, day after day, to satisfy basic nutrition needs, the gnawing emptiness that creates a constant focus on eating and how to obtain food. In contrast to the hunger dieters feel from cutting calories, this deprivation is involuntary and unwanted.

Technically speaking, *malnutrition* can be any kind of unhealthy nutritional status, including the result of imbalance and excess—obesity or toxicity from oversupplementation, for example. And although we touch on obesity as an emerging issue, even in developing countries, in this chapter, *malnutrition* generally refers to undernutrition resulting from hunger.

Along the spectrum of malnutrition and hunger is the less extreme condition of **food insecurity**, the ongoing worry about having enough to eat. At the opposite end of the spectrum is **food security**, access to nutritionally adequate and safe food. Most people in the industrialized world are food-secure. Overabundance and obesity are the primary problems in these populations, but malnutrition is a serious problem among certain groups, such as the homeless and urban poor.

Malnutrition in the United States

Why Is This Important? Malnutrition and hunger are invisible to many of us. We may think it exists only in poor countries, or only among people who look sick. Understanding that malnutrition and hunger exist everywhere and can affect anyone will help you see how communities might work together to bring resources to those in need.

Malnutrition and hunger are serious problems not only in developing countries, but also in the United States and other industrialized countries. Among those who suffer the worst malnutrition are the homeless, children, older adults, the working poor, and the rural poor.

The Face of American Malnutrition

Even in the food-rich United States, food insecurity remains a problem.[4] (See **FIGURE SW.2**.) It is characterized by anxiety about having enough to eat and about running out of food and having no money to purchase more. Some people actually go hungry in the United States: During 2015, 42.2 million Americans, including more than 13 million children, lived in households experiencing food insecurity.[5]

Households that are struggling to meet basic food needs tend to follow a typical pattern as their plight worsens. First, adults worry about having enough food. Then, they stretch resources and juggle other necessities, with more of the budget going for fixed expenses than for food. The quality and variety of the diet decline. Next, the adults eat less and less often. And finally, as food becomes more limited, the children also eat less. When there is not enough food, common strategies include eating less varied diets and participating in local and federal emergency relief and food assistance programs.[6]

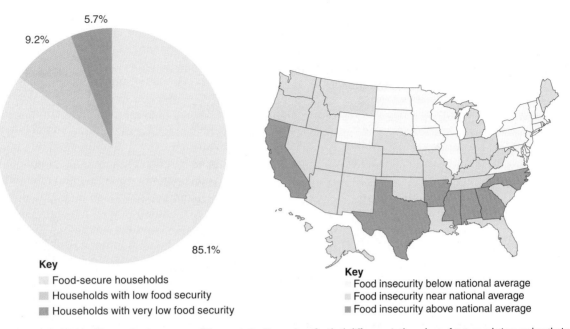

5.7%

9.2%

85.1%

Key
Food-secure households
Households with low food security
Households with very low food security

Key
Food insecurity below national average
Food insecurity near national average
Food insecurity above national average

FIGURE SW.2 Prevalence of food insecurity. State-to-state differences in food insecurity reflect both differences in the makeup of state populations, such as the income, employment, age, education, and family structure of their residents, and differences in state characteristics, such as economic conditions, the accessibility and use of food assistance programs, and tax policies.

Pie graph: Reproduced from ERS using data from the Current Population Survey Food Security Supplement; Map: Reproduced from ERS using data from the Current Population Survey Food Security Supplement.

Surprisingly, obesity is more prevalent among low-income, food-insecure groups than among those with higher incomes. To stave off hunger, households with little money often rely on cheaper, high-calorie foods. Those who live in a state of food insecurity consume significantly fewer healthful foods and micronutrients.[7] Although such suboptimal diets usually do not lead to overt deficiency diseases, more subtle effects are serious and costly, showing up years later as chronic illness or more immediately as reduced immune function.

Prevalence and Distribution

How much hunger and food insecurity exists in the United States? Many people with limited financial resources manage to eat well. However, under certain circumstances, such as loss of a job, people who live well above the poverty line (see **TABLE SW.1**) may be food-insecure.

The U.S. Department of Agriculture (USDA) tracks hunger with an annual **Food Security Supplement Survey**, which asks about food availability and hunger in the household. (See **TABLE SW.2**.) In a recent survey, food insecurity was strongly associated with poverty and was interlinked with economic and social factors. Food insecurity and hunger were highest in households headed by single women with children and in Hispanic and African American households.[8] Geographically, food insecurity is more common in rural areas and large inner cities and, regionally, is more prevalent in the South. (See **FIGURE SW.3**.) To combat food insecurity and hunger effectively, nutrition programs must be accompanied by social and economic efforts.

The Working Poor

Employment does not guarantee that families always have enough to eat. Often the pay is too little to lift households out of poverty, and

▶ **Food Security Supplement Survey** A federally funded survey that measures the prevalence and severity of food insecurity and hunger.

TABLE SW.1

Poverty Guidelines: Income Levels Defined as Poverty for a Given Household Size

Persons in Family	48 Contiguous States and Washington, DC	Alaska	Hawaii
1	$11,880	$14,840	$13,670
2	16,020	20,020	18,430
3	20,160	25,200	23,190
4	24,300	30,380	27,950
5	28,440	35,560	32,710
6	32,580	40,740	37,470
7	36,730	45,920	42,230
8	40,890	51,120	47,010
For each additional person, add:	4,160	5,200	4,780

Note: Despite the limits to the use of household income as a proxy for estimating food insecurity, poverty remains an intuitively reasonable indicator. Keep in mind that, in addition to food, income must cover housing, clothing, transportation, medical care, and other essentials.

Reproduced from U.S. Department of Health and Human Services, Office of the Secretary. Annual update of the HHS poverty guidelines. Federal Register. 2016;81(15):4036–3637. https://www.federalregister.gov/documents/2016/01/25/2016-01450/annual-update-of-the-hhs -poverty-guidelineshttp://aspe.hhs.gov/poverty/13poverty.cfm. Accessed September 21, 2017.

TABLE SW.2

Sample Questions from the Food Security Questionnaire

Light Food Insecurity

"We worried whether our food would run out before we got money to buy more." Was that often, sometimes, or never true for you in the last 12 months?
"The food that we bought just didn't last and we didn't have money to get more." Was that often, sometimes, or never true for you in the last 12 months?

Moderate Food Insecurity

In the last 12 months did you or other adults in the household ever cut the size of your meals or skip meals because there wasn't enough money for food?
In the last 12 months, were you ever hungry but didn't eat because you couldn't afford enough food?

Severe Food Insecurity

In the last 12 months did you or other adults in the household ever not eat for a whole day because there wasn't enough money for food?
(For households with children) In the last 12 months did any children ever not eat for a whole day because there wasn't enough money for food?

Reproduced from Coleman-Jensen A, Rabbitt M, Gregory C, and Singh A. Household Food Security in the United States in 2015. USDA; September 2016. Economic Research Service. Report No. 215. https://www.ers.usda.gov/publications/pub-details/?pubid=79760. Accessed February 22, 2017.

work-related expenses, such as transportation or child care, further deplete family budgets. Food insecurity can be as common among the working poor as the unemployed. Low-paid workers may be unaware that they still qualify for food-assistance programs. However, their work hours may preclude program participation.

Migrant farm workers may have access to plenty of fresh produce but are poorly paid and may not have the money to buy other foods. Farm workers and undocumented workers (illegal aliens) may not qualify for government programs to help the poor or may not sign up for fear of deportation.

Food Deserts

Areas where people lack access to affordable healthy foods such as low-fat milk products, whole grains, fruits, and vegetables are termed

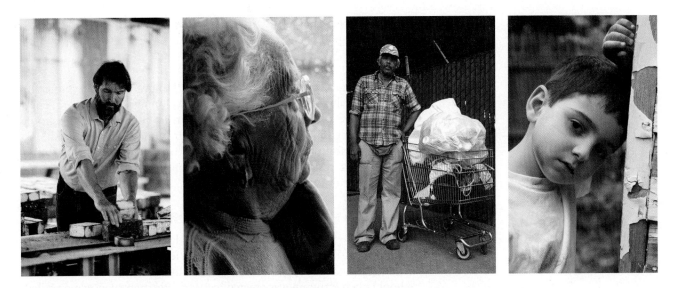

FIGURE SW.3 Americans at risk. Americans most at risk for hunger include the working poor, older adults, homeless people, and children.
Working poor: © Photodisc; Older adults: © Photodisc; Homeless people: © Jack Star/PhotoLink/Photodisc; Children: © Jaimie Duplass/Shutterstock, Inc.

food deserts.[9] Access is defined by distance to supermarkets or grocery stores that offer affordable food, individual-level resources such as personal wealth, and neighborhood-level characteristics such as availability of public transportation.[10] Approximately 54.4 million people in the United States live in a low-income and low-access area, where low access is measured by the proximity to the nearest supermarket. In urban areas, low access is defined as being greater than ½ to 1 mile away from a supermarket; in rural areas it is defined as being greater than 10 to 20 miles away.[11]

The Isolated

Some people become isolated despite living in populated cities. Even though they live in a crowded neighborhood or apartment building, they are alone and are physically or mentally unable to obtain adequate food.

Older Adults

The infirmities of age, along with feelings of vulnerability, keep some older adults homebound and lonely. Physical ailments may make cooking and eating difficult, while actually increasing nutrient needs. Like others with limited resources, older adults cut food purchases to pay for other necessities. Although food assistance may be available, pride or shame may keep an older person from participating in such programs.

The Homeless or Inadequately Housed

The homeless rely on soup kitchens and other public programs for much of their food. Some resort to handouts and even forage through garbage. Many are mentally ill or substance abusers. The addict often has little interest in eating and may sell available food to buy more drugs. Many other people live in welfare hotels, single-room-occupancy facilities, or rooming houses without storage or cooking facilities.

▶ **food deserts** Urban neighborhoods and rural towns without ready access to fresh, healthy, and affordable food.

Quick **Bite**

Is There a Food Desert Near You?
The USDA's Economic Research Service created the Food Access Research Atlas to track indicators of food deserts using mapping and spatial technology. To find food deserts, you can access the map on the USDA website at www.ers.usda.gov.

As the monthly budget dwindles, they often rely on fast-food meals and then soup kitchens.

Children

Perhaps no group is more vulnerable to hunger than the young. In poorly nourished children, growth and development are delayed. They get sick more often. It is harder for them to concentrate in school. Children are captives of their family circumstances; poverty and lack of nutritious food in the household are beyond a child's control. In the United States, roughly 12.7 percent of households were food-insecure at some time during 2015.[12]

Attacking Hunger in the United States

Government efforts to fight hunger began during the Great Depression of the 1930s. From that modest beginning, federal efforts have grown to include at least 14 programs that address hunger. (See **TABLE SW.3**.) The School Lunch Program was created in 1946 after many young men failed the physical requirements for military service in World War II because of poor nutrition. The Supplemental Nutrition Assistance Program (SNAP, formerly called the Food Stamp Program), begun on a small scale years earlier, was greatly expanded in the early 1970s following an exposé on hunger in Appalachia and the Mississippi Delta and the television documentary "Hunger in America." The federal government initiated the Special Supplemental Nutrition Program for Women, Infants, and Children (WIC) in the 1970s in response to concerns about maternal and child health. Other government programs have since been added to meet the special needs of the young, the elderly, the disadvantaged, and the disabled. The **Food Research and Action Center** is a national nonprofit advocacy group that fights hunger and undernutrition at the national, state, and local levels.

▶ **Food Research and Action Center**   A nonprofit child advocacy group that works to improve public policies to eradicate hunger and undernutrition in the United States; founded in 1970 as a public interest law firm.

TABLE SW.3

USDA Food and Nutrition Service Food Assistance Programs

- Supplemental Nutrition Assistance Program (SNAP)
- Women, Infants, and Children (WIC) Program
- Farmers' Market Nutrition Program
- Senior Farmers' Market Nutrition Program
- School meals
- National School Lunch Program
- School Breakfast Program
- Fresh Fruit and Vegetable Program
- Special Milk Program
- Team Nutrition
- Summer Food Service Program
- Child and Adult Care Food Program
- Food assistance for disaster relief
- Food distribution
- Commodity Supplemental Food Program
- Food Distribution Program on Indian Reservations
- The Emergency Food Assistance Program

Data from U.S. Department of Agriculture, Food, and Nutrition Service. Nutrition assistance programs. http://www.fns.usda.gov/fns. Accessed February 25, 2017.

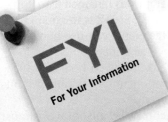

Hungry and Homeless

A shabbily dressed man slowly pushes a shopping cart along the sidewalk. It is laden with bottles and cans that he can redeem for cash. In front of a supermarket, a woman and child clutch a sign scrawled with the words "Hungry. Please help." On a street corner, a man confronts every passing car with a sign that says "Will work for food." When confronted by a homeless person, do you feel uncomfortable? Do you turn away? Or, do you try to help?

In the 2016 Annual Report on Hunger and Homelessness, from the U.S. Conference of Mayors and National Alliance to End Homelessness, 14.3 percent of the homeless population were chronically homeless.[a] Request for food assistance rose approximately 2 percent among 41 percent of the cities surveyed. Mayors reported the top causes of hunger to be lack of affordable housing and poverty, unemployment, and medical/healthcare costs.[b]

Who are the homeless? On any given night in the United States, approximately 560,000 people are homeless.[c] According to 2014 statistics on the sheltered homeless population, 62.3 percent are male, 40.6 percent are African American, 20.8 percent are age 62 or older, 63.9 percent are single individuals (rather than members of homeless families), and 42.2 percent are physically disabled.[d] Homelessness is also a concern among youth. It is estimated that approximately 380,000 youth under 18 years old experience homelessness of longer than one week per year.[e] Furthermore, mental illness and substance abuse are also highly prevalent among homeless populations.[f]

Complex challenges face the homeless, who may sleep in the streets or in emergency shelters. The homeless get food from many sources—shelters, drop-in centers, fast-food restaurants, and garbage bins. According to the Hunger in America studies, the number of clients the Feeding America network served between years 2006 and 2010 increased by 46 percent.[g] Yet, only 27 percent of clients who reported using a food pantry recurrently did not own or rent a home, compared to 43 percent of clients that owned a home and 35 percent that rented a home.[h] Soup kitchens are a primary source of meals, yet navigating this system to obtain adequate food can be a formidable and time-consuming task. Also, although homeless people often are eligible for food stamps, they are extremely limited in their ability to store and prepare food, and few restaurants are authorized to accept SNAP benefits.

Homeless families and individuals rely on emergency food assistance facilities not only during emergencies, but also for extended periods. Unfortunately, these facilities are strained beyond their capacities. Due to limited space, emergency shelters must turn away families with children experiencing homelessness. Some shelters have resorted to rationing to extend their food resources to a greater number of people. Because of a lack of resources, over half may be forced to turn people away. Addressing hunger is a top priority. Once access to food is secure, obtaining a nutritionally adequate diet and dealing with health issues become reasonable goals.

a National Low Income Housing Coalition. U.S. Conference of Mayors and NAEH release hunger and homelessness report. December 2016. http://nlihc.org/article/us-conference-mayors-and-naeh-release-hunger-and-homelessness-report. Accessed October 3, 2017.

b Ibid.

c National Alliance to End Homelessness. Homelessness statistics. http://www.endhomelessness.org/pages/faqs. Accessed September 21, 2017.

d Ibid.

e Ibid.

f Ibid.

g Research Brief Food Banks: Hunger's New Staple. Hunger in America 2011. http://www.feedingamerica.org/research/hungers-new-staple/hungers-new-staple-full-report.pdf. Accessed October 23, 2017.

h Ibid.

THINK About It 2

Nonprofit community agencies, charities, religious organizations, and similar groups create a large network of food pantries, soup kitchens, and services for home-delivered meals. (See the FYI feature "Hungry and Homeless.") Most federal government programs for direct distribution of food or meals operate at the local level through these networks. Both laypeople and public health professionals, such as dietitians, work in these programs, either as volunteers or as staff, to fight hunger and malnutrition.

Food assistance programs have greatly reduced the prevalence of hunger, but not of food insecurity, which requires social and economic change. The following are among the federal government's most far-reaching programs against hunger.

The Supplemental Nutrition Assistance Program

On October 1, 2008, the Food Stamp Program was renamed the Supplemental Nutrition Assistance Program (SNAP). SNAP is the main food security program in the United States. Recipients can use benefits to purchase food but not nonfood items such as paper goods, pet food, and alcohol. The benefit amount varies according to household size and income level. In 2014, SNAP participation among eligible persons living in the U.S. was estimated at 83 percent.[13]

Actually, the term *food stamp* is becoming a misnomer. Almost half the people who receive benefits use **Electronic Benefits Transfer (EBT)** cards. (See **FIGURE SW.4**.) The card resembles and functions like a debit card. Each month the household's benefit amount is credited to the card, which is then used at participating retailers and farmers' markets.

Supplemental Nutrition Assistance Program Education (SNAP-Ed) provides nutrition education and obesity prevention programs among SNAP recipients. Each state offers SNAP-Ed programs that focus on improving healthy food choices on a limited food budget and encourage active lifestyles that are consistent with the *2015–2020 Dietary Guidelines for Americans* and MyPlate. The Healthy, Hunger-Free Kids Act of 2010 established SNAP-Ed as the Nutrition Education and Obesity Prevention Grant Program.[14]

Special Supplemental Nutrition Program for Women, Infants, and Children

The WIC program provides food to pregnant and breastfeeding women, infants, and preschoolers. More than 8 million women and children receive WIC benefits each month.[15] To be eligible for WIC services, the participant must be at nutritional risk and the household's income must be less than the federal definition of poverty level. For a family of four in fiscal year 2016–2017, the eligibility cut-off point is an annual income of no more than $44,955.[16]

Nutrition assessment and nutrition education are important components of the WIC program. In most states, participants receive coupons, "checks," or EBT cards for specific categories of healthful foods, and they use them at participating grocery stores. Unlike SNAP benefits, the amount of the WIC benefit varies with nutritional need, not income.

National School Lunch Program

The National School Lunch Program (NSLP), established in 1946 through the National School Lunch Act, is administered by USDA's Food and Nutrition Service. The purpose of the NSLP is to safeguard the health and nutrition of children; it allows schools to receive federal assistance to serve nutritious meals to children living in homes with limited income. For a family of four for the 2017–2018 school year, the child's meals are free if the household income is less than $31,980; the allotment for meals is reduced if the household income exceeds $31,980 but is less than $45,510.[17] School lunches must comply with the *2015–2020 Dietary Guidelines for Americans* and provide one-third or more of dietary requirements for key nutrients. The program operates in more than 100,000 public and nonprofit private schools

▶ **Electronic Benefits Transfer (EBT)** Electronic delivery of government benefits by a single plastic card that allows access to food benefits at point-of-sale locations.

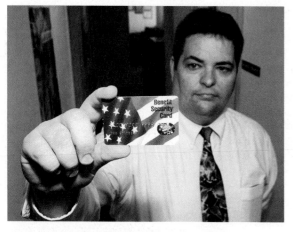

FIGURE SW.4 Electronic Benefits Transfer card. Electronic Benefits Transfer (EBT) is an electronic system that allows recipients to authorize transfer of their government benefits from a federal account to a retailer account to pay for products received.

© Danny Johnston/AP Photos.

and residential child-care institutions. It provides nutritionally balanced, low-cost or free lunches to more than 31 million children each schoolday.[18] (See **FIGURE SW.5**.)

Child and Adult Care Food Program

The **Child and Adult Care Food Program** provides funds for children's meals and snacks at nonprofit licensed child-care centers, day care homes, after-school programs, and similar settings. Nutritious meals for older adults or disabled people are also funded at nonprofit facilities such as adult day care centers and recreation centers. This program serves more than 3.3 million children and 120,000 adults each day. On April 25, 2016, the USDA's Food and Nutrition Service updated the meal pattern requirements to be consistent with the *2015–2020 Dietary Guidelines for Americans* and major public health and scientific organizations' recommendations.[19]

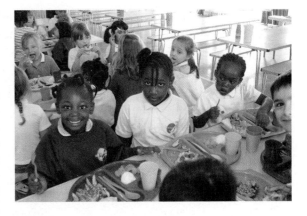

FIGURE SW.5 National School Lunch Program.
© Mike Booth/Alamy Images.

Feeding America

Feeding America, formerly known as America's Second Harvest, is the largest charitable hunger-relief organization in the United States. This network of more than 200 member food banks and food-rescue organizations secures and distributes more than 3 billion pounds of donated food and groceries throughout the United States. Each year, Feeding America provides food assistance to more than 46 million hungry people, including 12 million children and 7 million seniors.[20]

Feeding America focuses on nutritious products such as fresh produce, seafood, meat, cereal, rice, and pasta. The organization also works to effect changes in public attitudes and laws that assist Americans who are hungry or at risk of being hungry. Feeding America works to educate the general public and keep them informed about hunger in America.

▶ **Child and Adult Care Food Program** A federally funded program that reimburses approved family child-care providers for USDA-approved foods served to preschool children; also provides funds for meals and snacks served at after-school programs for school-age children and to adult day care centers serving chronically impaired adults or people over age 60.

▶ **Feeding America** The largest charitable hunger-relief organization in the United States. Its mission is to feed America's hungry through a nationwide network of member food banks and to engage the country in the fight to end hunger.

Key Concepts Although overt malnutrition in the United States is uncommon, more than 8.3 million U.S. households experience food insecurity at some time during the year. Food insecurity and hunger are interlinked with poverty. Groups at risk include the working poor, the isolated, the homeless, children, and older adults. A large network of individual volunteers, nonprofit agencies, and charities, together with major government programs such as SNAP, WIC, the National School Lunch Program, and the Child and Adult Care Food Program have done much to reduce hunger. However, food insecurity, which continues among an unacceptably large number of people, must be overcome by social and economic improvements. Feeding America is the largest charitable hunger-relief organization in the United States.

Malnutrition in the Developing World

🍎 **Why Is This Important?** Millions of people around the world do not have access to clean water and healthy, affordable, and safe food. How can this be? Understanding the major factors affecting global health is essential for reversing malnutrition in the developing world.

According to the **World Health Organization (WHO)**, "The enjoyment of the highest attainable standard of health is one of the fundamental rights of every human being without distinction of race, religion, political belief, economic, or social condition." Director Dr. Margaret Chan identified that, "The world needs a global health guardian, a custodian of values, a protector and defender of health, including the right to health."[21]

▶ **World Health Organization (WHO)** A global organization that directs and coordinates international health work. Its goal is the attainment by all peoples of the highest possible level of health, defined as a state of complete physical, mental, and social well-being and not merely the absence of disease or infirmity.

▶ **Food and Agriculture Organization (FAO)** The largest autonomous United Nations agency; the FAO works to alleviate poverty and hunger by promoting agricultural development, improved nutrition, and the pursuit of food security.

Position Statement: Academy of Nutrition and Dietetics

Nutrition Security in Developing Nations: Sustainable Food, Water, and Health

It is the position of the Academy of Nutrition and Dietetics that all people should have consistent access to an appropriately nutritious diet of food and water, coupled with a sanitary environment, adequate health services, and care that ensure a healthy and active life for all household members. The Academy supports policies, systems, programs, and practices that work with developing nations to achieve nutrition security and self-sufficiency while being environmentally and economically sustainable.

Reprinted from *Journal of the Academy of Nutrition and Dietetics*, 113(4), Stacia M. Nordin, Marie Boyle, Teresa M. Kemmer, Position of the Academy of Nutrition and Dietetics: Nutrition Security in Developing Nations: Sustainable Food, Water, and Health, Page no. 581-595, 2013, with permission from Elsevier.

Quick Bite

Where Were You Born?

Location of birth greatly influences an infant's chance of survival. Angola has the highest infant mortality rate (96 deaths per 1,000 live births), according to estimates for 2015. Other countries with high infant mortality rates include Sierra Leone (87 per 1,000), Afghanistan (66 per 1,000), and Liberia (53 per 1,000). At the other end of the spectrum are Norway, Estonia, Japan, and several other countries (2 per 1,000). Canada (4 per 1,000) has a lower infant mortality rate than the United States (6 per 1,000).

United Nations Inter-agency Group for Child Mortality Estimation. Levels and trends in child mortality. Report 2015. http://www.childmortality.org/files_v20/download/IGME%20Report%202015_9_3%20LR%20Web.pdf. Accessed September 21, 2017.

Hunger is a global problem. (See **FIGURE SW.6**.) "The number and the proportion of undernourished people have declined, but they remain unacceptably high. Undernourishment remains higher than before the food and economic crises, making it ever more difficult to achieve international hunger targets," says the **Food and Agriculture Organization (FAO)** of the United Nations.[22] (See **FIGURE SW.7**.)

THINK About It 3

The World Food Equation

Soaring food prices are hitting the world's most vulnerable—those who must spend a substantial part of their income on food. Changes in food availability, rising commodity prices, and new producer–consumer linkages have crucial implications for the livelihoods of poor and food-insecure people.[23] Today the world consumes more than it produces, and the cost of food has been rising steadily, reversing a downward trend of more than four decades. Food stocks are at a low, and the food supply is vulnerable to unpredictable factors, such as adverse weather. During a disaster, food prices rise rapidly while family incomes decline, thus producing an economic mismatch that is the root cause of most famines.[24]

Global Economic Boom

Some developing countries are undergoing rapid economic expansion. People in emerging economies, such as China, India, Brazil, and at least 10 African countries, have become more prosperous and are changing their diets. Since 1990, China has nearly doubled its consumption of meat, fish, and dairy products. Because it takes 7 pounds of grain to produce 1 pound of meat, this shift removes grain from the global marketplace. In just the past few years, China has changed from being one of the largest corn exporters to importing corn.[25]

Global Climate Change and Severe Weather Events

As a consequence of climate change, farmers will face growing unpredictability and variability in water supplies and increasing frequency of droughts and floods. However, these impacts will vary tremendously from place to place. According to a recent report from the FAO, climate change already affects food security and puts millions of people at risk for hunger and poverty, but these effects may be even more catastrophic in tropical, developing regions where households and communities are already vulnerable to food insecurity.[26]

Water is fundamental to the stability of global food production. Reliable access to water increases agricultural yields, and a lack of sustainable water management places global food security at risk. In developing countries, drought is the single most common natural cause of severe food shortages. Floods are another major cause of food emergencies. To the extent that climate change increases rainfall variability and the frequency of extreme weather events, it will threaten food security.

The Fight Against Global Hunger

International relief agencies and government programs help combat food shortages and hunger. Some U.S. agencies involved in the fight against global hunger are the USDA; the U.S. State Department, through its Agency for International Development; and the Centers for Disease Control and Prevention (CDC), through the Center for Communicable Diseases. These agencies offer both short-term emergency efforts and long-term programs for repair and rebuilding.

THINK About It 4

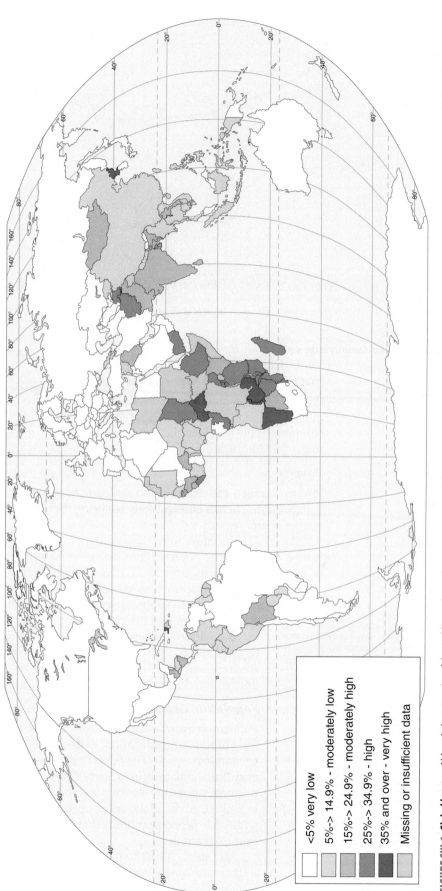

FIGURE SW.6 Global hunger. Although the proportion of the world's population that is chronically undernourished has been decreasing over the last few decades, undernutrition is still widespread, particularly in certain regions. As of 2015, 73 out of 129 developing countries achieved the goal of halving the proportion of chronically undernourished people.

Food and Agriculture Organization of the United Nations, 2015, The FAO Hunger Map 2015, http://www.fao.org/hunger/en/. Reproduced with permission.

Legend:
- <5% very low
- 5%–>14.9% - moderately low
- 15%–>24.9% - moderately high
- 25%–>34.9% - high
- 35% and over - very high
- Missing or insufficient data

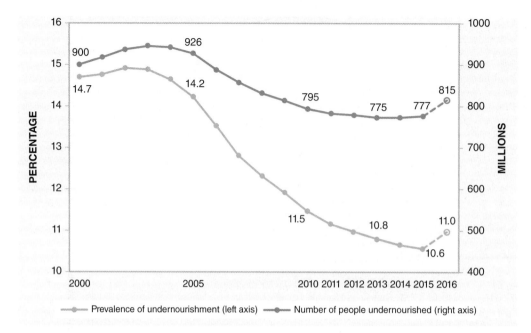

FIGURE SW.7 The state of food insecurity in the world.

Social and Economic Factors

Poverty, overpopulation, and migration to overcrowded cities are closely interrelated causes of hunger. (See **FIGURE SW.8**.) Each of those situations compounds the effects of the others as they steadily drive a population toward malnutrition.

Poverty

Poverty, hunger, and malnutrition stalk one another in a vicious circle, compromising health and wreaking havoc on the development of entire countries and regions.

Poverty is the most important underlying reason for persistent hunger.[27] Obviously, poverty limits access to food. It limits purchase of farming supplies to grow food, boats and equipment to fish, and storage equipment to prevent spoilage. It limits access to medical care. It compromises efforts at sanitation. It discourages education and the chance for personal advancement.

For nations, poverty means paralyzed economic development and too few jobs; inadequate investments in infrastructure and basic housing; and too few resources to train doctors, nutritionists, nurses, and other healthcare workers.

Population Growth

Population growth in many regions is outstripping gains in food production, education, employment, health care, and economic progress. The burgeoning numbers stress limited environmental resources, contributing to environmental degradation and pollution. In rural areas where farmland is limited, each small parcel of family land is subdivided with each generation, until there is too little land to support each family.

You might think that poverty would pressure parents to limit family size, but, ironically, poverty and sickness do just the reverse. Where child mortality rates are high, having

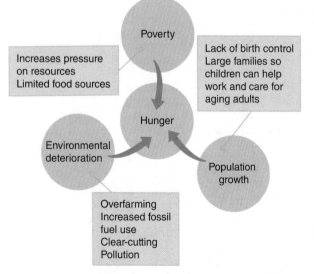

FIGURE SW.8 Major problems causing hunger. Poverty, population growth, and environmental degradation interact to make hunger worse.

many babies guarantees some children will survive. In countries that have no economic safeguards for disability, unemployment, or old age, parents consider their children a source of security and support in times of need. Many other factors contribute to large families, from ignorance of birth control methods to the attitude that big families reflect the father's masculinity. Some political and religious groups also encourage high birth rates and fast population growth as a way to achieve political or military dominance. To slow population growth, socioeconomic and cultural changes that make smaller family size acceptable, even desirable, must accompany access to birth control.

Urbanization

As rural lands become too crowded or exhausted farmland no longer supports good crops, rural people migrate to the city in hopes of jobs and a better life. Unfortunately, in fast-growing cities, social disorder, sanitary conditions, and living standards may be much worse. Hunting, fishing, foraging, and gardening—sources of accessible food in the rural setting—are seldom an option in the city. Breastfeeding becomes impractical for many mothers who could nurse their babies while doing farm work but cannot do so with jobs in the city.

Infection and Disease

Infection interacts with malnutrition, each making its victim more vulnerable to the other, each making the other worse, in a downward spiral. Nutrient deficiencies lower resistance to infections. In turn, the fever of infection speeds depletion of calories and nutrients. Other symptoms (e.g., loss of appetite, weakness, nausea, mouth lesions) limit ability to eat. Infectious diarrhea is especially dangerous, quickly wasting what few nutrients are consumed; infants and young children can die quickly from loss of electrolytes. Programs that prevent or control infection (e.g., immunizations, improvements in hygiene and sanitation, safe water supplies, access to medicine and medical care) all indirectly improve nutrition status.

Infection with the human immunodeficiency virus (HIV) provides a dramatic demonstration of the interaction between malnutrition and infection. (See the FYI feature "AIDS and Malnutrition.") Transmission of the virus from mother to fetus is more likely when the mother is deficient in vitamin A. Among those who are afflicted, the infection progresses fastest in people who are poorly nourished. Severe loss of weight and muscle are hallmarks of the advanced disease, acquired immune deficiency syndrome (AIDS). AIDS is the fourth leading cause of death among low- and middle-income countries. More than 36 million people are living with HIV, partly because infected people are living longer than before, and AIDS-related deaths have declined in recent years.[28] Ninety-seven percent of people living with HIV/AIDS live in low- and middle-income countries, and an estimated 66 percent of all people living with HIV worldwide live in sub-Saharan Africa, where it is the leading cause of death.[29] Other areas experiencing severe epidemics include Eastern Europe, Latin America, Asia, and Central Asia. In 2015, an estimated 150,000 people newly infected with HIV were children, and the majority contracted it during birth or while breastfeeding.[30] Despite the recent prevention of 1.6 million new pediatric infections due to drug access, children under 4 years of age still have the highest rates of AIDS-related deaths among all ages.[31]

Quick **Bite**

Is Enough Food Produced in the World to Feed Everyone?

World agriculture produces enough food to feed us all. Seventeen percent more calories per person are being produced today compared to 30 years ago, even despite a 70 percent increase in population. Food production worldwide can provide at least 2,720 kilocalories per person per day. The problem, however, is that many people in the world do not have sufficient land to grow food or income to purchase enough food to keep them from being hungry.

Quick **Bite**

Food Supply Versus Food Safety

Sometimes obtaining food is more important than food safety. Food from street vendors is important in the diets of many urban populations, particularly the socially disadvantaged. Health authorities responsible for food safety should balance their risk management with issues of food availability and hunger. Rigorous application of codes and regulations suited to larger and permanent food-service establishments may cause the disappearance of the street vendors, with consequent aggravation of hunger and malnutrition. The WHO encourages the development of regulations that empower vendors to take greater responsibility for the preparation of safe food.

Quick **Bite**

Rehydration Therapy for Diarrhea

Simple and inexpensive packets of carbohydrate and salts diluted with sterile water replace lost fluids and electrolytes. These packets are saving thousands of people's lives each year.

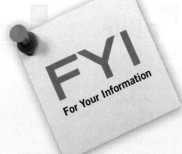

AIDS and Malnutrition

Like other infections, HIV interacts with malnutrition in a vicious, devastating cycle. Left untreated, HIV infection progresses to acquired immune deficiency syndrome (AIDS). The virus attacks by destroying its victim's immune system. When a person is unable to fight infections and malignancies, the disease quickly depletes marginal nutrient stores, speeding the way to severe malnutrition and death. But malnutrition and HIV interact on several levels, as well[a]:

- Poor nutrition contributes to declining immune function, HIV progression, and further deterioration in health.
- HIV can be transmitted to infants in breast milk; but in impoverished regions substitutions for breast milk typically increase infantile diarrhea, malnutrition, and death.
- AIDS leaves mothers too weak to feed and care for their children. Eventually, AIDS turns children into orphans.
- AIDS disables parents so they cannot work to support and feed their families.
- Among those who are afflicted, the infection progresses faster in people who are poorly nourished.

- Weight loss and muscle wasting in an infected person are associated with faster progression of HIV and AIDS.
- Infections that accompany AIDS cause fever and diarrhea, making malnutrition worse. Nausea and loss of appetite also contribute to malnutrition.
- Severe protein-energy malnutrition (PEM) is characteristic of untreated AIDS and frequently is the ultimate cause of death.
- Adequate dietary intake and nutrient absorption are essential to achieving the maximum benefit of drug treatment for HIV/AIDS.

More than 36 million people worldwide were living with HIV in 2010.[b] Sub-Saharan Africa, Southeast and Central Asia, Latin America, and Eastern Europe continue to be areas with a high prevalence of HIV. Without treatment, these people are doomed to death, usually within 10 years of the initial infection. The fate of severe PEM in millions of people appears unavoidable. If we do not arrest the continued transmission of HIV, the number of PEM victims will climb even higher.

a U.S. Agency for International Development. Multi-sectoral nutrition strategy 2014–2025. Technical guidance brief. https://www.usaid.gov/sites/default/files/documents/1864/nutrition-food-security-HIV-AIDS-508_cbt_2.pdf. Accessed September 21, 2017.
b Joint United Nations Programme on HIV/AIDS (UNAIDS). AIDS by the numbers—AIDS is not over, but it can be. November 2016. http://www.unaids.org/en/resources/documents/2016/AIDS-by-the-numbers. Accessed October 4, 2017.

Quick Bite

To Breastfeed or Not?

A common practice among mothers with HIV is to avoid breastfeeding entirely or end it early out of concern that they will pass the virus to their infants. However, new research has shown that although the virus can be transmitted through breastmilk, a combination of exclusive breastfeeding and use of drug treatment can significantly reduce the risk of transmitting HIV to infants. The World Health Organization in 2010 for the first time recommended drug treatment for either the HIV-infected mother or HIV-exposed infant to reduce risk of transmission of HIV to breastfeeding infants. According to a recent report, "the scale-up of prevention of mother-to-child transmission, particularly in the past five years, is one of the greatest public health achievements of recent times."

World Health Organization. Antiretroviral drugs for treating pregnant women and preventing HIV infection in infants: recommendations for a public health approach—2010 version. http://apps.who.int/iris/bitstream/10665/75236/1/9789241599818_eng.pdf. Accessed October 23, 2017.

Political Disruptions

Social upheavals and natural disasters such as floods and drought can leave famine in their wake. The resulting displacement of populations and inequitable food distribution usually lead to hunger and malnutrition.

War

Whereas poverty is the underlying cause of chronic mild to moderate malnutrition, war and its aftermath cause severe malnutrition and famine. War diverts limited financial resources from development efforts to expenditures for fighting and destruction. Men and women no longer farm, fish, or bring home a paycheck—they are in the army. Households become fatherless and sometimes motherless, often permanently. Crops and croplands are destroyed, along with irrigation systems, food-processing facilities, and transportation infrastructure, which may have taken decades to develop.

Refugees

Masses of refugees—many very young, old, infirm, and already weakened by chronic hunger—find themselves without the basic elements of sustenance. The resulting famine has become an all too common sight on the evening news. International relief agencies have learned to respond to these emergencies quickly and with great determination, but logistical difficulties (e.g., mobilizing manpower, obtaining food, transporting supplies, setting up feeding stations) may slow relief until it is too late for the sickest or weakest. Some refugee groups are inaccessible, hidden, or intentionally kept hungry as part of a political plan; emergency food may never reach many of them.

Sanctions

International sanctions and embargoes create food shortages, both directly and indirectly, by limiting access to agricultural supplies, fuel, and food-processing supplies. Some people argue that shortages created by embargoes hurt powerless people rather than government officials; others say that such actions are preferable to war.

Agriculture and the Environment: A Tricky Balance

Advances in agriculture increase food supplies and reduce food costs. Because the economies of most developing countries are based on agriculture, improvements boost rural incomes and buying power, increase demand for agricultural labor, stimulate commerce among small vendors and food processors, and ultimately help a nation's economy.

Dramatic gains in agricultural productivity took place in the 1960s and 1970s with the development of new seed varieties, especially rice and corn. The seeds greatly increased crop yields. Expectations were so strong that these seeds would finally solve the world's food shortage that their development and use was dubbed the "Green Revolution." Despite its successes, the Green Revolution had limitations. The seeds required irrigation and heavy use of pesticides and fertilizers, which poor farmers could not afford. (See the FYI feature "Tough Choices.") The farming techniques were sometimes hard on the environment. Gains from the Green Revolution have now about reached their limit and, if current trends continue, threaten to be lost to the population explosion.

Proponents of agricultural biotechnology see it as another step along the continuum of plant-breeding techniques and a promising tool to increase crop production. Some uses of biotechnology are well accepted—for example, diagnostic kits that identify plants and insects by DNA and tissue culture for plant reproduction, a technique already in widespread commercial use. More controversial is the modification of plant genetic material. The technology has the potential to improve plants' resistance to disease, tolerance to adverse conditions, yield, and nutritional quality.

At the other end of the technology spectrum is a renewed appreciation for and conservation of traditional seed varieties, those selected over the generations by local farmers because they do well in local conditions. In developing countries, farmers typically save some of these seeds at each harvest to use in the next planting season. The seeds grow well in the regions where they've evolved, whereas imported seeds, no matter how carefully bred, often fail.

In addition to seed selection, strategies to optimize agriculture include irrigation, soil preparation, improved planting and harvest methods, erosion prevention, fertilization, pest control, and flood control. The methods should be affordable, suitable for the level of local development, and protective of the environment. For example, where there is an abundant supply of willing farm laborers and gasoline is

---

Position Statement: Academy of Nutrition and Dietetics

Nutrition Intervention and Human Immunodeficiency Virus Infection

It is the position of the American Dietetic Association that efforts to optimize nutritional status through individualized medical nutrition therapy, assurance of food and nutrition security, and nutrition education are essential to the total system of health care available to people with human immunodeficiency virus (HIV) infection throughout the continuum of care.

Reprinted from *Journal of the American Dietetic Association*, 110(7), Cade Fields-Gardner, Position of the American Dietetic Association: Nutrition Intervention and Human Immunodeficiency Virus Infection, Page no.1105-1119, 2010, with permission from Elsevier.

Quick **Bite**

Emergency Management

Imagine a civil war in a developing country that displaces tens of thousands of people. What are the most important measures for preventing sickness and death among these refugees? Protection from violence heads the list, closely followed by adequate food rations, clean water and sanitation, diarrheal disease control, measles immunization, and maternal and child health care.

Quick **Bite**

Who Produces the World's Soybeans?

Before 1900, the soybean was rarely grown in the United States. Today, the United States is the world's largest soybean producer. According to the USDA, 90 percent of the nation's oil seed production comes from soybeans; the United States accounts for 34 percent of the world's soybean production.

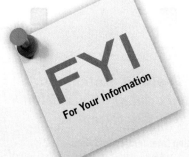

Tough Choices

Imagine you live in a poor village of a developing country. How would you make these choices?

- You've learned you must boil your drinking water to prevent diarrhea. But that means cutting young trees for firewood. You recently planted those trees to stop erosion. What do you do?

- You've recently given birth to your fourth child. Your husband was injured in an accident and is unable to work. But, you can work at a nearby factory and use your pay to buy food and clothes for the older children. How would you feed the new baby?
- Your small herd of goats provides milk for your young children. You like the goats because they can survive in the rough, hilly countryside, but the goats are overgrazing the grasses on the hillside. What can you do?
- Insects have destroyed your crop. In the past, you burned fields after harvest to control insects, but you've learned that "slash and burn" is bad for the land. You've thought about using a chemical pesticide, but it is too expensive. You could clear the jungle for another growing field. Do you have other choices? What should you do?
- You can grow either vegetables to feed your family or a "cash crop" to sell for export. The cash crop would help pay for medicine and other necessities. Which should you grow?

expensive, using heavy-duty farm machinery makes little sense. Other examples include mulching to conserve water and control weeds, and using manure (after composting to kill pathogens) to reduce the need for fertilizer.

Environmental Degradation

Environmental degradation is a growing concern in both the developing and the industrialized world. In developing countries, there is pressure for more land to support rapidly expanding populations. In industrialized countries, there is pressure from the affluent for more land, more houses, larger properties, more recreation areas, and so on. Residents of the industrialized world consume vast amounts of resources (e.g., water, fuel, wood, paper, textiles, food) without a thought and often without making the small effort to conserve or recycle. Residents of the developing world consume much less per person, but the impact of their numbers is greater.

Environmental degradation has nutritional consequences because it threatens food production. Urbanization and the expansion of cities reduce acreage available for farming. The pressure to supply food to growing populations leads to clear-cutting marginal land, eventually eroding hilly terrain or quickly exhausting fragile rain forest soils. Overdependence on irrigation can drain water, eventually creating deserts. The destruction of vast areas of natural ground cover can lead to global climate changes. Overuse of pesticides and fertilizers pollutes waterways, destroying fish and seafood.

Key Concepts Despite gains in eradicating malnutrition, almost all undernourished people in the world live in developing countries. Factors that allow hunger to continue include rising food prices, poverty, poor sanitation, urbanization, and inefficient food distribution. Infection, especially AIDS; rapid population growth; wars; and environmental degradation threaten to reverse hard-won gains.

Malnutrition: Its Nature, Its Victims, and Its Eradication

Most diseases of nutritional deficiency exist throughout the developing world, but seldom in isolation. Typically, the malnourished person has two or more coexisting deficiencies, each increasing the severity of the other. Keep the potential for this deadly synergy in mind as we discuss some major categories of malnutrition.

Protein-Energy Malnutrition

Lack of protein and also energy can have devastating consequences, especially on the young. In kwashiorkor, the body and face swell with excess fluid, the hair turns wispy and red, and a terrible rash develops; without treatment, the person dies. Marasmus paints an even more dramatic picture of sunken eyes, shriveled limbs, and a clearly visible outline of the skeleton; it is as deadly as kwashiorkor.

Protein-energy malnutrition (PEM) is by far the most lethal form of malnutrition, and children are its most visible victims.[32] Their fast growth creates high nutrient demands, leaving them especially vulnerable to inequitable food distribution in the family, inappropriate infant and child feeding practices, and interactions of infection with malnutrition. PEM typically develops after a child is weaned from the breast. Men in the household may have priority for nutritious food. In big families, the young child must also compete for food with many siblings.

In the developing world, breastfeeding is almost always essential to an infant's survival. Inappropriate bottle-feeding puts a baby at grave risk. Relative to income, formula is usually very expensive and often is diluted to make it "stretch." Contaminated water and lack of other hygienic requirements for bottle preparation cause diarrhea. The combination of diarrhea and nutritional deficiency from watered-down formula often is fatal.

A tremendous educational effort, including promotion of breastfeeding, has reduced the global prevalence and severity of infant and childhood PEM. Severe PEM typified by kwashiorkor or marasmus has become more sporadic, occurring mainly as a result of war or natural disaster. However, mild to moderate PEM continues to pose a grave problem in the developing world, putting children at risk of delayed growth, impaired psychological development, and the deadly interactions of disease and malnutrition.

Iodine Deficiency Disorders

Iodine deficiency is the world's most common cause of preventable brain damage and a main cause of impaired cognitive development in children.[33] Its impairment of intellectual ability and work performance is potentially so widespread that **iodine deficiency disorders** can actually slow a nation's social and economic development.

Iodine deficiency is most devastating during pregnancy, causing spontaneous abortions, stillbirths, and birth defects, including cretinism, a disease of mental retardation that is often severe. Deafness and spastic paralysis are likely to accompany the retardation. In regions of Africa, dwarfism also occurs where diets rich in goitrogen-containing vegetables (e.g., cassava, cabbage) make the deficiency worse. Moreover, iodine deficiency is damaging at all ages, limiting mental development in infants and children and producing apathy and marginal mental function in adults.

▶ **iodine deficiency disorders** A wide range of disorders due to iodine deficiency that affect growth and development.

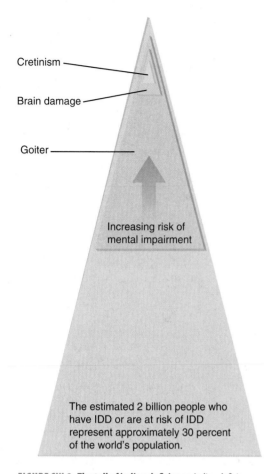

Cretinism

Brain damage

Goiter

Increasing risk of
mental impairment

The estimated 2 billion people who
have IDD or are at risk of IDD
represent approximately 30 percent
of the world's population.

FIGURE SW.9 The toll of iodine deficiency. Iodine deficiency remains the single greatest cause of preventable brain damage and mental retardation worldwide.

Iodine deficiency disorders are endemic throughout much of the developing world where the soil is low in iodine. These areas typically are mountainous or far from the oceans. They often are isolated and impoverished. Fifty-four countries are still iodine-deficient.[34] The WHO estimates that 36.5 percent of school-age children (285.4 million) have insufficient iodine intake.[35] (See **FIGURE SW.9.**)

Disturbing though these figures are, great strides have been made in the prevention of these disorders, mainly through iodizing salt. More than two-thirds of households throughout the world now use iodized salt, and in countries with salt iodization programs in place for five years or more, the improvement in iodine status has been dramatic.[36] The cost is merely 5 cents per person per year.

Vitamin A Deficiency

Vitamin A deficiency is the leading cause of preventable blindness in children. It also increases the risk of disease and death from severe infections. Vitamin A deficiency causes night blindness and may increase the risk of maternal mortality in pregnant women.

Vitamin A deficiency is a public health problem in more than half of all countries, especially those in Africa and Southeast Asia, hitting young children and pregnant women in low-income countries the hardest. The nutrient is crucial for maternal and child survival, and supplying adequate vitamin A in high-risk areas can significantly reduce mortality. Conversely, its absence causes a needlessly high risk of disease and death. An estimated 250 million preschool children are vitamin A–deficient. Of the estimated 250,000 to 500,000 children who become blind every year from vitamin A deficiency, one-half will die within 12 months of losing their sight.[37]

Vitamin A deficiency often coexists with marginal PEM. The vitamin deficiency predisposes infants and children to diarrheal diseases, which, in turn, worsen the child's nutritional status, leading to severe PEM. Common childhood infections, most notably measles, are much more serious in vitamin A–deficient children, with a much greater risk of death or permanent damage from complications.

In communities where vitamin A deficiency exists, pregnant and breastfeeding women often experience night blindness, an early symptom of deficiency. Maternal death, poor pregnancy outcome, and failure to lactate are all increased with vitamin A deficiency. Vitamin A levels in the breast milk of these women are likely to be low as well, putting their infants at later risk of deficiency.

Many countries are taking a multipronged approach to vitamin A deficiency that includes promotion of breastfeeding, fortification of foods, supplementation, and nutrition education. Foods such as eggs, dairy foods, and liver are promoted as important for women and children; educational programs also encourage growing and eating fruits and vegetables high in beta-carotene. However, dietary change can be difficult and slow. The best sources of vitamin A often are the most expensive or inaccessible. For absorption and conversion to vitamin A, beta-carotene requires dietary fat—another expensive item in many areas—and other factors not completely understood. Meanwhile, periodic single, large-dose vitamin A supplements, often given in tandem with maternal–child immunizations, are proving an effective short-term measure.

Biotechnology may have a significant impact on vitamin A deficiency. Through genetic engineering, scientists have developed a new strain of rice that is rich in beta-carotene. When these rice plants are crossed with locally grown strains of rice, they become suited to a particular region's climate and growing conditions. If local farmers and consumers accept such crops, bioengineered rice may play a critical role in feeding the world's burgeoning population and alleviating widespread vitamin A deficiency.[38]

Iron-Deficiency Anemia

Iron deficiency is the most common nutritional disorder in the world. The numbers are staggering: 2 billion people—over 30 percent of the world's population—are anemic, mainly due to iron deficiency. In resource-poor areas, the condition frequently is worsened by infectious diseases, including malaria, HIV/AIDS, and hookworm infestation.[39] Although iron deficiency occurs in all age groups, fast growth in young children and reproductive blood loss in women make them especially vulnerable to low-iron diets. Anemia impairs childhood development, work capacity, learning capacity, and resistance to disease.[40] Anemia during pregnancy increases illness and death rates for mother and baby. For all groups of people, anemia can cause profound fatigue, and severe anemia causes death.

The anemias of the developing world demonstrate the interaction of multiple nutrient deficiencies, which, in turn, interact with infection, sanitation, and poverty. Supplying iron alone is seldom enough to correct the problem. Iron-deficient diets are typically high in starch and cereal grains. During digestion, cereals may bind with the very limited iron the diet provides, preventing its absorption. Other blood-building nutrients, such as vitamins B_6 and B_{12} and folate, are in short supply as well.

Anemia-producing parasites are common in areas of iron deficiency, aggravating the effects of poor diet. Blood cells are destroyed by malarial infections. Intestinal malabsorption and intestinal bleeding are caused by hookworm, which is prevalent where human waste contaminates the fields where people walk barefoot, and by other parasites, acquired when human waste contaminates the water people drink or in which people bathe.

People debilitated by anemia may be too weak to build outhouses, too poor to buy shoes or fuel to boil water, or too apathetic to clear standing water where malaria-carrying mosquitoes breed. Moreover, they often do not understand the connection among sanitation, infection, and malnutrition. Added to this mix are excessive blood loss from repeated pregnancies, inherited blood disorders such as sickle cell disease, and chronic bacterial or viral infections such as HIV.

Timely treatment can restore personal health and raise national productivity levels by as much as 20 percent.[41] The WHO has developed a comprehensive package of public health measures based on a three-pronged approach:

1. *Increase iron intake:* Dietary diversification, including iron-rich foods and enhancement of iron absorption, food fortification, and iron supplementation
2. *Control infection:* Immunization and control programs for malaria and parasitic worm diseases
3. *Improve nutritional status:* Prevention and control of other nutritional deficiencies, such as vitamin B_{12}, folate, and vitamin A

Quick **Bite**

The Importance of Rice
Rice is the principal food crop for one-half of the world's population.

Deficiencies of Other Micronutrients

Deficiencies of zinc and calcium often coexist with other deficiencies, contributing to illness and death during periods of growth and threatening immune function and skeletal health in people who survive to old age.

Selenium deficiency, although limited to only a few countries, has serious consequences. It occurs where the soil is selenium-poor, in distinct regional patterns in China and Russia. In China, where the deficiency is most severe, it predisposes individuals to the fatal Keshan disease, in which heart muscle is destroyed. Keshan disease affects mainly women and children. The condition can be prevented by selenium supplementation or by fortification, as in programs undertaken in New Zealand, where soil is also low in selenium.

The classical deficiency diseases beriberi, pellagra, and scurvy still occur among the world's poorest and most underprivileged people. Most often, however, these diseases strike the victims of war and political strife—the refugees. Diets based on milled cereals and starchy roots, all poor thiamin sources, predispose refugee populations to beriberi. People who rely on corn-based diets low in niacin and tryptophan are susceptible to pellagra. The disruption of refugee life can easily tip the balance from marginal deficiency to overt deficiency disease.

Overweight and Obesity

Obesity is a growing health problem worldwide and is increasingly being recognized as a form of malnutrition.[42] Obesity has reached epidemic proportions globally. In 2014, more than 1.9 billion adults were overweight—and at least 600 million of them clinically obese. Obesity also reaches across the lifespan, beginning early in life. Approximately 42 million children under the age of 5 years were overweight or obese in 2014.[43] Obesity is a major contributor to the global burden of chronic disease and disability.[44] In developing countries, obesity can exist alongside undernutrition. Obesity also occurs in areas of economic advancement and in urban areas. Its prevalence is rising rapidly in Latin America and the Caribbean, but obesity still is relatively uncommon in Asia and Africa.

Societal changes and the worldwide nutrition transition are driving the obesity epidemic. Economic growth, modernization, urbanization, and globalization of food markets are just some of the forces thought to underlie the epidemic.

As incomes rise and populations become more urban, diets high in complex carbohydrates give way to more varied diets with a higher proportion of fats, saturated fats, and sugars. Calorie-dense foods that have few other nutrients often are cheap, satisfying, convenient, and heavily promoted; some are foreign brands that have become affordable status symbols. In poor communities, cultural attitudes toward overweight may be more accepting and even admired.

At the same time, large shifts toward less physically demanding work have been observed worldwide. Moves toward less physical activity are also found in the increasing use of automated transport, technology in the home, and more passive leisure pursuits. The reductions in energy expenditure can be dramatic.

If an individual is overweight, can we assume that the person is well nourished? Not necessarily. A new trend in developed countries is the presence of malnutrition with obesity. With too little physical activity, obese individuals may be eating too many calories of poor-nutrient foods and not enough nutritious foods such as vegetables and fruit. The availability of an overabundance of inexpensive, poor food choices in combination with lack of accessible opportunities for physical activity are just some of the factors contributing to the obesogenic environment in which many people are currently living.[45]

Key Concepts The most critical nutritional deficiencies in today's developing world are deficiencies of protein, calories, iodine, vitamin A, and iron. There have been gains in reducing the severity and prevalence of protein-energy malnutrition through breastfeeding promotion, nutrition education, and improvements in food supplies. Fortification and supplementation programs are effectively attacking iodine and vitamin A deficiencies but have had less success overcoming iron deficiency. All the underlying causes of malnutrition must be addressed to reduce and eliminate these and other deficiencies.

Learning Portfolio

Key Terms

Study Points

- Hunger and malnutrition continue to be problems in both industrialized and developing countries.

- Although most people in the United States are food-secure, malnutrition is a serious problem among the working poor, the rural poor, the homeless, older adults, and children.

- Many federal programs address hunger in the United States. Among them are the Supplemental Nutrition Assistance Program (SNAP); the Special Supplemental Nutrition Program for Women, Infants, and Children (WIC); the National School Lunch and Breakfast Programs; and the Child and Adult Care Food Program. Feeding America is the largest charitable hunger-relief organization in the United States.

- Progress against global hunger and malnutrition is slow and uneven. It is estimated that more than 795 million people in the developing world do not have enough to eat.

- Social and economic factors, infection, disease, political disruptions, natural disasters, and inequitable food distribution all contribute to hunger in the developing world.

- Advances in agricultural practices have increased food supplies and reduced food costs in the developing world; however, the increase in production has led to environmental degradation as a result of urbanization, clear-cutting, overirrigation, and soil erosion.

- Protein-energy malnutrition (PEM) refers to physical conditions, such as kwashiorkor and marasmus, that result from not having enough to eat.

- Infants and children are most likely to suffer from PEM. However, nutrition education efforts, including promotion of breastfeeding, have reduced the severity and prevalence of PEM.

- Iodine deficiency is the largest cause of preventable brain damage and impaired cognitive development in the developing world. It can cause damage to people of all ages.

- Great strides have been made in preventing iodine deficiency disorders through salt iodization programs. More than two-thirds of households in countries affected by these disorders now use iodized salt.

- Vitamin A deficiency is the leading cause of preventable childhood blindness. It also makes its victims more vulnerable to infection, diarrheal diseases, and PEM.

- Pregnant and breastfeeding women with vitamin A deficiency are at increased risk of death, poor pregnancy outcomes, and lactation failure.

- Many countries are taking a multipronged approach to vitamin A deficiency that includes promotion of breastfeeding, fortification of foods, supplementation, and nutrition education.

- The best sources of vitamin A often are expensive and inaccessible to people in developing countries. Scientists have developed new bioengineered strains of rice that are rich in beta-carotene and that may play a critical role in alleviating widespread vitamin A deficiency.

- The anemias of the developing world demonstrate the interaction of multiple nutrient deficiencies, which, in turn, interact with infection, poor sanitation, and poverty.

- Food fortification and iron supplementation for women and children are the mainstays of anemia prevention and treatment, along with efforts to overcome poverty and improve sanitation.

- The classical deficiency diseases beriberi and pellagra still occur among the world's poorest and most underprivileged people.

- In some developing countries, obesity exists right alongside undernutrition.

Study Questions

1. What is the difference between food insecurity and hunger?

2. What is food security?

3. What groups are most at risk for food insecurity in the United States?

4. List some organizations and programs that fight hunger and food insecurity in the United States.

5. List four causes of malnutrition worldwide.

6. List four common nutritional deficiencies worldwide.

7. What populations are at increased risk of nutritional deficiencies, and why?

Try This

Try Giving Up Your Stove and Refrigerator

A homeless person has no kitchen facilities to store or prepare food. For one day, eat a balanced diet without resorting to cooking or using your refrigerator. Some foods you could eat include the following:

Breads, bagels, tortillas, rolls
Cereals
Crackers
Milk—canned, evaporated, or aseptically packaged
Cheese—hard cheeses keep well

Pudding cups (single-serve, nonrefrigerated type)
Tuna/chicken—canned
Sardines, salmon—canned
Nuts, peanut butter
Beans—canned
Fruits and vegetables—fresh, canned, dried fruits

How satisfying did you find this eating pattern? What did you miss most? What would it be like to eat this way for an extended time?

Community Food Programs

The purpose of this exercise is to see how you can contribute to decreasing or eliminating food insecurity in your community. Look in the phone book (under "Food Programs" and "Human Services") to see what programs are available. Consider volunteering at your local food bank or another community program to help feed people who do not have the means to feed themselves.

Getting Personal

Food Insecurity Where You Live

Find out the current state of food insecurity where you live. Go to map.FeedingAmerica.org and use the map features to look up your state. Look at the data provided on the number of people who are food-insecure, program eligibility among food-insecure people, food budget shortfall, and cost of one meal.

Questions to ask yourself:

1. Were the rates of food insecurity higher or lower than you expected?

2. Was food insecurity higher or lower in certain regions? Were these urban or rural areas?

3. What are some factors that might be contributing to food insecurity?

4. What are potential opportunities for you to take action against hunger in your state?

Learning Portfolio (continued)

References

1. World Hunger Education. 2016 world hunger and poverty facts and statistics. http://www.worldhunger.org/2015-world-hunger-and-poverty-facts-and-statistics/. Accessed September 21, 2017.

2. Ibid.

3. Ibid.

4. Position of the American Dietetic Association: food insecurity and hunger in the United States. *J Am Diet Assoc.* 2010;110(9):1368-1377.

5. Coleman-Jensen A, Rabbitt MP, Gregory C, Singh A. Household food security in the United States in 2015. U.S. Department of Agriculture, Economic Research Service. https://www.ers.usda.gov/publications/pub-details/?pubid=79760. Accessed September 21, 2017.

6. Position of the American Dietetic Association. Op. cit.

7. Finkelstein EA, Strombotne KL. The economics of obesity. *Am J Clin Nutr.* 2010;91(5):1520S-1524S.

8. Coleman-Jensen A, Rabbitt MP, Gregory C, Singh A. Op. cit.

9. Centers for Disease Control and Prevention. A look inside food deserts. http://www.cdc.gov/features/fooddeserts. Accessed September 21, 2017.

10. Rhone A, Ver Ploeg M, Dicken C, Williams R, Breneman V. Low-income and low-supermarket-access census tracts, 2010-2015, EIB-165. U.S. Department of Agriculture, Economic Research Service. January 2017. https://www.ers.usda.gov/publications/pub-details/?pubid=82100. Accessed September 21, 2017.

11. Ibid.

12. Coleman-Jensen A, Rabbitt MP, Gregory C, Singh A. Op. cit.

13. Gray F, Cunnyham K. Supplemental Nutrition Assistance Program participation rates: fiscal year 2014. https://www.fns.usda.gov/snap/trends-supplemental-nutrition-assistance-program-participation-rates-fiscal-year-2010-fiscal-year. Accessed October 4, 2017.

14. U.S. Department of Agriculture. SNAP-Ed connection. About. https://snaped.fns.usda.gov/about. Accessed September 21, 2017.

15. U.S. Department of Agriculture, Food and Nutrition Service. Special Supplemental Nutrition Program for Women, Infants, and Children (WIC) data as of February 2017. https://www.fns.usda.gov/pd/wic-program. Accessed October 4, 2017.

16. U.S. Department of Agriculture, Food and Nutrition Service. WIC eligibility requirements. https://www.fns.usda.gov/wic/wic-eligibility-requirements. Accessed September 21, 2017.

17. U.S. Department of Agriculture. Child nutrition programs: income eligibility guidelines. *Fed Reg.* 2017;82(67). http://www.gpo.gov/fdsys/pkg/FR-2017-04-10/pdf/2017-07043.pdf. Accessed September 21, 2017.

18. U.S. Department of Agriculture, Food and Nutrition Service. National School Lunch Program (NLSP). http://www.fns.usda.gov/cnd/lunch. Accessed September 21, 2017.

19. U.S. Department of Agriculture, Food and Nutrition Service. Child and Adult Care Food Program (CACFP). https://www.fns.usda.gov/cacfp/child-and-adult-care-food-program. Accessed September 21, 2017.

20. Feeding America. About us. http://feedingamerica.org/about-us/. Accessed September 21, 2017.

21. World Health Organization. Health and Human Rights. Fact Sheet No. 323. December 2015. http://www.who.int/mediacentre/factsheets/fs323/en/. Accessed October 4, 2017.

22. Food and Agriculture Organization of the United Nations. The state of food insecurity in the world 2017. http://www.fao.org/publications/sofi/en. Accessed October 4, 2017.

23. Cohen MJ. The world food situation. International Food Policy Research Institute. 2007. http://www.ifpri.org/publication/world-food-situation-2. Accessed September 21, 2017.

24. Sheeran J. The new face of hunger. Keynote address. Center for Strategic and International Studies. Washington, DC. April 18, 2008.

25. Ibid.

26. Food and Agricultural Organization of the United Nations. The state of food and agriculture: climate change, agriculture and food security. 2017. Available at http://www.fao.org/publications/card/en/c/15718990-8d8d -427c-ad0f-782c10e52a13/. Accessed September 21, 2017.

27. Hunger Notes. 2016 World Hunger and Poverty Facts and Statistics. http://www.worldhunger.org/2015-world-hunger-and-poverty-facts-and -statistics/. Accessed October 4, 2017.

28. Joint United Nations Programme on HIV/AIDS (UNAIDS). AIDS by the numbers—AIDS is not over, but it can be. November 2016. http:// www.unaids.org/en/resources/documents/2016/AIDS-by-the-numbers. Accessed October 4, 2017.

29. Ibid.

30. Ibid.

31. United Nations Children's Fund. *For Every Child, End AIDS*. Seventh Stocktaking Report. New York: UNICEF; December 2016.

32. World Health Organization, Nutrition for Health and Development. Nutrition for Health and Development: a global agenda for combating malnutrition. http://apps.who.int/iris/bitstream/10665/66509/1 /WHO_NHD_00.6.pdf. Accessed September 21, 2017.

33. World Health Organization. Micronutrient deficiencies: iodine deficiency disorders. http://www.who.int/nutrition/topics/idd/en. Accessed September 21, 2017.

34. Ibid.

35. World Health Organization. Proportion of school-age children population with insufficient iodine intake. http://www.who.int/vmnis/iodine/status /summary/iodine_data_status_summary_t1/en/. Accessed September 21, 2017.

36. World Health Organization. Micronutrient deficiencies: iodine deficiency disorders. Op. cit.

37. World Health Organization. Micronutrient deficiencies: vitamin A deficiency. http://www.who.int/nutrition/topics/vad/en/. Accessed September 21, 2017.

38. Tang G, Qin J, Dolnikowski GG, Russell RM, Grusak MA. Golden rice is an effective source of vitamin A. *Am J Clin Nutr*. 2009;89(6):1776-1783.

39. World Health Organization. Micronutrient deficiencies: iron deficiency anemia. http://www.who.int/nutrition/topics/ida/en/index.html. Accessed September 21, 2017.

40. Ibid.

41. Ibid.

42. Hunger Notes. Op. cit.

43. World Health Organization. Obesity and overweight: fact sheet. June 2016. http://www.who.int/mediacentre/factsheets/fs311/en. Accessed September 21, 2017.

44. Ibid.

45. U.S. Department of Agriculture, U.S. Department of Health and Human Services. *2015–2020 Dietary Guidelines for Americans*. 8th ed. December 2015. http://health.gov/dietaryguidelines/2015/guidelines. Accessed September 21, 2017.

Chapter 13

Food Safety and Technology: Microbial Threats and Genetic Engineering

Revised by Paul Insel

THINK About It

1   Do you worry about getting sick from the food you eat?

2   To what extent do you rely on organically grown food to avoid pesticides?

3   What food safety measures, such as thawing meat in the refrigerator, do you practice at home?

4   Would genetically engineered rice be welcome at your dinner table?

LEARNING Objectives

1   Identify common food pathogens and related illnesses.

2   Identify common food contaminants and related health concerns.

3   Discuss governmental agencies and their strategies that help keep food safe in the United States.

4   Compare food technology methods and their impact when used on the food supply in the United States.

5   List the issues related to genetically engineered foods.

The newspaper headline screams, "Contaminated Peanut Butter Proves Fatal." You read further and discover that a child's death has been traced to bacteria thriving in improperly packaged peanut butter that has since been recalled. Additionally, several adults have become ill from the same source. This worries you; the peanut butter is your favorite brand, and several jars are in your pantry. The lot numbers on your jars don't match what was recalled. "I think I'll throw them away anyway," you decide, and wonder if you should change brands. Have you made the right choice? Or should you investigate this issue further?

Although once confined mainly to cookbooks and textbooks, today food safety advice shows up in many places—the popular press, the classroom, the Internet, even the *2015–2020 Dietary Guidelines for Americans*. What has prompted such concern? Among other things, the public's interest springs from the potentially wide-ranging and serious effects of inadequate food preparation, and from the liability of food processing companies. Recent headlines show how serious this issue is. Microbial contamination of such foods as hamburger, apple juice, eggs, raw sprouts, peanuts, pistachios, melon, and both fresh and frozen berries has seriously sickened thousands and killed many, especially those most susceptible: young children, people with compromised immune systems, and seniors.

Consumers are voicing concerns about other food safety issues as well—including fears about excessive pesticide residues in plant foods, antibiotics and hormones in animals used for food, and hidden food allergens (e.g., nuts, milk, eggs) in prepared foods. Increasingly, they are checking prepared foods for ingredients to which they are allergic (e.g., caseinates as milk protein) and questioning preparation methods to avoid an allergen that might be an unintentional food additive (e.g., peanut material found in milk chocolate candy might be residue left on machinery from earlier processing of peanut butter cups). Other, less frequently discussed food hazards include physical contamination with glass

Quick Bite

A Morbid Marginal Note
Every year, more than 48 million Americans get sick from something they ate. Three thousand of them die.

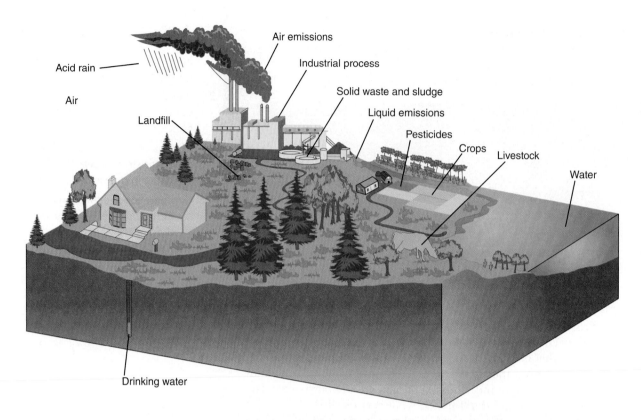

FIGURE 13.1 **Heavy metals and other contaminants can be found in foods.** Industrial plants and automobiles release heavy metals and other contaminants into the air. Rainfall carries these contaminants to the soil. Plants for food crops and animal feed absorb contaminants from the soil. Runoff can pick up contaminants from pesticides, fertilizers, and animal manure. This pollutes surface water (lakes and streams), groundwater, and coastal water. Polluted water contaminates seafood and other fish that people eat.

fragments and other sharp objects, heavy metals, and naturally occurring toxins in seafood and some agricultural products. (See **FIGURE 13.1**.)

This chapter reviews major food safety hazards and examines controversial issues such as the merits of organic foods, the use of food irradiation, and the production of genetically engineered foods.

Food Safety

🍎 **Why Is This Important?** Consider the process of getting food from where it is manufactured, or produced, to the consumer. A number of factors that are a part of the food production and delivery process can make each of the foods we eat harmful in some way. Understanding possible risks to food safety can help prevent food waste, as well as unnecessary food contamination.

Harmful Substances in Foods

In the United States and Canada, most foodborne diseases are caused by microorganisms and can be prevented by cleaning hands and surfaces, cooking raw foods sufficiently, and refrigerating foods promptly.

Pathogens

In North America, most food safety experts agree that the chief cause of **foodborne illness** is pathogenic (disease-causing) microorganisms, including bacteria, viruses, and parasites. See **TABLE 13.1** for a list of common foodborne microbes and the serious illnesses they

▶ **foodborne illness** A sickness caused by food contaminated with microorganisms, chemicals, or other substances hazardous to human health.

cause. Each year in the United States, approximately 48 million Americans (that's 1 in 6) become sick, 128,000 are hospitalized, and 3,000 die from foodborne illnesses, according to researchers at the Centers for Disease Control and Prevention (CDC).[1] Illness can range from relatively mild stomach upset to severe symptoms that can be fatal. Foodborne illnesses cost the United States about $15 billion annually.[2]

THINK About It 1

TABLE 13.1
Common Foodborne Pathogens and Illnesses

Organism	Sources	Diseases and Symptoms
Bacteria		
Campylobacter jejuni	Raw poultry and meat and unpasteurized milk © Purestock/Getty Images.	Campylobacteriosis **Onset:** Usually 2 to 5 days after eating **Symptoms:** Diarrhea, stomach cramps, fever, bloody stools; lasts 2 to 10 days
Clostridium botulinum—illness is caused by a toxin produced by this organism	Improperly canned foods, such as corn, green beans, soups, beets, asparagus, mushrooms, tuna, and liver pate; also, luncheon meats, ham, sausage, garlic in oil, lobster, and smoked and salted fish © Evlakhov Valeriy/Shutterstock.	Botulism **Onset:** 18 to 36 hours after eating **Symptoms:** Nerve dysfunction, such as double vision, inability to swallow, speech difficulty, and progressive paralysis of respiratory system; can lead to death
Escherichia coli 0157:H7	Raw or undercooked meat, raw vegetables, unpasteurized milk, minimally processed ciders and juices, contaminated water © Ana Blazic Pavlovic/Shutterstock.	*E. coli* infection **Onset:** 2 to 5 days after eating **Symptoms:** Watery and bloody diarrhea, severe stomach cramps, dehydration, colitis, neurological symptoms, stroke, and hemolytic uremic syndrome (HUS), a particularly serious disease in young children that can cause kidney failure and death
Listeria monocytogenes	Soft cheeses, unpasteurized milk, hot dogs, luncheon meats, cold cuts, other deli-style meat and poultry **Note:** Resists salt, heat, nitrites, and acidity better than most microorganisms © kaband/Shutterstock.	Listeriosis **Onset:** From 7 to 21 days after eating, but symptoms have been reported 9 to 48 hours after eating **Symptoms:** Fever, headache, nausea, and vomiting; primarily affects pregnant women and their fetuses, newborns, older adults, and people with cancer and compromised immune systems; can cause death in fetuses and babies

(continues)

TABLE 13.1 (*continued*)
Common Foodborne Pathogens and Illnesses

Organism	Sources	Diseases and Symptoms
Salmonella	Raw or undercooked meats, poultry, eggs; raw milk and other dairy products; seafood; fresh produce, including raw sprouts; coconut; pasta; chocolate; foods containing raw eggs © Supattra Luasook/Shutterstock.	Salmonellosis **Onset:** 1 to 3 days after eating **Symptoms:** Nausea, abdominal cramps, diarrhea, fever, and headache
Shigella	Undercooked liquid or moist food that has been handled by an infected person © Hirurg/Shutterstock.	Shigellosis (bacillary dysentery) **Onset:** 12 to 50 hours after eating **Symptoms:** Stomach cramps; diarrhea; fever; sometimes vomiting; and blood, pus, and mucus in stools
Staphylococcus aureus—illness is caused by a toxin produced by this organism	Meat and poultry; egg products; tuna, potato, and macaroni salads; cream-filled pastries and other foods left unrefrigerated for long periods **Note:** *S. aureus* is frequently found in cuts on skin and in nasal passages. © Rohit Seth/Shutterstock.	Staphylococcal food poisoning **Onset:** 1 to 6 hours after eating **Symptoms:** Diarrhea, vomiting, nausea, stomach pain, and cramps; lasts 1 to 2 days
Vibrio vulnificus	Raw seafood, especially raw oysters © gori910/Shutterstock.	*Vibrio* infection **Onset:** 1 to 7 days **Symptoms:** Chills, fever, nausea and vomiting, and possibly death, especially in people with underlying health problems
Viruses		
Hepatitis A	Raw shellfish from polluted water, food handled by an infected person © Ewan Loughlin/iStock/Getty Images.	Hepatitis A **Onset:** Averages about 1 month after exposure **Symptoms:** At first, malaise, loss of appetite, nausea, vomiting, and fever; after 3 to 10 days, jaundice and darkened urine; severe cases can result in liver damage and death

TABLE 13.1 (*continued*)
Common Foodborne Pathogens and Illnesses

Organism	Sources	Diseases and Symptoms
Noroviruses Norwalk-like virus	Raw shellfish from polluted water; salads, sandwiches, and other ready-to-eat foods handled by an infected person. Noroviruses are highly contagious and spread rapidly from person to person because of the ease of transmission by touch. © MaraZe/Shutterstock.	Gastroenteritis **Onset:** 1 to 3 days **Symptoms:** Nausea, vomiting, diarrhea, stomach pain, headache, and low-grade fever
Protozoa		
Anisakis	Raw fish © Abramova Elena/Shutterstock.	Anisakiasis **Onset:** 12 to 24 hours **Symptoms:** Abdominal pain, can be severe
Cryptosporidium	Food that comes in contact with sewage-contaminated water; foods handled by a person who did not wash hands after using the toilet © wk1003mike/Shutterstock.	Cryptosporidiosis **Onset:** 1 to 12 days **Symptoms:** Profuse, watery stools; stomach pain; loss of appetite; vomiting; and low-grade fever
Giardia lamblia	Consumption of contaminated water, contamination of food by an infected person © dominique landau/Shutterstock.	Giardiasis **Onset:** 1 to 3 days **Symptoms:** Diarrhea, abdominal cramps, nausea
Toxoplasma gondii	Raw or undercooked meat and, under certain conditions, unwashed fruits and vegetables; also, cats shed cysts in their feces during acute infection—organism may be transmitted to humans, if feces are handled © TAGSTOCK1/Shutterstock.	Toxoplasmosis **Onset:** 10 to 13 days **Symptoms:** Fever, headache, rash, sore muscles, diarrhea; can kill a fetus or cause severe defects, such as mental retardation

▶ **botulism** An often-fatal type of food poisoning caused by a toxin released from *Clostridium botulinum*, a bacterium that can grow in improperly canned low-acid foods.

▶ **Salmonella** Rod-shaped bacteria responsible for many foodborne illnesses.

▶ **Escherichia coli (E. coli)** Bacteria that are the most common cause of urinary tract infections. Because they release toxins, some types of *E. coli* can rapidly cause shock and death.

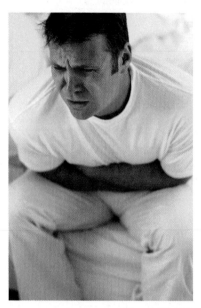

© Bananastock/Thinkstock.

Quick Bite

Flesh-Eating Bacteria?

An estimated 80,000 infections are caused by species of *Vibrio* bacteria (vibriosis) in the United States each year; 52,000 are caused by eating raw or undercooked seafood, especially oysters. Because oysters feed by filtering water, bacteria can concentrate in their tissues. One species, *V. vulnificus*, which can enter the body through wounds on the skin exposed to seawater containing the bacteria, is often described in the media as "flesh-eating." This is because *Vibrio* skin infections can lead to necrotizing fasciitis, a rare but serious, and often deadly, condition that spreads quickly and destroys the body's soft tissue.

Quick Bite

Sticky *Salmonella*

One in six Americans suffers a foodborne illness each year. In 2013, 818 foodborne disease outbreaks resulted in 13,360 people reporting illness, 1,062 people going to the hospital, and 16 people dying. What made all these people sick? The most common causes were norovirus in fruits and *Salmonella* in chicken and pork.

Development of foodborne illness results from the interaction of three factors: the pathogen, the host, and the environment in which they exist and interact.[3] Foodborne illnesses can result directly from infection with a pathogen or from toxins produced by a pathogenic microorganism. For example, the bacterium *Staphylococcus aureus*, a common bacterium found on the skin of many healthy people, creates havoc in the gastrointestinal tract by producing a toxin. When food containing *S. aureus* stands unrefrigerated, the bacteria begin multiplying. After several hours, the expanding bacterial population can produce enough of a nasty toxin to cause nausea, vomiting, and abdominal cramps. Staphylococcal food poisoning is common and causes approximately 241,148 illnesses each year.[4] Fortunately, the illness usually resolves after a day or so of a person vomiting and feeling miserable, with no further harmful effects.

Another toxin-producing bacterium, *Clostridium botulinum*, causes the rare but deadly illness **botulism**. Improperly canned foods, as well as garlic-in-oil preparations, are sources of botulism. Honey can be contaminated with *C. botulinum*, but the acid in adult stomachs kills the bacteria. Infants produce insufficient amounts of stomach acid to kill botulinum, so even small amounts of contaminated honey can be fatal.

Salmonella causes more than 1 million cases of foodborne illness and almost 400 deaths each year, according to CDC estimates.[5] *Salmonella* bacteria are prevalent on poultry and in eggs as well as in a wide variety of other foods. Choosing eggs cooked "over easy" is potentially disastrous because inadequate cooking can leave you vulnerable to the misery of salmonellosis. (See the FYI feature "Safe Food Practices" later in this chapter for more information on how to protect yourself from foodborne illness.)

Escherichia coli (E. coli) are a diverse group of bacteria. Although most varieties are harmless, others can make you sick. Some types cause diarrhea, whereas others cause more serious illnesses, even death. Many foods, including eggs, dairy products, meat and poultry, seafood, fresh produce, unpasteurized juices, and cereal grains, can harbor these disease-causing bacteria.

Because bacteria and other infectious organisms are pervasive in the environment, the contamination of food can occur anywhere from the farm to your plate. Many organisms capable of causing foodborne illness in humans are naturally present in food-producing animals and their environment. For example, *Salmonella enteritidis* bacteria enter eggs directly from the egg-laying hen, and *E. coli* are normally present in the intestines of cattle. Microorganisms natural to the marine environment, but toxic to humans, can contaminate seafood. (See the FYI feature "Seafood Safety.")

Exposure to animal manure or sewage runoff can contaminate crops. Sewage runoff into rivers and streams also can contaminate fish that live there. In the food-processing stage, contamination can occur from dirty equipment, rodent droppings, improper food storage, and infectious employees who fail to wash their hands adequately or take proper precautions when handling food. Poor food safety practices in retail facilities and at home also can contaminate food.

Patterns of foodborne illness have changed dramatically over the last several decades as our food production has become more centralized. When food animals and produce were grown, prepared, and eaten on the family farm, the consequences of errors in food handling were generally limited to a single family. Now, much of the food we eat is

Seafood Safety

Seafood can be a delicious and heart-healthy part of our diets. However, as with all food, contamination can have serious consequences. Seafood is one of the most rapidly perishable foods, so proper refrigeration and rapid processing and transport to the consumer are essential. Although certain types of microbial contaminants and toxins are unique to seafood, properly handled and cooked seafood is as safe to eat as most other foods. To kill seafood parasites, fully cook fish prior to eating, or freeze it for at least 72 hours.

Eating raw seafood is risky business. Despite the popularity of such dishes as sashimi, sushi, and raw oysters, uncooked fish, no matter how carefully prepared, poses a risk for infection. People with liver disease, diabetes, cancer, or other diseases that impair immune function should be especially careful to stay away from raw seafood. Pregnant women also should avoid uncooked seafood; some physicians recommend that pregnant women avoid seafood altogether. The rest of us should think twice before enjoying those raw oysters and sashimi and, at the very least, should make sure they are fresh and from a reliable source before letting those slippery delicacies pass our lips.

Seafood-related illness falls into several categories (see **TABLE A**). Sources of infection include bacteria, viruses, and parasites. Toxins occur naturally in some fish, and human pollution can contaminate seafood. The following are several examples of seafood-caused illness:

- Raw or undercooked shellfish such as oysters, clams, and mussels can be contaminated with bacteria such as *Salmonella*, *Vibrio* species, and *Staphylococcus aureus*. Hepatitis A (caused by a virus) and gastroenteritis are other illnesses that can be contracted by eating uncooked shellfish from polluted waters.
- Fish such as mahi-mahi, tuna, and bluefish that have begun to spoil can cause scombroid poisoning. A toxin in these decomposing fish causes flushing, itching, and headache. Cooking does not destroy the toxin, so the best prevention is proper refrigeration and rapid use of fresh fish.

- Some tropical fish, such as red snapper and barracuda, might contain ciguatera toxin, which can cause gastrointestinal and neurological problems in humans. Larger warm-water fish are most often implicated in this illness. The toxin is actually produced by tiny plants that are eaten by small fish. When larger fish consume many small fish, the toxin can accumulate. The flesh of these large fish can contain enough of the toxin to make humans very ill. Heating or freezing does not destroy this toxin.
- *Anisakis* is a parasite found in raw fish. After a person eats an infected fish, the larvae of this roundworm can invade the human stomach, causing severe abdominal pain. Thoroughly cooking the fish, or freezing it for at least 72 hours, can kill this parasite.
- Red tide is a well-known phenomenon in which huge numbers of tiny, toxic organisms called dinoflagellates infest seawater. Shellfish in the area become poisonous as a result. Respiratory paralysis and death are possible effects of eating shellfish from red tide areas.
- Human pollution is a serious problem, especially near population centers where industrial wastes and human sewage flow into the water. Heavy metals such as mercury can accumulate in larger fish (e.g., sharks, swordfish) that have been exposed to mercury in their environment for long periods.
- Dioxin and polychlorinated biphenols (PCBs) also can accumulate in fish living in polluted water. Commercial seafood companies tend to avoid contaminated areas, but local fishers who frequently catch and eat fish from these waters may be at some risk.

TABLE A
Understanding Seafood Safety

Condition	Explanation
Scombroid poisoning	Scombroid poisoning is a type of food intoxication caused by the consumption of scombroid and scombroid-like marine fish species that have begun to spoil with the growth of particular types of food bacteria. Fish most commonly involved are members of the *Scombridae* family (tunas and mackerels) and a few nonscombroid relatives (bluefish, mahi-mahi, and amberjacks). The suspect toxin is an elevated level of histamine generated by bacterial degradation of substances in the muscle protein.
Anisakis	*Anisakis simplex* (herring worm) and *Pseudoterranova* (*Phocanema*, *Terranova*) *decipiens* (cod or seal worm) are anisakid nematodes (roundworms) that have been implicated in human infections caused by the consumption of raw or undercooked seafood. *Anisakiasis* is the term generally used to refer to the acute disease in humans.
Red tide	When temperature, salinity, and nutrients reach certain levels, algae grow very fast or "bloom" and accumulate into dense, visible patches near the surface of the water. *Red tide* is a common name for such a phenomenon where certain species of phytoplankton contain reddish pigments and bloom such that the water appears to be colored red. The term *red tide* is a misnomer, however, because the reddish color is not associated with tides. A small number of species produces potent neurotoxins that can cause illness and even death.
Polychlorinated biphenols (PCBs)	Polychlorinated biphenols are a group of toxic, persistent chemicals used as insulation for electrical transformers and capacitors and as lubricants in gas pipeline systems. PCBs are a serious health problem because of their persistence in the environment, accumulation in the body, and potential for a long-term negative effect on health. In the United States, their manufacture was stopped in 1976.

mass-produced at central locations and distributed widely to restaurant chains and supermarkets. Although most food poisoning cases arise from poor food handling in homes and restaurants, contamination at a processing plant can make hundreds or even thousands of people ill. This can have nationwide implications and therefore receives intense national media attention.

Prions and Mad Cow Disease

Bovine spongiform encephalopathy (BSE), known popularly as **mad cow disease**, is a chronic degenerative disease that affects the central nervous system of cattle. Once thought to infect only cows, scientists have found that BSE can cause a rare, but fatal, brain-wasting disease in humans called Creutzfeldt-Jakob disease.

Researchers believe that **prions**—proteins found in the cells of humans and other mammals—are responsible. When mammals eat tissues contaminated with abnormal prions, they can develop BSE. Cooking and irradiation do not kill or deactivate abnormal prions.

The skull, brain, eyes, vertebral column, and spinal cord of cows at least 30 months of age are most likely to harbor abnormal prions. The tonsils and a portion of the small intestine of all cattle also can contain the agent. To protect the safety of meat, milk, and dairy products, Canadian and U.S. agencies prohibit these cow parts in the human food supply. Government agencies also regulate and provide guidance to manufacturers who produce cow-derived foods, such as gelatin and some dietary supplements.

> **Key Concepts** Foodborne pathogens are a major cause of illness in the United States and Canada. Pathogenic (disease-causing) agents include bacteria, viruses, parasites, and prions. Contamination of food can occur at many points along the chain from farm to table.

Chemical Contamination

To avoid foods exposed to chemicals, more and more people are turning to **organic foods**. (See the section "Organic Alternatives" later in this chapter.) Yet food safety experts consider contamination by pathogenic microorganisms to be a much greater risk to public health than contamination by chemicals. Chemical contaminants include pesticides, drugs, pollutants, and natural toxins.

Pesticides   **Pesticides** play an important role in food production—controlling plant diseases, weeds, insects, and other pests. Pesticides protect crops and ensure a substantial yield, thus ensuring that consumers have a wide variety of foods at affordable prices. Without these chemicals, many argue that crop production would fall and prices for food would rise.

Every year, the U.S. Food and Drug Administration (FDA) collects thousands of domestic and imported food samples and analyzes them for pesticide residues.[6] Nearly two-thirds of produce samples tested by the U.S. Department of Agriculture (USDA) in 2013 contained pesticide residues; however, according to the USDA, the levels were not high enough to pose a safety concern.[7] The FDA also samples and analyzes domestic and imported animal feeds for pesticide residues. This monitoring focuses on feeds for livestock and poultry—animals that become or produce foods for human consumption. Processing methods can either reduce or concentrate pesticide residues in foods.

▶ **bovine spongiform encephalopathy (BSE)** A chronic degenerative disease, widely referred to as "mad cow disease," that affects the central nervous system of cattle.

▶ **mad cow disease** See *bovine spongiform encephalopathy (BSE)*.

▶ **prions** Short for *proteinaceous infectious particle*. Self-reproducing protein particles that can cause disease.

▶ **organic foods** Foods that originate from farms or handling operations that meet the standards set by the USDA National Organic Program.

▶ **pesticides** Chemicals used to control insects, diseases, weeds, fungi, and other pests on plants, vegetables, fruits, and animals.

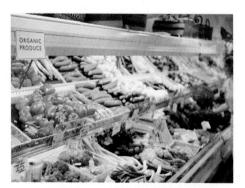
© Jupiterimages/Creatas/Thinkstock.

Pickling and canning cucumbers to make pickles reduces pesticide residues by washing and dilution.

Milling grain to make flour has no effect on pesticide residues.

Washing lettuce and tomatoes reduces pesticide residues.

Drying corn to make feed corn for cattle concentrates pesticide residues, which are further concentrated in beef (particularly in the fat).

Washing and peeling potatoes for potato chips reduces pesticide residues. However, extracting oil from corn and using it to deep fry the potato chips concentrates pesticide residues.

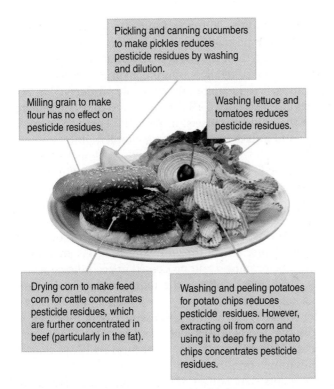

FIGURE 13.2 Pesticide pathways to dinner. Food processing and preparation methods can either reduce or concentrate pesticide residues in foods.

Photo of Hamburger on plate with potato chips: © Photodisc.

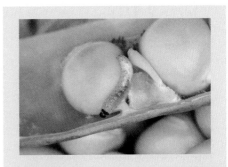

1. **Legal control**
   State and federal guidelines are designed to limit the spread of pests.

2. **Biological control**
   Beneficial organisms, such as predators, parasites, and viruses, are released into the environment to suppress pest organisms.

3. **Cultural control**
   Rotation, sanitation, and other good farming techniques are employed to help reduce pest populations.

4. **Physical control**
   Barriers, traps, and the location and timing of planting are all used to control pest infestations.

5. **Genetic control**
   Resistant plant strains are developed to reduce the impact of pests.

6. **Chemical control**
   Conventional pesticides, biopesticides, pheromones, and other chemicals are used to prevent or suppress pest outbreaks. The chemical controls are specific to a pest species and are ideally short-lived in the environment. In addition, the chemicals are used at their lowest effective rate and may be alternated to help prevent the development of pest resistance.

FIGURE 13.3 Integrated pest management. Integrated pest management is a sustainable approach that combines prevention, avoidance, monitoring, and suppression strategies in a way that minimizes economic, health, and environmental risks. It minimizes pesticide use and promotes economically sound practices.

Caterpillar on Peas: © Ivaschenko Roman/Shutterstock, Inc.

(See **FIGURE 13.2.**) Despite these results that reassure consumers about low pesticide residues, concerns about pesticides in food persist. According to a 2014 survey by *Consumer Reports*' Food Safety and Sustainability Center, 85 percent of Americans worry about pesticide exposure in food.[8]

Infants and young children are particularly susceptible to the hazards of pesticides. Their small size and rapid growth make them especially vulnerable to pesticide residues, which can accumulate in their bodies over their lifetimes. Enacted in 1996, the Food Quality Protection Act includes landmark protections for the young. For the first time, manufacturers had to show that pesticide levels are safe for infants and children. In addition, when determining a safe level for a pesticide in a food, the U.S. Environmental Protection Agency (EPA) must account for the cumulative effect of exposures to similar pesticides and toxic chemicals.[9]

Excessive use of synthetic pesticides, herbicides, and fertilizers contributes substantially to the pollution of soil and water. Overuse can be particularly hazardous to farm workers, whose exposure to these chemicals typically is much higher than that of consumers. Overuse also threatens wildlife. Today, many farmers use **integrated pest management (IPM)** to reduce pesticide use. (See **FIGURE 13.3.**) IPM methods include crop rotation, use of natural rather than synthetic pesticides, and planting nonfood crops nearby that lure pests away from food crops. Releasing sterile fruit flies into orchards also allows reductions in pesticide use. Because fruit flies produce no offspring when they mate with sterile partners, the overall fruit fly population drops.

▶ **integrated pest management (IPM)** Economically sound pest control techniques that minimize pesticide use, enhance environmental stewardship, and promote sustainable systems.

Quick Bite

How Many *Salmonella* Does It Take?

As backyard chicken coops become more common across the United States, so too do salmonella outbreaks linked to contact with live poultry. Since January 2017, state and federal agencies have been investigating eight outbreaks across 47 states that, as of May 2017, had infected 372 people and hospitalized 71; one-third of the victims were children under 5 years of age. The previous year (2016) saw eight outbreaks across 48 states, with 895 infections and three deaths.

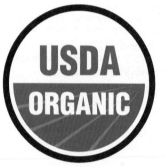

Courtesy of the USDA.

Organic Alternatives   Organic foods are grown or produced without most synthetic pesticides and without synthetic fertilizers. In the United States, growth of the organic food industry can be seen in the expanding number of retailers offering a variety of organic foods and the widespread introduction of new organic products.[10] In 2015, sales of organic foods exceeded $43.3 billion, and they continue to grow.[11] Growth of the industry reflects, in part, the United States' distrust of technology and a desire to return to a simpler, more "natural" way of food production.

The Organic Foods Production Act and the National Organic Program (NOP) are intended to assure U.S. consumers that the organic foods they purchase are produced, processed, and certified to consistent national standards. The labeling requirements of this program apply to raw meats, fresh produce, and processed foods that contain organic ingredients. Foods that are sold, labeled, or represented as organic must be produced and processed in accordance with the NOP standards.[12] **TABLE 13.2** outlines the requirements for labeling a food product as being organic.

Under the NOP, farm and processing operations that grow and process organic foods must be certified by the USDA. The certification process includes an on-site inspection to verify that the applicant's operation complies with strict national organic standards. Certifying agents may collect and test soil, water, waste, plant and

TABLE 13.2
Labeling Requirements for Organic Food

Organic products have strict production and labeling requirements. Unless noted below, organic products must meet the following requirements:
- Produced without excluded methods (e.g., genetic engineering), ionizing radiation, or sewage sludge
- Produced per the National List of Allowed and Prohibited Substances (National List)
- Overseen by a USDA National Organic Program–authorized certifying agent, following all USDA organic regulations

100 PERCENT ORGANIC: Raw or processed agricultural products in the "100 percent organic" category must meet these criteria:
- All ingredients must be certified organic.
- Any processing aids must be organic.
- Product labels must state the name of the certifying agent on the information panel.
- May include USDA organic seal and/or 100 percent organic claim.
- Must identify organic ingredients by name (e.g., organic dill) or via asterisk or other mark.

ORGANIC: Raw or processed agricultural products in the "organic" category must meet these criteria:
- All agricultural ingredients must be certified organic, except where specified on National List.
- Non-organic ingredients allowed per National List may be used, up to a combined total of 5 percent of non-organic content (excluding salt and water).
- Product labels must state the name of the certifying agent on the information panel.
- May include USDA organic seal and/or organic claim.
- Must identify organic ingredients by name (e.g., organic dill) or via asterisk or other mark.

"MADE WITH" ORGANIC: Multi-ingredient agricultural products in the "made with" category must meet these criteria:
- At least 70 percent of the product must be certified organic ingredients (excluding salt and water).
- Any remaining agricultural products are not required to be organically produced but must be produced without excluded methods.
- Non-agricultural products must be specifically allowed on the National List.
- Product labels must state the name of the certifying agent on the information panel.
- May state "made with organic (insert up to three ingredients or ingredient categories)." Must not include USDA organic seal anywhere, represent finished product as organic, or state "made with organic ingredients."
- Must identify organic ingredients by name (e.g., organic dill) or via asterisk or other mark.

SPECIFIC ORGANIC INGREDIENTS: Multi-ingredient products with less than 70 percent certified organic content (excluding salt and water) don't need to be certified. Any non-certified product:
- Must not include USDA organic seal anywhere or the word "organic" on principal display panel.
- May only list certified organic ingredients as organic in the ingredient list and the percentage of organic ingredients. Remaining ingredients are not required to follow the USDA organic regulations.

USDA National Organic Program, Agricultural Marketing Service. Organic Labeling. https://www.ams.usda.gov/rules-regulations/organic/labeling. Accessed May 23, 2017.

animal tissues, and processed products. A certified operation may label its products or ingredients as organic and may use the "USDA Organic" seal.[13]

Organic farming has its drawbacks. The use of manure as a natural fertilizer raises food safety concerns. The organic producer must manage animal and plant waste materials so they do not contribute to contamination of crops, soil, or water. Manure runoff can pollute nearby lakes and streams. Some critics charge that organic farming is "elitist" and that synthetic fertilizers and pesticides are necessary to meet the food needs of an expanding world population. They also point out that complete freedom from pesticides cannot be guaranteed, no matter how carefully a food is produced, because pesticide residues may still exist in soil, water, and air.

Organic foods are not pesticide-free foods. Organic farmers can use natural and approved synthetic pesticides to control weeds and insects.[14,15] A 2012 audit by the USDA's National Organic Program revealed that 43 percent of organic produce had some degree of prohibited pesticides.[16] Microbial contaminants that cause foodborne illness can be found in organic as well as conventional foods. Consumers must handle all food appropriately, whether organically or conventionally grown.

THINK About It 2

Animal Drugs   Current agricultural practice depends heavily on the use of drugs in food animals and food-producing animals raised specifically to provide meat, milk, and eggs. Producers use drugs to maintain animal health and well-being as well as to increase production. Keeping animals in good health reduces the chance that disease will spread from animals to humans, and healthy animals can use nutrients for growth and production rather than to fight infection. But there is a possibility that drugs used in animals could enter human food and possibly increase the risk of ill health in humans.[17]

Can drugs used to raise animals for food affect your health? The FDA is responsible for ensuring that drugs approved for use in animals are safe not only for the animals, but also for humans who eat food produced from the animals. Because antibiotics used in both humans and animals contribute to the development of antimicrobial resistance, in 2013 the FDA implemented a voluntary plan working with industry to phase out the use of certain antibiotics for enhanced food production in farm animals.[18] The FDA recommends that use of medically important antimicrobial drugs in food-producing animals be limited to situations where the use of these drugs is necessary for ensuring animal health, and their use includes veterinary oversight or consultation.

Pollutants   **Pollutants** from animal manure and other wastes, factories, human sewage, and industrial runoff can contaminate food-production areas. For example, some scientists theorize that dioxin contamination of foods can cause human cancer. **Dioxins** are chemical compounds created in the manufacturing, combustion, and chlorine bleaching of pulp and paper and in other industrial processes.[19] Dioxins can accumulate in the food chain and are potent animal carcinogens.[20]

Mercury both occurs naturally in the environment and is produced by human activities. It is not soluble in water or most other liquids, but it will dissolve in lipids (fats and oils). Bacteria can cause chemical changes that transform mercury to **methylmercury**, a more toxic

Quick **Bite**

A Not So Dirty Dozen
The Environmental Working Group (EWG), an environmental advocacy organization, publishes an annual list of the "Dirty Dozen"—fruits and vegetables suspected of having the greatest potential for contamination with pesticide residues. According to UC Davis researchers, however, "findings conclusively demonstrate that consumer exposures to the ten most frequently detected pesticides on EWG's 'Dirty Dozen' commodity list are at negligible levels and that the EWG methodology is insufficient to allow any meaningful rankings among commodities."

Quick **Bite**

Is It Stomach Flu or Food Poisoning?
Both can have similar symptoms—miserable vomiting, abdominal cramping, and diarrhea. Although we often do not know the exact cause, stomach flu tends to occur in the winter months and is preceded by other symptoms, such as sore throat. Food poisoning tends to occur in summer months, and symptoms usually appear suddenly without warning. Symptoms may not begin until 12 to 72 hours after eating tainted food. If many people who ate the same food get sick around the same time, it's probably food poisoning.

Quick **Bite**

Community Supported Agriculture
How about having direct access to high-quality, fresh produce grown locally by regional farmers? You can have it by becoming a member. Community Supported Agriculture (CSA) has become a popular way for consumers to buy local, seasonal food directly from a farmer. As a member of the nearest CSA, you are able to choose the box type, size, and delivery frequency that best fits your lifestyle. The delivery day usually depends on your zip code, and the delivery frequency can be weekly, every other week, or every 3 or 4 weeks. You can find a CSA farmer on the Internet or through organizations like Local Harvest, which maintains a list of CSA farms and current information.

▶ **pollutants** Gaseous, chemical, or organic waste that contaminates air, soil, or water.

▶ **dioxins** Chemical compounds created in the manufacturing, combustion, and chlorine bleaching of pulp and paper and in other industrial processes.

▶ **methylmercury** A toxic compound that results from the chemical transformation of mercury by bacteria. Mercury is water-soluble in trace amounts and contaminates many bodies of water.

Quick Bite

Well-Traveled Dioxin

In Nunavut, a Canadian province, the breast milk of native Inuits has twice the average concentration of dioxin—a highly toxic compound produced in herbicide production and paper bleaching—as does the milk of women in southern Quebec. Native Inuits primarily eat fatty animals high on the food chain. These animals accumulate dioxin, but where did the dioxin originate? Not Canada. Carried by the wind, most comes from industrial combustion in the eastern and midwestern United States, and some originates as far away as Mexico.

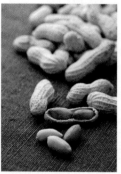

© matin/Shutterstock, Inc.

▶ **natural toxins** Poisons that are produced by or naturally occur in plants or microorganisms.

form. Fish absorb methylmercury from water passing over their gills and by eating other contaminated aquatic species. Larger predatory fish can consume many contaminated smaller fish, thereby accumulating higher levels of methylmercury. (See **FIGURE 13.4**.) People are making more informed seafood choices; even so, shark, swordfish, king mackerel, and tilefish contain high levels of mercury, and therefore the FDA and EPA continue to recommend that women who may become pregnant, pregnant women, nursing mothers, and young children avoid eating these fish.[21]

Natural Toxins   Other chemical contamination of food can occur from **natural toxins**. Examples include the following:

- **Aflatoxins**, found in contaminated food or animal feed: Aflatoxins are produced by certain strains of *Aspergillus* fungi under certain conditions of temperature and humidity. The most pronounced contamination has been found in tree nuts, peanuts, and other oilseeds, such as corn and cottonseed.
- **Ciguatera** and other marine toxins: These toxins can accumulate in seafood (mainly in large tropical fish) and, when ingested,

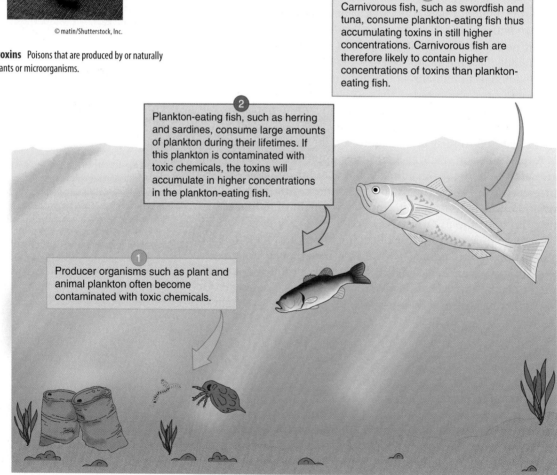

Carnivorous fish, such as swordfish and tuna, consume plankton-eating fish thus accumulating toxins in still higher concentrations. Carnivorous fish are therefore likely to contain higher concentrations of toxins than plankton-eating fish.

Plankton-eating fish, such as herring and sardines, consume large amounts of plankton during their lifetimes. If this plankton is contaminated with toxic chemicals, the toxins will accumulate in higher concentrations in the plankton-eating fish.

Producer organisms such as plant and animal plankton often become contaminated with toxic chemicals.

FIGURE 13.4 Toxins in the food chain. As toxins travel up the food chain, they become concentrated in larger fish. The longer a fish lives, the higher the level of toxins it will accumulate.

cause serious problems, including paralysis, amnesia, and nerve toxicity. Cooking does not destroy these toxins.

- **Poisonous mushrooms**: These plants produce toxic substances that can cause stomach upset, dizziness, hallucinations, and other neurological symptoms. The more lethal mushroom species can cause liver and kidney failure, coma, and death.
- **Solanine**, a toxic substance in raw potato skins: Solanine develops in the greenish layer of improperly stored potatoes. It can be removed by thoroughly peeling the potato.

A variety of compounds in herbs and spices also can be toxic. However, foodborne illness caused by these and other natural toxins is relatively rare compared with illness from pathogenic microorganisms.

Food Allergens   In the United States, about 4 percent of adults and 8 percent of infants and young children (nearly 15 million people) have food allergies.[22] Eight major foods or food groups—milk, eggs, fish, shellfish, tree nuts, peanuts, wheat, and soybeans—account for 90 percent of allergic reactions. (See **FIGURE 13.5**.) Whenever these foods (or ingredients derived from them) are present in a food product, food labels must identify them.[23] In an allergic person, these foods can cause a variety of reactions, including gastrointestinal problems, skin irritation, breathing difficulty, shock, and even death.

Contaminants, such as glass, metal, and other objects, can be introduced unintentionally during food production. Improper use of cleaning agents in food-contact areas can add these undesirable substances to food. Insects, dirt, and other undesirable items, although generally not a health hazard, also can find their way into food.

▶ **aflatoxins** Toxins produced by a mold that grows on crops, such as peanuts, tree nuts, corn, wheat, and oil seeds (like cottonseed).

▶ **ciguatera** A toxin found in more than 300 species of Caribbean and South Pacific fish. It is a nonbacterial source of food poisoning.

▶ **poisonous mushrooms** Mushrooms that contain toxins that can cause stomach upset, dizziness, hallucinations, and other neurological symptoms.

▶ **solanine** A potentially toxic alkaloid that is present with chlorophyll in the green areas on potato skins.

> **Key Concepts** Chemical contaminants in foods include pesticides, natural toxins, and contamination related to pollution. Although organic foods are grown without synthetic pesticides or fertilizers, they still can contain chemical contaminants. Other potential food hazards are allergens and nonfood contaminants.

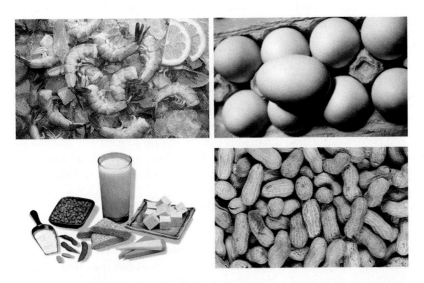

FIGURE 13.5 Foods that commonly cause allergic reactions. In sensitive people, an allergic reaction to food can be life threatening.

Shellfish: © Michael Lamotte/Cole Group/Photodisc/Getty Images; Eggs: © Photodisc; Soy products: © Photodisc; Peanuts: © LiquidLibrary.

Food Additives

🍎 **Why Is This Important?** Getting the most out of foods that we eat, such as preserving freshness and extending shelf life, or adding vitamins or minerals that would otherwise be underconsumed to commonly eaten foods, are important practices in food manufacturing. Not all food additives are the same, and in an effort to make healthy food choices, it is important to understand the potential risks of some additives, as well as the benefits of others.

▶ **direct additives** Substances that are added to a food for a specific reason.

▶ **indirect additives** Substances that unintentionally become part of the food in trace amounts

Food additives work in many different ways to give us a safe, plentiful, varied, and relatively inexpensive food supply. Food additives can be either direct or indirect. **Direct additives** are added to a food for a specific reason. Aspartame, saccharin, and sucralose are direct food additives, used instead of sugar to sweeten. Direct additives are identified in the ingredient list on the food label. **Indirect additives** are substances that unintentionally become part of the food in trace amounts—for example, chemicals from a food's packaging can become part of the food. The FDA evaluates both direct and indirect additives for safety.

Direct additives are used in foods for five main reasons:

1. *To maintain product consistency:* Emulsifiers give products such as peanut butter a consistent texture and prevent them from separating. Stabilizers and thickeners give ice cream a smooth, uniform texture. Anticaking agents help substances such as salt to flow freely.
2. *To improve or maintain nutritional value:* Vitamins and minerals are added to many common foods such as milk, flour, cereal, and margarine to make up for elements likely to be lacking in a person's diet, replace those lost in processing, or improve shelf life.
3. *To keep the food appetizing and wholesome:* Preservatives help protect against mold, air, bacteria, fungi, or yeast, which all can cause food to spoil.
4. *To provide leavening or control acidity and alkalinity:* Leavening agents help cakes, biscuits, and other baked goods to rise during baking. Other additives modify the acidity and alkalinity of foods for flavor, taste, and color.
5. *To enhance flavor or give a desired color:* Many spices and added flavors enhance the taste of foods. Colors, likewise, enhance the appearance of certain foods to make them more appealing or meet consumer expectations.

Although most people think additives are complex chemicals with unfamiliar names, three of the most common additives are sugar, salt, and corn syrup. These three, plus citric acid (found naturally in oranges and lemons), baking soda, vegetable colors, mustard, and pepper account for more than 98 percent by weight of all food additives used in the United States and Canada.

Regulation by the FDA

Although additives serve important functions (see **FIGURE 13.6**), you might be skeptical about their safety. Additives fall into four regulatory categories: food additives, color additives, Generally Recognized as Safe (GRAS) substances, and prior-sanctioned substances. The FDA must approve a new food additive before it can be put on the market. The manufacturer must provide convincing research evidence that

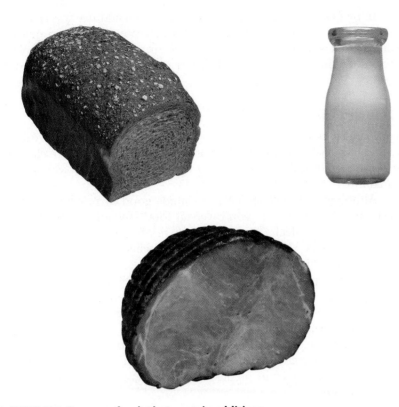

FIGURE 13.6 Common foods that contain additives.
Loaf of bread: © Digital Stock; Bottle of milk: © Photodisc; Half of a cooked ham: © Photodisc.

the additive not only performs its intended function, but also is not harmful at expected consumption levels. Based on this and other scientific information, the FDA decides whether to approve the additive and determines the types of foods that may contain the additive, the quantities that can be used, and the way the substance will be identified on labels.

A **color additive** is any dye, pigment, or substance that can give color when added to a food, drug, or cosmetic or to the human body. Colors allowed for use in food are classified as either certified or exempt from certification. Certified colors are synthetic. The manufacturer and the FDA test each batch to ensure their purity. Certified colors added to a food must be listed on the food's ingredient list by common name. Colors exempt from certification include natural substances derived from vegetables, minerals, or animals. These colors also must be produced according to specifications that ensure purity.

A third type of additive falls under the category **Generally Recognized as Safe (GRAS)**. Congress first defined GRAS substances in 1958 when it passed the Food Additives Amendment to the Food, Drug, and Cosmetic Act. If a substance is classified as GRAS, experts generally consider it safe to use, either because it was safely used in food before 1958 or because there is published scientific evidence for its safety. Salt, sugar, spices, vitamins, and monosodium glutamate (MSG), along with several hundred other substances, are considered GRAS. Manufacturers themselves may assert that a food has GRAS status or petition the FDA to have a new additive be considered GRAS. In either case, the manufacturer must have evidence of safety and a basis for concluding that this evidence is known and accepted by qualified experts.

▶ **color additives** Any dye, pigment, or substance that can give color when added to a food, drug, or cosmetic or to the human body.

▶ **Generally Recognized as Safe** A classification for substances which is assigned when experts generally consider a substance safe to use.

▶ **prior-sanctioned substance** An additive which was determined by the FDA or USDA to be safe for use in a specific food before the 1958 legislation.

▶ **Delaney Clause** A legal provision stating that food or color additives cannot be approved if they cause cancer in humans or animals.

If the FDA or USDA had determined that an additive was safe for use in a specific food before the 1958 legislation, then it is a **prior-sanctioned substance**, the fourth category of additives. Examples include sodium nitrite and potassium nitrite to preserve luncheon meats.

Delaney Clause

Food additives and color additives cannot be approved if they cause cancer in humans or animals. This provision of the law is often referred to as the **Delaney Clause**, named for the congressman who sponsored it.

Although the Delaney Clause sounds good in principle, it has become one of the most controversial food laws on the books. To determine a chemical's safety, researchers often administer massive doses to rodents. Many experts question whether an additive that causes cancer in laboratory animals at extremely high levels should be banned from use in foods at low levels. They argue that feeding animals large doses of a substance over their entire lifetimes may have little relevance to human consumption of trace amounts of that same substance.

For now, the Delaney Clause remains part of our food safety laws. Future scientific techniques might decrease reliance on animal testing and improve accuracy in predicting the effects of food additives on human health.

> **Key Concepts** Direct additives are used for specific purposes. Indirect additives become part of the food in trace amounts when the food comes in contact with the substance. Additives are used for many reasons; these include improving product quality, maintaining freshness, and improving nutritional value. Unless a new additive meets the requirements to be considered GRAS or is a prior-sanctioned ingredient, the FDA demands that it undergo extensive testing to be proved safe and effective. The FDA is responsible for approving and regulating additives. The Delaney Clause prohibits the approval of an additive if it is found to cause cancer in humans or animals.

Keeping Food Safe

🍎 **Why Is This Important?** Foodborne illness can be costly; yet in many cases, it can also be prevented. Understanding proper food handling techniques is an important step in preventing foodborne illness.

Having safe foods to eat requires the efforts of a great many people along the way from the farm to your plate. Imagine yourself enjoying a piece of broiled chicken. Consider that harmful contamination of that chicken could have occurred at the farm, in the processing plant, or during transportation to the supermarket. Once at the supermarket, the chicken might have been under-refrigerated or kept too long before being sold. After buying the chicken, you might have left it in a warm car or kept it in a refrigerator that was not cold enough. Your kitchen hygiene might not have been the best; finally, you could have undercooked the chicken. Considering the many opportunities for contamination, it is truly amazing that most of the time our food does not make us sick.

Keeping foods free from contamination is a job that falls to many parties. It is the responsibility not only of government officials at the

Quick Bite

Chill Out!

In 1939, Fred McKinley Jones, a prolific African American inventor, and Joe Numero received a patent for a vehicle refrigeration device for large trucks. Their invention eliminated the problem of food spoilage during long shipping times and permitted year-round delivery of fresh produce across the country. Refrigerated shipping launched international markets for food; helped create new industries such as frozen foods, fast foods, and container shipping; and forever altered consumers' eating habits.

national, state, and local levels, but also of everyone who comes in contact with food—the producer, the manufacturer, the retailer, and ultimately, the consumer.

Government Agencies

The basis of modern U.S. food law is the Federal Food, Drug, and Cosmetic (FD&C) Act of 1938, which gives the Food and Drug Administration authority over food and food ingredients and defines requirements for truthful labeling of ingredients.

To update and reform the food safety system in the United States, the FDA Food Safety Modernization Act (FSMA) was signed into law on January 4, 2011. The primary objective of FSMA is to ensure that the U.S. food supply is safe by enabling the FDA to increase its focus on preventing food safety problems rather than primarily reacting after problems occur. Under this law, the FDA has higher authority to enforce compliance with prevention- and risk-based food safety standards and to better respond to and contain problems when they do occur. The law also enables the FDA to better ensure the safety of imported foods and build an integrated national food safety system in partnership with state and local authorities.[24] Under direction of the FDA, the Coordinated Outbreak Response and Evaluation (CORE) Network is in place to strengthen and streamline efforts to prevent, investigate, and control outbreaks of foodborne illnesses.

THINK About It 3

To help reduce food contamination and foodborne illnesses in the home, the *2015–2020 Dietary Guidelines for Americans* offers the following food safety principles and guidance, which are also the cornerstones of Fight BAC!, a food safety education campaign. When preparing food:

- *Clean* hands, food contact surfaces, and food.
- *Separate* raw, cooked, and ready-to-eat foods while shopping, storing, and preparing foods.
- *Cook* foods to safe temperatures to kill microorganisms.
- *Chill* (refrigerate) perishable food promptly.

At the federal level, six agencies (see **FIGURE 13.7**) share responsibility for food safety.

1. The Food and Drug Administration (FDA) enforces laws governing the safety of domestic and imported food, except meat and poultry.
2. The Centers for Disease Control and Prevention (CDC) monitors outbreaks of foodborne diseases, investigates their causes, and determines proper prevention.
3. The USDA Food Safety and Inspection Service (FSIS) enforces laws governing the safety of domestic and imported meat and poultry products.
4. The USDA Cooperative State Research, Education, and Extension Service (CSREES) develops research and education programs on food safety for farmers and consumers.
5. The USDA Agricultural Research Service (ARS) conducts research to extend knowledge of various agricultural practices, including those involving animal and crop safety.
6. The Environmental Protection Agency (EPA) regulates public drinking water and approves pesticides and other chemicals used in the environment.

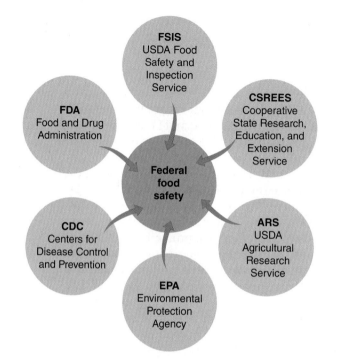

Other Agencies with food safety responsibilities

Federal Trade Commission (FTC)
· Regulates the advertising and marketing of food products.
· Has the authority to take legal action against unwarranted advertising claims.

Department of Justice
· Seizes products when federal food safety laws are violated.
· Prosecutes suspected violators of food safety laws.

Bureau of Alcohol, Tobacco, and Firearms (BATF)
· Enforces laws that involve the production, distribution, and labeling of most alcoholic beverages.
· Sometimes shares responsibilities with FDA when alcoholic beverages are adulterated or contain food or color additives, pesticides, or contaminants.

National Marine Fisheries Service (NMFS)
· Responsible for seafood quality and identification, fisheries management and development, habitat conservation, and aquaculture production.

State and local governments
· Inspect restaurants, retail food outlets, dairies, grain mills, and other food establishments within their areas of jurisdiction.
· Embargo illegal food products in many situations.

FIGURE 13.7 **Government agencies that help protect our food supply.** Although the FDA has primary responsibility for the safety of much of our food supply, many government agencies provide oversight.

Quick **Bite**

Wood vs. Plastic: The Cutting Controversy

Which type of cutting board is safer to use while cutting meat: wood or plastic? Both have drawbacks. A wood cutting board tends to absorb bacteria, sucking them down into the wood fibers. This may be safer than a plastic board, which keeps bacteria on the surface, in an easy position to rub off onto food and other objects. But with use, wooden cutting boards tend to keep more on the surface than new wooden boards, acting more like plastic boards. What's the solution? Keep cutting boards clean by heating wooden boards in the microwave or putting plastic boards in the dishwasher.

▶ **critical control points (CCPs)** Operational steps or procedures in a process, production method, or recipe at which control can be applied to prevent, reduce, or eliminate a food safety hazard.

State and local health and agricultural departments oversee food safety in their jurisdictions, often in conjunction with federal agencies.

Hazard Analysis Critical Control Point

Hazard Analysis Critical Control Point (HACCP) is a food industry program that focuses on preventing contamination by identifying areas in food production and retail where contamination could occur. HACCP also is an important line of defense against intentional contamination by bioterrorists. (See the FYI feature "At War with Bioterrorism.")

Companies and retailers analyze their food-production processes and determine **critical control points (CCPs)**—points at which hazards could occur. They then determine measures that they can institute at these points to prevent, control, or eliminate the hazards.[25]

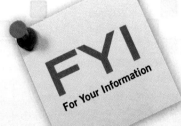

At War with Bioterrorism

Late one afternoon, restaurant owner Dave Lutgens first felt nauseated, and then experienced mild stomach cramps. By evening he was dizzy and disoriented. Suffering from diarrhea, he had to crawl to reach the toilet. Weak and dehydrated, he was wracked with chills, fever, and vomiting. Two days later his wife became ill with the same symptoms. By the end of the week, 13 employees were sick as well as dozens of customers. The culprit was *Salmonella typhimurium*, a rod-shaped bacterium responsible for many foodborne illnesses. But this was not a simple case of food poisoning. Occurring in 1984, this was a criminal assault on the small Oregon town of Dalles. The Rajaneesh religious cult attempted to sway local election results by poisoning people to keep them away from the polls. The cult deliberately perpetrated this terrifying food experience by contaminating a number of self-service salad bars and coffee creamers with home-grown *Salmonella*. Ten restaurants were affected, and more than 700 people fell ill from the biological attack.

Bioterrorism is a deliberate attack using agents typically found in nature, such as viruses, bacteria, or other germs, to cause illness or death.[a] Biological agents can be spread through food or water and could be used by terrorists because they can be difficult to detect and might not cause illness for hours or days.

After September 11, 2001, food bioterrorism received a surge of attention, and efforts focused on protecting against a large-scale terrorist attack on the nation's food or water supply.[b]

Food and water poisonings can be divided into three categories[c]:

1. *Bioterrorism and biowarfare:* Terrorist acts by state-sponsored organizations or hate groups. Few such events have occurred to date.
2. *Biocrime:* Intent to harm for personal gain or revenge. A few dozen events have occurred during recent decades.
3. *Biomisfortune:* Naturally occurring foodborne disease. Virtually all foodborne disease falls into this category, which is a daily concern for public health agencies everywhere.

Americans enjoy one of the safest food supplies in the world; however, our food supply is an obvious route for the delivery of chemical and biological agents. Food production and distribution form a complex system not protected easily from the deliberate introduction of toxic agents. The attacks on the World Trade Center and Pentagon and the anthrax assaults increased the concern and vigilance of the U.S. and Canadian governments, which are acutely aware that public food and water supplies are among the most vulnerable avenues for terrorist attacks.

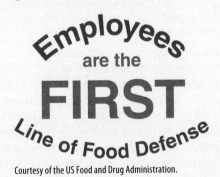

Courtesy of the US Food and Drug Administration.

At ports of entry, food inspection facilities, and research labs and buildings, government personnel are at a heightened state of alert. To prevent the entry of animal or plant pests and diseases, product and cargo inspections of travelers and baggage are intensified. Food safety inspectors have been given a mandate to be alert to any irregularities at food-processing facilities. If not already in place at processing facilities, specific plans for security should be developed to reduce the risk of tampering and other malicious, criminal, or terrorist actions. Employees FIRST is an initiative from the FDA designed to educate food industry workers about the risk of intentional food contamination and identify actions to reduce risk.[d] (See **TABLE A**.)

TABLE A	
Employees FIRST	
F	FOLLOW company food defense plans and procedures.
I	INSPECT your work area and surrounding areas.
R	RECOGNIZE anything out of the ordinary.
S	SECURE all ingredients, supplies, and finished product.
T	TELL management if you notice anything unusual or suspicious.

Courtesy of the US Food and Drug Administration.

The Public Health Security and Bioterrorism Preparedness and Response Act of 2002 (called the Bioterrorism Act) mandated that the FDA take numerous steps to protect the safety and security of the food and drug supply. Since then, the FDA has developed additional food safety regulations, increased domestic and foreign surveillance, and continued to work toward reducing threats and vulnerabilities. To protect the nation's food supply from both unintentional contamination and deliberate attack, the Food Protection Plan (2007) was developed by the FDA to address changes in food sources, production, and consumption as a strategy.[e]

What can consumers do to protect themselves from food contamination? We must be the final judges of the safety of the food we buy. At a minimum, we should:

- Make sure the food package or can is intact before opening it. If it has been damaged or dented or opened prior to purchase, call it to the attention of the appropriate person.
- Be alert to abnormal color, taste, and appearance of a food item. If you have any doubt, don't eat it.
- If the food appears to be tampered with, report it immediately.
- Follow safe food-handling practices. (See the FYI feature "Safe Food Practices.")

a Centers for Disease Control and Prevention. Bioterrorism. https://emergency.cdc.gov/bioterrorism/index.asp. Accessed September 19, 2017.
b Position of the Academy of Nutrition and Dietetics: food and water safety. *J Acad Nutr Diet.* 2014;114:1819-1129.
c Sobel J. Epidemiologic preparedness and response to terrorist events involving the nation's food supply. Paper presented at Centers for Disease Control and Prevention's Health Preparedness Conference; February 2005.
d U.S. Food and Drug Administration. Employees FIRST. Food defense awareness for front-line food industry workers. June 2016. https://www.fda.gov/food/fooddefense/toolseducationalmaterials/ucm295997.htm. Accessed September 19, 2017.
e U.S. Food and Drug Administration. Food: food protection plan 2007. http://www.fda.gov/Food/GuidanceRegulation/FoodProtectionPlan2007/. Accessed September 19, 2017.

TABLE 13.3
HACCP: Hazard Analysis and Critical Control Point

Step 1: Analyze hazards.	Identify the potential hazards associated with a food. The hazard could be biological (e.g., a microbe), chemical (e.g., mercury), or physical (e.g., ground glass, metal).
Step 2: Identify critical control points (CCPs).	Identify points in a food's production path—from its raw state through processing and shipping to consumption—where a potential hazard can be controlled or eliminated. Examples of CCPs are cooking, chilling, handling, cleaning, and storage.
Step 3: Establish preventive measures with critical limits for each control point.	An example is setting the minimum cooking temperature and time to ensure safety for a particular food. (The temperature and time are critical limits.)
Step 4: Establish procedures to monitor the control points.	Such procedures might include determining how and by whom cooking time and temperature should be monitored.
Step 5: Establish corrective actions to be taken when a critical limit has not been met.	For example, food should be reprocessed or disposed of if the minimum cooking temperature is not met.
Step 6: Establish effective record keeping to document the HACCP system.	For example, record hazards and their control methods, monitor safety requirements, and take action to correct potential problems.
Step 7: Establish procedures to verify that the system is working consistently.	For example, test time-recording and temperature-recording devices to verify that a cooking unit is working properly.

Modified from U.S. Food and Drug Administration. Hazard Analysis and Critical Control Point principles and application guidelines. https://www.fda.gov/Food/GuidanceRegulation/HACCP/ucm2006801.htm. Accessed May 31, 2017.

▶ **Food Code** A reference published periodically by the Food and Drug Administration for restaurants, grocery stores, institutional food services, vending operations, and other retailers on how to store, prepare, and serve food to prevent foodborne illness.

Position Statement: Academy of Nutrition and Dietetics

Food and Water Safety

It is the position of the Academy of Nutrition and Dietetics that all people should have access to a safe food and water supply. The Academy supports science-based food regulations and recommendations that are applied consistently across all foods and water regulated by all agencies and that incorporate traceability and recall to limit food and waterborne outbreaks. Registered dietitian nutritionists and dietetic technicians are encouraged to participate in policy decisions, program development, and implementation of a global food safety culture.

Reprinted from *Journal of the Academy of Nutrition and Dietetics*, 114(11), Mildred M. Cody, Theresa Stretch, Position of the Academy of Nutrition and Dietetics: Food and Water Safety, Page no. 1819-1829, 2014, with permission from Elsevier.

(See **TABLE 13.3**.) Critical control points can occur anywhere in a food's production—from its raw state through processing and shipping to purchase by the consumer. Preventive measures can include proper cooking, chilling, and sanitizing, as well as preventing cross-contamination and improving employee hygiene.

The USDA requires HACCP for the food products it regulates—meat and poultry. The FDA, which regulates all other foods, requires HACCP in the seafood and low-acid canned-food industries and the juice industry.[26] Also, the FDA has incorporated HACCP principles in its *Food Code*, a reference for restaurants, grocery stores, institutional food services, vending operations, and other retailers on how to store, prepare, and serve food to prevent foodborne illness.[27] The FDA updates and publishes the *Food Code* periodically as a model for states to adopt and use to regulate retail food establishments in their jurisdictions.

Key Concepts Food safety is the responsibility of many agencies at the federal and state levels. The use of the Hazard Analysis Critical Control Point system allows government and industry to identify possible sites of food contamination and correct problems before they occur.

Some food-handling practices are so important that the federal government requires specific instructions or warnings on labels of certain foods. Following outbreaks of illness from *E. coli* O157:H7 in contaminated hamburger in 1993, the USDA mandated instructions on labels of raw meat and poultry to encourage consumers to follow recommendations for safe handling and cooking of these products.

Labels of unpasteurized or otherwise untreated, packaged juice products carry a warning statement about the product's possible danger to children, older adults, and people with weakened immune systems. The warning states that the product has not been pasteurized and therefore might contain harmful bacteria that can cause serious illness in these high-risk groups. This requirement was made after a number of people became seriously ill from drinking unpasteurized apple juice that was contaminated with *E. coli*.

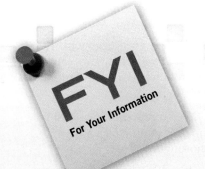

Safe Food Practices

Because bacteria grow rapidly between 40°F and 140°F (4–60°C), most food should be kept out of this temperature range, known as the Danger Zone. Cold temperatures keep bacteria from multiplying; the fewer bacteria, the lower the risk of illness. Proper cooking (or other heat treatment, such as pasteurization) kills the bacteria. These principles serve as the basis for many of the following recommended food-handling practices.

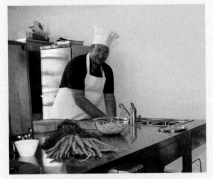

© Simone van den Berg/Shutterstock.

Buying Food

- Buy from reputable dealers and grocers who keep their selling areas and facilities clean and sanitary and maintain food at the appropriate temperature—for example, holding dairy foods, eggs, meats, seafood, and certain produce such as cut melons and raw sprouts at refrigerator temperatures.
- Don't buy canned goods with dents or bulges. Avoid torn, crushed, or open food packages. Also, avoid buying packages that are above the frost line in the store's freezer. If the package cover is transparent, look for frost or ice crystals, signs that the product has been stored for a long time or thawed and refrozen.

Storing Food

- Separate raw, cooked, and ready-to-eat foods while shopping, preparing, and storing.
- Refrigerate perishable items as quickly as possible after purchase. The refrigerator temperature should be 40°F or colder. Check it periodically with a thermometer to make sure the correct temperature is being maintained.
- Keep eggs in their original carton and store them in the refrigerator itself, not the door, where the temperature is warmer.
- If raw meat, poultry products, or fresh seafood will be used within two days, store them in the coldest part of the refrigerator, usually under the freezer compartment or in a special "meat keeper." Store the

packages loosely to allow air to circulate freely around each package, and be sure to wrap them tightly so raw juices can't leak out and contaminate other foods.

- If raw meat, poultry, and seafood will not be used within two days, store them in the freezer, which should have a temperature of 0°F. Check this temperature periodically, too, and adjust as needed.
- Read label directions for storing other foods; for example, mayonnaise and ketchup need to be refrigerated after they have been opened.
- Store potatoes and onions in a cool dark place, but not under the sink because leakage from pipes can contaminate and damage them. Keep them away from household cleaning products and other chemicals as well.

Preparing Food

- Wash hands thoroughly with warm, soapy water for at least 20 seconds before beginning food preparation and every time you handle raw foods, including fresh produce.
- Defrost meat, poultry, and seafood products in the refrigerator, microwave oven, or a watertight plastic bag submerged in cold water. (The water must be changed every 30 minutes.) Never defrost at room temperature—an ideal temperature for bacteria to grow and multiply.
- Marinate foods in the refrigerator. Discard the marinade after use because it contains raw juices, which can harbor bacteria; make a separate batch for basting food while cooking.
- Always use a clean cutting board. Wash cutting boards with hot water, soap, and a scrub brush. Then sanitize them in an automatic dishwasher or by rinsing with a solution of 5 milliliters (1 teaspoon) chlorine bleach to about 1 liter (1 quart) of water. If possible, use one cutting board for fresh produce and a separate one for raw meat, poultry, and seafood. Once cutting boards become excessively worn or develop hard-to-clean grooves, you should replace them.
- Before opening canned foods, wash the top of the can to prevent dirt from coming in contact with the food.

- Wash fresh fruits and vegetables thoroughly with cold water. It is not necessary to wash or rinse meat or poultry.
- Avoid eating dough or batter containing raw eggs because of the risk of *Salmonella enteritidis*, a bacterium that can live in eggs.

Cooking Food

- Cook foods to the USDA Recommended Safe Minimum Internal Temperatures.[a]
  - 145°F for whole meats with a three-minute rest period after cooking
  - 160°F for ground meats
  - 165°F for all poultry
- The only safe way to know whether food is "done" is to use a food thermometer. According to the USDA, one of every four hamburgers turns brown before reaching a safe internal temperature.
- During the three-minute rest period after meat is removed from the heat source, the internal temperature remains constant or continues to rise, which destroys pathogens.
- Never place cooked food on a plate that previously held raw meat, poultry, or seafood.
- When microwaving foods, rotate the dish and stir its contents several times to ensure even cooking. Follow recommended standing times, then check meat, poultry, and seafood products with a thermometer to make sure they have reached the correct internal temperature.
- Cook eggs until the white and the yolk are both firm.

Serving Food

- Keep hot foods at 140°F (60°C) or higher and cold foods at 40°F (4°C) or lower.
- Refrigerate or freeze leftovers and perishables within two hours or sooner.
- Date and label leftovers so they can be used within a safe time—generally, three to five days in the refrigerator.

a U.S. Department of Agriculture, Food Safety and Inspection Service. Safe minimum internal temperature chart. https://www.fsis.usda.gov/wps/portal /fsis/topics/food-safety-education/get-answers /food-safety-fact-sheets/safe-food-handling/safe -minimum-internal-temperature-chart/ct_index. Accessed September 19, 2017.

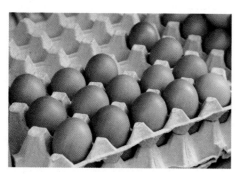

© evilbeau/Shutterstock.

Quick **Bite**

How Good Are Your Food Safety Habits?

Do Americans practice food safety in their own kitchens? Apparently not. A study conducted by the FDA and the Centers for Disease Control and Prevention showed that one-half of people surveyed ate undercooked eggs in the past year. Twenty percent of people ate undercooked hamburger, and 25 percent of men and 14 percent of women failed to wash their hands with soap after handling raw meat.

Fresh eggs must be handled carefully, and even eggs with clean, uncracked shells occasionally contain *Salmonella* that can cause an intestinal infection. The FDA requires the following safe handling statement on egg cartons[28]:

SAFE HANDLING INSTRUCTIONS: To prevent illness from bacteria: keep eggs refrigerated, cook eggs until yolks are firm, and cook foods containing eggs thoroughly.

Food manufacturers may voluntarily place other safe handling instructions on the label, such as those for proper cooking and storage of the item. Consumers should always follow these instructions.

Who Is at Increased Risk for Foodborne Illness?

Although everyone should follow safe food practices, infants and young children, pregnant women, older adults, and those who are immuno-compromised or have certain chronic conditions must be especially careful. In particular, they should not eat or drink raw (unpasteurized) milk or any products made from raw milk. They also should not eat raw or partially cooked eggs or foods containing raw eggs, raw or undercooked meat and poultry, raw or undercooked fish or shellfish, unpasteurized juices, and raw sprouts.

A Final Word on Food Safety

The United States and Canada enjoy a reputation as having food supplies that are among the safest in the world, but a totally risk-free system of food production is an unattainable goal. To keep our food clean, fresh, and uncontaminated with debris, chemicals, or organisms that cause sickness or discomfort, food safety experts are continually trying to ensure that every participant in the food production chain—the farmer, the manufacturer, the retailer, and the consumer—undertakes measures to help reduce and perhaps even eliminate foodborne disease. That's one reason food safety advice today is turning up in so many places—to ensure that everyone gets the word on food safety.

Key Concepts Consumers play a huge role in food safety. They can avoid foodborne illness by following a few simple food-handling and preparation rules: Keep hands and food-preparation areas clean; avoid cross-contamination of foods; cook foods adequately; refrigerate foods promptly. People who have weak or less-developed immune systems are at higher risk for foodborne illnesses.

Food Technology

🍎 **Why Is This Important?** Our food system has changed over time, from one originally centered around a family producing all of the food that they ate, to the modern system of today. Food science and technology are an important component in feeding the world's population.

Technology increasingly impacts the food we eat. Our use of preservatives, other preservation techniques, and genetic engineering has implications for our food supply in the years to come and has triggered debates about the risks and benefits of such practices.

Food Preservation

In our modern society, few people grow their own vegetables, fruits, and grains, or keep livestock as a source of meat and milk. Rather, we shop for our food, typically at a large, full-service supermarket. Because we don't often consume our food at the point of harvest or slaughter, we use food preservation methods to help maintain the quality of the foods we purchase. Among food preservation methods are the addition of chemical preservatives, canning or freezing, **pasteurization**, and irradiation.

Preservatives

Preservatives are added to foods to prevent spoilage and increase shelf life. The most common antimicrobial agents are salt and sugar. Other preservatives, such as potassium sorbate and sodium propionate, extend the shelf life of baked goods and many other products. Antioxidants are a type of preservative that prevents the changes in color and flavor caused by exposure to air. Common antioxidants include vitamin C and vitamin E, sulfites, and BHA and BHT.

Preparation for Preservation

Some preservation techniques, such as salting and fermenting, date to ancient times and are still practiced along with their modern counterparts—freezing, canning, pasteurization, and the like. Salting, drying, or fermenting foods creates an environment in which bacteria cannot multiply and therefore cannot cause food spoilage. Canned foods are heated quickly to a temperature that kills microbes and then are sealed airtight to prevent both contamination and oxidative damage. Freezing temperatures not only keep bacteria from multiplying, but also prevent normal enzymatic changes in food that would cause spoilage. Pasteurization of milk or other beverages uses a very high temperature for a very short time to kill bacteria but minimizes changes that would result from longer heating. The food industry and the North American public readily accept these food preservation methods. One of the most modern preservation techniques—irradiation—also is the most controversial, in part because of our fear of anything that has to do with radiation.

Irradiation

Before it received official approval, food **irradiation** underwent more than 40 years of scientific research and testing—more than any other food technology.[29] During irradiation, foods are exposed to a measured dose of radiation to reduce or eliminate pathogenic bacteria, including *E. coli* O157:H7, *Salmonella*, and *Campylobacter*, the chief causes of foodborne illness today. Irradiation also can destroy insects and parasites, reduce spoilage, and inhibit sprouting and delay ripening of certain fruits and vegetables. Irradiated strawberries, for example, stay unspoiled for up to three weeks versus three to five days for untreated berries. Irradiation also is effective in raw poultry and meat, where it can reduce levels of many pathogens significantly. Although some people fear irradiation will make the food radioactive, the energy used to irradiate foods passes through the food and leaves no residue—in the same way that microwaves pass through food. Despite its benefits, use of irradiation remains rare in North America.

Because food manufacturers fear consumer rejection, they have been reluctant to use irradiation on their products. Some consumers and advocacy groups protest its use because they are concerned that irradiation may compromise a food's nutritional value and change its texture, taste, or appearance. In fact, irradiation may cause less nutritive loss than conventional methods of food preservation.[30] At appropriate doses, irradiation of food does not significantly change its flavor, texture,

▶ **pasteurization** A process for destroying pathogenic bacteria by heating liquid foods to a prescribed temperature for a specified time.

▶ **preservatives** Chemicals or other agents that slow the decomposition of a food.

▶ **irradiation** A food preservation technique in which foods are exposed to measured doses of radiation to reduce or eliminate pathogens and kill insects, reduce spoilage, and, in certain fruits and vegetables, inhibit sprouting and delay ripening.

Quick **Bite**

Where Do *E. coli* Hang Out?
Ground beef is the most common source of *E. coli* bacteria, but *E. coli* also have been found on apples, spinach, and lettuce.

Quick **Bite**

Bacteria at the Supermarket
Bacteria abound on the surface of supermarket meat. A piece of pork, on average, can harbor a few hundred bacteria per cubic centimeter, and a piece of chicken might have 10,000 in the same area (not all of these bacteria are illness-causing). Most people have no response to these bacteria.

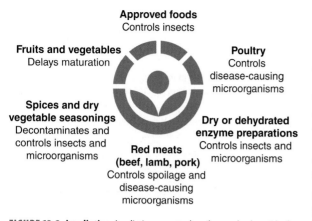

Approved foods
Controls insects

Fruits and vegetables
Delays maturation

Poultry
Controls
disease-causing
microorganisms

**Spices and dry
vegetable seasonings**
Decontaminates and
controls insects and
microorganisms

**Dry or dehydrated
enzyme preparations**
Controls insects and
microorganisms

**Red meats
(beef, lamb, pork)**
Controls spoilage and
disease-causing
microorganisms

FIGURE 13.8 Irradiation. Irradiation can retard spoilage and reduce risk of foodborne illness.

▶ **bacteriophages** Viruses that infect bacteria.

▶ **genetically engineered (GE) foods** Foods produced using plant or animal ingredients that have been modified using gene technology.

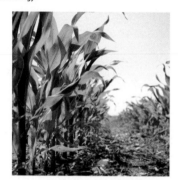

© ryasick photography/Shutterstock, Inc.

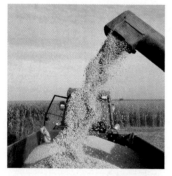

© sima/Shutterstock, Inc.

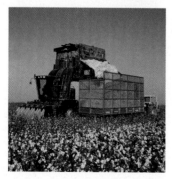

© Alaettin YILDIRIM/Shutterstock, Inc.

or appearance.[31] Many organizations, including the Academy of Nutrition and Dietetics, the American Medical Association, and the World Health Organization, endorse irradiation as a means of providing the public with a safer food supply.

The FDA requires labels of irradiated foods to state that the product was "treated with irradiation" or "treated by irradiation" and display the international symbol for irradiation, the radura. (See **FIGURE 13.8**.)

Bacteriophages

The Food and Drug Administration has approved a mixture of viruses as a food additive to protect people from bacterial infections. The viruses used in the additive are called **bacteriophages** ("bacteria eaters"). A bacteriophage is any virus that infects bacteria.

Bacteriophages are common in soil, water, and our bodies. In the human gut and oral cavity, bacteriophages are normal and beneficial microbial inhabitants. Bacteriophages infect only bacteria and do not bother mammalian or plant cells. The increase in concern regarding antibiotic-resistant and virulent bacteria has renewed scientific interest in bacteriophages for use in clinical and medical settings and commercial food safety.[32,33]

Under the Federal Meat Inspection Act and the Poultry Products Inspection Act, both administered by the USDA, the use of the bacteriophage preparation must be declared on labeling as an ingredient. Consumers will see "bacteriophage preparation" on the label of meat or poultry products that have been treated with the additive.[34]

> **Key Concepts** Various processing methods help protect us from contamination of food by pathogens. Drying, salting, canning, freezing, and pasteurizing are methods that consumers accept. Irradiation is a process in which foods are exposed to a measured dose of radiation to reduce or eliminate pathogenic bacteria. Although government and professional organizations deem irradiation a safe procedure, consumers are still wary. The FDA has also approved spraying ready-to-eat meats and poultry products with bacteriophages, viruses that infect bacteria.

Genetically Engineered Foods

Genetically engineered (GE) foods have arrived, and most of us are already dining on them. When you prepare a dinner of broccoli and tofu, some of the soybeans used to make the tofu probably came from plants genetically engineered to resist herbicide sprays or insect pests or both. And although your broccoli is currently "natural," you can be sure that in a lab somewhere genetically engineered broccoli seeds are sprouting, perhaps with enhanced nutrient or other phytochemical levels. If you are eating tenderloin tonight, the steak probably came from a steer fed on genetically engineered corn that had its DNA altered by the addition of foreign genes to allow the plant to resist insect pests and herbicides.

Should you be indignant that these new foods are showing up on your table without any indication on the label, or should you be grateful that these high-tech methods are keeping crop yields high and food costs low? An informed answer to this question requires some understanding of how genetic engineering works, how new crops and foods are regulated, and how gene modification of crops and animals differs from the classical methods of agricultural breeding that have been practiced for thousands of years.

THINK
About It

4

A Short Course in Plant Genetics

How do GE plants differ from those developed through traditional cross-pollination and hybridization? The answer, surprisingly, is that most crop modifications achieved by DNA manipulation and associated techniques of **biotechnology** also could be achieved with classical techniques, but the time scale and expense are very different. (See **FIGURE 13.9.**)

The classical techniques for breeding a plant with new characteristics have been practiced for hundreds of years. They involve crossing two plants with different characteristics, and then growing the resulting hybrid seeds and looking for plants with the desired combination of characteristics. Hybrid plants get half their genes from one parent and half from the other. Though the hybrid might combine favorable qualities from both parents, a lot of undesirable genetic baggage must be sorted out after formation of such a hybrid. It usually takes dozens of additional crosses, and many years, to separate the desirable genes from the undesirable, and the process has a large element of chance. As a result of human intervention, today virtually every crop plant species differs greatly from its original, wild form.

Genetic engineering, in contrast, allows scientists to transform a plant one gene at a time, using well-established methods for manipulating DNA sequences and integrating them into the plant **genome** (its set of genes). In some cases, a gene can be selected and introduced into plant cells, and new GE seeds can be prepared within a year or two. When we consider that it took centuries of selection and breeding to transform the weedy wild maize plant of pre-Columbian Mexico into our modern varieties of corn, the scale and speed of the gene revolution in agriculture are astounding.

Genetically Engineered Foods: An Unstoppable Experiment?

Concern about antimicrobial resistance in the food industry has been growing in recent years and has contributed to the advancement of genetically engineered crops, designed to be antibiotic resistant and have potentially transferrable antimicrobial genes.[35] In the United States, the number of GE crops has grown rapidly in the past decade. Common GE crops grown by U.S. farmers include corn, cotton, soybeans, canola, squash, and papaya. (See **FIGURE 13.10.**) About 94 percent of the U.S. soybean crop and 93 percent of the cotton crop are genetically modified.[36] Already, an estimated 70 percent of processed foods contain at least one ingredient from a GE plant.[37] Internationally, biotech crops are grown by more than 17 million farmers in 28 countries.[38] The increased yields and lower costs associated with GE crops make them attractive to farmers. There is now strong, perhaps unstoppable, momentum to continue and expand GE crop plantings.

Some farmers are concerned about possible ecological damage from such crops and fear potential unintended consequences of genetic "tampering" with the food supply. Although some U.S. consumer groups voice similar concerns, agribusiness, the Academy of Nutrition and Dietetics, the American Medical Association, the National Academy of Sciences, and the Food and Agriculture Organization of the United Nations have been supportive of the trend toward GE foods.[39]

The GE crops mentioned earlier are just the tip of the genetic-modification iceberg; hundreds more are under development in university laboratories and in the labs of giant agribusinesses. Research in plant biotechnology has focused primarily on characteristics that

▶ **biotechnology** The set of laboratory techniques and processes used to modify the genome of plants or animals and thus create desirable new characteristics. The means used to genetically engineer cells.

▶ **genetic engineering** Manipulation of the genome of an organism by artificial means for the purpose of modifying existing traits or adding new genetic traits.

▶ **genome** The total genetic information of an organism, stored in the DNA of its chromosomes.

Quick **Bite**

Biotechnology in the 1930s
One of the first examples of genetic theory successfully applied to food production was hybrid corn. When first introduced, it seemed miraculous and convinced skeptical farmers of the potential benefits of this emerging agricultural science. To this day, tougher and healthier new hybrids continue to exceed the yield of their predecessors.

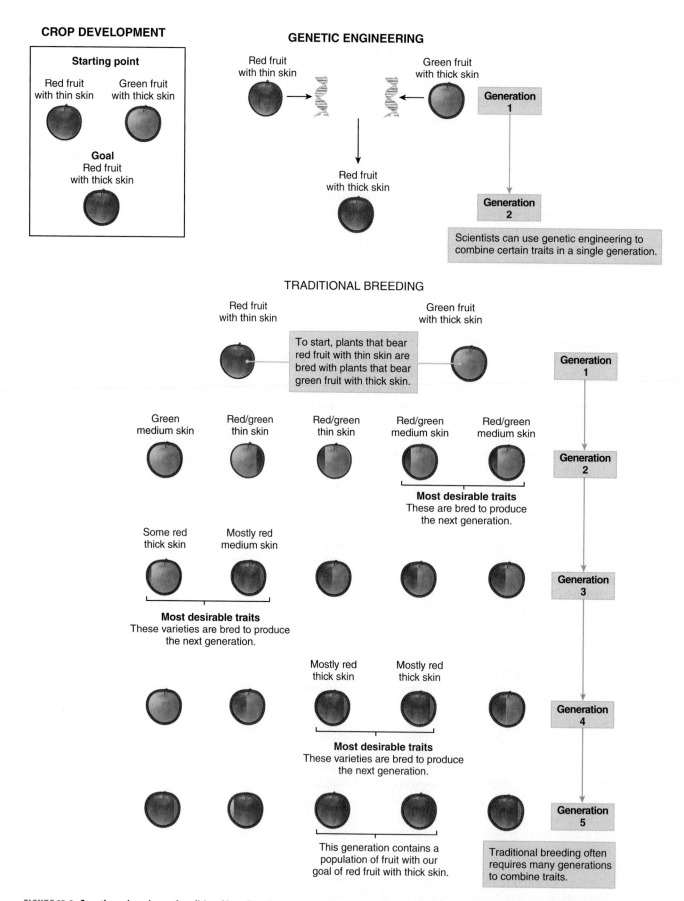

FIGURE 13.9 Genetic engineering and traditional breeding. Genetic engineering can fast-track crop development that can take years with traditional breeding practices.

improve resistance to pests, reduce the need for pesticides, and increase the ability of the plant to survive adverse growing conditions such as drought, soil salinity, and cold. Many of these goals would be achievable with classical selection techniques, but with genetic engineering, they move from laboratory to table in decades rather than centuries.

If only plant genes were involved in GE food production, there would be much less controversy. However, *any* gene, including genes from bacteria and animals, can be introduced into a plant genome. Some people find this frightening, and an imaginative term, *Frankenfoods*, has been coined to express the "unnatural" nature of some GE products. But how unnatural is the exchange of DNA between species? It may be reassuring to realize that organisms have been swapping DNA for eons, with no help from humans. Foreign DNA can be carried from one species to another by a variety of viruses, for example. Nature has already performed millions of "gene modifications" on its own, and exchange of DNA is an established part of the evolutionary process. Now that we can do our own experiments with DNA manipulation, we hope the benefits will be increased.

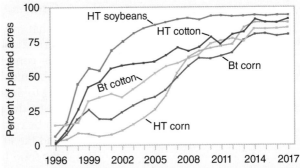

FIGURE 13.10 Adoption of genetically engineered crops in the United States, 2017.

USDA, Economic Research Service using data from Fernandez-Cornejo and McBride (2002) for the years 1996-99 and USDA, National Agricultural Statistics Service, June Agricultural Survey for the years 2000-17.

Benefits of Genetic Engineering

Whatever the risks, no one can argue with the success of these GE techniques. For instance, a bacterial gene was used to create insect-resistant varieties of corn, potatoes, and soybeans. This gene, the **Bt gene**, was taken from the soil bacterium *Bacillus thuringiensis*. When inserted into a plant genome, the *Bt* gene directs the plant to produce a protein that makes the plant toxic to insects. Such crops have been extremely successful and produce high yields without use of insecticides.

Bt-modified crops, which are now grown in the United States over an area larger than Rhode Island, are a boon to both the economy and the environment. Because chemical insecticides are not necessary, many benign insects are spared, and insect **biodiversity** is preserved. Similarly, other plants can be genetically engineered to resist the effects of common herbicides. Chemical sprays that are lethal to most plant life have no effect on these GE plants. The crop plant grows larger in the absence of weeds, and the farmer gets a better yield with less effort and expense.

The economic benefits of GE foods are clearly substantial. Increased yields of important food plants can help feed increasing populations without the need for putting more land under the plow or increasing the use of toxic insecticides. This might be the difference between starvation and adequate nutrition in many developing countries.

It is easy to imagine how manipulating plant amino acids and plant oils could yield superior foods, which not only would be able to satisfy calorie requirements, but also would address protein and vitamin needs. A strain of rice genetically engineered to be rich in beta-carotene, known as Golden Rice, could benefit the more than 1 million children in developing countries who die or are weakened by vitamin A deficiency.[40] In developed countries, where heart disease and cancer loom as greater risks than malnutrition, the ability to adjust the saturation level of plant lipids or to boost beneficial phytochemicals would be of great value to public health. But do these undoubted benefits outweigh the risks?

▶ **Bt gene** *Bacillus thuringiensis (Bt)* is a bacterium that produces a protein called the *Bt* toxin. One of the bacterium's genes, the *Bt* gene, carries the information for the *Bt* toxin. Inserting a copy of the *Bt* gene into plants enables them to produce *Bt* toxin protein and resist some insect pests. The *Bt* protein is not toxic to humans.

▶ **biodiversity** The countless species of plants, animals, and insects that exist on the earth. An undisturbed tropical forest is an example of the biodiversity of a healthy ecosystem.

© Anderl/Shutterstock, Inc.

Position Statement: Academy of Nutrition and Dietetics

Agricultural and Food Biotechnology

It is the position of the Academy of Nutrition and Dietetics that agricultural and food biotechnology techniques can enhance the quality, safety, nutritional value, and variety of food available for human consumption and increase the efficiency of food production, food processing, food distribution, and environmental and waste management. The ADA (for American Dietetic Assoc) encourages the government, food manufacturers, food commodity groups, and qualified food and nutrition professionals to work together to inform consumers about this new technology and encourage availability of these products in the marketplace.

Reprinted from *Journal of the American Dietetic Association*, 106(2), Position of the American Dietetic Association: Agricultural and Food Biotechnology, Page no. 285-293, 2006, with permission from Elsevier.

Risks

What are the specific risks of GE foods? Many consumers are concerned about whether these new foods are safe to eat. The answer to this concern is a fairly unequivocal "yes." When a new protein or other substance is introduced into a food, the FDA requires substantial testing to demonstrate its safety. With GE foods, the potential risk appears to be the possibility of introducing a new allergen into a GE food.[41] To be cautious, the FDA has focused on allergy issues. Under the law and the FDA's biotech food policy, companies must tell consumers on the food label when a product includes a gene from a food that commonly causes an allergic reaction.

Of greater concern, and more difficult to predict, are environmental effects, although no ecological disasters have occurred thus far. For example, what if the *Bt*-containing plants lead to the development of insects resistant to *Bt*-modified plants and to other insecticides? Another concern is the development of herbicide-resistant weeds, or "superweeds." When herbicide-resistant crops are planted in proximity to related wild plants, pollen can drift from food plant to weed, and the resistant genes might be passed to the weedy cousins of the GE plants. In the presence of herbicide, this might lead to the rapid selection of herbicide-resistant weeds.

A final concern is that the herbicide-resistant food plants might become so successful that they are planted over a vast acreage. In the worst-case scenario, this could lead to a loss of many species of unmodified plants as well as the insect and animal communities that depend on them. Many scientists feel that the loss of biodiversity is one of the greatest threats to the planet today. Because of the complexity and interdependence of the biosphere, this is perhaps the greatest unknown and the greatest danger of unmonitored use of GE crops. **TABLE 13.4** summarizes benefits and current controversies.

Regulation

The FDA regulates foods and food safety, and it oversees genetically engineered foods and animals as well as conventional foods. For foods derived from new varieties of plants, the FDA takes the position that whether modified by traditional breeding or genetic engineering, testing for safe human consumption is the legal responsibility of the producer or manufacturer of the foods.

Some consumer groups are pushing for mandatory labeling of GE foods. They believe consumers have the right to know whether a food is bioengineered. Other groups desire labeling so they can adhere to cultural or religious beliefs that might ban certain animal foods.

The FDA supports the voluntary labeling of products that contain genetically engineered ingredients and requires that food labels disclose any significant difference between the bioengineered food and its conventional counterpart.[42] Such differences would include changes in nutritional properties, the presence of an allergen that consumers would not expect in the food, or any property that would require special handling, storage, cooking, or preservation.

Similar to U.S. regulations, Health Canada requires special labeling for genetically engineered foods when there is a potential for allergic reactions or a difference in composition or nutritional value. Voluntary positive ("does contain") and voluntary negative ("does not contain") labeling is permitted, provided the statements are factual and not misleading or deceptive.[43]

TABLE 13.4
GE Products: Benefits and Controversies

Benefits

Crops
- Enhanced taste and quality
- Reduced maturation time
- Increased nutrients, yields, and stress tolerance
- Improved resistance to diseases, pests, and herbicides
- New products and growing techniques

Animals
- Increased resistance, productivity, hardiness, and feed efficiency
- Better yields of meat, eggs, and milk
- Improved animal health and diagnostic methods

Environment
- "Friendly" bioherbicides and bioinsecticides
- Conservation of soil, water, and energy
- Bioprocessing for forestry products
- Better natural waste management
- More efficient processing

Society
- Increased food security for growing populations

Controversies

Safety
- Potential human health impacts, including allergens, transfer of antibiotic resistance markers, and unknown effects
- Potential environmental impacts, including unintended transfer of transgenes through cross-pollination, unknown effects on other organisms (e.g., soil microbes), and loss of flora and fauna biodiversity

Access and Intellectual Property
- Domination of world food production by a few companies
- Increasing dependence on industrialized nations by developing countries
- Biopiracy, or foreign exploitation of natural resources

Ethics
- Violation of natural organisms' intrinsic values
- Tampering with nature by mixing genes among species
- Objections to consuming animal genes in plants and vice versa
- Stress for animals

Labeling
- Not mandatory in some countries (e.g., United States)
- Mixing GE crops with non-GE products confounds labeling attempts

Society
- New advances might be skewed to interests of rich countries

Reproduced from U.S. Department of Energy, Human Genome Project. Genetically modified foods and organisms. November 2008. fog.ccsf.edu/~cpogge/Bio41L/GMfoods.pdf. Accessed June 2, 2017.

Many groups (government agencies, such as the FDA; professional organizations, such as the ADA; and consumer advocacy groups) are monitoring developments in biotechnology. Websites for these organizations can be a source of policy statements and breaking news in this area. Regardless of our views on genetic manipulation of food plants, research and development will continue.

Key Concepts Genetic engineering allows scientists to transform a plant one gene at a time, using well-established methods for manipulating DNA sequences. The goals of genetic modification of foods are higher yields, lower costs, increased amounts of critical nutrients, and a healthier mix of plant oils. Because of the complexity and interdependence of the biosphere, loss of genetic biodiversity is perhaps the greatest unknown and the greatest danger of unmonitored GE crops.

Learning Portfolio

Key Terms

	page
aflatoxins	705
bacteriophages	716
biodiversity	719
biotechnology	717
botulism	698
bovine spongiform encephalopathy (BSE)	700
Bt gene	719
ciguatera	705
color additive	707
critical control points (CCPs)	710
Delaney Clause	708
dioxins	703
direct additives	706
Escherichia coli (E. coli)	698
Food Code	712
foodborne illness	694
Generally Recognized as Safe	707
genetic engineering	717
genetically engineered (GE) foods	716
genome	717
indirect additives	706
integrated pest management (IPM)	701
irradiation	715
mad cow disease	700
methylmercury	703
natural toxins	704
organic foods	700
pasteurization	715
pesticides	700
poisonous mushrooms	705
pollutants	703
preservatives	715
prior-sanctioned substance	708
prions	700
Salmonella	698
solanine	705

Study Points

- Foodborne illness is extremely common; it affects millions of Americans each year. Estimates of the frequency of foodborne illness are difficult because the vast majority of foodborne illnesses go unreported.

- The incidence of foodborne illness may be on the rise in the United States and Canada. Many factors are responsible, including the increased centralization of food preparation, food imports, an increasing population of especially susceptible individuals (such as older adults and those with weakened immune systems), and failure of consumers and retail establishments to follow appropriate food safety measures.

- Microorganisms cause most foodborne diseases in the United States and Canada. Most of these illnesses are preventable.

- *Staphylococcus aureus* is one of the most common causes of foodborne illness. Onset of illness is rapid, typically occurring between 30 minutes and a few hours after consuming the contaminated food.

- Common symptoms of foodborne illness are diarrhea, nausea, abdominal cramps, and sometimes fever. The severity of the illness depends on the type of organism and the amount of contaminant eaten.

- Ensuring a safe food supply is a farm-to-table continuum involving producers, manufacturers, retailers, and consumers.

- Pesticides, animal drugs, natural toxins, and pollutants are the major forms of chemical food contamination.

- The government monitors imported and domestic foods for pesticide residues by testing food samples for both amounts and types of pesticides. Efforts are under way to reduce the allowable amounts of certain pesticides to avoid harm to infants and children.

- The FDA evaluates drugs used in food-producing animals for safety in both animals and humans. Overuse of animal antibiotics could contribute to the emergence of antibiotic-resistant microorganisms that could threaten human health.

- The government and the food industry use the Hazard Analysis Critical Control Point system to prevent food contamination.

- Consumers must take responsibility for food safety in their homes. Cleaning hands and surfaces, avoiding cross-contamination, cooking adequately, and refrigerating foods promptly are important steps that prevent foodborne illness.

- Food preservation techniques inhibit growth of microorganisms. Canning, drying, freezing, fermentation, and pasteurization are common methods.

- Although the FDA has approved food irradiation for numerous uses, it is rarely used, mostly because of consumer fears. Food irradiation does not make foods radioactive. It can kill insects and most microorganisms. Appropriate doses of radiation extend the shelf life of many foods.

■ Genetically engineered (GE) foods are most likely already on your table. Soybeans, corn, and potatoes are some of the GE foods being commercially produced. Concerns about GE foods include worries about decreasing biodiversity and the development of herbicide-resistant weeds.

Study Questions

1. What are the two main ways that pathogenic bacteria can cause foodborne illness?

2. Why shouldn't your 97-year-old great-grandmother drink homemade eggnog made from raw eggs?

3. List four naturally occurring toxins.

4. What does HACCP stand for, and what is its purpose?

5. What are some ways to keep food safe at home?

6. List the most common food preservation techniques.

7. What are scientists' two major concerns about genetically engineered crops?

Try This

Bacterial Detective

What sources of bacteria do you encounter in your everyday activities? Here's an experiment to find out. First, you'll need the following:
■ Cotton swabs
■ Six or more Petri dishes with agar

If you are unable to obtain a set of agar-filled Petri dishes from your school or local health department, you can make your own culture medium. Here's how:

1. Add 2 teaspoons of unflavored gelatin (1 packet) and 2 teaspoons of sugar to one cup of water.

2. Bring the solution to a boil and stir for 1 minute until everything is dissolved. Pour ¼ inch of the solution into each Petri dish or other suitable container.

Then, using separate Petri dishes,

1. Pluck a hair and lay it in one Petri dish, labeled "Hair."

2. Sneeze or cough into another Petri dish, labeled "Cough."

3. Run a cotton swab around a nostril and carefully zigzag it across the agar in another Petri dish, labeled "Nose."

4. Run a cotton swab across a dampened kitchen sink sponge and carefully zigzag it across the agar in another Petri dish, labeled "Sponge."

5. Run a cotton swab around a clean kitchen countertop and carefully zigzag it across the agar in another Petri dish, labeled "Countertop."

6. Use the same procedure to collect additional samples from any other area in which bacteria might be present.

7. Store the Petri dishes in a warm environment, at a constant temperature around 80°F.

Check your specimens periodically. Within a week, you should see something growing! What do you observe? Which Petri dishes show the most growth? Which show the least? Does this change your ideas about cleaning habits?

Organic Foods

Organic foods are increasing in popularity. Are organic foods widely available in your neighborhood? What types of organic produce can you find? Go to either a natural food store or the local grocery store and look at the array of organic produce. Compare the prices of organic produce and nonorganic produce. Do you think the cost differences outweigh possible benefits? Compare the look of the organic and nonorganic produce. Do you see any differences? What other organic products can you find?

Getting Personal

Using the numbers shown, please indicate how often you engage in the following food safety practices:

1. Rarely or never
2. Sometimes
3. Frequently
4. Always

___ Wash hands before handling food and after touching raw meat.

___ Reheat leftovers to 165°F.

___ Refrigerate leftovers within two hours of preparation.

___ Avoid using food products whose use-by date has expired.

Learning Portfolio (continued)

___ Do not eat foods containing uncooked eggs.

___ Wash fresh produce including prepackaged greens.

___ Avoid eating fish high in mercury levels.

___ Defrost food in the refrigerator, the microwave, or cold water, not on the counter.

___ Use separate cutting boards for raw meat, poultry, and fish.

___ Wash cutting boards after use before putting them away.

Total the numbers you have selected. If your score is less than 20, you should revisit the items to which you assigned a number less than 2 and consider a plan to incorporate a food safety practice that will raise your total score.

References

1. Centers for Disease Control and Prevention. Foodborne germs and illnesses. https://www.cdc.gov/foodsafety/foodborne-germs.html. Accessed September 19, 2017.

2. U.S. Department of Agriculture. Cost estimates of foodborne illnesses. https://www.ers.usda.gov/data-products/cost-estimates-of-foodborne-illnesses.aspx#48446. Accessed September 19, 2017.

3. Institute of Food Technologists. IFT expert report on emerging microbiological food safety issues: implications for control in the 21st century. April 2010. http://www.ift.org/knowledge-center/read-ift-publications/science-reports/expert-reports/~/media/Knowledge%20Center/Science%20Reports/Expert%20Reports/Emerging%20Microbiological/Emerging%20Micro.pdf. Accessed September 19, 2017.

4. Centers for Disease Control and Prevention. Burden of foodborne illness: findings. https://www.cdc.gov/foodborneburden/2011-foodborne-estimates.html. Accessed September 19, 2017.

5. Ibid.

6. U.S. Food and Drug Administration. Pesticide residue monitoring program. https://www.fda.gov/Food/FoodborneIllnessContaminants/Pesticides/ucm2006797.htm. Accessed September 19, 2017.

7. Ibid.

8. Zuraw L. *Consumer Reports* guides shoppers through produce pesticide residues. *Food Safety News.* March 19, 2015. http://www.foodsafetynews.com/2015/03/consumer-reports-guides-shoppers-through-produce-pesticide-residues/#.VnCUn79URMc. Accessed September 19, 2017.

9. U.S. Environmental Protection Agency. Overview of risk assessment in the pesticide program. http://www.epa.gov/pesticide-science-and-assessing-pesticide-risks/overview-risk-assessment-pesticide-program. Accessed September 19, 2017.

10. Dimitri C, Oberholtzer L. Marketing U.S. organic foods: recent trends from farms to consumers. September 2009. *Economic Information Bulletin* No. 58. https://www.ers.usda.gov/webdocs/publications/44430/11009_eib58_1_.pdf?v=41055. Accessed September 19, 2017.

11. Organic Trade Association. U.S. organic sales post new record of $43.3 billion in 2015. May 19, 2016. https://www.ota.com/news/press-releases/19031. Accessed September 19, 2017.

12. U.S. Department of Agriculture, Agricultural Marketing Service. National organic program. https://www.ams.usda.gov/about-ams/programs-offices/national-organic-program. Accessed September 19, 2017.

13. Ibid.

14. Ibid.

15. U.S. Department of Agriculture, Agricultural Marketing Service. NOSB meetings. http://www.ams.usda.gov/AMSv1.0/nosbmeetings. Accessed September 19, 2017.

16. Porterfield A. Fraud or drift? USDA finds 43 percent of organic foods contain 'prohibited' substances. Genetic Literacy Project. July 2015. http://www.geneticliteracyproject.org/2015/07/22/fraud-or-drift-usda-finds-43-percent-of-organic-foods-contain-prohibited-substances/. Accessed September 19, 2017.

17. National Research Council, Committee on Drug Use in Food Animals, Panel on Animal Health, Food Safety, and Public Health. *The Use of Drugs in Food Animals.* Washington, DC: National Academies Press; 1999.

18. U.S. Food and Drug Administration. Phasing out certain antibiotic use in farm animals. http://www.fda.gov/forconsumers/consumerupdates/ucm378100.htm. Accessed September 19, 2017.

19. Food and Agriculture Organization of the United Nations. Fact sheet: dioxins in the food chain: prevention and control of contamination. April 2008. http://www.fao.org/AG/AGAINFO/PROGRAMMES/documents/VPH_factsheets/FAO_Fact_Sheet_020408.pdf. Accessed September 19, 2017.

20. Food and Agriculture Organization of the United Nations. Dioxins: food safety—needs a solid food chain approach. http://www.fao.org/food/food-safety-quality/a-z-index/dioxins/en/. Accessed September 19, 2017.

21. U.S. Food and Drug Administration, Environmental Protection Agency. Eating fish: what pregnant women and parents should know. https://www.fda.gov/Food/FoodborneIllnessContaminants/Metals/ucm393070.htm. Accessed September 19, 2017.

22. Food Allergy Research & Education. Food allergy facts and statistics for the U.S. https://www.foodallergy.org/file/facts-stats.pdf. Accessed September 19, 2017.

23. U.S. Food and Drug Administration. Food allergies: what you need to know. http://www.fda.gov/Food/ResourcesForYou/Consumers/ucm079311.htm. Accessed September 19, 2017.

24. U.S. Department of Health and Human Services. FDA Food Safety Modernization Act (FSMA). http://www.fda.gov/Food/FoodSafety/FSMA/default.htm. Accessed September 19, 2017.

25. U.S. Food and Drug Administration. HACCP principles and application guidelines. http://www.fda.gov/Food/GuidanceRegulation/HACCP/ucm2006801.htm. Accessed September 19, 2017.

26. U.S. Food and Drug Administration. Hazard Analysis Critical Control Point (HACCP). http://www.fda.gov/Food/GuidanceRegulation/HACCP/. Accessed September 19, 2017.

27. U.S. Food and Drug Administration. FDA food code. https://www.fda.gov/Food/GuidanceRegulation/RetailFoodProtection/FoodCode/default.htm. Accessed September 19, 2017.

28. Food labeling, safe handling statements, labeling of shell eggs; refrigeration of shell eggs held for retail distribution, final rule. *Federal Register.* 2000;65:76091-76114.

29. U.S. Food and Drug Administration. Food irradiation: what you need to know. http://www.fda.gov/Food/ResourcesForYou/Consumers/ucm261680.htm. Accessed September 19, 2017.

30. Iowa State University. Consumer questions about food irradiation. June 2010. www.sciencedirect.com/science/article/pii/B9781845695514500198

31. U.S. Food and Drug Administration. Food irradiation: what you need to know. Op. cit.

32. Maura D, Debarbieux L. Bacteriophages as twenty-first century antibacterial tools for food and medicine. *Appl Microbiol Biotechnol.* 2011;90(3):851-859. doi: 10.1007/s00253-011-3227-1. Epub March 29, 2011.

33. Lu TK, Koeris MS. The next generation of bacteriophage therapy. *Curr Opin Microbiol.* 2011;14(5):524-531. doi: 10.1016/j.mib.2011.07.028. Epub August 23, 2011.

34. Bren L. Bacteria-eating virus approved as food additive. *FDA Consumer.* January–February 2007.

35. Capita R, Alonso-Calleja C. Antibiotic-resistant bacteria: a challenge for the food industry. *Crit Rev Food Sci Nutr*. 2013;53(1):11-48. doi: 10.1080/10408398.2010.519837.

36. U.S. Department of Agriculture, Economic Research Service. Adoption of genetically engineered crops in the U.S. https://www.ers.usda.gov /data-products/adoption-of-genetically-engineered-crops-in-the-us.aspx. Accessed September 19, 2017.

37. U.S. Department of Agriculture. Biotechnology frequently asked questions (FAQs). https://www.usda.gov/topics/biotechnology/biotechnology -frequently-asked-questions-faqs. Accessed September 19, 2017.

38. U.S. Department of Agriculture. Biotechnology frequently asked questions (FAQs). Op. cit.

39. Position of the American Dietetic Association: agricultural and food biotechnology. *J Am Diet Assoc*. 2006;106(2):285-293.

40. Tang G, Qin J, Dolnikowski GG, et al. Golden rice is an effective source of vitamin A. *Am J Clin Nutr*. 2009;89(6):1776-1783.

41. Selgrade MK, Bowman CC, Ladics GS, et al. Safety assessment of biotechnology products for potential risk of food allergy: implications of new research. *Toxicol Sci*. 2009;110(1):31-39.

42. U.S. Food and Drug Administration. FDA's role in regulating safety of GE foods. https://njfb.org/wp-content/uploads/2013/07/FDA-GE-Answers .pdf. Accessed September 19, 2017.

43. Health Canada. The regulation of genetically modified food. http://www .hc-sc.gc.ca/sr-sr/pubs/biotech/reg_gen_mod-eng.php. Accessed September 19, 2017.

Appendix A   Dietary Reference Intakes

The Food and Nutrition Board of the National Academy of Sciences determines recommended nutrient intakes that apply to healthy individuals. Beginning in 1997, the Food and Nutrition Board (with the involvement of Health Canada) began releasing updated recommendations under a new framework called the Dietary Reference Intakes (DRIs). In these revisions, target intake levels for healthy individuals in the U.S. and Canada are listed as either Adequate Intake (AI) levels or Recommended Dietary Allowances (RDAs). Also, the DRI values include a set of Tolerable Upper Intake Levels (ULs), which are levels of nutrient intake that should not be exceeded due to the potential for adverse effects from excessive consumption.

Dietary Reference Intakes (DRIs)

Life stage group	Vitamin A (µg/d)[1]	Vitamin D (IU/d)[2]	Vitamin E (mg/d)[3]	Vitamin K (µg/d)	Thiamin (mg/d)	Riboflavin (mg/d)	Niacin (mg/d)[4]	Pantothenic Acid (mg/d)	Biotin (µg/d)	Vitamin B6 (mg/d)	Folate (µg/d)[5]	Vitamin B12 (µg/d)	Vitamin C (mg/d)	Choline (mg/d)	Sodium (g/d)
Infants															
0-6 mo	400*	400*	4*	2.0*	0.2*	0.3*	2*	1.7*	5*	0.1*	65*	0.4*	40*	125*	0.12*
6-12 mo	500*	400*	5*	2.5*	0.3*	0.4*	4*	1.8*	6*	0.3*	80*	0.5*	50*	150*	0.37*
Children															
1-3 y	300	600	6	30*	0.5	0.5	6	2*	8*	0.5	150	0.9	15	200*	1.0*
4-8 y	400	600	7	55*	0.6	0.6	8	3*	12*	0.6	200	1.2	25	250*	1.2*
Males															
9-13 y	600	600	11	60*	0.9	0.9	12	4*	20*	1.0	300	1.8	45	375*	1.5*
14-18 y	900	600	15	75*	1.2	1.3	16	5*	25*	1.3	400	2.4	75	550*	1.5*
19-30 y	900	600	15	120*	1.2	1.3	16	5*	30*	1.3	400	2.4	90	550*	1.5*
31-50 y	900	600	15	120*	1.2	1.3	16	5*	30*	1.3	400	2.4	90	550*	1.5*
51-70 y	900	600	15	120*	1.2	1.3	16	5*	30*	1.7	400	2.4[7]	90	550*	1.3*
>70 y	900	800	15	120*	1.2	1.3	16	5*	30*	1.7	400	2.4[7]	90	550*	1.2*
Females															
9-13 y	600	600	11	60*	0.9	0.9	12	4*	20*	1.0	300	1.8	45	375*	1.5*
14-18 y	700	600	15	75*	1.0	1.0	14	5*	25*	1.2	400[6]	2.4	65	400*	1.5*
19-30 y	700	600	15	90*	1.1	1.1	14	5*	30*	1.3	400[6]	2.4	75	425*	1.5*
31-50 y	700	600	15	90*	1.1	1.1	14	5*	30*	1.3	400[6]	2.4	75	425*	1.5*
51-70 y	700	600	15	90*	1.1	1.1	14	5*	30*	1.5	400	2.4[7]	75	425*	1.3*
>70 y	700	800	15	90*	1.1	1.1	14	5*	30*	1.5	400	2.4[7]	75	425*	1.2*
Pregnancy															
≤18 y	750	600	15	75*	1.4	1.4	18	6*	30*	1.9	600	2.6	80	450*	1.5*
19-30 y	770	600	15	90*	1.4	1.4	18	6*	30*	1.9	600	2.6	85	450*	1.5*
31-50 y	770	600	15	90*	1.4	1.4	18	6*	30*	1.9	600	2.6	85	450*	1.5*
Lactation															
≤18 y	1,200	600	19	75*	1.4	1.6	17	7*	35*	2.0	500	2.8	115	550*	1.5*
19-30 y	1,300	600	19	90*	1.4	1.6	17	7*	35*	2.0	500	2.8	120	550*	1.5*
31-50 y	1,300	600	19	90*	1.4	1.6	17	7*	35*	2.0	500	2.8	120	550*	1.5*

This table presents Recommended Dietary Allowances (RDAs) and Adequate Intakes (AIs). An asterisk (*) indicates AI. RDAs and AIs may both be used as goals for individual intake.

[1] As retinol activity equivalents (RAE).

[2] As cholecalciferol.

[3] As α-tocopherol.

[4] As niacin equivalents (NE).

[5] As dietary folate equivalents (DFE).

[6] In view of evidence linking folate intake with neural-tube defects in the fetus, it is recommended that all women capable of becoming pregnant consume 400 µg of folic acid from supplements or fortified foods in addition to intake of food folate from a varied diet.

[7] Because 10 to 30% of older people may malabsorb food-bound vitamin B12, it is advisable for those older than 50 years to meet their RDA mainly by consuming foods fortified with vitamin B12 or a supplement containing vitamin B12.

[8] The AI for water represents total water from drinking water, beverages, and moisture from food.

Life stage group	Potassium (g/d)	Chloride (g/d)	Calcium (mg/d)	Phosphorus (mg/d)	Magnesium (mg/d)	Iron (mg/d)	Zinc (mg/d)	Selenium (µg/d)	Iodine (µg/d)	Copper (µg/d)	Manganese (mg/d)	Fluoride (mg/d)	Chromium (µg/d)	Molybdenum (µg/d)	Water (L/d)[8]
Infants															
0-6 mo	0.4*	0.18*	200*	100*	30*	0.27*	2*	15*	110*	200*	0.003*	0.01*	0.2*	2*	0.7*
6-12 mo	0.7*	0.57*	260*	275*	75*	11	3*	20*	130*	220*	0.6*	0.5*	5.5*	3*	0.8*
Children															
1-3 y	3.0*	1.5*	700	460	80	7	3	20	90	340	1.2*	0.7*	11*	17	1.3*
4-8 y	3.8*	1.9*	1,000	500	130	10	5	30	90	440	1.5*	1*	15*	22	1.7*
Males															
9-13 y	4.5*	2.3*	1,300	1,250	240	8	8	40	120	700	1.9*	2*	25*	34	2.4*
14-18 y	4.7*	2.3*	1,300	1,250	410	11	11	55	150	890	2.2*	3*	35*	43	3.3*
19-30 y	4.7*	2.3*	1,000	700	400	8	11	55	150	900	2.3*	4*	35*	45	3.7*
31-50 y	4.7*	2.3*	1,000	700	420	8	11	55	150	900	2.3*	4*	35*	45	3.7*
51-70 y	4.7*	2.0*	1,000	700	420	8	11	55	150	900	2.3*	4*	30*	45	3.7*
>70 y	4.7*	1.8*	1,200	700	420	8	11	55	150	900	2.3*	4*	30*	45	3.7*
Females															
9-13 y	4.5*	2.3*	1,300	1,250	240	8	8	40	120	700	1.6*	2*	21*	34	2.1*
14-18 y	4.7*	2.3*	1,300	1,250	360	15	9	55	150	890	1.6*	3*	24*	43	2.3*
19-30 y	4.7*	2.3*	1,000	700	310	18	8	55	150	900	1.8*	3*	25*	45	2.7*
31-50 y	4.7*	2.3*	1,000	700	320	18	8	55	150	900	1.8*	3*	25*	45	2.7*
51-70 y	4.7*	2.0*	1,200	700	320	8	8	55	150	900	1.8*	3*	20*	45	2.7*
>70 y	4.7*	1.8*	1,200	700	320	8	8	55	150	900	1.8*	3*	20*	45	2.7*
Pregnancy															
≤18 y	4.7*	2.3*	1,300	1,250	400	27	12	60	220	1,000	2.0*	3*	29*	50	3.0*
19-30 y	4.7*	2.3*	1,000	700	350	27	11	60	220	1,000	2.0*	3*	30*	50	3.0*
31-50 y	4.7*	2.3*	1,000	700	360	27	11	60	220	1,000	2.0*	3*	30*	50	3.0*
Lactation															
≤18 y	5.1*	2.3	1,300	1,250	360	10	13	70	290	1,300	2.6*	3*	44*	50	3.8*
19-30 y	5.1*	2.3	1,000	700	310	9	12	70	290	1,300	2.6*	3*	45*	50	3.8*
31-50 y	5.1*	2.3	1,000	700	320	9	12	70	290	1,300	2.6*	3*	45*	50	3.8*

Data compiled from *Dietary Reference Intakes for Calcium, Phosphorus, Magnesium, Vitamin D, and Fluoride*. Washington, DC: National Academies Press; 1997. *Dietary Reference Intakes for Thiamin, Riboflavin, Niacin, Vitamin B₆, Folate, Vitamin B₁₂, Pantothenic Acid, Biotin, and Choline*. Washington, DC: National Academies Press; 1998. *Dietary Reference Intakes for Vitamin C, Vitamin E, Selenium, and Carotenoids*. Washington, DC: National Academies Press; 2000. *Dietary Reference Intakes for Vitamin A, Vitamin K, Arsenic, Boron, Chromium, Copper, Iron, Manganese, Molybdenum, Nickel, Silicon, Vanadium, and Zinc*. Washington, DC: National Academies Press; 2000. *Dietary Reference Intakes for Water, Potassium, Sodium, Chloride, and Sulfate*. Food and Nutrition Board. Washington, DC: National Academies Press; 2005. *Dietary Reference Intakes for Calcium and Vitamin D*. Washington, DC: National Academies Press; 2011. These reports may be accessed via http://nap.edu.

Tolerable Upper Intake Levels (ULs[1])

Life stage group	Vitamin A[2] (µg/d)	Vitamin D (µg/d)	Vitamin E[3,4] (mg/d)	Niacin[4] (mg/d)	Vitamin B_6 (mg/d)	Folate[4] (µg/d)	Vitamin C (mg/d)	Choline (g/d)	Calcium (g/d)	Phosphorus (g/d)	Magnesium[5] (mg/d)	Sodium (g/d)
Infants												
0-6 mo	600	25	ND[7]	ND	ND	ND	ND	ND	ND	ND	ND	ND
7-12 mo	600	25	ND	ND	ND	ND	ND	ND	ND	ND	ND	ND
Children												
1-3 y	600	50	200	10	30	300	400	1.0	2.5	3	65	1.5
4-8 y	900	50	300	15	40	400	650	1.0	2.5	3	110	1.9
Males, females												
9-13 y	1,700	50	600	20	60	600	1,200	2.0	2.5	4	350	2.2
14-18 y	2,800	50	800	30	80	800	1,800	3.0	2.5	4	350	2.3
19-70 y	3,000	50	1,000	35	100	1,000	2,000	3.5	2.5	4	350	2.3
>70 y	3,000	50	1,000	35	100	1,000	2,000	3.5	2.5	3	350	2.3
Pregnancy												
≤18 y	2,800	50	800	30	80	800	1,800	3.0	2.5	3.5	350	2.3
19-50 y	3,000	50	1,000	35	100	1,000	2,000	3.5	2.5	3.5	350	2.3
Lactation												
≤18 y	2,800	50	800	30	80	800	1,800	3.0	2.5	4	350	2.3
19-50 y	3,000	50	1,000	35	100	1,000	2,000	3.5	2.5	4	350	2.3

Life stage group	Iron (mg/d)	Zinc (mg/d)	Selenium (µg/d)	Iodine (µg/d)	Copper (µg/d)	Manganese (mg/d)	Fluoride (mg/d)	Molybdenum (µg/d)	Boron (mg/d)	Nickel (mg/d)	Vanadium[6] (mg/d)	Chloride (g/d)
Infants												
0-6 mo	40	4	45	ND	ND	ND	0.7	ND	ND	ND	ND	ND
7-12 mo	40	5	60	ND	ND	ND	0.9	ND	ND	ND	ND	ND
Children												
1-3 y	40	7	90	200	1,000	2	1.3	300	3	0.2	ND	2.3
4-8 y	40	12	150	300	3,000	3	2.2	600	6	0.3	ND	2.9
Males, females												
9-13 y	40	23	280	600	5,000	6	10	1,100	11	0.6	ND	3.4
14-18 y	45	34	400	900	8,000	9	10	1,700	17	1.0	ND	3.6
19-70 y	45	40	400	1,100	10,000	11	10	2,000	20	1.0	1.8	3.6
>70 y	45	40	400	1,100	10,000	11	10	2,000	20	1.0	1.8	3.6
Pregnancy												
≤18 y	45	34	400	900	8,000	9	10	1,700	17	1.0	ND	3.6
19-50 y	45	40	400	1,100	10,000	11	10	2,000	20	1.0	ND	3.6
Lactation												
≤18 y	45	34	400	900	8,000	9	10	1,700	17	1.0	ND	3.6
19-50 y	45	40	400	1,100	10,000	11	10	2,000	20	1.0	ND	3.6

[1] UL = The maximum level of daily nutrient intake that is likely to pose no risk of adverse effects. Unless otherwise specified, the UL represents total intake from food, water, and supplements. Due to lack of suitable data, ULs could not be established for vitamin K, thiamin, riboflavin, vitamin B_{12}, pantothenic acid, biotin, or carotenoids. In the absence of ULs, extra caution may be warranted in consuming levels above recommended intakes.

[2] As preformed vitamin A (retinol) only.

[3] As α-tocopherol; applies to any form of supplemental α-tocopherol.

[4] The ULs for vitamin E, niacin, and folate apply to synthetic forms obtained from supplements, fortified foods, or a combination of the two.

[5] The ULs for magnesium represent intake from a pharmacological agent only and do not include intake from food and water.

[6] Although vanadium in food has not been shown to cause adverse effects in humans, there is no justification for adding vanadium to food and vanadium supplements should be used with caution. The UL is based on adverse effects in laboratory animals and these data could be used to set a UL for adults but not children or adolescents.

[7] ND = Not determinable due to lack of data on adverse effects in this age group and concern with regard to lack of ability to handle excess amounts. Source of intake should be from food only to prevent high levels of intake.

Daily Values for Food Labels

The Daily Values are standard values developed by the Food and Drug Administration (FDA) for use on food labels.

Nutrient[1]	Amount
Protein[1]	50 g
Thiamin	1.5 mg
Riboflavin	1.7 mg
Niacin	20 mg
Pantothenic Acid	10 mg
Biotin	300 μg
Vitamin B_6	2 mg
Folate	400 μg
Vitamin B_{12}	6 μg
Vitamin C	60 mg
Vitamin A[2]	5,000 IU
Vitamin D[2]	400 IU
Vitamin E[2]	30 IU
Vitamin K	80 μg
Chloride	3,400 mg
Calcium	1,000 mg
Phosphorus	1,000 mg
Magnesium	400 mg
Iron	18 mg
Zinc	15 mg
Selenium	70 μg
Iodine	150 μg
Copper	2 mg
Manganese	2 mg
Chromium	120 μg
Molybdenum	75 μg

[1] The Daily Values for protein vary for different groups of people: pregnant women, 60 g; nursing mothers, 65 g; infants under 1 year, 14 g; children 1 to 4 years, 16 g.

[2] The Daily Values for fat-soluble vitamins are expressed in International Units (IU), an old system of measurement.

Food Component	Amount	Calculation Factors
Fat	65 g	30% of kcalories
Saturated fat	20 g	10% of kcalories
Cholesterol	300 mg	Same regardless of kcalories
Carbohydrate (total)	300 g	60% of kcalories
Fiber	25 g	11.5 g per 1,000 kcalories
Protein	50 g	10% of kcalories
Sodium	2,400 mg	Same regardless of kcalories
Potassium	3,500 mg	Same regardless of kcalories

Note: Daily Values were established for adults and children over 4 years old. The values for energy-yielding nutrients are based on 2,000 kcalories a day.

Dietary Reference Intakes (DRIs) for Carbohydrates, Fiber, Fat, Fatty Acids, and Protein

Life stage group	Carbohydrate (g/d)	Fiber (g/d)	Fat (g/d)	Linoleic Acid (g/d)	α-Linolenic Acid (g/d)	Protein[1] (g/d)
Infants						
0-6 mo	60*	ND[2]	31*	4.4*	0.5*	9.1*
7-12 mo	95*	ND	30*	4.6*	0.5*	11
Children						
1-3 y	130	19*	ND	7*	0.7*	13
4-8 y	130	25*	ND	10*	0.9*	19
Males						
9-13 y	130	31*	ND	12*	1.2*	34
14-18 y	130	38*	ND	16*	1.6*	52
19-30 y	130	38*	ND	17*	1.6*	56
31-50 y	130	38*	ND	17*	1.6*	56
51-70 y	130	30*	ND	14*	1.6*	56
> 70 y	130	30*	ND	14*	1.6*	56
Females						
9-13 y	130	26*	ND	10*	1.0*	34
14-18 y	130	26*	ND	11*	1.1*	46
19-30 y	130	25*	ND	12*	1.1*	46
31-50 y	130	25*	ND	12*	1.1*	46
51-70 y	130	21*	ND	11*	1.1*	46
> 70 y	130	21*	ND	11*	1.1*	46
Pregnancy						
≤ 18 y	175	28*	ND	13*	1.4*	71
19-30 y	175	28*	ND	13*	1.4*	71
31-50 y	175	28*	ND	13*	1.4*	71
Lactation						
≤ 18 y	210	29*	ND	13*	1.3*	71
19-30 y	210	29*	ND	13*	1.3*	71
31-50 y	210	29*	ND	13*	1.3*	71

This table presents Recommended Dietary Allowances (RDAs) and Adequate Intakes (AIs). An asterisk (*) indicates AI. RDAs and AIs may both be used as goals for individual intake.

[1] Based on 1.52 g/kg/day for infants 0-6 mo, 1.2 g/kg/day for infants 7-12 mo, 1.05 g/kg/day for 1-3 y, 0.95 g/kg/day for 4-13 y, 0.85 g/kg/day for 14-18 y, 0.8 g/kg/day for adults, and 1.3 g/kg/day for pregnant women (using pre-pregnancy weight) and lactating women.

[2] ND = Not determinable due to lack of data on adverse effects in this age group and concern with regard to lack of ability to handle excess amounts. Source of intake should be from food only to prevent high levels of intake.

Data compiled from *Dietary Reference Intakes for Calcium, Phosphorus, Magnesium, Vitamin D, and Fluoride.* Washington, DC: National Academies Press; 1997. *Dietary Reference Intakes for Thiamin, Riboflavin, Niacin, Vitamin B_6, Folate, Vitamin B_{12}, Pantothenic Acid, Biotin, and Choline.* Washington, DC: National Academies Press; 1998. *Dietary Reference Intakes for Vitamin C, Vitamin E, Selenium, and Carotenoids.* Washington, DC: National Academies Press; 2000. *Dietary Reference Intakes for Vitamin A, Vitamin K, Arsenic, Boron, Chromium, Copper, Iron, Manganese, Molybdenum, Nickel, Silicon, Vanadium, and Zinc.* Washington, DC: National Academies Press; 2000. *Dietary Reference Intakes for Water, Potassium, Sodium, Chloride, and Sulfate.* Food and Nutrition Board. Washington, DC: National Academies Press; 2005. Dietary Reference Intakes for Calcium and Vitamin D. Washington, DC: National Academies Press; 2011.

These reports may be accessed via http://nap.edu.

Appendix **B**   **USDA Food Intake Patterns**

The table below shows suggested amounts of food to consume from the basic food groups, subgroups, and oils to meet recommended nutrient intakes at 12 different calorie levels. Nutrient and energy contributions from each group are calculated according to the nutrient-dense forms of foods in each group (e.g., lean meats and fat-free milk). The table also shows the empty calories that can be accommodated within each calorie level, in addition to the suggested amounts of nutrient-dense forms of foods in each group.

Daily Amount of Food from Each Group

Calorie Level[1]	1,000	1,200	1,400	1,600	1,800	2,000	2,200	2,400	2,600	2,800	3,000	3,200
Fruits[2]	1 cup	1 cup	1.5 cups	1.5 cups	1.5 cups	2 cups	2 cups	2 cups	2 cups	2.5 cups	2.5 cups	2.5 cups
Vegetables[3]	1 cup	1.5 cups	1.5 cups	2 cups	2.5 cups	2.5 cups	3 cups	3 cups	3.5 cups	3.5 cups	4 cups	4 cups
Grains[4]	3 oz-eq	4 oz-eq	5 oz-eq	5 oz-eq	6 oz-eq	6 oz-eq	7 oz-eq	8 oz-eq	9 oz-eq	10 oz-eq	10 oz-eq	10 oz-eq
Protein foods[5]	2 oz-eq	3 oz-eq	4 oz-eq	5 oz-eq	5 oz-eq	5.5 oz-eq	6 oz-eq	6.5 oz-eq	6.5 oz-eq	7 oz-eq	7 oz-eq	7 oz-eq
Dairy[6]	2 cups	2.5 cups	2.5 cups	3 cups	3 cups	3 cups	3 cups	3 cups	3 cups	3 cups	3 cups	3 cups
Oils[7]	15 g	17 g	17 g	22 g	24 g	27 g	29 g	31 g	34 g	36 g	44 g	51 g
SoFAs limit[8]	137	121	121	121	161	258	266	330	362	395	459	596

Vegetable Subgroup Amounts per Week

Calorie Level	1,000	1,200	1,400	1,600	1,800	2,000	2,200	2,400	2,600	2,800	3,000	3,200
Dark-green veg.	0.5 c/wk	1 c/wk	1 c/wk	1.5 c/wk	1.5 c/wk	1.5 c/wk	2 c/wk	2 c/wk	2.5 c/wk	2.5 c/wk	2.5 c/wk	2.5 c/wk
Red and orange veg.	2.5 c/wk	3 c/wk	3 c/wk	4 c/wk	5.5 c/wk	5.5 c/wk	6 c/wk	6 c/wk	7 c/wk	7 c/wk	7.5 c/wk	7.5 c/wk
Beans and peas (legumes)	0.5 c/wk	0.5 c/wk	0.5 c/wk	1 c/wk	1.5 c/wk	1.5 c/wk	2 c/wk	2 c/wk	2.5 c/wk	2.5 c/wk	3 c/wk	3 c/wk
Starchy veg.	2 c/wk	3.5 c/wk	3.5 c/wk	4 c/wk	5 c/wk	5 c/wk	6 c/wk	6 c/wk	7 c/wk	7 c/wk	8 c/wk	8 c/wk
Other veg.	1.5 c/wk	2.5 c/wk	2.5 c/wk	3.5 c/wk	4 c/wk	4 c/wk	5 c/wk	5 c/wk	5.5 c/wk	5.5 c/wk	7 c/wk	7 c/wk

[1] **Calorie Levels** are set across a wide range to accommodate the needs of different individuals. The following table, "USDA Food Intake Pattern Calorie Levels," can be used to help assign individuals to the food intake pattern at a particular calorie level.

[2] **Fruit Group** includes all fresh, frozen, canned, and dried fruits and fruit juices. In general, 1 cup of fruit or 100% fruit juice or 1/2 cup of dried fruit can be considered as 1 cup from the fruit group.

[3] **Vegetable Group** includes all fresh, frozen, canned, and dried vegetables and vegetable juices. In general, 1 cup of raw or cooked vegetables or vegetable juice or 2 cups of raw leafy greens can be considered as 1 cup from the vegetable group.

[4] **Grains Group** includes all foods made from wheat, rice, oats, cornmeal, and barley, such as bread, pasta, oatmeal, breakfast cereals, tortillas, and grits. In general, 1 slice of bread, 1 cup of ready-to-eat cereal, or 1/2 cup of cooked rice, pasta, or cooked cereal can be considered as 1 ounce equivalent from the grains group. *At least half of all grains consumed should be whole grains.*

[5] **Protein Foods Group** in general, 1 ounce of lean meat, poultry, or fish; 1 egg; 1 Tbsp. peanut butter; 1/4 cup cooked dry beans; or 1/2 ounce of nuts or seeds can be considered as 1 ounce equivalent from the protein foods group.

[6] **Dairy Group** includes all fluid milk products and foods made from milk that retain their calcium content, such as yogurt and cheese. Foods made from milk that have little to no calcium, such as cream cheese, cream, and butter, are not part of the group. Most milk group choices should be fat-free or low-fat. In general, 1 cup of milk or yogurt, 1 1/2 ounces of natural cheese, or 2 ounces of processed cheese can be considered as 1 cup from the dairy group.

[7] **Oils** include fats from many different plants and from fish that are liquid at room temperature, such as canola, corn, olive, soybean, and sunflower oil. Some foods are naturally high in oils, like nuts, olives, some fish, and avocados. Foods that are mainly oil include mayonnaise, certain salad dressings, and soft margarine.

[8] **SoFAs** are calories from solid fats and added sugars. The limit for SoFAs is the remaining amount of calories in each food pattern after selecting the specified amounts in each food group in nutrient-dense forms (forms that are fat-free or low-fat and with no added sugars). The number of SoFAs is lower in the 1,200-, 1,400-, and 1,600-calorie patterns than in the 1,000-calorie pattern. The nutrient goals for the 1,200- to 1,600-calorie patterns are higher and require that more calories be used for nutrient-dense foods from the food groups.

Reproduced from *Dietary Guidelines for Americans 2010*, 7th ed., U.S. Government Printing Office, 2010. Courtesy of U.S. Department of Agriculture and U.S. Department of Health and Human Services.

USDA Food Intake Pattern Calorie Levels

USDA food patterns assign individuals to a calorie level based on their sex, age, and activity level. The chart below identifies the calorie levels for males and females by age and activity level. Calorie levels are provided for each year of childhood, from 2–18 years, and for adults in five-year increments. The estimates are rounded to the nearest 200 calories. An individual's calorie needs may be higher or lower than these average estimates.

	Males				Females		
Activity level	Sedentary*	Moderately Active*	Active*	Activity level	Sedentary*	Moderately Active*	Active*
Age				Age			
2	1,000	1,000	1,000	2	1,000	1,000	1,000
3	1,200	1,400	1,400	3	1,000	1,200	1,400
4	1,200	1,400	1,600	4	1,200	1,400	1,400
5	1,200	1,400	1,600	5	1,200	1,400	1,600
6	1,400	1,600	1,800	6	1,200	1,400	1,600
7	1,400	1,600	1,800	7	1,200	1,600	1,800
8	1,400	1,600	2,000	8	1,400	1,600	1,800
9	1,600	1,800	2,000	9	1,400	1,600	1,800
10	1,600	1,800	2,200	10	1,400	1,800	2,000
11	1,800	2,000	2,200	11	1,600	1,800	2,000
12	1,800	2,200	2,400	12	1,600	2,000	2,200
13	2,000	2,200	2,600	13	1,600	2,000	2,200
14	2,000	2,400	2,800	14	1,800	2,000	2,400
15	2,200	2,600	3,000	15	1,800	2,000	2,400
16	2,400	2,800	3,200	16	1,800	2,000	2,400
17	2,400	2,800	3,200	17	1,800	2,000	2,400
18	2,400	2,800	3,200	18	1,800	2,000	2,400
19–20	2,600	2,800	3,000	19–20	2,000	2,200	2,400
21–25	2,400	2,800	3,000	21–25	2,000	2,200	2,400
26–30	2,400	2,600	3,000	26–30	1,800	2,000	2,400
31–35	2,400	2,600	3,000	31–35	1,800	2,000	2,200
36–40	2,400	2,600	2,800	36–40	1,800	2,000	2,200
41–45	2,200	2,600	2,800	41–45	1,800	2,000	2,200
46–50	2,200	2,400	2,800	46–50	1,800	2,000	2,200
51–55	2,200	2,400	2,800	51–55	1,600	1,800	2,200
56–60	2,200	2,400	2,600	56–60	1,600	1,800	2,200
61–65	2,000	2,400	2,600	61–65	1,600	1,800	2,000
66–70	2,000	2,200	2,600	66–70	1,600	1,800	2,000
71–75	2,000	2,200	2,600	71–75	1,600	1,800	2,000
76 and up	2,000	2,200	2,400	76 and up	1,600	1,800	2,000

*Calorie levels are based on the Estimated Energy Requirements (EER) and activity levels from the Institute of Medicine *Dietary Reference Intakes Macronutrients Report*, 2002. *Sedentary* means a lifestyle that includes only the light physical activity associated with typical day-to-day life. *Moderately active* means a lifestyle that includes physical activity equivalent to walking about 1.5 to 3 miles per day at 3 to 4 miles per hour, in addition to the light physical activity associated with typical day-to-day life. *Active* means a lifestyle that includes physical activity equivalent to walking more than 3 miles per day at 3 to 4 miles per hour, in addition to the light physical activity associated with typical day-to-day life.

Reprinted from *Journal of Nutrition Education and Behavior*, 38(6), Patricia Britten, Kristin Marcoe, Sedigheh Yamini & Carole Davis, Development of food intake patterns for the MyPyramid Food Guidance System, Page no. S78-S92, 2006, with permission from Elsevier.

Appendix C   Nutrition Assessment Methods

Nutrition Assessment: Determining Nutritional Health

In a nutritional sense, what does it mean to be healthy? Nutritional health is quite simply obtaining all the nutrients in amounts needed to support body processes. We can measure nutritional health in a number of ways. Taken together, such measurements can give you much insight into your current and long-term well-being. The process of measuring nutritional health is usually termed **nutrition assessment**.

Nutrition assessment serves a variety of purposes. It may help evaluate nutrition-related risks that may jeopardize a person's current or future health. Nutrition assessment is a routine part of the nutritional care of hospitalized patients. In this setting, nutrition assessment not only identifies risks, but also measures the effectiveness of treatment. In public health, nutrition assessment helps identify people in need of nutrition-related interventions and monitors the effectiveness of intervention programs. Sometimes, assessments determine the nutritional health of an entire population—identifying health risks common in a population group so specific policy measures can be developed to combat them.

► **nutrition assessment** Measurement of the nutritional health of the body. It can include anthropometric measurements, biochemical tests, clinical observations, and dietary intake, as well as medical histories and socioeconomic factors.

Nutrition Assessment of Individuals

In healthcare settings, a registered dietitian or physician may do an individual nutrition assessment of a patient or client. Depending on the purpose of the nutrition assessment, the measures may be very comprehensive and detailed. A dietitian can then use this information to plan individualized nutrition counseling. Nutrition assessment measures often are repeated in order to assess the effectiveness of nutrition counseling or a change in diet.

Nutrition Assessment of Populations

Population-based nutrition assessment is done in conjunction with programs to monitor the status of nutrition in the United States or Canada or as part of large-scale epidemiological studies. Typically, nutrition assessment of populations is not as comprehensive as an assessment of an individual. One of the largest ongoing nationwide surveys of dietary intake and health status is the National Health and Nutrition Examination Survey (NHANES). To date, four of these surveys have been completed, and they have told us a great deal about the nutritional status of our population. Another tool for monitoring the dietary intake of Americans is the Continuing Survey of Food Intake by Individuals (CSFII).

Nutrition Assessment Methods

Just as there is not one measure of physical fitness, there is not just one indicator of nutritional health. Nutrients play many roles in the body, so measures of nutritional status must look at many factors. Often these factors are termed the **ABCDs of nutrition assessment**: Anthropometric measurements, Biochemical tests, Clinical observations, and Dietary intake (see **TABLE C.1**).

Anthropometric Measurements

Anthropometric measurements are physical measurements of the body, such as height and weight, head circumference, waist circumference, or skinfold thickness.

Height and Weight

To provide useful information, height and weight must be measured accurately. For infants and very young children, measurement of height is really measurement of recumbent length (that is, when they are lying down). Careful measurement of length at each checkup gives a clear indication of a child's growth rate. Standard growth charts show how the child's growth compares with that of others of the same age and gender. For children 2 to 20 years old, charts illustrating growth are based on standing height, or stature.

The standing height of older children and adults can be determined with a tape measure fixed to a wall and a sliding right-angle headboard for reading the measurement. Aging adults lose some height due to bone loss and curvature, so it is important to measure height and not simply rely on remembered values. Because many calculations/standards use metric measures, it's important to be familiar with standard conversion factors.

Weight is a critical measure in nutrition assessment. It is used to assess children's growth, predict energy expenditure and protein needs, and determine body composition. Weight should be measured using a calibrated scale. For assessments that need a high degree of precision, subtract the weight of the clothing.

For the anthropometric assessment of infants and young children, a third measurement is common: head circumference. This is measured using a flexible tape measure, put snugly around the head. Head circumference measures are another useful indicator of normal growth and development, especially during rapid growth from birth to age 3.

▶ **ABCDs of nutrition assessment** Nutrition assessment components: Anthropometric measurements, Biochemical tests, Clinical observations, and Dietary intake.

▶ **anthropometric measurements** Measurements of the physical characteristics of the body, such as height, weight, head circumference, waist circumference, and skinfold thickness. Anthropometric measurements are particularly useful in evaluating the growth of infants, children, and adolescents and in determining body composition.

To convert inches to centimeters, multiply the number of inches by 2.54

$$\text{inches} \times 2.54 = \text{centimeters}$$

To convert pounds to kilograms, divide the number of pounds by 2.2

$$\text{pounds} \div 2.2 = \text{kilograms}$$

To calculate BMI

$$BMI = \frac{\text{weight (kg)}}{\text{height (m)}^2}$$

$$BMI = \frac{\text{weight (lb)}}{\text{height (in)}^2} \times 704.5$$

TABLE C.1
The ABCDs of Nutrition Assessment

Assessment Method	Why It's Done
Anthropometric measures	Measure growth in children; show changes in weight that can reflect diseases (e.g., cancer or thyroid problems); monitor progress in fat loss
Biochemical tests	Measure blood, urine, and feces for nutrients or metabolites that indicate infection or disease
Clinical observations	Assess change in skin color and health, hair texture, fingernail shape, etc.
Dietary intake	Evaluate diet for nutrient (e.g., fat, calcium, protein) or food (e.g., number of fruits and vegetables) intake

▶ **skinfold measurements** A method to estimate body fat by measuring the thickness of a fold of skin and subcutaneous fat.

▶ **biochemical assessment** Assessment by measuring a nutrient or its metabolite in one or more body fluids such as blood and urine, and in feces. Also called laboratory assessment.

Skinfolds

Skinfold measurements serve a variety of purposes. Because a significant amount of the body's fat stores are right beneath the skin (subcutaneous fat), the sizes of skinfolds at various sites around the body can give a good indication of body fatness. This information may be used to evaluate the physical fitness of an athlete or predict the risk of obesity-related disorders. Skinfold measurements are also useful in cases of illness; the maintenance of fat stores in a patient's body may be a valuable indicator of dietary adequacy. Skinfold measurements are done with special calipers (see **FIGURE C.1**). For reliable measurements, training in the use of calipers is essential. Skinfold measurements can be used to estimate the percentage of body fat, or can be compared with percentile tables for specific gender and age categories.

Biochemical Tests

Because of their relation to growth and body composition, anthropometric measurements give a broad picture of nutritional health—whether the diet contains enough calories and protein to maintain normal patterns of growth, normal body composition, and normal levels of lean body mass. However, anthropometric measures do not give specific information about *nutrients*. For that information, a variety of biochemical tests are useful.

Biochemical assessment measures a nutrient or metabolite (a related compound) in one or more body fluids such as blood and urine, or in feces. For example, the concentration of albumin (an important transport protein) in the blood can be an indicator of the

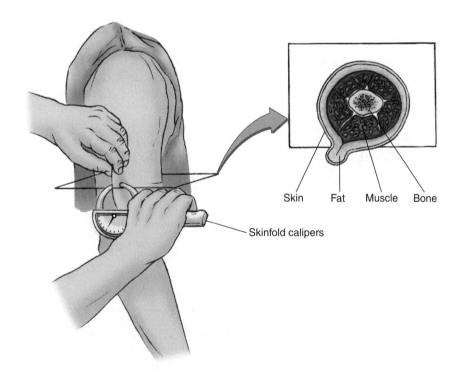

FIGURE C.1 Skinfold measurements. A significant amount of the body's fat stores lie just beneath the skin, so when done correctly, skinfold measurements can provide an indication of body fatness. An inexperienced or careless measurer, however, can easily make large errors. Skinfold measurements usually work better for monitoring malnutrition than for identifying overweight and obesity. They also are widely used in large population studies.

body's protein status. If little protein is eaten, the body produces smaller amounts of body proteins such as albumin.

Biochemical assessment may include measurements of a nutrient metabolite, a storage or transport compound, an enzyme that depends on a vitamin or mineral, or another indicator of the body's functioning in relation to a particular nutrient. These measures usually are a better indicator of nutritional status than directly measuring blood levels of nutrients such as vitamin A or calcium. The levels of nutrients excreted in the urine or feces also provide valuable information.

Clinical Observations

Clinical observations—the characteristics of health that can be seen during a physical exam—help complete the picture of nutritional health. Although often nonspecific, clinical signs are clues to nutrient deficiency or excess that can be confirmed or ruled out by further testing. In a clinical nutrition examination, a clinician observes the hair, nails, skin, eyes, lips, mouth, bones, muscles, and joints. Specific findings, such as cracking at the corners of the mouth (suggestive of riboflavin, vitamin B_6, or niacin deficiency) or petechiae (small, pinpoint hemorrhages on the skin indicative of vitamin C deficiency) need to be followed by other assessments.

Dietary Intake

A picture of nutritional health would not be complete without information about dietary intake. Dietary information may confirm the lack or excess of a dietary component suggested by anthropometric, biochemical, or clinical evaluations.

There are a number of ways to collect dietary intake data. Each has strengths and weaknesses. It is important to match the method to the type and quantity of data needed. Remember, too, that the quality of information obtained about people's diets often relies heavily on people's memories, as well as their honesty in sharing those recollections. How well do you remember *everything* you ate yesterday?

Diet History

The most comprehensive form of dietary intake data collection is the **diet history**. In this method, a skilled interviewer finds out not only what the client has been eating in the recent past but also the client's long-term food consumption habits. The interviewer's questions also may address other risk factors for nutrition-related problems, such as economic issues.

Food Record

Food records, or diaries, provide detailed information about day-to-day eating habits. Typically, a person records all foods and beverages consumed during a defined period, usually three to seven consecutive days. Because food records are recorded concurrently with intake, they are less prone to inaccuracy from lapses in memory. Because the data are completely self-reported, however, food records will not be accurate if the person fails to record all items. To make food records more precise, the items in a meal can be weighed before consumption. Remaining portions are weighed at the end of the meal to determine exactly how much was eaten. **Weighed food records** are much more time consuming to complete.

▶ **clinical observations** Assessment by evaluating the characteristics of well-being that can be seen in a physical exam. Nonspecific, clinical observations can provide clues to nutrient deficiency or excess that can be confirmed or ruled out by biochemical testing.

▶ **diet history** Record of food intake and eating behaviors that includes recent and long-term habits of food consumption. Done by a skilled interviewer, the diet history is the most comprehensive form of dietary intake data collection.

▶ **food records** Detailed information about day-to-day eating habits; typically includes all foods and beverages consumed for a defined period, usually three to seven consecutive days.

▶ **weighed food records** Detailed food records obtained by weighing foods before eating, and then weighing leftovers to determine the exact amount consumed.

Food Item	Average use during past year					
	<1 serving per month	1–3 servings per month	1–4 servings per week	5–7 servings per week	2–4 servings per day	5+ servings per day
Coffee					√	
Dark bread	√					
Ice cream				√		

Food Item	Your serving size				How often?				
	Medium Serving	S	M	L	Day	Week	Month	Year	Never
Coffee	(1 cup)			√	2				
Dark bread	(1 slice)								√
Ice cream	(1/2 cup)		√			3			

FIGURE C.2 Examples of food frequency questionnaire formats.

Modified from Lee RD, Nieman DC. *Nutritional Assessment.* 2nd ed. St Louis: Mosby; 1996.

▶ **food frequency questionnaire (FFQ)** A questionnaire for nutrition assessment that asks how often the subject consumes specific foods or groups of foods, rather than what specific foods the subject consumes daily. Also called food frequency checklist.

▶ **24-hour dietary recall** A form of dietary intake data collection. The interviewer takes the client through a recent 24-hour period (usually midnight to midnight) to determine what foods and beverages the client consumed.

Food Frequency Questionnaire

A **food frequency questionnaire (FFQ)** asks how often the subject consumes specific foods or groups of foods, rather than what specific foods the subject consumes daily. A food frequency questionnaire may ask, for example, "How often do you drink a cup of milk?" with response options of daily, weekly, monthly, and so on (see **FIGURE C.2**). This information is used to estimate that person's average daily intake.

Although food frequency questionnaires do not require a trained interviewer and can be completed relatively quickly, there are disadvantages to this method of data collection. One problem is that it is often difficult to translate a person's response to how often they drink milk, or how many cups of milk they drink per week, into specific nutrient values without more detailed information. More importantly, food frequency questionnaires require a person to average, over a long period, foods that may be consumed erratically in portions that are sometimes large and sometimes small.

24-Hour Dietary Recall

The **24-hour dietary recall** is the simplest form of dietary intake data collection. In a 24-hour recall, the interviewer takes the client through a recent 24-hour period (usually midnight to midnight) to determine what foods and beverages the client consumed. To get a complete, accurate picture of the subject's diet, the interviewer must ask probing questions like, "Did you put anything on your toast?" but not leading questions like, "Did you put butter and jelly on your toast?" Comprehensive population surveys frequently use 24-hour recalls as the main method of data collection. Although a single 24-hour recall is not very useful for describing the nutrient content of an individual's overall diet (there's too much day-to-day variation), in large-scale studies it gives a reasonably accurate picture of the average nutrient intake of a population. Multiple diet recalls also are useful for estimating nutrient intake of individuals.

Methods of Evaluating Dietary Intake Data

Once the data are collected, the next step is to determine the nutrient content of the diet and evaluate that information in terms of dietary standards or other reference points. This is commonly done using nutrient analysis software. Computer programs remove the tedium of looking up foods in tables of nutrient composition; large databases allow for simple access to food composition, and the computer does the math automatically.

Comparison to Dietary Standards

It is possible to compare a person's nutrient intake to dietary standards such as the RDA or AI values. Although this will give a qualitative idea of dietary adequacy, it cannot be considered a definitive evaluation of a person's diet, because we don't know that individual's specific nutrient requirements. Comparisons of individual diets to RDA or AI values should be interpreted with caution.

Comparison to MyPlate

Another type of dietary analysis compares a person's food intake to the recommendations in MyPlate. This involves categorizing foods into the various groups and determining the number of servings the subject has eaten. Making these comparisons can be difficult because many common foods (e.g., pizza, sandwiches, casseroles) contain servings or partial servings from multiple food groups. Using the MyPlate SuperTracker feature on the www.ChooseMyPlate.gov website makes comparing food intake to MyPlate guidelines and customizing food plans straightforward and easy.

Comparison to Dietary Guidelines for Americans

For a general picture of the subject's dietary habits, the evaluator can compare the person's diet to the *Dietary Guidelines for Americans.* While these evaluations usually are not specific, they give a general idea of whether the subject's diet is high or low in saturated fat, or whether the subject is eating enough fruits and vegetables.

Outcomes of Nutrition Assessment

When taken together, anthropometric measures, biochemical tests, clinical exams, and dietary evaluation, along with the individual's family history, socioeconomic situation, and other factors give a complete picture of nutritional health. A client's assessment may lead to a recommendation for a diet change to reduce weight or blood cholesterol, the addition of a vitamin or mineral supplement to treat a deficiency, the identification of abnormal growth due to inadequate infant feeding, or simply the affirmation that dietary intake is adequate for current nutrition needs. Reviewing a client's BMI is another important step (see **TABLE C.2**). BMI can play a critical role in a person's lifespan (see **FIGURE C.3**).

TABLE C.2
Adult BMI Chart

BMI	19	20	21	22	23	24	25	26	27	28	29	30	31	32	33	34	35
Height								Weight in pounds									
4'10"	91	96	100	105	110	115	119	124	129	134	138	143	148	153	158	162	167
4'11"	94	99	104	109	114	119	124	128	133	138	143	148	153	158	163	168	173
5'	97	102	107	112	118	123	128	133	138	143	148	153	158	163	158	174	179
5'1"	100	106	111	116	122	127	132	137	143	148	153	158	164	169	174	180	185
5'2"	104	109	115	120	126	131	136	142	147	153	158	164	169	175	180	186	191
5'3"	107	113	118	124	130	135	141	146	152	158	163	169	175	180	186	191	197
5'4"	110	116	122	128	134	140	145	151	157	163	169	174	180	186	192	197	204
5'5"	114	120	126	132	138	144	150	156	162	168	174	180	186	192	198	204	210
5'6"	118	124	130	136	142	148	155	161	167	173	179	186	192	198	204	210	216
5'7"	121	127	134	140	146	153	159	166	172	178	185	191	198	204	211	217	223
5'8"	125	131	138	144	151	158	164	171	177	184	190	197	203	210	216	223	230
5'9"	128	135	142	149	155	162	169	176	182	189	196	203	209	216	223	230	236
5'10"	132	139	146	153	160	167	174	181	188	195	202	209	216	222	229	236	243
5'11"	136	143	150	157	165	172	179	186	193	200	208	215	222	229	236	243	250
6'	140	147	154	162	169	177	184	191	199	206	213	221	228	235	242	250	258
6'1"	144	151	159	166	174	182	189	197	204	212	219	227	235	242	250	257	265
6'2"	148	155	163	171	179	186	194	202	210	218	225	233	241	249	256	264	272
6'3"	152	160	168	176	184	192	200	208	216	224	232	240	248	256	264	272	279
	Healthy weight						Overweight					Obese					

Locate the height of interest in the leftmost column and read across the row for that height to the weight of interest. Follow the column of the weight up to the top row that lists the BMI. BMI of 19 to 24 is the healthy weight range, BMI of 25 to 29 is the overweight range, and BMI of 30 and above is in the obese range. Due to rounding, these ranges vary slightly from the NHLBI values.

Clinical Guidelines on the Identification, Evaluation, and Treatment of Overweight and Obesity in Adults—The Evidence Report. National Institutes of Health, National Heart, Lung, and Blood Institute. September 1998.

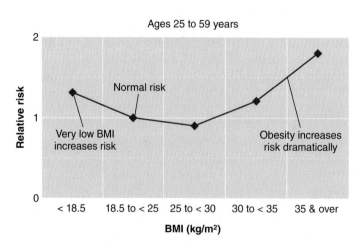

Ages 25 to 59 years

FIGURE C.3 BMI and mortality. People with a high or very low BMI have a higher relative mortality rate.
Modified from Flegal KM, Graubard BI, Williamson DF, Gail MH. Excess deaths associated with underweight, overweight and obesity. *JAMA*. 2005; 293:1861-1867.

Appendix **D**   **Vitamin and Mineral Summary Tables**

Fat-Soluble Vitamins		
Name	**Main Roles**	**Recommended Intake (Adult)**

Vitamin A (retinol, retinal, and retinoic acid)
 	
Provitamin A carotenoids
	Regulates cell growth and cell death. Growth/maintenance of bones/teeth; skin, mucous membranes, and other epithelial cells. Required for reproduction, immune function, vision/night vision, wound healing.	**RDA**
		Men: 900 µg RAE
		Women: 700 µg RAE
		
		RAE is retinol activity equivalent
		
		1 RAE = 1 µg retinol
		       = 12 µg beta-carotene
		       = 24 µg alpha-carotene, beta-cryptoxanthin, other provitamin A carotenoids
		       = 2 µg beta-carotene in oil base/supplements

Vitamin D (cholecalciferol and calcitriol; ergocalciferol is D$_2$, cholecalciferol is D$_3$)	Regulates calcium and phosphorus levels by regulating their intestinal absorption, retention by the kidneys, deposition into bone, and absorption from bone when calcium and phosphorus blood levels dip. Required for bone/teeth growth and maintenance.	**Update Vitamin D to an RDA** Ages 19–70: 600 IU >70: 800 IU
Vitamin E (alpha-tocopherol) (Includes natural alpha-tocopherol and several, but not all, synthetic variations)	As a fat-soluble antioxidant, it protects unsaturated fats, phospholipids, and other fat-soluble substances; discourages oxidation of blood lipids and their subsequent deposition in arteries; and helps prevent oxygen damage in the lungs, skin, eyes, liver, and other organs. Helps maintain red blood cell integrity, nervous system function.	**RDA** Adults: 15 mg
Vitamin K (phylloquinone and menaquinone)	Required in production of thrombin for blood clotting. Involved in bone formation and maintenance.	**RDA** Men: 120 µg Women: 90 µg

AI, Adequate Intake; RDA, Recommended Dietary Allowance; UL, Tolerable Upper Intake Level.

(continues)

Fat-Soluble Vitamins (*continued*)

Deficiency	Good Food Sources	Toxicity
Eyes: Night blindness, Bitot's spots (foamy deposits on cornea), keratomalacia (corneal dryness, itching), progressing to xerophthalmia (corneal scarring and degeneration, blindness). Skin, mucous membranes: Hyperkeratosis (bumpy dry skin from clogged hair follicles); compromised linings of respiratory, digestive, and reproductive systems. Impaired immunity, growth, and reproduction.	Vitamin A (animal sources): Liver, egg yolk, butterfat, cream, cheese, whole milk, fortified low-fat milks, fortified margarine. Provitamin A (vegetable sources): Spinach, collards, and other dark-green vegetables; pumpkin, sweet potato, carrots, apricots, peaches, cantaloupe, mango, and other orange or dark yellow fruits and vegetables (the carotenoid in oranges/tangerines is not converted to vitamin A).	**UL:** 3,000 µg Teratogenic (birth defects from excessive use during pregnancy). Dry, itchy skin. Hair loss. Bone/joint pain. Bone abnormalities. Loss of appetite. Liver abnormalities/damage. (UL does not apply to provitamin carotenoids.)
Growth retardation. Rickets (bowed legs, knocked knees, other skeletal deformities) develop in childhood. Adults develop osteomalacia (excessive loss of calcium from bones) with risk of bone fracture. Severe deficiency due to illness or metabolic error causes twitching and muscle spasms.	Synthesis by the body when skin is exposed to sunlight is the most important source of vitamin D. Vitamin D–fortified milk. Fish liver oils. Salmon, mackerel, and other fatty fish; egg yolk; butter; and liver. (Vitamin D levels in foods vary widely.)	**UL:** 50 µg Impairs kidney function; excessive urination and thirst. Kidney stones and calcium deposition in other soft tissues—heart, blood vessels, and membranes in bone joints. Joint pain. Bone loss. Growth retardation.
Hemolysis (breaking) of red blood cells and hemolytic anemia, especially in premature babies. Retinopathy of prematurity. Neurological problems.	Wheat germ. Nuts and seeds such as pumpkin, sunflower, sesame. Vegetable oils, margarine, salad dressings.	**UL:** 1,000 µg Interferes with blood clotting. (UL applies only to vitamin E in supplements or fortified foods; includes natural-form alpha-tocopherol and all synthetic versions.)
Hemorrhage. Possible decrease in bone density.	Synthesis by intestinal bacteria. Vegetable sources (phylloquinone): Dark-green leafy vegetables, vegetables in cabbage family. Animal sources (menaquinone): Egg yolk, butterfat, liver.	Possible interference with anticoagulation medication. No UL has been set.

Water-Soluble Vitamins and Choline		
Name	**Main Roles**	**Recommended Intake (Adult)**
Thiamin (vitamin B$_1$)	As part of coenzyme TPP (thiamin pyrophosphate), it functions in several energy-producing pathways, is required for RNA and DNA synthesis, and is involved in nervous system function.	**RDA** Men: 1.2 mg Women: 1.1 mg
Riboflavin (vitamin B$_2$)	As part of coenzymes FMN (flavin mononucleotide) and FAD (flavin adenine dinucleotide), it functions in energy production and metabolism of amino acids. Involved in oxidation/reduction reactions. Required for vision.	**RDA** Men: 1.3 mg Women: 1.1 mg
Niacin (vitamin B$_3$, niacinamide, nicotinic acid, nicotinamide)	As part of coenzymes NAD and NADP (nicotinamide adenine dinucleotide/phosphate), it functions in energy metabolism and synthesis of fatty acids, steroid hormones, DNA, and amino acids.	**RDA** Men: 16 mg NE Women: 14 mg NE NE is niacin equivalent 1 NE = 1 mg niacin = 60 mg tryptophan
Pantothenic acid	As part of coenzyme A, it has many metabolic activities, including energy production and synthesis of lipids, steroid hormones, and proteins.	**AI** Adults: 5 mg
Biotin	As part of several coenzymes, it has many metabolic activities, including DNA and lipid synthesis, and energy production from carbohydrates, proteins, and fats.	**AI** Adults: 30 μg

AI, Adequate Intake; RDA, Recommended Dietary Allowance; UL, Tolerable Upper Intake Level.

(continues)

Water-Soluble Vitamins and Choline (*continued*)

Deficiency	Good Food Sources	Toxicity
Beriberi deficiency disease: Painful leg muscles, overall muscle weakness and wasting, loss of reflexes, and ultimately paralysis; edema, enlarged heart, and heart failure; loss of appetite; depression, mental confusion; death. When complicated by alcoholism, Wernicke/Korsakoff syndrome with mental/emotional symptoms, involuntary eye movements, or eye paralysis.	Pork. Organ meats. Enriched or fortified bread, pasta, rice, and breakfast cereals; whole grain products. Nuts, seeds, and legumes. (Widely distributed in small amounts in most fruits, vegetables, animal products, and dairy foods.)	Not determined. No UL has been set.
Ariboflavinosis deficiency disease: Glossitis and stomatitis (inflamed tongue and mouth), cheilosis (fissures at corners of mouth), seborrheic dermatitis (inflammation of skin's oil-producing glands). Sensitivity to light. Ariboflavinosis usually coexists with other vitamin deficiencies.	Milk, and other dairy products. Liver, and other organ meats. Enriched or fortified grain products; whole-grain products. Dark-green vegetables.	Not determined. No UL has been set.
Pellagra deficiency disease: The 4 Ds—dementia, diarrhea, dermatitis, death. Rough, darkened skin rash where exposed to sun. Inflamed mouth and tongue. Neuritis, confusion, anxiety.	Eggs, organ meats, meats, poultry, and fish. Peas, peanuts, and soybeans. Enriched or fortified grain products; whole-grain products. Milk, cheese, and yogurt. (Tryptophan can be converted to niacin; 60 mg tryptophan provides 1 NE.)	**UL:** 35 mg >35 mg may cause flushing. >250 mg may cause itching, rash, headache, nausea; glucose intolerance; blurred vision. Extremely high doses (over 3 g/d) are associated with liver damage. (UL applies only to niacin in supplements and fortified foods.)
Irritability, fatigue, apathy, nausea, vomiting, tingling, muscle cramps. (Deficiency symptoms seen only in experimental settings.)	Widely distributed in most foods. Eggs, milk, and yogurt. Fish, shellfish, meat, and poultry. Peas, potatoes, and winter squash.	Not determined. No UL has been set.
Hair loss, rash, convulsions, impaired growth. (Deficiency symptoms seen in infants with rare genetic error of biotin metabolism.)	Cauliflower, liver, nuts, peanuts, cheese, and egg yolks (raw egg whites interfere with biotin absorption). Little information is available on food sources.	Not determined. No UL has been set.

Name	Main Roles	Recommended Intake (Adult)
Vitamin B$_6$ (pyridoxine, pyridoxal, pyridoxamine)	As part of PLP (pyridoxal phosphate) and other coenzymes, it functions in amino acid, carbohydrate, and fatty acid metabolism; red and white blood cell synthesis; conversion of tryptophan to niacin; synthesis of several neurotransmitters.	**RDA** Ages 19–50 years: 1.3 mg Men >51 years: 1.7 mg Women >51 years: 1.5 mg
Folate (folic acid, folacin)	As the coenzyme THFA (tetrahydrofolic acid), involved in DNA and RNA synthesis, red blood cell maturation, synthesis of neurotransmitters, and metabolism of homocysteine and other amino acids. Important for reproduction.	**RDA** Adults: 400 µg DFE DFE is dietary folate equivalent 1 µg DFE = 1 µg food folate = 0.5 µg supplemental folic acid on empty stomach = 0.6 µg supplemental folic acid taken with food or folic acid from fortified food
Vitamin B$_{12}$ (cobalamin)	As part of cobalamin coenzymes, involved in cell synthesis, red blood cell maturation. Regeneration of folate. Maintenance of protective sheath around nerve fibers. Involved in fatty acid metabolism.	**RDA** Adults: 2.4 µg
Vitamin C (ascorbic acid)	An antioxidant. Needed for collagen synthesis: wound healing, blood vessel integrity, maintenance of gums, bone growth, and maintenance. Aids iron absorption. Involved in thyroxin metabolism; synthesis of neurotransmitters, carnitine, and amino acids.	**RDA** Men: 90 mg Women: 75 mg Smokers: add 35 mg to above
Choline	A methyl donor. A component of bile, and of the neurotransmitter acetylcholine. As part of the phospholipid lecithin, it is an emulsifier and functions in cell membranes.	**AI** Men: 550 mg Women: 425 mg

AI, Adequate Intake; RDA, Recommended Dietary Allowance; UL, Tolerable Upper Intake Level.

(continues)

Water-Soluble Vitamins and Choline (*continued*)

Deficiency	Good Food Sources	Toxicity
Anemia. Depression, confusion, headache, convulsions. Seborrheic dermatitis. Possible relation to cardiovascular disease from homocysteine buildup.	Fortified breakfast cereals. Liver, other meat, poultry, seafood, and fish. Bananas, avocados, green and leafy vegetables, legumes, and potatoes.	**UL:** 100 mg Nerve damage causing weakness, numbness, inability to walk. At high doses, damage may be irreversible.
Anemia. Impaired immunity. Diarrhea. Neuropathy, depression, confusion, fatigue. Sore, inflamed mouth and tongue. Possible relation to cardiovascular disease from homocysteine buildup. Inadequate folate early in pregnancy related to neural tube birth defects such as spina bifida.	Fortified breakfast cereals, wheat germ, and enriched grain products. Leafy green vegetables, asparagus, broccoli, and cauliflower. Oranges. Peanuts, legumes, and seeds such as pumpkin or sunflower. Liver.	**UL:** 1,000 μg Masks vitamin B_{12} deficiency. Allergic reactions possible. May interfere with antiseizure medications. (UL applies only to folic acid in supplementsand fortified foods.)
Anemia. Impaired immunity. Diarrhea. Neuropathy, which becomes irreversible. Possible relation to cardiovascular disease from homocysteine buildup.	Liver and other meats, poultry, fish, and seafood. Milk, cheese, and eggs. Only vegetable sources are fortified foods and Cyanobacteria (blue-green algae). (For adults >51 years, B_{12} supplements or fortified foods are recommended.)	Not determined. No UL has been set.
Scurvy deficiency disease: Broken blood vessels with tiny hemorrhages; easily bruised; bleeding gums and loose or missing teeth; pain in joints, bones, muscles; nonhealing wounds, bedsores; delayed bone growth, bone fragility; anemia. Severe scurvy can be fatal.	Citrus fruits, kiwi, strawberries, peppers, cabbage-family vegetables, dark leafy greens, potatoes, melon, and papaya.	**UL:** 2,000 mg May cause diarrhea. Tooth erosion. Excessive iron absorption. Buildup of oxalates and uric acid may cause kidney stones. Interference with diagnostic testing and with some medications.
Fatty liver and liver damage.	Egg yolk, liver, milk and dairy products, soybeans, and peanuts.	**UL:** 3,500 mg Fishy body odor, vomiting, excess sweating and salivation, liver damage, digestive disturbance, low blood pressure.

Major Minerals		
Name	**Main Roles**	**Recommended Intake (Adult)**
Sodium	Major cation in extracellular fluid. Involved in regulating body water distribution, blood pressure, acid–base balance, and nerve and muscle function.	**AI** 19–50 years: 1,500 mg 51–70 years: 1,300 mg >70 years: 1,200 mg
Potassium	Major intracellular cation. Involved in transmitting nerve impulses, regulating blood pressure, and controlling muscle contractility.	**AI** Adults: 4,700 mg
Chloride	Major anion in extracellular fluid. Involved in maintaining fluid and electrolyte balance. Component of gastric juice.	**AI** 19–50 years: 2,300 mg 51–70 years: 2,000 mg >70 years: 1,800 mg
Calcium	Structural material for bones and teeth. Involved in regulating nerve conduction, blood clotting, membrane permeability, nerve irritability, and muscle contraction.	Ages 19–50 years: 1,000 mg 51–70 years: men 1,000 mg 51–70 years: women 1,200 mg >70 years: 1,200 mg
Phosphorus	Structural material for bones and teeth. Component of nucleic acids, of phospholipids, of numerous enzymes, and of high-energy compounds such as ATP.	**RDA** Adults: 700 mg
Magnesium	Participates in hundreds of enzyme reactions. Regulates muscle contractility. Involved in nerve function and blood clotting, release of energy from ATP.	**RDA** 19–30 years: men 400 mg 19–30 years: women 310 mg >30 years: men 420 mg >30 years: women 320 mg
Sulfur (sulfate)	Component of some amino acids and the vitamins biotin and thiamin. Used to make many essential compounds.	Not established. Adequate intake of sulfur-containing amino acids provides ample amounts for the body.

AI, Adequate Intake; RDA, Recommended Dietary Allowance; UL, Tolerable Upper Intake Level.

(*continues*)

Major Minerals (*continued*)

Deficiency	Good Food Sources	Toxicity
Muscle cramps, fatigue.	Salt (sodium chloride), salty snacks and condiments (e.g., ketchup, pickles, sauerkraut, soy sauce), processed meats, canned vegetables, cheeses, prepackaged entrees, and flavored salts.	**UL:** 2,300 mg Excess consumption of sodium chloride is associated with high blood pressure and its consequences. High intake of sodium chloride can also increase calcium excretion, which in turn may affect bone health and kidney stone formation.
Muscle cramps, heartbeat irregularities, glucose intolerance, elevated blood pressure.	Bananas, potatoes, avocados, oranges, and other fruits and vegetables; meats, fish, seafood, and poultry; milk and dairy products.	Excess intake from food unlikely in healthy people. Supplemental potassium should be used only under medical supervision. Acute hyperkalemia can cause cardiac arrest. No UL has been set.
Hypochloremic metabolic alkalosis, confusion, stupor.	Added to foods as sodium chloride (salt).	**UL:** 3,600 mg Excess consumption of sodium chloride is associated with high blood pressure and its consequences. High intake of sodium chloride can also increase calcium excretion, which in turn may affect bone health and kidney stone formation.
Slow, stunted growth; osteoporosis (bone loss) with dowager's hump, bone fractures, bone pain. Tooth loss. Muscle cramping.	Milk, cheese, yogurt, and ice cream; canned fishes with bones; tofu made with calcium carbonate; fortified fruit juices; broccoli, kale, and almonds.	**UL:** 2,500 mg May interfere with absorption of iron, zinc, magnesium, and other minerals. May cause kidney stones; may be constipating. Very high blood calcium levels cause coma and cardiac arrest.
Weakness, muscle loss, bone loss and pain, anorexia. (Deficiency is rare. Most likely in people taking phosphorus-binding drugs.)	Protein-rich foods. Cereal grains. Soft drinks. Present in most foods.	**UL:** 4,000 mg Contributes to osteoporosis. Lowers blood calcium levels. Severe calcium depletion causes convulsions, muscle spasms.
Weakness, confusion. Constipation. Disturbed heart rhythm.	Whole-grain products; green vegetables; nuts; legumes; bananas; seafood; molasses; cocoa and chocolate.	**UL:** 350 mg Nausea, vomiting, low blood pressure, diarrhea. Severe hypermagnesemia (from magnesium-containing drugs) depresses breathing, causes coma, cardiac arrest. (UL applies only to magnesium in supplements and drugs.)
None reported.	All protein-rich foods, drinking water.	No UL has been set. Diarrhea may result for high levels in drinking water.

Trace and Ultra-Trace Minerals		
Name	**Main Roles**	**Recommended Intake (Adult)**
Iron	Component of hemoglobin, which transports oxygen in blood; component of myoglobin, which holds oxygen for muscle use. Required for energy utilization, immune function.	**RDA** Men: 8 mg Women: 19–50 years: 18 mg >50 years: 8 mg
Zinc	As a cofactor in many enzymes, it is involved with gene expression, protein metabolism, sexual maturation, sperm production, fetal development, and bone health. It is needed for vitamin A metabolism, wound healing, and taste perception.	**RDA** Men: 11 mg Women: 8 mg
Selenium	Component of the antioxidant enzyme glutathione peroxidase. Works synergistically with vitamin E. Involved in immune function and thyroid metabolism.	**RDA** Adults: 55 μg
Iodine	As a component of thyroid hormones, it is involved with regulating body temperature, metabolic rate, reproduction, and growth.	**RDA** Adults: 150 μg
Copper	Functions of copper-containing enzymes include antioxidant activity; participation in electron transport, synthesis of connective tissue, synthesis of melanin; myelination of nerve tissue. It is involved with immune function and heart health. The copper-containing enzyme ceruloplasmin catalyzes oxidation of ferrous to ferric iron.	**RDA** Adults: 900 μg

AI, Adequate Intake; RDA, Recommended Dietary Allowance; UL, Tolerable Upper Intake Level.

(continues)

Trace and Ultra-Trace Minerals (*continued*)

Deficiency	Good Food Sources	Toxicity
Anemia with weakness, fatigue, reduced learning ability, impaired reactivity and coordination, pale skin or pallor, intolerance of cold. Slowed wound healing. Lowered resistance to infection.	Liver, gizzards, red meat, seafood, and fish; enriched grain products; dark-green leafy vegetables; nuts, legumes, and dried fruits.	**UL:** 45 mg Gastric distress. Accidental iron poisoning in children can cause death. People with hemochromatosis are at risk of toxicity: fatigue; joint pain; liver, kidney, and heart damage; increased oxidation of blood lipids.
Growth retardation, delayed puberty, hypogonadism; loss of taste sensations, anorexia, weight loss, diarrhea; hair loss; delayed wound healing; night blindness; impaired immunity.	Protein-rich foods, especially oysters, red meat, and other seafood; whole-grain products.	**UL:** 40 mg Impaired immunity, impaired copper absorption. Acute toxicity (2,000–4,000 mg zinc intake) causes nausea, vomiting, cramping.
Impaired immunity. Susceptibility to Keshan disease (a heart disorder).	Brazil nuts; tuna fish, seafood, meats and poultry, and other fish; whole-grain products.	**UL:** 400 µg Fatigue, "garlic body odor," irritability, abnormal fingernails, hair loss, skin lesions.
Simple goiter is deficiency disease: enlargement of the thyroid gland, cold intolerance, weight gain, sluggishness, decreased body temperature. Cretinism is deficiency disease caused by inadequate iodine intake during pregnancy: mental retardation, stunted growth, deafness.	Iodized salt; ocean fish and seafood; seaweed; foods produced on iodine-rich soils (usually near an ocean); bread made with dough conditioners; dairy products (if iodine-containing disinfectants are used to clean processing areas).	**UL:** 1,100 µg Toxicity produces goiter.
Anemia, bone abnormalities, immune impairment. Menkes' syndrome is a rare, usually fatal genetic disorder that causes copper deficiency.	Liver, seafood, nuts, whole-grain products, seeds, and legumes.	**UL:** 10 mg Wilson's disease is a genetic disorder of copper retention; untreated it causes nerve and liver problems.

Name	Main Roles	Recommended Intake (Adult)
Manganese	As a cofactor for many enzymes, it assists in energy metabolism, urea synthesis, growth, and reproduction.	**AI** Men: 2.3 mg Women: 1.8 mg
Fluoride	A component of bones and teeth; promotes bone and tooth formation; discourages tooth decay; may reduce risk of osteoporosis.	**AI** Men: 4 mg Women: 3 mg
Chromium	Assists in glucose metabolism.	**AI** 19–50 years: men 35 µg 19–50 years: women 30 µg >50 years: men 25 µg >50 years: women 20 µg
Molybdenum	Enzyme cofactor.	**RDA** Adults: 45 µg
Arsenic	Function unclear.	None set.
Boron	Appears to be involved in bone metabolism.	Probable need of ~1 mg
Nickel	Enzyme cofactor.	Probable need of ~100–300 µg
Silicon	Appears to be involved in bone metabolism.	None set.
Vanadium	Function unclear.	None set.

AI, Adequate Intake; RDA, Recommended Dietary Allowance; UL, Tolerable Upper Intake Level.

(continues)

Trace and Ultra-Trace Minerals (*continued*)

Deficiency	Good Food Sources	Toxicity
None identified in humans.	Whole-grain and cereal products; tea and coffee; cloves; fruits, dried fruits, and vegetables.	**UL:** 11 mg Toxicity is likely to occur from breathing manganese-containing dust, not from diet. Impaired coordination and memory.
Increased tooth decay; possibly increased risk of bone fractures from osteoporosis.	Water, fluoridated or with naturally occurring fluoride. Beverages and foods made with fluoride-containing water.	**UL:** 10 mg Chronic excessive consumption causes fluorosis: discoloration of the teeth, kidney problems, possible muscle or nerve problems. Chronic intake of 2–8 mg daily can mottle children's teeth. Acute fluoride toxicity causes headaches, nausea, abnormal heart rhythm.
Neurological disorders from long-term chromium-free total parenteral nutrition.	Nuts, chocolate, whole grains, mushrooms, asparagus.	Airborne chromium is toxic, but toxicity of dietary sources is unclear.
Weakness, confusion from long-term molybdenum-free total parenteral nutrition.	Peas, beans, organ meats, cereals.	**UL:** 2 mg Possible reproductive problems.
None reported.		Not determined. Excess is clearly toxic. No UL has been set.
None reported.		**UL:** 20 mg Poor appetite, nausea.
None reported.		**UL:** 1 mg Possible delayed growth. Airborne nickel is toxic.
None reported.		Not determined. Airborne silicon causes lung disease. No UL has been set.
None reported.		**UL:** 1.8 mg Possible kidney problems.

Appendix E   The Gastrointestinal Tract

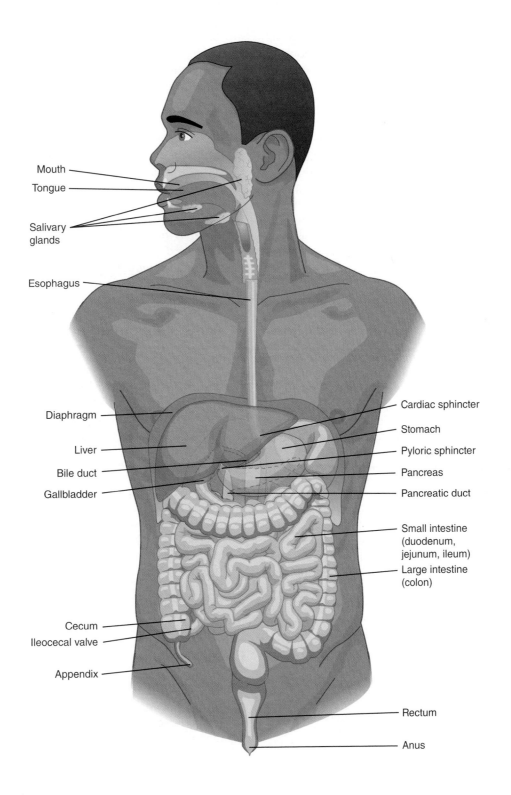

Mouth

Tongue

Salivary glands

Esophagus

Diaphragm

Liver

Bile duct

Gallbladder

Cecum

Ileocecal valve

Appendix

Cardiac sphincter

Stomach

Pyloric sphincter

Pancreas

Pancreatic duct

Small intestine (duodenum, jejunum, ileum)

Large intestine (colon)

Rectum

Anus

Mouth

- In the mouth, food is broken up by chewing with the teeth and tongue. Saliva lubricates food and makes swallowing easier. Salivary amylase begins the digestion of starch. The mouth warms or cools the food so that it is closer to body temperature. When the food bolus (a fairly liquid ball of food) is ready, swallowing is consciously initiated.

Tongue

- The tongue is a mobile mass of muscle that helps teeth tear food into pieces by forcing it against the bony palate. The tongue contains receptors for sweet, salty, sour, and bitter tastes. Umami, a fifth taste elicited by monosodium glutamate, is a meaty, savory sensation. Flavor is a complex combination of taste, smells (the nose has about 6 million olfactory receptor cells), physical sensations (e.g., spicy foods), and food texture.

Salivary Glands

- The three pairs of salivary glands produce saliva. The water in saliva helps dissolve food particles, facilitating taste sensations. The mucus in saliva lubricates food for swallowing and transport. Digestive enzymes begin breaking down foodstuffs. Salivary amylase begins the chemical breakdown of starches into simple sugars. Lingual lipase initiates the breakdown of fat. The mineral sodium and the enzyme lysozyme in the saliva act as disinfectants, destroying bacteria and other microorganisms in food.

Epiglottis

- The epiglottis is a flap of tissue that acts as a valve during swallowing. It closes the entrance to the larynx and prevents food from entering the respiratory passages.

Trachea

- These tubes allow air to pass to and from the lungs.

Esophagus

- The esophagus is the tube that connects the mouth to the stomach. Wavelike muscle action (peristalsis) moves food through the esophagus to the stomach. The upper one-third of the muscles of the esophagus are under voluntary control, the middle third are a mixture of voluntarily controlled muscle and automatically controlled smooth muscle, and the lower third is smooth muscle alone.

Cardiac Sphincter

- The cardiac sphincter is a muscular valve at the lower end of the esophagus. This control valve relaxes to allow food to pass into the stomach. When contracted, it prevents backflow (reflux) of stomach contents into the esophagus. Named for its proximity to the heart, a malfunction can cause painful esophageal reflux (heartburn), which can be so severe that it is mistaken for a heart attack.

Stomach

- The upper bag-like portion of the stomach acts as a hopper to receive and hold the food prior to delivery to the lower two-thirds. Three layers of smooth muscle surround this lower portion of the stomach. Muscular contractions churn the food, so the solids can ferment and mix with acids, fluid, and protein-splitting enzymes. The result is a sticky semiliquid, called chyme, that is gradually released into the duodenum (the first part of the small intestine). Stomach acid halts the digestion of starch, but the stomach also produces gastric lipase, an enzyme that acts on fat.

Pyloric Sphincter

- The pyloric sphincter is a muscular valve that controls passage of chyme from the stomach to the small intestine. When contracted, it prevents backflow from the small intestine into the stomach.

Liver

- The liver is the body's chemical factory and detoxification center. It has many functions in controlling metabolism and deactivating hormones, drugs, and toxins. It also produces bile—a mixture of bile salts, phospholipids, cholesterol, pigments, proteins, and inorganic ions such as sodium. The detergent-like action of bile emulsifies fat, facilitating fat digestion.

Gallbladder

- The gallbladder stores and concentrates bile. The arrival of fatty food in the duodenum stimulates the release of the duodenal hormone CCK, which signals the gallbladder to contract. The bile is then released into the duodenum, where it aids fat digestion.

Bile Duct

- The bile duct carries bile from the gallbladder to the duodenum.

Pancreas

- The pancreas is a complex gland that produces a pancreatic juice rich in bicarbonate and enzymes. The pancreatic juice is released into the duodenum where it does its work. Pancreatic amylase breaks down starch into maltose. Lipase splits fats into monoglycerides, fatty acids, and glycerol. The pancreatic proenzyme trypsinogen is converted to the enzyme trypsin. Trypsin splits polypeptides and proteins into amino acids. Bicarbonate produced by the pancreas neutralizes the acid chyme that enters the small intestine. In addition, the pancreas produces insulin and glucagon—hormones that have important roles in regulating carbohydrate metabolism and blood sugar.

Pancreatic Duct

- The pancreatic duct carries pancreatic juice from the pancreas to the duodenum.

Small Intestine

- The small intestine is a tube approximately 10 feet long that is divided into three parts: the duodenum (the first 10 to 12 inches), the jejunum (about 4 feet), and the ileum (about 5 feet). Whereas the duodenum is mainly responsible for breaking down food, the jejunum and ileum primarily deal with the absorption of food. The duodenum secretes mucus, enzymes, and hormones to aid digestion. Most digestion and absorption occur in the small intestine. Intestinal cells secrete disaccharidases and peptidases to help complete carbohydrate and protein digestion. The intestinal lining is highly folded to increase its surface area and is richly supplied with circulatory vessels, which carry away absorbed nutrients in the blood and lymph. Undigested material is passed on to the large intestine.

Ileocecal Valve (sphincter)

- The ileocecal valve is the sphincter at the lower end of the small intestine. When open, it permits food residue to move from the small intestine to the large intestine. When closed, it prevents backflow from the large intestine.

Large Intestine

- The large intestine is made up of the appendix, cecum, colon, rectum, and anus. The colon is about 2.5 inches in diameter and about 4 feet long. In the large intestine, bacteria break down dietary fiber and other undigested carbohydrates, releasing acids and gas. The large intestine absorbs water and minerals while dehydrating and processing the remaining undigested material into solid feces. The colon walls secrete a viscous mucus to help lubricate and mold the feces. This mucus also helps protect the colon wall from mechanical damage.

Appendix

- The appendix is a fingerlike appendage attached to the cecum, the first part of the colon. The appendix has no known function.

Cecum

- The cecum is the pouchlike beginning of the large intestine. The small intestine's ileum empties into the cecum.

Rectum

- The rectum stores waste prior to elimination.

Anus

- The anal sphincter holds the rectum closed. Either voluntary or involuntary control may open it to allow elimination.

Appendix F ATP Produced from Macronutrients

Pathway	ATP formed by pathway	ATP formed by electron transport chain
Glycolysis (1 glucose)		
Net 2 ATP (4 produced − 2 used)	2	
2 NADH[a]		3 to 5
Pyruvate to Acetyl CoA (2 pyruvate)		
First pyruvate → Acetyl CoA		
1 NADH		2.5
Second pyruvate → Acetyl CoA		
1 NADH		2.5
Citric Acid Cycle (twice)		
First acetyl CoA → Citric acid cycle		
1 GTP (ATP)	1	
1 FADH$_2$		1.5
3 NADH		7.5
Second acetyl CoA → Citric acid cycle		
1 GTP (ATP)	1	
1 FADH$_2$		1.5
3 NADH		7.5
Subtotal	4	26 to 28
	Total = 30 to 32	

FIGURE F.1 The complete breakdown of glucose. These metabolic pathways and molecules move energy from glucose to ATP. Complete breakdown of one glucose molecule yields 30 to 32 ATP.

Note: [a] Each NADH molecule formed in the cytosol by glycolysis will produce either 2.5 or 1.5 ATP molecules in the electron transport chain. NADH formed by the citric acid cycle will produce 2.5 ATP molecules in the electron transport chain.

Pathway	ATP yield
Beta Oxidation (stearic acid C18:0)	
8 NADH	20
8 FADH$_2$	12
Citric Acid Cycle (9 acetyl CoA)	
1 GTP x 9 = 9 GTP	9
1 FADH$_2$ x 9 = 9 FADH$_2$	13.5
3 NADH x 9 = 27 NADH	67.5
Subtotal	122
ATP needed to start beta-oxidation	−2
Net Yield	**120**

The Grand Total:
120 ATP molecules from one molecule of stearic acid

FIGURE F.2 The complete breakdown of stearic acid. The complete breakdown of one 18-carbon fatty acid yields about four times as much ATP as the complete breakdown of one glucose molecule.

Pathway		ATP yield
Alanine to Pyruvate		0
Pyruvate to Acetyl CoA		
1 NADH		2.5
Citric Acid Cycle		
1 GTP (ATP)		1
1 FADH$_2$		1.5
3 NADH		7.5
	Total	12.5

FIGURE F.3 The complete breakdown of alanine. The complete breakdown of the amino acid alanine yields about one-third the ATP of the complete breakdown of one glucose molecule.

Pathway		ATP yield
Methionine to Succinyl CoA[a]		0
Citric Acid Cycle (partial)		
1 GTP (ATP)		1
1 FADH$_2$		1.5
1 NADH		2.5
	Total	5

FIGURE F.4 The complete breakdown of methionine. The complete breakdown of the amino acid methionine yields about one-sixth the ATP of one glucose molecule.

Note: [a] Succinyl CoA is an intermediate of the citric acid cycle.

Appendix G   Major Metabolic Pathways

- ▸ **Glycolysis**
- ▸ **Citric Acid Cycle**
- ▸ **Electron Transport Chain**
- ▸ **Urea Cycle**

Glycolysis

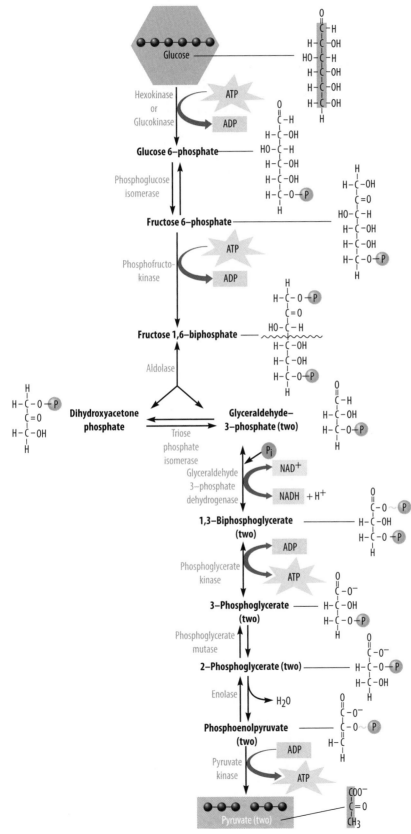

Glycolysis is the first step in metabolizing glucose and other monosaccharides for energy. Unlike the reaction that converts blood glucose to glucose 6-phosphate, the reaction that converts glucose from glycogen to glucose 6-phosphate does not require ATP. Thus the glycolysis of glucose from glycogen directly yields 3 ATP as compared to the 2 ATP from blood glucose. Additional ATP is produced from glycolytic NADH in the electron transport chain.

The reactions that convert fructose to fructose 6-phosphate require ATP so fructose produces the same amount of ATP as blood glucose. The same is true for galactose, which enters at glucose 6-phosphate.

Citric Acid Cycle

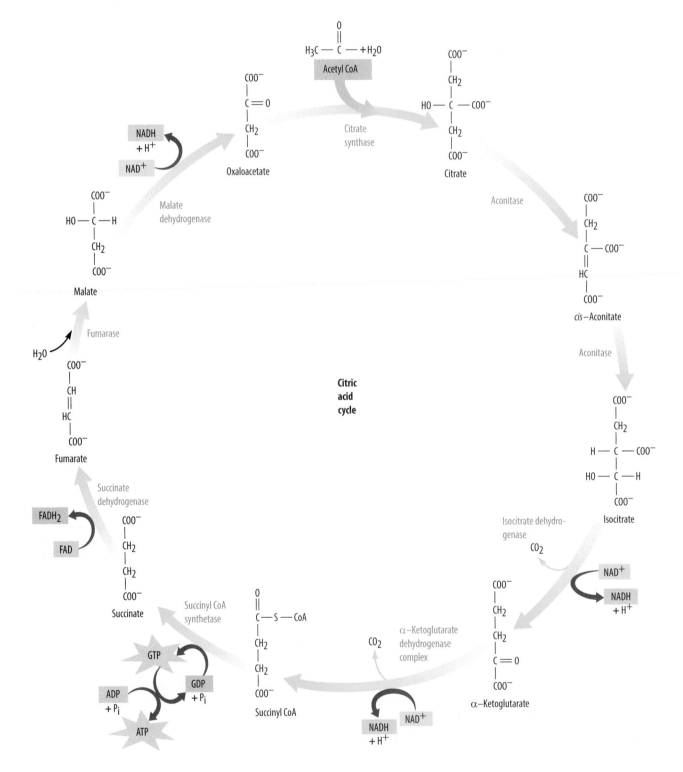

Electron Transport Chain

(site of oxidative phosphorylation)

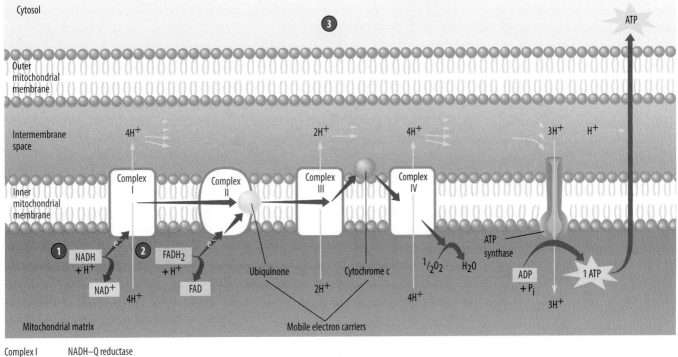

Complex I	NADH–Q reductase
Complex II	Succinate–Q reductase
Complex III	Cytochrome reductase
Complex IV	Cytochrome oxidase

Complexes I, III, and IV are proton (H$^+$) pumps. Complex II does not pump protons. The three proton pumps are linked by the mobile electron carriers ubiquinone and cytochrome c.

NADH

1 A pair of electrons from NADH enters the chain at complex I (NADH-Q reductase). The flow of electrons from NADH to ubiquinone leads to the pumping of 4 H$^+$ from the matrix to the intermembrane space. The flow of electrons from ubiquinone to cytochrome c through complex III (cytochrome reductase) pumps another 2 H$^+$ into the intermembrane space. As complex IV (cytochrome oxidase) catalyzes the transfer of electrons from cytochrome c to O$_2$, it pumps another 4 H$^+$. (Complex IV actually uses 4 electrons to produce 2 H$_2$O from a single O$_2$.) The transit of the NADH electron pair through the electron transport chain pumps a total of 10 H$^+$ into the intermembrane space. Each 3 H$^+$ returning to the matrix through the ATP synthase produces 1 ATP. Another H$^+$ is consumed in transporting ATP from the matrix to the cytosol. Thus the two electrons from NADH produce about 2.5 ATP (10 pumped ÷ 4 = 2.5).

FADH$_2$

2 A pair of electrons from FADH$_2$ enter the chain at complex II (succinate-Q), which is the non-pumping complex. The flow of electrons from FADH$_2$ to ubiquinone does not pump any protons to the intermembrane space. The flow of electrons through complexes III and IV is the same as for NADH. Thus the transit of the two FADH$_2$ electrons through the electron transport chain pumps a total of 6 H$^+$ into the intermembrane space and produces about 1.5 ATP (6 ÷ 4 = 1.5).

Cytosolic NADH

3 Glycolysis forms NADH in the cytosol, but the outer mitochondrial membrane is impervious to NADH. How can NADH deliver its electrons to the electron transport chain? NADH transfers its pair of electrons to special carriers that can cross the mitochondrial membrane. One carrier, glycerol 3-phosphate, shuttles the electrons to the matrix and delivers them to FAD, thereby forming FADH$_2$. This FADH$_2$ delivers the electrons to the chain where they form 1.5 ATP. In the heart and liver, malate shuttles the electrons from cytosolic NADH to the matrix. Malate crosses the mitochondrial membrane and delivers the electrons to NAD$^+$, thereby forming NADH inside the mitochondrion. This NADH delivers the electron pair to the chain where they form 2.5 ATP. Depending on the carrier, cytosolic NADH may produce 1.5 or 2.5 ATP.

Urea Cycle

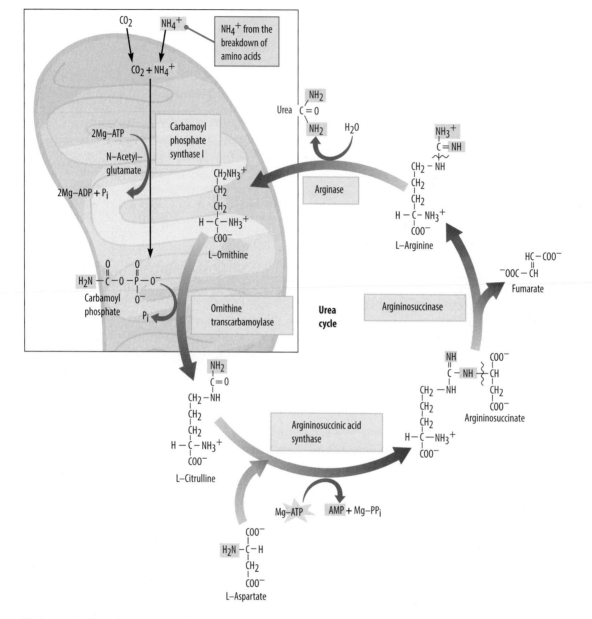

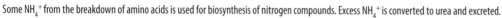

Some NH_4^+ from the breakdown of amino acids is used for biosynthesis of nitrogen compounds. Excess NH_4^+ is converted to urea and excreted.

Appendix **H**   **Food Safety Tables**

▶ **Minimum Internal Cooking Temperatures**
▶ **Cold Storage Chart**

Minimum Internal Cooking Temperatures

Beef, veal, lamb (steaks and roasts) .... 145°F (63°C)
Fish .... 145°F (63°C)
Pork .... 160°F (71°C)
Beef, veal, lamb (ground) .... 160°F (71°C)
Egg dishes .... 160°F (71°C)
Turkey, chicken, and duck
(whole, pieces, and ground) .... 165°F (74°C)
Casseroles and leftovers .... 165°F (74°C)

USDA Food Safety and Inspection Service.

Cold Storage Chart

Because product dates are not a guide for safe use of a product, consult this chart and follow these tips. These short but safe time limits will help keep refrigerated food (40°F) from spoiling or becoming dangerous.

- Purchase the product before "sell-by" or expiration dates.
- Follow handling recommendations on product.
- Keep meat and poultry in its package until just before using.
- If freezing meat and poultry in its original package longer than two months, overwrap these packages with airtight heavy-duty foil, plastic wrap, or freezer paper, or place the package inside a plastic bag.

Because freezing (0°F) keeps food safe indefinitely, recommended freezer storage times are for quality only.

Product	Refrigerator	Freezer
Eggs		
Fresh, in shell	3 weeks	Don't freeze
Raw yolks, whites	2 to 4 days	1 year
Hard cooked	1 week	Doesn't freeze well
Liquid pasteurized eggs or egg substitutes		
Opened	3 days	Don't freeze
Unopened	10 days	1 year
Cooked egg dishes	3 to 4 days	Doesn't freeze well
Dairy Products		
Swiss, brick, processed cheese	3 to 4 weeks	Can be frozen, but freezing can affect texture and taste
Mayonnaise, Commercial		
Refrigerate after opening	2 months	Don't freeze
TV Dinners, Frozen Casseroles		
Keep frozen until ready to heat	Keep frozen	3 to 4 months

Product	Refrigerator	Freezer
Deli and Vacuum-Packed Products		
Store-prepared (or homemade) egg, chicken, tuna, ham, macaroni salads	3 to 5 days	Doesn't freeze well
Pre-stuffed pork and lamb chops, chicken breasts stuffed with dressing	1 day	Doesn't freeze well
Store-cooked convenience meals	3 to 4 days	Doesn't freeze well
Commercial brand vacuum-packed dinners with USDA seal, unopened	2 weeks	Doesn't freeze well
Raw Hamburger, Ground and Stew Meat		
Hamburger and stew meats	1 to 2 days	3 to 4 months
Ground turkey, veal, pork, lamb, and mixtures of them	1 to 2 days	3 to 4 months
Ham, Corned Beef		
Corned beef in pouch with pickling juices	5 to 7 days	Drained, 1 month
Ham, canned, labeled "Keep Refrigerated"		
Opened	3 to 5 days	1 to 2 months
Unopened	6 to 9 months	Don't freeze
Ham, fully cooked, whole	7 days	1 to 2 months
Ham, fully cooked, half	3 to 5 days	1 to 2 months
Ham, fully cooked, slices	3 to 4 days	1 to 2 months
Hot Dogs and Lunch Meats (in freezer wrap)		
Hot dogs		
Opened package	1 week	1 to 2 months
Unopened package	2 weeks	1 to 2 months
Lunch meats		
Opened package	3 to 5 days	1 to 2 months
Unopened package	2 weeks	1 to 2 months
Soups and Stews		
Vegetable or meat-added	3 to 4 days	2 to 3 months
Bacon and Sausage		
Bacon	7 days	1 month
Sausage, raw from pork, beef, chicken, or turkey	1 to 2 days	1 to 2 months
Smoked breakfast links, patties	7 days	1 to 2 months
Summer sausage labeled "Keep Refrigerated"		
Opened	3 weeks	1 to 2 months
Unopened	3 months	1 to 2 months
Fresh Meat (Beef, Veal, Lamb, and Pork)		
Steaks	3 to 5 days	6 to 12 months
Chops	3 to 5 days	4 to 6 months
Roasts	3 to 5 days	4 to 12 months
Variety meats (tongue, kidneys, liver, heart, chitterlings)	1 to 2 days	3 to 4 months

Product	Refrigerator	Freezer
Meat Leftovers		
Cooked meat and meat dishes	3 to 4 days	2 to 3 months
Gravy and meat broth	1 to 2 days	2 to 3 months
Fresh Poultry		
Chicken or turkey, whole	1 to 2 days	1 year
Chicken or turkey, parts	1 to 2 days	9 months
Giblets	1 to 2 days	3 to 4 months
Cooked Poultry, Leftover		
Fried chicken	3 to 4 days	4 months
Cooked poultry dishes	3 to 4 days	4 to 6 months
Pieces, plain	3 to 4 days	4 months
Pieces covered with broth, gravy	1 to 2 days	6 months
Chicken nuggets, patties	1 to 2 days	1 to 3 months
Fish		
Lean (such as cod)	1 to 2 days	Up to 6 months
Fatty (such as blue, perch, salmon)	1 to 2 days	2 to 3 months

Reproduced from USDA Food Safety and Inspection Service with data from Food Marketing Institute for fish and dairy products only.

Appendix I   Information Resources

Academic

www.mayoclinic.com/findinformation
   /healthylivingcenter/index.cfm
Mayo Clinic nutrition information

www.navigator.tufts.edu
Tufts University Nutrition Navigator

Aging

www.aoa.gov
Administration on Aging
330 Independence Avenue SW
Washington, DC 20201
1-202-619-7501

www.aarp.org
American Association of Retired Persons (AARP)
601 E Street NW
Washington, DC 20049
1-800-424-3410

www.americangeriatrics.org
American Geriatrics Society
The Empire State Building
350 Fifth Avenue, Suite 801
New York, NY 10118
1-212-308-1414

www.aoa.gov/naic
National Aging Information Center
330 Independence Avenue SW
Washington, DC 20201
1-202-619-7501

www.ncoa.org
National Council on the Aging
1828 L Street NW
Washington, DC 20036

www.nia.nih.gov
National Institute on Aging
Building 31, Room 5C27
31 Center Drive, MSC 2292
Bethesda, MD 20892
1-301-496-1752

www.nof.org
National Osteoporosis Foundation
1232 22nd Street NW
Washington, DC 20037-1292
1-202-223-2226

Alcohol and Drug Abuse

www.al-anon.alateen.org
Al-Anon/Alateen
1600 Corporate Landing Parkway
Virginia Beach, VA 23154-5617
1-888-425-2666; 1-757-563-1600

www.aa.org
Alcoholics Anonymous (AA)
General Service Office
Grand Central Station
P.O. Box 459
New York, NY 10163
1-212-870-3400

http://prevention.samhsa.gov/
Center for Substance Abuse Prevention
Substance Abuse and Mental Health Services
   Administration
1 Choke Cherry Road
Room 8-1054
Rockville, MD 20857
1-240-276-2420; fax: 1-240-276-2430

www.wsoinc.com
Narcotics Anonymous (NA)
P.O. Box 9999
Van Nuys, CA 91409
1-818-773-9999; fax: 1-818-700-0700

www.health.org
National Clearinghouse for Alcohol and Drug
   Information (NCADI)
P.O. Box 2345
Rockville, MD 20847-2345
1-800-729-6686

Alcohol and Drug Abuse (*continued*)

www.ncadd.org
National Council on Alcoholism and Drug
 Dependence (NCADD)
20 Exchange Place
Suite 2902
New York, NY 10005
1-800-622-2255; 1-212-269-7797; fax: 1-212-269-7510

Canadian Government: Federal

www.agr.gc.ca
Agriculture and Agri-Food Canada
Public Information Request Services
Sir John Carling Building
930 Carling Avenue
Ottawa, ON K1A 0C7
1-613-759-1000; fax: 1-613-759-6726

www.hc-sc.gc.ca/food-aliment/ns-sc/e_nutrition.html
Bureau of Nutritional Sciences
Nutrition Evaluation Division
Sir Fredrick G. Banting Research Center
Tunney's Pasture (2203A)
Ottawa, ON K1A 0L2
1-613-957-0352; fax: 1-613-941-6636

www.hc-sc.gc.ca/food-aliment/ns-sc/e_nutrition.html
Bureau of Nutritional Sciences
Nutrition Research Division
Sir Fredrick G. Banting Research Center
Tunney's Pasture (2203C)
Ottawa, ON K1A 0L2
1-613-957-0919; fax: 1-613-941-6182

www.inspection.gc.ca
Canadian Food Inspection Agency
59 Camelot Drive
Ottowa, ON K1A 0Y9
1-800-442-2342; 1-613-225-2342; fax: 1-613-228-6653

www.cihi.ca
Canadian Institute for Health Information
377 Dalhousie Street
Suite 200
Ottawa, ON K1N 9N8
1-613-241-7860; fax: 1-613-241-8120

www.cpha.ca
Canadian Public Health Association
400-1565 Carling Avenue
Ottawa, ON K1Z 8R1
1-613-725-3769; fax: 1-613-725-9826

www.agr.gc.ca/misb/fb-ba/nutra/index_e.php?
 page=intro
Functional Foods and Nutraceuticals
Food Bureau
597-930 Carling Avenue
Ottawa, ON K1A 0C5

www.hc-sc.gc.ca
Health Canada

www.ccfn.ca
The Canadian Council of Food and Nutrition
3800 Steeles Avenue West, Suite 301A
Woodbridge, ON L4L 4G9
1-905-265-1349

Canadian Government: Provincial and Territorial

Consultant, Nutrition
Health and Wellness Promotion, Population Health,
 Department of Health and Social Services, Government
 of the Northwest Territories
Center Square Tower, 6th Floor
P.O. Box 1320
Yellowknife, NT X1A 2L9

Coordinator, Health Information
 Resource Center
Department of Health and Social Services
1 Rochford Street, Box 2000
Charlottetown, PEI C1A 7N8

Director, Health Promotion
Department of Health, Government of Newfoundland
 and Labrador
P.O. Box 8700
Confederation Building, West Block
St. John's, NF A1B 4J6
Director, Nutrition Services
Yukon Hospital Corporation
#5 Hospital Road
Whitehorse, YT Y1A 3H7

Executive Director
Health Programs
2nd Floor 800 Portage Avenue
Winnipeg, MB R3G 0P4

Health Promotion Unit
Population Health Branch
Saskatchewan Health
3475 Albert Street
Regina, SK S4S 6X6

Canadian Government: Provincial and Territorial (*continued*)

Nutritionist
Preventive Services Branch
Ministry of Health
1520 Blanshard Street
Victoria, BC V8W 3C8

Population Health Strategies Branch
Alberta Health
23rd Floor, TELUS Plaza, North Tower
10025 Jasper Avenue
Edmonton, AB T5J 2N3

Project Manager, Public Health Management Services
Health and Community Services
P.O. Box 5100
520 King Street
Fredericton, NB E3B 5G8

Public Health Nutritionist
Central Health Region
201 Brownlow Avenue, Unit 4
Dartmouth, NS B3B 1W2

Responsables de la santé cardiovasculaire et de la
  nutrition
Ministère de la Santé et des Services sociaux, Service
  de la Prévention en Santé
3e étage, 1075, chemin Sainte-Foy
Québec (Québec) G1S 2M1

Senior Consultant, Nutrition
Public Health Branch
Ministry of Health, 8th Floor
5700 Yonge St.
New York, ON M2M 4K5

Complementary and Alternative Nutrition

http://nccam.nih.gov/
National Center for Complementary and Alternative
  Medicine, NIH
Bethesda, MD 20892
(888) 644-6226

www.hc-sc.gc.ca/hpb/onhp/
Office of Natural Health Products
171 Slater Street
9th Floor
Ottawa, ON K1P 5H7
1-613-946-1615

Consumer Organizations

www.diabetes.ca
Canadian Diabetes Association

15 Toronto Street
Suite 800
Toronto, ON M5C 2E3
1-800-226-8464; 1-416-363-3373

www.cspinet.org
Center for Science in the Public Interest (CSPI)
1875 Connecticut Ave NW, Suite 300
Washington, DC 20009-5728
1-202-332-9110; fax: 1-202-265-4954

www.consumersunion.org
Consumers Union
101 Truman Avenue
Yonkers, NY 10703-1057
1-914-378-2000

www.pueblo.gsa.gov
Federal Consumer Information Center
Pueblo, CO 81009
1-800-688-9889; 1-888-878-3256

www.ncahf.org
National Council Against Health Fraud, Inc. (NCAHF)
119 Foster Street
Peabody, MA 01960
1-978-532-9383

www.quackwatch.com
Stephen Barrett, MD
P.O. Box 1747
Allentown, PA 18105
1-610-437-1795

Eating Disorders

www.anred.com
Anorexia Nervosa and Related Eating Disorders
  (ANRED)
P.O. Box 5102
Eugene, OR 97405
1-541-344-1144

www.anad.org
National Association of Anorexia Nervosa and Associated
  Disorders, Inc. (ANAD)
P.O. Box 7
Highland Park, IL 60035
1-847-831-3438; fax: 1-847-433-4632

www.nedic.ca
National Eating Disorder Information Centre
200 Elizabeth Street, CW 1-211
Toronto, Ontario M5G 2C4
1-866-633-4220; 1-416-340-4156; fax: 1-416-340-4736

Eating Disorders (*continued*)

www.nationaleatingdisorders.org
National Eating Disorders Association
603 Stewart Street, Suite 803
Seattle, WA 98101
1-206-382-3587

Food Safety

www.foodandfarming.info
The Alliance for Food & Farming
P.O. Box 2747
Watsonville, CA 95077
1-831-786-1666; fax: 1-831-786-1668

www.cfsan.fda.gov
FDA Center for Food Safety and Applied Nutrition
5100 Paint Branch Parkway
College Park, MD 20740
1-888-723-3366

www.epa.gov/opptintr/lead/nlic.htm
National Lead Information Center
1-800-424-5323

www.npic.orst.edu/index.html
National Pesticide Information Center
Oregon State University
333 Weniger Hall
Corvallis, OR 97331-6502
1-800-858-7378

Seafood Safety Hotline
1-800-332-4010; 1-202-205-4314

U.S. EPA Safe Drinking Water Hotline
1-800-426-4791

www.fsis.usda.gov
USDA Food Safety and Inspection Service
Food Safety Education Office
Room 1180-S
Washington, DC 20250
1-202-720-3333

USDA Meat and Poultry Hotline
1-800-535-4555

Infancy, Childhood, and Adolescence

www.aap.org
American Academy of Pediatrics
141 Northwest Point Boulevard
Elk Grove Village, IL 60007-1098
1-847-434-4000; fax: 1-847-434-8000

www.birthdefects.org
Birth Defect Research for Children, Inc.
930 Woodcock Road
Suite 225
Orlando, FL 32803
1-407-895-0802

www.cps.ca
Canadian Paediatric Society
100-2204 Walkley Road
Ottawa, ON K1G 4G8
1-613-526-9397; fax: 1-613-526-3332

www.childrensfoundation.net
Children's Foundation
725 Fifteenth Street NW
Suite 505
Washington, DC 20005-2109
1-202-347-3300; fax: 1-202-347-3382

www.KidsHealth.org
KidsHealth
The Nemours Foundation

www.ncemch.org
National Center for Education in Maternal &
   Child Health
2000 15th Street North
Suite 701
Arlington, VA 22201-2617
1-703-524-7802

International Agencies

www.fao.org
Food and Agriculture Organization of the United
   Nations (FAO)
Liaison Office for North America
2175 K Street, Suite 300
Washington, DC 20437
1-202-653-2400

www.ific.org
International Food Information Council Foundation
1100 Connecticut Avenue NW
Suite 430
Washington, DC 20036
1-202-296-6540

www.unicef.org
UNICEF
3 United Nations Plaza
New York, NY 10017
1-212-326-7000; fax: 1-212-887-7465

International Agencies (*continued*)

www.who.int/home-page
World Health Organization (WHO)
Regional Office
525 23rd Street NW
Washington, DC 20037
1-202-974-3000; fax: 1-202-974-3663

Pregnancy and Lactation

www.acog.org
American College of Obstetricians and Gynecologists
   Resource Center
409 12th Street SW
Washington, DC 20024-2188
1-202-638-5577

www.lalecheleague.org
La Leche League International, Inc.
1400 N. Meacham Road
Schaumburg, IL 60173-4048
1-847-519-7730

www.modimes.org
March of Dimes Birth Defects Foundation
1275 Mamaroneck Avenue
White Plains, NY 10605
1-888-663-4637

Professional Nutrition Organizations

ADA, The Nutrition Line
1-800-366-1655

www.eatright.org
Academy of Nutrition and Dietetics
216 West Jackson Boulevard
Suite 800
Chicago, IL 60606-6995
1-800-877-1600; 1-312-899-0040

www.ascn.org
American Society for Clinical Nutrition
9650 Rockville Pike
Bethesda, MD 20814-3998
1-301-530-7110; fax: 1-301-634-7350

www.asns.org
American Society for Nutritional Sciences
9650 Rockville Pike
Suite 4500
Bethesda, MD 20814
1-301-634-7050; fax: 1-301-634-7892

Canadian Dietetic Association
480 University Avenue
Suite 601
Toronto, ON M5G 1V2

Canadian Society for Nutritional Sciences
Department of Food and Nutrition
University of Manitoba
Winnipeg, MB R3T 2N2

www.dietitians.ca
Dietitians of Canada
480 University Avenue, Suite 604
Toronto, ON M5G 1V2
1-416-596-0857; fax: 1-416-596-0603

http://hni.ilsi.org
ILSI Human Nutrition Institute (HNI)
One Thomas Circle
Washington, DC 20005
1-202-659-0524; fax: 1-202-659-3617

www.ift.org
Institute of Food Technologists
525 West Van Buren
Suite 1000
Chicago, IL 60607
1-312-782-8424; fax: 1-312-782-8348

www.nationalacademies.org/nrc
National Academy of Sciences/National Research
   Council (NAS/NRC)
2101 Constitution Avenue NW
Washington, DC 20418
1-202-234-2000

www.sne.org
Society for Nutrition Education
9202 North Meridian
Suite 200
Indianapolis, IN 46260
1-800-235-6690

Sports Nutrition

www.acsm.org
American College of Sports Medicine (ACSM)
401 W. Michigan Street
Indianapolis, IN 46202-3233
1-317-637-9200; fax: 1-317-634-7817

www.acefitness.org
American Council on Exercise (ACE)

Sports Nutrition (*continued*)

4851 Paramount Drive
San Diego, CA 92123
1-800-825-3636

www.cahperd.ca
Canadian Association for Health, Physical Education,
    Recreation, and Dance
403-2197 Riverside Drive
Ottawa, ON K1H 7X3
1-613-523-1348

www.csep.ca
Canadian Society for Exercise Physiology
185 Somerset St. West
Suite 202
Ottawa, ON K2P 0J2
1-613-234-3755; fax: 1-613-234-3565

www.fitness.gov
President's Council on Physical Fitness and Sports
Humphrey Building, Room 738
200 Independence Avenue SW
Washington, DC 20201
1-202-690-9000; fax: 1-202-690-5211

www.runnersworld.com
Runners World
Rodale, Inc.
Emmaus, PA 18098
1-610-967-8809

Sports Medicine and Science Council of Canada
1600 James Naismith Drive
Suite 306
Gloucester, Ontario K1B 5N4
1-613-748-5671; fax: 1-613-748-5729

Sports Safety Board of Quebec
100 Laviolette
Bureau 306
Trois-Riveres, Quebec G9A 5S9
1-819-371-6033

www.scandpg.org
Sports, Cardiovascular and Wellness Nutritionists
    (SCAN)

www.ideafit.com
The International Association for Fitness Professionals
    (IDEA)
6190 Cornerstone Court East # 204

San Diego, CA 92121-3773
1-800-999-4332 ext 7; fax: 1-858-535-8234

www.veggie.org
Veggie Sports Association

Supplements

http://dietary-supplements.info.nih.gov/databases/ibids
.html
International Bibliographic Information on Dietary
    Supplements (IBIDS)
http://dietary-supplements.info.nih.gov
Office of Dietary Supplements
National Institutes of Health
Building 31, Room 1B29
31 Center Drive, MSC 2086
Bethesda, MD 20892-2086
1-301-435-2590; fax: 1-301-480-1845

Trade and Industry Organizations

www.aibonline.org
American Institute of Baking
1213 Bakers Way
P.O. Box 3999
Manhattan, KS 66505-3999
1-800-633-5137; 1-785-537-4750; fax: 1-785-537-1493

www.meatami.org
American Meat Institute
1700 North Moore Street
Suite 1600
Arlington, VA 22209
1-703-841-2400; fax: 1-703-527-0938

www.beechnut.com
Beech-Nut Nutrition Corporation
100 S. 4th Street
St. Louis, MO 63102
1-800-233-2468

www.gssiweb.com
Gatorade Sports Science Institute
617 West Main Street
Barrington, IL 60010
1-800-616-4774

www.generalmills.com/corporate
General Mills, Inc.
Number One General Mills Boulevard
Minneapolis, MN 55426
1-800-328-6787

Trade and Industry Organizations (*continued*)

www.gerber.com
Gerber Products Co.
445 State Street
Fremont, MI 49413-0001
1-800-443-7237

www.heinz.com
H.J. Heinz Company
World Headquarters
P.O. Box 57
Pittsburgh, PA 15230-0057
1-412-456-5700

www.kelloggs.com
Kellogg Company
P.O. Box 3599
Battle Creek, MI 49016-3599
1-616-961-2000

www.kraftfoods.com
Kraft Foods
Consumer Response and Information Center
One Kraft Court
Glenview, IL 60025
1-800-323-0768

www.nationaldairycouncil.org
National Dairy Council
10255 West Higgins Road
Suite 900
Rosemont, IL 60018-5616
1-847-803-2000

www.pillsbury.com
Pillsbury Company
2866 Pillsbury Center
Minneapolis, MN 55402
1-800-775-4777

www.pg.com
Procter & Gamble Company
One Procter and Gamble Plaza
Cincinnati, OH 45202
1-513-983-1100

www.sunkist.com
Sunkist Growers
Consumer Affairs, Fresh Fruit Division
14130 Riverside Drive
Sherman Oaks, CA 91423
1-800-248-7875

www.dannon.com
The Dannon Company
120 White Plains Road
Tarrytown, NY 10591-5536
1-877-326-6668

www.nutrasweet.com
The NutraSweet Company
P.O. Box 2986
Chicago, IL 60654-0986
1-800-323-5316

www.uffva.org
United Fresh Fruit and Vegetable Association
727 North Washington Street
Alexandria, VA 22314
1-703-836-3410

www.usarice.com
USA Rice Federation
4301 North Fairfax Drive
Suite 305
Arlington, VA 22203
1-703-351-8161

www.cognis.com/veris/verisdefault.htm
VERIS Online Research Information Service

Weight Management

http://nutrition.uvm.edu/bodycomp/
Body Composition Analysis Tutorials

www.overeatersanonymous.org
Overeaters Anonymous (OA)
World Service Office
6075 Zenith Court NE
Rio Rancho, NM 87124
1-505-891-2664; fax: 1-505-891-4320

www.shapeup.org
Shape Up America!
6707 Democracy Boulevard
Suite 306
Bethesda, MD 20817
1-301-493-5368

www.tops.org
TOPS (Take Off Pounds Sensibly)
4575 South Fifth Street
P.O. Box 07360
Milwaukee, WI 53207-0360
1-800-932-8677; 1-414-482-4620

Weight Management (*continued*)

www.niddk.nih.gov/index.htm
Weight-control Information Network
1 WIN Way
Bethesda, MD 20892-3665
1-877-946-4627; 1-202-828-1025;
    fax: 1-202-828-1028

www.weightwatchers.com
Weight Watchers International
Consumer Affairs Department/IN
175 Crossways Park West
Woodbury, NY 11797
1-516-390-1400; fax: 1-516-390-1632

World Hunger

www.bread.org
Bread for the World
50 F Street, NW
Suite 500
Washington, DC 20001
1-800-822-7323; 1-202-639-9400

http://hunger.tufts.edu
Center on Hunger, Poverty, and Nutrition Policy
Tufts University School of Medicine
11 Curtis Avenue
Medford, MA 02155
1-617-627-6223; fax: 1-617-627-3688

www.freefromhunger.org
Freedom from Hunger
1644 DaVinci Court
Davis, CA 95616
1-800-708-2555; fax: 1-530-758-6241

www.oxfamamerica.org
Oxfam America
26 West Street
Boston, MA 02111-1206
1-800-776-9326; fax: 1-617-728-2594

www.worldwatch.org
Worldwatch Institute
1776 Massachusetts Avenue NW
Suite 800
Washington, DC 20036
1-202-452-1999

U.S. Government

www.nutrition.gov
Online federal government information on nutrition

www.cdc.gov
Centers for Disease Control and Prevention
1600 Clifton Road
Atlanta, GA 30333
1-800-311-3435; 1-404-639-3534

FDA Consumer Information Line
(301) 827-4420
FDA Office of Nutritional Products, Labeling, and
    Dietary Supplements
HFS-800
200 C Street SW
Washington, DC 20204
1-202-205-4561; fax: 1-202-205-4594

FDA Office of Plant and Dairy Foods and Beverages
HFS-300
200 C Street SW
Washington, DC 20204
1-202-205-4064; fax: 1-202-205-4422

www.ftc.gov
Federal Trade Commission (FTC)
CRC-240
Washington, DC 20580
1-877-382-4357

www.fda.gov
Food and Drug Administration (FDA)
Office of Consumer Affairs, HFE 1
Room 16-85
5600 Fishers Lane
Rockville, MD 20857
1-888-463-6332; 1-301-443-1544

www.nal.usda.gov/fnic
Food and Nutrition Information Center
National Agricultural Library, Room 105
10301 Baltimore Avenue
Beltsville, MD 20705-2351
1-301-504-5719; fax: 1-301-504-6409

www.frac.org
Food Research and Action Center (FRAC)
1875 Connecticut Avenue NW
Suite 540
Washington, DC 20009
1-202-986-2200; fax: 1-202-986-2525

www.healthfinder.gov
Gateway for Health and Nutrition Information

U.S. Government (*continued*)

www.nidr.nih.gov
National Institute of Dental and Craniofacial Research (NIDCR)
National Institutes of Health
Bethesda, MD 20892-2190
1-301-496-4261

www.niddk.nih.gov
National Institute of Diabetes & Digestive & Kidney Diseases
Office of Communications and Public Liaison
NIDDK, NIH
Building 31, Room 9A04 Center Drive, MSC 2560
Bethesda, MD 20892-2560

www.nih.gov/health
National Institutes of Health search engine and free access to MEDLINE and PubMed databases

www.usda.gov
U.S. Department of Agriculture (USDA)
14th Street SW and Independence Avenue
Washington, DC 20250
1-202-720-2791

www.dhhs.gov
U.S. Department of Health and Human Services

200 Independence Avenue SW
Washington, DC 20201
1-877-696-6775; 1-202-619-0257

www.epa.gov
U.S. Environmental Protection Agency (EPA)
1200 Pennsylvania Avenue NW
Washington, DC 20460
1-202-260-2090

www.pueblo.gsa.gov
U.S. General Services Administration
Federal Communication Information Center
Pueblo, CO 81009

www.bookstore.gpo.gov
U.S. Government Online Bookstore
U.S. Government Printing Office
701 N. Capitol Street, NW
Washington, DC 20401
1-202-512-0132; fax: 1-202-512-1355

www.usda.gov/cnpp
USDA Center for Nutrition Policy and Promotion
3101 Park Center Drive
Room 1034
Alexandria, VA 22302-1594
1-703-305-7600; fax: 1-703-305-3400

Appendix J Calculations and Conversions

Energy from Food

grams carbohydrate × 4 kcal/g
grams protein × 4 kcal/g
grams fat × 9 kcal/g
grams alcohol × 7 kcal/g

---

total = energy from food

Example:

Carbohydrate	275 g × 4 kcal/g = 1,100 kcal
Protein	64 g × 4 kcal/g = 256 kcal
Fat	60 g × 9 kcal/g = 540 kcal
Alcohol	15 g × 7 kcal/g = 105 kcal

TOTAL ENERGY 2,001 kcal

Calculating the percentage of calories for each:

Carbohydrate	(1,100 kcal ÷ 2,001 kcal) × 100 = 54.97% (55%)
Protein	(256 kcal ÷ 2,001 kcal) × 100 = 12.79% (13%)
Fat	(540 kcal ÷ 2,001 kcal) × 100 = 26.99% (27%)
Alcohol	(105 kcal ÷ 2,001 kcal) × 100 = 5.25% (5%)

1 kilocalorie = 4.184 kilojoules
1 kilojoule = 0.239 kilocalories

Recommended Protein Intake for Adults

grams of recommended protein = weight in kilograms × 0.8 g/kg

Example:

A 70-kg (154-lb) person
grams of recommended protein = 70 kg × 0.8 g/kg = 56 grams protein, or
grams of recommended protein = (154 lb ÷ 2.2) × 0.8 g/kg = 56 grams protein

Note: Endurance athletes involved in heavy training may require 1.2 to 1.4 grams of protein per kilogram of body weight per day.

Niacin Equivalents (NE)

Determining the amount of niacin from tryptophan:

NE = milligrams niacin
NE from tryptophan = grams excess protein ÷ 6
NE from tryptophan = (grams dietary protein − protein RDA) ÷ 6

Example:

Assume dietary protein = 86 g and protein RDA = 56 g
NE from tryptophan = (86 g − 56 g) ÷ 6
NE from tryptophan = 5

Dietary Folate Equivalents (DFE)

Dietary folate equivalents account for differences in the absorption of food folate, synthetic folic acid in dietary supplements, and folic acid added to fortified foods. Food in the stomach also affects bioavailability. Folic acid taken as a supplement when fasting is two times more bioavailable than food folate. Folic acid taken with food and folic acid in fortified foods are 1.7 times more bioavailable than food folate.

1 µg DFE = 1 microgram of food folate
          = 0.5 µg of folic acid supplement taken on an empty stomach
          = 0.6 µg of folic acid supplement consumed with meals
          = 0.6 µg of folic acid in fortified foods

1 µg folic acid as a fortificant   = 1.7 µg DFE
1 µg folic acid as a supplement, fasting   = 2.0 µg DFE

Example:

Food folate in cooked spinach	100 µg = 100 µg DFE
Ready-to-eat cereal fortified with folic acid	100 µg = 170 µg DFE
Supplemental folic acid taken without food	100 µg = 200 µg DFE

Estimating DFE from Daily Value:

DFE = %DV × DV × bioavailability factor

Example:
Assume that a serving of fortified breakfast cereal contains 10% of the Daily Value for folate

Daily Value = 400 µg folic acid

DFE = %DV × DV × bioavailability factor
DFE = 0.10 × 400 µg × 1.7
DFE = 68 µg, which can be rounded to 70 µg DFE

Retinol Activity Equivalents (RAE)

Retinol activity equivalents are a standardized measure of vitamin A activity that account for differences in the bioavailability of different sources of vitamin A. Of the provitamin A carotenoids, beta-carotene produces the most vitamin A.

1 µg RAE = 1 µg retinol
          = 12 µg beta-carotene
          = 24 µg of other vitamin A precursors

Many vitamin supplements still report vitamin A content as International Units (IU).

1 µg RAE = 3.33 IU from retinol
          = 10 IU from beta-carotene in supplements
          = 20 IU from beta-carotene in foods

Vitamin D

Many vitamin supplements still report vitamin D content as International Units (IU).

$$1 \text{ IU} = 0.025 \text{ μg cholecalciferol}$$
$$\text{μg cholecalciferol} = \text{IU} \div 40$$

Example:

A vitamin supplement contains 100 IU vitamin D

μg cholecalciferol = 100 ÷ 40 = 2.5

Vitamin E

Although outdated, many vitamin supplements still report vitamin E content as International Units (IU) rather than as milligrams of α-tocopherol. Two conversion factors are used to convert IU to milligrams of α-tocopherol. If the form of the supplement is "natural" or RRR-α-tocopherol (historically labeled as *d*-alpha-tocopherol), the conversion factor is 0.67 mg/IU. If the form of the supplement is *all rac*-α-tocopherol (historically labeled *dl*-α-tocopherol), the conversion factor is 0.45 mg/IU.

Examples:

A multivitamin supplement contains 30 IU of *d*-α-tocopherol

30 IU × 0.67 = 20 mg α-tocopherol

A multivitamin supplement contains 30 IU of *dl*-α-tocopherol

30 IU × 0.45 = 13.5 mg α-tocopherol

Estimating Energy Expenditure

The Estimated Energy Requirement (EER) is defined as the dietary energy intake (in kilocalories per day) that is predicted to maintain energy balance in a healthy adult of a defined age, gender, weight, height, and level of physical activity consistent with good health.* The EER equations predict Total Energy Expenditure (TEE). Adult men (age 19 and older):

$$\text{EER} = 662 - 9.53 \times \text{Age [yr]} + \text{PA} \times (15.91 \times \text{Weight [kg]} + 539.6 \times \text{Height [m]})$$

PA is the Physical Activity coefficient that represents physical activity level.

Sedentary	PA = 1.0
Low active	PA = 1.11
Active	PA = 1.25
Very active	PA = 1.48

Adult women (age 19 and older):

$$\text{EER} = 354 - 6.91 \times \text{Age [yr]} + \text{PA} \times (9.36 \times \text{Weight [kg]} + 726 \times \text{Height [m]})$$

PA is the Physical Activity coefficient that represents physical activity level.

Sedentary	PA = 1.0
Low active	PA = 1.12
Active	PA = 1.27
Very active	PA = 1.45

Example:

A 21-year-old woman, 5'4" (1.6 m) tall, who weighs 120 pounds (54.5 kilograms) and is active

$$= 354 - 6.91 \times 21 \text{ yr} + 1.27 \times$$
$$(9.36 \times 54.5 \text{ kg} + 726 \times 1.6 \text{ m})$$
$$= 354 - 145.11 + 1.27 \times (510.12 + 1{,}161.6)$$
$$= 354 - 145.11 + 1.27 \times 1{,}671.72$$
$$= 354 - 145.11 + 2{,}123.08$$
$$= 2{,}331.97$$
$$= 2{,}332 \text{ kcal/day}$$

*Institute of Medicine, Food, and Nutrition Board. *Dietary Reference Intakes for Energy, Carbohydrate, Fiber, Fat, Fatty Acids, Cholesterol, Protein, and Amino Acids.* Washington, DC: National Academy Press; 2005.

Total energy expenditure can also be estimated by first estimating resting energy expenditure (REE) and then adding additional energy to account for physical activity and the thermic effect of food.

Resting Energy Expenditure (REE)

Harris-Benedict Equations

Adult men	$\text{REE} = 66 + 13.7W + 5.0H - 6.8A$
Adult women	$\text{REE} = 655 + 9.6W + 1.8H - 4.7A$

(W = weight in kilograms, H = height in centimeters, A = age)

Note: Harris-Benedict equations may overestimate resting energy expenditure, especially for obese people.

Quick Estimate

Adult men	$\text{REE} = \text{weight (kg)} \times 1.0 \text{ kcal/kg} \times 24 \text{ hours}$
	$\text{REE} = \text{weight (kg)} \times 1.0 \times 24$
Adult women	$\text{REE} = \text{weight (kg)} \times 0.9 \text{ kcal/kg} \times 24 \text{ hours}$
	$\text{REE} = \text{weight (kg)} \times 0.9 \times 24$

Physical Activity (PA)

Physical activity can be estimated as a percentage of the resting energy expenditure (REE) based on the frequency and intensity of physical activity.

Percentage of REE	Activity Level	Descriptor
20–30%	Sedentary	Mostly resting, with little or no activity
30–45%	Light	Occasional unplanned activity (e.g., going for a stroll)
45–65%	Moderate	Daily planned activity, such as brisk walks
65–90%	Heavy	Daily workout routine requiring several hours of continuous exercise
90–120%	Exceptional	Daily vigorous workouts for extended hours; training for competition

Thermic Effect of Food (TEF)

The thermic effect of food can be estimated as 10% of the sum of REE + PA.

Total energy expenditure (TEE) = REE + PA + TEF

Example using quick estimate of REE:

A 175-pound (79.5 kg), 30-year-old man engages in moderate activity (60% of REE).

REE = 79.5 kg × 1.0 kcal/kg/hr × 24 hr/day
= 1,908 kcal/day

PA = 60% of REE
= 0.60 × 1908 kcal/day
= 1144.8 kcal/day

TEF = 10% of REE + PA
= 0.10 × (1908 + 1144.8 kcal/day)
= 0.10 × 3052.8 kcal/day
= 305.3 kcal/day

TEE = REE + PA + TEF
= 1908 + 1144.8 + 305.3 kcal/day
= 3358 kcal/day

Body Mass Index (BMI)

U.S. Formula

BMI = [weight in pounds ÷ (height in inches)^2] × 703

Example:

A 154-pound man is 5 ft 8 inches (68 inches) tall
BMI = [154 ÷ (68 in × 68 in)] × 703
BMI = (154 ÷ 4,624) × 703
BMI = 23.41

Metric Formula

BMI = weight in kilograms ÷ [height in meters]^2
or
BMI = [weight in kilograms ÷ (height in cm)^2] × 10,000

Example:

A 70-kg man is 1.75 meters tall
BMI = 70 kg ÷ (1.75 m × 1.75 m)
BMI = 70 ÷ 3.0625
BMI = 22.86

Metric Prefixes

giga-	G	1,000,000,000
mega-	M	1,000,000
kilo-	k	1,000
hecto-	h	100
deka-	da	10
deci-	d	0.1
centi-	c	0.01
milli-	m	0.001
micro-	μ	0.000001
nano-	n	0.000000001

Length: Metric and U.S. Equivalents

1 centimeter	0.3937 inch
1 decimeter	3.937 inches
1 foot	0.3048 meter
1 inch	2.54 centimeters
1 meter	39.37 inches
	1.094 yards
1 micron	0.001 millimeter
	0.00003937 inch
1 millimeter	0.03937 inch
1 yard	0.9144 meter

Capacities or Volumes

1 cup, measuring	8 fluid ounces
	1/2 liquid pint
1 gallon (U.S.)	231 cubic inches
	3.785 liters
	0.833 British gallon
	128 U.S. fluid ounces
1 gallon (British Imperial)	277.42 cubic inches
	1.201 U.S. gallons
	4.546 liters
	160 British fluid ounces
1 liter	1.057 liquid quarts
	0.908 dry quart
	61.024 cubic inches
1 milliliter	0.061 cubic inches
1 ounce, fluid or liquid (U.S.)	1.805 cubic inches
	29.574 milliliters
	1.041 British fluid ounces
1 pint, dry	33.600 cubic inches
	0.551 liter
1 pint, liquid	28.875 cubic inches
	0.473 liter
1 quart, dry (U.S.)	67.201 cubic inches
	1.101 liters
	0.969 British quart
1 quart, liquid (U.S.)	57.75 cubic inches
	0.946 liter
	0.833 British quart
1 quart (British)	69.354 cubic inches
	1.032 U.S. dry quarts
	1.201 U.S. liquid quarts
1 tablespoon, measuring	3 teaspoons
	1/2 fluid ounce
1 teaspoon, measuring	1/3 tablespoon
	1/6 fluid ounce
1 kilogram	2.205 pounds
1 microgram (μg)	0.000001 gram

Food Measurement Equivalents

16 tablespoons = 1 cup
12 tablespoons = 3/4 cup

10 tablespoons + 2 teaspoons = 2/3 cup
8 tablespoons = 1/2 cup
6 tablespoons = 3/8 cup
5 tablespoons + 1 teaspoon = 1/3 cup
4 tablespoons = 1/4 cup
2 tablespoons = 1/8 cup
2 tablespoons + 2 teaspoons = 1/6 cup
1 tablespoon = 1/16 cup
2 cups = 1 pint
2 pints = 1 quart
3 teaspoons = 1 tablespoon
48 teaspoons = 1 cup

Food Measurement Conversions: U.S. to Metric

Capacity

1/5 teaspoon.............1 milliliter
1 teaspoon ....5 milliliters
1 tablespoon ....15 milliliters
1 fluid ounce ....30 milliliters
1/5 cup......................47 milliliters

1 cup ....237 milliliters
2 cups (1 pint).........473 milliliters
4 cups (1 quart).......0.95 liter
4 quarts (1 gal.) ......3.8 liters

Weight

1 ounce ....28 grams
1 pound.................454 grams

Food Measurement Conversions: Metric to U.S.

Capacity

1 milliliter ....1/5 teaspoon
5 milliliters..........1 teaspoon
15 milliliters........1 tablespoon
100 milliliters......3.4 fluid oz
240 milliliters......1 cup
1 liter ....34 fluid oz
.................4.2 cups
.................2.1 pints
.................1.06 quarts
.................0.26 gallon

Weight

1 gram ....0.035 ounce
100 grams...................3.5 ounces
500 grams ....1.10 pounds
1 kilogram......................2.205 pounds
.................................35 ounces

Conversion Factors

To change	To	Multiply by
centimeters	inches	0.3937
centimeters	feet	0.03281
cubic feet	cubic meters	0.0283
cubic meters	cubic feet	35.3145
cubic meters	cubic yards	1.3079
cubic yards	cubic meters	0.7646
feet	meters	0.3048
gallons (U.S.)	liters	3.7853
grams	ounces avdp	0.0353
grams	pounds	0.002205
inches	millimeters	25.4000
inches	centimeters	2.5400
inches	meters	0.0254
kilograms	pounds	2.2046

liters	gallons (U.S.)	0.2642
liters	pints (dry)	1.8162
liters	pints (liquid)	2.1134
liters	quarts (dry)	0.9081
liters	quarts (liquid)	1.0567
meters	feet	3.2808
meters	yards	1.0936
millimeters	inches	0.0394
ounces avdp	grams	28.3495
ounces	pounds	0.0625
pints (dry)	liters	0.5506
pints (liquid)	liters	0.4732
pounds	kilograms	0.4536
pounds	ounces	16
quarts (dry)	liters	1.1012
quarts (liquid)	liters	0.9463

Fahrenheit and Celsius (Centigrade) Scales

°Celsius	°Fahrenheit
−273.15	−459.67
−250	−418
−200	−328
−150	−238
−100	−148
−50	−58
−40	−40
−30	−22
−20	−4
−10	14
0	32
5	41
10	50
15	59
20	68
25	77
30	86
35	95
40	104
45	113
50	122
55	131
60	140
65	149
70	158
75	167
80	176
85	185
90	194
95	203
100	212

Zero on the Fahrenheit scale represents the temperature produced by the mixing of equal weights of snow and common salt.

	°Fahrenheit	°Celsius
Boiling point of water	212°	100°
Freezing point of water	32°	0°
Normal body temperature	98.6°	37°

Comfortable room temperature .... 68–77° .... 20–25°
Absolute zero .... −459.6° .... −273.1°

Absolute zero is theoretically the lowest possible temperature, the point at which all molecular motion would cease.

To Convert Temperature Scales

To convert Fahrenheit to Celsius (Centigrade), subtract 32 and multiply by $\frac{5}{9}$.

$$°C = \frac{5}{9}(°F - 32)$$

To convert Celsius (Centigrade) to Fahrenheit, multiply by $\frac{9}{5}$ and add 32.

$$°F = (\frac{9}{5} \times °C) + 32$$

Do You Speak Metric?

Although the metric system isn't really a language like English or Spanish, in some sense it is the language of science. Nutritionists must be fluent in metrics. Pick up any nutrition journal and you will find units of measurement expressed in terms like kilograms and liters.

The metric system is a decimal-based system of measurement units. Like our monetary system, units are related by factors of 10. There are 10 pennies in a dime, and 10 dimes equal 1 dollar. Calculations involve the simple process of moving the decimal point to the right or to the left.

There are only seven basic units in the metric system. The most common units are the meter (m) to measure length, the gram (g) for mass, the liter (L) for volume, and degree Celsius (°C) for temperature. The metric system avoids the confusing dual use of terms, such as the current use of ounces to measure both weight and volume.

One strategy for learning metric is to find common or familiar associations. For example, when using degrees Celsius you should equate 22 degrees Celsius (22°C) with room temperature, 37 degrees Celsius (37°C) with body temperature, and 0 and 100 degrees Celsius with the freezing and boiling points of water, respectively. A millimeter (1 mm) is about the thickness of a dime, and 2 centimeters (2 cm) is about the diameter of a nickel. When you pick up a 2-pound box of sugar, you are holding about 900 grams.

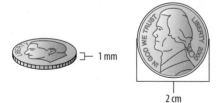

A fluid ounce can be tricky because it's a measure of liquid volume, not weight. Most people already recognize 1-liter and 2-liter soft-drink bottles. A 1-liter bottle equals 33.8 fluid ounces.

The United States is the only industrialized country in the world not officially using the metric system. Because of its many advantages (e.g., easy conversion

between units of the same quantity), the metric system has become the internationally accepted system of measurement.

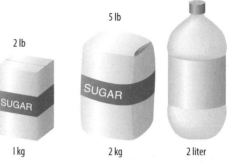

Many members of the international scientific community use the International System of Units (SI). The SI is the modern metric system and has adopted the joule rather than the calorie to measure food energy. Although we think of the calorie as a measure of energy, it is more accurately a measure of heat. Joules are a measure of work, not heat, and the amount of energy potential in foods is expressed best in kilojoules (kjoules). Each kilocalorie is equivalent to approximately 4.2 (4.184) kilojoules. For example, a 100-kilocalorie glass of juice provides about 420 kilojoules.

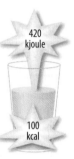

The Celsius (C) temperature scale should be used instead of the Fahrenheit (F) scale. The following are familiar points:

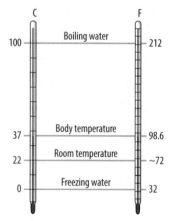

TABLE J.1
Measures Commonly Used in Nutrition

	Metric	English
Length	1 meter (m)	39.4 inches (in)
	1 centimeter (cm)	0.394 inch (in)
	2.54 centimeters (cm)	1 inch (in)
Weight (mass)	1 kilogram (kg)	2.2 pounds (lb)
	454 grams (g)	1 pound (lb)
	5 grams (g) of salt	about 1 teaspoon (tsp)
Volume	1 liter (L)	1.057 quarts (about 4 cups)
	236 milliliters (mL)	about 1 cup (c)
	15 milliliters (mL)	about 1 tablespoon (Tbsp)
	5 milliliters (mL)	about 1 teaspoon (tsp)

Note:
1 gram = 1,000 milligrams
1 milligram = 1,000 micrograms (μg or mcg)

Glossary

2015–2020 Dietary Guidelines for Americans The foundation of federal nutrition policy; they are developed by the U.S. Department of Agriculture (USDA) and the U.S. Department of Health and Human Services (DHHS). These science-based guidelines are intended to reduce the number of Americans who develop chronic diseases such as hypertension, diabetes, cardiovascular disease, obesity, and alcoholism.

ABC model of behavior A behavioral model that includes the external and internal events that precede and follow the behavior. The "A" stands for antecedents, the events that precede the behavior ("B"), which is followed by consequences ("C") that positively or negatively reinforce the behavior.

absorption The movement of substances into or across tissues; in particular, the passage of nutrients and other substances into the walls of the gastrointestinal tract and then into the bloodstream.

Acceptable Macronutrient Distribution Ranges (AMDRs) Range of intakes for a particular energy source that are associated with reduced risk of chronic disease while providing adequate intakes of essential nutrients.

accessory organs Organs that assist in the digestion and absorption of foods and nutrients.

acesulfame K [ay-see-SUL-fame] An artificial sweetener that is 200 times sweeter than common table sugar (sucrose). Because it is not digested and absorbed by the body, acesulfame contributes no calories to the diet and yields no energy when consumed.

acetaldehyde A toxic intermediate compound formed by the action of the alcohol dehydrogenase enzyme during the metabolism of alcohol.

acetyl CoA A key intermediate product in the metabolic breakdown of carbohydrates, fatty acids, and amino acids. It consists of a two-carbon acetate group linked to coenzyme A, which is derived from pantothenic acid.

acidosis An abnormally low blood pH (below about 7.35) resulting from increased acidity.

acne An inflammatory skin eruption that usually occurs in or near the sebaceous glands of the face, neck, shoulders, and upper back.

acrolein A pungent decomposition product of fats, generated from dehydrating the glycerol component of fats; responsible for the coughing attacks caused by the fumes released by burning fat. This toxic water-soluble liquid vaporizes easily and is highly flammable.

active transport The movement of substances into or out of cells against a concentration gradient. Active transport requires energy (ATP) and involves carrier (transport) proteins in the cell membrane.

adenosine diphosphate (ADP) [ah-DEN-oh-seen di-FOS-fate] A molecule composed of adenosine and two phosphate groups.

adenosine triphosphate (ATP) [ah-DEN-oh-seen try-FOS-fate] A high-energy compound composed of adenosine and three phosphate groups. ATP is the main direct fuel that cells use to synthesize molecules, contract muscles, transport substances, and perform other tasks. Breaking down ATP to adenosine diphosphate (ADP) releases energy, and forming ATP from ADP captures energy.

Adequate Intake (AI) The nutrient intake that appears to sustain a defined nutritional state or some other indicator of health (e.g., growth rate or normal circulating nutrient values) in a specific population or subgroup. AI is used when there is insufficient scientific evidence to establish an EAR.

adipocytes Fat cells.

adipose tissue Body fat tissue.

adolescence The period between onset of puberty and adulthood.

aerobic [air-ROW-bic] Referring to the presence of or need for oxygen. The complete breakdown of glucose, fatty acids, and amino acids to carbon dioxide and water occurs only via aerobic metabolism. The citric acid cycle and electron transport chain are aerobic pathways.

aerobic endurance The ability of skeletal muscle to obtain a sufficient supply of oxygen from the heart and lungs to maintain muscular activity for a prolonged time.

aflatoxins Toxins produced by a mold that grows on crops, such as peanuts, tree nuts, corn, wheat, and oil seeds (like cottonseed).

albumin A protein that circulates in the blood and helps transport many minerals and some drugs.

alcohol Common name for ethanol or ethyl alcohol. As a general term, it refers to any organic compound with one or more hydroxyl (–OH) groups.

alcohol dehydrogenase (ADH) The enzyme that catalyzes the oxidation of ethanol and other alcohols.

alcohol poisoning An overdose of alcohol. The body is overwhelmed by the amount of alcohol in the system and cannot metabolize it fast enough.

aldehyde dehydrogenase (ALDH) The enzyme that catalyzes the conversion of acetaldehyde to acetate, which forms acetyl CoA.

aldosterone [al-DOS-ter-own] A hormone secreted from the adrenal glands that acts on the kidneys to regulate electrolyte and water balance. It raises blood pressure by promoting retention of sodium (and thus water) and excretion of potassium.

alkalosis An abnormally high blood pH (above about 7.45) resulting from increased alkalinity.

alpha (α) bonds Chemical bonds linking monosaccharides, which can be broken by human intestinal enzymes, releasing the individual monosaccharides. Starch, maltose, and sucrose contain alpha bonds.

alpha-linolenic acid [al-fah-lin-oh-LEN-ik] An essential omega-3 fatty acid that contains 18 carbon atoms and 3 carbon–carbon double bonds (18:3).

Alzheimer's disease (AD) A presenile dementia characterized by accumulation of plaques in certain regions of the brain and degeneration of a certain class of neurons.

amenorrhea [A-men-or-EE-a] Absence or abnormal stoppage of menses in a female; commonly indicated by the absence of three to six consecutive menstrual cycles.

amino acid pool The amino acids in body tissues and fluids that are available for new protein synthesis.

amino acids Compounds that function as the building blocks of protein.

amniotic fluid The fluid that surrounds the fetus; contained in the amniotic sac inside the uterus.

amylopectin [am-ih-low-PEK-tin] A branched-chain polysaccharide composed of glucose units.

amylose [AM-ih-los] A straight-chain polysaccharide composed of glucose units.

anabolic steroids Several compounds derived from testosterone or prepared synthetically. They promote body growth and masculinization and oppose the effects of estrogen.

anabolism [an-A-bol-iz-um] Any metabolic process whereby cells build complex substances from simple, smaller units.

anaerobic [AN-ah-ROW-bic] Referring to the absence of oxygen or the ability of a process to occur in the absence of oxygen. Glycolysis is an anaerobic pathway.

android obesity [AN-droyd] Excess storage of fat located primarily in the abdominal area.

anemia Abnormally low concentration of hemoglobin in the bloodstream; can be caused by impaired synthesis of red blood cells, increased destruction of red blood cells, or significant loss of blood.

anencephaly A type of neural tube birth defect in which part or all of the brain is missing.

anions Ions that carry a negative charge.

anorexia athletica A generic term used to describe athletes with eating disorders.

anorexia nervosa [an-or-EX-ee-uh ner-VOH-sah] An eating disorder marked by prolonged refusal to eat, self-starvation and excessive weight loss, distorted body image, and an intense and irrational fear of becoming fat.

anorexia of aging Loss of appetite and wasting associated with old age.

antibodies [AN-tih-bod-eez] Infection-fighting protein molecules in blood or secretory fluids that tag, neutralize, and help destroy pathogenic microorganisms (e.g., bacteria, viruses) or toxins.

antidiuretic hormone (ADH) A hormone secreted by the pituitary gland that increases blood pressure and prevents fluid excretion by the kidneys. Also called *vasopressin*.

antioxidant A substance that combines with or otherwise neutralizes a free radical, thus preventing oxidative damage to cells and tissues.

appetite A psychological desire to eat that is related to the pleasant sensations often associated with food.

aspartame [AH-spar-tame] An artificial sweetener composed of two amino acids. It is 200 times sweeter than sucrose and sold under the trade name NutraSweet.

atherosclerosis A type of "hardening of the arteries" in which cholesterol and other substances in the blood build up in the walls of arteries. As the process continues, the arteries to the heart may narrow, cutting down the flow of oxygen-rich blood and nutrients to the heart.

ATP–CP energy system A simple and immediate anaerobic energy system that maintains ATP levels. Creatine phosphate is broken down, releasing energy and a phosphate group, which is used to form ATP.

atrophic gastritis An age-related condition in which the stomach loses its ability to secrete acid. In severe cases, ability to make intrinsic factor is also impaired.

autonomic nervous system (ANS) The part of the central nervous system that regulates the automatic responses of the body; consists of the sympathetic and parasympathetic systems.

avidin A protein in raw egg whites that binds biotin, preventing its absorption. Avidin is denatured by heat.

bacteriophages Viruses that infect bacteria.

bariatric surgery An operation that helps a person lose weight by altering the structure of the digestive system.

base pair Two nitrogenous bases (adenine and thymine or guanine and cytosine), held together by weak bonds, that form a "rung" of the "DNA ladder." The bonds between base pairs hold the DNA molecule together in the shape of a double helix.

benign Not cancerous; does not invade nearby tissue or spread to other parts of the body.

beriberi Thiamin-deficiency disease. Symptoms include muscle weakness, loss of appetite, nerve degeneration, and edema in some cases.

beta (β) bonds Chemical bonds linking monosaccharides, which sometimes can be broken by human intestinal enzymes. Lactose contains digestible beta bonds, and cellulose contains nondigestible beta bonds.

beta-glucan Functional fiber, consisting of branched polysaccharide chains of glucose, that helps lower blood cholesterol levels; found in barley and oats.

beta-oxidation The breakdown of a fatty acid into numerous molecules of the two-carbon compound acetyl coenzyme A (acetyl CoA).

bile An alkaline, yellow-green fluid that is produced in the liver and stored in the gallbladder. Bile emulsifies dietary fats, aiding fat digestion and absorption.

binge drinking Consuming excessive amounts of alcohol in short periods of time.

binge eaters Individuals who routinely consume a very large amount of food in a brief period of time (e.g., two hours) and lose control over how much and what is eaten.

binge-eating disorder An eating disorder marked by repeated episodes of binge eating and a feeling of loss of control. The diagnosis is based on a person's having an average of at least one binge-eating episode per week for three months.

bingeing Eating, in a discrete period of time (e.g., within a 2-hour period), an amount of food that is larger than most people would eat during a similar period of time and under similar circumstances, while simultaneously experiencing a loss of control or feeling that one cannot stop eating or control what or how much one is eating.

bioavailability A measure of the extent to which a nutrient becomes available to the body after ingestion and thus is available to the tissues.

biodiversity The countless species of plants, animals, and insects that exist on the earth. An undisturbed tropical forest is an example of the biodiversity of a healthy ecosystem.

bioelectrical impedance analysis (BIA) Technique to estimate amounts of total body water, lean tissue mass, and total body fat. It uses the resistance of tissue to the flow of an alternating electric current.

bioflavonoids Naturally occurring plant chemicals, especially from citrus fruits, that reduce the permeability and fragility of capillaries.

biosynthesis Chemical reactions in which complex biomolecules, especially carbohydrates, lipids, and proteins, are formed from simple molecules.

biotechnology The set of laboratory techniques and processes used to modify the genome of plants or animals and thus create desirable new characteristics. Genetic engineering in the broad sense.

blastogenic stage The first stage of gestation, during which tissue proliferation by rapid cell division begins.

bleaching process A complex light-stimulated reaction in which rod cells lose color as rhodopsin is split into retinal and opsin.

blood pressure The pressure of blood against the walls of a blood vessel or heart chamber. Unless there is reference to another location, such as the pulmonary artery or one of the heart chambers, this term refers to the pressure in the systemic arteries, as measured, for example, in the forearm.

BodPod A device used to measure the density of the body based on the volume of air displaced as a person sits in a sealed chamber of known volume.

body composition The chemical or anatomical composition of the body. Commonly defined as the proportions of fat, muscle, bone, and other tissues in the body.

Body dissatisfaction Body dissatisfaction is defined as a negative subjective evaluation of the weight and shape of one's own body.

body fat distribution The pattern of fat distribution on the body.

body image A person's internal view of their own outer appearance.

body mass index (BMI) Body weight (in kilograms) divided by the square of height (in meters), expressed in units of kg/m².

bolus [BOH-lus] A chewed, moistened lump of food that is ready to be swallowed.

botulism An often-fatal type of food poisoning caused by a toxin released from *Clostridium botulinum*, a bacterium that can grow in improperly canned low-acid foods.

bovine spongiform encephalopathy (BSE) A chronic degenerative disease, widely referred to as "mad cow disease," that affects the central nervous system of cattle.

bran The layers of protective coating around the grain kernel that are rich in dietary fiber and nutrients.

***Bt* gene** *Bacillus thuringiensis (Bt)* is a bacterium that produces a protein called the *Bt* toxin. One of the bacterium's genes, the *Bt* gene, carries the information for the *Bt* toxin. Inserting a copy of the *Bt* gene into plants enables them to produce *Bt* toxin protein and resist some insect pests. The *Bt* protein is not toxic to humans.

buffers Compounds that can take up and release hydrogen ions to keep the pH of a solution constant. The buffering action of proteins and bicarbonate in the bloodstream plays a major role in maintaining the blood pH at 7.35 to 7.45.

built environment Any human-formed, developed, or structured areas, including the urban environment that consists of buildings, roads, fixtures, parks, and all other human developments that form its physical character.

bulimia nervosa [bull-EEM-ee-uh ner-VOH-sah] An eating disorder marked by binge eating followed by compensatory behaviors such as self-induced vomiting, use of laxatives or other drugs, excessive exercise, fasting, or other practices to avoid weight gain.

calcitonin A hormone secreted by the thyroid gland in response to elevated blood calcium. It stimulates calcium deposition in bone and calcium excretion by the kidneys, thus reducing blood calcium.

calcitriol The active form of vitamin D; an important regulator of blood calcium levels.

calmodulin A calcium-binding protein that regulates a variety of cellular activities, such as cell division and proliferation.

calorie The general term for energy in food and used synonymously with the term *energy*. Often used instead of kilocalorie on food labels, in diet books, and in other sources of nutrition information.

Canada's Guidelines for Healthy Eating Key messages that are based on the 1990 *Nutrition Recommendations for Canadians* and that provide positive, action-oriented, scientifically accurate eating advice to Canadians.

cancer A term for diseases in which abnormal cells divide without control. Cancer cells can invade nearby tissues and can spread through the bloodstream and lymphatic system to other parts of the body.

carbohydrate loading Changes in dietary carbohydrate intake and exercise regimen before competition to maximize glycogen stores in the muscles. It is appropriate for endurance events lasting 60 to 90 consecutive minutes or longer. Also known as *glycogen loading*.

carbohydrates Compounds, including sugars, starches, and dietary fibers, that usually have the general chemical formula (CH₂O)ₙ, where *n* represents the number of CH₂O units in the molecule. Carbohydrates are a major source of energy for body functions.

carcinogens [kar-SIN-o-jins] Any substances that cause cancer.

cardiac output The amount of blood expelled by the heart.

cardiovascular disease (CVD) Any abnormal condition characterized by dysfunction of the heart and blood vessels. CVD includes atherosclerosis (especially coronary heart disease, which can lead to heart attacks), cerebrovascular disease (e.g., stroke), and hypertension (high blood pressure).

carnitine [CAR-nih-teen] A compound that transports fatty acids from the cytosol into the mitochondria, where they undergo beta-oxidation.

carotenoids A group of yellow, orange, and red pigments in plants. Many of these compounds are precursors of vitamin A.

case control studies Investigations that use a group of people with a particular condition rather than a randomly selected population. These cases are compared with a control group of people who do not have the condition.

catabolism [ca-TA-bol-iz-um] Any metabolic process whereby cells break down complex substances into simpler, smaller ones.

catalyze To speed up a chemical reaction.

cations Ions that carry a positive charge.

cecum The blind pouch at the beginning of the large intestine into which the ileum opens from one side and that is continuous with the colon.

celiac disease [SEA-lee-ak] A disease that involves an inability to digest gluten, a protein found in wheat, rye, and barley. If untreated, it causes flattening of the villi in the intestine, leading to severe malabsorption of nutrients. Symptoms include diarrhea, fatty stools, swollen belly, and extreme fatigue.

cells The basic structural units of all living tissues. Cells have two major parts—the nucleus and the cytoplasm.

cellulose [SELL-you-los] A straight-chain polysaccharide composed of hundreds of glucose units linked by beta bonds. It is nondigestible by humans and is a component of dietary fiber.

central nervous system (CNS) The brain and the spinal cord. The central nervous system transmits signals that control muscular actions and glandular secretions along the entire GI tract.

ceruloplasmin A copper-dependent enzyme that enables iron to bind to transferrin. Also known as *ferroxidase I*.

chain length The number of carbons that a fatty acid contains. Foods contain fatty acids with chain lengths of 4 to 24 carbons, and most have an even number of carbons.

chemical energy Energy contained in the bonds between atoms of a molecule.

Child and Adult Care Food Program A federally funded program that reimburses approved family child-care providers for USDA-approved foods served to preschool children; also provides funds for meals and snacks served at after-school programs for school-age children and to adult day care centers serving chronically impaired adults or people over age 60.

childhood The period of life from age 1 to the onset of puberty.

chitin A long-chain structural polysaccharide of slightly modified glucose. Found in the hard exterior skeletons of insects, crustaceans, and other invertebrates; also occurs in the cell walls of fungi.

chitosan Polysaccharide derived from chitin.

cholesterol [ko-LES-te-rol] A waxy lipid (sterol) whose chemical structure contains multiple hydrocarbon rings.

choline A nitrogen-containing compound that is part of phosphatidylcholine, a phospholipid. Choline also is part of the neurotransmitter acetylcholine. The body can synthesize choline from the amino acid methionine.

chylomicron [kye-lo-MY-kron] A large lipoprotein formed in intestinal cells following the absorption of dietary fats. A chylomicron has a central core of triglycerides and cholesterol surrounded by phospholipids and proteins.

chyme [KIME] A mass of partially digested food and digestive juices moving from the stomach into the small intestine.

ciguatera A toxin found in more than 300 species of Caribbean and South Pacific fish. It is a nonbacterial source of food poisoning.

ciliary action Wave-like motion of small hair-like projections on some cells.

circular muscle Layers of smooth muscle that surround organs, including the stomach and the small intestine.

circulation Movement of substances through the vessels of the cardiovascular or lymphatic system.

cis fatty acid An unsaturated fatty acid with a bent carbon chain. Most naturally occurring unsaturated fatty acids are cis fatty acids.

citric acid cycle The metabolic pathway occurring in mitochondria in which the acetyl portion ($CH_3COO–$) of acetyl CoA is oxidized to yield two molecules of carbon dioxide and one molecule each of NADH, $FADH_2$, and GTP. Also known as the *Krebs cycle* and the *tricarboxylic acid cycle*.

clinical trials Studies that collect large amounts of data to evaluate the effectiveness of a treatment.

coenzyme A A cofactor derived from the vitamin pantothenic acid.

coenzymes Organic compounds, often derived from B vitamins, that combine with inactive enzymes to form active enzymes.

cofactors Compounds required for an enzyme to be active. Cofactors include coenzymes and metal ions such as iron, copper, and magnesium.

colic Periodic inconsolable crying in an apparently healthy infant that appears to result from abdominal cramping and discomfort.

collagen The most abundant fibrous protein in the body. Collagen is the major constituent of connective tissue, forms the foundation for bones and teeth, and helps maintain the structure of blood vessels and other tissues.

colon The portion of the large intestine extending from the cecum to the rectum. It is made up of four parts: the ascending, transverse, descending, and sigmoid colons.

color additives Any dye, pigment, or substance that can give color when added to a food, drug, or cosmetic or to the human body.

colostrum A precursor of breast milk; a thick, yellow fluid rich in immune factors and secreted during pregnancy and the first days after delivery.

complementary and integrative health care A broad range of healing philosophies, approaches, and therapies that include treatments and healthcare practices not taught widely in medical schools, not generally used in hospitals, and not usually reimbursed by medical insurance companies.

complementary foods Any foods or liquids other than breast milk or infant formula fed to an infant.

complementary protein An incomplete food protein whose assortment of amino acids makes up for, or complements, another food protein's lack of specific essential amino acids so that the combination of the two proteins provides sufficient amounts of all the essential amino acids.

complementary sequence Nucleic acid-base sequence that can form a double-stranded structure with another DNA fragment by following base-pairing rules (A pairs with T, and C pairs with G). The complementary sequence to GTAC, for example, is CATG.

complete proteins Proteins that supply all of the indispensable amino acids in the proportions the body needs. Also known as *high-quality proteins*.

complex carbohydrates Chains of more than two monosaccharides. May be oligosaccharides or polysaccharides.

compulsive overeating An eating disorder marked by repeated episodes of binge eating and a feeling of loss of control. The diagnosis is based on a person's having an average of at least one binge-eating episode per week for three months.

concentration gradients Differences between the solute concentrations of two solutions.

conditionally essential amino acids Amino acids that are normally made in the body (nonessential) but become essential under certain circumstances, such as during critical illness.

conditioning The body's adaptations to exercise and activity. Endurance (aerobic) conditioning is the strengthening of the heart and lungs (cardiovascular system) through the rhythmic movement of large muscle groups. Strength conditioning is the strengthening of skeletal muscle through resistance training. To maintain or increase the level of conditioning, athletes must maintain or progressively increase their training level.

cone cells Cells in the retina that are sensitive to bright light and translate it into color images.

congeners Biologically active compounds in alcoholic beverages that include nonalcoholic ingredients as well as other alcohols such as methanol. Congeners contribute to the distinctive taste and smell of the beverage and may increase intoxicating effects and subsequent hangover.

conjugated linoleic acid (CLA) A polyunsaturated fatty acid in which the position of the double bonds has moved so that a single bond alternates with two double bonds.

connective tissues Tissues composed primarily of fibrous proteins, such as collagen, and that contain few cells. Their primary function is to bind together and support various body structures.

constipation Infrequent and difficult bowel movements, followed by a sensation of incomplete evacuation.

control group A set of people used as a standard of comparison to the experimental group. The people in the control group have characteristics similar to those in the experimental group and are selected at random.

cornea The transparent outer surface of the eye.

coronary heart disease (CHD) A type of heart disease caused by narrowing of the coronary arteries that feed the heart, which needs a constant supply of oxygen and nutrients carried by the blood in the coronary arteries. When the coronary arteries become narrowed or clogged by fat and cholesterol deposits and cannot supply enough blood to the heart, CHD results.

correlations Connections co-occurring more frequently than can be explained by chance or coincidence but without a proven cause.

creatine An important nitrogenous compound found in meats and fish and synthesized in the body from amino acids (glycine, arginine, and methionine).

creatine phosphate An energy-rich compound that supplies energy and a phosphate group for the formation of ATP. Also called *phosphocreatine*.

cretinism A congenital condition often caused by severe iodine deficiency during gestation; characterized by arrested physical and mental development.

critical control points (CCPs) Operational steps or procedures in a process, production method, or recipe at which control can be applied to prevent, reduce, or eliminate a food safety hazard.

critical period of development Time during which body structures are forming and environmental influences, such as drugs and infections, have the greatest impact on the developing embryo.

cytoplasm The material of the cell, excluding the cell nucleus and cell membranes. The cytoplasm includes the semifluid cytosol, the organelles, and other particles.

cytosol The semifluid inside the cell membrane, excluding organelles. The cytosol is the site of glycolysis and fatty acid synthesis.

Daily Values (DVs) A single set of nutrient intake standards developed by the Food and Drug Administration to represent the needs of the "typical" consumer; used as standards for expressing nutrient content on food labels.

dark adaptation The process that increases the rhodopsin concentration in your eyes, allowing them to detect images in the dark better.

DASH (Dietary Approaches to Stop Hypertension) An eating plan low in total fat, saturated fat, and cholesterol and rich in fruits, vegetables, and low-fat dairy products that has been shown to reduce elevated blood pressure.

deamination The removal of the amino group (–NH₂) from an amino acid.

Delaney Clause A legal provision stating that food or color additives cannot be approved if they cause cancer in humans or animals.

denaturation A change in the three-dimensional structure of a protein resulting in an unfolded polypeptide chain that cannot fulfill the protein's function. Treatment with heat, acid, alkali, or extreme agitation can denature most proteins.

dental caries [KARE-ees] Destruction of the enamel surface of teeth caused by acids resulting from bacterial breakdown of sugars in the mouth.

diabetes mellitus A chronic disease in which uptake of glucose into body cells is impaired, resulting in higher glucose levels in blood and urine. Type 1 is caused by impaired insulin release from the pancreas. Type 2 occurs when body cells, such as fat and muscle cells, have an impaired response to insulin.

diarrhea Watery stools due to reduced absorption of water.

diastolic Pertaining to the time between heart contractions, a period known as diastole. Diastolic blood pressure is measured at the point of maximum cardiac relaxation.

dietary fiber Carbohydrates and lignins that are naturally in plants and are nondigestible; that is, they are not digested and absorbed in the human small intestine.

dietary folate equivalents (DFEs) A measure of folate intake used to account for the high bioavailability of folic acid taken as a supplement compared with the lower bioavailability of the folate found in foods.

Dietary Reference Intakes (DRIs) A framework of dietary standards that includes Estimated Average Requirement (EAR), Recommended Dietary Allowance (RDA), Adequate Intake (AI), and Tolerable Upper Intake Level (UL).

dietary standards A set of values for the recommended intake of nutrients.

Dietary Supplement Health and Education Act (DSHEA) Legislation that regulates dietary supplements.

dietary supplements Products taken by mouth in tablet, capsule, powder, gelcap, or other nonfood form that contain one or more of the following: vitamins, minerals, amino acids, herbs, enzymes, metabolites, or concentrates.

digestion The process of transforming the foods we eat into units for absorption.

digestive secretions Substances released at different places in the GI tract to speed the breakdown of ingested carbohydrates, fats, and proteins.

diglyceride A molecule of glycerol combined with two fatty acids.

dioxins Chemical compounds created in the manufacturing, combustion, and chlorine bleaching of pulp and paper and in other industrial processes.

dipeptide Two amino acids joined by a peptide bond.

direct additives Substances that are added to a food for a specific reason.

disaccharides [dye-SACK-uh-rides] Carbohydrates composed of two monosaccharide units linked by a glycosidic bond. They include sucrose (common table sugar), lactose (milk sugar), and maltose.

disease A particular quality, habit, or disposition regarded as adversely affecting a person or group of people.

disordered eating An abnormal change in eating pattern related to an illness, a stressful event, or a desire to improve one's health, appearance, or athletic performance. If it persists it can lead to an eating disorder.

diuresis The formation and secretion of urine.

diuretics [dye-u-RET-iks] Drugs or other substances that promote the formation and release of urine. Diuretics are given to reduce body fluid volume in treating such disorders as high blood pressure, congestive heart disease, and edema. Both alcohol and caffeine act as diuretics.

diverticulitis [dy-vur-tik-yoo-LY-tis] A condition that occurs when small pouches in the colon (diverticula) become infected or irritated. Also called *left-sided appendicitis*.

diverticulosis [dy-vur-tik-yoo-LOH-sis] A condition that occurs when small pouches (diverticula) push outward through weak spots in the colon.

double-blind study A research study set up so that neither the subjects nor the investigators know which study group is receiving the placebo and which is receiving the active substance.

duodenum [doo-oh-DEE-num] The portion of the small intestine closest to the stomach. The duodenum is 25 to 30 cm (10 to 12 in.) long and wider than the remainder of the small intestine.

eating disorders Psychiatric disorders that include extreme emotional distress, disordered self-evaluation based primarily on faulty perceptions of one's body size or shape, and abnormal eating and compensatory behaviors performed in an attempt to alter body shape. Currently, the American Psychiatric Association recognizes three eating disorders: anorexia nervosa, bulimia nervosa, and binge-eating disorder. Several other unhealthy patterns of eating have been identified, but sufficient evidence does not yet exist to classify these as psychiatric disorders.

Eating Well with Canada's Food Guide Recommendations to help Canadians select foods to meet energy and nutrient needs while reducing the risk of chronic disease. The *Food Guide* is based on the *Nutrition Recommendations for Canadians* and *Canada's Guidelines for Healthy Eating* and is a key nutrition education tool for Canadians age 4 years or older.

eclampsia The occurrence of seizures in a pregnant woman that are unrelated to brain conditions.

edema Swelling caused by the buildup of fluid between cells.

eicosanoids A class of hormone-like substances formed in the body from long-chain essential fatty acids.

electrolytes [ih-LEK-tro-lites] Substances that separate into charged particles (ions) when dissolved in water or other solvents and thus become capable of conducting an electrical current. The terms *electrolyte* and *ion* often are used interchangeably.

Electronic Benefits Transfer (EBT) Electronic delivery of government benefits by a single plastic card that allows access to food benefits at point-of-sale locations.

electron transport chain An organized series of protein carrier molecules located in mitochondrial membranes. As high-energy electrons delivered by NADH and FADH$_2$ traverse the electron transport chain to oxygen, it produces ATP and water.

elimination The removal of undigested food from the body.

embryonic stage The developmental stage between the time the egg implants in the uterine wall (about two weeks after fertilization) through the eighth week; the stage of major organ system differentiation and development of main external features.

emetics Agents that induce vomiting.

emulsifiers Agents that blend fatty and watery liquids by promoting the breakup of fat into small particles and stabilizing their suspension in a watery solution.

endosperm The largest, middle portion of a grain kernel. The endosperm is high in starch to provide food for the growing plant embryo.

endothelial cells Thin, flattened cells that line internal body cavities in a single layer.

endothelium See *endothelial cells*.

enemas Infusions of fluid into the rectum, usually for cleansing or other therapeutic purposes.

energy The capacity to do work. The energy in food is chemical energy, which the body converts to mechanical, electrical, or heat energy.

energy availability (EA) The energy intake needed for optimal health and fitness, rather than energy balance. EA is the amount of energy available to the body to perform all functions after the energy cost of exercise is subtracted.

energy balance The balance in the body between amounts of energy consumed and expended.

energy equilibrium A balance of energy intake and output that results in little or no change in weight over time.

energy intake The caloric or energy content of food provided by the sources of dietary energy: carbohydrate (4 kcal/g), protein (4 kcal/g), fat (9 kcal/g), and alcohol (7 kcal/g).

energy output The use of calories or energy for basic body functions, physical activity, and processing of consumed foods.

enrich To add vitamins and minerals lost or diminished during food processing, particularly the addition of thiamin, riboflavin, niacin, folic acid, and iron to grain products.

enteric nervous system A network of nerves located in the gastrointestinal wall.

enterohepatic circulation [EN-ter-oh-heh-PAT-ik] Recycling of certain compounds between the small intestine and the liver.

enzymes [EN-zimes] Proteins in the body that speed up the rate of chemical reactions but are not altered in the process.

epinephrine A hormone released in response to stress or sudden danger, epinephrine raises blood glucose levels to ready the body for "fight or flight." Also called *adrenaline*.

epiphyses The heads of the long bones that are separated from the shaft of the bone until the bone stops growing.

epithelial cells The millions of cells that line and protect the external and internal surfaces of the body. Epithelial cells form epithelial tissues such as skin and mucous membranes.

epithelial tissues Closely packed layers of epithelial cells that cover the body and line its cavities.

ergogenic aids Substances that can enhance athletic performance.

Escherichia coli (E. coli) Bacteria that are the most common cause of urinary tract infections. Because they release toxins, some types of *E. coli* can rapidly cause shock and death.

esophageal sphincter The opening between the esophagus and the stomach that relaxes and opens to allow the bolus to travel into the stomach, and then closes behind it. Acts as a barrier to prevent the reflux of gastric contents. Also called the *cardiac sphincter*.

esophagitis Inflammation of the esophagus.

esophagus [ee-SOFF-uh-gus] The food pipe that extends from the pharynx to the stomach.

essential amino acids Amino acids that the body cannot make at all or cannot make enough of to meet physiological needs. Essential amino acids must be supplied in the diet.

essential fatty acids (EFAs) Fatty acids that the body needs but cannot synthesize and must obtain from the diet.

essential hypertension Hypertension for which no specific cause can be identified. Ninety to 95 percent of people with hypertension have essential hypertension.

essential nutrients Substances that must be obtained in the diet because the body either cannot make them or cannot make adequate amounts of them.

Estimated Average Requirement (EAR) The intake value that meets the estimated nutrient needs of 50 percent of individuals in a specific life-stage and gender group.

Estimated Energy Requirement (EER) Dietary energy intake that is predicted to maintain energy balance in a healthy adult of a defined age, gender, weight, height, and level of physical activity consistent with good health.

ethanol Chemical name for drinking alcohol. Also known as *ethyl alcohol*.

ethyl alcohol See *ethanol*.

excretion The process of separating and removing waste products of metabolism.

experimental group A set of people being studied to evaluate the effect of an event, substance, or technique.

extracellular fluid The fluid located outside of cells. It is composed largely of the liquid portion (plasma) of the blood and the fluid between cells in tissues (interstitial fluid), with fluid in the GI tract, eyes, joints, and spinal cord contributing a small amount. It constitutes about one-third of body water.

extreme obesity Obesity characterized by body weight exceeding 100 percent of normal; a condition so severe it often requires surgery.

extrusion reflex A young infant's response when a spoon is put in its mouth; the tongue is thrust forward, indicating that the baby is not ready for spoon feeding.

facilitated diffusion A process by which carrier (transport) proteins in the cell membrane transport substances into or out of cells down a concentration gradient.

FAD Flavin adenine dinucleotide (FAD), a coenzyme derived from the B vitamin riboflavin, becomes $FADH_2$ as it accepts a pair of high-energy electrons for transport in cells.

failure to thrive (FTT) Abnormally low gains in length (height) and weight during infancy and childhood; can result from physical problems or poor feeding, but many affected children have no apparent disease or defect.

fast-twitch (FT) fibers Muscle fibers that can develop high tension rapidly. These fibers can fatigue quickly but are well suited to explosive movements in sprinting, jumping, and weight lifting.

fat replacers Compounds that imitate the functional and sensory properties of fats but contain less available energy than fats.

fatty acids Compounds containing a long hydrocarbon chain with a carboxyl group (–COOH) at one end and a methyl group (–CH_3) at the other end.

fatty liver Accumulation of fat in the liver, a sign of increased fatty acid synthesis.

Feeding America The largest charitable hunger-relief organization in the United States. Its mission is to feed America's hungry through a nationwide network of member food banks and to engage the country in the fight to end hunger.

female athlete triad A syndrome in young female athletes that involves disordered eating, amenorrhea, and lowered bone density.

fermentation The anaerobic conversion of various carbohydrates to carbon dioxide and an alcohol or organic acid.

ferritin A major storage form of iron.

fetal alcohol syndrome A set of physical and mental abnormalities observed in infants born to women who abuse alcohol during pregnancy. Affected infants exhibit poor growth, characteristic abnormal facial features, limited hand–eye coordination, and mental retardation.

fetal stage The period of rapid growth from the end of the embryonic stage, starting in the ninth week and lasting until birth.

fibrin A stringy, insoluble protein that is the final product of the blood-clotting process.

flatulence The presence of excessive amounts of air or other gases in the stomach or intestines.

flatus Lower intestinal gas that is expelled through the rectum.

flavor The collective experience that describes both taste and smell.

fluorosis Mottled discoloration and pitting of tooth enamel caused by prolonged ingestion of excess fluoride that is characterized in children by discoloration and pitting of the teeth.

Food and Agriculture Organization (FAO) The largest autonomous United Nations agency; the FAO works to alleviate poverty and hunger by promoting agricultural development, improved nutrition, and the pursuit of food security.

Food and Drug Administration (FDA) The federal agency responsible for ensuring that foods sold in the United States (except for eggs, poultry, and meat, which are monitored by the U.S. Department of Agriculture [USDA]) are safe, wholesome, and labeled properly. The FDA sets standards for the composition of some foods, inspects food plants, and monitors imported foods. The FDA is an agency of the U.S. Department of Health and Human Services (DHHS).

Food and Nutrition Board A board within the Institute of Medicine of the National Academy of Sciences. It is responsible for assembling the group of nutrition scientists who review available scientific data to determine appropriate intake levels of the known essential nutrients.

foodborne illness A sickness caused by food contaminated with microorganisms, chemicals, or other substances hazardous to human health.

Food Code A reference published periodically by the Food and Drug Administration for restaurants, grocery stores, institutional food services, vending operations, and other retailers on how to store, prepare, and serve food to prevent foodborne illness.

food deserts Urban neighborhoods and rural towns without ready access to fresh, healthy, and affordable food.

food groups Categories of similar foods, such as fruits or vegetables.

food insecurity (1) Limited or uncertain availability of nutritionally adequate and safe foods or (2) limited or uncertain ability to acquire acceptable foods in socially acceptable ways.

food label Label required by law on virtually all packaged foods and having five requirements: (1) a statement of identity; (2) the net contents (by weight, volume, or measure) of the package; (3) the name and address of the manufacturer, packer, or distributor; (4) a list of ingredients; and (5) nutrition information.

Food Research and Action Center A nonprofit child advocacy group that works to improve public policies to eradicate hunger and undernutrition in the United States; founded in 1970 as a public interest law firm.

food security Access to enough food for an active, healthy life, including (1) the ready availability of nutritionally adequate and safe foods and (2) an assured ability to acquire acceptable foods in socially acceptable ways.

Food Security Supplement Survey A federally funded survey that measures the prevalence and severity of food insecurity and hunger.

fortify Refers to the addition of vitamins or minerals that were not originally present in a food.

free radicals Short-lived, highly reactive chemicals often derived from oxygen-containing compounds, which can have detrimental effects on cells, especially DNA and cell membranes.

French paradox The phenomenon observed in the French, who have a lower incidence of heart disease than people whose diets contain comparable amounts of fat. Part of the difference has been attributed to the regular and moderate drinking of red wine.

fructose [FROOK-tose] A common monosaccharide containing six carbons that is naturally present in honey and many fruits; often added to foods in the form of high-fructose corn syrup. Also called *levulose* or *fruit sugar*.

full-term baby A baby delivered during the normal period of human gestation, between 38 and 41 weeks.

functional dyspepsia Pain in the upper abdomen not due to any obvious physical cause.

functional fiber Isolated nondigestible carbohydrates, including some manufactured carbohydrates, that have beneficial effects in humans.

functional food A food that may provide a health benefit beyond basic nutrition.

galactose [gah-LAK-tose] A monosaccharide containing six carbons that can be converted into glucose in the body. In foods and living systems, galactose usually is joined with other monosaccharides.

gallbladder A pear-shaped sac that stores and concentrates bile from the liver.

galvanized Describes iron or steel with a thin layer of zinc plated onto it to protect against corrosion.

gastric lipase An enzyme in the stomach that primarily breaks down butterfat.

gastrin [GAS-trin] A hormone released from the walls of the stomach and duodenum that stimulates gastric secretions and motility.

gastritis Inflammation of the stomach.

gastroesophageal reflux disease (GERD) A backflow of stomach contents into the esophagus, accompanied by a burning pain because of the acidity of the gastric juices.

gastrointestinal (GI) tract [GAS-troh-in-TES-tin-al] The connected series of organs and structures used for digestion of food and absorption of nutrients. Also called the *alimentary canal* or the *digestive tract*.

gene expression The process by which proteins are made from the instructions encoded in DNA.

Generally Recognized as Safe A classification for substances which is assigned when experts generally consider a substance safe to use.

genes Sections of DNA that contain hereditary information. Most genes contain information for making proteins.

genetically engineered (GE) foods Foods produced using plant or animal ingredients that have been modified using gene technology.

genetic code The instructions in a gene that tell the cell how to make a specific protein. A, T, G, and C are the "letters" of the DNA code; they stand for the chemicals adenine, thymine, guanine, and cytosine, respectively, which make up the nucleotide bases of DNA. Each gene's code combines the four chemicals in various ways to spell out three-letter "words" that specify which amino acid is needed at every step in making a protein.

genetic engineering Manipulation of the genome of an organism by artificial means for the purpose of modifying existing traits or adding new genetic traits.

genome The total genetic information of an organism, stored in the DNA of its chromosomes.

geophagia Ingestion of clay or dirt.

germ The innermost part of a grain, located at the base of the kernel, that can grow into a new plant. The germ is rich in protein, oils, vitamins, and minerals.

gestational diabetes A condition that results in high blood glucose levels during pregnancy.

ghrelin A hormone produced by the stomach that stimulates feeding by increasing release of neuropeptide Y.

glucagon [GLOO-kuh-gon] Produced by alpha cells in the pancreas, this polypeptide hormone promotes the breakdown of liver glycogen to glucose, thereby increasing blood glucose. Glucagon secretion is stimulated by low blood glucose levels and by growth hormone.

glucogenic A term describing an amino acid whose carbon skeleton can be used in gluconeogenesis to form glucose.

gluconeogenesis [gloo-ko-nee-oh-JEN-uh-sis] Synthesis of glucose within the body from noncarbohydrate precursors such as amino acids, lactic acid, and glycerol. Fatty acids cannot be converted to glucose.

glucose [GLOO-kose] A common monosaccharide containing six carbons that is present in the blood. It is a component of the disaccharides sucrose, lactose, and maltose and various complex carbohydrates. Also known as *dextrose* or *blood sugar*.

glutathione peroxidase A selenium-containing enzyme that reduces toxic hydrogen peroxide formed within cells; works with vitamin E to reduce free radical damage.

glycerol [GLISS-er-ol] The backbone of mono-, di-, and triglycerides; alone, it is a thick, smooth liquid.

glycogen [GLY-ko-jen] A very large, highly branched polysaccharide composed of multiple glucose units. Sometimes called *animal starch*, glycogen is the primary storage form of glucose in animals.

glycogenesis The formation of glycogen from glucose.

glycogen loading See *carbohydrate loading*.

glycolysis [gligh-COLL-ih-sis] The anaerobic pathway that breaks down a glucose molecule into two molecules of pyruvate and yields two molecules of ATP and two molecules of NADH. Glycolysis occurs in the cytosol of a cell.

goiter A chronic enlargement of the thyroid gland, visible as a swelling at the front of the neck; usually associated with iodine deficiency.

goitrogens Compounds that interfere with iodine absorption and can induce goiter.

growth charts Charts that plot the weight, length, and head circumference of infants and children as they grow.

guanosine triphosphate (GTP) A high-energy compound, similar to ATP but with three phosphate groups linked to guanosine.

gums Dietary fibers, which contain galactose and other monosaccharides, found between plant cell walls.

gut microbiota The population of microorganisms living in the digestive tract.

gynoid obesity Excess storage of fat located primarily in the buttocks and thighs. Also called *gynecoid obesity*.

hangover The collection of symptoms experienced by someone who has consumed a large quantity of alcohol. Symptoms can include pounding headache, fatigue, muscle aches, nausea, stomach pain, heightened sensitivity to light and sound, dizziness, and possibly depression, anxiety, and irritability.

head circumference Measurement of the largest part of the infant's head (just above the eyebrows and ears); used to determine brain growth.

health claim Any statement that associates a food or a substance in a food with a disease or health-related condition. The FDA authorizes health claims.

health disparities Differences in health outcomes and their determinants between segments of the population, as defined by social, demographic, environmental, and geographic attributes.

heartburn Burning pain behind the breastbone area caused by acidic stomach contents backing up into the esophagus.

heat capacity The amount of energy required to raise the temperature of a substance 1°C.

heme A chemical complex with a central iron atom that forms the oxygen-binding part of hemoglobin and myoglobin.

heme iron The iron found in the hemoglobin and myoglobin of animal foods.

hemicellulose [hem-ih-SELL-you-los-es] A group of large polysaccharides in dietary fiber that are fermented more easily than cellulose.

hemochromatosis A hereditary disorder in which excessive absorption of iron results in abnormal iron deposits in the liver and other tissues.

hemoglobin [HEEM-oh-glow-bin] The oxygen-carrying protein in red blood cells that consists of four heme groups and four globin polypeptide chains. The presence of hemoglobin gives blood its red color.

hemosiderin An insoluble form of storage iron.

herbal therapy (phytotherapy) The therapeutic use of herbs and other plants to promote health and treat disease.

high-density lipoproteins (HDLs) The blood lipoproteins that contain high levels of protein and low levels of triglycerides. Synthesized primarily in the liver and small intestine, HDL picks up cholesterol released from dying cells and other sources and transfers it to other lipoproteins. HDL cholesterol sometimes is called "good cholesterol."

high-fructose corn syrup Sweetener made from corn commonly added to food products and beverages in the United States. It is composed of either 42 percent or 55 percent fructose, with the remaining sugar being glucose.

hormones Chemical messengers that are secreted into the blood by one tissue and act on cells in another part of the body.

Human Genome Project An effort coordinated by the Department of Energy and the National Institutes of Health to map the genes in human DNA.

hunger The internal, physiological drive to find and consume food. Unlike appetite, hunger is often experienced as a negative sensation, often manifesting as an uneasy or painful sensation; the recurrent and involuntary lack of access to food that may produce malnutrition over time.

husk The inedible covering of a grain kernel. Also known as the *chaff*.

hydrochloric acid (gastric acid) A very strong acid of chloride and hydrogen atoms made by stomach glands and secreted into the stomach. Also called *gastric acid*.

hydrogenation [high-dro-jen-AY-shun] A chemical reaction in which hydrogen atoms are added to a fat; hydrogenation produces more saturated fatty acids and converts some unsaturated fatty acids from a cis form to a trans form.

hydrolysis A reaction that breaks apart a compound through the addition of water.

hydrostatic weighing See *underwater weighing*.

hydroxyapatite A crystalline mineral compound of calcium and phosphorus that makes up bone.

hyperactivity A maladaptive and abnormal increase in activity that is inconsistent with developmental levels. Includes frequent fidgeting, inappropriate running, excessive talking, and difficulty engaging in quiet activities.

hypercellular obesity Obesity due to an above-average number of fat cells.

hypercholesterolemia The presence of greater than normal amounts of cholesterol in the blood.

hyperglycemia [HIGH-per-gly-SEE-me-uh] Abnormally high concentration of glucose in the blood.

hyperplastic obesity (hyperplasia) Obesity due to an increase in both the size and number of fat cells.

hypertension Condition in which resting blood pressure persistently exceeds 140 mm Hg systolic or 90 mm Hg diastolic.

hyperthermia A much higher than normal body temperature.

hypertrophic obesity Obesity due to an increase in the size of fat cells.

hypervitaminosis High levels of vitamins in the blood, usually a result of excess supplement intake.

hypoglycemia [HIGH-po-gly-SEE-mee-uh] Abnormally low concentration of glucose in the blood; any blood glucose value below 40 to 50 mg/dL of blood.

hypogonadism Decreased functional activity of the gonads (ovaries or testes) with retardation of growth and sexual development.

hypothalamus [high-po-THAL-ah-mus] A region of the brain involved in regulating hunger and satiety, respiration, body temperature, water balance, and other body functions.

hypothesis A supposition or proposed explanation made on the basis of limited evidence as a starting point for further investigation.

hypothyroidism The result of a lowered level of circulating thyroid hormone, with slowing of mental and physical functions.

ileum [ILL-ee-um] The terminal segment (about 5 feet or 152 cm) of the small intestine, which opens into the large intestine.

immune response A coordinated set of steps, including production of antibodies, that the immune system takes in response to an antigen.

incomplete proteins Proteins that lack one or more indispensable amino acids. Also called *low-quality proteins*.

indirect additives Substances that unintentionally become part of the food in trace amounts.

infancy The period between birth and 12 months of age.

inorganic Any substance that does not contain carbon, excepting certain simple carbon compounds such as carbon dioxide and carbon monoxide. Common examples include table salt (sodium chloride) and baking soda (sodium bicarbonate).

insensible water loss The continual loss of body water by evaporation from the respiratory tract and diffusion through the skin.

insoluble fiber Nondigestible carbohydrates that do not dissolve in water.

insulin [IN-suh-lin] Produced by beta cells in the pancreas, this polypeptide hormone stimulates the uptake of blood glucose into muscle and adipose cells, the synthesis of glycogen in the liver, and various other processes.

insulin resistance State in which enough insulin is produced but cells do not respond to the action of insulin. Also called *insulin insensitivity.*

integrated pest management (IPM) Economically sound pest control techniques that minimize pesticide use, enhance environmental stewardship, and promote sustainable systems.

intermediate-density lipoproteins (IDLs) The lipoproteins formed when lipoprotein lipase strips some of the triglycerides from VLDL.

interstitial fluid [in-ter-STISH-ul] The fluid between cells in tissues, usually high in sodium and chloride. Also called *intercellular fluid.*

intervention studies See *clinical trials.*

intracellular fluid The fluid in the body's cells. It usually is high in potassium and phosphate and low in sodium and chloride. It constitutes about two-thirds of total body water.

intravascular fluid The fluid portion (plasma) of the blood contained in arteries, veins, and capillaries. It accounts for about 15 percent of the extracellular fluid.

intrinsic factor A glycoprotein released from parietal cells in the stomach wall that binds to and aids in absorption of vitamin B_{12}.

iodine deficiency disorders A wide range of disorders due to iodine deficiency that affect growth and development.

iodopsin Color-sensitive pigment molecules in cone cells that consist of opsin-like proteins combined with retinal.

ions Atoms or groups of atoms with an electrical charge resulting from the loss or gain of one or more electrons.

iron overload Toxicity from excess iron.

irradiation A food preservation technique in which foods are exposed to measured doses of radiation to reduce or eliminate pathogens and kill insects, reduce spoilage, and, in certain fruits and vegetables, inhibit sprouting and delay ripening.

irritable bowel syndrome (IBS) A disruptive state of intestinal motility with no known cause. Symptoms include constipation, abdominal pain, and episodic diarrhea.

isoflavones Plant chemicals that include genistein and daidzein and may have positive effects against cancer and heart disease. Also called *phytoestrogens.*

jejunum [je-JOON-um] The middle section (about 4 feet or 122 cm) of the small intestine, lying between the duodenum and ileum.

keratin A water-insoluble fibrous protein that is the primary constituent of hair, nails, and the outer layer of the skin.

Keshan disease Selenium-deficiency disease that impairs the structure and function of the heart.

ketoacidosis Acidification of the blood caused by a buildup of ketone bodies. It is primarily a consequence of uncontrolled type 1 diabetes mellitus and can be life threatening.

ketogenesis The process in which excess acetyl CoA from fatty acid oxidation is converted into ketone bodies.

ketogenic A term describing an amino acid broken down to acetyl CoA (which can be converted into ketone bodies).

ketone bodies Molecules formed when insufficient carbohydrate is available to completely metabolize fat. Formation of ketone bodies is promoted by a low glucose level and high acetyl CoA level within cells. Acetone, acetoacetate, and beta-hydroxybutyrate are ketone bodies. Beta-hydroxybutyrate is sometimes improperly called a ketone.

ketones [KEE-tonez] Organic compounds that contain a chemical group consisting of C=O (a carbon–oxygen double bond) bound to two hydrocarbons. Pyruvate and fructose are examples of ketones. Acetone and acetoacetate are both ketones and ketone bodies. Although beta-hydroxybutyrate is not a ketone, it is a ketone body.

ketosis [kee-TOE-sis] Abnormally high concentration of ketone bodies in body tissues and fluids.

kilocalories (kcal) [KILL-oh-kal-oh-rees] Units used to measure food energy (1,000 calories = 1 kilocalorie).

Krebs cycle See *citric acid cycle.*

kwashiorkor A type of malnutrition that occurs primarily in young children who have an infectious disease and whose diets supply marginal amounts of energy and very little protein. Common symptoms include poor growth, edema, apathy, weakness, and susceptibility to infections.

lactate A three-carbon compound that is produced when insufficient oxygen is present in cells to break down pyruvate to acetyl CoA. Often called *lactic acid.*

lactation The process of synthesizing and secreting breast milk.

lactation consultants Health professionals trained to specialize in education about and promotion of breastfeeding; can be certified as an International Board Certified Lactation Consultant (IBCLC).

lacteal A small lymphatic vessel in the interior of each intestinal villus that picks up chylomicrons and fat-soluble vitamins from intestinal cells.

lactic acid energy system Anaerobic energy system; using glycolysis, the process rapidly produces energy (ATP) and lactate. Also called *anaerobic glycolysis.*

lactose [LAK-tose] A disaccharide composed of glucose and galactose. Also called *milk sugar* because it is the major sugar in milk and dairy products.

lactose intolerance The inability to digest lactose, leading to diarrhea, bloating, and gas whenever lactose-containing foods are consumed.

large intestine The tube (about 5 feet or 152 cm long) extending from the ileum of the small intestine to the anus. The large intestine includes the appendix, cecum, colon, rectum, and anal canal.

laxatives Substances that promote evacuation of the bowel by increasing the bulk of the feces, lubricating the intestinal wall, or softening the stool.

lean body mass The portion of the body exclusive of stored fat, including muscle, bone, connective tissue, organs, and water.

lecithin In the body, a phospholipid with the nitrogen-containing component choline. In foods, lecithin is a blend of phospholipids with different nitrogen-containing components.

legumes A family of plants with edible seed pods, such as peas, beans, lentils, and soybeans. Also called *pulses.*

leptin A hormone produced by adipose cells that signals the amount of body fat content and influences food intake.

let-down reflex The release of milk from the breast tissue in response to the stimulus of the hormone oxytocin. The major stimulus for oxytocin release is the infant suckling at the breast.

leukemia [loo-KEE-mee-a] Cancer of blood-forming tissue.

lignin [LIG-nin] Insoluble fiber composed of multi-ring alcohol units that constitute the only noncarbohydrate component of dietary fiber.

limiting amino acid The amino acid in shortest supply during protein synthesis. Also the amino acid in the lowest quantity when evaluating protein quality.

lingual lipase A fat-splitting enzyme secreted by cells at the base of the tongue.

linoleic acid [lin-oh-LAY-ik] An essential omega-6 fatty acid that contains 18 carbon atoms and 2 carbon–carbon double bonds (18:2); a thin liquid at room temperature.

lipids A group of fat-soluble compounds that includes triglycerides, sterols, and phospholipids.

lipogenesis [lye-poh-JEN-eh-sis] Synthesis of fatty acids from acetyl CoA derived from the metabolism of fats, alcohol, and some amino acids.

lipoprotein A complex that transports lipids in the lymph and blood. Lipoproteins consist of a central core of triglycerides and cholesterol surrounded by a shell composed of proteins, cholesterol, and phospholipids. The various types of lipoproteins differ in size, composition, and density.

lipoprotein a [Lp(a)] A substance that consists of an LDL "bad cholesterol" part plus a protein (apoprotein a), whose exact function is currently unknown.

lipoprotein lipase The major enzyme responsible for the breakdown of lipoproteins and triglycerides in the blood.

liver The largest glandular organ in the body, it produces and secretes bile, detoxifies harmful substances, and helps metabolize carbohydrates, lipids, proteins, and micronutrients.

longitudinal muscle Muscle fibers aligned lengthwise.

Lou Gehrig's disease A syndrome marked by muscular weakness and atrophy due to a degeneration of motor neurons of the spinal cord. Technically known as *amyotrophic lateral sclerosis (ALS)*.

low-birth-weight infant A newborn who weighs less than 2,500 grams (5.5 pounds) as a result of either premature birth or inadequate growth in utero.

low-density lipoproteins (LDLs) The cholesterol-rich lipoproteins that result from the breakdown and removal of triglycerides from intermediate-density lipoprotein. LDL cholesterol sometimes is called "bad cholesterol."

lumen Cavity or hollow channel in any organ or structure of the body.

lycopene One of a family of plant chemicals, the carotenoids. Others in this big family include alpha-carotene and beta-carotene.

lymph Fluid that travels through the lymphatic system, made up of fluid drained from between cells and large fat particles.

lymphatic system A system of small vessels, ducts, valves, and organized tissue (e.g., lymph nodes) through which lymph moves from its origin in the tissues toward the heart.

lymph nodes [limf nodes] Rounded masses of lymphatic tissue that are surrounded by a capsule of connective tissue. Lymph nodes filter lymph (lymphatic fluid), and they store lymphocytes (white blood cells). They are located along lymphatic vessels. Also called *lymph glands*.

lymphocytes White blood cells that are primarily responsible for immune responses. Present in the blood and lymph.

lymphoma [lim-FO-ma] Cancer that arises in cells of the lymphatic system.

macrominerals Major minerals required in the diet and present in the body in large amounts compared with trace minerals.

macronutrients Nutrients, such as carbohydrate, fat, or protein, that are needed in relatively large amounts in the diet.

macrophages Large immune system cells that function as patrol cells and engulf and kill foreign invaders.

macular degeneration Progressive deterioration of the macula, an area in the center of the retina, that eventually leads to loss of central vision.

mad cow disease See *bovine spongiform encephalopathy (BSE)*.

major minerals Minerals that are required in the diet and are present in the body in large amounts compared with trace minerals. Also known as *macrominerals*.

malabsorption syndromes Conditions that result in imperfect, inadequate, or otherwise disordered gastrointestinal absorption.

malignant [ma-LIG-nant] Cancerous; a growth with a tendency to invade and destroy nearby tissue and spread to other parts of the body.

malnutrition Failure to achieve nutrient requirements, which can impair physical and/or mental health. It may result from consuming too little food or from a shortage or imbalance of key nutrients.

maltose [MALL-tose] A disaccharide composed of two glucose molecules. Maltose seldom occurs naturally in foods but is formed whenever long molecules of starch break down. Sometimes called *malt sugar*.

marasmus A type of malnutrition resulting from chronic inadequate consumption of protein and energy that is characterized by wasting of muscle, fat, and other body tissue.

Meals on Wheels A voluntary, not-for-profit organization established to provide nutritious meals to homebound people (regardless of age) so they can maintain their independence and quality of life.

megadoses Doses of a nutrient that are 10 or more times the recommended amount.

megaloblastic anemia Excess amounts of megaloblasts (immature red blood cells) in the blood caused by deficiency of folate or vitamin B_{12}.

melanocytes [mel-AN-o-sites] Cells in the skin that produce and contain the pigment called melanin.

melanoma A form of skin cancer that arises in melanocytes, the cells that produce pigment. Melanoma usually begins in a mole.

menadione A medicinal form of vitamin K. Also known as *vitamin K_3*.

menaquinones The form of vitamin K that comes from animal sources or is produced by intestinal bacteria. Also known as *vitamin K_2*.

menarche First menstrual period.

Menkes syndrome A genetic disorder that results in copper deficiency.

metabolically healthy obesity A condition of reduced risk for obesity-related metabolic diseases.

metabolic pathway A series of chemical reactions that either break down a large compound into smaller units (catabolism) or synthesize more complex molecules from smaller ones (anabolism).

metabolic syndrome A cluster of at least three of the following risk factors for heart disease: hypertriglyceridemia (high blood triglycerides), low HDL cholesterol, hyperglycemia (high blood glucose), hypertension (high blood pressure), and excess abdominal fat.

metabolism All chemical reactions within organisms that enable them to maintain life. The two main categories of metabolism are catabolism and anabolism.

metabolites Substances produced during metabolism.

metastasis [meh-TAS-ta-sis] The spread of cancer from one part of the body to another. Tumors formed from cells that have spread are called "secondary tumors" and contain cells that are like those in the original (primary) tumor. The plural is *metastases*.

methylmercury A toxic compound that results from the chemical transformation of mercury by bacteria. Mercury is water-soluble in trace amounts and contaminates many bodies of water.

micelles Tiny emulsified fat packets. They are composed of emulsifier molecules (phospholipids) oriented with their fat-soluble part facing inward and their water-soluble part facing outward toward the surrounding aqueous environment.

microencephaly A type of neural tube birth defect in which the brain is abnormally small.

microminerals See *trace minerals*.

micronutrients Nutrients, such as vitamins and minerals, that are needed in relatively small amounts in the diet.

microsomal ethanol-oxidizing system (MEOS) An energy-requiring enzyme system in the liver that normally metabolizes drugs and other foreign substances. When the blood alcohol level is high, alcohol dehydrogenase cannot metabolize it fast enough, and the excess alcohol is metabolized by MEOS.

microvilli Minute, hairlike projections that extend from the surface of absorptive cells facing the intestinal lumen.

mineralization The addition of minerals, such as calcium and phosphate, to bones and teeth.

minerals Inorganic compounds needed for growth and for regulation of body processes.

mitochondria (mitochondrion) The sites of aerobic production of ATP, where most of the energy from carbohydrate, protein, and fat is captured. Called the "power plants" of the cell, the mitochondria are where the citric acid cycle and electron transport chain are located. A human cell contains about 2,000 mitochondria.

mitochondrial membrane The mitochondria are enclosed by a double shell separated by an intermembrane space. The outer membrane acts as a barrier and gatekeeper, selectively allowing some molecules to pass through while blocking others. The inner membrane is where the electron transport chain is located.

monoglyceride A molecule of glycerol combined with one fatty acid.

monosaccharides [mon-uh-SACK-uh-rides] Any sugars that are not broken down further during digestion and have the general formula $C_nH_{2n}O_n$, where $n = 3$ to 7. The common monosaccharides glucose, fructose, and galactose all have six carbon atoms ($n = 6$).

monounsaturated fatty acid (MUFA) A fatty acid in which the carbon chain contains one double bond.

morbid obesity See *extreme obesity*.

morning sickness A persistent or recurring nausea that often occurs in the morning during early pregnancy.

motor proteins Proteins that use energy and convert it into some form of mechanical work. Motor proteins are active in processes such as cell division, muscle contraction, and sperm movement.

mucilage Gelatinous soluble fiber containing galactose, mannose, and other monosaccharides; found in seaweed.

mucosa [myu-KO-sa] The innermost layer of a cavity. The inner layer of the gastrointestinal tract (the intestinal wall). It is composed of epithelial cells and glands.

mucus A slippery substance secreted in the GI tract (and other body linings) that protects cells from irritants.

multiple sclerosis A progressive disease that destroys the myelin sheath surrounding nerve fibers of the brain and spinal cord.

muscle fibers Individual muscle cells.

mutation A permanent structural alteration in DNA. In most cases, DNA changes either have no effect or cause harm. Occasionally, a mutation can improve an organism's chance of surviving and passing the beneficial change on to its descendants. Certain mutations can lead to cancer or other diseases.

myelin sheath The protective coating that surrounds nerve fibers.

myoglobin The oxygen-transporting protein of muscle that resembles blood hemoglobin in function.

MyPlate The current nutrition guide published by the United States Department of Agriculture, presented in the format of an easy-to-understand visual image intended to empower people with the information they need to make healthy food choices and create eating habits consistent with the *Dietary Guidelines for Americans, 2015–2020*.

NAD+ Nicotinamide adenine dinucleotide (NAD+), a coenzyme derived from the B vitamin niacin, becomes NADH as it accepts a pair of high-energy electrons for transport in cells.

National Center for Complementary and Integrative Health (NCCIH) An NIH organization established to stimulate, develop, and support objective scientific research on complementary and integrative health for the benefit of the public.

National Institutes of Health (NIH) A U.S. Department of Health and Human Services agency composed of 27 separate institutes and centers with a mission to advance knowledge and improve human health.

natural killer cells Nonspecific lymphocytes that spontaneously attack and kill cancer cells and cells infected by microorganisms. They are "natural" killers because they do not need to recognize a specific antigen in order to attack and kill.

natural sweeteners Sweeteners such as honey and maple syrup that contain monosaccharides and disaccharides that make them taste sweet. Honey contains a mix of fructose and glucose—the same two monosaccharides that make up sucrose. Bees make honey from the sucrose-containing nectar of flowering plants. Real maple syrup contains primarily sucrose and is made by boiling and concentrating the sap from sugar maple trees. Most maple-flavored syrups sold in grocery stores, however, are made from corn syrup with maple flavoring added.

natural toxins Poisons that are produced by or naturally occur in plants or microorganisms.

negative energy balance Energy intake is lower than energy expenditure, resulting in a depletion of body energy stores and weight loss.

negative nitrogen balance Nitrogen intake is less than the sum of all sources of nitrogen excretion.

negative self-talk Mental or verbal statements made to one's self that reinforce negative or destructive self-perceptions.

neonate An infant less than four weeks old.

neophobia A dislike for anything new or unfamiliar.

neural tube defects (NTDs) Birth defects resulting from failure of the neural tube to develop properly during early fetal development.

neuropeptide Y (NPY) A neurotransmitter widely distributed throughout the brain and peripheral nervous tissue. NPY activity has been linked to eating behavior, depression, anxiety, and cardiovascular function.

neurotransmitters Substances released at the end of a stimulated nerve cell that diffuse across a small gap and bind to another nerve cell or muscle cell, stimulating or inhibiting it.

niacin equivalents (NEs) A measure that includes preformed dietary niacin as well as niacin derived from tryptophan; 60 milligrams of tryptophan yield about 1 milligram of niacin.

night blindness The inability of the eyes to adjust to dim light or to regain vision quickly after exposure to a flash of bright light.

nitrogen balance Intake minus the sum of all sources of nitrogen excretion.

nitrogen equilibrium Nitrogen intake equals the sum of all sources of nitrogen excretion; nitrogen balance equals zero.

nonessential amino acids Amino acids that the body can make if supplied with adequate nitrogen. Nonessential amino acids do not need to be supplied in the diet.

nonessential fatty acids Fatty acids that your body can make when they are needed. It is not necessary to consume them in the diet.

nonessential nutrients Those nutrients that can be made by the body.

nonexercise activity thermogenesis (NEAT) The output of energy associated with fidgeting, maintenance of posture, and other minimal physical exertions.

nonheme iron The iron in plants and animal foods that is not part of hemoglobin or myoglobin.

non-nutritive sweeteners Substances that impart sweetness to foods but supply little or no energy to the body. They include acesulfame, aspartame, saccharin, and sucralose. Also called *artificial sweeteners* or *alternative sweeteners*.

normal weight BMI at or above 18.5 kg/m² and less than 25 kg/m².

nucleic acids A family of more than 25,000 molecules found in chromosomes, nucleoli, mitochondria, and the cytoplasm of cells.

nucleotides Subunits of DNA or RNA consisting of a nitrogenous base (adenine, guanine, thymine, or cytosine in DNA; adenine, guanine, uracil, or cytosine in RNA), a phosphate molecule, and a sugar molecule (deoxyribose in DNA and ribose in RNA). Thousands of nucleotides are linked to form a DNA or RNA molecule.

nucleus The primary site of genetic information in the cell, enclosed in a double-layered membrane.

nutrient content claims These claims describe the level of a nutrient or dietary substance in the product, using terms such as *good source*, *high*, or *free*.

nutrient density A description of the healthfulness of foods. Foods high in nutrient density are those that provide substantial amounts of vitamins and minerals and relatively few calories; foods low in nutrient density are those that supply calories but relatively small amounts of vitamins and minerals (or none at all).

nutrients Any substances in food that the body can use to obtain energy, synthesize tissues, or regulate functions.

nutrigenomics The study of how nutrition interacts with specific genes to influence a person's health.

nutrition The science of foods and their components (nutrients and other substances), including the relationships to health and disease (actions, interactions, and balances); processes within the body (ingestion, digestion, absorption, transport, functions, and disposal of end products); and the social, economic, cultural, and psychological implications of eating.

Nutrition Facts panel A portion of the food label that states the content of selected nutrients in a food in a standard way prescribed by the Food and Drug Administration. By law, Nutrition Facts must appear on nearly all processed food products in the United States. The new Nutrition Facts panel is intended to make it easier for consumers to make informed decisions about the foods they are eating. For example, the new panel includes nutrients that better reflect people's adequate consumption, overconsumption, or underconsumption of nutrients and vitamins such as added sugar, vitamin D, and potassium.

nutrition informatics "The effective retrieval, organization, storage, and optimum use of information, data, and knowledge for food and nutrition related problem solving and decision-making. Informatics is supported by the use of information standards, processes, and technology." (Academy of Nutrition and Dietetics)

Nutrition Recommendations for Canadians A set of scientific statements that provide guidance to Canadians for a dietary pattern that will supply recommended amounts of all essential nutrients while reducing the risk of chronic disease.

nutritive sweeteners Substances that impart sweetness to foods and that can be absorbed and yield energy in the body. Simple sugars, sugar alcohols, and high-fructose corn syrup are the most common nutritive sweeteners used in food products.

obesity Excessive accumulation of body fat leading to a body weight in relation to height that is substantially greater than some accepted standard. A BMI at or above 30 kg/m².

obesogenic environment Circumstances in which a person lives, works, and plays in a way that promotes the overconsumption of calories and discourages physical activity and calorie expenditure.

obsessive-compulsive disorder A psychiatric disorder in which a person attempts to relieve anxiety by ritualistic behavior and continuous repetition of certain acts.

Older Americans Act Nutrition Program A federally funded program (formerly known as the Elderly Nutrition Program) that provides older persons with nutritionally sound meals through home-delivered nutrition services, congregate nutrition services, and the nutrition services' incentive.

oligopeptide Four to 10 amino acids joined by peptide bonds.

oligosaccharides Short carbohydrate chains composed of 3 to 10 sugar molecules.

omega-3 fatty acid An essential fatty acid; alpha-linolenic acid is the primary type.

omega-6 fatty acid An essential fatty acid; linoleic acid is the primary type.

opsin A protein that combines with retinal to form rhodopsin in rod cells.

organelles Various membrane-bound structures that form part of the cytoplasm. Organelles perform specialized metabolic functions.

organic In chemistry, any compound that contains carbon, except carbon oxides (e.g., carbon dioxide) and sulfides and metal carbonates (e.g., potassium carbonate). The term *organic* also is used to denote crops that are grown without synthetic fertilizers or chemicals.

organic foods Foods that originate from farms or handling operations that meet the standards set by the USDA National Organic Program.

organogenesis The period when organ systems are developing in a growing fetus.

orthomolecular medicine The preventive or therapeutic use of high-dose vitamins to treat disease.

osmosis The movement of a solvent, such as water, through a semi-permeable membrane from the dilute to the concentrated side until the concentrations on both sides of the membrane are equal.

osteoblasts Bone cells that synthesize and excrete the extracellular matrix that forms the structure of bone.

osteoclasts Bone cells that break down bone structure and release calcium and phosphate into the blood.

osteomalacia A disease in adults that results from vitamin D deficiency; it is marked by softening of the bones, leading to bending of the spine, bowing of the legs, and increased risk for fractures.

osteoporosis A bone disease characterized by a decrease in bone mineral density and the appearance of small holes in bones due to loss of minerals.

overnutrition The long-term consumption of an excess of nutrients. The most common type of overnutrition in the United States results from the regular consumption of excess calories, fats, saturated fats, and cholesterol.

overweight BMI at or above 25 kg/m^2 and less than 30 kg/m^2.

oxalate (oxalic acid) An organic acid in some leafy green vegetables, such as spinach, that binds to calcium to form calcium oxalate, an insoluble compound the body cannot absorb.

oxaloacetate A four-carbon intermediate compound in the citric acid cycle. Acetyl CoA combines with free oxaloacetate in the mitochondria, forming citric acid and beginning the cycle.

oxidation Occurs when oxygen attaches to the double bonds of unsaturated fatty acids. It causes fats to become rancid.

oxygen energy system A complex energy system that requires oxygen. To release ATP, it completes the breakdown of carbohydrate and fatty acids via the citric acid cycle and electron transport chain.

oxytocin A pituitary hormone that stimulates the release of milk from the breast.

palatable Pleasant tasting.

pancreas An organ that secretes enzymes that affect the digestion and absorption of nutrients and that releases hormones, such as insulin, that regulate metabolism as well as the way nutrients are used in the body.

pancreatic amylase Starch-digesting enzyme secreted by the pancreas.

parathyroid hormone (PTH) A hormone secreted by the parathyroid glands in response to low blood calcium. It stimulates calcium release from bone and calcium absorption by the intestines, while decreasing calcium excretion by the kidneys. It acts in conjunction with 1,25(OH)$_2$D$_3$ to raise blood calcium. Also called *parathormone*.

passive diffusion The movement of substances into or out of cells without the expenditure of energy or the involvement of transport proteins in the cell membrane. Also called *simple diffusion*.

pasteurization A process for destroying pathogenic bacteria by heating liquid foods to a prescribed temperature for a specified time.

pathogenic Capable of causing disease.

pectin A type of dietary fiber found in fruits.

peer review An appraisal of research against accepted standards by professionals in the field.

pepsin A protein-digesting enzyme produced by the stomach.

pepsinogen The inactive form of the enzyme pepsin.

peptide bond The bond between two amino acids formed when a carboxyl (–COOH) group of one amino acid joins an amino (–NH$_2$) group of another amino acid, releasing water in the process.

perceived exertion The subjective experience of how difficult an effort is.

peristalsis [per-ih-STAHL-sis] The wavelike, rhythmic muscular contractions of the GI tract that propel its contents down the tract.

pernicious anemia A form of anemia that results from an autoimmune disorder that damages cells lining the stomach and inhibits vitamin B$_{12}$ absorption; causes vitamin B$_{12}$ deficiency.

pesticides Chemicals used to control insects, diseases, weeds, fungi, and other pests on plants, vegetables, fruits, and animals.

pH A measurement of the hydrogen ion concentration, or acidity, of a solution.

phenylketonuria (PKU) An inherited disorder caused by a lack or deficiency of the enzyme that converts phenylalanine to tyrosine.

phosphate group A chemical group that contains phosphate (–PO$_4$) attached to a larger molecule. Attaching a phosphate group, along with two fatty acids, to a glycerol backbone forms a phospholipid.

phosphocreatine See *creatine phosphate*.

phospholipids Compounds that consist of a glycerol molecule bonded to two fatty acid molecules and a phosphate group with a nitrogen-containing component. Phospholipids have both water-soluble and fat-soluble regions, which makes them good emulsifiers.

photosynthesis The process by which green plants use light energy from the sun to produce carbohydrates from carbon dioxide and water.

phylloquinone The form of vitamin K that comes from plant sources. Also known as *vitamin K$_1$*.

phytate (phytic acid) A phosphorus-containing compound in the outer husks of cereal grains that binds with minerals and inhibits their absorption.

phytochemicals Substances in plants that may possess health-protective effects, even though they are not essential for life.

phytoestrogens Compounds that have weak estrogen activity in the body.

phytosterols Sterols found in plants. Phytosterols are poorly absorbed by humans and reduce intestinal absorption of cholesterol. They recently have been introduced as a cholesterol-lowering food ingredient.

placebo An inactive substance that is outwardly indistinguishable from the active substance whose effects are being studied.

placebo effect A physical or emotional change that is not due to properties of an administered substance. The change reflects participants' expectations.

placenta The organ formed in the mother's uterus during pregnancy that produces hormones to maintain the pregnancy, and across which the fetus receives oxygen and nutrients from the mother and empties its waste materials via the mother's circulatory system.

plaque A buildup of substances that circulate in the blood (e.g., calcium, fat, cholesterol, cellular waste, fibrin) on a blood vessel wall, making it vulnerable to blockage from blood clots.

plasma The fluid portion of the blood that contains blood cells and other components.

platelets Tiny disk-shaped components of blood that are essential for blood clotting.

poisonous mushrooms Mushrooms that contain toxins that can cause stomach upset, dizziness, hallucinations, and other neurological symptoms.

pollutants Gaseous, chemical, or organic waste that contaminates air, soil, or water.

polyols See *sugar alcohols.*

polypeptide More than 10 amino acids joined by peptide bonds.

polyphenols Organic compounds that may produce bitterness in coffee and tea.

polysaccharides Long carbohydrate chains composed of more than 10 sugar molecules. Polysaccharides can be straight or branched.

polyunsaturated fatty acid (PUFA) A fatty acid in which the carbon chain contains two or more double bonds.

positive energy balance Energy intake exceeds energy expenditure, resulting in an increase in body energy stores and weight gain.

positive nitrogen balance Nitrogen intake exceeds the sum of all sources of nitrogen excretion.

positive self-talk Constructive mental or verbal statements made to one's self to change a belief or behavior.

prebiotics Natural, nondigestible components of food that promote the growth of healthy bacteria in the gut and overall health.

precursor A substance that is converted into another active substance. Enzyme precursors also are called *proenzymes.*

pre-diabetes Blood glucose levels higher than normal but not high enough to warrant a diagnosis of diabetes.

preeclampsia A condition of late pregnancy characterized by maternal hypertension, edema, and proteinuria.

preformed vitamin A Retinyl esters, the main storage form of vitamin A. About 90 percent of dietary retinol is in the form of esters, mostly found in foods from animal sources.

prematurity Birth before 37 weeks of gestation.

preservatives Chemicals or other agents that slow the decomposition of a food.

preterm delivery A delivery that occurs before the thirty-seventh week of gestation.

prions Short for *proteinaceous infectious particle.* Self-reproducing protein particles that can cause disease.

prior-sanctioned substance An additive which was determined by the FDA or USDA to be safe for use in a specific food before the 1958 legislation.

probiotics Living microorganisms that provide health benefits when ingested, either directly through interactions with host cells or indirectly through effects on other bacterial species. Also known as *live cultures.*

proenzymes Inactive precursors of enzymes.

prolactin A pituitary hormone that stimulates the production of milk in breast tissue.

proteases [PRO-tea-aces] Enzymes that break down protein into peptides and amino acids.

protein digestibility-corrected amino acid score (PDCAAS) A measure of protein quality that takes into account the amino acid composition of the food and the digestibility of the protein.

protein-energy malnutrition (PEM) A condition resulting from long-term inadequate intakes of energy and protein that can lead to wasting of body tissues and increased susceptibility to infection.

protein hydrolysates Proteins that have been treated with enzymes to break them down into amino acids and shorter peptides.

proteins Large, complex compounds consisting of many amino acids connected in varying sequences and forming unique shapes.

protein turnover Constant breakdown and synthesis of proteins in the body.

provitamin A Carotenoid precursors of vitamin A in foods of plant origin, primarily deeply colored fruits and vegetables.

provitamins Inactive forms of vitamins that the body can convert into active usable forms. Also referred to as *vitamin precursors.*

psyllium The dried husk of the psyllium seed.

puberty The period of life during which the secondary sex characteristics develop and the ability to reproduce is attained.

purging Emptying the gastrointestinal (GI) tract by self-induced vomiting and/or misuse of laxatives, diuretics, or enemas.

pyloric sphincter A circular muscle that forms the opening between the duodenum and the stomach. It regulates the passage of food into the small intestine.

pyruvate The three-carbon compound that results from glycolysis. Cells also can make glucose from pyruvate, but this process requires energy and several enzymes not involved in glycolysis. Pyruvate also can be derived from glycerol and some amino acids.

reactive hypoglycemia A type of hypoglycemia that occurs about one hour after eating carbohydrate-rich food. The body overreacts and produces too much insulin in response to food, rapidly decreasing blood glucose.

Recommended Dietary Allowances (RDAs) The nutrient intake levels that meet the nutrient needs of almost all (97 to 98 percent) individuals in a life-stage and gender group.

Recommended Nutrient Intakes (RNIs) Canadian dietary standards that have been replaced by Dietary Reference Intakes.

rectum The muscular final segment of the intestine, extending from the sigmoid colon to the anus.

refined sweeteners Composed of monosaccharides and disaccharides that have been extracted and processed from other foods, such as high-fructose corn syrup and agave syrup.

requirement The lowest continuing intake level of a nutrient that prevents deficiency in an individual.

resistant starch A starch that is not digested.

resting energy expenditure (REE) The minimum energy needed to maintain basic physiological functions (e.g., heartbeat, muscle function, respiration). The resting metabolic rate (RMR) extrapolated to 24 hours.

resting metabolic rate (RMR) A clinical measure of resting energy expenditure performed three to four hours after eating or performing significant physical activity.

restrained eaters Individuals who routinely avoid food as long as possible, and then gorge on food.

retina A paper-thin tissue that lines the back of the eye and contains cells called rods and cones.

retinal The aldehyde form of vitamin A; one of the retinoids; the active form of vitamin A in the retina; interconvertible with retinol.

retinoic acid The acid form of vitamin A; one of the retinoids; formed from retinal but not interconvertible; helps growth, cell differentiation, and the immune system; does not have a role in vision or reproduction.

retinoids Compounds in foods that have chemical structures similar to vitamin A. Retinoids include the active forms of vitamin A (retinol, retinal, and retinoic acid) and the main storage forms of retinol (retinyl esters).

retinol The alcohol form of vitamin A; one of the retinoids; the main physiologically active form of vitamin A; interconvertible with retinal.

retinol activity equivalent (RAE) A unit of measurement of the vitamin A content of a food. One RAE equals 1 microgram of retinol.

rhodopsin Found in rod cells, this light-sensitive pigment molecule consists of a protein called opsin combined with retinal.

rickets A bone disease in children that results from vitamin D deficiency.

risk factors Anything that increases a person's chance of developing a disease, including substances, agents, genetic alterations, traits, habits, or conditions.

rod cells Light-sensitive cells in the retina that react to dim light and transmit black-and-white images.

saccharin [SAK-ah-ren] An artificial sweetener that tastes about 300 to 700 times sweeter than sucrose.

salivary amylase [AM-ih-lace] An enzyme that catalyzes the hydrolysis of amylose, a starch. Also called *ptyalin*.

salivary glands Glands in the mouth that release saliva.

Salmonella Rod-shaped bacteria responsible for many foodborne illnesses.

salts Compounds that result when the hydrogen of an acid is replaced with a metal or a group that acts like a metal.

satiation Feeling of satisfaction and fullness that terminates a meal.

satiety The effects of a food or meal that delay subsequent intake. Feeling of satisfaction and fullness following eating that quells the desire for food.

saturated fatty acid A fatty acid completely filled by hydrogen, with all carbons in the chain linked by single bonds.

secondary hypertension Hypertension caused by an underlying condition such as a kidney disorder. Once the underlying condition is treated, the blood pressure usually returns to normal.

segmentation Periodic muscle contractions at intervals along the GI tract that alternate forward and backward movement of the contents, thereby breaking apart chunks of the food mass and mixing in digestive juices.

simple carbohydrates Sugars composed of a single sugar molecule (a monosaccharide) or two joined sugar molecules (a disaccharide).

skeletal muscles Muscles composed of bundles of parallel, striated muscle fibers under voluntary control. Also called *voluntary muscle* or *striated muscle*.

skinfold measurements A method to estimate body fat by measuring the thickness of a fold of skin and subcutaneous fat.

sleep apnea Periods of absence of breathing during sleep.

slow-twitch (ST) fibers Muscle fibers that develop tension more slowly and to a lesser extent than fast-twitch muscle fibers. ST fibers have high oxidative capacities and are slower to fatigue than fast-twitch fibers.

small intestine Where the digestion of protein, fat, and carbohydrate is completed and where the majority of nutrients are absorbed. The small intestine is approximately 3 meters [10 ft] long and is divided into three parts: the duodenum, the jejunum, and the ileum.

solanine A potentially toxic alkaloid that is present with chlorophyll in the green areas on potato skins.

soluble fiber Nondigestible carbohydrates that dissolve in water.

Special Supplemental Nutrition Program for Women, Infants, and Children (WIC) A USDA program that provides federal grants to states for supplemental foods, healthcare referrals, and nutrition education for low-income pregnant, breastfeeding, and nonbreastfeeding postpartum women, and to infants and children at nutritional risk.

sphincters [SFINGK-ters] Circular bands of muscle fibers that surround the entrance or exit of a hollow body structure (e.g., the stomach) and act as valves to control the flow of material.

sphygmomanometer [sfig-mo-ma-NOM-ehter] An instrument for measuring blood pressure and especially arterial blood pressure.

spina bifida A type of neural tube birth defect.

sports anemia A lowered concentration of hemoglobin in the blood due to dilution. The increased plasma volume that dilutes the hemoglobin is a normal consequence of aerobic training.

squalene A cholesterol precursor found in whale liver and plants.

standard drink One serving of alcohol (about 15 grams) is equal to 12 ounces of beer, 4 to 5 ounces of wine, or 1.5 ounces of liquor.

starch The major storage form of carbohydrate in plants; starch is composed of long chains of glucose molecules in a straight (amylose) or branching (amylopectin) arrangement.

statement of identity A mandate that commercial food products prominently display the common or usual name of the product or identify the food with an "appropriately descriptive term."

stem cells A formative cell whose daughter cells can differentiate into other cell types.

sterols A category of lipids that includes cholesterol. Sterols are hydrocarbons with several rings in their structures.

stomach The enlarged, muscular, saclike portion of the digestive tract between the esophagus and the small intestine, with a capacity of about 1 quart.

structure/function claims These statements may claim a benefit related to a nutrient-deficiency disease (e.g., Vitamin C prevents scurvy) or describe the role of a nutrient or dietary ingredient intended to affect a structure or function in humans (e.g., Calcium helps build strong bones).

subcutaneous fat Fat stores under the skin.

sucralose An artificial sweetener made from sucrose; it was approved for use in the United States in 1998 and has been used in Canada since 1992. Sucralose is non-nutritive and about 600 times sweeter than sugar.

sucrose [SOO-crose] A disaccharide composed of one molecule of glucose and one molecule of fructose joined together. Also known as *table sugar*.

sugar alcohols Compounds formed from monosaccharides by replacing a hydrogen atom with a hydroxyl group (–OH); commonly used as nutritive sweeteners. Also called *polyols*.

Supplemental Nutrition Assistance Program (SNAP) A USDA program that helps single people and families with little or no income to buy food. Formerly known as the Food Stamp Program.

Supplement Facts panel Content label that must appear on all dietary supplements.

systolic Pertaining to a heart contraction. Systolic blood pressure is measured during a heart contraction, a time period known as systole.

taste threshold The minimum amount of flavor that must be present for a taste to be detected.

teratogen Any substance that causes birth defects.

thermic effect of food (TEF) The energy used to digest, absorb, and metabolize energy-yielding foodstuffs. It constitutes about 10 percent of total energy expenditure but is influenced by various factors.

thiamin pyrophosphate (TPP) A coenzyme of which the vitamin thiamin is a part. It plays a key role in removing carboxyl groups in chemical reactions and helps drive the reaction that forms acetyl CoA from pyruvate during metabolism.

thyroid-stimulating hormone (TSH) Hormone secreted from the pituitary gland at the base of the brain; regulates synthesis of thyroid hormones.

tissue A group or layer of cells that are alike and that work together to perform a specific function.

tocopherol The chemical name for vitamin E. There are four tocopherols (alpha, beta, gamma, and delta), but only alpha-tocopherol is active in the body.

tocotrienol Four compounds (alpha, beta, gamma, and delta) chemically related to tocopherols. The tocotrienols and tocopherols are collectively known as vitamin E.

toddler A child between 12 and 36 months of age.

Tolerable Upper Intake Levels (ULs) The maximum levels of daily nutrient intakes that are unlikely to pose health risks to almost all of the individuals in the group for whom they are designed.

total energy expenditure (TEE) The total of the resting energy expenditure (REE), energy used in physical activity, and energy used in processing food (TEF); usually expressed in kilocalories per day.

trace minerals Those minerals present in the body and required in the diet in relatively small amounts compared with major minerals. Also known as *microminerals*.

trans fatty acid An unsaturated fatty acid with a straighter chain than a cis fatty acid, usually as a result of hydrogenation; trans fatty acids are more solid than cis fatty acids.

transferrin A protein synthesized in the liver that transports iron in the blood to the red blood cells for use in heme synthesis.

tricarboxylic acid (TCA) cycle See *citric acid cycle*.

triglycerides Fats composed of three fatty acid chains linked to a glycerol molecule.

trimesters Three equal time periods of pregnancy, each lasting approximately 13 to 14 weeks, that do not coincide with specific stages in fetal development.

tripeptide Three amino acids joined by peptide bonds.

tryptophan An amino acid that serves as a niacin precursor in the body. In the body, 60 milligrams of tryptophan yield about one milligram of niacin, or 1 niacin equivalent (NE).

tumor An abnormal mass of tissue that results from excessive cell division. Tumors perform no useful body function. They can be benign (not cancerous) or malignant (cancerous).

type 1 diabetes Diabetes that occurs when the body's immune system attacks beta cells in the pancreas, causing them to lose their ability to make insulin.

type 2 diabetes Diabetes that occurs when target cells (e.g., fat and muscle cells) lose the ability to respond normally to insulin.

ulcer A craterlike lesion that occurs in the lining of the stomach or duodenum; also called a *peptic ulcer* to distinguish it from a skin ulcer.

umami [ooh-MA-mee] A Japanese term that describes a delicious meaty or savory sensation. Chemically, this taste detects the presence of glutamate.

undernutrition Poor health resulting from depletion of nutrients caused by inadequate nutrient intake over time. It is now most often associated with poverty, alcoholism, and some types of eating disorders.

underwater weighing Determining body density by measuring the volume of water displaced when the body is fully submerged in a specialized water tank. Also called *hydrostatic weighing*.

underweight BMI less than 18.5 kg/m^2.

unsaturated fatty acid A fatty acid in which the carbon chain contains one or more double bonds.

urea The main nitrogen-containing waste product in mammals. Formed in liver cells from ammonia and carbon dioxide, urea is carried via the bloodstream to the kidneys, where it is excreted in urine.

urinary tract infection (UTI) An infection of one or more of the structures in the urinary tract; usually caused by bacteria.

U.S. Department of Agriculture (USDA) The government agency that monitors the production of eggs, poultry, and meat for adherence to standards of quality and wholesomeness. The USDA also provides public nutrition education, performs nutrition research, and administers the WIC program.

U.S. Department of Health and Human Services (DHHS) The principal federal agency responsible for protecting the health of all Americans and providing essential human services. The agency is especially concerned with those Americans who are least able to help themselves.

U.S. Pharmacopeia (USP) Established in 1820, the USP is a nonprofit healthcare organization that sets quality standards for a range of healthcare products.

vascular system A network of veins and arteries through which the blood carries nutrients. Also called the *blood circulatory system*.

very-low-density lipoproteins (VLDLs) The triglyceride-rich lipoproteins formed in the liver. VLDL enters the bloodstream and is gradually acted upon by lipoprotein lipase, releasing triglyceride to body cells.

villi Small fingerlike projections that blanket the folds in the lining of the small intestine. Singular is *villus*.

visceral fat Fat stores that cushion body organs.

vitamin precursors See *provitamins*.

vitamins Organic compounds necessary for reproduction, growth, and maintenance of the body. Vitamins are required in miniscule amounts.

waist circumference The waist measurement, as a marker of abdominal fat content, that can be used to indicate health risks.

wasting The breakdown of body tissue, such as muscle and organ, for use as a protein source when the diet lacks protein.

weight cycling Repeated periods of gaining and losing weight. Also called *yo-yo dieting*.

weight management The adoption of healthful and sustainable eating and exercise behaviors that reduce disease risk and improve well-being.

Wilson's disease Genetic disorder of increased copper absorption, which leads to toxic levels in the liver and heart.

World Health Organization (WHO) A global organization that directs and coordinates international health work. Its goal is the attainment by all peoples of the highest possible level of health, defined as a state of complete physical, mental, and social well-being and not merely the absence of disease or infirmity.

xerophthalmia A condition caused by vitamin A deficiency that dries the cornea and mucous membranes of the eye.

zoochemicals The animal equivalent of phytochemicals in plants that are believed to provide health benefits beyond the traditional nutrients that foods contain.

Index

Note: Page numbers followed by *f* or *t* indicate materials in figures or tables respectively.

toxicity
  biotin, 280
  folate, 276
  riboflavin, 268
  thiamin, 267
  vitamin A, 249f, 250
  vitamin B$_6$, 273
  vitamin B$_{12}$, 278
  vitamin C, 283
  vitamin D, 257
  vitamin E, 261
  vitamin K, 263, 264t
toxins, natural, 704–705
Toxoplasma gondii, 697t
trace minerals, 16, 346, 346f, 367–371, D-9–D-12
trachea, E-2
trans fatty acids, 165, 165f, 172, 175
transferrin, 349, 350f
transport, protein functions, 207
tricarboxylic acid (TCA) cycle, 390
triglycerides, 15
  digestion and absorption, 176–178, 177f
  energy from, 392, 400
  in food, 169–172, 169f
  functions of, 167–169, 167f–169f
  insulation and protection, 168
  lipoprotein, 182
  metabolism, 382f
  structure, 166–167, 167f
trimesters, 591
tripeptide, 201
tryptophan, 269
tumor, 513
type 1 diabetes, 522–524, 524t
type 2 diabetes, 116, 522–524, 524t
tyrosine, 200

U

ulcers, 95
ultra-trace minerals, D-9–D-12
umami, 5
underwater weighing, 421
underweight, 419, 575–576, 590–591, 658. *See also* eating disorders
  anorexia nervosa, 469
United States, malnutrition in
  description, 638
  hunger in, 675–679, 678f

prevalence and distribution, 669–672, 670t, 671f
unsaturated fatty acids, 164
urbanization, 679, 682
urea, 213–214
urea cycle, G-6
urinary tract infection (UTI), 646
urine, 86
U.S. Department of Agriculture (USDA)
  food assistance programs, 672t
  food intake patterns calorie levels, B-2–B-3
  food labels, 38, 56
  food safety, 708, 709, 712
  organic foods, 702–703, 702t
  role of, 38
U.S. Department of Health and Human Services (DHHS), 38
U.S. Government, I-9–I-10
U.S. Pharmacopeia (USP) verification mark, 308, 308f, 309
U.S. Preventive Services Task Force, 153

V

valerian, 297t
vanadium, 371, D-11
variety, food choices, 33
vascular system, 84–85, 85f
vegan/vegetarian diet
  children, 636–637
  dietary recommendations for, 225–227, 226t
  health benefits of, 224
  health risks of, 225
  iron, 224–225, 594
  pregnancy, 594
  protein sources, 218–219
  religious groups and vegetarian practices, 223, 223t
  sports performance, 454–455
  types of, 223t, 224
  vitamin B$_{12}$, 225, 226, 277
vegetable oil, 175–176
vegetables
  American diet, 10, 11t
  carbohydrates, 15
  Dietary Guidelines for Americans, 2015-2020, 41
  Eating Well with Canada's Food Guide, 47
  fiber, 108, 108t
  and fruits, 503–504, 517–518

heart disease and, 190–191
  MyPlate, 33, 44t–45t, 48t
  preparation, 242
  proteins, 16, 222, 222t
vegetarian athlete, 454–455
very-low-calorie diets (VLCDs), 571
very-low-density lipoproteins (VLDLs), 181
Vibrio vulnificus, 696t
villi, 80
visceral fat, 168
vision
  carotenoids, 251–252
  macular degeneration, 252
  older adults, 657
  vitamin A, 245–246, 246f, 684–685
vitamin A, 15, 16, 244–250, D-1
  absorption, 240, 241f
  adolescent intake, 639, 639f
  alcohol use and, 150
  deficiency, 249–250, 249f, 684–685
  dietary recommendations for, 247–248, 247f
  forms of, 244, 244f
  functions of, 245–247, 245f, 247f
  osteoporosis, dietary and lifestyle factors, 530
  pregnancy and, 586, 593t, 595
  sources of, 248–249, 248f
  toxicity, 249f, 250
  transport of, 207
  vision, 245–246, 246f, 684–685
vitamin B$_1$ (thiamin), 16, 265–267, 593t, D-3
vitamin B$_2$ (riboflavin), 16, 267–268, 268f, 593t, D-3
vitamin B$_3$ (niacin), 16, 269–270, 269f, D-3
vitamin B$_5$ (pantothenic acid), 16, 279, 279f, 593t
vitamin B$_6$ (pyridoxine), 16, 284t, 300, D-5
  alcohol use and, 150
  functions and sources, 271–272, 271f–272f
  pregnancy, 593t
vitamin B$_7$ (biotin), 16, 279–280, 593t
vitamin B$_9$ (folate), 16, 273–276, 274f, 275f, 593t, 595
vitamin B$_{12}$ (cobalamin), 276–278, 277f, 278f, 284t, 300, D-5
  absorption, 82
  alcohol use and, 150